nutrition
in health
and disease

Helen S. Mitchell

A.B., Ph.D., Sc.D., Formerly Research Consultant, Harvard School of Public Health; Dean Emeritus of the School of Home Economics and formerly Research Professor of Nutrition, University of Massachusetts, Amherst; Exchange Professor Hokkaido University, Sapporo, Japan; Formerly Principal Nutritionist, Office of Defense, Health and Welfare; Professor of Physiology and Nutrition, Battle Creek College

Henderika J. Rynbergen

B.S., M.S., Professor of Science, Emeritus, Cornell University-New York Hospital School of Nursing; Formerly Director of Dietetics, American University Hospital, Beirut, Lebanon; Food Clinic Dietitian, Vanderbilt Clinic, Presbyterian Hospital, New York; Food Clinic Dietitian, Barnes Hospital, St. Louis; Nutritionist, Community Health Association, Boston

Linnea Anderson

R.D., M.P.H., Associate Professor of Medical Dietetics, School of Allied Medical Professions, The Ohio State University; Formerly Associate Professor of Nutrition, School of Nursing and College of Home Economics, Syracuse University

Marjorie V. Dibble

R.D., M.S., Chairperson and Professor, Department of Human Nutrition; Formerly Nutrition Supervisor, Family Development Research Program, Children's Center, College for Human Development, Syracuse University

nutrition in health and disease

sixteenth edition

Mitchell

Rynbergen

Anderson

Dibble

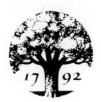

J. B. Lippincott Company
Philadelphia
New York / San Jose / Toronto

Sixteenth Edition

Copyright © 1976, 1968, by J. B. Lippincott Company

Copyright 1963, 1958, 1953, 1950, 1947, 1943, 1941, 1938, 1935, 1933, 1931, 1930, 1929, 1928, by J. B. Lippincott Company

Distributed in Great Britain by
Blackwell Scientific Publications, Oxford, London, and Edinburgh

ISBN-0-397-54177-5

Library of Congress Catalog Card Number 63-20822

Printed in the United States of America

57986

preface

"Medicine arose from dietetics: the Pythagoreans (including Hippocrates) used diet to prevent and cure diseases, and drugs only if these failed."

H. M. Sinclair*

This book has been revised for the members of the health services professions—physicians, and their assistants, dietitians/nutritionists, and nurses—who share the responsibility for the nutritional care and counseling of individuals and their families. The central focus is the client with emphasis on those knowledges, attitudes, and abilities required of the professional person to be an effective nutrition counselor. The reader is reminded that professional practice in the late twentieth century is related to basic biomedical and psychosocial principles and that the nutritional component of practice derives not only from genetics, nutritional biochemistry, anatomy, physiology, and food science, but also from sociology, psychology, and anthropology. Pertinent principles from these disciplines are repeated only for clarity where these are essential for bridging the gap between theory and practice.

As in previous editions the text presents a comprehensive overview of the principles of nutrition as they apply to individuals and groups throughout the life span as well as the dietary needs of individuals with metabolic aberrations due to pathological conditions.

In Section One, Principles of Nutrition, Chapter 1 has been completely revised to introduce the concept of nutrition counseling and the roles of the various

*In *Health and Food*, G. G. Birch, et al., eds. New York, John Wiley & Sons, 1972, p. 23.

health professions in providing nutritional services. It includes a general overview of national and international nutrition problems. Chapters 2 through 9, in Section One, present the functions and food sources of nutrients, energy metabolism, and nutrient utilization. The information on the vitamins and trace minerals has been extensively revised to reflect current knowledge of these nutrients. Chapter 8, Energy, has been revised to reflect more appropriately the relationship of this subject to Nutrient Utilization, Chapter 9. Chapter 9 has been expanded significantly to further emphasize the importance of the complex interrelationships of nutrients in human metabolic processes.

Chapter 10 presents the guidelines used in the assessment of food practices such as the NAS-NRC Recommended Dietary Allowances, and the U.S.D.A. Food Guide. Information about food composition tables, nutrient composition of food, effect of food processing on nutrient composition, and enrichment and fortification programs has been added. The U.S. Recommended Dietary Allowances and current information on nutrition labeling are included. A new chapter, Meal Management, Chapter 11, includes discussions on food budgeting, the U.S.D.A. Weekly Food Plans, food planning, storage, and preparation. Chapter 12, The Helping Process in Nutrition Services, is also new. It presents a theory of the helping process as applied to nutrition counseling. The new information in Chapter 13, Regional, Cultural, and Religious Food Practices covers such topics as factors influencing food habits, American Indian foods, and unusual dietary practices.

Section Two, Application of Nutrition to Critical Periods Throughout the Life Span, represents a reorganization of material on the maternity-infancy cycle, childhood, adolescence and the aging process. A new chapter, Growth and Development, Chapter 15, is a general overview of the relationship of nutrition to the growth process, the growth cycle and nutrition, and brain growth and behavior. Chapter 20, Malnutrition—A World Problem, discusses human nutrition problems throughout the world.

Section Three, Diet in Disease, incorporates the content of Part II, Diet in Disease, and Part III, Modification of Food for Therapeutic Diets, from the 15th Edition of this text. Recipes are not included in this edition, but sources of recipes are listed where appropriate and available.

While the chapters in Section Three continue to have titles which describe disease processes, the sequence of chapters has been rearranged to reflect related metabolic problems. For instance, Chapter 27, Weight Control, Chapter 28, Diabetes Mellitus, and Chapter 29, Atherosclerosis, are in sequence because the metabolic problem shared by these clinical entities is energy metabolism, particularly carbohydrate and lipid metabolism. Similarly, Cardiovascular Disease, Chapter 30, Renal Disease; Nephrolithiasis, Chapter 31, and Liver Disease, Chapter 32, share a common requirement, manipulation of fluid and electrolyte intake; and also, in renal and liver disease, protein (nitrogen) intake. At the beginning of most chapters the reader is advised to review basic principles in the related chapter or chapters in Section One. Hopefully, this arrangement of material will help the user of the book to approach diet therapy from the metabolic viewpoint and not, as in the past, as "a diet for a disease."

Wherever appropriate, exchange systems, comparable to that used for diabetic diets, have been designed for calculating diet patterns to meet other diet prescriptions. The discussion of the foods used in the various exchange systems has been expanded over that in the previous edition.

In Chapter 25, the dietary treatment in peptic ulcer disease has been extensively revised, based on current research in this area. However, the traditional diet plans are still included for the reader's convenience. In Chapter 26, Nutritional Care—Surgical and Burn Therapy, information on elemental diets and hyperalimentation is included. A table on the energy and nutrient composition per 100 ml. of a variety of commercial tube feedings has been added. In Chapter 33, Special Problems, food-drug interactions are discussed.

Chapter 34, Nutrition in Diseases of Infancy and Childhood, has been expanded to include a discussion of the problems of the critically ill infant, including a table of the ingredients in and the uses of special infant formulas. In this edition the inborn errors of metabolism, especially inborn errors of amino acid metabolism, are discussed in Chapter 35.

Section Four, as in previous editions, includes various reference tables, extensive bibliographies, and a glossary of terms. Table 1 is a general food composition table. The cholesterol values in Table 2, Selected Fatty Acids and Cholesterol in Common Foods, include the revised figures published in 1972 by the U.S.D.A. Table 5, Zinc Content of Foods, and Table 10, Current Guidelines for Criteria of Nutritional Status for Laboratory Evaluation, are new in this edition.

An extensive and current bibliography, classified by subjects, will be of special help to instructors and others wishing to pursue certain subjects in greater depth than is possible in the text. The Glossary of terms has also been expanded and brought up to date.

The Authors

acknowledgments

The authors wish to express their deep appreciation to their colleagues and friends for the generous help given during the preparation of the 16th edition of Nutrition in Health and Disease. One of the compensations for the arduous work involved in such a revision is the contact with and the courtesy extended by investigators, associates, and other authors for permission to use material from their research and work.

In this edition the authors are indebted to: Pirkko Turkki, R.D., Ph.D., College of Human Development, Syracuse University, for writing Chapter 8, Energy, and Chapter 9, Nutrient Utilization; to Clair Agresti Johnson, R.D., Ph.D., Medical Dietetics Division, School of Allied Medical Professions, The Ohio State University, for writing Chapter 12, The Helping Process in Nutrition Services; and to the late Nancy D. Herrick, M.S., M.P.H., and Marian F. Chase, M.S., L.P.T., Chief of Physical Therapy, Nisonger Center, The Ohio State University Center for Mental Retardation, for writing Chapter 24, Handicapping Problems.

Miss Diane Kopetz, R.D., Metabolic Unit, and Mrs. Marilyn Stevenson, R.D., Out-Patient Services, Columbus Children's Hospital, Columbus, Ohio, assisted the authors with the revision of Chapter 34, Nutrition in Diseases of Infancy and Childhood, and, based on their clinical experience, organized the information in Chapter 35, Inborn Errors of Metabolism.

Special thanks are due to: Dr. Moises Behar for the photographs in Chapter 20; Dr. Marvin H. Sleisenger, University of California School of Medicine, San Francisco, who gave permission to use the photographs of the mucosa of the jejunum in celiac disease before and after treatment; and to Miss Geraldine Getty of the Arkansas Children's Hospital for obtaining the photograph which was used in Chapter 34 of hospitalized children eating together at the table.

Lastly, the authors wish to acknowledge the patience and skill of their editors, David T. Miller, Bernice Heller, Elaine Terranova, and Joyce Mkitarian in converting the manuscript into a book.

To these persons as well as to others who have assisted in the preparation of this textbook, the authors express gratitude and recognize that factual errors which may appear in the text are solely their own responsibility.

contents

principles of nutrition

introduction to nutrition counseling

1

WHY DO WE NEED NUTRITION COUNSELING?
Evidence that Adequate Diets Affect Health

Early in this century the application of nutrition research demonstrated the importance of adequate nutrient intake to the promotion of normal growth and development in infants and young children and to the protection of all segments of society against deficiency diseases. In 1932 Bowles, an anthropologist, showed that freshmen students entering Harvard College were taller and heavier than their fathers were on admission to the same school in the early 1900s. Better food intake during infancy and childhood was one factor accounting for the difference between these two generations. Control of acute and chronic infectious diseases and better obstetrical care were also important factors.

In another study Ito[1] demonstrated that Japanese women born and reared in California were taller and heavier than relatives born and reared in Hawaii, while those born and reared in Japan were smaller and lighter than the other two groups. The differences in these three groups could be accounted for in part by the quantity and quality of the food consumed during infancy and childhood. More recently Mitchell[2] has observed that when the nutritional needs of the adolescent are not met, stature potential is not realized. In Japan during World War II, food shortages resulted in a reduction in height among Japanese youth at all ages, compared to the prewar stature of that age group. With increased prosperity resulting in more and better food after 1950, Japanese youth have grown taller than they have ever been before.

These and similar observations have demonstrated to health workers that an adequate intake of nutrients during infancy and childhood is required if any healthy individual is to achieve his growth potential.

In 1915, Goldberger reported on his success in curing and preventing pellagra, a deficiency of the B vitamin niacin, by adding animal and leguminous protein foods to a diet of cereals and vegetables served to an institutionalized population. Prior to World War I, workers in England and the United States showed that the addition of cod-liver oil to an infant's diet protected against rickets. The factor in the cod-liver oil was later proven to be vitamin D.

The Importance of Nutrition Counseling

Throughout this century and up to the present day, many other studies have continued to demonstrate the importance of an adequate diet to health. Unfortunately, however, even today medical, dietetic, and nursing students can observe the effects of inadequate feeding on the growth and development of infants in the pediatric units of general and teaching hospitals. The infant admitted with the diagnosis of failure to thrive (FTT), who is shown to have no organic disease and who, following treatment in the hospital, gains weight daily in excess of any norm, is seen too frequently in U.S. hospitals. If the knowledge of the relationship of adequate diet to health, discovered in the past, is to benefit today's infants and children and their families, it is accepted that each generation requires nutrition counseling.

Dietary modification is also an important factor in both the prevention and treatment of many diseases. There are still unsolved nutritional problems such as obesity and atherosclerosis. Diet therapy is important in the treatment of diabetes mellitus and in other metabolic and endocrine disorders. Diseases affecting the gastrointestinal tract, the kidney, and certain

inborn errors of metabolism require nutritional management as a major part of the treatment.

NUTRITIONAL STATUS IN THE UNITED STATES
Nutritional Status Surveys

A comprehensive nutritional status survey must be so designed that it reflects the relationship between the intake of food, the utilization of the nutrients in the food, and the total health status of the subjects studied. The components of a comprehensive nutritional status survey are: the clinical assessment of the individuals being studied, including medical history, physical examination, anthropometric studies, and x-ray measurements; biochemical measurements performed on samples of blood and urine collected under standard conditions; dental examinations; evaluation of dietary intake to obtain information on the level of nutrients, food habits, food preparation practices, and food attitudes; and socioeconomic data including such items as income, availability of food and government food distribution programs, health and education facilities and their use, and the ethnic and cultural characteristics of the subjects. To determine the nutritional status of any population requires an adequate number of cooperative subjects; a representative sample of the population as a whole; a team of knowledgeable investigators; and the appropriate equipment for both the collection and analysis of the data.

The U.S. Public Health Service conducted nutritional status surveys in the late 1940s in various parts of the country. From 1947 to 1958 several studies were sponsored by the Cooperative State Agriculture Experiment Stations and the Agricultural Research Service of the U.S. Department of Agriculture (USDA). These surveys indicated that the population as a whole consumed diets adequate in essential nutrients and was free from symptoms of frank deficiency diseases. There were signs, however, that the nutritional status of pregnant women, infants, preschool children, and adolescent girls merited special concern.

In 1967, a group of concerned citizens raised the question of hunger "in our midst." Congressional hearings pointed to the probability of problems of serious hunger and malnutrition in the United States. In December of 1967, Congress directed the Secretary of Health, Education, and Welfare to make a comprehensive survey of the incidence and location of hunger and malnutrition and related health problems in the U.S. The survey undertaken to carry out this mandate is known as the *Ten-State Nutrition Survey*,

1968-1970. At approximately the same time the Maternal and Child Health Service in the Health Services and Mental Health Administration, Public Health Service, contracted with a research team for a *Preschool Nutrition Survey* to study a cross-sectional sample of children one to six years of age in the United States.

TEN-STATE NUTRITION SURVEY (TSNS), 1968-1970: The TSNS[3] was conducted in low income areas in ten states widely distributed throughout the nation and reflects the nutritional problems related to specific ethnic groups and income levels. The Poverty Income Ratio (PIR) was calculated for each family according to certain characteristics of the family (size, farm or nonfarm, sex of the head of the household) as compared with family income. A PIR of 1.0 indicated that a family was living at the poverty line. Although all the subjects studied had low incomes, those who lived in Texas, Louisiana, South Carolina, Kentucky, and West Virginia had a median PIR below the overall median for the ten states, while those who resided in Massachusetts, New York, Michigan, Washington, and California had a median PIR above the overall median. Therefore, the first five states are referred to as low income states and the other five as high income states in the survey reports.

The outcomes of the TSNS indicate that the growth and development of children 0 to 9 years of age appears to present a relatively important problem for both sexes in all ethnic groups (white, black, Spanish-Americans in Texas) regardless of income ratio. Obesity was an important nutritional problem in women 17 years of age and older in all ethnic groups. The black female population seems to present a greater problem than the white population in this regard. Iron nutriture was a problem in all age and ethnic groups, with the black population in the low income ratio states and the pregnant and lactating women in all states presenting a more important problem than the rest of the survey sample. The Spanish-American population (primarily the Mexican-Americans residing in Texas) presented an important problem in vitamin A nutriture.

PRESCHOOL NUTRITION SURVEY (PNS), 1968-1970: The subjects in this study[4] represented all socioeconomic and ethnic groups in the U.S. The outcomes of this survey also indicate that it is the children in the lowest socioeconomic group who are most at risk as demonstrated by their lower dietary intakes, lower biochemical indices, and smaller physical size for age compared with the rest of the subjects. It was concluded that the major nutritional problem is insufficient food for the children in the lowest socioeconomic group. The nutritional quality of the intakes might have been adequate if the quantity of food eaten had been sufficient. Approximately one third of the children in the lowest socioeconomic group consumed diets inadequate in total calories. Their intake of protein was not a problem. The level of ascorbic acid intake was also related to the socioeconomic status of the family. More than half of all children in the survey consumed diets inadequate in iron.

In the fifteenth edition of this book the authors stated:

> For pregnant women, infants and preschool children socioeconomic factors may be affecting food intake. At the same time we are faced with a problem of overnutrition: obesity and, possibly, certain chronic diseases are the results of too much food (p. 5).

The outcomes of the Ten-State Nutrition Survey and the Preschool Nutrition Survey would appear to support the speculations of the authors in 1968.

Nutritional Status Surveillance

Since 1956, the National Center for Health Statistics in the Department of Health, Education, and Welfare (DHEW) has been responsible for the Health Examination Survey. Recently, nutritional status surveillance has become a component of the Health Examination Survey, and the program is now known as the Health and Nutrition Examination Survey (HANES).[5] At this time HANES is collecting data in various areas throughout the United States. The survey equipment is housed in three large trailers which can be stationed in supermarket parking lots or other places close to the population to be studied. It can be anticipated that the data collected by HANES will be analyzed and reported by DHEW or by the areas surveyed (such as a city or a county) and will be available for the planning of health services of that area.

Although nutritional status surveys are useful to the nutrition counselor in that they indicate nutrition problems or the lack of them in general, the data derived from them cannot be used to predict the nutritional status of any individual client or group of clients.

TRENDS IN FOOD CONSUMPTION

Information about trends in food consumption in the United States are also available to the nutrition counselor. There are two methods of collecting these data: (1) household food consumption surveys, and (2) statistics on the availability of food for civilian consumption. These data give us information about what the public eats but no information about nutritional status. The information has been used to identify areas where improvement in nutrition is needed and gives direction to programs to improve the national food supply. For example, the data from one of the household food consumption surveys were responsible for the initiation of bread and flour enrichment (see Chapter 10).

Household Food Consumption Surveys

A nationwide survey of food consumption was made in the United States in 1965-1966. Earlier surveys were made in 1936, 1942, 1948, and 1955. In 1965-1966, data on household usage of foods were collected from 15,000 homes during the four seasons of the year and in different sections of the country. Some of the changes in food consumption between 1955 and 1965 reflect a shift to foods requiring less preparation in the home, for example, more frozen and chilled than fresh citrus juices; more processed than fresh potatoes; and more commercial bakery products. A greater use of foods associated with snacking was also observed.[6]

These changes resulted in a decrease in the number of "good" diets—from 60 percent in 1955 to 50 percent in 1965—and an increase in the number of "poor" diets—from 15 percent in 1955 to 21 percent in 1965. Diets were classified as "good" if seven nutrients (protein, calcium, iron, vitamin A, thiamine, riboflavin, ascorbic acid) were supplied in amounts that met the recommended dietary allowances. If one or more nutrients were supplied in amounts equaling less than two thirds of the recommended dietary allowances, the diet was classified as "poor." The nutrients most frequently found to be supplied in amounts below two thirds of the recommended dietary allowances were ascorbic acid, vitamin A, and calcium. The recommended dietary allowances for iron were changed in 1968, and if the revised allowances were applied to these data, iron too would be a nutrient which is frequently not supplied in amounts adequate to meet allowances.

Food Available for Civilian Consumption

Table 1-1 shows the trends in U.S. consumption of nutrients from 1957-1959 to 1974. These trends are derived by the Agricultural Research Service of the U.S. Department of Agriculture from the statistics on the quantities of foods that are available in the retail markets each year. It is interesting to note the increase in all nutrients except calcium. The decrease in consumption of fluid whole milk is primarily responsible for the decrease in calcium. The increased consumption of citrus fruits, particularly the frozen concentrates, accounts for the increased ascorbic acid; increased meat consumption, especially poultry, has increased the amounts of protein, niacin, vitamin B_6, and vitamin B_{12} in the diet. Increased consumption of salad and cooking oils accounts for the increased fat (Fig. 1-1).

NUTRITION CANADA

A national survey of the nutritional status of Canadians has recently been completed.[7] Among the findings of the survey were a general problem of obesity among the adult population, high prevalence of elevated cholesterol among both men and women, low intakes of protein among preschool children and pregnant women, and shortage of calcium and vitamin D in the diets of many infants, children, and adolescents. Eskimos and Indians were found to be at higher risk than the general population in terms of ascorbic acid and vitamin A deficiencies. To meet the problems identified in this survey, priorities dealing

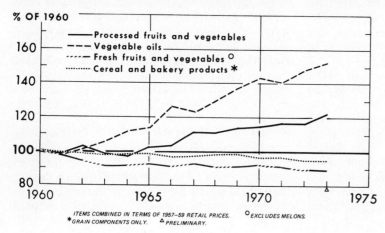

Fig. 1-1. Per capita consumption of selected crop products. (U.S. Department of Agriculture, Economic Research Service)

with government policies, industry's action, and consumer attitudes were recommended.

WORLD NUTRITION PROBLEMS

Ever since World War II scientists in technically advanced countries have become increasingly aware of world food problems. Surveys have been made in many of the developing countries in an effort to understand their specific problems of food production, distribution, conservation, and nutrient content of the local food supply. The public press has repeatedly commented that the world food supply is not keeping pace with the population explosion. There is a growing awareness that

> A global effort is essential to increase food production and to distribute it more equitably, to provide technical assistance for agricultural and economic development, to educate professional and lay personnel in nutrition, to provide nutritional health services for those in need and to control the rapid expansion of the world's population.[8]

It is generally agreed that the realistic approach is to give the kind of aid that will help the developing countries to help themselves. In the United States, the Agricultural Extension Service worked with rural families during the 1920s and 1930s to increase food production by improving agricultural procedures. The lessons learned in this country from extension methods, an example of nutrition counseling of groups of people, could be more effectively applied

Table 1–1. Nutrients Available for Civilian Consumption, Per Capita Per Day, Selected Periods*

Nutrient	Unit	Average 1957–1959	1967	1972	1973	1974 preliminary	1974 as a percentage of 1957–1959
Food energy	cal.	3140	3210	3320	3300	3350	107
Protein	g.	95	98	101	99	101	106
Fat	g.	143	150	158	155	158	110
Carbohydrate	g.	374	373	381	385	388	104
Calcium	g.	0.98	0.94	0.94	0.95	0.95	97
Phosphorus	g.	1.51	1.52	1.54	1.52	1.54	102
Iron	mg.	16.1	17.2	18.0	17.9	18.3	114
Magnesium	mg.	348	343	346	346	348	100
Vitamin A value	IU	8000	7900	8100	8100	8200	103
Thiamine	mg.	1.84	1.91	1.94	1.90	1.94	105
Riboflavin	mg.	2.28	2.33	2.35	2.32	2.33	102
Niacin	mg.	20.6	22.4	23.4	22.9	23.4	114
Vitamin B₆	mg.	2.01	2.18	2.29	2.24	2.28	113
Vitamin B₁₂	mcg.	8.9	9.5	9.8	9.5	9.7	109
Ascorbic acid	mg.	105	108	115	118	119	113

*Adapted from Friend, B., and Marston, R., Nutritional Review, National Food Situation. U.S. Department of Agriculture, Economic Research Service, November, 1974.

than at present among rural and village people in many underdeveloped countries.

There is reason to believe that if an all-out international effort were made to improve conventional agriculture, annual food production could be doubled throughout the world, and if at the same time an equal effort were made to achieve zero population growth, the food gap between the have and have-not nations could be reduced with all of society reaping the benefits.[9]

Research and development of nonconventional methods of providing additional food sources should also be encouraged. These include aquaculture and organized fishing systems, utilization of solar and geothermal energy, genetic improvement of biological species, creation of new biological species through genetic manipulations, control of pests and pathogens, and utilization of single cell protein.

In considering world nutrition problems today, one must recognize the many complex factors which enter into the current world food crisis. Although the "green revolution" (see p. 20) sharply increased grain production, especially in certain Asian nations, stores of grains are currently at their lowest level in years. Increased food production in the developing countries, while occurring as rapidly as in the developed countries, has not yielded any appreciable improvement in the per capita food available because rampant population growth has offset the gains (Fig. 1–2). At the same time, the increasing affluence of Western Europe, Japan, and the Soviet Union has put heavier demands on the world's food supplies. Since more of these peoples expect animal rather than vegetable protein, the demand for grain for increasing numbers of livestock has increased at a rapid rate.

Adverse weather conditions in recent years have drastically reduced crops in Africa, India, the Philippines, Australia, and the Soviet Union. These crop losses have not only increased the price of cereal grains but have caused famines in those countries too poor to buy grain in the world market. Some forecasters are predicting that changing climatic conditions threaten to cause a dry-weather pattern from the sub-Sahara drought belt through the Middle East to India, South Asia, and North China. Drought could even return the U.S. Great Plains to "dust bowl" conditions with ensuing crop losses in this country.

Because petroleum is a major source of fertilizer, the petroleum shortage is having a drastic impact on the price and availability of commercial fertilizers, essential items for modern agricultural production. As a result of the increased cost of fertilizer, grain production in the developing countries may decrease.

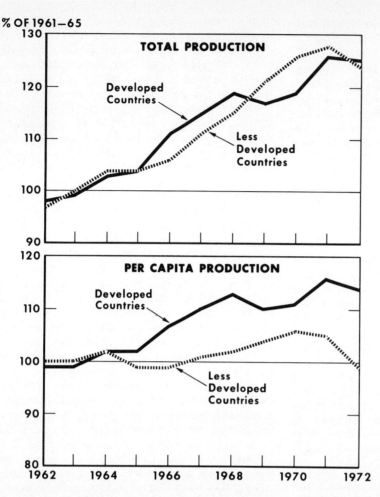

% OF 1961—65

TOTAL PRODUCTION

Developed
Countries

Less
Developed
Countries

PER CAPITA PRODUCTION

Developed
Countries

Less
Developed
Countries

Fig. 1–2. Indices of food production in the developed and less developed countries. North America, Europe, U.S.S.R., Japan, Republic of South Africa, Australia, and New Zealand. (U.S. Department of Agriculture, Economic Research Service)

The United States, which has supplied billions of dollars worth of food to needy countries under the Food for Peace program, now tends to view agricultural products as sources of foreign exchange needed to pay for American imports. Thus, the U.S. food surpluses will be committed more to trade than to relieving food shortages in low income countries.

Over-fishing and pollution are also reducing the supply of fish which in the past has contributed significantly to meeting the world's food needs. International regulations and conservation techniques must be applied to the sea and inland waterways if these sources are to continue their yields in the future.

To help formulate a world food plan which will deal effectively with the present food crisis, a World Food Conference was held in Rome in November 1974. Action was called for on five fronts: accelerating food production in developing countries, improving distribution and financing, enhancing food quality, increasing the production of present food exporters, and insuring security against food emergencies.

NATIONAL NUTRITION POLICY

In the U.S., the National Nutrition Consortium has recently published its proposed Guidelines for a National Nutrition Policy.[10] Since nutrition counselors will function more effectively if they understand their role in terms of the overall nutrition policy, counselors are urged to review the following guidelines carefully.

The goals of a national nutrition policy should be to:

1. assure an adequate wholesome food supply at reasonable cost to meet the needs of all segments of the population, this supply being available at a level consistent with the affordable life style of the area;
2. maintain food resources sufficient to meet emergency needs and to fulfill a responsible role as a nation in meeting world food needs;
3. develop a level of sound public knowledge and responsible understanding of nutrition and foods that will promote maximal nutritional health;

4. maintain a system of quality and safety control that justifies public confidence in its food supply;
5. support research and education in foods and nutrition with adequate resources and reasoned priorities to solve important current problems and to permit exploratory basic research.

To attain these goals, it is essential to:
1. maintain surveillance of the nutritional status of the population and determine the nature of nutritional problems observed;
2. develop programs within the health care system that will prevent and rectify nutritional problems;
3. assist the health professions in coordinated efforts to improve the nutritional status of the population through the life cycle;
4. develop programs for nutrition education for both health professionals and the general public;
5. identify areas in which nutrition knowledge is inadequate and foster research to provide this knowledge;
6. assemble information on the food supply, including food production and distribution, and provide a nutritional input in the regulation of foreign agricultural trade;
7. determine the nutrient composition of foods and promote and monitor food quality and safety;
8. cooperate with other nations and international agencies in developing measures for solving the world food and nutrition problems.

DEFINITION OF NUTRITION

Although one may find nutrition defined in a variety of ways, the following definition by the American Medical Association is used because it covers the broad scope of the term as it is referred to in the text.

Nutrition is the science of food, the nutrients and other substances therein, their action, interaction, and balance in relation to health and disease, and the process by which the organism ingests, digests, absorbs, transports, utilizes and excretes food substances. In addition, nutrition must be concerned with social, economic, cultural, and psychological implications of food and eating.[11]

THE NUTRITION COUNSELOR
Role of the Nutrition Counselor

The nutrition counselor is responsible for guiding the food choices of people, either as individuals or as members of a group, wherever they enter the health care system. Within our present health care system, nutrition counseling may take place in a community health agency, a maternity and infant care project, a children and youth project, a health maintenance organization, a pediatrician's or other physician's office, a general hospital or its ambulatory care facilities, an extended care facility, or a rehabilitation institute for the handicapped.

Nutrition counseling focuses on the promotion of normal growth and development in infants, children, and adolescents; on the health maintenance of adults, including the special needs of the pregnant and lactating woman; and on the modifications of food intake in the treatment or rehabilitation of the acutely or chronically ill in any age group. To be effective in guiding individuals and groups, the nutrition counselor must be truly committed not only to the doing aspect of professional practice, but also to the knowing and caring which underlie effective doing.

KNOWING: Basic to effective nutrition counseling—as to any professional practice—is that body of knowledge which is unique to the discipline. In this case, it is a knowledge of the sciences of food and human nutrition as well as the biomedical sciences, coupled with a comprehension of fundamental concepts from the behavioral and social sciences and of the limitations of the individual and his circumstances.

The science of human nutrition provides the counselor with an understanding of the qualitative and quantitative nutrient needs of people at any point in their life-spans under a wide variety of conditions. Food science provides an understanding of the qualitative and quantitative components of the nutrient composition of foods and the ways in which societies make food available to their consumers. From the biomedical sciences the nutrition counselor gains knowledge of the utilization of nutrients at the cellular level and the effect of diseases on nutrient utilization. The social and behavioral sciences help the counselor to understand the psychosocial conditions which affect food choices and to perceive ways of influencing these choices.

CARING: The nutrition counselor enters into a helping relationship with an individual or with a group to assist people to meet their health needs. To establish this relationship, the counselor must accept the client as a human being with rights, values, and a life-style which may be similar to or different from the counselor's, and with the potential to achieve reasonable progress toward his (the client's) goals. To be effective, the counselor must be sensitive to age, sex, and social class differences and to various life-styles in order to avoid setting up barriers to communication with clients. The counselor must not only accept the client but must perceive the situation as the client sees it and work in partnership with him. In other words, the counselor makes a commitment to assist the client to meet his needs, not to meet the counselor's needs.

DOING: The counselor applies both knowing and caring abilities in guiding and teaching the client. Recognizing that behavioral changes are made slowly, the counselor plans *with* the client and offers him alternative solutions to his problems in an effort to move the client toward reasonable practices. The client participates by accepting the alternative which most nearly meets his need. Evaluation of the client's progress is a very important aspect of the helping process and implies continuity of client-counselor contact. It also implies a team approach, by which various members can share the client's progress and give support to each other's roles. The helping process in nutrition counseling is discussed in more detail in Chapter 12.

Who Is the Nutrition Counselor?

THE PHYSICIAN: As the individual responsible for health care, the physician identifies and makes recommendations concerning the nutritional component of health counseling. He may undertake the role of nutrition counselor, or more frequently he refers the client to the appropriate team member.

THE DIETITIAN-NUTRITIONIST: The dietitian-nutritionist is the primary nutrition counselor on the health care team. The Study Commission on Dietetics has described the dietitian as the "translator of the science of nutrition into the skill of furnishing optimal nourishment to people."[12] Through education and supervised clinical experience, she becomes the member of the team who is the specialist in applied human nutrition. She may share these functions with another member of the health team such as the nurse, social worker, dietetic technician, or dietetic assistant. However, the ultimate responsibility for the quality of the nutritional care rendered by any health care team rests with the physician and the dietitian-nutritionist.

THE NURSE: The nurse in any health care delivery setting may be of great assistance in helping a client understand and accept his nutritional care plan. She may consult with the dietitian-nutritionist when she is assisting a client to establish his plan or she may be the member of the team who refers the client to the dietitian-nutritionist. The nurse working in the community health agency has many opportunities to carry nutrition services into clients' homes where these services would not otherwise be available. Her function may be largely educational, or it may involve giving bedside care or directing the home health aide.

THE SOCIAL WORKER: In many health care settings, the social worker is concerned with the socioeconomic functioning of clients. She is frequently as involved with the socioeconomic and psychological aspects of nutritional care as any other member of the health care team.

OTHER MEMBERS OF THE TEAM: Health educators and health or nutrition aides supplement and extend the nutrition counseling services to the client, while health planners help to identify needs and resources and to structure the environment for the delivery of all health care services, including nutrition.

How Does The Nutrition Counselor Function?

ESTABLISHING AND MAINTAINING THE RELATIONSHIP: The first task of the nutrition counselor is to establish communication with the client. This is a talking *with* process, not a talking *to* process. Establishment of communication leads to the next task, gathering and assessing information.

COLLECTING AND ASSESSING INFORMATION: The nutrition counselor is responsible for collecting accurate data regarding the client's food practices in relation to his needs. In many instances the counselor will also need to collect the same information about the client's family. Since there are many patterns of eating that can provide adequate nutrient intake, dietary practices which do not conform to established food guides should not be judged inappropriate without careful estimation of their actual nutrient value.

Estimating the nutrient value of a client's usual daily intake is a particularly difficult task today when food processors remove, replace, and add nutrients to basic foods during processing, as well as fabricate new foods from resources not formerly used. For example, a TV dinner may have more or less calories as the same dinner prepared at home from the same foods. Or the same sized serving of breaded veal cutlet may contain 200 calories in one restaurant and 300 calories in another (see Table 10-6, p. 168).

Not only is the total daily nutrient intake of concern to the counselor but also the distribution of the nutrient intake throughout the day. Recent research indicates that nutrient utilization by the body is more consistent when meals of relatively equal value are consumed throughout the day rather than when one large meal per day is consumed.

An assessment of a client's nutritional needs should also take into consideration information about height and weight and any laboratory data such as hemoglobin, hematocrit, glucose, cholesterol, and triglycerides. Also, it must be recognized that any indication of less than adequate nutritional status may be secondary to an acute or chronic disease which prevents an appropriate nutrient intake or adversely affects nutrient utilization.

Essential to any nutritional care planning is the knowledge of the client's economic resources, living situation, daily routines, emotional maturity, and ability to learn. All of these factors have an important impact on what and when an individual eats.

The same elements of the assessment process used to identify an individual client's nutritional needs are applicable to identifying those of a group. The counselor's next step is planning with the individual and his family or with the group to meet these needs.

PLANNING WITH THE CLIENT: In many instances the first step in the planning process is to give priority to the client's needs. Dibble and Lally[13] showed that the problem for one mother was not what to feed her infant as much as it was the money to purchase food. Also, the client's involvement in the assessment process can result in his identifying his own needs.

Planning with the client demonstrates to him that the counselor does accept him as an individual with rights, and does respect his values and life-style. It is during the planning stage that the counselor must be capable of offering the client viable alternatives.

IMPLEMENTATION—TEACHING THE CLIENT: The client who has been involved in assessment and planning is more likely to recognize his need for information to solve his nutritional problem, and the counselor who has involved him in the processes is better able to provide him with specific information. All the information which most clients need to achieve reasonable performance cannot be given in one contact with the nutrition counselor. Continuity of contact is required to give the client the information he needs in the proper sequence at the right time. For example, the mother of a two-week-old infant, her first, will want to know today what and how to feed him next week, not what to feed him when he is one year old.

EVALUATION: In the evaluation, the nutrition counselor will identify the client's progress toward the achievement of his goals. Evaluation also leads to reassessment, replanning, and reteaching as the client's situation changes. At the same time evaluation of the client's progress can help the counselor to evaluate her own effectiveness.

See Chapter 12 for more detail on these functions.

RESOURCES FOR THE NUTRITION COUNSELOR

Numerous federal, state, and local government agencies, private agencies, and industrial and educational institutions are engaged in various phases of nutrition research and education. Their publications are generally available, and many of them are valuable aids to professional education, or for use in educational programs with the lay public. A few of the groups from which reliable information can be obtained are listed in the following paragraphs.

Official Agencies

The U.S. Department of Agriculture (USDA) has many divisions concerned with food and nutrition. Of particular interest are two sections of the Agricultural Research Service: the Consumer and Food Economics Research Division and the Human Nutrition Research Division. They conduct research and surveys, such as those referred to earlier in this chapter, and also publish numerous bulletins which serve as references for everyone working in the field. For example, the Consumer and Food Economics Research Division publishes Agriculture Handbook No. 8, "Composition of Foods: Raw, Processed, and Prepared," which is widely used as a reference. Table 1, Section 4 in this book was compiled primarily from this reference. The Department of Agriculture, through the state educational agencies, also administers the school lunch program, which feeds millions of children in a school day.

The Department of Health, Education, and Welfare (HEW) has several units involved in nutrition research or service. The Maternal and Child Health Service is concerned with health services to mothers and children, including the nutritional needs of pregnant women, infants, and children. The Food and Drug Administration (FDA) through its regulations is involved in protecting the safety of our food and drugs. The Public Health Service (PHS) is involved both in nutrition research and service. It carries on and supports research through the National Institutes of Health, and, through state and local health agencies, is involved in service programs.

The nutrition activities of these and other agencies are coordinated at the federal level by the Interagency Committee on Nutrition Education. Their Nutrition Committee News is a valuable source of information for nutrition counselors.

The U.S. Government Printing Office prints numerous publications for a variety of U.S. government agencies and makes them available at nominal charge through its Public Documents Department. The monthly publication, Selected U.S. Government Publications, which is free of charge and includes an order form, makes it convenient for health workers to acquire a wide variety of materials as they are published.

Other Agencies, Professional Societies, and Institutions

The Food and Nutrition Board of the National Academy of Sciences—National Research Council was established in 1940 to consider questions pertaining to nutrition measures necessary during World War II. The Academy is a quasigovernmental agency. The Food and Nutrition Board has taken the leadership in promoting nutrition research and its application to health. The Recommended Dietary Allowances, the yardstick to good nutrition, was one of their first accomplishments and has been revised at about five-year intervals since it was first published in 1941.

The American Institute of Nutrition (AIN) is a professional society for nutrition scientists and publishes the *Journal of Nutrition*. The American Society of Clinical Nutrition, a division of the AIN, publishes the *American Journal of Clinical Nutrition*.

The Nutrition Today Society was initiated in 1974 to disseminate reliable nutrition information to various professional groups interested in nutrition.

For those persons who are interpreters of nutritional sciences and motivators for the development of good nutritional practices, the Society for Nutrition Education publishes the Journal of Nutrition Education.

The Nutrition Foundation, Inc., established in 1941 by the food and allied industries, "seeks to make essential contributions to the advancement of nutrition knowledge and its effective application, and thus serve the health and welfare of the public." Since 1942 the Foundation has published Nutrition Reviews—abstracts of current scientific literature in nutrition. Throughout the years the Foundation has also published semipopular brochures on nutrition topics of current interest.

The American Dietetic Association (ADA), the professional society for dietitians, was founded in 1917 during World War I by pioneers in the then-emerging profession of dietetics. The Association began publication of the *Journal of the American Dietetic Association* in 1925, and continues to report research and studies in food and nutrition and in the administration of food service. In addition, the Association publishes educational materials which are as useful to nurses, doctors, teachers, and others in related professions as to dietitians.

Unreliable Organizations

In recent years several widely advertised organizations, which were deliberately given names similar to those of organizations mentioned above, have issued unreliable publications in the field of nutrition and dietetics. They have even led some professionally trained people to accept fads and false ideas about food requirements, vitamin and mineral supplements, and the "dangers" of commercial fertilizers and food additives. Food fads and unreliable sources are discussed more fully in Chapter 13.

STUDY QUESTIONS AND ACTIVITIES

1. What are the components of a nutritional status survey?
2. What evidence do we have that nutrition influences the physical growth of population groups?
3. List the specific population groups which are at greatest risk of nutritional inadequacies in the United States and Canada. Indicate the nutrient or nutrients which present the greatest problem for each group.
4. Explain the present trend in food consumption in the United States as it affects the nutrients available in the diet.
5. Collect articles from newspapers and magazines on the world food situation during the next month. Post them on the bulletin board.
6. Define nutrition and the role of the nutrition counselor. Explain what is meant by "doing," "knowing," and "caring" as they relate to nutrition counseling.
7. Describe your role as a nutrition counselor. What other professional or paraprofessional workers share your responsibility for providing nutritional care? What do they do?
8. Begin compiling a list of reliable source material for nutrition information. Start with the suggestions in this chapter and add to it during the term.
9. Select a recent pamphlet or popular book concerned with nutrition and evaluate its content and appropriateness for the lay public.

SUPPLEMENTARY READINGS

The American Dietetic Association Position Paper on the nutrition component of health services delivery systems. J. Am. Dietet. A. 58:538, 1971.

The American Dietetic Association Position Paper on nutrition services in health maintenance organizations. J. Am. Dietet. A. 60:317, 1972.

Cason, D., and Wagner, M. G.: The changing role of the service professional within the ghetto. J. Am. Dietet. A. 60:21, 1972.

Cottam, H. R.: The world food conference. J. Am. Dietet. A. 66:333, 1975.

Egan, M. C., and Hallstrom, B. J.: Building nutrition services in comprehensive health care. J. Am. Dietet. A. 61:491, 1972.

Goldsmith, G. A.: Nutrition and world health. J. Am. Dietet. A. 63:513, 1973.

Harrar, J. G.: Nutrition and numbers in the Third World. Nutr. Rev. 32:97, 1974.

Hueneman, R. L.: Interpretation of nutritional status. J. Am. Dietet. A. 63:123, 1973.

Johnson, D.: The dietitian—nutritional information translator. J. Am. Dietet. A. 64:608, 1974.

National Nutrition Consortium: Guidelines for a national nutrition policy. Nutr. Rev. 32:153, 1974.

Preliminary Findings of the First Health and Nutrition Examination Survey, United States, 1971-1972: Dietary Intake and Biochemical Findings. Department of Health, Education, and Welfare Publ. No. (HRA) 74-1219-1, 1974.

Sabry, Z. I., Campbell, E. E., Campbell, J. A., and Forbes, A. L.: Nutrition Canada. Nutrition Today 9:5 (Jan.-Feb.), 1974.

Ten-State Nutrition Survey in the United States, 1968—1970. Washington, D.C., U.S. Department of Health, Education, and Welfare, 1972.

For further references see Bibliography in Section 4.

REFERENCES

1. Ito, P. K.: Human Biol. 14:279, 1942.
2. Mitchell, H. S.: J. Am. Dietet. A. 44:165, 1966.
3. Highlights, Ten-State Nutrition Survey, DHEW Pub. No. (HSM) 72-8134, 1972.
4. Owen, G. M., et al: Pediatrics 53, Supplement, April 1974.
5. Plan and Operation of the Health and Nutrition Examination Survey, U.S., 1971-1973, DHEW Publ. No. (HSM) 73-1310, 10a & b.
6. Household Food Consumption Survey, Report No. 1, 1965-1966.
7. Nutrition: A National Priority, Report by Nutrition Canada to the Department of National Health and Welfare, Ottawa, Information Canada, 1973.
8. Goldsmith, G. A.: J. Am. Dietet. A. 63:513, 1973.
9. Hammar, J. G.: Nutr. Rev. 32:97, 1974.
10. National Nutrition Consortium: Nutr. Rev. 32:153, 1974.
11. Council on Food and Nutrition: JAMA 183:955, 1963.
12. Study Commission on Dietetics: *The Profession of Dietetics.* Chicago, Am. Dietet. A., 1972.
13. Dibble, M. V., and Lally, J. R.: J. Nutr. Educa. 5:200, 1973.

2 carbohydrates

MAN'S MAJOR SOURCE OF ENERGY

Carbohydrates, chiefly in the form of cereal grains and root vegetables, are the major sources of energy for most peoples of the world. They provide from 45 to 50 percent of the calories of the American diet and a far higher percentage for many other peoples. They are the cheapest and the most easily digested form of human and animal energy. The protein-sparing function of carbohydrates, whereby they supply the energy needs and "spare" protein for other purposes, is an important consideration if the supply of protein is limited. "Carbohydrate, the fuel of life" applies to more people than does the more common phrase, "Bread, the staff of life."

The proportion of total calories derived from common carbohydrate foods around the world throws light on the respective standards of living in various countries. Most of the peoples of Asia, the Middle Eastern countries, Africa, and Latin America derive over 80 percent of their calories from grains and potatoes or other root vegetables.

As economic standards have gone up,

especially in the United States and Great Britain, the amount of sugar in the diet has increased while the amount of starch from cereal grains has decreased proportionately. The consumption of sugar in the United States increased until about 1925, but since that time has remained stable at 16 to 17 percent of total energy. The percentage of total energy consumed as starch has decreased from 43 percent in 1909 to 29 percent in the 1970s.[1] The grains and other carbohydrate foods used typically in different countries will be mentioned as the food sources are discussed. (Energy metabolism is discussed in Chapter 8.)

PHOTOSYNTHESIS

Carbohydrates are the chief form in which plants store potential energy. They are compounds of carbon, hydrogen, and oxygen which, with the aid of the sun, are synthesized from the water in the soil and the carbon dioxide in the air by the chlorophyll in the chloroplasts of green plants (Fig. 2-1). This process, which converts solar energy into chemical energy, is known as photosynthesis. The reaction is so complex that science has yet to fully understand and duplicate the chemical laboratory of the green leaf.

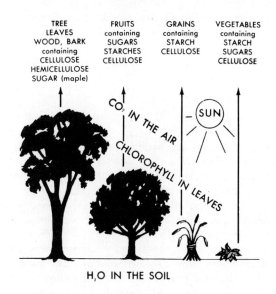

Fig. 2-1. Synthesis of carbohydrates in plants.

The largest proportion of the sun's energy which is transformed into potential energy by plants appears in some form of carbohydrate. Monosaccharides, particularly glucose, are synthesized first, and then com-

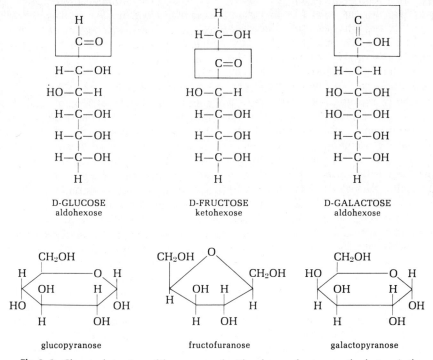

Fig. 2-2. Chemical structure of the monosaccharides glucose, fructose, and galactose in the straight chain form (above) and the ring form (below). Each of these sugars is a hexose containing 6 carbon atoms, 12 hydrogen atoms, and 6 oxygen atoms. Glucose and galactose are aldoses and fructose is a ketose (boxed-in areas). Glucose and galactose are shown below in the pyranose ring form and fructose in the furanose ring form.

bined to form disaccharides and polysaccharides. The chemical energy formed in this process can be utilized for the biosynthesis of fat, certain amino acids, and other essential substances in the plant.

SIMPLE SUGARS

Monosaccharides (Fig. 2-2) are the simplest carbohydrate units and are classified according to (1) whether they are aldehyde or ketone derivatives and (2) the number of carbon atoms in the molecule. Hexoses, sugars containing six carbon atoms, are the nutritionally significant sugars found in foods, while others, particularly the pentoses, ribose and deoxyribose, which contain five carbon atoms, are produced in the metabolism of foodstuffs. The single hexoses, glucose, fructose, and galactose, require no digestion and are readily absorbed from the intestine directly into the bloodstream (see Chapter 9).

Glucose, also called dextrose, is a moderately sweet sugar found in fruits and vegetables. Linked with another molecule of a monosaccharide it is a component of all the disaccharides and is the basic structural unit of the polysaccharides starch and cellulose. It is prepared commercially as corn syrup by the acid hydrolysis of starch. Fermentation of glucose by the enzyme zymase in yeast results in the formation of carbon dioxide and ethyl alcohol. Glucose is the form of carbohydrate to which all other carbohydrates are converted eventually for transport in the blood and for utilization by the cells of the body. The following terms are used to describe the blood glucose level in the body: *normoglycemia* refers to a blood glucose level within normal range (60 to 100 mg. percent), *hyperglycemia* indicates a blood glucose level above normal range, and *hypoglycemia* means a blood glucose level below normal range.

Fructose, also called levulose or fruit sugar, is found associated with glucose in many fruits and vegetables, and especially in honey. It is a highly soluble sugar and the sweetest of the simple sugars. It is fermented by yeast. It is combined with glucose to form sucrose and is the structural unit in inulin, a polysaccharide found in certain roots (Jerusalem artichoke) and bulbs (onions and garlic). Inulin, however, has limited dietary significance since very little is digested in the gastrointestinal tract.

Galactose is seldom found free in nature but is derived chiefly by hydrolysis from the disaccharide lactose, found in milk. It is less soluble in water and less sweet than glucose. Some galactosans, also called galactans, occur in food. Since little is known about the digestibility of these galactose-containing polysaccharides, they are frequently excluded in the dietary treatment of galactosemia (Chapter 35). Galactose is also a constituent of the glycolipids and glycoproteins found in many tissues. In the body, glucose can be changed to galactose so that the mammary glands can produce lactose.

Sugar alcohols called sorbitol and mannitol have a sweetening effect similar to glucose. *Sorbitol,* which is made commercially from glucose by hydrogenation and also is found in many fruits and vegetables, is very slowly absorbed into the bloodstream and can apparently be metabolized without insulin. It has the same caloric value as glucose, the sugar from which it is derived. *Mannitol,* obtained commercially by hydrogenation of mannose, occurs naturally in pineapples, olives, asparagus, and carrots, and may also be added as a drying agent to other foods. Since it is poorly absorbed, mannitol supplies about one half the energy value of glucose.

Inositol occurs in many foods, especially in the bran of cereal grains. Inositol when combined with certain phosphate groups forms phytic acid which reduces the absorption of calcium and iron from the intestines. *Dulcitol*, obtained from galactose by hydrogenation, is sometimes added to foods.

Alcohol or **ethanol** is produced from the fermentation of glucose by the enzymes in yeast and may, for certain individuals consuming large quantities of alcoholic beverages, represent a significant part of the total energy intake. One gram of alcohol yields 7 kilocalories (kcal.). One jigger, approximately 1 ounce (30 ml.), of 100-proof alcohol (50 percent alcohol) contains about 15 g. of alcohol which contributes 105 kcal. (see Table 6, Section 4).

Ethanol requires no digestion and can be absorbed throughout the gastrointestinal tract. Its concentration in the body is in proportion to the water content of the tissue, and hence the blood can contain large amounts of alcohol while bone and adipose tissue have little. Alcohol is metabolized primarily in the liver where the enzyme alcohol dehydrogenase, essential for the conversion of ethanol to acetaldehyde, is found. Since alcohol also requires NAD^+ (nicotinamide adenine dinucleotide) (see Chapter 9) for this reaction, the rate of alcohol metabolism is increased by the simultaneous metabolism of carbohydrate (pyruvate). For the same reason, fasting or starvation decreases the rate of alcohol metabolism.

The **disaccharides** (Fig. 2-3)—sugars containing two hexose units—that are commonly encountered in foods are sucrose (cane or beet sugar), maltose (malt sugar), and lactose (milk sugar). Disaccharides are hydrolyzed by specific enzymes in the digestive tract into monosaccharides, or commercially by acid hydrolysis. Each of the three disaccharides has distinct characteristics of interest in human nutrition.

Sucrose—ordinary granulated, powdered, or brown sugar and molasses—is one of the sweetest forms of sugar. It is also found free in most fruits and vegetables. It is very soluble and on hydrolysis yields equal amounts of fructose and glucose, or invert sugar, as this mixture is commonly called.

Maltose, or malt sugar, does not occur free in nature but is manufactured from starch by enzyme or acid hydrolysis. It is less sweet than sucrose and very soluble in water. Two molecules of glucose are formed by the hydrolysis of maltose. In the body it is an intermediate product in starch digestion.

Maltose, easily utilized by the body, is sometimes used in combination with dextrin, a polysaccharide, as an ingredient in home-prepared infant formulas where it is desirable to have a soluble form of carbohydrate which does not readily ferment in the digestive tract.

Lactose, or milk sugar, is the only one of the common sugars not found in plants. It is not very soluble and is the least sweet of the sugars, only about one-sixth as sweet as sucrose; hence it is responsible for the blandness of milk. It is formed only in the mammary glands of lactating mothers, animal or human. When lactose is hydrolyzed, a molecule of glucose and a molecule of galactose are formed.

A **trisaccharide** called *raffinose*, containing the three hexoses, glucose, fructose, and galactose, is found along with sucrose in molasses. *Maltotriose*, an intermediate product formed during the digestion of starch, contains three glucose units.

COMPLEX CARBOHYDRATES

For more stable and efficient storage of potential energy, plants and animals pack carbohydrate energy in units much larger than the sugars—i.e., dextrin, starch, cellulose, and glycogen. All of these are **polysaccharides,** the molecules of which may contain several hundred times as many glucose units as those of the sugars. Consequently they are much less soluble and more stable but differ markedly among themselves as to digestibility and resistance to spoilage. Since there is so much moisture in all growing plants, one essential characteristic of a storage material is insolubility. To be suitable for human food, however, a carbohydrate must be subject to digestion by the enzymes of the digestive tract. Starches and dextrins fall into this category, but celluloses and hemicelluloses, which also occur in food, are not digested by humans.

Dextrins occur mostly as intermediate products in

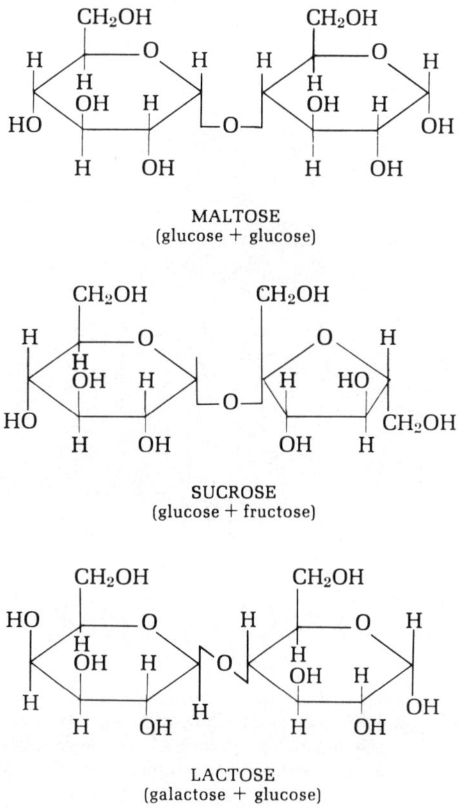

Fig. 2-3. Disaccharides in their ring forms. Maltose contains two glucose molecules, sucrose one glucose and one fructose molecule, and lactose one glucose and one galactose molecule.

the partial hydrolysis of starch by enzymatic action or in cooking. They are made up of many glucose units joined together with the same linkages as starch. The individual molecules are smaller than starch, and they do not have the thickening property of starch. They are water soluble and, depending on their color reaction with iodine, are classified as soluble starch (blue), amylodextrin (purple), erythrodextrin (red), and achroodextrin (colorless). Dextrins are formed when bread or cereals are toasted or flour is browned. They are also used in some infant formula preparations and in products used in soda fountain beverages.

α-Limit dextrins are formed in the digestion of the amylopectin form of starch since beta-amylase cannot split the branched chain linkage.[1,6]

Starch, the chief form of carbohydrate in the diet, occurs in two forms (Fig. 2-4): (1) amylose, a straight chain polysaccharide of glucose units linked together the same as maltose (1,4 glucosidic bonds) and (2) amylopectin, a branched structure of glucose units

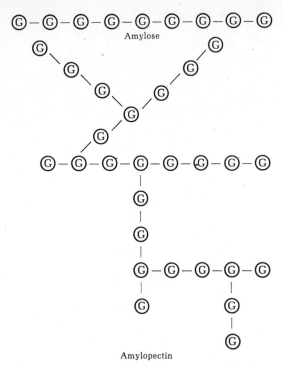

Amylose

Amylopectin

Fig. 2-4. Simplified diagrams of amylose and amylopectin, the two forms of starch found in foods. Amylose molecules consist of 250 to 300 units of glucose in a straight chain. Amylopectin in addition to containing the straight chain units of amylose also has branched chains and is composed of over 1000 glucose units.

ENDOSPERM

. . . about 83% of the kernel

Source of white flour. Of the nutrients in the whole kernel the endosperm contains about:

70-75% of the protein
43% of the pantothenic acid
32% of the riboflavin
12% of the niacin
6% of the pyridoxine
3% of the thiamine

} B-complex vitamins

Enriched flour products contain added quantities of riboflavin, niacin and thiamine, plus iron, in amounts equal to or exceeding whole wheat—according to a formula established on the basis of popular need of those nutrients.

BRAN . . . about 14½% of the kernel

Included in whole wheat flour. Of the nutrients in whole wheat, the bran, in addition to indigestible cellulose material contains about:

86% of the niacin
73% of the pyridoxine
50% of the pantothenic acid
42% of the riboflavin
33% of the thiamine
19% of the protein

GERM . . . about 2½% of the kernel

The embryo or sprouting section of the seed, usually separated because it contains fat which limits the keeping quality of flours. Available separately as human food. Of the nutrients in whole wheat, the germ contains about:

64% of the thiamine
26% of the riboflavin
21% of the pyridoxine
8% of the protein
7% of the pantothenic acid
2% of the niacin

with a linkage different from maltose at the branchings (1,6 glucosidic bonds) but similar throughout the rest of the chain. Starch is found in cereal grains, vegetables, and other plants. The starch of the grain is mostly in the endosperm (Fig. 2-5), encased in a protective covering of cellulose (the bran or the husk). The starch granule in the endosperm consists of tiny particles of starch usually arranged in concentric layers in a pattern of characteristic shape and appearance. The starch granules in turn may be enclosed in cells of larger size. This storage of starch in plants may be compared to warehouse storing of small packages of prepared cereal in cartons, with the cartons in turn packed in larger containers for ease in handling.

Before starch can be used readily by the body, the outer membrane must be broken, either by grinding or cooking. By the application of heat and moisture the outer cellulose envelope is ruptured, and the moisture permeates the starch granules themselves. Starch granules have an affinity for water, absorbing it like a

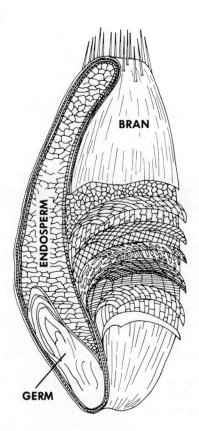

Fig. 2-5. A cross section of a kernel of wheat and the nutrients in each of the three parts—endosperm, bran, and germ (Kansas Wheat Commission)

sponge and increasing greatly in volume. The thickening property of a starch varies according to the source: for example, that of potato starch is greater than those of corn or wheat. After rupture of the cellulose wall by cooking, the starch is in a form that can be acted on more easily by digestive enzymes.

Cooking may carry the breakdown of starch to the dextrin stage if continued long enough. Starch granules break down most rapidly when moisture is present. Long application of dry heat, such as in baking or toasting, will also change starch to soluble dextrins. The palatable flavor of the brown crust of rolls or bread or the brown part of toast or of toasted cereals is due partly to forms of dextrin.

Modified food starches are natural starches which have been chemically and/or physically modified to provide special properties desirable in food processing. The types of modification include cross-bonding with phosphates, derivatization such as esterification, conversion by acid or enzyme activity, and pregelatinization. Thus depending on their treatment modified starches may have greater viscosity, more resistance to syneresis (weeping or leaking), improved clarity, and/or the ability to be dispersed in cold water. They are used in the processing of sauces for canned and frozen foods, frozen fruit pies, infant foods, canned and instant puddings, and gumdrops.

Cellulose, found in the framework of plants, is also a polysaccharide of glucose units but with linkages different from maltose and starch. It is the chief constituent of wood, stalks and leaves of all plants, and the outer coverings of seeds and cereals. Cellulose forms the more or less porous walls of cells in which water, starch, minerals, and other substances are stored in the plant much as honey is held in the comb.

No cellulose-splitting enzyme is secreted by the mucosa of the human gastrointestinal tract, but bacterial fermentation or disintegration may play a role in dissolving the substances that bind the cellulose fibers or particles together.

The indigestibility of cellulose is its major asset, since the undigested fiber furnishes the bulk necessary for efficient and normal peristaltic action (muscular contraction) of the intestines. Research has demonstrated that the normal colon performs better when a reasonable amount (4 to 7 g.) of bulk or residue is present.

Methylcellulose and other cellulose derivatives which absorb large quantities of water may be used in manufacturing low calorie foods such as imitation syrups and salad dressings.

Glycogen, or "animal starch" is the form in which the animal stores carbohydrate. It is a polysaccharide similar to amylopectin but with more branched chains and higher molecular weight. When more glucose than can be immediately metabolized enters the bloodstream, the normal individual combines many glucose molecules (up to 30,000) to form glycogen. By the same token, when glucose is needed, glycogen is broken down and glucose becomes quickly available for energy (see Chapter 8). In the living mammal both the liver and muscle store glycogen. Approximately three quarters of a pound of glycogen can be stored by the adult male, one quarter pound in the liver and one half pound in muscles. The liver glycogen is the more quickly available for replenishing blood sugar. The muscle glycogen is used primarily as fuel for the muscles. In muscle meat as purchased little glycogen is present because it disappears during rigor mortis. Scallops, oysters, and other shellfish contain significant amounts of glycogen.

Other polysaccharides, such as the pectic substances, agar, alginates, carrageenans (Irish moss), and vegetable gums, cannot be digested but are used in various foods because of their colloidal property, i.e., the ability to absorb water and form a gel. Commercial pectin, prepared from cull apple peels and cores or the albedo of lemons and available as liquid or powder, is used primarily for making fruit jellies. Agar is used as a thickening agent in candy manufacturing and in processing meats; the alginates and carrageenans are used in the manufacture of ice cream to give body and smooth consistency and as stabilizing agents in other food processing. Carrageenans have the unique ability to stabilize milk proteins and hence are used in evaporated and flavored milks. Vegetable gums, including arabic, tragacanth, guar, and xanthan, are also used in a variety of products as waterbinders, thickeners, and stabilizers.

In the process of human metabolism *mucopolysaccharides* such as hyaluronic acid and chondroitin sulfate are synthesized and found in the ground substance of connective tissue where they have structural importance.

ROLE OF CARBOHYDRATES IN HEALTH
Energy

Carbohydrates are a major source of energy in the human diet; approximately 4 kcal. are provided by each gram of carbohydrate. Although fat and protein can replace carbohydrate as a source of energy for most of the cells of the body, some carbohydrate is essential for humans. Brain, nerve, and lung tissue require glucose as their source of energy. If the blood glucose level falls (hypoglycemia) and the brain is deprived of glucose, convulsions may result. It should be pointed out, however, that certain amino acids and part of the fat molecule can also contribute to the total amount of glucose available in the body and thus provide a source of energy for these tissues. Also, as will be discussed in Chapter 9, carbohydrates, especially sugars, are converted to fats (triglycerides) in the liver and become available to cells for energy or storage in adipose tissue. In transamination reactions intermediary products of carbohydrate metabolism can be converted into amino acids and used for protein synthesis.

Although we very seldom find a diet free of carbohydrate, persons who, as participants in experimental studies, have consumed such diets have developed many of the same symptoms as persons on a starvation regimen. These symptoms include abnormal fat metabolism, breakdown of body protein, increased sodium excretion, loss of energy, and fatigue. Relatively small amounts (50 to 100 g.) of carbohydrate appear to prevent these symptoms.[2]

Detoxification

Glucuronic acid, an oxidation product of glucose metabolism, is important in the detoxification of a number of intermediary products of normal metabolism and of certain drugs. Morphine, salicylic acid, and the sulfa drugs are but a few of the drugs that are detoxified by combining with and being excreted as glucuronic acid derivatives.

Dental Caries

Carbohydrates, primarily sugars, are easily fermented and can produce weak inorganic acids capable of dissolving the mineral constituents of the enamel and dentin of the teeth. The combination of sugar and certain bacteria found in plaque, a sticky, colorless film of nonpathogenic oral bacteria that forms on teeth, results in the production of acids which can attack the tooth and lead to decay. Foods which adhere to the teeth and sticky sweets, such as caramels, pastries, and candied apples, are the most damaging. However, soft drinks and sweetened juices can also be harmful to dental health. Good oral hygiene, less frequent consumption of sweets, and limiting certain forms of snack foods are practices that will help reduce the incidence of dental caries.[3]

Fiber in the Diet

Scala has estimated that during this century in the United States the consumption of fiber from fresh and processed fruits and vegetables has declined by 20 percent, and from cereals and grain, by 50 percent.[4] Fiber or bulk in the diet promotes more frequent bowel movements and softer stools having increased weight. Diets high in cereal fibers, because of the effect that the looser, softer stools have on the intestines, have been shown to reduce the symptoms of diverticulosis, a disease of the large intestines. In rural Africa, where the amount of fiber in the diet is four to six times higher than in the typical American diet, diverticular disease is unknown. However, in urban Africa, where fiber consumption is similar to that of the United States, the incidence of the disease is comparable.

Persons who consume high fiber diets also excrete more fat, sterols, and bile acids in their stools and have been shown to have lower blood cholesterol levels. Thus it has been suggested that the amount of fiber in the diet may be a factor in the prevention of atherosclerosis.

It has also been postulated that the reduction of fiber in the American diet may be a factor in the increased incidence in the United States of cancer of the colon. If a foreign material, a virus or a chemical, causes the cancer, this substance would be in the intestinal tract longer and hence could do more harm in individuals consuming low fiber diets.

Although the nutrition counselor should be aware of the possible roles of fiber in the maintenance of positive health, specific application of these findings to nutrition counseling awaits further study.

PLANT SOURCES OF CARBOHYDRATES
Cereal Grains

The ancient Romans called Demeter, the Greek goddess of the grains and harvests, Ceres, and from her name the word cereal is derived. Because of their wide cultivation, good keeping qualities, bland flavor, and great variety, cereals have continued to be the staple of the human diet from prehistoric times to the present. Most of them belong to the botanic family of grasses, with the exception of buckwheat. Each of the cereals has characteristic properties and uses.

The "green revolution," which combined modern agricultural methods with new high-yielding varieties of cereals, has produced a dramatic increase in cereal grain production throughout certain areas of the world. Asian countries, particularly India, have benefited most. In 1973, 40 percent of India's grain production came from new varieties and was grown on only 20 percent of the total grain acreage.[5] The continuation and spread of the "green revolution" offers great hope that more and more of the developing nations can become self-sufficient in their food production. Unfortunately, recent shortages of fertilizers, made from petrochemicals at present expensive and in short supply, have counteracted some of the benefits of the "green revolution."

Rice has the widest use of any cereal in the world. It is the staple food for Asia, the Near East, some Latin American countries and some African countries and is widely used elsewhere. It provides as much as 70 to 80 percent of the calories for the larger part of the population of these areas.

About 80 percent of the billion and a half Asians are involved in the production and distribution of rice. To meet the ever increasing demand for rice, the International Rice Research Institute in the Philippines directs work on improving rice production and was involved in the development of a new strain with improved yield and drastically reduced growing time. Rice production in Ceylon increased over 30 percent in three years and for the first time in 70 years the Philippines are self-sufficient in rice.[6]

Rice is usually milled as *regular* white rice, the form preferred by most people, although much of the vitamin and mineral content is lost in the milling. When the ancient home milling process, which involves parboiling or steaming before polishing, is used, some of the vitamins and minerals are forced into the center of the kernel and thus are conserved. The *parboiled* or converted rice available in the United States is commercially parboiled by special steam processing before milling and retains a somewhat higher vitamin and mineral content than regular white rice. Parboiled rice supplies about twice as much calcium, phosphorus, and potassium per serving as regular. However, enriched regular and enriched parboiled rice contain approximately the same amounts of iron, thiamine, and niacin. These amounts are based on minimum levels of enrichment as specified by U. S. government regulations. Enriched *precooked* (instant) rice, which requires a minimum of preparation time, is also available in the United States and contains the same level of enrichment as regular and parboiled rice.

A high-vitamin "premix" is being used in Japan and the Philippines. The "premix," which is heavily fortified with certain B vitamins, is applied to the white rice together with a protective coating that is highly resistant to cooking losses.

Unpolished brown rice and "wild rice," both of which contain more of the original minerals and vitamins than does white rice, have limited use because of their different flavor, poor keeping quality, and high price. Rice-eating countries do not use rice for bread making but use it in place of bread. Rice flour is used in making a wide variety of delectable snack foods in some of the Oriental countries.

Wheat is the next most common cereal used throughout the world and the most widely used in the Americas and Europe. High-yielding varieties of wheat have been developed through research sponsored by the Rockefeller and Ford Foundations at the International Maize and Wheat Improvement Center in Mexico. When the new Mexican wheat was planted in India and Pakistan the annual increase in yield per acre was doubled and wheat production increased by 50 percent in four years.[7]

Wheat can be milled for a variety of uses—as breakfast cereals, as flour for bread, cakes, pastries, and crackers, and for macaroni products. It lends itself to bread making better than other grains because of its high gluten content, which is necessary for yeast breads that demand kneading. Wheat flour is equally good for baking-powder breads, cakes, and cookies. Certain varieties of wheat are preferred for bread flour, others for cake flour, but for both the flour is manufactured by roller- or impact-milling—complicated processes designed to produce a pure white flour containing none of the bran or the germ. The final product represents 70 percent or less of the wheat kernel. The outer coatings and the germ, which contain the bulk of the minerals and vitamins, are sold mostly as stock feed. A small amount of pure wheat germ is processed for human consumption. Some bran is also processed for use as high-roughage breakfast cereals.

A small proportion of our wheat crop in the United States is milled as whole-wheat or Graham flour and some as whole-wheat breakfast cereal. Hard winter wheat is milled as semolina for the manufacture of macaroni, spaghetti, vermicelli, and noodles. A wide variety of these products are used in Italy and elsewhere in Europe as well as in the Americas and the Orient.

Rye is similar to wheat in many respects; rye flour may be used with wheat or by itself for bread making. Rye breads such as pumpernickel or Swedish rye are used in northern and central Europe and in Russia more commonly than in the United States.

Triticale, a hybrid cereal produced by crossbreeding wheat and rye, has been known since the late 1880s but has not been grown to any extent until recently. Research at the International Maize and Wheat Improvement Center in cooperation with the University of Manitoba has led to the development of high-yielding varieties of triticale which can be milled into flour to make bread, rolls, and pasta products such as macaroni, noodles, and spaghetti.[8] In the future we may have in the United States a very mild rye-flavored white bread made from triticale.

Corn (or maize) is used for human food in many countries of the world; some areas, for example in Central and South America, depend on corn as the staple food. To people in these areas the research currently being done in Mexico City at the International Maize and Wheat Improvement Center to develop new varieties of corn is especially important. By genetic manipulation a new maize variety with increased amounts of the essential amino acid lysine has been developed, thereby improving the protein quality of the corn (see Chapter 4).[9]

Corn is processed from several different varieties of mature field corn into many forms: cornmeal, white and yellow; hominy grits; samp, or hulled corn; popcorn; cornflakes or similar ready-to-eat cereals; and as a source of cornstarch, corn syrup, and corn oil. Yellow or white cornmeal is cooked as mush or grits and is used in pancakes or in cornmeal breads, corn pone, muffins, johnnycakes and, in Central and South America, for tamales and tortillas. Cornstarch is sold commercially as a thickening agent used in cooking. Waxy cornstarch which contains only the branched or amylopectin fraction, provides thickening without retrogradation. Since it is relatively stable to freezing and thawing it can be used as a thickening agent in prepared frozen dishes.

New high-amylose cornstarches are also now available to food processors and because of their unique properties are being used in a variety of food products. Due to their linear structure they have the ability to form films which act as oxygen and fat barriers on food and packaging materials, to form quick-setting structurally stable gels, and to bind other materials into stable extruded shapes. The consumer will find increased use of these starches in partially fried foods such as french-fried potatoes; textured protein products (see Chapter 4); gelatin molds; gumdrops; textured pastes, e.g., tomato paste; applesauce; and edible or readily biodegradable food packaging.

Enzymatically produced cornstarch hydrolysates having properties intermediate between cornstarch and corn syrup are also available to the food processor for use in fabricated foods. They are soluble, nonsweet, and easily digestible, and may be used to improve the body and texture of certain food items.

Corn sugar and syrup are made by hydrolyzing the starch in the corn, i.e., breaking it down into dextrins, maltose, and glucose. A new dextrose (glucose)-levulose (fructose) syrup is now being manufactured from corn syrup by enzymatically (glucose isomerase) converting dextrose to levulose. The syrup contains approximately 45 percent fructose and 53 percent glucose, has a sweet flavor, and is highly fermentable.

Corn oil is extracted from the corn germ by a carefully controlled commercial process. The special properties of corn oil will be discussed in Chapter 3.

Oats are used chiefly in the form of rolled oats or oatmeal in the United States and western Europe. In recent years some ready-to-eat cereals have been processed from oats. Oat products carry more of the original kernel than do most other processed cereals and thus lose fewer nutrients between field and table than products of any other cereal.

Granola-type cereals are usually mixtures of whole oats and wheat with brown sugar, raisins, nuts, and other ingredients added.

Barley is used mostly as "pearled" barley, which is the kernel left after the bran and the germ have been removed. Barley flour is made by grinding the "pearls." In the United States pearl barley has limited use in soups. In some other countries such as Korea and Japan barley is raised and used as a low-cost substitute for rice.

Buckwheat is not a true cereal botanically, i.e., it does not belong to the grasses as do the other cereals, but it serves the same purpose for human food. The bran, or the husk, is removed and the rest of the kernel is rolled and bolted to produce buckwheat flour. In the United States its most common use is in buckwheat pancakes, waffles, and ready-to-eat cereals; in Japan buckwheat is used in noodles. In Europe buckwheat is used in making heavy breads, puddings, cakes, and beer.

Millet is a staple food for millions of people in India, Russia, China, and Africa but is little known in the United States. It can be raised where land is too poor and the climate too dry to grow wheat, rice, corn, or most other grains. Millet is used in eastern Europe for making flat bread and porridge. Russian "kasha" (cereal), often made from millet, may also be made from wheat or buckwheat.

MILLING OF GRAINS. Natural grains carry not only the store of carbohydrates already mentioned but also protein and certain minerals and vitamins essential for good nutrition. The vitamin-B-complex factors present in the natural whole grains are usually sufficient in amount to help form the enzymes necessary for the metabolism of the carbohydrate of the grain. The balance of nature is upset when we find it desirable to modify natural grains by milling them to produce a whiter, more easily digested flour with better keeping qualities. In so doing some of the minerals and vitamins are lost or discarded in the millings. It is interesting to note that the latter find excellent use as animal feed. Attempts to educate people accustomed to white-flour products to return to the use of whole-grain products have never been successful. Consequently, the expedient of enrichment of bread and flour was initiated in the United States during World War II, with other cereal products of various types added to the list later. Thiamine, riboflavin, niacin, and iron are the factors added (see Chapter 10). Bread and flour enrichment is of first importance because bread and products made from flour constitute some of the main sources of energy in the American diet.

Fruits

Fruits and vegetables constitute a less concentrated source of carbohydrates than do the cereals because of their high water content. In fruits the carbohydrate is mostly in the form of the monosaccharides glucose and fructose. The disaccharide, sucrose, may be found in a few fresh fruits, and most canned fruits contain added sucrose or glucose unless specifically labeled "canned without added sugar." The soluble sugars along with the fruits' acids and traces of volatile oils give fruits their odor and appetite appeal, which is further enhanced by color and texture.

The sugar content of fresh fruits may vary from 6 to 20 percent, those of cantaloupe and watermelon being the lowest and that of banana one of the highest. Of course, dried fruits such as prunes, apricots, raisins, dates, and figs have a much higher sugar content (near 70 percent) due to their low moisture content. The energy value of fruits—fresh, canned, or frozen—is determined largely by their sugar content.

Although most fruits are considered highly desirable raw, plantains, which are related to but larger than the banana, are not palatable unless cooked. Because of their high starch content these fruits are an important source of carbohydrates in many tropical countries and when boiled, baked, or fried are frequently used in the main course of the meal.

The avocado pear and the olive are different from all other fruits because of their high fat content, which gives them a comparatively high energy value in spite of their low carbohydrate content.

Most fresh fruits also contain some cellulose or hemicellulose. This type of bulk, along with the fruit acids, seems to serve as a stimulant to intestinal motility for many people.

Vegetables

Under the term *vegetables* are grouped foods representing practically every part of the plant—leaves, stems, seeds, seed pods, flowers, fruits, roots, and tubers. They vary as widely in composition as they do in function in the plant and may contain anywhere from 3 to 35 percent of carbohydrate in the forms of starch, sugars, cellulose, and hemicellulose.

Obviously, the energy value of vegetables varies with the percentage of carbohydrate present, but, in general, the high water and cellulose content of leaf, flower, and stem vegetables puts them in the low calorie class. These include all the green leafy vegetables, plus celery, asparagus, cauliflower, broccoli, and Brussels sprouts. The roots, the tubers, and the seeds of plants have a higher starch and sugar content and less water and, therefore, provide more calories per unit of weight. These include all kinds of potatoes, beets, carrots, turnips, parsnips, peas, beans, and lentils.

The cellulose and hemicellulose found typically in vegetables also vary in amount and digestibility. Some forms of cellulose such as that in certain leafy and stem vegetables and in sweet corn are so resistant even to bacterial digestion and so frequently irritating that they may not be tolerated by some adults or by young children.

Root vegetables often provide much of the carbohydrate in the diets of certain African, Latin American, and Asian peoples. Since they are for the most part very poor in protein, their wide use creates certain nutrition problems, particularly in infant feeding where they may take the place of more nutritious foods. Cassava, also called manioc or yuca, has a long root which is 1 to 3 inches thick. It is frequently grated, dried, and powdered as a "meal"—tapioca or arrowroot. Taro, which is also grown in tropical and subtropical countries, can be baked or boiled like a potato. The Hawaiians boil the eddoes (as the roots are called), then peel and grind them with water to make *poi*, the sticky pastelike food so popular in the Islands. Other roots and tubers such as sweet potatoes, yams, turnips, and Jerusalem artichokes may also be used as staple foods at certain times by

Table 2-1. Carbohydrates in Common Foods

STARCHES	Percent
Barley, pearled	79
Breads, all types	52-58
Cassava, meal and flour	85
Cornmeal and grits	74-78
Crackers	71-74
Macaroni, spaghetti, and noodles	73-77
Oatmeal or oat cereals	70
Potatoes, cooked	19
Rice or rice cereals	79
Rye flour	68-78
Wheat flour	69-79
Wheat cereals	72-80

SUGARS	Percent
Cakes*	56-62
Candies	56-99
Cookies*	60-80
Dried fruits	75-88
Honey	80
Jams and jellies	65-71
Syrups	74
Cane or beet sugar	100

*Also include starch

various peoples. To improve agricultural production of certain tropical crops the International Center of Tropical Agriculture in Colombia and the International Institute of Tropical Agriculture in Nigeria have been established.

Nuts

Nuts seldom are thought of as a source of carbohydrate because of their high content of fat and protein. However, because of their low moisture content, they contain from 10 to 27 percent total carbohydrate. They also contain from 1 to 2 percent fiber. Peanuts, which are really legumes, are usually classed with the nuts because of their composition and common usage.

Because of the high fat content, nuts digest slowly. Chopping or grinding improves digestibility. In the form of nut butter and combined with other foods, there is usually no digestive difficulty. Peanut butter may be used in sandwiches or as an ingredient of a recipe.

Other Plant Sources of Carbohydrates

Common table sugar—the refined white granulated or powdered sugar or brown sugar—is processed from either sugar cane or sugar beets.

Sucrose is the chief source of sweetening used in most desserts, ice creams, candies, and soft drinks. The average per capita consumption of sugar in the United States is estimated at approximately two pounds per week. This means, of course, that some persons use much more than this, and others consume far less. Since sugar is 99.9 percent carbohydrate and furnishes almost 4 calories to the gram, those who use the average amount or more are getting more than 3,500 empty calories per week. Sugar is concentrated fuel but furnishes no other nutrients. Furthermore, candies and other sweets are reputed to aggravate dental caries, a major health problem. Sugar consumption in the form of candies, soft drinks and rich desserts is certainly a contributing factor to the great American problem of obesity (Chapter 27).

Molasses is a by-product of sugar refining and carries more of the mineral content of the original plant than do the refined sugars.

Maple syrup and sugar are made by boiling down the sap from sugar maples. This was one of the kinds of sugar used earliest in America—its source known to the Indians and taught to the early settlers by them. Regardless of flavor or color, which are due to traces of other factors, the sugar in all of the above products is the disaccharide sucrose.

Corn syrup, made from field corn by hydrolysis of the starch, is mostly glucose and maltose.

Honey, made by bees from flower nectars, contains a mixture of the two monosaccharides, glucose and fructose. The fructose in honey makes it taste sweeter than corn syrup because fructose has a sweeter taste then either glucose or maltose.

Sorghum syrup is made from the sweet juice of the grain sorghum stem, and its use is confined largely to the southeastern and south central states. Grain sorghums are also used for food in parts of India, China, and Africa.

Other forms of plant life not usually classed as vegetables are the seaweeds used for food in many countries, notably Japan. Certain varieties of seaweed are sources of *agar, alginates,* and *carrageenans*.

Change of Form

Interchanges among the different forms of carbohydrate in the plant world are interesting and significant factors in food quality and keeping properties. As growth proceeds, there is constant exchange from one form to another. In fruits such as the banana the carbohydrate is in the form of starch in the maturing fruit, but some of it is changed to sugar as the fruit ripens. In some vegetables sugar synthesized by the leaves is stored as starch, as in potatoes and in mature beans, peas, and corn. Connoisseurs of fresh garden vegetables are aware of how quickly the sugar of corn and green peas disappears after harvesting, and how much more delicious they are when used immediately after picking. This change is due to the enzymes that are present in the vegetables, and the change is stopped as soon as the enzymes are destroyed by heating. Thus, frozen vegetables that have been blanched promptly after harvesting and before freezing may have better flavor than do so-called fresh vegetables that have been shipped long distances and stored before appearing at market.

Animal Sources of Carbohydrates

Most animal foods, such as meats, poultry, and fish, contain only traces of carbohydrate in the form of *glycogen* used for muscle contraction. Eggs also contain only traces of carbohydrate. Only liver contains an appreciable amount, and this is in the form of glycogen. In all animals the liver serves as a temporary storehouse for quickly available fuel for the body, and it may contain from 2 to 6 percent of glycogen. Another source of glycogen in foods is the seafood, scallops, which are the muscles of shellfish and contain about 3 percent of glycogen.

Fresh milk contains about 5 percent of carbohydrate in the form of *lactose*, a disaccharide. When consumed in amounts greater than those ordinarily present in milk, some lactose may not be digested. An undigested residue of lactose in the large intestine has a laxative action which may be desirable in certain instances but in excess causes diarrhea. Lactose is an excellent medium for the growth of certain useful acid-tolerant bacteria and has been used therapeutically to increase this type of bacterial flora in the large intestines. Lactose also seems to increase the absorption or utilization of calcium, and often this finding is cited as the reason for the efficient utilization of calcium from milk. Sometimes lactose is given as an accompaniment of calcium salts prescribed for persons who have an allergy to milk and must obtain their calcium in another form.

A summary of the types and amounts of carbohydrates found in various foods was compiled by Hardinge et al.[10]

STUDY QUESTIONS AND ACTIVITIES

1. Name the monosaccharides and give some food sources of each. What are their chemical similarities and differences?
2. What are the two forms of starch? How do they differ in structure and in use?
3. Why is it important to include alcohol consumption when food intake is calculated?
4. What kind of sugar is made from cane or sugar beets? Where else may this same sugar be found in nature?
5. In what way is the sugar of milk unique? How is it classified chemically?
6. Which carbohydrates are most common in fruits? In root vegetables?
7. What type of food provides the most common source of carbohydrate and energy for the world's people? What are some of the regional or national preferences?
8. What is another name for "animal starch"? Where is it found? Of what significance is it in animal nutrition?
9. Certain polysaccharides are not digested by intestinal enzymes. Which are they? In which foods do we find them? What is their function?
10. Compare the sweetness of the sugars. Why does honey taste sweeter than cane syrup?
11. List the carbohydrate foods you consumed in the past 24 hours. How wide a variety of plant sources is represented?
12. How does your sugar intake compare with that of other carbohydrate sources? If it seems high, how can you replace it with more nutritious but equally desirable foods?
13. Glance at the "ready-to-eat" cereal shelf in the local supermarket. How many cereal grains are represented? What added ingredients do some of them have? Do you consider this beneficial? What would you judge to be the difference in cost between a serving (1 ounce) of ready-to-eat cereal and a cooked cereal?

SUPPLEMENTARY READINGS

Hodges, R. E.: Present knowledge of carbohydrates. Nutr. Rev., 24:65, 1966.
Macdonald, I.: Symposium on dietary carbohydrates in man. Am. J. Clin. Nutr. 20:65, 1967.
Mendeloff, A. I.: Dietary fiber. Nutr. Rev. 33:321, 1975.
Review: Frequency of eating and dental caries prevalence. Nutr. Rev. 32:139, 1974.
Scala, J.: Fiber—the forgotten nutrient. Food Tech. 28:34, 1974.
Shaw, J. H.: Diet regulations for caries prevention. Nutrition News 36, No. 1 (Feb.) 1973.

For further references see Bibliography in Section 4.

REFERENCES

1. Friend, B.: National Food Situation, USDA No. 142, PP22–28, 1972.
2. Council on Foods and Nutrition: JAMA 224:1415, 1973.
3. Nizel, A. E.: Today's Health, October, 1973.
4. Scala, J.: Food Tech. 28:34, 1974.
5. Schertz, L. P.: Nutr. Rev. 31:201, 1973.
6. Goldsmith, G. A.: J. Am. Dietet. A. 63:513, 1973.
7. Ibid.
8. Lorenz, K.: Food Tech. 26:66, 1972.
9. Mertz, E. T.: Nutr. Rev. 32:129, 1974.
10. Hardinge, M. G., et al: J. Am. Dietet. A. 46:197, 1965.

3

fats and
other lipids

FATS IN THE HUMAN DIET

Fats are a form of stored energy in animals as important as carbohydrates are in plants. They serve multiple purposes in the diet. In addition to their high energy value, they contain essential fatty acids and act as carriers for the fat-soluble vitamins. That fat makes a meal more satisfying is due partially to its slow gastric emptying time and therefore its satiety value, and to the flavor it gives to other foods.

There is no physiological evidence that the human body needs as much fat as Americans consume, and many experts recommend a moderate reduction of fat in the diet. In many countries of the Orient, the Middle East, and Africa the average diet provides less than 20 percent of the total calories in the form of fat, as compared with over twice that amount in the American diet.

Because Americans differ so widely in their patterns of food preparation and in their eating practices in regard to fat, reliable information as to the actual individual consumption of this nutrient is difficult for the nutrition counselor to obtain. Some homemakers use considerable amounts of fat

26

for frying and flavoring foods; others may use methods of preparation, especially in the cooking of meats and poultry, which markedly reduce the amount of fat in the cooked food. Habits vary in regard to the eating or discarding of fat on meat, the use of table fats on breads and cream on cereals, and the use of salad dressings. Thus, people who are made aware of the amount of fat that they are consuming and of its caloric value frequently modify their intake without making major adjustments in their eating habits.

STRUCTURE AND CHARACTERISTICS OF LIPIDS

Fats, oils, and fatlike substances, because of similar solubilities, are classified as lipids (Table 3-1). They are insoluble in water and soluble in one or more of the so-called fat solvents, ether, chloroform, benzene, and acetone. Like carbohydrates, fats are composed of carbon, hydrogen, and oxygen but in proportions that greatly increase their energy value. Fats that are fluid at room temperature are usually called oils, while those that are solid are called fats. Both are primarily mixtures of triglycerides.

Triglycerides are esters of glycerol with three fatty acids (Fig. 3-1). They usually contain a mixture of two or three different fatty acids rather than three identical ones. The large number of fatty acids in natural foods and the mixing of them makes possible a large number of different triglycerides in any individual fat. Milk fat is said to have the possibility of containing almost 125,000 different triglycerides.

There is current interest in the positioning of the fatty acids in the triglyceride molecule since the position, as well as the chain length and degree of saturation of the fatty acids, affects the melting point and hence the digestibility and absorption of the fat. The

Table 3–1. Classification of Lipids

1. **Simple Lipids**
   - A. Triglycerides—esters of fatty acids with glycerol
   - B. Esters of fatty acids with high-molecular-weight alcohols
     - Waxes
     - Cholesterol esters
     - Vitamin A and D esters
2. **Compound Lipids**
   - A. Phospholipids—phosphorus-containing lipids
     - Lecithins
     - Cephalins
     - Sphingomyelins
   - B. Glycolipids—sugar-containing lipids
     - Cerebrosides
     - Gangliosides
   - C. Sulfolipids—sulfur-containing lipids
   - D. Lipoproteins—protein-containing lipids
   - E. Lipopolysaccharides—polysaccharide-containing lipids
3. **Derived Lipids**
   - A. Fatty acids
   - B. Alcohols
     - Glycerol
     - High-molecular-weight alcohols
   - C. Mono- and diglycerides
   - D. Sterols
     - Cholesterol
     - Ergosterol
     - Bile acids
     - Steroid hormones
     - Vitamin D
   - E. Hydrocarbons
     - Squalene
     - Carotenoids
     - Aliphatic hydrocarbons
   - F. Fat-soluble vitamins
     - Vitamin A
     - Vitamin E
     - Vitamin K

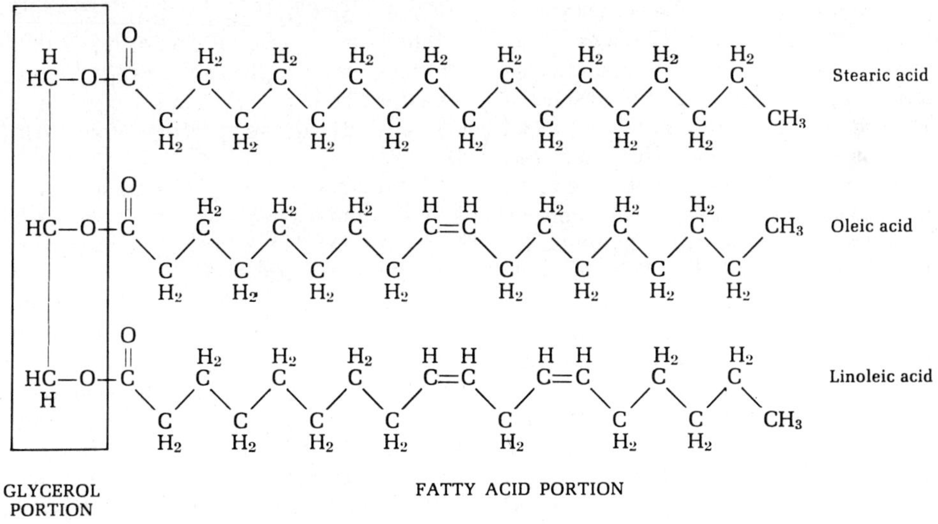

GLYCEROL PORTION

FATTY ACID PORTION

Fig. 3–1. The three fatty acids, stearic (saturated), oleic (monounsaturated), and linoleic (polyunsaturated), combined in ester linkage with glycerol to form a triglyceride or fat.

number 2 position on the triglyceride molecule is the central position and is occupied by different types of fatty acids depending on the origin of the fat. Seed fats, such as cottonseed oil, usually have unsaturated fatty acids (oleic or linoleic acids) in this position.

Hydrolysis of triglycerides by heat or by the fat-splitting enzymes, lipases, yields glycerol, fatty acids, diglycerides, and monoglycerides. If an alkali agent (NaOH) is used, soaps are formed; this process is called *saponification*.

Glycerol is an alcohol containing three carbon atoms and three hydroxyl groups. The latter are the reactive groups which can combine with fatty acids to form mono-, di-, and triglycerides (Fig. 3-1).

Fatty Acids. The type and configuration of the fatty acids in fats are responsible for differences in flavor, texture, melting point, absorption, essential fatty acid activity, and other characteristics. Fatty acids vary in length from four to about 24 carbon atoms including, with few exceptions, only the even-numbered members of the series. They are referred to as short chain (4 to 6 carbons), medium chain (8 to 12 carbons) and long chain (more than 12 carbons). Reference may also be made to extra long chain fatty acids, or those over 20 carbons. Natural fats contain 16 and 18 carbon fatty acids in the largest quantities, athough short chain fatty acids are found in butterfat and coconut oil. In addition to being present in relatively small amounts in natural fats, triglycerides containing medium chain fatty acids are commercially prepared from such fats as coconut oil. The ease with which fats with medium chain fatty acids are hydrolyzed, absorbed, and transported has made them useful in treating patients with certain types of malabsorption syndromes (see Chapters 9 and 25).

Fatty acids are also classified as saturated or unsaturated, depending on the presence or absence of double bonds. A double bond occurs when two adjoining carbons each have one less hydrogen atom than they normally hold. Then a double bond between the two carbons satisfies the carbon valence of 4. Fatty acids such as oleic are called monounsaturated because they contain one double bond, while linoleic, linolenic, and arachidonic acids, which contain 2, 3, and 4 double bonds respectively, are called polyunsaturated (Fig. 3-1.) The polyunsaturated fatty acids have been shown in certain instances to lower blood cholesterol level, whereas saturated fatty acids tend to raise the serum cholesterol level. Table 3-2 shows the fatty acid composition of some common animal and vegetable fats. Saturated fatty acids, particularly the long chain fatty acids and their glycerides, have higher melting points and hence tend to be solid in form at room temperature. These fats are found in greater amounts in animal sources. Oils for the most part contain large amounts of unsaturated fatty acids, have lower melting points, and are chiefly of vegetable origin. Coconut oil is a notable exception, however, since it is almost 90 percent saturated; short and medium chain acids account for its being an oil. Animals, including man, are able metabolically to increase or decrease the chain length of fatty acids by the addition or removal of 2 carbon fragments and can convert the saturated fatty acid stearic to the monounsaturated fatty acid oleic by removal of 2 hydrogens. Man cannot, however, synthesize the polyunsaturated fatty acid, linoleic; hence, this is considered to be an essential fatty acid (EFA).

In addition to the length of the fatty acid chain and the degree of saturation, the *configuration* of the fatty acid at the double bond as well as the position of the double bonds are factors which determine the role of fats in nutrition. The fatty acids in most natural fats are in the *cis* form, which means that at the double bond the molecule turns back on itself ⌐⎯. In processed fats such as margarine much of the fatty acid has been changed into the *trans* form, whereby the chain is stretched out ⎯⎯⎿⎯⎯. For example, the trans form (isomer) of oleic acid is elaidic acid. This increases the melting point so that a desirable consistency for a table or cooking fat is accomplished with a low degree of saturation.

Hydrogenation, the addition of hydrogen atoms to unsaturated fats, increases the degree of saturation and changes a liquid oil to a solid fat. These changes in the configuration and degree of saturation of fats have been found not to affect their energy value.

Mono- and *diglycerides* are esters of glycerol containing one and two fatty acids respectively and are produced from triglycerides in the process of digestion (see Chapter 9). They are also used commercially in prepared baked and processed foods to improve the texture.

Nonnutritive Oils. A clear distinction should be kept in mind between oils which are true fats and the hydrocarbons derived from petroleum, such as lubricating oil or purified mineral oil. The latter contain carbon and hydrogen but no oxygen. Mineral oil is completely indigestible in the animal body and cannot be classified as a food. Formerly, it was used in place of true fats in certain low calorie diets. This procedure is generally discouraged because mineral oil tends to interfere with the absorption of the fat-soluble vitamins. It is particularly detrimental when used in a food such as in salad dressing and when taken with meals. Vegetable gums are now frequently used in low calorie salad dressings to achieve the desired consistency.

Table 3-2. Analyses of Major Fatty Acids Typical of Some Fats of Animal and Plant Origin*†

	SATURATED				MONOUNSATURATED		POLYUNSATURATED			
	Lauric 12:0	Myristic 14:0	Palmitic 16:0	Stearic 18:0	Palmitoleic 16:1	Oleic 18:1	Linoleic 18:2	Linolenic 18:3	Arachidonic 18:4	Other Polyenoic Acids
ANIMAL FATS										
Lard	....	1.5	27.0	13.5	3.0	43.5	10.5	0.5	....	....
Chicken	2.0	7.0	25.0	6.0	8.0	36.0	14.0	....	....	....
Egg	....	....	25.0	10.0	....	50.0	10.0	2.0	3.0	....
Beef	....	3.0	29.0	21.0	3.0	41.0	2.0	0.5	0.5	....
Butter	3.5	12.0	28.0	13.0	3.0	28.5	1.0	....	....	....
Human Milk	7.0	8.5	21.0	7.0	2.5	36.0	7.0	1.0	0.5	....
Menhaden (fish)	....	9.0	19.0	5.5	16.0	....	....	....	....	48.5
VEGETABLE OILS										
Corn	....	....	12.5	2.5	....	29.0	55.0	0.5	....	....
Peanut	....	....	11.5	3.0	....	53.0	26.0	....	....	....
Cottonseed	....	1.0	26.0	3.0	1.0	17.5	51.5	....	....	....
Soybean	....	....	11.5	4.0	....	24.5	53.0	7.0	....	....
Olive	....	....	13.0	2.5	1.0	74.0	9.0	0.5	....	....
Coconut	49.5	19.5	8.5	2.0	....	6.0	1.5	....	....	....

*Adapted from Dietary Fat and Human Health, National Research Council Publication 1147, Washington, D. C., 1966.
†Composition is given in weight percentages of the component fatty acids (rounded to nearest 0.5) as determined by gas chromatography. The number of carbon atoms: number of double bonds are indicated under the common name of the fatty acid. These data were derived from a variety of sources. They are representative determinations, rather than averages, and considerable variation is to be expected in individual samples from other sources.

Phospholipids, structural compounds found in cell membranes, are essential components of certain enzyme systems, are involved in the transport of lipids in the plasma, and are a source of energy. Their chemical structure is similar to that of fats except that a phosphoric acid radical and a nitrogen-containing base have replaced one of the fatty acids.

Lecithins are the most abundant of the phospholipids in both tissues and foods where, because of their emulsifying properties, they serve as solubilizers and stabilizers. Lecithins are made commercially from soybeans and egg yolks and may be added as emulsifiers to margarines, cheese products, and other processed foods. There is no justification for the food faddists' recommendation of dietary supplements of lecithins. They are found in a wide variety of foods from both animal and vegetable sources—liver, egg yolks, and soybeans are especially rich in lecithins. Of even more importance, the cells of the body are capable of synthesizing lecithins as needed.

Choline, a part of the lecithin molecule, prevents the accumulation of fat in the liver. Other substances, such as the essential amino acid methionine and its derivatives, also have a function in preventing fatty liver. Such substances are called lipotropic because they have the ability to move or mobilize fat.

Other phospholipids, cephalin and sphingomyelin, are also present in most tissues, the latter primarily in brain and nerve tissue as a constituent of the myelin sheaths.

Cholesterol and other sterols. The two most common sterols are ergosterol, found in plants, and cholesterol, found in animal tissues. Cholesterol, an essential constituent of many cells, especially the myelin sheath around nerve fibers and in glandular tissues, is found in high concentration in the liver, where it is synthesized and stored. Cholesterol, both free and esterified, is also present in the plasma lipoproteins.

Egg yolks and brains are particularly rich sources of cholesterol in the diet. Other important food sources include butter, cream, cheese, heart, kidneys, liver, sweetbreads, lobster, shrimp, crab, and fish roe. For additional food sources, see Table 2, Section 4.

In normal individuals the body compensates for the level of cholesterol intake in the diet through changes in the synthesis, degradation, and excretion of the compound. Cholesterol synthesis may vary from 0.5 g. to 2 g. per day. Conversion in the liver to bile acids, which appears to require adequate tissue levels of ascorbic acid, is the chief method of degradation and excretion, but cholesterol as such may also leave the body through the feces by excretion into the bile. Although as much as 50 percent of the cholesterol synthesized each day in the body may be secreted with the bile into the intestines, after having been temporarily stored in the gallbladder, much of it may also be reabsorbed in the process of fat absorption.

The maintenance of a normal level of blood cholesterol is of great physiological importance. It is a precursor of vitamin D (see Chapter 6) and closely related to the steroid hormones in the body, the corticoids, androgens, and estrogens. It should not therefore be considered an abnormal substance in the body but one that has vital functions to perform. The Food and Nutrition Board's Report on Dietary Fat and Human Health states:

Evidence to support the concept that increased plasma concentrations of cholesterol are atherogenic is considerable but not conclusive. The type and quantity of dietary fat and the amount of cholesterol eaten influence the cholesterol concentration in the blood. Fats high in saturated fatty acids support a somewhat higher plasma cholesterol concentration than do those rich in polyunsaturated fatty acids. Many, but not all, population studies indicate that diets high in fat, among other nutrients, are correlated with higher concentrations of plasma cholesterol and with increased prevalence of cardiovascular disease. However, proof of a causal relationship is lacking.[1]

Further discussion of the relationship of blood cholesterol levels to atherosclerotic disease is included in Chapter 29.

LIPOPROTEINS. Since lipids are insoluble in water, they are transported in the blood in the form of lipoproteins, water-soluble fat-protein complexes. Lipoproteins are classified according to their density as alpha-lipoproteins or high-density lipoproteins (HDL), beta-lipoproteins or low-density lipoproteins (LDL), prebeta-lipoproteins or very low-density lipoproteins (VLDL), and chylomicrons. They all contain protein, triglycerides, phospholipids, and cholesterol but in varying amounts (Table 3-3). Two procedures are used most frequently for the separation and classification of the plasma lipoproteins: ultracentrifugation and electrophoresis. Ultracentrifugation separates them according to their weight or rate of flotation, which is designated as Svedberg flotation units, S_f. The lower the density the higher the S_f, hence chylomicrons which consist primarily of triglycerides have S_f values of 400 or above. In an electrophoretic technique a drop of plasma is placed on a filter paper and put into an electrophoretic cell containing buffer solution with albumin. The electric field causes the lipoproteins to migrate on the paper strip at different rates. Distinct bands are formed as a result of differences in the migration rates of the various lipoproteins and hence the expression prebeta-, beta-, and alpha-lipoprotein bands.

Chylomicrons consist primarily of triglycerides from dietary fat, and the creamy layer which their presence produces in the plasma disappears in the normal individual's blood 12 hours after a meal when the triglycerides have been hydrolyzed into free fatty acids and oxidized or stored in tissue.

Prebeta-lipoproteins (VLDL) are the result of endogenous synthesis of triglycerides from carbohydrate in the diet, and these too tend to disappear in the normal person's blood in the fasting state as evidenced by the loss of turbidity in the plasma sample.

Table 3-3. The Percent Composition (Dry Weight) of Plasma Lipoproteins

Lipoproteins	Protein	Phospho- lipids	Cholesterol	Triglycerides
Chylomicrons S_f 400* and above	0.5-2.5	3-15	2-12	79-95
Very low-density (VLDL) S_f 20-400 (prebeta-)	2-13	10-25	9-24	50-80
Low-density (LDL) S_f 0-20 (beta-)	20-25	22	43	10
High-density (HDL) (alpha-)	45-55	30	18	5-8

*S_f refers to flotation rate–Svedberg units.

The alpha- (HDL) and beta- (LDL) lipoproteins change less readily in relationship to food intake and are the lipoproteins most reflective of the plasma cholesterol level.

Free fatty acids are transported in the blood bound to plasma albumin.

FOOD SOURCES OF LIPIDS
Animal Sources (See Fig. 3–2)

The body fat of each form of animal life is typical of the species but varies with function in the body and temperature of the environment. The fat of cold-blooded animals—fish, for example—is a soft fat which remains plastic in the low temperature environment in which the fish live. The fats of warm-blooded animals have higher melting points but are also plastic at the body temperature of each species. As a rule, the fat of herbivorous animals is harder than the fat of carnivorous animals. When adipose tissue of animals is subjected to heat, the fat liquefies and separates from the connective-tissue cells in which it was stored. Thus pork fat is "tried out" in the manufacture of lard. Sheep have the hardest body fat of any domestic animal; when extracted, it is known as mutton tallow. Poultry fats are intermediate between meat and fish fats both in hardness and in the content of polyunsaturated fatty acids.

The quantity of fat in meat also varies with different animals. Beef, pork, and lamb are approximately equal in fat content (15 to 30 percent); veal is lower and is comparable to chicken (6 to 15 percent). If all visible fat is trimmed from lean cuts of meat and a cooking method such as broiling or roasting, which increases fat losses, is employed, the amount of fat consumed from meat can be reduced considerably.

The fat of fish is always fluid at cold temperatures and is therefore called an oil. Fish fats can contain a higher proportion of polyunsaturated extra long chain fatty acids than do the meat or poultry fats (See Table 3-2). However, there is a great difference in the fat content of fish, which varies from less than 1 percent to more than 12 percent. Thus fish are classified either as low in fat or high in fat. The amount in all fish varies somewhat with the season of the year, with the time of spawning, and with changes in feeding conditions. It may be noted that certain fish which have very little fat in the edible portion have a comparatively large amount in the liver. Fish liver oils are extracted and refined for use as rich sources of vitamins A and D.

Milk fat is in an unstable emulsion which breaks (i.e., separates) on standing and allows the cream to rise. Homogenization of milk produces a more stable emulsion with smaller fat globules, and, therefore, the cream does not separate. Butter is the milk fat plus some moisture and milk solids separated by churning; the finished product contains about 85 percent of fat. Butter contains very little polyunsaturated fatty acid, as will be noted in Table 3–2. Butter is valued as a good source of vitamin A.

Plant Sources (See Fig. 3–2)

All fats in the plant kingdom are oils at room temperature. Most vegetables and fruits contain less than 1 percent of fat, with the exception of avocados and olives, as may be seen in Figure 3–2. The nuts and

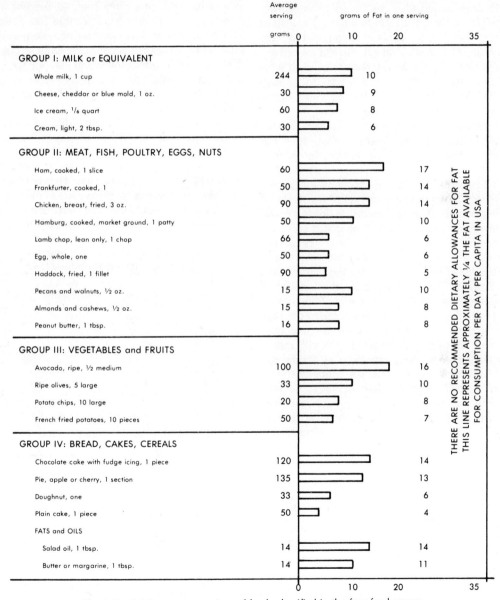

Fig. 3–2. Fat in average servings of foods classified in the four food groups.

the seeds have a higher fat content. Seed oils are mostly extracted or expressed for use as salad and cooking oils. Many of these have a high proportion of linoleic acid, as may be seen in Table 3-2. Olive and peanut oils are exceptions since both contain more oleic acid than the other salad and cooking oils.

Margarines and cooking fats are usually made from vegetable oils, cottonseed, safflower, soybean, and corn oils by the process of hydrogenation. This chemical process involves the introduction of hydrogen into the fat molecule under carefully controlled conditions to produce a fat with exactly the right melting point and other properties for culinary purposes. Hydrogenation also results in transforming part of the fat to the *trans* form to obtain the desired consistency. Fat thus treated is homogenized to form a creamy smooth product, but evidence of its being a mixture is given by the grainy texture of such a fat once it has been melted and allowed to harden again—the high and the low melting point ingredients are no longer evenly mixed.

The public demand for unsaturated fat has prompted margarine manufacturers to reduce the amount of hydrogenation to a minimum in order to retain as much of the polyunsaturated fatty acid as possible. Margarines are manufactured by either partially hydrogenating the total amount of vegetable oil to the desired consistency or by adding liquid vegetable oil to a more completely hydrogenated solid fat. The latter type contains approximately twice the amount of linoleic acid. Certain of the "soft" margarines marketed in bowllike containers rather than in sticks contain two to four times the amount of polyunsaturated as saturated fatty acids. The first ingredient named on the label of the margarine package tells consumers which product they are selecting: "liquid corn oil plus hydrogenated corn oil" means that the margarine has been processed by the second method and hence would have a higher ratio of polyunsaturated to saturated fatty acids (Table 3-4). The fat thus prepared is churned with cultured milk and other ingredients to give the product the flavor of butter. All brands are now fortified with vitamin A to the equivalent of average butter, and some have vitamin D added. Therefore, margarine is nutritionally the equivalent of butter and is frequently preferred because of the higher content of unsaturated fatty acids and usually slightly lower cost. All states now permit the sale of margarine to which coloring has been added; Wisconsin in 1967 was the last state to legalize such sales.

TRENDS IN FAT CONSUMPTION IN THE UNITED STATES

Although there are wide differences among individuals and regions, surveys indicate that Americans as a group consume more than 42 percent of their calories as fat (Table 3-5). Visible fats from such sources as butter, lard, margarine, shortening, and salad and cooking oils account for about 43 percent of the fat intake, whereas the fats of meats, eggs, cheese, nuts, and cereals, often referred to as invisible fats, contribute about 57 percent of the total fat in the diet (Table 3-6).

In the last 25 years the percentage of fat available to the American consumer from animal sources has decreased (75 percent in 1947-1949; 60 percent in 1973), while that from vegetable sources has increased (25 percent in 1947-1949; 40 percent in 1973). This change is due in large measure to the significant increase in the use of salad and cooking oils. Twice as much salad and cooking oils were used in 1967 as in

Table 3-5. Trends in Fat Consumption During Selected Periods—U. S.*

Period	Calories Per Capita Per Day	Fat Per Capita Per Day (g.)	Fat Calories (Percent)
1909-13	3490	125	32.2
1935-39	3270	133	36.6
1964	3170	147	41.4
1973	3290	156	42.4

*Figures adapted from Nutritive Value of Food for Consumption, United States, 1909-64, Friend, B., Agricultural Research Service 62-14, Washington, D.C., USDA, 1966, and Nutritional Review, National Food Situation, Economic Research Service, Washington, D.C., USDA, 1973.

Table 3-6. Percent of Total Fat Contributed by Each Food Group in 1973—U. S.*

Food Group	Percent
Meat, poultry, fish	34.2
Eggs	3.0
Dairy products (excluding butter)	12.9
Fats and oils (including butter)	42.7
Fruits	0.4
Vegetables	0.5
Dried beans, peas, nuts, soya flour	3.7
Flour and cereal products	1.3
Sugars and sweeteners	0.0
Miscellaneous	1.3

*Figures adapted from Nutritional Review, National Food Situation, Economic Research Service, Washington, D.C., USDA, 1973.

Table 3-4. Selected Fatty Acids in Margarines*

TYPES OF MARGARINE (FIRST INGREDIENT NAMED ON LABEL)	AMOUNT IN 100 GRAMS			
			Unsaturated Fatty Acids	
	Total Fat (g.)	Total Saturated Fatty Acids (g.)	Oleic (g.)	Linoleic (g.)
Hydrogenated or hardened fat	81	18	47	14
Liquid oil	81	19	31	29

*Figures from Composition of Foods: Raw, Processed and Prepared. Agriculture Handbook No. 8. USDA, Washington, D. C., 1963.

	ANIMAL SOURCES (GRAMS)				VEGETABLE SOURCES (GRAMS)			
PERIOD	Butter	Lard	Edible Beef Fats	Total	Margarine	Shortening	Salad and Cooking Oils	Total
1947-49	10.6	16.4	0.5	27.5	5.5	10.6	9.1	25.2
1957-59	8.2	14.5	1.8	24.5	8.7	9.7	13.5	31.9
1967	5.5	11.1	3.0	19.6	9.7	13.2	18.8	41.6
1971	5.1	9.4	3.0	17.6	10.0	14.9	22.4	47.3
1973	4.7	7.2	2.8	14.7	10.6	15.6	25.5	51.7

*Figures adapted from Nutritional Review, National Food Situation, Economic Research Service, Washington, D.C., USDA, 1973.

1947-1949, and since 1967, their use has again increased by one third. Although the combined use of butter and margarine in the U.S. remains relatively constant, the amount of margarine used daily has doubled, whereas that of butter has decreased by 50 percent (Table 3-7).

There are other trends in the American food consumption pattern of which the nutrition counselor should be aware today. Americans as a group are consuming more beef, poultry, and fish in the 1970s than they did in the 1960s, and less veal, lamb, and pork. Among the dairy products more cheese and less milk is being consumed. Fewer eggs also appear in the market basket in this decade as compared to the last (Fig. 3-3).

These changes have led to differences in the composition of total fat in the diet. Although the amount of saturated fatty acids (55 g. per capita) has increased only one gram since 1947-1949, a marked change occurred for linoleic acid, with an increase from 15 to 24 g. per capita during this period. At the same time the amount of oleic acid available increased from 58 to 62 g. per capita. Of the 156 g. of fat available per person per day in 1973, saturated fat contributed 35 percent, oleic acid (monounsaturated) 40 percent, and linoleic acid (polyunsaturated) 15 percent. The ratio of polyunsaturated to saturated fatty acids (P/S) has increased from 0.33 in 1963 to 0.43 in 1973.

ROLE OF LIPIDS IN HEALTH

Essential Fatty Acids (EFA)

An essential fatty acid is one which is necessary for normal nutrition and which cannot be synthesized by the body from other substances. Linoleic acid, the polyunsaturated fatty acid most abundant in nature, is the main essential fatty acid to be considered. Linolenic acid, which was at first classed as one of the essential fatty acids, is not active in relieving the dermatitis of essential fatty acid deficiency; arachidonic acid, which is effective in curing the deficiency, can be synthesized in the body from linoleic acid. Only minute quantities of arachidonic acid occur naturally in food fats.

The exact function of linoleic acid and its derivatives in the body is not well understood, but such acids are known to be essential structural elements for synthesis of tissue lipids and hence should receive particular attention in infant feeding.[2] Alfin-Slater in discussing dietary fat allowances states that,

> Essential fatty acids are important because they seem to play a role in the regulation of several aspects of cholesterol metabolism, transport, transformation into metabolic products, and the ultimate excretion of some of these products. Diets high in essential fatty acids reduce hypercholesteremia in experimental animals and in

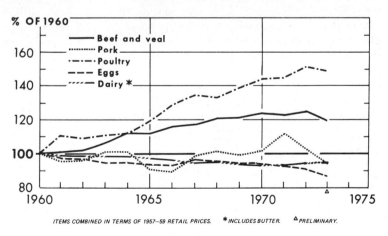

Fig. 3-3. Per capita consumption of selected livestock products. Consumption of eggs, dairy products, and pork decreased in 1973 as compared to 1960, while that of beef and veal and poultry increased. (U.S. Department of Agriculture, Economic Research Service)

ITEMS COMBINED IN TERMS OF 1957-59 RETAIL PRICES.   *INCLUDES BUTTER.   △ PRELIMINARY.

fats and other lipids   33

man, although the ultimate fate of the cholesterol removed from the circulation is still a controversial subject.[3]

Essential fatty acids are also precursors of prostaglandins, hormonelike compounds widely distributed in tissues, which produce various metabolic effects.

Demonstration of an essential fatty acid deficiency in animals requires the rigid exclusion of fat from the diet. Therefore, it is not surprising that evidence of essential fatty acid deficiencies in adult humans has not been recognized except in hospitalized patients maintained exclusively on intravenous feeding for long periods of time.[4,5] However, Hansen, Wiese, and associates[6,7] have demonstrated a fatty acid deficiency in infants, which proves beyond a doubt that essential fatty acids (EFA) are required by humans. After normal blood levels for 2, 3, and 4 double bond fatty acids were established by surveying healthy infants and children,[8] the same serum levels in poorly nourished children were studied. In the latter group the researchers found not only decreased blood levels of the fatty acids containing 2 and 4 double bonds—i.e., those with EFA activity— but also many cases of dermatitis similar to the symptoms of essential fatty acid deficiency seen in animals. Blood levels of fatty acids with three double bonds which are inactive physiologically were increased. These investigators also have been able to evaluate over 400 infants fed formulas containing varying amounts of linoleic acid. Again the dry and scaly skin of dermatitis was the most frequent finding among the infants receiving formulas low in linoleic acid. Infants also seemed to grow better and required fewer calories for growth when there was an adequate supply of EFA.

Although evaporated milk has proved satisfactory in infant feeding, Wiese et al[9] suggest that the amount of linoleic acid supplied by evaporated milk formulas (1 to 2 percent of total calories) may be considered minimal, whereas breast milk, which is four to five times higher in linoleic acid, contains optimal amounts of EFA. Attention was called by these authors to the infrequent incidence of eczema and other skin manifestations in breast-fed infants when compared with those on cow's milk. Analysis of the linoleic acid content of commercial infant formulas and precooked cereals indicates that these also make an important contribution of EFA to the infant diet.[10]

Although the adult human requirement of essential fatty acids is not known, the Food and Nutrition Board of the National Research Council states that, "to prevent deficiency, the required intake of essential fatty acid lies within the range of 1 to 2 percent of total calories."[11]

Fats as a Concentrated Source of Energy

Fats are the most concentrated source of energy for the human body; 1 g. of fat yields 9 cal., as compared to 4 cal. per gram from carbohydrate and protein. Thus, relatively small amounts of high-fat foods contribute large amounts of calories to the diet. The percentage of total calories derived from fat in the American diet has increased to 42 percent; this increase was accompanied by a similar increase in total calories consumed. These trends are of concern to the nutrition counselor, since any excess energy consumed is stored as adipose tissue and eventually leads to obesity. To avoid excessive weight gain and its accompanying health risks, it is necessary to balance energy needs with food intake carefully. This implies for most Americans who have sedentary living patterns only moderate consumption of fried foods, pies, pastries, and cakes, butter, margarine, and cream. When weight gain is a problem, it is often indicative that the amount of fat in the diet is higher than desirable. Obesity and its dietary treatment are discussed in Chapter 27.

For those individuals who are underweight, a moderate increase in the amount of fat in the diet would help achieve desirable weight status.

Lipids and Cardiovascular Disease

Since there is evidence of increased susceptibility to coronary heart disease among individuals with elevated levels of cholesterol and/or triglycerides, attention is focused on those food constituents which appear to affect these levels—the total fat and sugar intake and the proportion of saturated to polyunsaturated fatty acids and cholesterol. Although there is reasonable agreement among most medical authorities about the treatment of the hyperlipoproteinemias (elevated lipid levels in the blood), discussed in Chapter 29, there is still much controversy among nutrition scientists as to the kind and amount of diet modification which should be recommended for the population as a whole. The Committee on Dietary Allowances of the Food and Nutrition Board recommended that "the proportion of energy derived from fat should not exceed 35 percent." They also endorsed the additional recommendation of the American Heart Association that less than 10 percent of total calories should come from saturated fatty acids and up to 10 percent from polyunsaturated fatty acids which "would probably provide a diet conducive to better health in the United States population."[12] Complex carbohydrates rather than simple sugars should replace the fat in the diet, and weight reduction for overweight individuals is desirable to reduce serum triglyceride levels. In order to apply these recommendations, the foods selected will need to include more cereal grains, legumes, vegetables, fish, and vegetable oils and less animal fats and sugar. Nutrition counselors should continue to emphasize the need for a diet adequate in all the essential nutrients.

STUDY QUESTIONS AND ACTIVITIES

1. What can be said about the human requirement for fat in the diet? How does American consumption compare with that of some other countries?
2. What changes have occurred in the consumption and selection of fats by American consumers? Explain why there may be large differences in the amount of fat consumed by individual families.
3. What is meant by saturated and polyunsaturated fatty acids? Give illustrations of each.
4. Which of the polyunsaturated fatty acids is most widely distributed in foods? What types of foods contribute the most of this factor?
5. From what sources are margarine and some of the cooking fats manufactured and by what process?
6. Is there evidence that the level of fat in the diet of Americans may be a hazard to health? In what way?
7. Name the essential fatty acid. Why is it called essential?
8. Besides its use for energy, what other functions does fat perform in the body?
9. What are phospholipids? Sterols? Where are they found in the body? Which sterols may be converted to vitamin D?
10. What are the normal functions of cholesterol in the body? How is the excess excreted?
11. Name the plasma lipoproteins. What lipids do they contain? Which one contains the most cholesterol; triglycerides from dietary fat; triglycerides from liver synthesis?

SUPPLEMENTARY READINGS

Alfin-Slater, R. B.: Three essential nutrients—fats, essential fatty acids and ascorbic acid. J. Am. Dietet. A. 64:168, 1974.

Connor, W. E., and Connor, S. L.: The key role of nutritional factors in the prevention of coronary heart disease. Prev. Med. 1:49, 1972.

Feeley, R. M., Criner, P. E., and Watt, B. K.: Cholesterol content of foods. J. Am. Dietet. A. 61:134, 1972.

McIntyre, N., and Isselbacher, K. J.: Role of small intestine in cholesterol metabolism. Am. J. Clin. Nutr. 26:647, 1973.

National Research Council and American Medical Association: Diet and coronary heart disease. J. Am. Dietet. A. 61:379, 1972.

National Research Council Publication 1147. *Dietary Fat and Human Health*. Washington, D.C., 1966.

Reiser, R.: Saturated fat in the diet and serum cholesterol concentration: A critical examination of the literature. Am. J. Clin. Nutr. 26:524, 1973.

Review: Essential fatty acid deficiency in continuous-drip alimentation. Nutr. Rev. 33:329, 1975.

For further references see Bibliography in Section 4.

REFERENCES

1. National Research Council Publication 1147. *Dietary Fat and Human Health*. Washington, D.C., 1966.
2. Holman, R. T.: JAMA 178:930, 1961.
3. Alfin-Slater, R. B.: J. Am. Dietet. A. 64:168, 1974.
4. Collins, F. D., et al: Nutr. Metab., 13:150, 1971.
5. Paulrud, J. R., et al: Am. J. Clin. Nutr. 25:897, 1972.
6. Hansen, A. E., and Wiese, H. F.: J. Nutr. 52:367, 1954.
7. Hansen, A. E., et al: Pediatrics 31:171, 1963.
8. Wiese, H. F., et al: J. Nutr. 52:355, 1954.
9. Wiese, H. F., et al: J. Nutr. 66:345, 1958.
10. Hughes, G., et al: Clin. Pediat. 2:555, 1963.
11. Food and Nutrition Board: *Recommended Dietary Allowances*, 8th rev. Washington, D.C., National Academy of Sciences—National Research Council, 1974.
12. Ibid.

4 proteins

VITAL IMPORTANCE AND WORLD USE

Every animal, including man, must have an adequate source of protein in order to grow and maintain itself.

Proteins have long been recognized as the fundamental structural element of every cell of the body. More recently, specific proteins and protein derivatives have been identified as the functional elements in certain specialized cells, glandular secretions, enzymes, and hormones. In their role as enzymes, proteins control the breakdown of food for energy and the synthesis of new compounds for maintenance and repair of body tissues. When they are supplied in amounts greater than necessary for growth and maintenance, proteins contribute to the energy pool of the body and, similarly, if carbohydrates and fats are not sufficient to meet energy demands, protein will be diverted for this purpose. Thus, protein well deserves its name, which is of Greek derivation, meaning "of first importance." Since proteins are the principal constituents of the active tissues of the body and the body is, in turn, dependent upon food protein for these indispensable substances, the quality and the quantity in the daily diet are of prime importance.

In many parts of the world, the developing coun-

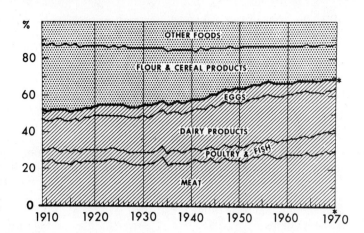

Fig. 4-1. Sources of protein in the diet of the U. S. population from 1910 to 1970. *—Total animal sources. (U. S. Department of Agriculture, Agricultural Research Service)

tries particularly, food sources of protein, especially proteins of good quality, are extremely scarce. There is some evidence that in countries where the quality and the quantity of protein and other nutrients are inadequate, the stature of whole groups of people may be affected. When height and weight growth curves of groups of preschool children in Mexico, Lebanon (Arab refugees), Hong Kong, and Thailand were compared with those of United States (Iowa) children, growth retardation was evident in the former groups. Children in Ethiopia, Jordan, and Vietnam were also shorter and weighed less than Iowa children between the ages of 1 and 17 years.[1] The increased stature of Japanese youths has paralleled increases in the Japanese diet of both total protein and protein from animal sources[2] (see Chapter 18). Similarly, Japanese who have lived in the U.S. for a generation or more have shown a marked increase in stature—clear evidence that heredity was not the determining factor;[3] and Australians and New Zealanders, perhaps the heaviest meat eaters on the globe, have large physiques.

The United States has ample sources of protein available (approximately 100 g. per capita per day), and more than two thirds of it comes from meat, fish, poultry, eggs, and dairy products (Fig. 4-1). Although surveys indicate that most of the North American population consumes an adequate amount, there are still people who, for economic or other reasons, may not get enough protein.

CLASSIFICATION AND STRUCTURE OF PROTEINS AND OTHER NITROGEN-CONTAINING COMPOUNDS
Proteins

Proteins, like fats and carbohydrates, are composed of carbon, hydrogen, and oxygen, and, in addition, they must contain nitrogen. Often sulfur and phosphorus and sometimes other elements such as

iron (in hemoglobin) and iodine (in thyroxine) are incorporated into the protein molecule.

Molecular nitrogen is "fixed" or converted into nitrogen compounds by certain bacteria living on the root nodules of plants such as clover or peas. The reaction produces ammonia which is converted into more complex nitrogen-containing molecules by the plant. Plants that do not themselves have nitrogen-fixing bacteria need to be fertilized with ammonia or nitrates.

Plants can then synthesize proteins from the nitrates and the ammonia in soil and decaying vegetable matter. Water and carbon dioxide from the air provide the necessary carbon, hydrogen, and oxygen. Animals are dependent on plants for this synthesis because animal cells cannot utilize to any great extent simpler forms of nitrogen, and animal metabolism of protein, in turn, eventually yields the forms of nitrogen which only plant life and microorganisms can utilize. This sequence of events is called the *nitrogen cycle*.

Proteins are made up of some 22 or more nitrogen-containing compounds known as amino acids. These amino acids are joined together by chemical linkages called peptide bonds in which the acid group of the first amino acid is attached to the nitrogen group of the next amino acid (Fig. 4-2). Two amino acids so linked are called a dipeptide; three amino acids, tripeptides. Polypeptides are composed

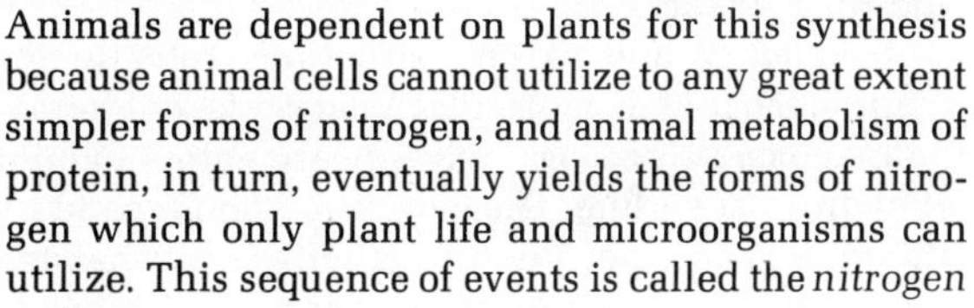

Fig. 4-2. Amino acids glycine and alanine joined by peptide linkage to form the dipeptide glycylalanine.

of 10 to 100 amino acids. Those polypeptide molecules containing over 100—sometimes several thousand—amino acids are referred to as proteins. The order in which all these amino acids are arranged is determined by the genetic code—the DNA (deoxyribonucleic acid) found in the nucleus of every cell (see Chapter 9).

CLASSIFICATION. Proteins may be classified according to their chemical structure.

Simple proteins yield only amino acids or their derivatives when they are hydrolyzed by acids, alkalies, or enzymes, e.g., albumins.

Conjugated proteins are polypeptides that contain some nonprotein parts called prosthetic groups, e.g., nucleoproteins.

Derived proteins are substances which result from the breakdown, such as hydrolysis, of simple or conjugated proteins, e.g., dipeptides.

STRUCTURE. The first step in determining the structure of a protein is to hydrolyze it and determine the kind and amount of amino acids which it contains. Since some proteins consist of more that one polypeptide chain, it is necessary to find out the number of these chains in each protein molecule. The final step is to determine the sequence of amino acids in each polypeptide chain. Thus, the *primary structure* refers to the ordinary structural formula, which includes the sequence of amino acids linked by peptide bonds and any other additional prosthetic groups and their linkages.

Secondary and *tertiary structures* refer to the shape of the protein molecule. A particular conformation is preferred because it gives rise to a great amount of hydrogen bonding. The most important secondary structure is the alpha-helix, a right- or left-handed spiral made rigid by intramolecular hydrogen bonds between carbonyl oxygen and amide nitrogen. In more complex proteins it is not unusual to find several helixes. The spatial arrangement of these helixes in relationship to one another is called the tertiary structure. Tertiary structures may be stabilized by other types of bonds, especially sulfide bonds. Proteins are classed as fibrous or globular depending on the tertiary spatial arrangement. Fibrous proteins such as those in muscle fiber (myosin), hair (keratin), and connective tissue (collagen and elastin) tend to be formed into relatively long molecules. The globular proteins are spherical and include hemoglobin, myoglobin, albumins, and globulins.

The *quaternary structure* is the aggregation of subunits in the final protein particle, maintained by electrostatic attraction. The oxygen-binding activity of hemoglobin is indicative of the biological activity of the quaternary structure.

Denaturation of proteins is any alteration from the naturally ordered conformation to a randomly structured molecule. Denaturation occurs before proteins coagulate and is caused by the application of heat, the addition of acids or alkalies, or mechanical action. The changes that occur in the protein when an egg is cooked or an acid is added to milk are examples of denaturation.

Because protein molecules are so large, with molecular weights ranging from 5,000 to several million, they have certain properties in common with colloidal solutions; the fact that protein molecules are too large to pass through cell membranes is important in physiology. For example, plasma proteins, because they cannot penetrate the capillary membranes, remain in the blood vessels and have an important effect on regulating water balance in the body (see Chapter 5).

Amino Acids

All the amino acids are organic acids containing at least one acid group (COOH) and one amino group (NH$_2$) (Fig. 4-2). Certain amino acids, however, have two acid groups (acidic), others have two amino groups (basic), and still others may contain ring structures (aromatic) or sulfur groups.

The first of the amino acids to be identified was discovered over 130 years ago; the last of the 22 listed in Table 4-1 was isolated and identified in 1935 by W. C. Rose. During the century between these discoveries much of the basic chemistry and physiological significance of proteins came to be understood. With the realization that the constituent amino acids were important factors in determining the nutritive value of a protein, many investigations were conducted to find out which of them were indispensable and which could be excluded safely from the diet without interfering with normal growth and body function.

Table 4-1. Classification of Amino Acids with Respect to Their Essentiality

Essential	Nonessential
Histidine*	Alanine
Isoleucine	Arginine
Leucine	Asparagine
Lysine	Aspartic acid
Methionine	Cysteine
Phenylalanine	Cystine
Threonine	Glutamic acid
Tryptophan	Glutamine
Valine	Glycine
	Hydroxyproline
	Proline
	Serine
	Tyrosine

*Histidine is required for infants but its essentiality for adults has not been clearly established.

Other Nitrogen-Containing Compounds

Ammonia (NH$_3$) is formed as a result of deamination (removal of the amino group) of amino acids in the liver and to some extent in the kidneys. The ammonia formed by deamination is converted to urea—(NH$_2$)$_2$CO$_2$—in the liver and excreted in the urine. It is the chief end product of protein metabolism and for individuals on a normal or high-protein diet comprises 85 to 92 percent of the total urinary nitrogen. On a low-protein diet the amount may be decreased to 60 percent. In acidosis the kidney converts part of the urea back to ammonia and the nitrogenous wastes are excreted as ammonium salts to neutralize the excess acids that are present.

Creatine and *creatinine* are also nitrogen-containing compounds found in the urine. Most of the creatine is synthesized in the body but it also may be obtained from creatine in food. It is found chiefly in the muscle, where part of it is converted to creatinine and later excreted in the urine. The amount of creatinine varies in proportion to the amount of muscle in the individual.

Purines (C$_5$H$_4$N$_4$) are nitrogen-containing ring structures widely distributed in nature, especially in nucleic acids.

Uric acid, an end product of purine metabolism, is excreted in the urine. It is formed from purines consumed in the diet (exogenous) and from body purines as a result of the breakdown of nucleic acids (endogenous). Abnormal uric acid metabolism is called gout.

PROTEIN REQUIREMENTS

It is necessary to separate consideration of protein needs into two categories. One is the requirement for the essential amino acids. The other is the requirement for total protein—or total nitrogen, as it is sometimes called—which must be available to the body for the synthesis of the nonessential amino acids and for other nitrogen-containing tissue constituents.

Essential Amino Acids

Amino acids that the body cannot synthesize in adequate amounts are called essential or indispensable because they must be supplied by the diet in proper proportions and amounts to meet the requirements for maintenance and growth of tissue. Nonessential or dispensable amino acids are those the body can synthesize in sufficient amounts to meet its needs if the total amount of nitrogen supplied by protein is adequate (Table 4-1).

Nitrogen balance studies have been used to determine the amounts of essential amino acids required by various groups. An individual is in nitrogen equilibrium or balance when the nitrogen intake from protein is approximately equal to the nitrogen lost in the feces and urine. An adult consuming a diet that contains sufficient amounts of the essential amino acids will be in nitrogen equilibrium. If an essential amino acid is removed from the diet, negative nitrogen balance results. This means more nitrogen is being lost than is consumed because tissues requiring the essential amino acid cannot be maintained and hence are broken down and their nitrogen excreted. Nitrogen equilibrium will again be attained when the lacking essential amino acid is supplied in amounts adequate to maintain tissues. Positive nitrogen balance, i.e., nitrogen intake from protein greater than nitrogen loss in urine and feces, occurs only when new tissues are synthesized such as in growth and pregnancy, or in replacement of tissue loss due to injury or disease.

Nine amino acids are essential for maintenance of nitrogen equilibrium in humans. The estimated essential amino acid requirements for infants, children, and adults are given in Table 4-2. Men in an older age group who were studied by Tuttle and associates[4] appear to differ in their requirements; studies thus far indicate an increased need for methionine and lysine. Infants[5] and children[6] have proportionally greater demands for essential amino acids than adults. In addition, infants require histidine as an essential amino acid.[7]

Factors in addition to the age, sex, and physiological condition of an individual influence the requirements for specific amino acids. If total protein intake is low, small surpluses of certain amino acids can increase the need for others.

The nonessential amino acids in protein also affect the quality of the protein. For example, the amount of the sulfur-containing essential amino acid methionine required may be somewhat reduced if cystine, a sulfur-containing nonessential amino acid, is supplied in the diet. Likewise, the presence in the diet of tyrosine, a nonessential amino acid similar in structure to phenylalanine, may reduce the requirement for phenylalanine. Thus, much definitive work on amino acid requirements has been accomplished, but pieces of the puzzle are still missing.

Quality of Protein

Osborne and Mendel in their pioneer work with rats showed that individual proteins differed in their ability to maintain life and support the growth of their animals (Fig. 4-3). Casein (milk protein), when fed at a level of 18 percent of the total calories, both maintained life and supported growth and hence was clas-

Table 4-2. Estimated Amino Acid Requirements of Man*

AMINO ACID	REQUIREMENT (MG./KG. OF BODY WEIGHT/DAY)			Amino Acid Pattern for High Quality Proteins, mg./g. of protein†
	Infant (3-6 mo.)	Child (10-12 yr.)	Adult	
Histidine	33	?	?	17
Isoleucine	80	28	12	42
Leucine	128	42	16	70
Lysine	97	44	12	51
Total S-containing amino acids	45	22	10	26
Total aromatic amino acids	132	22	16	73
Threonine	63	28	8	35
Tryptophan	19	4	3	11
Valine	89	25	14	48

*From Food and Nutrition Board, National Research Council: Improvement of protein nutriture. Washington, D.C., National Academy of Sciences, 1973.

†2 g. per kg. of body weight per day of protein of the quality listed in column 4 would meet the amino acid needs of the infant.

sified as a complete protein. Gliadin (wheat protein), since it maintained life but did not support growth, was called a partially incomplete protein. Incomplete proteins such as zein (corn protein) were those which could not even maintain life because they were lacking in one or more of the essential amino acids. Since casein was found to be only half as effective in supporting growth when fed at the 9 percent level as it was at the 18 percent level, it was recognized that quality and quantity were both important in determining the effectiveness of proteins.

As a result of early research, proteins were classed as complete, partially incomplete, and incomplete. These terms are still used by some authors to describe protein quality. Animal proteins, such as meats, poultry, fish, eggs, milk, and cheese, provide good quality protein in liberal amounts and are termed complete proteins. The exception to this is gelatin, the protein derived from animal connective tissue, which, because of its lack of tryptophan, is classified as an incomplete protein. Proteins from plant sources are usually not of as good quality as those from animal sources because one or more of the following essen-

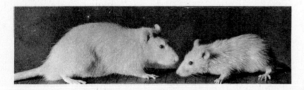

Fig. 4-3. Adequate and inadequate protein (18 percent vs. 4 percent). Rats of the same litter. This deficiency produces stunted growth but no deformities.

tial amino acids are in short supply: lysine, methionine, threonine, and tryptophan. They are therefore incomplete or partially incomplete. The best quality plant proteins are found in legumes, such as beans, peas, lentils, and peanuts, and in nuts. The proteins in bread and cereals and in vegetables other than those mentioned and in fruit are all incomplete. These proteins are nevertheless an important part of the food intake, since their amino acids contribute to the total nitrogen of the body which must be available for nonessential amino acids and other nitrogen-containing compounds in the tissues.

Protein quality is a measure of the efficiency with which a protein is used for growth or maintenance and depends primarily on the essential amino acid composition of the protein. When the diet is adequate in energy and total nitrogen (protein), protein quality can be calculated by comparing the essential amino acids in an unknown protein with those in a reference protein. The amino acid score (chemical score) can be calculated as follows:

$$\text{amino acid score} = \frac{\text{mg. of amino acid in 1 g. of test protein}}{\text{mg. of amino acid in reference protein}} \times 100$$

The amino acid score for the protein would be the score for the most limiting essential amino acid. If the most limiting essential amino acid is 80 percent of the reference pattern, then the amino acid score is considered to be 80. The proteins in egg and human milk have been used as the protein reference patterns, but the most recent report of the Joint FAO/WHO Committee also suggests a theoretical protein pattern (Table 4-3).[8]

The FAO/WHO 1973 recommendations[9] for protein requirements make adjustments of the "safe level of protein intake" according to the amino acid score of the protein in the diet. The committee also states that,

Available information on amino acid scores of national diets supports the assumption that the diets of rich countries have a quality relative to that of milk or eggs of about 80%, and those of poor countries about 70%. Situations may exist, particularly with diets in which 70-80% of the protein comes from such foods as cassava and maize and virtually none from animal foods, where the relative quality may be as low as 60%.[10]

Biological value (BV) is another term used to describe protein quality and is defined as the percentage of absorbed nitrogen *retained* by the body. This is determined by a carefully standardized assay using rats in which the nitrogen intake and losses are measured to determine the efficiency of utilization. Net protein utilization (NPU) is a measure of the effi-

Table 4-3. The FAO/WHO Pattern and the Proteins of Egg, Human Milk, and Cow's Milk (mg./g. of protein)*

Essential Amino Acids	1973 FAO/WHO Pattern	Egg	Human Milk	Cow's Milk
Histidine		22	26	27
Lysine	55	70	66	78
Leucine	70	86	93	95
Isoleucine	40	54	46	47
Methionine + cystine	35	57	42	33
Phenylalanine + tyrosine	60	93	72	102
Threonine	40	47	43	44
Tryptophan	10	17	17	14
Valine	50	66	55	64
Total	360	512	460	504

*Adapted from Report of a Joint FAO/WHO Committee: Energy and protein requirements. Tech. Rep. Series No. 522, World Health Organization, 1973.

ciency of utilization of the *ingested* protein. If proteins are completely digested, the biological value and net protein utilization are the same; for proteins less well digested the NPU will be less. Animal proteins in eggs, milk, cheese, meat, poultry, and fish have high biological values as compared with lower values for most of the vegetable proteins. The net protein utilization values vary from the biological values in terms of the coefficient of digestibility of the protein food. The amino acid score should correspond with the biological value for proteins that are completely digested.

Another method of evaluating protein quality is the protein efficiency ratio (PER). The PER is a measure of the weight gain per amount of protein consumed by a growing animal. It is the method used to determine protein quality for food labeling.

Fortunately, most of our foods contain a mixture of proteins, one of which often supplements another. More to the point, however, is the fact that we combine several different foods in a meal, the proteins of which tend to supplement one another because of their varying amino acid content. For instance, cereals which are low in lysine are usually eaten with milk, which provides a generous amount of this factor. Thus, cereal and milk or bread and cheese are good combinations. It is obvious that this type of complementary value among foods makes a varied diet more desirable than a restricted one.

The concept of protein supplementation has also been applied in areas where animal proteins are not readily available. Attempts to provide palatable low-cost foods with an adequate amino acid balance from inexpensive indigenous foods have resulted in combinations of various types of vegetable proteins. One such product is "Incaparina," developed by the Insti-

tute of Nutrition in Central America and Panama (INCAP). It consists of a mixture of ground maize, sorghum, cottonseed flour, torula yeast, and vitamin A.[11] A number of other countries in Asia, the Near East, and Africa have developed similar products from indigenous foods to meet the protein needs of young infants. Small amounts of animal protein such as skim milk or fish meal have also been added to mixtures of vegetable proteins to improve their quality. Another example is seen in the enrichment of cereal grains with one or more of the amino acids which are the limiting factors, such as the addition of lysine to wheat. These mixtures provide a relatively good source of protein, particularly for the growing child, who suffers the most from poor quality and inadequate protein intake.

The genetic improvement of plant crops both to increase the quality of their protein, such as the hybrid corn with increased lysine, and to increase their yield offers hope for the future.

Protein Allowances

Any quantitative estimate of protein requirement must take into account the quality of the proteins involved. The Food and Nutrition Board[12] recommends a daily intake of 0.8 g. of protein per kg. of body weight for adults consuming the mixed protein diet of the United States. Hence, the recommendation for the 70-kg. male is 56 g. of protein and for the 58-kg. female, 46 g.

The recommended dietary allowance of protein for infants is based upon the amount of milk protein which is known to produce a satisfactory growth rate. An additional amount of protein to allow for growth has been included in the allowance for children in age groups from 1 to 18 years.

An additional 30 g. per day has also been added for pregnancy from the second month to the end of gestation. The allowance for pregnant adolescents is proportionately higher depending on age. Twenty additional grams is recommended during lactation to cover the milk produced. As shown in Table 4-4, the Food and Nutrition Board's recommended dietary allowances are similar, except those for the pregnant woman, to the FAO/WHO "safe levels of intake" for individuals who consume diets with a protein score of 70 percent.[13] Both groups have emphasized that these recommendations for protein depend on energy needs being met.

In general, these protein allowances are much lower than the amounts consumed by most Americans, and may not be adequate if energy intakes are low. Calloway[14] also points out that, "the recommended allowances for protein are incompatible with

Table 4-4. Protein Standards of the Recommended Dietary Allowances and FAO/WHO*

| | RECOMMENDED DIETARY ALLOWANCES | | | | | FAO/WHO SAFE LEVEL OF INTAKE | | | |
Age (Years)	Body Weight kg.	Body Weight lbs.	Protein (g./day) per person	Protein (g./day) per kg.	Age (Years)	Body Weight kg.	Protein (g./kg./day) Reference†	Protein (g./kg./day) Score 70†
Infants								
0-0.5	6	14		2.2	0-0.5	breast-feeding recommended		
0.5-1	9	20		2.0	0.5-1	7.3	1.53	2.2
Children								
1-3	13	28	23	1.8	1-3	13.4	1.19	1.7
4-6	20	44	30	1.5	4-6	20.2	1.01	1.4
7-10	30	66	36	1.2	7-9	28.1	0.88	1.3
Males								
11-14	44	97	44	1.0	10-12	36.9	0.81	1.2
15-18	61	134	54	0.9	13-15	51.3	0.72	1.0
19-22	67	147	52	0.8	16-19	62.9	0.60	0.9
23-50	70	154	56	0.8	adult	65.0	0.57	0.8
51+	70	154	56	0.8				
Females								
11-14	44	97	44	1.0	10-12	38.0	0.76	1.1
15-18	54	119	48	0.9	13-15	49.9	0.63	0.9
19-22	58	128	46	0.8	16-19	54.4	0.55	0.8
23-50	58	128	46	0.8	adult	55.0	0.52	0.7
						per person per day		
pregnant			+30	1.3	pregnant		+9	+13
lactating			+20		lactating		+17	+24

*Adapted from Calloway, D.H.: Recommended dietary allowances for protein and energy, 1973. J. Am. Dietet. A. 64:157,1974.
†Reference protein is milk or egg; score 70 refers to protein utilized 70 percent as efficiently as the reference protein.

sound nutrition planning." By limiting the amount of protein-rich foods, trace minerals and vitamin B_6 may not be provided in adequate amounts in the diet, since only about 8 to 9 percent of the total calories in the diet will come from protein, as compared with the present 11 to 13 percent. This may be a particular problem when recommended dietary allowances are used by social welfare agencies to set family food allowances or to plan low-cost institutional menus. The assumption is that those Americans who can afford to will continue to consume amounts of protein in excess of recommended allowances and that this is probably a good practice until more is known about trace nutrients in food and their essentiality to good health. Thus, the calcium allowance set by the Food and Nutrition Board is based on a protein intake greater than the protein allowance for adults (Chapter 5).

It is highly desirable that at least one third of the daily protein intake be derived from animal sources, which is usually the case in the average diet in the United States. It is also strongly recommended that some good quality protein be included in every meal, since the tissues must have all of the essential amino acids present at one time for tissue synthesis. If they are not there when needed, those that are may be deaminized and oxidized for energy. This rule applies particularly to breakfast and lunch, for these are the meals that most often contain limited amounts of protein. It is also worth noting that, since protein foods with high protein scores are the most expensive

class of foods in the diet, there is a tendency among low income groups to consume less than recommended amounts of proteins, both quantitatively and qualitatively.

A basic dietary pattern for a day (Chapter 10) is useful in planning menus. This dietary pattern (Table 4-5) of approximately 1400 calories provides a liberal amount of protein, more than two thirds of which is derived from animal sources. Additional foods chosen to supply the extra calories would also provide more protein.

Protein requirement may be modified by certain pathological conditions. During convalescence from

Table 4-5. Protein in Pattern Dietary for One Day*

Food Group	Amount (g.)	Household Measure	Energy (kcal.)	Protein (g.)
Milk or equivalent	488	2 cups	320	17
Meat, fish, poultry, egg	120	4 ozs. cooked	376	30
Vegetables:				
Potato, cooked	100	1 medium	65	2
Green or yellow	75	1 serving	27	2
Other	75	1 serving	45	2
Fruits:				
Citrus	100	1 serving	43	1
Other	100	1 serving	85	—
Bread, white enriched	100	4 slices	270	9
Cereal, whole grain or enriched	30	1 oz. dry or		
	130	2/3 cup cooked	89	3
Butter or margarine	14	1 tbsp.	100	—
		Total	1420	66

*For basis of calculation, see Pattern Dietary in Chapter 10.

debilitating diseases or surgery, extra protein is required for nutritional rehabilitation. For this reason the earlier tendency to reduce protein intake in many diseases, with a few exceptions, has been reversed. The nutrition counselor should, however, recognize that certain diseases (see Chapters 31, 32, and 35) may require limiting the total amount of protein or the amount of a specific amino acid in a patient's diet.

FOOD SOURCES OF PROTEIN

From the bar chart of average servings (Fig. 4-4), it is evident that the first two food groups supply the most protein per serving and are also the best quality proteins. Dry legumes and nuts are included as meat alternates in Group II because they contain the best quality plant proteins.

Animal Sources of Protein

GROUP I. MILK AND MILK PRODUCTS. The foods listed in this group—milk, cheese, and ice cream—all derive their protein from milk. The proteins of milk are casein and lactalbumin, both complete, i.e., they contain a good balance of amino acids. Milk is the protein food that nature provides for the young of the

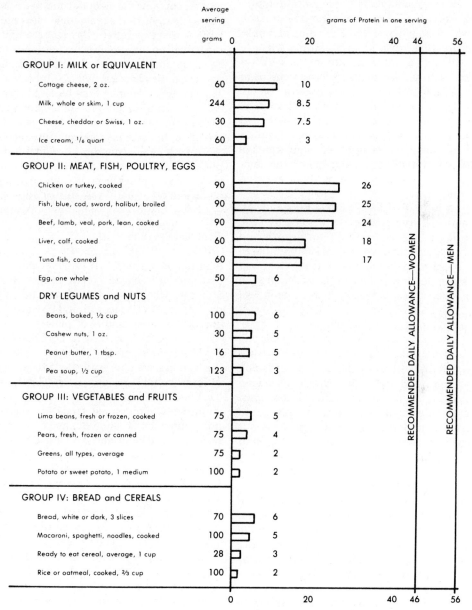

Fig. 4-4. Protein in average servings of foods classified in the four food groups.

species, and, around the world, milk from many different mammals is used for human food. Milk is almost essential for the infant; it is equally good as a source of protein for older children and adolescents during the growing years. Adults also should get some of their protein from milk and milk products. Nonfat dry milk, better known as dried skim milk, is an excellent source of milk protein and calcium at comparatively low cost.

Cheese is the term applied to any product made from the concentrated curd of milk. Cheese is thought to have been the first manufactured food, the process for which was probably discovered accidentally when milk was stored in a bag made from the stomach of a cow, which contains rennin. The action of rennin on milk causes the curds to form and the whey to separate. Although a certain amount of the milk nutrients remains in the whey, the majority remains in the curd, which provides a large amount of the natural food value in milk in concentrated form. The curd in cottage cheese is formed by the development of or addition of lactic acid bacteria to skimmed milk.

Both food value and flavor of the many kinds of cheese that are available today depend on the composition and the methods of ripening which are used in production.

GROUP II. MEAT, POULTRY, AND FISH are all forms of animal tissue protein synthesized by each species to meet its specific needs for growth and maintenance. Such proteins are remarkably similar in amino acid content to the amino acid requirements of humans. Meat, poultry, and seafoods vary in protein content in inverse ratio to the moisture content: veal 28, beef 25, lamb 24, poultry 20, and fish 15 to 20 g. of protein per 100 g. of fresh product.

Variety meats is a term applied to the organs and the glands of animals. They include tongue, liver, kidney, sweetbreads (thymus gland of calf or lamb), beef or calf heart, and beef brains. Organ meats tend to be much richer in vitamins and minerals than muscle meats. Popular luncheon meats such as spiced ham, pressed meat loaves, liverwurst, and various types of cold sausages such as bologna and frankfurters are sometimes classed as variety meats. They contain from 11 to 17 percent of protein in a convenient form for quick lunches.

Poultry is a general term covering a variety of domestic birds including chickens, turkeys, geese, and ducks. After roasting, the protein content of the lean meat of most poultry is about 30 percent; after frying or broiling the proportion of the protein content is slightly less than it is after roasting, because less moisture is lost.

Fish, including shellfish, compare favorably with meats and poultry as good sources of protein and in many countries are the chief source of animal protein. In the United States an effort is being made to stimulate the use of more varieties of both salt- and fresh-water fish. In other countries such products as fish sausage, fish flour and meal, and other processed fish foods of high protein value are being developed to improve the protein supply. Shellfish are low in fat and somewhat lower in protein ratio than fish because of their higher water content.

Eggs, a protein food of high nutritive value, are in a class by themselves. As mentioned previously, egg protein contains the essential amino acids in proportion so nearly like the theoretical ideal protein that it is often used experimentally as the reference standard in evaluating the protein of other foods (Table 4-2). Eggs contain 13 percent of protein—less than meats, poultry, or fish because of their higher water content. The egg white is one of the best examples of a pure colloidal solution of a protein (ovalbumin), containing 11 percent of protein and 89 percent of water. The protein of the yolk is more concentrated (16 percent) and much more complex. It contains lipoprotein, phosphoprotein, nucleoprotein, and possibly others, all of which provide nourishment for the embryo chick and are equally valuable as human food.

Plant Sources of Protein

GROUP III. VEGETABLES are poor sources of protein; the only group that provides more than 1 or 2 percent are the legumes. These may run as high as 5 or 6 percent when they are fresh and still higher in the dried form. For this reason, and because they provide one of the better quality of plant proteins, they are listed as meat alternates in the Four Food Group chart. Soybeans, which are the highest in protein content of the legumes, are now available in the U.S. in a variety of forms suitable for use in the fabrication of foods. They are also important sources of protein in many countries where animal foods are scarce. Soybean milk, curd, cheese, and flour are a few of the soybean products used by Orientals. In India, pulses (legumes) and beans could be produced and used more extensively than at present with great advantage because of their high nutritive value. They are especially important in a country where animal protein is scarce or the population is largely vegetarian.

Peanuts are really legumes although they are often classed as nuts. Roasted peanuts and peanut butter contain about 26 percent of protein, although roasting reduces the availability or destroys about 10 percent of three of the essential amino acids present. Peanuts—or groundnuts, as they are called in many countries—are often used without roasting or with much less heating than is common in the U. S.

Nuts in general are good sources of protein of fairly high quality. Because they are expensive they are seldom eaten in sufficient quantity to make an important contribution to the protein of the diet.

GROUP IV. BREADS AND CEREALS make an important contribution to the protein of the diet, not only because of their liberal consumption but also because many of their uses encourage or increase the consumption of animal proteins such as milk, eggs, meat, and fish. The protein of uncooked grains ranges from 7 to 14 percent. The grain proteins are low in one or more essential amino acids, e.g., wheat is low in lysine, corn in tryptophan, rice in tryptophan and the sulfur-containing amino acids, cystine and methionine. However, plant proteins may supplement each other in such a way that a combination may provide a better balance of amino acids than any one food alone.

A protein-fortified enriched macaroni product (wheat + soy flour) is now allowed to replace up to half the meat alternate requirement when served with meat, poultry, fish, or cheese in the School Lunch Program.

TEXTURED PROTEIN PRODUCTS are a new type of protein food made from one or more of the following sources: cottonseed, peanuts, sesame seed, soybeans, sunflower seed, and wheat. At the present time they are derived chiefly from soybeans. These products have similar appearance, taste, and texture to the foods they simulate—ground beef, ham, bacon, chicken, fish, cheese.

The textured protein products, also called analogs, are manufactured by making a fiber from one or more of the vegetable sources. Then the fiber can be spun into a form which simulates the texture of meat. Flavor additives are used to make them taste like the products they imitate. They may take the form of fiber, shred, chunk, bit, or slice. Some dehydrated forms are also available which may be rehydrated to serve as extenders to mix with ground meat.

The Food and Drug Administration has proposed the establishment of a definition and standard of identity for this new class of foods. Analogs have also been suggested as a food to be considered in nutritional guidelines to be set by the National Research Council. Because they may take the place of meat in the diet, their nutritional value should be comparable. They must supply a specific quantity and quality of protein as well as certain vitamins and minerals.

In 1971 the USDA authorized the use of textured vegetable protein fortified with vitamins and minerals in meals served under the School Lunch Program.

The ratio of hydrated vegetable protein to uncooked meat, poultry, or fish in combination must not exceed 30 parts to 70 parts respectively on a weight basis. Many supermarkets today sell a blend of ground meat and textured vegetable protein.

STABILITY OF PROTEINS IN FOODS

Bacterial Spoilage

Chemically pure proteins are fairly stable, but in the moist state in which they generally are found in foods they decompose readily at room temperature, owing to bacterial action, and may form substances toxic to the body. In this respect, nitrogenous foods are more unstable and will decompose more readily than carbohydrates and fats. Therefore, protein foods such as fresh meat, fish, milk, and eggs should be kept in the refrigerator to prevent or delay their decompositon.

Effect of Heat on Protein Foods

Proteins are modified (denatured) by heat, both in physical properties and in physiological availability. In ordinary cooking, proteins such as those in egg, meat, and fish are coagulated by heat, but the amino acid content is not changed.

STUDY QUESTIONS AND ACTIVITIES

1. Why is good quality protein important for breakfast as well as for other meals?
2. For what specific purposes are proteins used in the body?
3. What is meant by the terms nitrogen equilibrium, limiting factor, and polypeptide?
4. The structural components of proteins are amino acids. How many of these are known? Do tissues vary in the requirements for specific amino acids?
5. What is meant by "essential amino acids"? How is the amino acid score of a protein calculated?
6. Explain three ways that proteins may be supplemented to improve the quality of the diet. What is meant by net protein utilization? by biological value?
7. What theory is suggested as to why most Australians and New Zealanders are taller than people of similar racial strains living elsewhere?
8. What are the best food sources of complete proteins? Which food groups furnish the most protein? Compare the quality of protein from plant and animal foods.
9. What is the effect of heat on protein?
10. What are the National Research Council recom-

mendations for protein? Which foods must be included in the daily dietary, and how much of each, in order to ensure good nutrition?

11. The high-protein foods listed in Fig. 4-4 contain appreciable amounts of other food constituents. Look at the Pattern Dietary in Chapter 10 and see what each supplies.

12. What are textured protein products? How are they used to extend animal protein foods?

SUPPLEMENTARY READINGS

Altschul, A. M.: The revered legume. Nutrition Today 8:22 (March-April), 1973.

Calloway, D. H.: Recommended dietary allowances for protein and energy. J. Am. Dietet. A. 64:157, 1974.

Food and Nutrition Board: Improvement of Protein Nutriture. Washington, D.C., National Research Council, 1973.

Harper, E. A., Payne, P. R., and Waterlow, J. C.: Human protein needs. Lancet 1:1518, 1973.

Joint FAO/WHO Expert Comm.: Energy and Protein Requirements. Tech. Report Series No. 522, Geneva, World Health Organization, 1973.

For further references see Bibliography in Section 4.

REFERENCES

1. Pre-School Child Malnutrition—Primary Deterrent to Human Progress, NAS-NRC Publication No. 1282. Washington, D. C., 1966.
2. Mitchell, H. S.: J. Am. Dietet. A. 40:521, 1962.
3. Gruelich, W. W.: Science 127:515, 1958.
4. Tuttle, S. G., et al: Am. J. Clin. Nutr. 16:225, 1965.
5. Holt, L. E., and Snyderman, S. E.: Nutr. Abst. Rev. 35:1, 1965.
6. Nakagawa, I. T., et al: J. Nutr. 83:115, 1964.
7. Holt and Snyderman, op. cit.
8. Joint FAO/WHO Committee: Energy and Protein Requirements. Tech. Rep. Series 522, Geneva, World Health Organization, 1973.
9. Ibid.
10. Ibid., p. 73.
11. Scrimshaw, N. S., and Bressani, R.: Fed. Proc. 20:80, 1961.
12. Food and Nutrition Board: Recommended Dietary Allowances, 8th rev. Washington, D.C. National Academy of Sciences–National Research Council, 1974.
13. Joint FAO/WHO Committee, op. cit.
14. Calloway, D. H.: J. Am. Dietet. A. 64:157, 1974.

water and
mineral
metabolism

5

fluids and electrolytes

WATER AND BODY FUNCTION

Water is more essential to life than is food, for a person may live weeks without food but only days without water. It is an essential component of blood, lymph, the secretions of the body (extracellular fluid) and of every cell in the body (intracellular fluid). More than half the adult's weight is water, 60 percent for men, 54 percent for women. The internal environment of the body is bathed in fluids (which contain certain

47

electrolytes) held in compartments of the body (extracellular and intracellular spaces) divided by semipermeable membranes. The extracellular compartment (the space outside the cell membrane) accounts for 1/3 of the body water and includes the fluid in plasma and in interstitial spaces; intracellular fluid contains 2/3 of the body water.

Fluid is necessary for the functioning of every organ in the body. It is a structural component of cells. When cells lose their water they lose their shape. It is the universal medium in which the various chemical changes of the body take place. As a carrier it aids in digestion, absorption, circulation and excretion; it is essential in the regulation of body temperature; it plays an important part in mechanical functions, such as the lubrication of joints and the movement of the viscera in the abdominal cavity. Waste products from the tissues are transferred to the blood in watery solutions; they are carried by the blood, which is about 80 percent water; and they are excreted via the kidneys in urine, about 97 percent water (Fig. 5-1).

The same water is reused many times and for different purposes. Approximately 8 L. of digestive juices are produced and secreted by the glands in 24 hours (see Chapter 9). The water that carries the enzymes into the digestive tract is used during absorption to carry the digested nutrients into the blood and lymph. Over 4 L. of water are always circulating in the bloodstream. Water is the carrier of nutrients throughout the body. It is estimated that some 50 L. of water cross cell membranes in a day. In the kidney large volumes of water carry the dissolved waste material through the capsule of the uriniferous tubules, but, in passing through the tubules, most of the water, with some of its useful dissolved material, is reabsorbed. The urine which is excreted is the concentrated aqueous solution of the waste products.

Water Intake and Output

Normally, the body loses water through four routes: from the skin, as sensible and insensible perspiration; from the lungs, as water vapor in the expired air; from the kidneys, as urine; and from the intestines, in the feces. A minimum of 800 ml. of water is lost daily through the skin and lungs, and this amount may increase in hot, dry environments. The kidney eliminates approximately 1000 to 1500 ml. of water in the urine; fecal losses approximate 200 ml. daily but increase greatly when diarrhea occurs. Large water losses also result from excessive perspiration due to fever, vomiting, burns, or hemorrhage (Fig. 5-2).

Fluids are replaced by the ingestion of liquids and foods containing water. Although some water (14 ml. per 100 calories) is formed within the body as an end product of food metabolism, from 4 to 6 cups (1-1½ L.) of water or other liquids should be consumed daily in order to ensure a sufficient amount of water for body functions. Many foods contain a high percentage of water (Fig. 5-3) and may provide as much as 1 L. a day. Once ingested, water is absorbed rapidly from the digestive tract into the blood and lymph, although enough water is retained with food residues in the colon to produce a soft stool.

HOMEOSTASIS–WATER BALANCE. Water balance is carefully regulated within the body and normally a balance between intake and output is maintained, provided that there is free access to water. The weight of a man may vary by as much as 2 kg. in 48 hours due to changes in the amounts of water and salts.[1]

When water losses are increased due to excessive sweating or diarrhea, for example, the kidneys conserve water by making less urine. This action of the kidneys is under the control of the pituitary antidi-

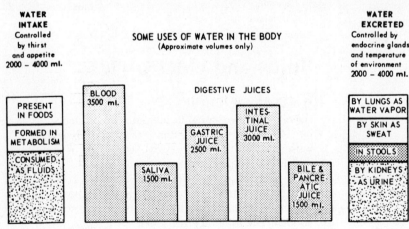

WATER INTAKE
Controlled by thirst and appetite
2000 – 4000 ml.

SOME USES OF WATER IN THE BODY
(Approximate volumes only)

PRESENT IN FOODS
FORMED IN METABOLISM
CONSUMED AS FLUIDS

BLOOD 3500 ml.

DIGESTIVE JUICES
SALIVA 1500 ml.
GASTRIC JUICE 2500 ml.
INTESTINAL JUICE 3000 ml.
BILE & PANCREATIC JUICE 1500 ml.

WATER EXCRETED
Controlled by endocrine glands and temperature of environment
2000 – 4000 ml.

BY LUNGS AS WATER VAPOR
BY SKIN AS SWEAT
IN STOOLS
BY KIDNEYS AS URINE

Fig. 5-1. Water in the body. Water functions in every tissue of the body. It constitutes 60 percent of body weight, one-half in muscles, two-thirds intracellular, one-third extracellular.

uretic hormone (ADH), which stimulates the renal tubules to increase the reabsorption of water.

Excessive loss of water results in sensations of extreme thirst. The mechanisms for stimulating thirst are located in the hypothalamus and are activated by an increase in the solute concentration in body fluid. Thirst is a sensation of dryness at the root of the tongue and the back part of the throat and is nature's signal that liquid intake must be increased.

DEHYDRATION. Dehydration may be fatal, a fact that further emphasizes the importance of water in the body. The German physiologist Rubner stated that we can lose all our reserve glycogen, all reserve fat, and about one-half of the body protein without great danger, but that a loss of 10 percent of the body water is serious and a loss of from 20 to 22 percent is fatal.

The term dehydration implies more than a change in water balance—there are always accompanying changes in electrolyte balance. When the water supply is restricted or when losses are excessive, the rate of water loss exceeds the rate of electrolyte loss. The extracellular fluid becomes concentrated, and osmotic pressure draws water from the cells into the extracellular fluid to compensate. This condition is called intracellular dehydration and is accompanied by extreme thirst and nausea. This is only one example of the 17 specific imbalances of body fluids that are recognized at present, according to Snively.[2]

The tremendous nutritional and physiologic importance of water is easy to demonstrate.[3] To evaluate the relative effect of water and carbohydrate supplements on work performance, six dogs were run to exhaustion on a treadmill. When they ran without food or water supplement 17 hours after the last meal, they were able to expend an average of 1190 cal. With a carbohydrate supplement without water they could expend 1300 cal. When allowed to drink while running, each dog consumed 1.5 L. of water during the run and increased his endurance until he expended 2140 cal. It has also been noted that Sir Edmund Hillary, the first person to climb Mt. Everest, attributed the success of his expedition during the last few days of the ascent to an adequate supply of water which other expeditions had lacked.

ELECTROLYTES AND NONELECTROLYTES

Chemical compounds that dissociate in water, breaking up into separate particles called ions, are known as electrolytes, and the process is referred to as ionization. Salts, acids, and bases are electrolytes; compounds such as glucose, urea, and protein are called nonelectrolytes because they are molecules that do not ionize.

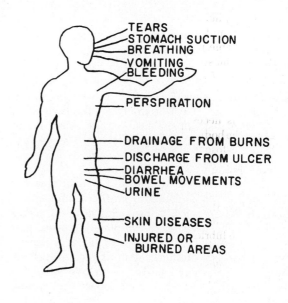

Fig. 5–2. Ways in which water and electrolytes may be lost.

Each ion, the dissociated particle of an electrolyte, carries an electric charge, either positive or negative. Positive ions (cations) in the body fluids include sodium ($Na+$), potassium ($K+$), calcium ($Ca++$), and magnesium ($Mg++$). The negative ions (anions) include chloride ($Cl-$), bicarbonate (HCO_3-), phosphate (HPO_4--), sulfate (SO_4--), ions of inorganic acids such as lactate, pyruvate, aceto-acetate, and many protein derivatives. Electrical balance is always maintained in the fluid compartments of the body. To measure the total combining power of electrolytes in solution, a unit of measure related to the number of electrical charges carried by the ions present in solution must be used. This unit is referred to as milliequivalents (mEq.). The cations and anions in each fluid compartment of the body, as measured in milliequivalents, are equal.

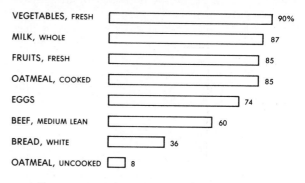

Fig. 5–3. Percentage of water in common foods.

Electrolyte Composition of the Body Fluids

Sodium is the major cation in plasma and interstitial fluid and chloride is the major anion. The major cation in intracellular fluid is potassium and the major anion is phosphate. Other ions are present in varying amounts in the different body fluids. Specific functions of these minerals will be discussed later in this chapter.

Osmotic Pressure

As previously stated, the fluid compartments of the body are separated by semipermeable membranes. These permit free exchange of water molecules but partially or completely prevent passage of dissolved particles such as glucose or electrolytes. If there is a solution containing a relatively large number of dissolved particles on one side of a semipermeable membrane and a solution containing a relatively small number of dissolved particles on the other, the force of osmosis is brought into play. Osmotic pressure causes water to pass across the semipermeable membrane from the less concentrated to the more concentrated solution, until the concentration of dissolved particles on both sides is equal.

Hence, exchanges of water between the various fluid compartments of the body occur as a result of osmotic pressure, which, in turn, is due chiefly to the concentration of electrolytes. Osmotic pressure in the cellular fluid is regulated mainly by the concentration of potassium and, in the extracellular fluid, by the concentration of sodium. If there is a loss or gain in either of these electrolytes in one compartment, the osmotic pressure is disturbed, and an increased amount of water will then be found in the compartment of greater osmotic pressure.

Plasma protein also plays an important role in maintaining osmotic equilibrium in the extracellular compartments. By remaining in the plasma it tends to prevent the leakage of water into the interstitial spaces, where an excess of extracellular fluid is known as *edema*.

Excess water losses may also result in excess loss of electrolytes. These are not always replaced through water intake, in which case serious problems may result. Moreover, as already noted, intracellular dehydration results when the rate of water loss from the body is greater than the rate of electrolyte loss.

ACID-BASE BALANCE

Electrolytes play an important part in maintaining the acid-base balance in the blood and throughout the tissues. The maintenance of this balance is a function of normal metabolism. The reaction of the blood is slightly alkaline (pH 7.3 to 7.45), varying only within narrow limits, regardless of the amount of acid products formed in metabolism. This equilibrium is maintained by a series of buffers in the blood and the tissue fluids. These buffers, which have a tendency to resist changes in their pH when treated with strong acids or bases, contain a weak acid or base and a salt of this acid or base. They have been likened to a chemical sponge in that they can soak up or release anions or cations as needed to maintain the normal pH. The principal buffers in the regulation of acid-base balance are the bicarbonate-carbonic acid system, the phosphate system, the hemoglobin-oxyhemoglobin system, and the proteins.

Acid products formed in metabolism are disposed of through either the lungs or the kidneys. The respiratory mechanism reacts quickly but the renal system adapts itself over longer periods of time. The respiratory system controls the removal of CO_2 from the blood and can either increase or decrease its loss by regulating the depth and rate of respiration. The kidneys, however, remove hydrogen ions from the body by excreting acids and, at the same time, return bicarbonate to the blood. This accounts for the urine's having a more acid reaction (pH 5.5 to 6.6) than the plasma. The reaction of the urine may vary widely in a normal individual because the amount of acid or base end-products of metabolism will vary and the excess must be eliminated.

When the supply of buffer susbtances becomes depleted due to starvation or inability to metabolize food properly, a condition known as acidosis may result. Actually, the blood does not become acid; rather, the term *acidosis* is used to indicate the lowered alkaline reserve which results when the basic elements are used up faster than they are replenished. This may happen in severe diabetes, when the organic acids from faulty fat metabolism accumulate.

Alkalosis is the opposite of acidosis. This may occur when severe vomiting over a period of time causes a great loss of hydrochloric acid. The body quickly adjusts when the acute condition is relieved.

Acid-Base Reaction of Foods

Conclusive evidence is not as yet available in regard to the practical importance of the acid-base balance of foods in relation to health. Experience and scientific evidence indicate a wide range of adaptability on the part of the human body and do not support the "scare" propaganda with which certain food faddists promote the sale of "alkalizing" compounds to prevent acidosis.

The usual mixed diet contains a good balance of acid and basic factors. The basic elements, sodium, potassium, magnesium, and calcium, may occur as salts of inorganic acids, such as phosphates, sulfates, or chlorides, or organic acids. The mineral elements are sometimes referred to as "ash" because they do not "burn" up. When foods are metabolized in the body, the mineral elements are released to function in maintaining the acid-base balance; the organic acids are oxidized mostly to carbon dioxide and water. Foods are said to be acid or basic according to whether the acid or the basic elements in the ash predominate. Most fruits contain organic acids combined with basic inorganic elements. When such compounds are oxidized in the body, they leave an alkaline ash. Some other foods, such as cereals and meats, not at all acid in taste, yield end products that are strongly acid. Thus, potential acidity or alkalinity of foods refers to the reaction that they will ultimately yield after being oxidized in the body.

Some workers have attempted to establish quantitative figures for the excess of acid or basic elements in foods, but the significance of these figures is now being questioned; therefore, they have been omitted.

minerals

ESSENTIAL MINERALS AND THEIR DISTRIBUTION

Although mineral elements constitute only a small proportion (4 percent) of the body tissue, they are essential as structural components and in many vital processes. Some form hard tissues such as bones and teeth; some are in the fluids and soft tissues. There are functions in which the balance of mineral ions is important—for example, for bone formation, the amount and the ratio of calcium and phosphorus, and for normal muscular acitvity, the ratio between potassium and calcium in the extracellular fluid. Electrolytes, of which sodium and potassium salts are the most important, are the major factors in the osmotic control of water metabolism as discussed earlier in this chapter. Other minerals may act as catalysts in enzyme systems, or as integral parts of organic compounds in the body, such as iron in hemoglobin, iodine in thyroxine, cobalt in vitamin B_{12}, zinc in insulin, and sulfur in thiamine and biotin.

Plant life and animals, as well as bacteria and other one-celled organisms, all require proper concentrations of certain minerals to make life possible.

Table 5-1. Mineral Composition of an Adult Human Body

Element	Percent of Total Ash	g./70-kg. Man
Calcium (Ca)	39	1160
Phosphorus (P)	22	670
Potassium (K)	5	150
Sulfur (S)	4	112
Chlorine (Cl)	3	85
Sodium (Na)	2	63
Magnesium (Mg)	0.7	21
Iron (Fe)	.15	4.5
Zinc (Zn)	.007	2.0
Iodine (I)	.0007	.02

In fact, changes in concentration of minerals, small in themselves, can be fatal to various forms of life. Thus, common salt, which in dilute solution is necessary for most forms of animal life, becomes a preservative when foods are salted or kept in brine because the salt concentration kills bacteria. On the other hand, marine forms (fish and shellfish) quickly die when subjected to fresh water. In the human body also, the maintenance of a normal concentration of minerals in body fluids is essential.

The mineral elements which the body requires are frequently classed as either macro- or micronutrients, depending on the amount of each that is needed in the diet. Calcium, phosphorus, potassium, sulfur, chlorine, sodium and magnesium are considered macronutrient elements. Iron, iodine, flourine, zinc, copper, chromium, selenium, cobalt, manganese, molybdenum, vanadium, tin, silicon, and nickel are often called micronutrient or trace elements. A comparison of the relative amounts of some of these minerals in the body is shown in Table 5-1. Cadmium, lead, mercury, arsenic, boron, lithium, aluminum, and other minerals may also be present in animal tissue as environmental contaminants but at this time they have no known essential nutritional role.

Mineral Content of Foods

In unrefined foods, minerals are present in various forms mixed or combined with proteins, fats and carbohydrates. Processed or refined foods, such as fats, oils, sugar and cornstarch, contain almost no minerals. The total mineral content of a food is determined by burning the organic or combustible part of a known amount of a food and weighing the resulting ash. The ash then is analyzed for individual mineral elements. Most foods have been analyzed for ten or more mineral elements, but in dietary practice the figures most commonly used are those for calcium, phosphorus, and iron and, for therapeutic purposes, sodium, potassium, and magnesium (Tables 1 and 4, Section 4).

Minerals such as iodine, copper, and other trace elements which are essential for life may be found abundantly in drinking water in certain areas or in foods grown in the soil of those areas, whereas in other parts of the country the same minerals are deficient in both soil and water. Still other mineral elements, such as sodium, potassium, chlorine, sulfur, and magnesium—all necessary in human nutrition—are so universally present in foods that we recognize no need to worry about deficiencies.

The question of relative availability of mineral elements for physiologic processes continues to stimulate new investigations in this field. Fifty or more years ago, the opinion prevailed that the organic forms of minerals found in plant and animal foods were utilized better than the inorganic forms. However, modern research has disproved this theory. Today we are aware that many minerals occur in inorganic form in natural foods and, as such, are absorbed from the digestive tract without change.

CALCIUM AND PHOSPHORUS
Functions of Calcium and Phosphorus
STRUCTURES OF BONES AND TEETH. Approximately 2 percent of the adult human body is calcium and 1 percent is phosphorus. Ninety-nine percent of the calcium and 75 percent of the phosphorus in our bodies are found as constituents of bone and teeth, giving them strength and rigidity.

Bone is made up of a flexible, extremely strong organic matrix plus bone salts which are deposited within the lattice-like framework of the matrix to make them hard and rigid. The bone matrix formed by the osteoblasts consists of protein collagen embedded in a gelatinous ground substance composed of mucopolysaccharides such as chondroitin sulfate. The ground substance varies in consistency from a relatively thin fluid to a thick gel, thus forming the interconnection with the tissue fluid that permits an exchange of ions and other elements in the blood. The bone salts or inorganic constituents of bone consist of small crystals of calcium phosphate in the form of hydroxyapatite ($3Ca_3(PO_4)_2 \cdot Ca(OH)_2$) and noncrystalline or amorphous calcium phosphate. Small amounts of magnesium, sodium, carbonate, citrate, chloride, and fluoride are also present in bone salts. The hydroxyapatite crystals, although relatively stable in structure, are extremely small, which gives them a large surface area, and can rapidly exchange ions at their surface. The intercrystalline fraction is more soluble and its elements can go back to the blood

by the simple process of solution. During early life the amorphous material predominates but it is replaced by the crystalline form in more mature bone. The size of the crystals also increases with maturity as does the calcium to phosphorus ratio[4]. Bones contain blood and lymph vessels, nerves, and bone marrow. The nutrients needed for bone metabolism pass from the blood vessels into the interstitial fluid that surrounds the crystals, so that exchanges between the tissues and the blood are easily accomplished.

There is constant deposition and resorption of bone. In children bone deposition, controlled by the activity of the osteoblasts, bone-forming cells, is greater than the resorption controlled by the osteoclasts, bone-destroying cells. On the other hand, the skeletal changes frequently observed in old age occur when bone resorption dominates and there is a decrease in the absolute amount of bone (osteoporosis). In the normal adult the two processes are equally balanced, with both calcification, or mineralization, and demineralization dependent on the level of calcium and phosphorus in the blood and extracellular fluids and on the normal functioning of the matrix cells. Approximately 600 to 700 mg. of calcium enter and leave the bones each day.

Hormones influence these processes. The parathyroid hormone controls the resorption of calcium from bone, and a thyroid hormone—thyrocalcitonin—inhibits calcium withdrawal from bone.

Bone, like other tissue, is in a state of dynamic equilibrium with the constituents of the plasma and other tissue. Calcium and phosphorus, when the food supply is abundant, can be stored in the trabeculae at the ends of the bones. From this storehouse these minerals are readily available to meet the needs of other tissues of the body when the dietary intake of calcium or phosphorus is inadequate. However, if calcium has not been stored in the trabeculae, calcium will be withdrawn from bone structure itself. Prolonged removal of calcium from bone naturally results in bones that are more easily bent or broken. When calcium phosphate is removed from bone, the remaining tissue is as flexible as cartilage; in fact, it is essentially the same as cartilage. Cartilage precedes bone in the development of the fetus and the young animal, and normally the calcium phosphate is deposited in it as growth and strain demand. The amount of calcium needed by the bones depends on the rate of skeletal development. The calcium content of the body increases from approximately 28 g. at birth to about 1200 g. at maturity. This is an average increase in body calcium of about 165 mg. per day. However, the variation of calcium deposition throughout the growth period is extremely great, with maximum needs of 300 to 400 mg. per day occurring in conjunction with the growth spurt in early adolescence. When nature's plan is thwarted by an inadequate supply of these minerals in food or by the body's inability to utilize them, growth may be retarded, or, as more often happens in young children, growth in size continues but the new bone is abnormal in structure and poorly calcified. This may result in the bowed legs, enlarged ankles and wrists, prolapsed thorax, and other bone deformities characteristic of rickets.

Tooth structures, particularly dentine and enamel, are metabolically more stable than the bones. The calcium phosphate in the teeth is in the same form, hydroxyapatite crystals, as in the bones. The protein matrix in the enamel is keratin and in the dentin is collagen. There is little turnover of calcium in the teeth.

The deciduous teeth begin to calcify in the fetus around the twentieth week of pregnancy and continue almost until they erupt into the mouth. Calcification of the permanent teeth may commence anywhere from three months to three years. Wisdom teeth begin around ten years of age. Teeth once formed do not require additional calcium since they cannot repair themselves after they have erupted.

However, poor tooth structure, reflected by increased susceptibility to dental caries, may be the result of inadequate calcium intake during the period of tooth formation.

FUNCTIONS OF CALCIUM AND PHOSPHORUS IN SERUM AND SOFT TISSUES. When compared with the amounts in bones and teeth, the concentrations of calcium and phosphorus in the blood are small, but their presence in normal amounts is essential for body function. Although they are often associated because they function together in the skeletal structures, elsewhere in the body their functions are quite distinct.

Bone calcium is in equilibrium with plasma calcium which is maintained at a relatively constant level of 10 mg. calcium/100 ml. (5 m Eq./L.) of blood approximately. Plasma calcium levels are regulated by both the physical equilibrium between the plasma and the soluble bone salts (noncrystalline form) and by the mobilization of calcium from the less soluble bone salts (crystalline form) under the control of parathormone (PTH). Physical equilibrium tends to keep the plasma calcium level up to about 70 percent of the normal content, while the remainder is supplied by a feedback mechanism under control of the parathyroid glands. When the plasma calcium level falls below about 7 mg. percent, the parathyroid

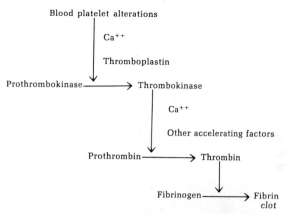

Fig. 5–4. The role of calcium in blood clot formation.

gland increases its secretion of parathormone which acts on the osteoclasts in bone to break down bone tissue and release calcium ions into the plasma; magnesium ions and citrate also seem to be involved in the process of calcium mobilization. PTH also increases the urinary excretion of phosphates. Vitamin D functions in maintaining plasma levels of calcium by promoting intestinal absorption of calcium.

A normal calcium level in the blood is necessary for blood clot formation. As shown in Fig. 5–4, when cells have been injured ionized calcium in the blood is responsible for stimulating release of various factors from the blood platelets which are effective in the activation of the enzyme thrombokinase. Thrombokinase, together with Ca^{++} and other accelerating factors, catalyzes the conversion of prothrombin to thrombin. The latter aids in the polymerization of fibrinogen to fibrin, the blood clot.

Calcium has a vital role in the contraction and relaxation of muscle. Its entrance into the muscle cell as a result of nerve stimulation sets in motion the biochemical processes which cause the proteins myosin and actin to be drawn together, thus contracting the cell, making it shorter and thicker. Since the so-called "relaxing factor" outside the cell has an affinity for calcium, calcium is quickly removed from the muscle cell, allowing the cell to relax.

Acetylcholine, the chemical transmitter of nerve impulses, is released upon stimulation of the nerve cell provided adequate amounts of calcium ions are present. In addition to being required for normal transmission, calcium also influences the permeability of cell membranes. The neuromuscular hyperirritability characteristic of tetany occurs when the blood calcium level falls below normal. Calcium is an activator of several enzymes including ATPase, lipase, and certain proteolytic enzymes. The absorp-

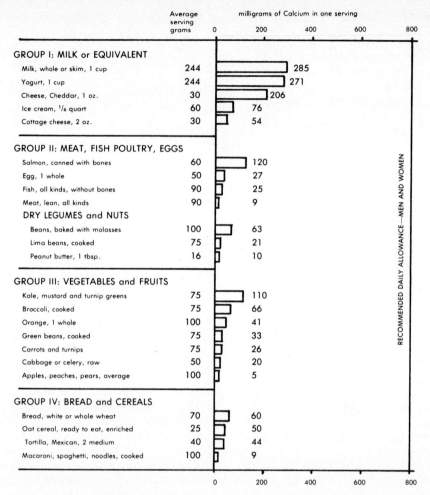

Fig. 5-5. Calcium in average servings of foods classified in the four food groups.

tion of vitamin B_{12} through the wall of the small intestine requires calcium.

Phosphorus is a necessary constituent of every cell in the body. It is part of the nucleic acids DNA (deoxyribonucleic acid) and RNA (ribonucleic acid) which determine the genetic code (see Chapter 9).

Phosphorus is part of the ATP (adenosine triphosphate)–ADP (adenosine diphosphate) energy-transporting systems in the cells (see Chapter 8) and is also a component of the phospholipids which are involved in the transport of fats and fatty acids. Phosphates, as previously mentioned, also assist in maintaining the acid-base balance of the blood.

Food Sources of Calcium and Phosphorus

It is apparent in Fig. 5-5 that milk and milk products are the most important sources of calcium in readily available form. A few of the green, leafy vegetables used commonly in the Southern states are good sources of calcium, but others such as spinach, chard, beet greens, and rhubarb contain sufficient oxalic acid to form insoluble calcium oxalate, thus rendering the calcium unavailable. In most sections of the country greens are not used regularly enough or in sufficient quantity to be relied upon to replace milk, but they are important when milk is scarce or unobtainable. Meats and poultry are poor sources of calcium. Cereal products contribute little, except where breads are enriched with calcium or are made with a high percentage of milk solids. The pattern dietary of 1400 cal. provides almost the recommended allowance of 800 mg. (0.8 g.), which will be supplemented by the calcium of the foods added to make up the needed calories (see Table 5-2 and Chapter 10.)

Phosphorus is more widely distributed than calcium and less likely to be deficient in the average diet. Poultry, fish, meats, cereals, nuts, and legumes, as well as milk and milk products, are all good sources.

Table 5–2. Calcium, Phosphorus, Magnesium, and Iron in Pattern Dietary for 1 Day*

Food Group	Amount in g.	Household Measure	Energy kcal.	Calcium mg.	Phosphorus mg.	Magnesium mg.	Iron mg.
Milk or equivalent	488	2 cups	320	576	452	63	.2
Meat, fish, poultry or egg	120	4 oz. cooked	376	13	212	104	3.3
Vegetables:							
Potato, cooked	100	1 medium	65	6	48	22	.5
Green, leafy, and yellow	75	1 serving	21	44	28	29	.9
Other	75	1 serving	45	16	41	18	.9
Fruits:							
Citrus	100	1 serving	44	18	16	12	.3
Other . .̇......................	100	1 serving	85	10	21	16	.8
Bread, white, enriched	100	4 slices	270	84	97	20	2.5
Cereal, whole grain or							
enriched	30	1 oz. dry or					
	130	2/3 c. cooked	89	12	95	34	.9
Butter or margarine	14	1 tbsp.	100	3	2	2	..
			1,415	782	1,012	335	10.3

*For basis of calculation, see Pattern Dietary in Chapter 10.

In the cooking of vegetables, there may be slight losses of calcium and phosphorus, especially if the cooking water is discarded.

Factors Affecting Absorption and Retention

Not all of the calcium and phosphorus in foods is available to the body. Approximately 20 to 40 percent of the calcium and 70 percent of the phosphorus consumed by an individual is absorbed from the intestinal tract into the bloodstream to become available. The amounts absorbed, however, may be greatly increased during periods of rapid growth when mineral needs are high. Individuals on limited intakes of calcium are also more efficient in their utilization of it than those on more liberal intakes. These factors help explain the following statement from the World Health Organization's Report on Calcium Requirements. "In general, children and adults in most countries can grow normally and live healthily on a daily calcium intake between 300 mg. and 1000 mg. or, in the absence of nutritional disorders and if their vitamin D status is adequate, on even somewhat lower or higher intakes."[5]

Various factors, in addition to need, influence the efficiency of calcium and phosphorus absorption. Adequate amounts of vitamin D, an acid pH in the upper part of the intestinal tract, and a normal motility of the gastrointestinal tract enhance the absorption of these minerals. On the other hand, large amounts of fats, phytates (phosphorus compounds found in cereals), or oxalates which can form insoluble compounds with calcium may interfere with intestinal absorption.

In cases of parathyroid disturbances variations in calcium absorption and retention are even greater than under normal conditions. Hypercalcemia (high serum calcium) may occur in hyperparathyroidism,

and hypocalcemia (serum calcium below normal) may result after operative removal of the parathyroid glands.

Dietary Requirements

The dietary requirements of calcium and phosphorus for children and adults have been investigated extensively. There is not, however, universal agreement among the experts on the interpretation of the findings.

Using balance studies to determine calcium and phosphorus requirements is a complicated procedure. As already mentioned, there are many factors which affect the amount of calcium absorbed and retained by the body. A person is said to be in equilibrium with respect to any nutrient if the intake approximately equals the output. The assumption that end products of metabolism appear in the urine and unabsorbed material in the feces does not hold for calcium and phosphorus. Some metabolized (endogenous) calcium and phosphorus may be excreted via the intestinal tract. Moreover, the evidence that man can maintain calcium balance over a wide range of calcium intakes (the amount required to maintain this balance is largely determined by past dietary history) has caused one authority to question the use of balance studies to estimate calcium requirements.[6] However, Table 5–3 indicates the method used to calculate the adult recommended allowance for calcium.

The Recommended Dietary Allowances (RDAs), as revised in 1974, continued the adult allowance for calcium and phosphorus at 800 mg. per day (0.8 g.). This allowance for calcium is considerably higher than the "suggested practical allowance" of 400 to 500 mg. per day recommended by the FAO/WHO Expert Committee on Calcium Requirements and re-

**Table 5–3. Bases for Calculating
the Adult Recommended Dietary Allowance
for Calcium***

Urinary calcium excretion	175 mg./day
Endogenous fecal calcium excretion	125 mg./day
Loss of calcium in sweat	20 mg./day
Total calcium losses	320 mg./day
Calcium absorbed from food 40 percent	

$$\frac{320}{x} \times \frac{100}{40} = 800 \text{ mg./day}$$

Recommended dietary allowance for adult	800 mg./day

*Figures from Recommended Dietary Allowances. National Academy of Sciences/National Research Council Publ. No. 1146. Washington, D.C., 1964.

ferred to by the Food and Nutrition Board's Committee on Dietary Allowances.[7] In setting the adult RDA at 800 mg. the Food and Nutrition Board recognized the effect which various levels of protein intake have on calcium metabolism.[8] The urinary loss of calcium when protein intake is high appears to be substantial and was a major consideration in the Board's decision to continue the adult allowance at the present level rather than adopting the FAO/WHO recommendation. However, the Board also states that "persons consuming less than the customary United States intake of protein will remain in calcium balance with intakes considerably below the allowance recommended."[9]

The calcium and phosphorus allowances during pregnancy and lactation are increased to 1200 mg. per day to cover fetal needs and the calcium and phosphorus required for producing human milk. These amounts are comparable to the FAO/WHO Committee's suggestion of 1000 to 1200 mg. each per day during these periods.

Except during infancy the calcium and phosphorus allowances are the same for all ages.

The calcium and phosphorus requirements for growth have been investigated in children of different ages by observing the level of intake at which maximum retention of calcium and phosphorus is attained. Growth of bone requires the storage of new calcium and phosphorus as well as replacement. The growth requirement varies with age, being highest in relation to weight in the infant, lower and fairly constant after the first year and until puberty, when there is a rise again during the period of rapid growth. The recommended allowances of calcium and phosphorus for children take into account different age needs. For ages one to ten allowances of 800 mg. per day of calcium and phosphorus are suggested, to be increased at preadolescence to 1200 mg. per day. A

calcium:phosphorus ratio of 1.5:1 is suggested for the first six months of life to more nearly approximate the calcium:phosphorus ratio in human milk.

A careful selection of foodstuffs rich in calcium and phosphorus is necessary to meet these needs. For infants, the intake requirements may well be stated in terms of the amount of milk, since this is the chief food source. For older children, the requirements for calcium and phosphorus are most easily met by including two to three cups of milk a day or its equivalent in milk products. The calcium and phosphorus contents of milk are not only high but in good proportion, and these minerals are more readily available from milk than from most other foods. During all periods of growth, vitamin D, or sunshine, is essential for the most efficient absorption and utilization of these two minerals. See Chapter 6, Fat-Soluble Vitamins.

The relationship between calcium intake and *osteoporosis* needs special consideration. There is good evidence that the condition of the bones in later life is related to the amount of bone present in early adult life and not primarily related to the calcium intake during adult life.[10] Furthermore it appears that the changes which occur in bone during adult life are a general phenomenon more pronounced in women than in men, and are not prevented by high intakes of calcium nor caused by low intakes.[11] Therefore it would appear to be impossible to prevent osteoporosis by dietary calcium alone. Guthrie[12] refers to "osteoporosities" because they seem to result from multiple origins. The decrease in bone mass characteristic of the disease may be the result of longstanding inadequate dietary intakes of calcium, increased parathormone activity stimulating bone resorption, failure to synthesize matrix protein, immobility, or low levels of estrogens. Assuming that bone formation is normal, bone resorption must occur at an accelerated rate. This could be in response to low dietary intake, poor absorption, or increased urinary loss. Thus the relationship between high protein intakes and low calcium intakes and its net effect on calcium balance needs to be examined further in terms of osteoporosis.

MAGNESIUM

Magnesium in the body (21 g.) (Table 5–1) is divided between the bone and other tissue; about 50 to 60 percent is combined with calcium and phosphorus in the structure of the bone, while most of the rest is found in the cells of the body. The highest concentration occurs in muscles and red blood cells. Magnesium is second to potassium as the chief cation in all living cells.

Absorption, Storage, and Excretion of Magnesium

Active absorption of magnesium occurs in the ileum. Magnesium may compete with and decrease calcium absorption from the intestines. The parathyroid hormone, parathormone, which controls serum calcium levels, has a similar effect on magnesium.

Magnesium is excreted in both stools and urine. Urinary excretion is reduced in magnesium depletion. Although almost twice the amount of magnesium is stored in bones as compared with soft tissues, bone magnesium is not readily exchanged with the magnesium of soft tissues.

Functions of Magnesium

Magnesium is an activator for most of the enzyme systems involving carbohydrate, fat, and protein in energy-producing reactions. It is necessary for the activation of alkaline phosphatase, an enzyme involved in calcium and phosphorus metabolism. It functions with other minerals such as calcium, sodium, and potassium in maintaining fluid and electrolyte balance. Proper levels of magnesium are necessary for normal neuromuscular contractions. The synthesis of proteins, nucleic acids, and fat also requires magnesium.

The homeostasis of potassium and calcium may be impaired by severe magnesium deficiency. Potassium is lost from the cell, resulting in an increase in urinary excretion. Serum calcium levels are also depressed. Magnesium depletion of iatrogenic origin may occur as a result of omitting magnesium in intravenous fluids or from extended periods of treatment with diuretics. There is a need for a better understanding of the relationships among magnesium, potassium, and calcium in clinical medicine.

The symptons of magnesium deficiency are similar to the tetany seen when blood levels of calcium are reduced. There is hyperneuromuscular activity which, if untreated, results in convulsive seizures as well as cardiac arrhythmia, or even cardiac arrest.

The relationships between high levels of magnesium intake and the decreased incidence of calcium deposits in soft tissues[13] and the reduced susceptibility to cardiovascular disease await further research on the functions of magnesium in metabolism.

Dietary Requirements and Food Sources of Magnesium

The recommended dietary allowances for magnesium are 350 mg. per day for adult men and 300 mg. per day for women. During pregnancy and lactation the recommended allowance is 450 mg. per day. Allowances based on the magnesium content of human milk and cow's milk were also established for infants and children.

Magnesium is widely distributed in foods: it is a part of the chlorophyll in green vegetables and is also found in cocoa, nuts, cereal grains, meat, milk, and seafood. Table 5, Section 4, gives the magnesium content of various foods.

The recommended dietary allowance of the adult woman for magnesium (300 mg.) is met by the pattern dietary of 1400 calories. The additional foods necessary to meet energy requirements will further supplement the magnesium intake of the adult man (see Table 5–2 and Chapter 10).

Seelig,[14] in reviewing the published data on magnesium, has suggested that diets in Western countries, which contain less magnesium (less than 5 mg. per kg. per day) than oriental diets (more than 6 mg. per kg. per day), may be marginal in their magnesium content. There is also evidence that bone magnesium is not readily available for replacement in soft tissues when dietary magnesium is severely reduced. These two factors have contributed, no doubt, to the magnesium deficiences observed in patients with certain clinical conditions where magnesium intake or absorption have been decreased or magnesium excretion has been increased. Among these conditions are chronic alcoholism, diabetes, malabsorption syndrome, renal disease, disorders of the parathyroid gland and postsurgical stress.[15]

MAGNESIUM SALTS taken by mouth are both diuretic and laxative. The cathartic action is due to the slow absorption of magnesium from the intestines and the consequent drawing of water into the gut.

SODIUM

Sodium is the most abundant cation in the extracellular fluid of the body. It acts with other electrolytes, especially potassium in the intracellular fluid, to regulate the osmotic pressure and maintain proper water balance within the body. Sodium is a major factor in maintaining acid-base equilibrium, in transmitting nerve impulses, and in relaxing muscle. Sodium is also required for glucose absorption and for the transport of other nutrients across cell membranes. One milliequivalent of sodium weighs 23 mg. An adult man (70 kg.) has 2700 to 3000 mEq. of sodium in his body. There is a concentration of 136 to 145 mEq./L. in the extracellular fluid and approximately 10 mEq./L. within the cells of the body. Bone contains 800 to 1000 mEq. of sodium of which about half is available if needed by the extracellular fluids.

The sodium intake of Americans has been estimated to be between 2 and 7 g. per day (equivalent to 6-18 g. of table salt/day), which is more than adequate for usual body needs. This amount may have to be reduced in certain diseases where water or electrolyte balance is disturbed. The sodium content of various foods is given in Table 5, Section 4, but it must be remembered that drinking water may be an important consideration in determining sodium intake.[16,17]

Most sodium consumed is excreted by the kidneys, with variable amounts lost through the skin and stools. In the normal individual, sodium is almost completely absorbed from the gastrointestinal tract but substantial losses may occur with vomiting and diarrhea. Sodium homeostasis is under the control of the hormone aldosterone secreted by the adrenal gland. When the need for sodium increases, increased amounts of aldosterone are secreted which increase the resorption of sodium ions by the kidney tubules.

Skin losses may increase greatly when there is profuse perspiration from strenuous physical exertion in a hot environment. Profuse sweating may cause losses of as much as 350 mEq. of sodium per day. Under such circumstances salt depletion may be accompanied by heat exhaustion. Salt tablets taken with a liberal amount of water may be advised.

POTASSIUM

Potassium is found principally in the intracellular fluid where it plays an important role as a catalyst in energy metabolism and in the synthesis of glycogen and protein. Potassium ions maintain osmotic equilibrium with the sodium ions in the extracellular fluid. However, a small amount of potassium in the extracellular fluid is necessary for normal muscular activity. Thirty-nine mg. of potassium equals 1 milliequivalent. The average adult man has about 3200 mEq. of potassium in his body; 125 mEq./L. within the cells and 3.5 to 5.0 mEq./L. in the plasma. Potassium levels in the body have been used to measure body composition. By estimating the amount of radioactive potassium-40 in the body (whole body counter) a determination of the lean body mass can be made and compared with weight to determine body fat.

Potassium requirements have not been established but an intake of 0.8 to 1.3 g. per day is estimated as approximately the minimum need. Potassium is widely distributed in our foods, the average intake varying from 50 to 150 mEq. per day. Although potassium deficiency is most unlikely in the healthy individual, medications such as certain diuretics and adrenal cortical hormones may cause potassium depletion if efforts are not made to replace potassium in the diet. As with sodium, potassium losses may also be increased with vomiting and diarrhea. Meats, cereals, fruits, fruit juices, and vegetables are good sources of potassium. Values for the potassium content of foods are given in Table 4, Section 4.

CHLORIDE

Chloride is the anion most commonly combined with sodium in the extracellular fluid and, to some extent, it is also found with potassium in the cells. But, unlike these bases, chlorine can pass freely between these two fluids through the cell membranes. The chlorides are among the electrolytes that help to maintain osmotic pressure and acid-base equilibrium in the body. During digestion some of the chloride of the blood is used for the formation of hydrochloric acid in the gastric glands; it is secreted into the stomach where it functions temporarily with the gastric enzymes and is then reabsorbed into the bloodstream along with other nutrients. The approximate intake of 3 to 9 g. daily from foods and from added table salt easily meets the requirement. The only time the body may be depleted of chloride is after the loss of gastric contents due to vomiting. Excess chloride is readily excreted by the kidneys and the skin, mostly as sodium chloride.

SULFUR

Sulfur is part of the protein in every cell of the body and occurs in most food proteins. Thus, sulfur intake is usually sufficient if protein is adequate. Sulfur occurs in a number of physiologically important organic compounds; in the amino acids methionine, cysteine and cystine; in insulin, glutathione, heparin, thiamine, biotin, and lipoic acid. Keratin (the protein of hair, fur, nails and hoofs) is rich in sulfur; thus, the sulfur-containing amino acid requirement of hairy animals tends to be higher than that of humans.

Sulfates formed in the metabolism of the sulfur-containing amino acids have a role in the detoxification of phenols, indoxyls, and other compounds which are excreted in the urine. They are also found as part of the sulfate mucopolysaccharides, chondroitin sulfate, and heparin.

ESSENTIAL TRACE ELEMENTS

Many inorganic elements occur in animal tissues in extremely small quantities and, in some instances, are detected only by spectrographic methods or by the use of radioactive elements. These are known as micronutrients, or trace elements, because they are found only in such minute quantities.

The essentiality of some micronutrients has been clearly established while that of others is under investigation. Mertz[18] has suggested a variety of criteria to determine essentiality, such as the presence of a trace mineral in healthy tissue. If the element also appears in the fetus and the newborn an even better case is made for its nutritional need. Additional evidence is provided if the body maintains homeostatic control over the rate of its excretion or uptake into blood or tissues. Consistent changes in blood levels, tissue concentrations, or distribution within a metabolic pool as a result of physiologic activity further affirm the concept of essentiality, as does the identification of the element in an enzyme or as the activator of an enzyme. Finally, animal studies allow for the most conclusive evidence. If specific symptoms can be produced as a result of the total or partial absence of the element and then alleviated by its addition to the diet, the element can then be considered essential.

As a result of changes in our food supply there is currently some concern about the adequacy of trace elements in the American diet. The increased consumption of highly refined, processed, and fabricated foods can reduce the amount of a trace mineral present in the diet. The development of new varieties of foods and changes in fertilization practices and in processing techniques and equipment can also alter the concentration of trace minerals; the net effect of such changes is unknown.

The interrelationships among these elements also present problems in assessing needs. Because they occur together in varying amounts in the diet, their absorption from the intestinal tract may be dependent on their relative concentrations, which could affect their excretion and their tissue concentration as well. The interactions of the trace minerals might be synergistic or antagonistic, and hence the amount of any one element could depend on the amount of other essential or nonessential elements or other constituents in the diet.

IRON

There is less than 5 g. of iron in the body of a normal healthy adult, but its importance to our well-being is strikingly out of proportion to the quantitative requirement. Sixty to 70 percent of the iron in the body is found in hemoglobin; iron stores in the liver, spleen, and bone marrow account for the next largest concentration of iron (30 to 35 percent). Small but essential amounts of iron are found in muscle myoglobin; in transport form (bound to protein-transferrin) in the blood serum; and in every cell as a constituent of certain enzymes, notably cytochrome oxidases and catalases, and in chromatin (colored) materials (see Fig. 5-6).

Hemoglobin Synthesis

Iron is a necessary constituent of hemoglobin, the coloring matter of the red blood cells, and as such is vital to the processes of nutrition. Hemoglobin is a conjugated protein composed of four iron-containing heme groups, each attached to four polypeptide chains which make up the globin moiety. The heme is responsible for the characteristic color and the oxygen-carrying capacity of blood. Hemoglobin combines with oxygen in the lung capillaries to form oxyhemoglobin, which travels in the bloodstream to the tissues where the oxygen is released to take part in oxidative processes. Part of the carbon dioxide formed is carried back by the same hemoglobin, which drops its load in the lungs and starts out with a new supply of oxygen. Hemoglobin values below 12 to 14 g./100 ml. of blood are considered low.

The synthesis of hemoglobin (approximately 800 g. in the adult man) proceeds concomitantly with the maturation of the red blood cell in the bone marrow, and lasts the "lifetime" of the cell—120 days. When the erythrocyte cell disintegrates, the reticuloendothelial cells, particularly those of the liver, spleen, and bone marrow, are responsible for the removal of the hemoglobin, the breakdown of the heme, and the release of the iron which is then made available for reuse.

Hemoglobin synthesis depends on the presence of copper. The discovery of the catalytic action of copper in the use of iron for elaboration of hemoglobin was dramatic because it supplied the first proof that one inorganic element can function in the utilization of another; copper is not present in the hemoglobin molecule but functions in the mobilization of iron for use in hemoglobin synthesis of heme. Adequate protein must also be available for synthesis of the globin fraction. Other dietary essentials, especially ascorbic acid, vitamin E, and vitamin B_{12}, influence the rate of destruction of the red blood cells.

MYOGLOBIN, found only in the muscle tissue, is related to blood hemoglobin in both structure and function. It is an oxygen carrier capable of supplying oxygen to the muscles and of removing carbon dioxide.

Cellular Iron

Iron has an important role in tissue respiration as part of the various enzymes, cytochrome oxidases, peroxidases, and catalases that catalyze oxidation-reduction processes in the cell.

Iron Absorption, Transport, Storage, and Losses

Physiologic control of iron balance is primarily achieved by regulating iron absorption from the gastrointestinal tract. Significant amounts of iron are absorbed into the intestinal (duodenum) mucosal cells within four hours after ingestion, probably by combining with an organic substance such as certain sugars, alcohols, or amino acids. It has recently been suggested that gastroferrin, a protein in normal gastric juice, is involved in the absorption of iron into the mucosal cell.[19] Once iron is inside the cell, some is released to transferrin in the plasma while another portion is transferred to the protein, apoferritin, thus forming ferritin, the storage form of iron. The precise mechanism for the release of iron from the mucosal cell into the plasma is not known but it appears that the unsaturated iron-binding capacity of the serum determines the rate of transfer. One theory is that the unsaturated transferrin molecule attaches to the epithelial cell and causes the release of iron from within the cell; once saturated by iron, the transferrin moves back into the plasma and transports iron to the bone marrow for hemoglobin synthesis, to the liver or spleen for storage, or to other tissues for their particular uses.[20] Normally, when transferrin is saturated up to about one-third of its total iron-binding capacity, no more iron is absorbed from the mucosal cells into the blood plasma. Instead, the iron remains in the mucosal cells which are sloughed from the wall of the intestine into the gut and excreted in the feces. In an iron deficiency or when there are increased demands for iron (as in pregnancy), the iron-binding capacity increases in an attempt to trap more iron for the body. On the other hand, in hemochromatosis (abnormal amounts of iron deposited in tissue) the iron-binding capacity is drastically reduced. To determine the iron status of individuals, assessments of plasma iron,

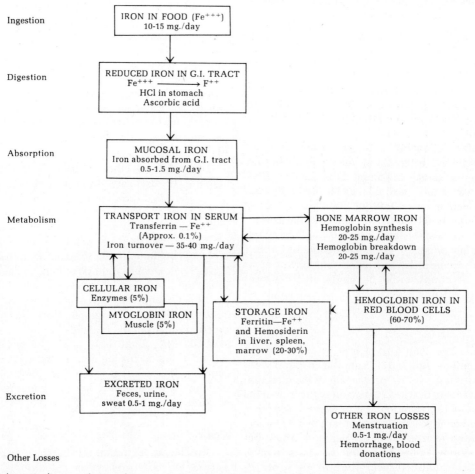

Fig. 5–6. Schematic diagram of iron pathways in the body. Figures in parentheses indicate approximate percent of total body iron in each compartment. Average amounts of iron consumed, absorbed, turned over in the body, and excreted per day are also included.

iron-binding capacity (percent transferrin satura-tion), bone marrow iron, and absorption of radioac-tive iron may be made.

Iron is stored as ferritin in the liver, spleen, intes-tinal mucosa, and in all reticuloendothelial cells. When iron is deposited in abnormally large amounts, such as in iron-loading or excessive blood transfu-sions, hemosiderin, a compound similar to ferritin but containing more iron, is formed in excess. The stores of iron, as well as the iron released from the disintegration of red blood cells, are available to the

body for hemoglobin synthesis. Hence, the iron of our bodies is used very efficiently and normally is not used up or destroyed but is conserved and utilized again and again. Thus, the iron actually used daily by an individual far exceeds that supplied by the dietary intake for the same period. Small amounts of unab-sorbed iron are lost in the stools together with the iron sloughed off from the mucosal cells. These losses amount to 0.5 to 1.0 mg. per day. Because of the loss of blood during menstruation the female of child-bearing age loses an additional 0.5 to 1.0 mg. of iron

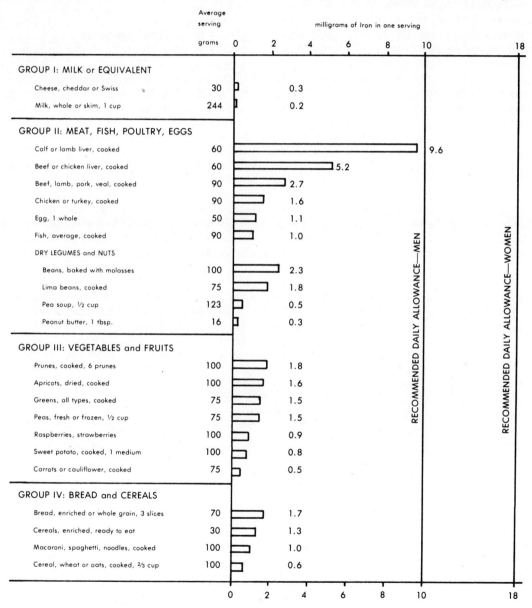

Fig. 5–7. Iron in average servings of foods classified in the four food groups.

per day. Major losses of iron also occur as a result of hemorrhage or blood donation. Fig. 5–6 illustrates the various pathways of iron in the body.

Food Sources of Iron

The best food sources of iron are found in the meat, fish, poultry, and egg group. Green, leafy vegetables, potatoes, dried fruits, and enriched bread and cereal products are the best plant sources. Milk and milk products are conspicuously low in iron (Fig. 5–7). Foods such as molasses and raisins, popularly featured as good sources of iron, are rich on a percentage basis, but small servings of these foods used infrequently do not constitute as important a source of food iron as some staple foods, for instance, whole grain or enriched breads and cereals (Fig. 5–8). The iron content of all common foods is given in Table 1, Section 4. Note that foods poor in iron have a noticeable lack of pigment, which is significant, since iron salts are all colored and usually lend color to a food rich in this element. Compare, for instance, egg yolk with egg white, molasses with white sugar, whole with milled grains, and spinach with celery.

The basic pattern dietary of 1400 calories provides 10.3 mg. of iron, which meets the RDA for the adult male. Additional foods to supply extra calories increase only slightly the amount of iron consumed by the menstruating woman for whom the recommended allowance is 18 mg. per day. Since usual food patterns will not supply this amount of iron, many suggestions have been made to insure an adequate intake of iron by women of child-bearing age, adolescents and children. They include: supplementation with an iron compound, of which there are a variety available; a return to iron cookware, which does not seem practical at the present time; and an increase in the use of whole grain flours, which also does not seem feasible in a country committed to white flour and its products. Increasing the levels of enrichment in cereal products has been proposed but has met with considerable opposition and postponement. If the proposed levels of flour enrichment are accepted, approximately 2 mg. per day of iron will be added, but the diet will still remain below the RDA for the menstruating woman. Mertz, in addition, suggests the application of an understanding of biologic availability of iron in various foods to the planning of meals.[21]

Factors Affecting Iron Absorption

As is the case with calcium and phosphorus, not all the iron present in foods is absorbed into the body. In fact, in the normal adult with adequate iron stores usually less than 10 percent of the iron in food is absorbed; infants and young children absorb greater amounts of iron from their food. Persons living at high altitudes absorb more iron than those at lower altitudes. Moore[22] and his associates, using radioactive iron, have shown that normal men and women absorb from 1 to 12 percent of food iron, whereas subjects with an iron deficiency absorbed 45 to 64 percent when fed the same amounts of iron.

The form of the iron in food also affects its biologic availability; ferrous (Fe^{++}) salts are absorbed more efficiently. Hence, since most food iron is in the form of ferric (Fe^{+++}) salts, they must be reduced for efficient absorption. Ascorbic acid and other reducing agents have been shown to enhance iron absorption.

Heme iron from animal meats is well absorbed and its availability depends less on the influence of other foods in the diet than does the availability of iron from eggs, cereal grains, vegetables, and fruits. Studies

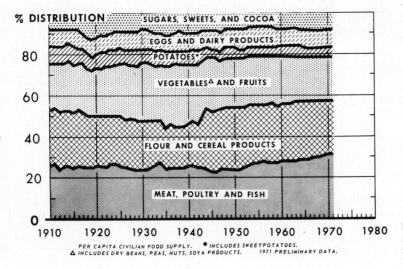

Fig. 5–8. Sources of iron. (U. S. Department of Agriculture, Agricultural Research Service)

have also indicated wide differences in the availability of iron from various compounds used for enrichment and supplementation. Iron is most available from ferrous sulfate and the ascorbate, fumarate, and citrate iron complexes. Iron is least available from iron phosphate, carbonate and EDTA complexes. (Ethylenediamine tetraacetic acid is a chelating and sequestering agent that forms water-soluble complexes with many different cations in solutions.) The availability of iron from reduced or metallic iron is intermediate—depending on the size of the particle in the preparation.[23]

Large amounts of fiber, or substances that form insoluble complexes with iron such as phytates and certain sulfur-containing compounds, reduce absorption. As might be expected, diarrhea also results in poor iron absorption.

Dietary Requirements for Iron

Iron requirements are determined by the demands for tissue growth and hemoglobin accretion and by replacement needs for iron lost in the urine, feces, and sweat and in the female in menstruation, pregnancy, and lactation. The three periods of greatest demand for iron are during (1) the first two years of life, (2) adolescence, especially girls and (3) the child-bearing period. Because of individual variation in absorptive capacity, the differences among foods in the availability of their iron for absorption, and the ability of the body to increase iron absorption during periods of deficiency, it is difficult to convert physiological requirements for iron into dietary allowances. Therefore, the United States recommendations for iron set by the Food and Nutrition Board of the National Research Council and those set by the Joint FAO/WHO Expert Group differ although based on the same considerations.

ADULTS. The 1974 National Research Council's recommended daily dietary allowance for women is 18 mg. of iron per day and for men, 10 mg. per day. After menopause in women, when menstruation has ceased, the sex difference in the iron requirement no longer exists. These recommendations assume that at least 10 percent of the iron will be absorbed from the diet (Table 5-4). The FAO/WHO Joint Committee based their recommendations for iron on the percent of calories in the diet from animal foods, since the availability of iron from these foods is in general greater than from vegetable sources.[24] See Table 5-5.

CHILDREN. During the period of rapid growth, when an increase in red cells and hemoglobin is taking place, provision for new material, as well as replacement of old, requires a more liberal supply of iron. The anemias of infancy and childhood are evidence of the

Table 5-4. National Research Council's Recommended Daily Dietary Allowances for Iron*

	AGE Years	IRON mg.
Infants	0.0-0.5	10
	0.5-1.0	15
Children	1-3	15
	4-10	10
Males	11-18	18
	19-51+	10
Females	11-50	18
	51+	10
	Pregnant	18+†
	Lactating	18

*From National Research Council: Recommended Dietary Allowances, Washington, D.C., 1974.
†This increased requirement cannot be met by ordinary diets: therefore, the use of supplemental iron is recommended.

shortage that frequently occurs, although nature seems to have provided for the period of nursing. Milk is essentially low in iron, but a reserve of this mineral provided by the high hemoglobin level of the infant at birth is economically conserved for repeated utilization. The potential shortage of iron that may occur by the sixth or the seventh month may be forestalled by the use of iron-fortified formulas and the introduction of fortified infant cereals and other suitable sources of iron into the infant's diet by his third month.

ADOLESCENTS. Few data are available for the requirements of this age group. The allowance of 18 mg. recommended was estimated on the assumption that

Table 5-5. Joint FAO/WHO Expert Group Recommended Daily Intakes of Iron*

		RECOMMENDED INTAKE ACCORDING TO TYPE OF DIET		
	Absorbed iron required (mg.)	Animal foods below 10% of calories (mg.)	Animal foods 10-25% of calories (mg.)	Animal foods over 25% of calories (mg.)
Infants: 0-4 months	0.5	[a]	[a]	[a]
5-12 months	1.0	10	7	5
Children: 1-12 years	1.0	10	7	5
Boys: 13-16 years	1.8	18	12	9
Girls: 13-16 years	2.4	24	18	12
Menstruating women[b]	2.8	28	19	14
Men	0.9	9	6	5

*From a Joint FAO/WHO Expert Group report: Requirements of Ascorbic Acid, Vitamin D, Vitamin B$_{12}$, Folate, and Iron, Tech. Report Series #452, Geneva, 1970.
[a]Breast-feeding is assumed to be adequate.
[b]For nonmenstruating women the recommended intakes are the same as for men.

an adolescent's needs are at least as great as the adult female's. Menstruation in adolescent girls means loss of hemoglobin and, consequently, an increased demand for all blood-building elements. Boys are growing rapidly at this age and also need iron for hemoglobin building.

Failure on the part of many people to meet these recommended allowances for iron was evident in the Ten-State Nutrition Survey which reported a high incidence of iron-deficiency anemia in the population surveyed.[25] See Chapters 20 and 33 for a discussion of anemias.

IODINE

Iodine was one of the first micronutrients to be recognized as vital to nutrition, and it is still considered one of the most important.

Common goiter has been known since prehistoric times, but it was not recognized as a deficiency disease until the late 19th century. Baumann discovered iodine in the thyroid gland in 1895, and from then on iodine was used more or less as a preventive or curative treatment for endemic goiter. Before that time burnt sponge (a good source of iodine) had been a popular remedy.

Not until 20 years after Baumann's discovery was serious attention given to iodine as prophylaxis against goiter in large population groups. No doubt action was stimulated by the high incidence of goiter among draftees from certain states during World War I.

Function of Iodine and Thyroid Activity

Before surveys were made of the iodine content of soil, it had been noted that the disease of common goiter was unevenly distributed over the United States and that it seemed to be most prevalent in the very regions where there was the least iodine. This early suspicion was confirmed, and we now recognize that common goiter is primarily an iodine deficiency disease.

An essential constituent of the thyroid gland in man and in animals, iodine in sufficient quantity must be supplied if that gland is to synthesize enough of the hormones thyroxine (T_4) and triiodothyronine (T_3) to function normally.

Dietary iodine is absorbed from the gastrointestinal tract into the blood; about 30 percent is removed by the thyroid gland for the synthesis of thyroid hormone and the rest is excreted by the kidneys. The amount of iodine present in the body of an adult is estimated to be about 25 mg., most of it concentrated in the thyroid, where it is stored in the form of thyroglobulin, a complex of protein and iodine. Proteolytic

enzymes break down this compound, and thyroxine and small amounts of triiodothyronine are excreted into the circulating blood. When the amount of thyroid hormone in the serum is decreased, the pituitary gland releases a thyroid-stimulating hormone (TSH) which causes the thyroid gland to produce more cells and increase in size in an attempt to manufacture more hormone. This results in enlargement of the thyroid gland, or simple goiter.

Thyroid hormone is recognized as essential in the regulation of energy; hyper- and hypothyroidism are reflected in increased or decreased basal metabolic rates. In addition, thyroxine influences protein synthesis, blood cholesterol levels, carbohydrate absorption, and the conversion of carotene to vitamin A.

Natural Food Sources of Iodine

The fact that goiter is not evenly distributed throughout the world or even within the United States indicates that some areas must provide natural protection through food or drinking water. People who live near the coasts and consume generous amounts of seafood get an adequate amount of iodine from these sources. In Japan, where seaweed as well as other seafoods in wide variety are popular, the iodine intake is estimated to be 0.5 to 1.0 mg. per day. The incidence of goiter in Japan is the lowest of any country in the world.

The iodine content of milk, other dairy products, and eggs varies with the composition of the animals' feed. The amount of iodine in bread varies with the mixing process used. One slice of bread made by the continuous mix process will supply the daily iodine requirement, while one slice made by the batch process contains very little. It is not easily determined which process has been used for any individual slice of bread.

Since growing plants pick up iodine when it is present in the soil, plant foods vary widely in iodine content according to the soil in which they are grown. Thus, plant foods grown near sea coasts and in our Southern states contain more iodine than those grown in the Great Lakes area or other regions where the surface soil is low in iodine. For this reason it is impossible to list the iodine content of foods in tables of food composition or to estimate the amount in the pattern dietary. Since our urban markets today abound in foods grown in many different regions there is less likely to be a severe iodine deficiency even in so-called goitrous regions. It is a very different situation where rural people confine their diet chiefly to home-grown products in mountainous regions where the soil is notably low in iodine. It should also be noted that iodized salt is not used in many commercially prepared foods; hence, the extensive use of these products may contribute to the problem of goiter. Similarly, when salt is purchased in bulk, as it is in many institutions including schools and hospitals, it is usually not iodized.

Dietary Allowances for Iodine

The recommended dietary allowances set for iodine in 1974 are 130 mcg. per day for adult males and 100 mcg. per day for adult females. An increase to 125 mcg. per day for pregnancy and to 150 mcg. per day during lactation is recommended. The need for iodine during growth is great, so that the recommendations for children are proportionately higher than for adults. (See Chapter 10.)

Goiter Prophylaxis

The suggestion was made by Marine and Kimball that iodine might be administered to children in goitrous regions as a preventive measure. Consequently, as an experiment, iodine was administered to school children in Akron, Ohio, with remarkably successful results. By a similar project, in three cantons in Switzerland the incidence of goiter was diminished during 3 years from 87 to 13 percent. These demonstrations suffice to show that the body requirements for iodine, although they are exceedingly small, must be met in order to prevent goiter. Many sections of the country, notably the East Coast and the Southern states, as well as California on the West Coast, need pay little attention to this factor because iodine is indigenous. However, in the goitrous regions this was a problem requiring attention, and Michigan led the way in its solution by promoting education in goiter therapy as a public health measure.

Administration of iodine as a prophylactic measure against goiter had to be planned as a public health activity so that it would reach all people in an area in safe but significant amounts. The use of tablets either at home or in school was impractical, and the addition of iodine to drinking water was too expensive. Common salt is used by nearly everyone in somewhat comparable amounts. Therefore, a small percentage of an iodine compound was added to table salt to be marketed in goitrous regions, and an educational campaign was conducted to inform people why they should buy and use iodized salt.

This plan was adopted by Michigan in 1924, and all salt manufacturers in the state put on the market a table salt containing 0.02 percent of sodium iodide. Eleven years later the results of this plan adopted by the Michigan Department of Health far exceeded the hopes of those who instigated it. Endemic goiter or enlarged thyroid had become nearly extinct.[26] The decrease in the sale of iodized salt that has occurred since publicity on the subject has fallen off is paralleled by a slight increase in the number of goiters in school children. The discontinuance of iodized salt in one county in Michigan was followed by a marked rise in the incidence of goiter within three years. A 1959-65 survey in Michigan found goiter in 6.6 percent of the 9000 people examined, and the incidence was higher in women than in men.[27]

In states where the use of iodized salt was not encouraged, the incidence of thyroid enlargement has remained fairly constant over the same period of years. The Ten-State Survey (1968-70) did not identify iodine deficiency as a significant problem in the populations surveyed.

In 1941, the National Study Committee on Endemic Goiter resolved that the content of potassium iodide in table salt and in salt for domestic animals should be 0.01 percent, provided that a suitable stabilizer was used. This amount was calculated from per capita consumption of salt to be sufficient for the prevention of endemic goiter and not great enough to cause harmful effects in other types of thyroid disorders. Iodized salt has since been continuously available in groceries in parts of the country where it is needed and at no increased cost to the consumer. However, education is still necessary if all people are to understand why it is desirable to choose iodized salt when shopping. Iodized salt is now being introduced into other countries where common goiter is endemic, probably as a result of its successful use in this country. (See Chapter 20.)

Goitrogens are substances that tend to produce goiters, and it has been demonstrated experimentally that such a substance is present in certain vegetables: cabbage, Brussels sprouts, cauliflower, rutabagas and peanuts. Goitrogenic action is prevented by cooking, and an adequate supply of iodine inhibits or prevents it.

ZINC

Functions

Zinc occurs in animal and plant tissue in slightly smaller amounts than iron. There are about 2 g. of zinc in the body where it is highly concentrated in the hair, skin, eyes, nails, and testes. It is a constituent of many enzymes involved in metabolism. Insulin is known to contain zinc, as does the enzyme carbonic anhydrase which plays an important role in the maintenance of equilibrium between carbon dioxide and carbonic acid. Zinc is an integral part of the alkaline phosphatases and alcohol dehydrogenases. There is also a concentration of zinc in the nucleic acids but its function there has not been identified. Animal studies have indicated that zinc plays an important role in growth and in appetite regulation. It is not easily mobilized in the body and the biologically available pool appears limited.

Studies in the Middle East[28,29] show that zinc deficiency does occur in humans. The deficiency symptoms found in the population where zinc intake was presumed inadequate were dwarfism, hypogonadism, and iron deficiency anemia. Less severe states of zinc deficiency have also been observed in the United States. The accelerated rate of wound healing[30] and the improved sense of taste[31] observed after zinc supplements were administered indicate that zinc nutriture in the subjects studied was less than optimum. In addition, marginal zinc deficiency was recently identified in a survey of children in Denver.[32] Of 150 apparently healthy children from middle income families, 8 percent displayed deficiency symptoms which included low levels of zinc in the hair (below 70 mcg./g.), impaired taste acuity, poor appetite, and suboptimal growth. When zinc intake was increased, the children showed improvement. In chronic alcoholism greatly increased zinc excretion may occur even when serum levels are low, and may result in zinc insufficiency.[33]

Requirement

In 1974 the Food and Nutrition Board set recommended dietary allowances for zinc for the first time. The average diet of the American adult contains approximately 10 to 15 mg. of zinc and metabolic studies indicate that this amount is adequate to maintain positive balance. Hence, the RDA for adult males and females was set at 15 mg. per day. An additional 5 mg. for pregnancy and 10 mg. for lactation were recommended. Allowances were also established for adolescents (15 mg. per day), children (10 mg. per day), and infants (3 mg., zero to six months; 5 mg., six months to one year). (See Chapter 10.)

Food Sources of Zinc

Animal products in general are important sources of zinc. Seafoods (especially oysters), meat, liver, eggs, and milk are good sources. Legumes and whole grain products such as whole wheat bread, rye bread, oatmeal, and whole corn also contribute zinc to the diet. About 20 to 30 percent of the zinc in food is absorbed by the body. Zinc from vegetable sources is less available to the body; hence, persons who consume primarily vegetable diets have more risk of zinc deficiency than those who include liberal amounts of animal foods. The zinc content of the pattern dietary has not been calculated because of the unavailability of adequate food analysis data for zinc. Recently the USDA published provisional tables on zinc in food (see Table 5, Section 4).

OTHER ESSENTIAL TRACE ELEMENTS
Copper

Copper is essential for the mobilization of iron in the synthesis of hemoglobin and as a constituent of many enzymes that function in tissue metabolism. Ceruloplasmin (CP), a copper-containing plasma enzyme, recently identified as ferroxidase-I, catalyzes the oxidation of the ferrous ion to ferric ion and thereby enables iron to be trapped by transferrin (ferri-transferrin) and transported to tissues for the synthesis of iron-containing compounds, especially hemoglobin.[34] It has now been determined that three other copper-containing proteins, at first designated as erythrocuprein, hepatocuprein, and cerebrocuprein, are identical and have an important enzymatic function. This conjugated protein, because of its biochemical function, has been termed "superoxide dismutase." It catalyzes the dismutation (simultaneous oxidation, reduction, and decarboxylation) of superoxide free radical anions, protecting the cell from their accumulation and potentially damaging effects.[35] Other copper-containing enzymes include tyrosinase, ascorbic acid oxidase, cytochrome oxidase, amine oxidase, delta aminolevulinic acid dehydrase, and dopamine beta hydroxylase. The ataxia seen in certain copper deficient animals (sheep, goats, pigs, guinea pigs, rats) has been attributed to cytochrome oxidase deficiency which prevents normal development of motor neurones. The synthesis of elastin and collagen has also been affected in various animals by low copper intakes, and this is related to the reduction in amine oxidase which is essential to the formation of intramolecular cross-linkages in the connective tissue.[36] The abnormal straight, stringy wool seen in copper deficient merino sheep indicates that copper is also essential in the synthesis of keratin.[37]

Although severe copper deficiencies are rare in humans, hypocupremia has been observed in protein-calorie malnutrition. Among malnourished children in Peru this was accompanied by anemia, neutropenia, and bone disease.[38] Some of the same symptoms have recently been observed in premature infants fed exclusively on modified cows' milk for two to three months and in infants during prolonged parenteral feeding.[39]

A genetically determined defect in copper absorption known as Menkes's "kinky hair" syndrome in infants has many of the symptoms of copper deficiency seen in animal studies. Progressive mental deterioration, defective keratinization of hair, low serum and liver copper levels, metaphyseal lesions, and degenerative changes in aortic elastin are characteristic features of the disease.[40]

Copper is absorbed from the duodenum. Metallothionein apparently mediates its absorption by binding it and other trace minerals prior to absorption into the plasma. The antagonism among copper, cadmium, and zinc probably results from competition for binding sites on this copper-containing protein. Since ascorbic acid decreases the amount of copper bound by metallothionein, it can contribute to copper deficiency. Large amounts of molybdenum and sulfate in the diet can also depress copper absorption. Approximately 32 percent of the copper in the diet is absorbed. Metallothionein in the liver and kidneys functions in the storage and detoxification of copper. Excess copper is excreted in the bile.

There are approximately 75 to 150 mg. of copper in the adult human body. Newborn infants have higher concentrations than adults, and the tissue distribution of the total body copper varies with age and copper status. Liver, brain, kidney, heart, and hair contain relatively high concentrations. Average serum copper levels are higher in adult females (114.0±4.67 mcg. Cu/100 ml.) than in males (105.5±5.03 mcg. Cu/100 ml.). Serum copper levels also increase significantly in women both during pregnancy and when taking oral contraceptives.

The average American diet contains about 2.5 to 5.0 mg. of copper, and it has been estimated that the human requirement may be 2.0 mg. or less per day. Requirements for infants and children have been calculated between 0.05 and 0.1 mg./kg. of body weight per day which is supplied by the mixed diet of later infancy. The FAO/WHO Joint Committee suggested an allowance of 80 mcg. per day for infants and young children.[41]

Copper intake is determined primarily by individual food selection. Crustaceans and shellfish, particularly oysters, and liver, kidney and brains, nuts, dried legumes, raisins, and cocoa are rich sources of copper. The amount of copper in green leafy vegetables, however, reflects to some degree the copper status of the soil. Copper contamination during processing, storage, and treatment of food also affects the total amount of copper ingested. Soft water contains more than hard water and water from the tap contains more than reservoir water. However, the latter is a better source of copper than water taken directly from the stream.

Manganese

Manganese plays essential roles in both plant and animal nutrition. The human body contains 10 to 20 mg. of manganese, widely distributed throughout the tissues. It is found in high concentration in the mitochondria of cells and is also associated with melanin. Homeostatic control of manganese is regulated chiefly by its excretion in the bile rather than by its absorption from the intestine. High calcium intakes have been shown to increase the fecal excretion and to reduce the retention of manganese in the liver.

Manganese is absorbed rapidly and transported in the blood bound to protein. The two manganese pools in the body—blood manganese and liver mitochondrial manganese—are in equilibrium and most of the body manganese is in a dynamic, highly mobile state.[42] Serum manganese levels are almost always elevated following a myocardial infarction.

Manganese is an important element in many enzyme systems. It is apparently a part of the enzyme arginase which is necessary for the formation of urea. It functions as a catalyst in the synthesis of mucopolysaccharides of cartilage.[43] Pyruvate carboxylase is a manganese-containing metalloprotein.[44] In addition, it has also been shown to be involved in glucose utilization.[45]

The manganese requirement of man is not known but neither is manganese deficiency in man; hence, the average daily intake of 2.5 to 7 mg. of manganese is probably adequate for adults. The Joint FAO/WHO Expert Group stated that an intake of 2 to 3 mg. per day can be assumed to be adequate for adults.[46] Although manganese deficiency in infants has never been reported, they have very low intakes while being fed exclusively on either breast or cows' milk.[47] When solid foods are introduced, the manganese intake increases greatly.[48] Nuts, whole grains, dried legumes, tea, and cloves are excellent sources of manganese. Fruits and vegetables are fair sources, depending on soil content. Blueberries tend to be the richest source in this group. Meat, fish, and dairy products are low in manganese.

Fluorine

Fluorine has long been recognized as a normal constituent of bones and teeth, with dental enamel especially rich in this element. The fluorine content of surface soils and water supplies varies widely; this, naturally, influences the fluorine content of food grown in the region and, in turn, the level of human consumption.

Excess fluorine is recognized as the cause of mottled enamel in the permanent teeth of children in certain areas of the world. This condition is endemic in limited areas—e.g., the Texas Panhandle and adjacent areas—and is commonly known as dental fluorosis. The mottling occurs when fluorine is present in the drinking water in concentrations of 1.5 ppm. (parts per million) or more. In these same areas the low incidence of dental caries attracted comment. Subsequently, the relation of traces of fluorine in local water supplies to the low incidence of dental caries has been studied extensively.[49, 50] The question of finding a level of fluorine in drinking water low enough to eliminate mottled enamel, but high enough to reduce the incidence of dental caries, had to be answered. It is now estimated that 1 ppm. is about the critical level and that water supplies can be standardized by adding fluorine to bring the concentration up to 1 mg. Fl/L. of water.

If this amount is added to the water in a community, a reduction of 50 to 60 percent in dental caries in children may be anticipated. Large-scale experiments in several communities pointed the way to effective use of fluorine prophylaxis. Mass control of dental caries in children is possible and has been recommended by medical and public health authorities.[51] See further discussion of this subject in Chapter 20.

It has been recognized for some time that optimal quantities of fluorides are required for maximal resistance to dental caries. Only recently, however, has fluorine been identified as essential to animal growth. Rats raised in an isolated environment and fed very low levels of fluorine demonstrated an increase in growth when fluorine was added to their diets.[52]

There is also some evidence that fluoride is effective in the treatment of osteoporosis. Increased retention of calcium accompanied by a reduction in bone demineralization was observed in patients receiving fluoride salts.[53] In addition, the incidence of osteoporosis in women and aortic calcification in men is less in areas where the drinking water has a high fluoride content.[54]

Fluoride is deposited in both bones and teeth when it replaces the hydroxyl ion in hydroxyapatite $(Ca_3P_3O_8 \cdot Ca(OH)_2)$ and forms fluorapatite $(Ca_3P_2O_8 \cdot Ca(F)_2)$. The fluoride-containing teeth are more caries resistant and the bone less prone to resorption.

Dietary intake of fluoride, exclusive of that from drinking water, ranges from 0.3 mg. in low fluoride areas to 3.1 mg. in high fluoride areas. The fluoride content of food varies widely according to where it is grown.

Chromium

Chromium is associated with glucose metabolism, possibly as a cofactor for insulin. When low chromium diets were fed to rats, they developed the symptoms of mild diabetes mellitus which disappeared when Cr(III) was supplied in drinking water.[55] Chromium seems to function by increasing the effectiveness of insulin, thereby facilitating the transport of glucose into the cell.

The adult male has less than 6 mg. of chromium in his body. Chromium levels are higher in human infants than in adults; the concentration in human tissues varies greatly in different parts of the world,

depending both on dietary habits and on the amount of chromium in water supplies. Injections of insulin or feeding of glucose leads to a rapid (30 to 120 min.) increase in serum chromium level. In chromium-supplemented subjects or in young persons the increase may be as much as five times the fasting level, while little or no increment may occur in the elderly. The failure to respond to this test may possibly be indicative of chromium deficiency. In studies with human diabetic subjects improved glucose tolerance tests (see Chapter 28) were reported following chromium supplementation for some subjects while others did not respond. Those who responded were, perhaps, chromium deficient, while nonresponding individuals were not.[56] Thus chromium is not a cure for diabetes nor a substitute for insulin.

The degree to which various forms of chromium can be converted into biologically active complexes is not well understood in man. The rat, for example, is very dependent on the organic form of chromium GTF (Glucose Tolerance Factor), and man may also be equally dependent.[57] Since little is known of the chemical forms in which chromium occurs in individual foods, no meaningful recommendations can be made for chromium at this time. Brewer's yeast, certain animal products (not fish), and whole grains contain good amounts of available chromium.

Molybdenum

Molybdenum is an essential micronutrient contained in the metalloenzyme, xanthine oxidase. The enzyme is dependent on the presence of this metal for its activity. Molybdenum has also been identified in the enzymes aldehyde oxidase and sulfite oxidase. No symptoms associated with molybdenum deficiency have been reported in humans. The Joint FAO/WHO Expert Group[58] suggests that a diet containing 2 mcg. of molybdenum per kg. of body weight will maintain equilibrium or slight positive balance. Beef kidney, certain cereals, and legumes appear to be good sources. The amount of molybdenum from vegetable sources varies depending on soil content. The estimated daily intake in the U.S. is 45 to 500 mcg. The relationship of molybdenum to dental caries needs further research before a possible role for this element can be determined.

Selenium

Selenium has been shown to protect rats against necrotic liver degeneration and to prevent degenerative changes of other types in the liver and muscle of lambs, pigs, chicks, turkeys, calves, mice, and mink. Recently an essential role for selenium distinct from its synergistic function with vitamin E (see Vitamin E, Chapter 6) was identified in chicks.[59] Selenium appears to be involved in the metabolism of sulfhydryl groups, and a relationship with glutathione has been postulated.[60]

Grains and onions grown on seleniferous soils may have a selenium level as high as 20 ppm., whereas meat, milk, and vegetables have levels of less than 0.5 ppm. Selenium deficiency in animals is prevented with a concentration of 1 mcg. of selenium per gram of diet, and this level is present in the average American diet. The effect of high dietary intakes of selenium on increased susceptibility to dental caries requires further study.

Cobalt

Cobalt is a component of vitamin B_{12}, a nutritional factor necessary for the formation of red blood cells. An overdose of cobalt given to animals experimentally has been shown to produce polycythemia, i.e., red cells in excess of normal. In human nutrition the cobalt problem is not primarily one of adequate intake but of absorption of vitamin B_{12}. (See Chapter 7.)

RECENTLY IDENTIFIED ESSENTIAL TRACE ELEMENTS

Nickel,[61] tin,[62] vanadium,[63] and silicon[64] have recently been identified as essential trace elements in laboratory animals raised in all-plastic isolated environments protected from metallic contamination. The implications of these findings in terms of human nutrition are not well understood at the present time. The prediction is that they will also turn out to be required by humans but that only under the most unusual conditions would human deficiencies be possible: for example, in the controlled environment of an extraterrestrial vehicle nickel deficiency might occur.

TOXICITY OF OTHER TRACE ELEMENTS

It is intriguing, says King, that eight of these trace elements "fit the pattern of discovery as an essential nutrient after several decades of biologic study that had been undertaken originally because in high concentrations [the element] had been dangerous" to some form of animal life. These findings of recent years "show how urgent the need is for the public as well as scientists to understand the concept that all nutrients are safe or useful to the body within a limited quantitative range."[65]

Boron has been shown to have an essential role in plants but there is no known biologically essential role for aluminum, arsenic, barium, bismuth, bromine, cadmium, germanium, gold, lead, lithium, mercury, rubidium, silver, strontium, titanium, or zirconium. However, traces of all of these may be found in animal and plant tissue. There is currently public concern regarding increased environmental exposure to several of the more toxic trace elements, such as lead, cadmium, mercury,[66] and arsenic. It is also important to emphasize that the safe level of an individual trace element can be affected by the amount of other trace minerals present in the environment. For example, zinc, copper, selenium, and calcium all appear to increase tolerance levels for cadmium.

Lead enters the body from air, food, and water, but home environment may contribute additional contamination. Lead paint on walls, woodwork, and toys, lead glazes on ceramics, and pewter containers may all contribute to the total lead intake and to the possibility of lead poisoning. Children between the ages of one and six years have been the main victims of lead poisoning, chiefly from the ingestion of flaking paint (pica) from old dilapidated houses.[67] Of the children who survive lead poisoning, many are left permanently retarded or with neurological handicaps.

Studies by Schroeder on trace metals implicate cadmium in the development of hypertension in the rat. This mineral is present in the kidneys in very small amounts at birth, gradually increasing with age. High levels were found in patients with high blood pressure.[68] Proof of the relationship between cadmium and human hypertension must await further studies on both animals and humans. An extreme manifestation of chronic cadmium poisoning was seen in Japan caused by excessive ingestion of cadmium from foods contaminated by industrial pollution. Itai-Itai disease, as this form of cadmium poisoning was called, resulted when a sensitive population, low in both calcium and vitamin D, consumed rice and drinking water from a river that had been polluted. The disease was characterized by multiple painful fractures as a result of severe osteomalacia.

Of the many forms of mercury, methylmercury found chiefly in fish is the most toxic. Mercury from industrial sources dumped into water can be changed into methylmercury and consumed by the fish. If fish with high mercury levels are in turn consumed by humans, mercury poisoning such as occurred in Minamata, Japan, can result. In this tragic incident of mercury poisoning from industrial pollution most of the survivors were left with permanent neurological damage.

Arsenic is another trace mineral which can be toxic in relatively small amounts. It is found in seafood and in the human body. It accumulates in hair and nails. The levels in food can be increased as a result of industrial contamination and from the use of arsenicals as insecticides and as additives to animal feeds.

Other trace minerals appear to be harmless in the amounts and forms found in foods.

Table 5-6. Summary of Mineral Elements in Nutrition
(The information summarized here is given in more detail in the text.)

ELEMENT	RICH SOURCES	DIETARY ALLOWANCE FOR ADULTS	FUNCTION IN THE BODY	ELIMINATION
Calcium	Milk, cheese, some green vegetables	0.8 g. daily, 1.2 g. in pregnancy and lactation	Bone and tooth formation; co-agulation of blood. Regulates muscle contractibility including heartbeat; activates enzymes.	Urine and feces; some in sweat
Phosphorus	Milk, poultry, fish meats, cheese, nuts, cereals, legumes	0.8 g. daily, 1.2 in pregnancy and lactation	Forms high-energy phosphate compounds for muscular and tissue cell activity, constituent of DNA, RNA, phospholipids, and buffer system.	Urine and feces
Magnesium	Nuts, cereals, legumes, green vegetables, milk, meat	Women, 300 mg; men, 350 mg	Constituent of bone; enzyme activator for, energy producing systems, regulates muscles and nerves.	Feces and urine
Sodium	Common salt, animal products	Estimated—about 0.5 g	In extracellular fluid, regulates electrolyte and water balance, muscle irritability.	Urine chiefly, and sweat
Potassium	Meats, cereals, vegetables, legumes, fruits	Estimated—0.8-1.3 g	In intracellular fluid, regulates electrolyte and water balance and cell metabolism.	Urine chiefly, and sweat
Chloride	Common salt, animal products	Estimated—about 0.5 g	Forms acid in gastric juice; helps to regulate electrolyte and water balance.	Urine chiefly, and sweat
Sulfur	Protein foods	Adequate if protein is adequate	Constituent of all body tissues—hair and nails especially—and of specific organic compounds.	Urine and feces
Iron	Liver, meat, legumes, whole or enriched grains, potatoes, egg yolk, green vegetables, dried fruits	Women, 18 mg; men, 10 mg	Constituent of hemoglobin, myoglobin, and tissue cells.	Feces, small amounts in urine and sweat; menstruation blood loss
Iodine	Seafoods, water and plant life in nongoitrous regions; sodium iodide in iodized salt	Women, 100 mcg; men, 130 mcg	Necessary for formation of thyroxine, a hormone of the thyroid gland.	Urine
Zinc	Seafoods, meat, liver, eggs, milk	15 mg daily	Constituent of insulin, carbonic anhydrase and other metalloenzymes; wound healing; taste acuity.	Urine and feces
Copper	Liver, nuts, legumes	Estimated—about 2.0 mg	Aids in utilization of iron in hemoglobin synthesis; constituent of many enzymes; electron transfer; connective tissue metabolism.	Feces chiefly—bile
Manganese	Nuts, whole grains, legumes, tea, cloves	2-3 mg/day	Synthesis of mucopolysaccharides, glucose utilization, constituent of several metalloenzymes.	Chiefly in feces—bile
Fluorine	Fluoridated water	unknown 1 ppm in water	Resistance to dental caries.	Urine, feces, and sweat
Chromium	Brewer's yeast, some animal products, whole grains	unknown	Glucose metabolism; cofactor for insulin.	Feces and urine
Other Micronutrients	Leafy foods, cereals, fruits, legumes, meats, seafoods	Minute traces	Enzyme, hormone or vitamin constituents; act as catalysts.	Urine and feces

STUDY QUESTIONS AND ACTIVITIES

1. How is water balance in the body maintained? If water in the body is not sufficient for metabolic needs, what makes a person aware of this particular need?

2. Explain the function of calcium in bones and teeth. What happens in growth if calcium and phosphorus are inadequate in the diet? Why are these two minerals usually discussed together?

3. Milk is the single best source of calcium in the diet. See if you can write a diet which meets the calcium allowance for the adult, allowing cheese but omitting milk. Repeat, omitting both cheese and milk. Calculate the amounts of phosphorus in both these diets and compare with the recommended dietary allowance for the adult (Chapter 10).

4. Explain the interrelationships of magnesium with other minerals in the body.

5. Explain the current concepts of iron balance control in the body. Give the reasons underlying the supposition that adult men need very little dietary intake of iron. Why do women need larger amounts? What situation results when the iron intake is low? Name four important food sources of iron other than liver.

6. How does iodine function in the body? Where in the United States and in the world is iodine lacking in surface soil and water? What is being done to overcome such shortages?

7. Compare the calcium, phosphorus, magnesium, and iron supplied by the 1400-calorie Pattern Dietary (Table 5-2) with recommended allowances for these minerals.

8. Which minerals are most important in maintaining the electrolyte balance in the body? How is this accomplished?

9. Which micronutrients are known to be essential for animal life? Discuss current interest and concern regarding trace minerals in the diet. Discuss the function of four of these nutrients.

10. For what tissues is fluoride important? How is this nutrient supplied to the body?

11. How may zinc status be assessed in children? Why are copper, cadmium, and zinc regarded as antagonistic to one another? What nutrients are involved in the synthesis of hemoglobin?

12. Are the blood and tissues basic or acidic in their reactions? How would you answer someone who said that she could not eat tomatoes "because they made her blood acid"? How does the body maintain its acid-base balance?

SUPPLEMENTARY READINGS

Bing, F. C.: Assaying the availability of iron. Techniques, interpretations and usefulness of the data. J. Am. Dietet. A. 60:114 1972

Carlisle, E. M.: Silicon. Nutr. Rev. 33:257, 1975.

Evans, G. W.: Function and nomenclature for two mammalian copper proteins. Nutr. Rev. 29:195, 1971.

FAO/WHO Expert Group: Calcium Requirements. WHO Tech. Report Series No. 230, Geneva, 1962.

_____: Evaluation of Mercury, Lead, Cadmium and the Food Additives Amaranth, Diethylpyrocarbonate and Actyl Gallate. WHO Food Additives Series No. 5, Geneva, 1972.

_____: Requirements of Ascorbic Acid. Vitamin D, Vitamin B_{12}, Folate and Iron. WHO Tech. Report Series No. 452, Geneva, 1970.

_____: Trace Elements in Human Nutrition. WHO Tech. Report Series No. 532, Geneva, 1973.

Finch, C. A.: Iron metabolism. Nutrition Today 4:2, (Summer) 1969.

Frieden, E.: Ceruloplasmin, a link between copper and iron metabolism. Nutr. Rev. 28:87, 1970.

Frieden, E.: The ferrous to ferric cycles in iron metabolism. Nutr. Rev. 31:41, 1973.

Irving, J. T.: *Calcium and Phosphorus Metabolism*. New York, Academic Press, 1973.

Kidd, P. S., et al: Sources of dietary iodine. J. Am. Dietet. A. 65:420, 1974.

Levander, O. A.: Selenium and chromium in human metabolism, J. Am. Dietet. A. 66:338, 1975.

Lin-Fu, J. S.: Lead poisoning in children. USDA, PHS publ. No. 2108, Washington, D.C. 1970.

Lowenstein, F. W.: Iodized salt in the prevention of endemic goiter: a world-wide survey of present programs. Am. J. Public Health 57:1815, 1967.

Lutwak, L.: Dietary calcium and the reversal of bone demineralization. Nutrition News 37:1, (Feburary) 1974.

Magnesium in Human Nutrition. National Dairy Council Digest 42:2, (March-April) 1971.

Mertz, W.: Effects and metabolism of glucose tolerance factor. Nutr. Rev. 33:129, 1975.

_____Recommended dietary allowances up to date—trace minerals. J. Am. Dietet. A. 64:163, 1974.

Norman, C.: Iron Enrichment. Nutrition Today 8:16, (November, December) 1973.

Pennington, J. T., and Calloway, D. H.: Copper content of foods. J. Am. Dietet. A. 63:143, 1973.

Review: Calcium utilization and requirement. Dairy Council Digest 44:5, (September, October) 1973.

Review: The role of essential trace elements in nutrition. Dairy Council Digest 44:4, (July, August) 1973.

Review: Absorption of dietary iron in man. Nutr. Rev. 29:113, 1971.

Review: Anemia and iron intake. Nutr. Rev. 29:246, 1971.

Review: Control of iron absorption by the gastrointestinal mucosal cell. Nutr. Rev. 30:168, 1972.

Review: The correlation of serum ferritin and body iron stores. Nutr. Rev. 33:11, 1975.

Review: Potassium and endocrine pancreatic function. Nutr. Rev. 32:9, 1974.

Review: Problems in iron enrichment and fortification of foods. Nutr. Rev. 33:46, 1975.

Review: The role of transferrin in iron absorption. Nutr. Rev. 31:131, 1973.

Review: Studies on selenium. Nutr. Rev. 33:138, 1975.

Review: Zinc homeostasis during pregnancy. Nutr. Rev. 29:253, 1971.

Robinson, J.: Water, the indispensable nutrient. Nutrition Today 5:16, (Spring) 1970.

Underwood, E. J.: *Trace elements in human and animal nutrition.* New York, Academic Press, 1971.

———: Cobalt. Nutr. Rev. 33:65, 1975.

Zinc in human medicine. Lancet 11:35, 1975.

For further references see Bibliography in Section 4.

REFERENCES

1. McCance, R. A.: Nutr. Abst. Rev. 42:1269, 1972.
2. Snively, W. D., Jr.: *Sea Within.* Philadelphia, Lippincott, 1960, p. 55.
3. Review: Nutr. Rev., 19:23, 1961.
4. Posner, A. S.: Responses of the Ultra-structure of Bone Mineral to Physiological Change in *Osteoporosis,* D. S. Barzel, ed. New York, Grune and Stratton, 1970, pp. 101-113.
5. FAO/WHO Expert Committee on Calcium Requirements: WHO Chronicle, 16:251, 1962.
6. Hegsted, D. M., JAMA 185:588, 1963.
7. FAO/WHO Expert Committee: Calcium Requirements. WHO Tech. Report Ser. No. 1230, Geneva, 1962.
8. Johnson, N. E., et al: J. Nutrition 100:1425, 1970.
9. Food and Nutrition Board: Recommended Dietary Allowances, 1974, National Academy of Sciences-National Research Council, Washington, D.C., 1974, p. 86.
10. Newton-John, H. F., and Morgan, D. B.: Lancet 1:232, 1968.
11. Garn, S. M., et al: Fed. Proc. 26:1729, 1967.
12. Guthrie, H. S.:*Introductory Nutrition.* St. Louis, Mosby, 1971, p. 123.
13. Hamuro, Y., et al: J. Nutrition 100:404, 1970.
14. Seelig, M. S.: Am. J. Clin. Nutr. 14:342, 1964.
15. Wacker, W. E. C. and Parisi, A. F.: N. Eng. J. Med. 278:658, 712, 772, 1968.
16. White, J. M., et al: J. Am. Dietet. A. 50:32, 1967.
17. Cooper, G. R., and Heap, B.: J. Am. Dietet. A. 50:37, 1967.
18. Mertz, W.: Fed. Proc. 29:1482, 1970.
19. Multani, J. S.: Biochem. 9:3970, 1970.
20. Levine, P. H., et al: J. Lab. Clin. Med. 80:333, 1972.
21. Mertz, W.: J. Am. Dietet. A. 64:163, 1974.
22. Moore, C. V. and Duback, R.: JAMA 162:197, 1956.
23. Fritz, J.: Measures to Increase Iron in Food and Diets. Proceedings of a workshop, Food and Nutrition Board, National Research Council-National Academy of Sciences, Washington, D.C., 1970.
24. Joint FAO/WHO Expert Committee: Requirements of Ascorbic Acid, Vitamin D, Vitamin B$_{12}$, Folate and Iron. WHO Tech. Rep. Ser. No. 1452, Geneva, 1970.
25. U.S. DHEW: Ten-State Nutrition Survey, 1968-70. Pub. No. 72-8132, Washington, D.C., 1972.
26. McClure, R. D.: JAMA 109:783, 1937.
27. Matovinovic, J., et al: JAMA 192:234, 1965.
28. Prasad, A. S., et al: Am. J. Clin. Nutr. 12:437, 1963.
29. Reinhold, J. B., et al: Am. J. Clin. Nutr. 18:294, 1966.
30. Pories, W. J., et al: Lancet 1:121, 1967.
31. Henkin, R. H., et al: JAMA 217:434, 1971.
32. Hambidge, K. M., et al: Pediat. Res. 6:868, 1972.
33. Sullivan, J. F., and Lankford, H. G.: Am. J. Clin. Nutr. 17:57, 1965.
34. Frieden, E.: Nutr. Rev. 31:41, 1973.
35. Evans, G. W.: Nutr. Rev. 29:195, 1971.
36. Bird, D. N., et al: Proc. Soc. Exp. Biol. Med. 123:250, 1966.
37. Underwood, E. J.: *Trace Element in Human and Animal Nutrition,* ed. 3. New York, Academic Press, 1971.
38. Cordano, A., et al: Pediatrics 34:324, 1968.
39. Al-Rashid, R. A., and Spangler, J.: N. Eng. J. Med. 285:841, 1971.
40. Danks, D. M., et al: Lancet 1:1100, 1972.
41. Joint FAO/WHO Expert Group: Trace Elements in Human Nutrition. WHO Tech. Report Ser. No. 1532, Geneva, 1973.
42. Underwood, op. cit.
43. Leach, R. M. and Muenster, A. M.: J. Nutrition 78:51, 1962.
44. Scrutton, M. C., et al: J. Biol. Chem. 241:3480, 1966.
45. Everson, G. J., and Shrader, R. E.: J. Nutrition 94:89, 1968.
46. Joint FAO/WHO Expert Group: Trace Elements in Human Nutrition. WHO Tech. Report Ser. No. 532, Geneva, 1973.
47. McLeod, B. E., and Robinson, M. F.: Brit. J. Nutr. 27:221, 229, 1972.
48. Joint FAO/WHO Expert Group, op. cit.
49. McClure, F. J.: JAMA 139:711, 1949.
50. Ast, A. B., et al: J. Am. Dent. A. 52:291, 296, 307, 1956.
51. American Academy of Pediatrics Committee on Nutrition: Pediatrics, 49:456, 1972.
52. Schwartz, K., and Milne, D. B.: Bioinorganic Chem. 1:331, 1972.
53. Bernstein, D. S., et al: J. Clin. Invest. 42:916, 1963.
54. Bernstein, D. S., et al: JAMA 198:439, 1966.
55. Underwood, op. cit.
56. Levine, R. A., et al: Metab., Clin. Exp. 17:114, 1968.
57. Underwood, op. cit.
58. Joint FAO/WHO Expert Group, op. cit.
59. Thompson, J. N., and Scott, M. L.: J. Nutrition 97:335, 1969; 100:797, 1970.
60. Rotruck, J. T., et al: Fed. Proc. 31:691, 1972.

61. Nielsen, F. H.: Studies on the Essentiality of Nickel, in *The New Trace Elements in Nutrition,* W. Mertz and Cornatzer, W. E., eds. New York, Dekker, 1971.
62. Schwartz, op. cit.
63. Hopkins and Mohr, op. cit.
64. Carlisle, E. M.: Fed. Proc. 31:700A, 1972.
65. King, C. G.: J. Am. Dietet. A. 38:223, 1961.
66. Joint FAO/WHO Expert Committee: Evaluation of Mercury, Lead, Cadmium, and the Food Additives Amaranth, Diethylpyrocarbonate and Octyl Gallate. WHO Food Additives Series No. 4, Geneva, 1972.
67. Lin-Fu, J. S.: Lead Poisoning in Children, U.S. DHEW, PHS Publ. No. 2108, Washington, D.C. 1970.
68. Schroeder, H. A.: J. Chron. Dis. 18:647, 1965.

6

fat-soluble vitamins

general discussion of all vitamins

The term *vitamine*, meaning a vital amine, was proposed by Funk in 1911 to designate a new food constituent necessary for life which he thought he had identified chemically. Other terminology was proposed as new factors were discovered, but the word *vitamin*, with the final "e" dropped to avoid any chemical significance, met with popular favor.

At first the individual vitamins were named by letter or according to their curative or preventive properties, but present opinion favors names descriptive of the substance itself. As its chemical structure is discovered, the vitamin is named appropriately, if it is not already a recognized compound. However, the lettered nomenclature may still be used to some extent, especially in popular discussions. From time to time new vitamins are postulated and are added to the accepted list after extensive research.

When a supposedly single vitamin proved to be more than one chemically and physiologically unrelated compound, the term *complex* was incorporated for additional identification, as in the B complex.

74

Sometimes it is convenient to group the vitamins according to solubility. Vitamins A, D, E, and K are fat-soluble. Two water-soluble groups are recognized—those having vitamin C activity and the large group known as the vitamin B complex.

Definitions

Vitamins are potent organic compounds that occur in small concentrations in foods; they perform specific and vital functions in the cells and the tissues of the body. They cannot be synthesized by the organism and their absence or improper absorption results in specific deficiency diseases. They differ from each other in physiologic function, in chemical structure, and in distribution in food.

As more knowledge of the vitamins has been gained, their classification according to function has been modified. Certain fat-soluble vitamins (i.e., vitamins A and D) are now classified by many authorities as hormones. Wolf and DeLuca[1] state, "By 'hormone' we mean a substance secreted into the bloodstream which influences tissues and organs to differentiate and elaborate new cell types and new enzymes. There is no *a priori* reason why a hormone should have to be made by the animal itself. It is quite conceivable that a hormone can be taken in the diet, stored in the liver, and secreted into the bloodstream when needed. The liver then acts as the endocrine organ."

Other vitamins (i.e., B complex) may be classified according to their function as biological catalysts or coenzymes in the many varied enzyme systems of the body.

A brief review of enzyme terminology is appropriate before specific functions of the various vitamins are discussed. Enzymes consist of at least two parts: the prosthetic group, or cofactor portion, and the protein portion. The specific amino acids which compose the protein part of the enzyme are determined by the genetic code (Chapter 9) and this portion is often referred to as the *apoenzyme*. Either mineral ions (such as Ca++, Mg++, Zn++) or vitamins or, in many instances, both, make up the cofactor portion of the complete enzyme (holoenzyme). The vitamin portion of the enzyme is usually called the *coenzyme* and the mineral, the *activator*,[2] hence the term coenzyme as applied to certain vitamins.

There are also terms that apply to vitamins in general. A *provitamin*, or *precursor*, is a compound structurally related to a vitamin which the body can convert to a vitamin active compound. The word *avitaminosis* literally means without vitamins, although it is generally used with a letter following (e.g., avitaminosis A) to indicate the specific deficiency of that factor. The word *deficiency* may be used to indicate varying degrees of shortage: mild, moderate, severe, or complete. The possibility of an excess intake of certain vitamins has been postulated, and in some instances a large excess has proved to be harmful; such a condition is termed *hypervitaminosis*. Early symptoms of vitamin deficiencies so vague that they are rarely noted except by a medical nutritionist are called *marginal*.

History

A few physicians early recognized the connection between food habits and the incidence of certain diseases. Beri-beri was described in the 7th century and scurvy in the 13th, but it was not until centuries later that certain foods were recommended as protective. The first vitamins were discovered as "accessory factors" in foods proven to be curative of specific deficiency diseases. In other words, vitamins were first recognized by their absence rather than by their presence.

In the early years of the 20th century, workers in Germany, the Netherlands, Great Britain, and the United States were beginning to use animals for nutrition experiments. A number of investigators showed that purified rations containing only protein, fat, carbohydrate, and minerals would not support growth. They observed that natural foods provided some substances other than the basal constituents which were essential for normal growth and well-being. These workers initiated the search for "accessory food factors," later called vitamins. Since then our knowledge of vitamins has grown rapidly.

There are still, however, wide gaps in our understanding of the total vitamin story. For instance, although we can recognize a specific vitamin deficiency and cure it with appropriate amounts of the vitamin, the actual roles of certain vitamins in metabolic processes remain to be defined.

Vitamin Units and Assay Methods

Feeding tests on animals at first offered the only device for testing foods for their vitamin content. This type of procedure, called the bio-assay method, is still the basis of comparison for the standardization of newer chemical or microbiologic methods of assay. After the chemists succeed in concentrating, identifying, and synthesizing a vitamin, its amount is expressed in metric weights of the pure crystalline substance.

The only vitamin values still given in International Units (IU) as originally defined by a League of Nations committee are vitamins A, D, and E. All others are given in milligrams (mg.) or micrograms (mcg.), whichever is appropriate. The FAO/WHO Expert Committee on Vitamin Requirements has suggested that vitamin A and D values also be given in micrograms (mcg.). The 1974 revision of the Recommended Dietary Allowances gives the Vitamin A recommendations in both IU and RE (retinol equivalent).

Vitamin Content of Foods

Determination of the specific vitamin activity of natural foods becomes an increasingly difficult task as the number and the complexity of vitamins increase. Table 1, Section 4, gives figures for many of the vitamins in foods. Vitamin losses in the cooking and storage of food will be mentioned more specifically under each vitamin, but, in general, certain principles of vitamin conservation are worth noting. Fat-soluble vitamins (A, D, E, K) are not easily lost by ordinary cooking methods and they do not dissolve out in the cooking water. Water-soluble vitamins (B complex and C) are dissolved easily in cooking water and a portion of the vitamins actually may be destroyed by heating; therefore, cooking food only until tender in as little water as possible is, in general, the best procedure. Vitamin losses due to storage of vegetables tend to parallel the degree of wilting; such losses are progressive in the long storage of fresh fruits and vegetables.

the fat-soluble group

The four vitamins A, D, E, and K are all soluble in fat and fat solvents and are therefore known as the fat-soluble group. Absorption from the intestinal tract follows the same path as the fats; thus, any condition that interferes with fat absorption may result in poor absorption of these vitamins. They can all be stored in the body to some extent, mostly in the liver, and as a consequence manifestation of deficiencies is likely to be slower than it is for most of the water-soluble group. In several instances, vitamin activity is not confined to a single substance and several related substances produce a similar effect on the body.

VITAMIN A
History

Vitamin A was the first fat-soluble vitamin to be recognized. This happened in 1913 when two groups of workers—McCollum and Davis, at the University of Wisconsin, and Osborne and Mendel, at Yale—demonstrated independently that rats fail to grow normally on diets deficient in natural fats. At about the time growth ceased, the eyes became inflamed and apparently infected. This characteristic eye disease, known as xerophthalmia, was relieved in a few days by the addition to the diet of a little butter fat or cod-liver oil which contained the protective or curative factor known as vitamin A.

Nomenclature

Today we recognize a group of structurally related compounds that have vitamin A activity. Those found in animal products are colorless or only slightly pigmented; the most common of these *preformed vitamins* are vitamin A_1 alcohol, or *retinol*, and vitamin A_2, 3-dehydroretinol. Other forms which have specific physiologic reactions include vitamin A al-

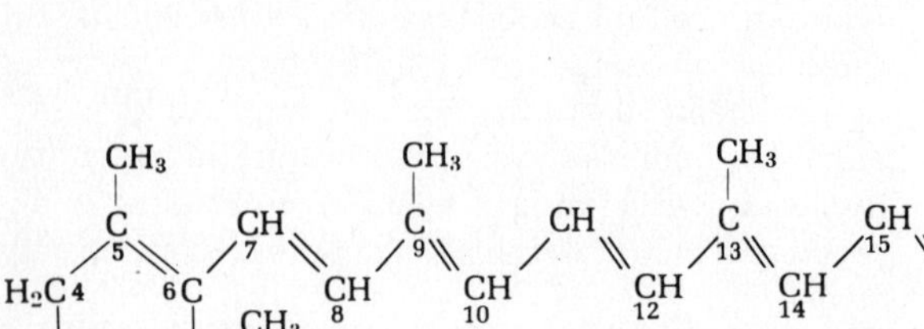

Vitamin A, retinol $C_{20}H_{30}O$

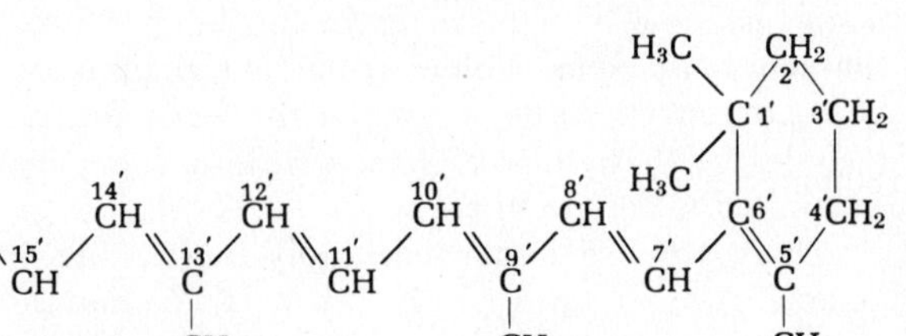

Vitamin A_2, 3-dehydroretinol $C_2H_{28}O$

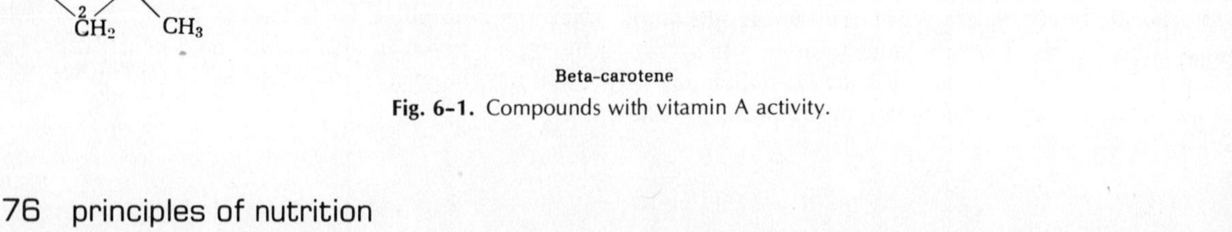

Beta-carotene

Fig. 6-1. Compounds with vitamin A activity.

dehyde, or *retinal*, and vitamin A acid, or *retinoic acid*.

A number of forms of *provitamin A* are found in the yellow carotenoid plant pigments. *Beta-carotene* has the highest biological activity of the carotenes, yielding two molecules of vitamin A per molecule of beta-carotene (Fig. 6–1).

Some animal products such as cream and butter may contain both preformed vitamin A and carotene, because some of the provitamin may remain unchanged.

Although vitamin A values in most food composition tables are given as International Units, the Report of the Joint FAO/WHO Expert Group on Requirements of Vitamin A, Thiamine, Riboflavine and Niacin, 1967, urges that this practice be changed and that units of weight be used.[3] This will necessitate that tables of food composition report separately the amounts of retinol, beta-carotene, and other mixed carotenoids in individual foods. The 1974 revision of the Recommended Dietary Allowances introduces the term "retinol equivalents."

International Units can be converted to micrograms as follows:[4]

1 ɪᴜ (or U.S.P. unit) of vitamin A
= 0.3 mcg. retinol
= 0.344 mcg. retinyl acetate
= 0.6 mcg. beta-carotene
= 1.2 mcg. other mixed carotene with vitamin A activity.

Vitamin A values can be converted to retinol equivalents as follows:[5]

1 retinol equivalent of vitamin A
= 1 mcg. retinol
= 6 mcg. beta-carotene (β-carotene)
= 12 mcg. other provitamin A carotenoids
= 3.33 ɪᴜ retinol
= 10 ɪᴜ beta-carotene

To calculate the retinol equivalents in a diet or foodstuff, one of the following equations should be used:[6]

a. If retinol and β-carotene are given in mcg., then:

$$\text{mcg. retinol} + \frac{\text{mcg. }\beta\text{-carotene}}{6} = \text{retinol equivalents}$$

EXAMPLE: A diet contains 500 mcg. retinol and 1800 mcg. β-carotene.

$$500 + \frac{1800}{6} = 800 \text{ retinol equivalents}$$

b. If both are given in ɪᴜ, then:

$$\frac{\text{ɪᴜ of retinol}}{3.33} + \frac{\text{ɪᴜ of }\beta\text{-carotene}}{10} = \text{retinol equivalents}$$

EXAMPLE: A diet contains 1666 ɪᴜ of retinol and 3000 ɪᴜ of β-carotene.

$$\frac{1666}{3.33} + \frac{3000}{10} = 800 \text{ retinol equivalents}$$

c. If β-carotene and other provitamin A carotenoids are given in mcg. then:

$$\frac{\text{mcg. }\beta\text{-carotene}}{6} + \frac{\text{mcg. other carotenoids}}{12}$$
$$= \text{retinol equivalents}$$

EXAMPLE: A 100-g sample of sweet potatoes contains 2400 ɪᴜ β-carotene and 480 ɪᴜ of other provitamin A carotenoids.

$$\frac{2400}{6} + \frac{480}{12} = 440 \text{ retinol equivalents}$$

This approach to evaluating the vitamin A content of foods is recommended because, as will be discussed later, the vitamin A requirement depends on the proportion of vitamin A (retinol) to provitamin A (carotene) in the diet.

Absorption, Transport, and Storage of Vitamin A and Carotene

VITAMIN A. Dietary vitamin A (i.e., retinyl esters) is hydrolyzed in the gastrointestinal tract to retinol and as such is absorbed across the mucosal cell membrane into the cell where it recombines with a fatty acid, usually palmitic. Vitamin A (retinyl) palmitate then travels in the chylomicrons by way of the lymphatic system and bloodstream to the liver, where it is stored.

Liver stores of vitamin A (retinyl esters) are hydrolyzed by enzymes to free retinol which is transported by a retinol-binding protein (RBP) complex to the tissues of the body wherever a metabolic requirement exits. The liver stores can maintain the blood at relatively constant vitamin A levels even when the diet is deficient. Hence, vitamin A deficiencies may not develop for long periods of time, depending on the reserve stores in the liver and the ability of the body to mobilize these reserves of vitamin A.

It is estimated that the liver may contain as much as 95 percent of the vitamin A of the entire body, with small amounts in adipose tissue, lungs, and kidneys. Infants and young animals probably have low reserves of vitamin A at birth but, if they are well fed, they store it rapidly. The liver gradually acquires, over a period of years, an increasing reserve of vitamin A which normally reaches its peak in adult life. The advantage of this reserve is chiefly to take care of temporary shortages or increased requirements. Obviously, an intake above minimum requirement must be maintained most of the time if such a reserve is to be built up. Reserve stores of vitamin A are evident even in young animals.

CAROTENE In the presence of fat and bile acids carotene is absorbed into the intestinal wall, where some is converted to vitamin A. The carotene that is not converted is absorbed into the lymph and carried to the bloodstream. Some carotene may be converted to vitamin A in the liver and some is stored in adipose tissue. According to the report of the FAO/WHO committee on vitamin requirements and the Food and Nutrition Board, approximately one third of the carotene in food is available to the body. Moreover, the amount of available carotene which is then converted to vitamin A varies considerably, but, in general, only about half is used this way. Thus, in the human the utilization efficiency of carotene is $1/6$; in other terms, 1 mcg. of beta-carotene would have the same biological activity as 0.167 mcg. of vitamin A alcohol, retinol. Other carotenoids have about $1/2$ the biological activity of beta-carotene (1 mcg. other carotenoids=0.0833 mcg. retinol).

Inadequate protein intakes decrease the absorption, transport and metabolism of both vitamin A and (to an even greater extent) carotene.

Functions of Vitamin A

CONSTITUENTS OF VISUAL PIGMENTS. The best-defined function of vitamin A is its role in the visual process. Vitamin A aldehyde, retinal, combines with the protein opsin, to form rhodopsin, or visual purple, in the rods of the retina of the eye which are responsible for vision in dim light (scotopic vision). When light strikes the eye, the rhodopsin is bleached to yield the original protein opsin and retinal. The retinal is converted to retinol and, although most of it is reconverted to retinal to combine again with opsin, some is lost and must be replaced. Adaptation to dim light depends on the completion of the cycle. When bright light has caused excessive bleaching of the visual purple, the eyes' ability to regenerate it appears to be directly related to the amount of vitamin A available. The "dark adaptation" test which measures the eyes' ability to recover visual acuity in dim light has been used as a means of determining vitamin A status. Insufficient vitamin A for the synthesis of rhodopsin results in night blindness, or nyctalopia. (See Fig. 6-2.)

The cones of the retina which are responsible for vision in bright light (photopic vision) also contain a light-sensitive vitamin A–protein complex, iodopsin (a photo-sensitive violet pigment).

MAINTENANCE OF EPITHELIAL TISSUE. Vitamin

A has long been associated with the maintenance of normal epithelial tissue but it is only recently that some metabolic explanations have been found for this function of vitamin A. Animal studies indicate that during cell differentiation the basal cells of the epithelia have two alternative pathways open to them depending on the availability of vitamin A. If adequate amounts of the vitamin are present they form columnar, mucus-secreting goblet cells, whereas, if vitamin A is lacking they keratinize. The effect of vitamin A on other types of epithelial tissue can be explained further by proposing that different tissues have varying threshold levels for vitamin A.

Wolf and DeLuca[7] suggest four types of epithelial tissue with different threshold levels for each. The lowest threshold is indicated for the simple columnar epithelium lining the gastrointestinal tract. During differentiation in the presence of vitamin A these basal cells will form mucus-secreting goblet cells. Squamous cells are formed in vitamin A deficiency. Next in order of threshold levels would be the epithelial cells lining the trachea; these also normally consist of simple columnar cells but in the absence of vitamin A they will differentiate into stratified squamous tissue. The corneal epithelium is an example of stratified squamous tissue which has a still higher threshold for the vitamin, but which in a vitamin A deficient state produces keratin. Lastly, the highest threshold level of vitamin A is proposed for the cells of the epidermis; normally they produce some keratin but, lacking vitamin A, increased amounts are produced. Although the mechanism for the role of vitamin A in modifying cell differentiation has not been identified, evidence indicates that "vitamin A is capable of influencing protein synthesis directly or indirectly. An effect that results in observable fine structural differences in many of the affected cells."[8]

Hence, in vitamin A deficiency, it has been observed that the membranes lining the nose, throat, trachea, and other air passages, the gastrointestinal tract, and the genitourinary tract show changes in the epithelial cells. A decrease in taste and smell thresholds has also been noted. Rough, dry, and scaly skin especially on the arms and thighs due to increased keratinization may occur with vitamin A deficiency as well.

Whenever these tissue changes occur, the natural mechanism for protection against bacterial invasion is impaired and the tissue may easily become infected. Clinical observations show that normal mucous membranes lining nose, throat, sinuses, and ear passages are the best defense against infections and that adequate vitamin A is an important factor in maintaining the normal functions of these mem-

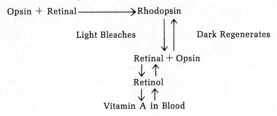

Fig. 6–2. Function of vitamin A in scotopic vision.

branes. Renal calculi may also be related to the keratinization of the urinary tract.

Damage to the epithelial layer of the eye is one of the most important clinical signs of vitamin A deficiency in humans, particularly children (see Chapter 20). There is a drying and thickening of the conjunctiva; the tear ducts fail to secrete; keratinization results, with the epithelial cells of the cornea becoming opaque and sloughing off. Infection and permanent blindness may follow if vitamin A is not administered.

MAINTENANCE OF BONE GROWTH. Bones also depend on vitamin A for normal growth and development, and this function of the vitamin is thought by several investigators to relate to cell changes that occur during differentiation. Hayes[9] suggests that when vitamin A is deficient, periosteal progenitor cells in bones and the fibroblasts in collagen have priority in synthesizing collagen fibers and ground substances at the expense of the remodeling osteoclasts and fibroclasts. Evidence of this defect is seen in the crippling which occurs in young rats fed a vitamin A deficient diet.

The nerve damage that frequently appears in vitamin A deficiency may be traced to the compression of growing tissue in a skeleton that ceases to grow rather than being a direct result of vitamin A deficiency.

GROWTH AND REPRODUCTION. Failure to grow is noted in vitamin A deficiency, as it is in many other nutrient deficiencies, before any other symptoms appear. The need for vitamin A for normal growth appears associated with protein utilization, weight gain and perhaps cell mitosis.[10]

Vitamin A is essential to normal reproduction in rats, pigs, and other animals. Studies have shown that for successful reproduction and lactation the diet must furnish more vitamin A than is needed for good growth. Female rats on a minimal supply of vitamin A intake may show no outward signs of vitamin A deficiency, yet they are not able to bear or rear vigorous young. With an outright deficiency there is an interference with the normal estrus cycle in the female and a testicular degeneration in the male rat. These symptoms appear related to cell changes which occur during differentiation. Sows deprived of adequate vitamin A may give birth to litters of pigs with defective eyes or without eyeballs. This finding was one of the first evidences that prenatal malnutrition might cause abnormalities in the fetus.

Dietary Requirement for Vitamin A

Human requirements for vitamin A are based on studies of two kinds: nutritional status studies on various population groups throughout the world and controlled depletion experiments carried out on man and other animals. Field studies have indicated that in countries where the vitamin A intake is 3000 to 9000 IU per person per day, vitamin A deficiency is rarely seen, whereas, in other countries, on intakes of 1000 to 2500 IU, vitamin A deficiency is known to occur in the population.

A recent study[11] has examined the amount of vitamin A necessary to relieve deficiency symptoms, such as impaired dark adaptation, loss of balance, decreased taste and smell thresholds, and skin lesions. Varying doses were required to relieve different symptoms; 150 mcg. of retinol per day reversed the changes in the eye; 300 mcg. per day of retinol resulted in normal balance as well as normal taste and smell thresholds; however, 600 mcg. per day of retinol were required to clear the skin lesions. Blood levels were also in the normal range when a 600 mcg. dose was given. Twice the amount of pure beta-carotene as compared to retinol was necessary to correct the symptoms.

The National Research Council's recommended allowance of 1000 RE (1000 mcg. retinol, 5000 IU vitamin A) for the male adult is in excess of the minimum to allow for some reserves of vitamin A to be stored in the body. The allowance for the adult female was set at 800 RE (800 mcg. retinol, 4000 IU vitamin A) or 80 percent of the male allowance because of the usually smaller body size of women. The allowances assume that the American diet provides half of the total vitamin A activity as retinol and half as provitamin A carotenoids. When calculated as International Units, this is 2500 IU as retinol and 2500 IU as provitamin A or a total of 5000 IU. In terms of retinol equivalents (RE), it is 750 mcg. retinol (1 RE = 3.33 IU retinol) and 250 retinol equivalents as beta-carotene (1 RE = 10 IU beta-carotene) for a total of 1000 RE.[12]

Allowances for infants are based on the amount of retinol in human milk, about 49 mcg./100 ml. An infant consuming 850 ml. of breast milk would receive approximately 420 mcg. (420 RE) of retinol; this amount was set as the recommendation for infants from birth to six months. It was reduced to 400 RE for infants six months to one year of age. Since no definite information is available regarding the actual requirements of children and adolescents, these recommendations were interpolated from the infant and the male adult allowances and are based on body weight and growth needs. The female allowance increases to 1000 RE during pregnancy and to 1200 RE during lactation.

The FAO/WHO committee on vitamin requirements adopted a recommended intake of 750 mcg. (2500 IU) of retinol per day for the normal adult. No

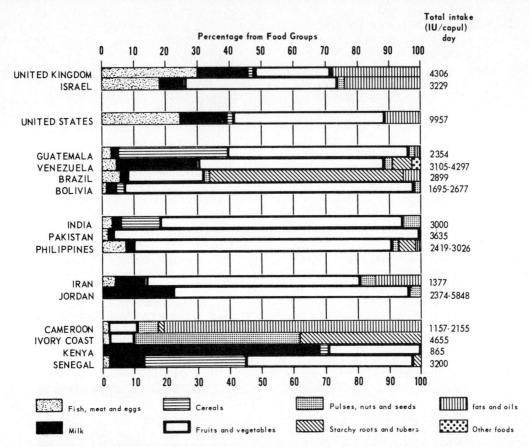

Fig. 6–3. Sources of vitamin A in the diets of population groups surveyed in some countries. (Report of a Joint FAO/WHO Expert Group: Requirements of Vitamin A, Thiamine, Riboflavin, and Niacin. FAO Nutrition Meetings Report Series No. 4. Rome)

additional recommendation for pregnancy was made, provided that the usual diet supplied the recommended adult intake. To cover the vitamin A secreted in milk, 1200 mcg. (4000 IU) of retinol was recommended during lactation. Recommendations for infants are based on the amount of vitamin A in breast milk. Suggested levels for children range from 300 mcg. (1000 IU) for the six-month-old to 750 mcg. (2500 IU) for the older adolescent.

Since carotene, which is less efficiently utilized ($\frac{1}{6}$) than retinol, is often the major source of vitamin A activity in the diet, the recommended intake of vitamin A is modified depending on the percent of vitamin A supplied by carotene.

Fig. 6–3 illustrates the percent of vitamin A supplied by various food groups in different countries throughout the world. Note the wide variation in sources of this vitamin. (For complete table of vitamin A allowances for all age and sex categories see Chapter 10.)

Hypervitaminosis A

An overdose of vitamin A may cause serious injury to health. It is most likely to happen when children are given too much of a high potency supplement. The symptoms of hypervitaminosis A are loss of appetite, abnormal skin pigmentation, loss of hair, dry skin (with itching), pain in long bones, and increased fragility of bones in general. Regular supplementation of more than 2000 RE (6700 IU) of retinol above that consumed in the diet should be carefully supervised by a physician.

In three cases of adolescent girls reported by Morrice and Havener,[13] massive doses of 90,000 and 200,000 IU of vitamin A caused symptoms of brain tumor (pseudotumor cerebri), along with most of the syndrome described above.

Carotene in large doses is not toxic but usually causes a yellow coloration of the skin which disappears when the carotene is discontinued.

Food Sources

The richest natural sources of vitamin A are the fish-liver oils, which are usually classed as food supplements rather than as foods. They vary according to the species and the season when caught, but commercial brands are well standardized for our convenience.

All animal livers are good sources of vitamin A, but they are not as rich as fish liver. All milk products that include milk fat, such as whole milk, butter, cream, or full cream cheese, are rich in vitamin A. The milk of cows on green pasture is usually higher in vitamin A than is the milk of stall-fed animals.

Carotene is abundant in carrots, from which it derives its name, but it is also present in even higher concentration in certain green, leafy vegetables and grasses in which the color of the chlorophyll masks the yellow of the carotene. In certain species such as corn there is more carotene—hence, more vitamin-A activity—in yellow varieties than in white. There are African countries where red palm oil is used extensively and contributes greatly to the carotene intake.

Animal foods that contain mostly preformed vitamin A seem to be more efficient sources of this factor for humans than are the precursors found in plants. However, the ample supply of carotenes in plant foods may well contribute a large share of the vitamin A requirement. Cooking, puréeing, or mashing of vegetables rupture the cell membranes and

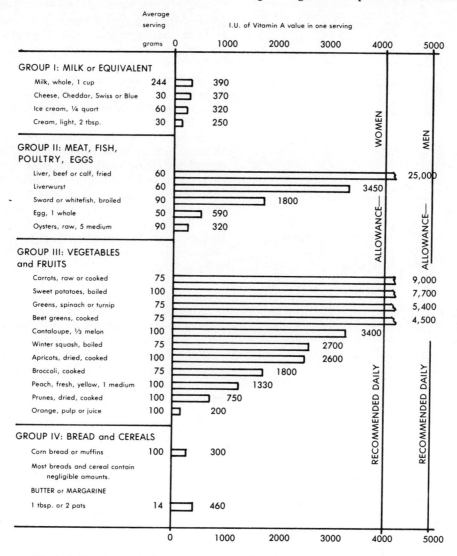

Fig. 6–4. Vitamin A value in average servings of foods classified in the four food groups.

thereby make the carotene more available. Fig. 6-4 shows the relative vitamin A values of some common foods in the four food groups.

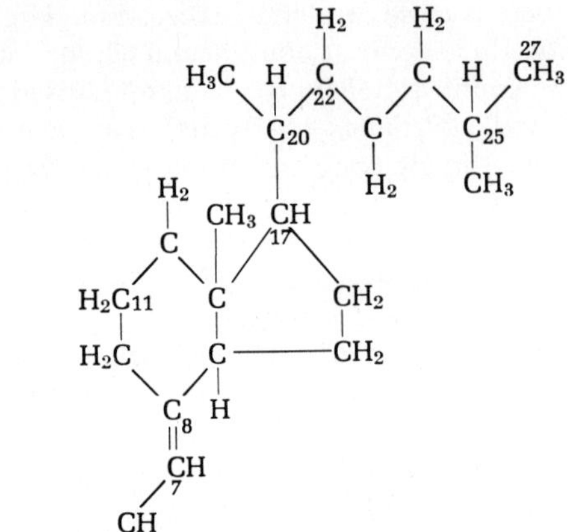

Vitamin D_3, cholecalciferol $C_{27}H_{44}O$

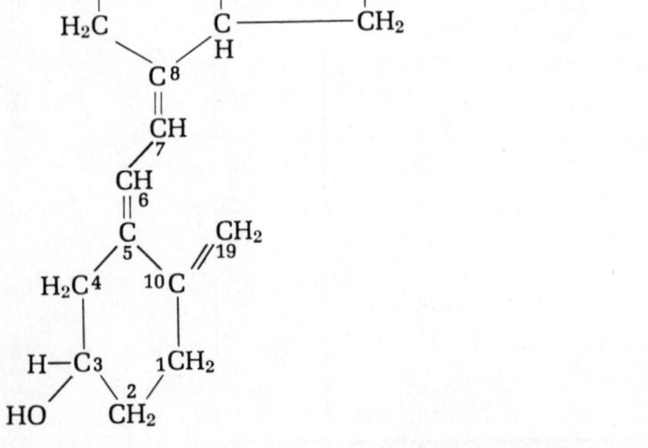

Vitamin D_2, ergocalciferol $C_{28}H_{44}O$

Fig. 6-5. Compounds with vitamin D activity.

VITAMIN D

History

Rickets has been known as a deficiency disease of infants for several centuries. Renaissance painters often depicted children with rachitic deformities, signs so common as to be considered normal. The history of rickets as a deficiency disease is much older than our knowledge of how to prevent it. In the early 19th century cod-liver oil was a well-known folk remedy in Holland; somewhat later it was accepted as a therapeutic agent for rickets by physicians in Holland, France and Germany. During the latter part of the 19th century cod-liver oil lost favor with the medical profession because physicians could not explain its action. It was not used extensively then for many years until the period of World War I, when active research on the prevention and the treatment of rickets was inaugurated.

Early workers recognized that normal bone growth apparently was controlled by some substance in natural fats. This unknown factor was credited with some control over the metabolism of calcium and phosphorus.

Research on the chemical nature of vitamin D was initiated in 1924, when Steenbock and Hess demonstrated independently that antirachitic activity could be induced in foods containing certain fat-soluble substances by exposure to ultraviolet light. This discovery of the activation of fat-like substances by ultraviolet rays permitted the manufacture of a concentrated vitamin D preparation such as viosterol long before the pure crystalline vitamin D, calciferol, was isolated in 1935.

Nomenclature

Although about ten compounds with vitamin-D activity have been identified the two most important are vitamin D_2, or *ergocalciferol*, and vitamin D_3, *cholecalciferol* (Fig. 6-5). As the names imply, these active vitamins are formed by the irradiation of two provitamins: ergosterol, found in lower forms of plants (such as yeast and fungi) and a form of cholesterol (7-dehydrocholesterol) found in the skin and other animal tissues. They appear to be equally effective in man.

Measurement of Vitamin D

The International Unit (IU) of vitamin D is the activity of 0.025 mcg. of pure crystalline vitamin D_3. One U.S.P. unit equals one IU, thus 2.5 mcg. equals 100 IU.

Criteria used for judging the severity of experimental rickets are roentgenograms (x-rays) showing the total mineral content of bone and the calcification of the metaphyses (the growing portion) of the long bones. The last observation was used in developing a standardized line test on rats which is employed for routine assays of vitamin D preparations. Rats are fed on a rickets-producing diet until a definite stage of early rickets occurs; the source of vitamin D (the product to be tested) is then fed and the animals are sacrificed on the eleventh day. Longitudinal sections of certain bones are stained in silver nitrate solution, which darkens only the calcified areas. Fig. 6–6 shows the progressive degrees in recalcification, or healing, that take place in rachitic bone when graded doses of vitamin D are administered. Other promising methods have been developed which shorten the time and the expense of vitamin D assays.

In spite of advances in the investigation of vitamin D—long recognized as necessary for the normal calcification of bones—many questions remain to be answered in regard to the mechanisms of action of this vitamin.

Absorption, Transport, Metabolism, Storage, and Excretion

Vitamin D is absorbed in the presence of bile from the jejunum and is transported like vitamin A in the lymph chylomicrons to the bloodstream. It is carried to the liver where it is hydroxylated to 25 hydroxycholecalciferol (25-HCC). This reaction is regulated by the level of 25-HCC present in the liver. In the liver it is transferred from the chylomicrons to a globulin protein which acts as a carrier for the vitamin. The kidney further hydroxylates 25-HCC to 1,25 dihydroxycholecalciferol, (1,25-DHCC) the most active metabolite (product of metabolism) of vitamin D and 24, 25 dihydroxycholecalciferol (24, 25-DHCC) whose function is unknown. Reserves of the vitamin are found in the liver, the skin, the brain, and the bones, in all of which it is stored for future use. Some vitamin D metabolites are excreted in the bile.

Functions

INCREASED ABSORPTION OF CALCIUM AND PHOSPHORUS FROM THE GASTROINTESTINAL TRACT. Current research on the action of vitamin D is rapidly unfolding the story of its relationship to calcium and phosphorus metabolism. Calcium is absorbed in the intestines by means of (1) an active cation pump which requires energy, a calcium binding protein (CaBP), and sodium, and which moves calcium from mucosal to serosal compartments in amounts resulting in a higher concentration in the serosal compartment; and (2) a passive transport system which moves calcium from the mucosal to the

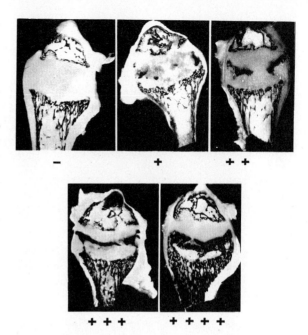

Fig. 6–6. Progressive degrees of recalcification or healing of rachitic bones due to graded doses of vitamin D. The increasing extent of the dark areas, where the white band appeared in the first photo, indicates mineral deposits. Photo marked + + + + represents one Steenbock or 2.7 U.S.P. units of vitamin D. (Wisconsin Alumni Research Foundation)

serosal compartments in the direction of the concentration difference and is also dependent on a calcium binding protein (CaBP).[14]

The vitamin D metabolite, 1,25-HDCC, formed in the kidney is transported in the blood and taken up by the intestines. It has been identified as the compound responsible for activating the synthesis of the calcium binding protein (CaBP) which binds and transports calcium across the intestinal mucosal cell in both active and passive transport systems. In the active pump transport, sodium ions are also necessary for the release of calcium from the mucosal cell into the serosal fluid. It has recently been postulated that the entrance of calcium into the mucosal cell across the brush border surface also requires vitamin D to activate the enzyme, ATPase.[15] Phosphate absorption, which is secondary to calcium absorption, is also enhanced by the presence of vitamin D.

There is evidence that the formation of 1,25-DHCC is under the influence of the parathyroid hormone, parathormone (PTH). A decrease in serum calcium levels stimulates PTH secretion (see Calcium, Chapter 5); this in turn stimulates production of the hydroxylating enzyme in the kidney which converts 25-HCC to 1,25-DHCC,[16] thus increasing the intestinal absorption of calcium into the blood. Thyrocalcitonin (thyroid hormone) inhibits the conversion of 25-HCC to 1,25-DHCC.[17]

BONE METABOLISM. Vitamin D (1,25-DHCC) is also involved in bone resorption which releases additional calcium and phosphorus into the blood to maintain normal serum levels of these minerals. Phosphate reabsorption by the kidney is also increased by vitamin D.

Although the mechanism is not clear, bone mineralization is probably directly influenced by vitamin D since, in the absence of the vitamin, bone mineralization is impaired and collagen synthesis is defective. Hence, rickets in children and osteomalacia in adults result from vitamin D deficiency.

Human Requirements

Since vitamin D may be supplied either by ingesting it in foods or supplements or by exposure to certain wavelengths of sunlight, its requirement has been difficult to determine.

In infants 100 IU (2.5 mcg.) of vitamin D per day will prevent rickets, and provide for adequate calcium absorption, normal bone mineralization, and a satisfactory growth rate. However, since increased growth and better calcium absorption resulted from feeding 300 to 400 IU (7.5 to 10.0 mcg.) daily, the National Research Council's Food and Nutrition Board and the Joint FAO/WHO Expert Committee[18] recommend 400 IU, or 10 mcg., of vitamin D per day for infants and young children, birth through six years of age. These recommendations apply to both formula-fed and breast-fed infants. The premature infant who is growing rapidly and is usually not exposed to sunlight for a considerable length of time is more prone to develop rickets than the full-term infant and hence, should be assured an adequate amount of vitamin D.

Because there is little information regarding vitamin D requirements in older children and adolescents and because rickets is practically nonexistent in this age group, the Joint FAO/WHO Expert Committee reduced their recommendation to 2.5 mcg. (100 IU) per day for individuals over the age of six, including adults.

The Food and Nutrition Board, recognizing the same situation, however, recommends a daily intake of 400 IU (10 mcg.) of vitamin D from birth through age 22. Although the adult requirement is not known it is assumed to be so small that the individual will receive sufficient vitamin D in the diet and by exposure to sunlight. However, small amounts of vitamin D may be desirable for adults who get little exposure to sunlight.

During pregnancy and lactation 400 IU (10 mcg.) daily are recommended by both the Food and Nutrition Board and by the Joint FAO/WHO Expert Committee.

Hypervitaminosis D

Vitamin D has been demonstrated to have specific toxicity when administered in overdosage. Usually toxicity is not manifest except after huge doses. Estimations are that 20 percent of adults receiving a daily dose of 100,000 IU of vitamin D for several weeks or months would develop hypercalcemia. A comparable amount for infants based on weight would be 10,000 to 30,000 IU per day. Cases of vitamin D toxicity occur "because of unjustified and indiscriminate medical use of the vitamin, lack of appreciation of its toxicity and the self-administration of highly concentrated preparations."[19] The maximum safe level of vitamin D for infants has yet to be precisely established, although intakes of 1600 IU—four times the recommended dietary allowance—have not interfered with the rate of growth in either length or weight of infants.[20] However, evidence that certain infants may be more sensitive to the toxic effects of vitamin D and may develop hypercalcemia on intakes of 2000 IU has caused considerable concern regarding the infant's total intake of this vitamin.[21] It is particularly important that the mother recognize the need for vitamin D, but, even more important, that she be aware of the harmful effects of overdosage. This means, of course, that the physician and the mother should be aware of the sources of vitamin D in the diet as well as in supplements.

In adults, hypercalcemia has been accompanied by symptoms such as anorexia, nausea, weight loss, polyuria, constipation, and azotemia. Similar symptoms are seen in infants, and, in certain rare severe forms, mental retardation also occurs.

Sources of Vitamin D

SUNSHINE. The low incidence of rickets in tropical climates suggested that sunshine might play a role in its prevention. Even after it had been demonstrated conclusively that the ultraviolet light from sunshine aided in the healing of rickets, it was difficult to understand the connection between this effect of light and the similar effect of vitamin D from sources such as cod-liver oil. Eventually, the puzzle was solved when it was discovered that vitamin D activity could be produced by irradiation. In the skin a form of cholesterol is activated to vitamin D_3 when exposed to sunlight; by absorption into the circulation, this cholecalciferol (vitamin D_3) protects the body against rickets. The amount of ultraviolet light in sunlight varies with the season and the locality, as does the total amount of sunlight. These rays are also filtered out by fog, smoke and ordinary window glass. It is obvious that an adequate natural source of ultraviolet light is impossible in northern climates during the winter months. Thus, some other source of vitamin D is needed.

Similarly, the pigments in the skin which protect against overproduction of vitamin D in dark-skinned peoples living in the tropics also reduce the effectiveness of the smaller amount of irradiation in temperate climates. As a result, the incidence of rickets is higher in dark-skinned babies living in temperate zones than in either light-skinned babies in this zone or dark-skinned infants in the tropics.

FOODS AND SUPPLEMENTS. The natural distribution of vitamin D in common foods is limited to small, often insignificant, amounts in fatty tissue, cream, butter, eggs and liver. Thus, we have come to depend on fortified foods, fish-liver oil, or concentrates for preventive and therapeutic use.

It was necessary to decide on one food, commonly used by children, to be fortified with a standard amount of vitamin D. Thus, the Council on Foods and Nutrition of the American Medical Association made the following decision:

"Of all the common foods available, milk is the most suitable as a carrier of added vitamin D. Vitamin D is concerned with the utilization of calcium and phosphorus, of which milk is an excellent source."[22]

Vitamin D milk now on the market is produced by adding a vitamin D concentrate to homogenized milk; the present standard of 400 IU per quart means that a quart of milk provides a day's requirement of vitamin D. All brands of evaporated milk also have vitamin D added, and strong recommendations to fortify nonfat milk solids with vitamins A and D have also been made by the American Medical Association.[23] Promiscuous fortification of a variety of other foods with vitamin D does not seem to be either necessary or desirable.

In the numerous fish-liver oils investigated there is a wide range of potency. This seems to vary with the season of the catch and the oil content of the livers. The highest potency oil is often yielded from fish that give the lowest amount of oil. Concentrates are made from the natural fish-liver oils or by irradiating pure ergosterol and cholesterol. Such preparations are labeled with the exact units per dose or per capsule and are prescribed accordingly. A protective dose to meet the daily requirement is considerably less than what may be prescribed as a curative dose.

In a study of the consumption of vitamin D by children (birth to 18 years) the average daily intake for all age groups was above 400 IU. Fortified milk

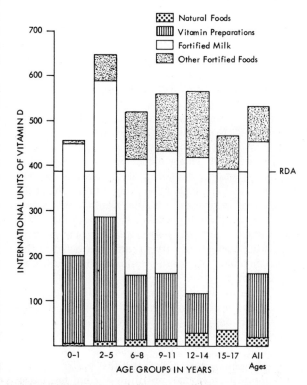

Fig. 6-7. Average daily intakes of vitamin D by age groups and sources. (Dale, A. E., and Lowenberg, M. E.: J. Pediat. 70:954)

supplied the largest amount of vitamin D, the percentage increasing with age. Vitamin preparations were more important in the infant and preschool groups than with older children. Fortified foods contributed to intakes of vitamin D over the recommended dietary allowance, particularly in the school age group (Fig. 6-7).[24]

Chemical synthesis of the metabolites of vitamin D, 25-HCC and 1,25-DHCC, may make it possible to replace the missing metabolite in kidney or liver disease when it cannot be synthesized in sufficient amounts. A recent study[25] has suggested that vitamin D dependent rickets is an inborn error of metabolism resulting from a genetic defect in 25-hydroxy-cholecalciferol-1-hydroxylase, the enzyme responsible for production of 1,25-HDCC, the active metabolite of vitamin D, and that patients with the disease respond to very small doses of 1,25-HDCC as compared with massive doses of vitamin D_2, D_3 and 25-HCC.

STABILITY. Vitamin D in foods and in food concentrates is remarkably stable to heating, aging, and storage. Vitamin D milk that is warmed for the baby is still a reliable source of this factor.

VITAMIN E
History

The existence of a dietary factor essential for reproduction in the rat was recognized in the early 1920s by Evans; it was given the name vitamin E, or antisterility factor, by Sure in 1924. Much of the experimental work has been done on rats, the males and the females being affected differently. Vitamin E deficiency leads to destruction of germ cells in the testes of the male and thus to permanent sterility. In a vitamin E deficient female mated with a normal male, ovulation and implantation of the ovum may take place normally, but about halfway through the gestation period resorption of the developing fetus occurs and no young are born. With less severe vitamin E deficiency, which may permit the birth of a weakling litter, the chances of survival are poor because this same deficiency seems to interfere with lactation or, later, with growth of the young.

Earlier work on nutritional muscular dystrophy in rabbits has been repeated with other animals, and the nutritional deficiency factor has been identified as vitamin E. However, clinical evidence fails to indicate that vitamin E is a significant factor in human reproduction or muscular dystrophy. In fact, the role of vitamin E in human nutrition has not been well defined.

Nomenclature

Eight naturally occurring compounds have vitamin E activity. They are fat-soluble alcohols of high molecular weight, closely related in structure, called tocopherols and tocotrienols. Alpha-tocopherol is the most active form (Fig 6-8). It deteriorates on exposure to light and decomposes upon irradiation with ultraviolet light. Contact with lead and iron hastens destruction. Tocopherols, because they are readily oxidized themselves, have antioxidant properties and prevent deterioration of certain foods by oxidation. This characteristic probably exerts a protective action on vitamin A.

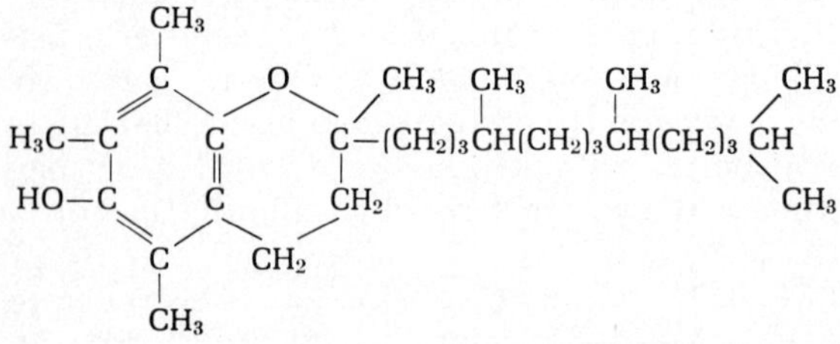

Vitamin E, alpha-tocopherol $C_{29}H_{50}O_2$

Fig. 6-8. Compound with vitamin E activity.

Conversion factors for vitamin E activity are as follows:

1 mg. dl-α-tocopheryl acetate (natural or synthetic) = 1 IU
1 mg. dl-α-tocopherol (synthetic free) = 1.1 IU
1 mg. d-α-tocopherol (natural occurring) = 1.49 IU
1 mg. d-α-tocopheryl acetate (natural occurring) = 1.36 IU

Food allowances are based on the alpha-tocopherol content of food. Other vitamin E active compounds may be assumed to contribute additional vitamin E activity equivalent to about 20 percent of the indicated alpha-tocopherol content of a mixed diet.[26]

Absorption, Transport, Storage, and Excretion

Approximately 50 to 85 percent of the vitamin E in the diet is absorbed in the intestines. It is carried in plasma, mainly in the lipoproteins, but quickly equilibrates between these and the red blood cell membranes. A plasma level of total tocopherols below 0.5 mg./100 ml. is considered undesirable. Factors that affect the plasma lipoprotein concentration also affect plasma tocopherol levels. The average intake of vitamin E will, over a time, be reflected in its levels in all the tissues of the body. Vitamin E is stored in adipose tissue and is mobilized with fat. Metabolites of vitamin E are excreted in urine and feces.

Functions and Physiologic Significance of Vitamin E in Humans

Although there is little agreement among investigators as to the mode of action of vitamin E, the function of the vitamin is to help protect the integrity of cellular and intracellular structures and to prevent destruction of certain enzymes and intracellular components. The controversy surrounding the biological role of vitamin E relates to the way this function is carried out.[27] There is no conclusive evidence at the present time as to the mode of action of vitamin E but each of the following theories have their advocates: Tappel[28] makes a strong case for the lipid antioxidant theory; Schwarz and Baumgartner[29] support the hypothesis that vitamin E is involved in an enzyme system related to the electron transfer chain, and Olson[30] suggests that vitamin E regulates the synthesis of specific proteins related to the differentiation or adaptation of certain tissues.

Vitamin E is found distributed throughout the fat-soluble portion of the membranous parts of the cell together with phospholipids, cholesterol and triglycerides. As an antioxidant vitamin E is said to react with free radicals formed from the oxidation of polyunsaturated fatty acids and to convert these free radicals into harmless compounds, thus preventing tissue damage. Investigators have also explained the vitamin's antioxidant function in terms of protecting other labile substances, such as vitamin A, sulfur-containing enzymes, ascorbic acid, and ATP, from peroxidative destruction in the tissues.[31]

In a recent review of vitamin E, Tappel[32] suggests that the nutritional relationships among the sulfur-containing amino acids, selenium, and vitamin E are based on the roles of these nutrients in the glutathione peroxidase system. According to this theory selenium is an essential nutrient for the functioning of glutathione peroxidase, an enzyme synthesized from sulfur-containing amino acids, whose function in the water-soluble portion of the cell is similar to that suggested for vitamin E in the fat-soluble portion, namely to protect against oxidation of polyunsaturated fatty acids and resultant tissue demage. This would, in fact, explain the observation of many workers that selenium may replace or spare vitamin E in certain of its functions.

The only apparent agreement among investigators at the present time, however, has to do with the need for vitamin E relative to the amount of polyunsaturated fatty acid (PUFA) in the tissues. Red blood cells from subjects on low vitamin E and high polyunsaturated fatty acid dietary intakes have less resistance to hemolysis in the presence of hydrogen peroxide than those from individuals on higher vitamin E and lower PUFA intakes. Although the clinical significance is not clear, this test is one of the measurements used to determine the vitamin E status of individuals. Vitamin E deficiencies in man are very rare; however, considerable interest has been shown in this area because of the relationship of vitamin E to PUFA and the present trend toward increasing PUFA in the diets of large segments of the population.

Newborn infants tend to have low plasma levels of vitamin E (approximately $1/3$ the adult level) due not only to lower concentrations of blood lipids in the newborn but also to limited transfer of the vitamin across the placenta. Plasma levels begin to rise after birth, more rapidly in the breast-fed infant, and reach normal concentrations by about one month of age. Low birth weight (LBW) infants have even lower levels of vitamin E at birth and vitamin E deficiency has been reported for infants fed commercial formulas low in vitamin E.[33]

The hemapoietic effect of vitamin E on children with protein-calorie malnutrition is not clear since different workers report varying results from the administration of this vitamin. Horwitt[34] suggests that they may have been treating patients whose vitamin E status was not comparable.

Human Requirement

The recommended dietary allowance of vitamin E was set at 15 IU for the adult male and 12 IU for the adult female. These allowances are based on the vitamin E content of average U. S. diets, assumed adequate since no biochemical or clinical evidence is available to indicate inadequate vitamin E intakes by the normal United States population. The allowance for infants (4 to 5 IU) is based on the vitamin E content of human milk, 2 to 5 IU per liter. Vitamin E allowances for children increase with increasing body weight. The adult female allowance for vitamin E is increased to 15 IU during pregnancy and lactation.

FOOD SOURCES. Wheat germ and wheat-germ oil afford the richest source of this factor, but it is so widely distributed in common foods that it is actually difficult to obtain a food mixture for experimental purposes that is deficient in vitamin E.

Animal foods are relatively poor sources of vitamin E although depot fat and liver contain moderate amounts. Some tocopherol is removed from oils in the purification process. When chlorine dioxide is used to bleach flour, tocopherol is lost.

Table 6–1. Food Sources of Vitamin E*

Food	Milligrams per 100 g.
FATS AND OILS	
Corn oil	
Unhydrogenated	100
Hydrogenated	105
Cottonseed oil	
Unhydrogenated	91
Hydrogenated	80
Soybean oil	
Unhydrogenated	101
Hydrogenated	73
Coconut oil	8
Mayonnaise	50
Margarine (made with corn oil)	47
Butter	1
FRUITS AND VEGETABLES	
Tomatoes, fresh	0.85
Green peas, frozen	0.65
Banana	0.42
Carrots	0.21
Orange juice, fresh	0.20
Potatoes, baked	0.085
CEREAL GRAINS	
Yellow cornmeal	3.4
Whole wheat bread	2.2
Cornflakes	0.43
White bread	0.23
MEAT, FISH, POULTRY, AND EGGS	
Beef liver, broiled	1.62
Egg	1.43
Filet of haddock, broiled	1.20
Ground beef	0.63
Pork chops, pan-fried	0.60
Chicken breast	0.58

*From Bunnel, R. H., et al: Am. J. Clin. Nutr. 17:1, 1965.

Herting[35] reported that, in individual vegetable oils and fats, the tocopherol levels varied according to source of the plant, time of harvest, stability after harvest, refining procedure, and commercial hydrogenation procedures. When estimates of man's requirement for vitamin E as related to PUFA were compared with the amount of both substances in common edible oils high in polyunsaturated fatty acids (cottonseed, corn, safflower and soybean), only cottonseed supplied sufficient vitamin E to counterbalance the effect of its PUFA content. Table 6–1 lists some common food sources of vitamin E. Satisfactory food tables for vitamin E in foods are not available, hence, this nutrient is not included in the pattern dietary.

There are no sound scientific experiments or clinical observations to support the misleading claims that vitamin E supplementation of the ordinary diet will cure or prevent human abnormalities such as sterility, lack of virility, abnormal termination of pregnancy, heart disease, muscle weakness, cancer, ulcers, skin disorders, or burns. Since nutrition surveys indicate that the United States population consumes adequate amounts of vitamin E in the usual diet, additional supplementation is unlikely to prove beneficial in alleviating any of the problems mentioned.[36]

VITAMIN K
History
In 1935 Dam recognized a severe deficiency disease in newly hatched chicks fed on a ration adequate in protein, minerals, and all known vitamins. Hemorrhage apparently was due to a fall in prothrombin, the clotting agent in the blood; normal clotting time was restored by administering hog-liver fat or by feeding alfalfa. The antihemorrhagic factor found in these

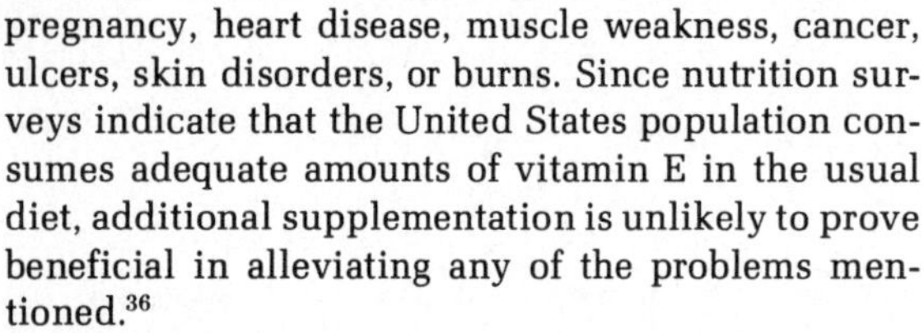

Vitamin K_1, phylloquinone

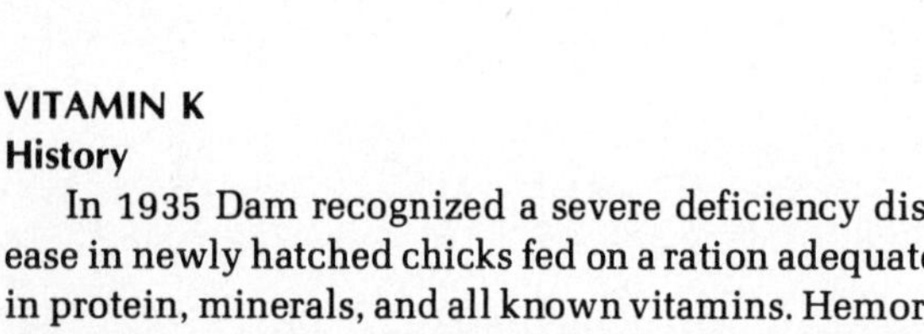

Vitamin K_2 series, menaquinone-n

Fig. 6–9. Compounds with vitamin K activity.

materials Dam called vitamin K—Koagulation Vitamin.

This discovery and the identification, isolation, and synthesis of compounds with vitamin K activity have made possible extensive clinical use of this vitamin for the control and the prevention of hemorrhages due to vitamin K deficiency.

Nomenclature
Vitamin K is a yellowish crystalline substance. At least two forms (K_1, phylloquinone, and K_2, menaquinone-n) occur naturally (Fig. 6–9). The menaquinone family (vitamin K_2) consists of a large series of vitamins containing unsaturated side chains which vary in the number of isoprenyl units. Animals synthesize menaquinone-4 from menadione, formerly known as vitamin K_3. Other menaquinones synthesized by bacteria include menaquinone-4 through menaquinone-13. The K vitamins are heat resistant but are destroyed by alkalis, strong acids, and certain oxidizing agents. In the concentrated form vitamin K seems to be sensitive to light.

Vitamin K can be measured in micrograms of the pure synthetic compound, and the vitamin K activity of other substances can be expressed in similar terms. One method of assay uses young chicks and is based on the minimum dose that will maintain the normal coagulation time of the blood at the end of one month.

Absorption, Transport, Synthesis, and Storage
Ingested vitamin K is absorbed by the intestines in much the same way as dietary fat. The absorption of vitamin K seems to be dependent on the presence of bile and pancreatic juice, and the percent (10 to 70 percent) absorbed depends on the vehicle used for its administration. It is carried first in the lymph chylomicrons and then transferred to the beta-lipoproteins. Large amounts appear in the liver shortly after ingestion (1 to 2 hours). Other tissues, kidney, heart, skin, and muscle, increase their concentration levels to a maximum over a 24-hour period and then decline. Some vitamin K is stored in the liver. Bacterial synthesis of vitamin K occurs in the intestines of man and provides an important source of the nutrient.

Function
Vitamin K is essential in blood coagulation for the maintenance of normal prothrombin time through its effect on factor II, prothrombin; factor VII, proconvertin; factor IX, Christmas factor; and factor X, Stuart-Prower factor. These four vitamin K-dependent factors are present in the extrinsic (activated by injury) and intrinsic (activated by platelets) coagulation systems and in the common pathway leading to clot

Table 6–2. Summary. Fat-Soluble Vitamins

	A	D	E	K
Active Chemical Forms	Retinol 3-dehydroretinol Retinal Retinoic acid Carotenoids	Cholecalciferol Ergocalciferol	Tocopherols α, β, γ etc. Tocotrienols	Vitamin K_1 phylloquinone and K_2 menaquinone
Important Food Sources	Liver Egg yolk Butter, cream Margarine Green and yellow vegetables Apricots Cantaloupe	Irradiated foods Small amounts in: Butter Egg yolk Liver Salmon Sardines Tuna fish	Wheat germ Leafy vegetables Vegetable oils Egg yolk Legumes Peanuts Margarine	Cabbage Cauliflower Spinach Other leafy vegetables Pork liver Soybean oil and other vegetables oils
Stability to Cooking, Drying, Light, etc.	Gradual destruction by exposure to air, heat, and drying, more rapid at high temperatures	Stable to heating, aging, and storage Destroyed by excess ultraviolet irradiation	Stable to methods of food processing Destroyed by rancidity and ultraviolet irradiation	Stable to heat, light, and exposure to air Destroyed by strong acids, alkalis, and oxidizing agents
Function	Maintains function of epithelial cells, mucous membranes, skin, bone, constituent of visual pigments	Calcium and phosphorus absorption and utilization in bone growth	Protects cell structures	Necessary in formation of 4 factors essential for clotting of blood
Deficiency: Signs and Symptoms	Night blindness Glare blindness Rough, dry skin Dry mucous membranes Xerophthalmia	Rickets Soft bones Bowed legs Poor teeth Skeletal deformities	Increased hemolysis of red blood cells	Slow clotting time of blood Some hemorrhagic disease of newborn Lack of prothrombin
Adult Human Requirement	Male 1000 RE (5000 IU); Female 800 RE (4000 IU)	Children and adolescents, 400 IU	Male 15 IU Female 12 IU	Unknown

formation by conversion of fibrinogen to fibrin. There is still uncertainty as to whether vitamin K regulates the synthesis of these coagulation factors at the ribosomal level in the liver[37], or if the vitamin acts in some way to convert precursor proteins, whose syntheses are not directly controlled by the vitamin, to active factors.[38] When their level in the blood is reduced as in vitamin K deficiency, blood coagulation time is depressed.

Dicumarol and warfarin (coumarin compounds) are used in anticoagulation therapy to prevent thrombus formation and act as vitamin K antagonists. Their concentration in the liver stops prothrombin synthesis and reduces blood coagulation.

Human Requirement

Studies of liver stores of vitamin K indicate that approximately 50 percent of the vitamin comes from the diet and 50 percent from bacterial synthesis in the intestines. The total daily requirement which has been postulated as approximately 2 mcg./kg. is met by a diet supplying 1 mcg./kg. Since the average diet in the U.S. contains 300 to 500 mcg. of vitamin K per day there is little danger of inadequate intakes under normal conditions.[39] A deficiency state would more likely be caused by a failure to absorb or utilize the vitamin. Low vitamin K intakes plus antibiotic therapy (neomycin), which reduces the bacterial synthesis, may result in lowered levels of the vitamin K dependent coagulation factors. The use of mineral oil in reducing diets or as a laxative interferes with the absorption of vitamin K as well as other fat-soluble vitamins and this is not recommended.

Infants represent a special situation in terms of vitamin K because of limited placental transfer of the vitamin and because the gut of the newborn is sterile and cannot synthesize the vitamin. Thus, some infants require vitamin K administration to prevent hemorrhage. It may be given in a water-soluble or fat-soluble form. If mothers have received anticoagulant therapy, their infants should be given 2 to 4 mg. of vitamin K immediately after birth.

Hypervitaminosis K

Vitamin K can be toxic if given in large doses over a prolonged period of time. Symptoms of vitamin K toxicity reported by Smith and Custer[40] are hypoprothrombinemia, petechial hemorrhages, and renal tubule degeneration, and, in premature infants, hemolytic anemia.

In 1963 the Food and Drug Administration recommended the removal of menadione from all food supplements. Vitamins K_1 and K_2 are still permitted in carefully regulated amounts.

Food Sources

Vitamin K is fairly widely distributed in foods. It appears abundantly in cauliflower, cabbage, spinach, pork liver, and soybeans and, to a lesser extent, in wheat and oats. Animal products contain little vitamin K; however, cows' milk is a better source than human milk.

STUDY QUESTIONS AND ACTIVITIES

1. How was the term vitamin arrived at? Can you define a vitamin as distinct from any other food nutrient?
2. Why are vitamins A and D referred to as hormones?
3. Give some events and names of people of interest in the history of vitamin discoveries.
4. Describe the function of each of the fat-soluble vitamins and good food sources for each, if there are any.
5. Does the depth of yellow color in butter or egg yolks indicate the vitamin A potency? Why, or why not?
6. Since the supply of vitamin D is small in natural foods, what commercial process is used to produce foods containing vitamin D? Which foods are commonly fortified with vitamin D?
7. Describe the two functions that have been postulated for vitamin E.
8. When is a deficiency of vitamin K most likely to occur and what prophylactic measures are sometimes recommended?
9. Are any of the fat-soluble vitamins toxic if used in too large quantities? For which one is special caution necessary when concentrates are administered to infants?

SUPPLEMENTARY READINGS

American Academy of Pediatrics, Committee on Nutrition. The relation between infantile hypercalcemia and vitamin D—public health implications in North America. Pediatrics 40:1050, 1967.
———, Vitamin K supplementation for infants receiving milk substitute infant formulas and for those with fat malabsorption. Pediatrics 48:483, 1971.
Avioli, L. V., and Haddad, J. G.: Vitamin D: Current Concepts. Metabolism 22:507, 1973.
Bieri, J. G.: Fat-soluble vitamins in the eighth revision of the Recommended Dietary Allowances. J. Am. Dietet. A. 64:171, 1974.

———: Vitamin E. Nutr. Rev. 33:161, 1975.
Bieri, J. G., and Evarts, R. P.: The recommended allowances for vitamin E: Tocopherols and fatty acids in American diets. J. Am. Dietet. A. 62:147, 1973.
———: Vitamin E adequacy of vegetable oils. J. Am. Dietet. A. 66:134, 1975.
Comm. on Nutritional Misinformation: Hazards of overdose of vitamin D. Nutr. Rev. 33:61, 1975.
DeLuca, H. F.: Vitamin D: a new look at an old vitamin. Nutr. Rev. 29:179, 1971.
Editorial. Supplementation of human diet with vitamin E. Statement of the Food and Nutrition Board, National Research Council. Nutr. Rev. 30:327, 1973.
Haussler, M. R.: Vitamin D: Mode of action and biomedical applications. Nutr. Rev. 32:257, 1974.
Hayes, K. C.: On the physiopathology of vitamin A deficiency. Nutr. Rev. 29:3, 1971.
Olson, R. E.: The mode of action of vitamin K. Nutr. Rev. 28:171, 1970.
———: Vitamin E and its relation to heart disease. Circulation 48:179, 1973.
Palmisano, P. A.: Vitamin D: A reawakening. JAMA 224:1526, 1973.
Review: A role of 1,25-dihydroxyvitamin D_3 in phosphate metabolism. Nutr. Rev. 32:247, 1974.
Review: Control of vitamin D metabolism. Nutr. Rev. 31-187, 1973.
Review: Effect of calcitonin on bone resorption induced by excess vitamins A and D. Nutr. Rev. 29:150, 1971.
Review: Two physiological forms of human retinol binding protein. Nutr. Rev. 30:90, 1972.
Roels, O. A.: Vitamin A physiology. JAMA 214:1097, 1970.
Suttie, J. W.: Vitamin K and prothrombin synthesis. Nutr. Rev. 31:105, 1973.
Sweeney, J. P., and Marsh, A. C.: Effect of processing on provitamin A in vegetables. J. Am. Dietet. A. 59:238, 1971.

For further references see Bibliography in Section 4.

REFERENCES

1. Wolf, G., and DeLuca, L.: Recent studies on some metabolic functions of vitamin A, in The Fat-Soluble Vitamins, H. F. DeLuca and J. W. Suttie, eds., Madison, University of Wisconsin Press, 1969, p. 257.
2. Wagner, A. F., and Folkers, K.: Vitamins and Coenzymes. New York, Wiley, 1964. p. 7.
3. Requirements of Vitamin A, Thiamine, Riboflavine and Niacin. WHO Tech. Report Series No. 362. Geneva, 1967.
4. Ibid.
5. Recommended Dietary Allowances. National Research Council. Washington, D.C., 1974.
6. Ibid.
7. Wolf and DeLuca, op. cit.
8. Hayes, K. C.: Nutr. Rev. 29:3, 1971.

9. Ibid.
10. Ibid.
11. Hodges, R. E., and Kolder, H.: Summary of proceedings. Workshop on biochemical and clinical criteria for determining human vitamin A nutriture. National Academy of Sciences. Washington, D.C., 1971, pp. 10-16.
12. Recommended Dietary Allowances. Washington, D.C., National Research Council, 1974.
13. Morrice, G., Jr., and Havener, W. H.: JAMA 173:1802, 1960.
14. Goodhart, R. S., and Shils, M. E.: *Modern Nutrition in Health and Disease*, ed. 5, Philadelphia, Lea and Febiger, 1973, p. 273.
15. Melancon, M. J., Jr., and DeLuca, H. F.: Biochem. 9:1658, 1970.
16. Fraser, D. R., and Kodicek, E.: Nature (New Biology) 241:163, 1973.
17. Rasmussen, H., et al: J. Clin. Invest. 51:2502, 1972.
18. Requirements of Ascorbic Acid, Vitamin D, Vitamin B_{12}, Folate and Iron. WHO Tech. Report Series No. 452, Geneva, 1970.
19. Fomon, S. J., et al: J. Nutrition 88:345, 1966.
20. Review: Nutr. Rev. 19:158, 1961.
21. Report: Pediatrics 31:512, 1963.
22. Council on Foods and Nutrition, AMA, Decision. JAMA 159:1018, 1955.
23. Council on Foods and Nutrition, AMA, Statement. JAMA 197:1107, 1966.
24. Dale, A. E., and Lowenberg, M. E.: J. Pediat. 70:954, 1967.
25. Fraser, D.: N. Eng. J. Med. 289:817, 1973.
26. Recommended Dietary Allowances. Washington, D.C., National Research Council, 1974.
27. Green, J.: Vitamin E and the biological antioxidant theory, in *The Fat-Soluble Vitamins*, ed. 4, H. F. DeLuca and J. W. Suttie, eds. Madison, University of Wisconsin Press, 1969, p. 293.
28. Tappel, A. L: Nutrition Today 8:4, (July, August) 1973.
29. Schwartz, K., and Baumgartner, W.: Kinetic studies on mitochondrial enzymes during respiratory decline relating to the mode of action of tocopherol, in *The Fat-Soluble Vitamins*, H. F. DeLuca and J. W. Suttie, eds. Madison, University of Wisconsin Press, 1969, p. 344.
30. Olson, R. E.: Food and Nutrition News 44:5-6 (February, March) 1973.
31. Tappel, A. L., op. cit.
32. Ibid.
33. Hussan, H. et al: Am. J. Clin. Nutr. 19:147, 1966.
34. Goodhart and Shils, op. cit., p. 180.
35. Herting, D. C., and Drury, E.-J. E.: J. Nutrition 81:335, 1963.
36. National Research Council: Nutr. Rev. 32:37 (July Supplement) 1974.
37. Olson, R. E.: Nutr. Rev. 28:171, 1970.
38. Suttie, J. W.: Nutr. Rev. 31:105, 1973.
39. Goodhart and Shils, op. cit., p.172.
40. Smith, A. M., Jr., and Custer, R. P.: JAMA 173:502, 1960.

7

water-soluble vitamins

ASCORBIC ACID

The history of scurvy as a deficiency disease in man is discussed in Chapter 20. Experimental scurvy was first induced in guinea pigs in 1907 by Holst and Frölich in Norway; these animals, unlike rats, chickens, dogs, and other domestic animals, develop characteristic hemorrhages around the joints, teeth, and other bony structures very similar to the symptoms of scurvy in man. Man, the primates, and guinea pigs do not possess the ability to synthesize vitamin C when this vitamin is missing from their diets and must rely totally on the vitamin C ingested with their food.

Properties

By 1932 the isolation of vitamin C in pure crystalline form had been accomplished independently by two groups of workers. The chemical structure was identified and the product synthesized in physiologically active form soon afterwards, and in 1938 "ascorbic acid" was officially accepted as the chemical name for vitamin C. It occurs naturally in foods in two forms, the reduced form (usually designated as *ascorbic acid*) and the oxidized form, (*dehydroascorbic acid*). They are shown in Fig. 7-1. Both are physiologically active and both are found in body tissues. The ascorbic acid in fruits and vegetables and the synthetic form are equally well utilized.

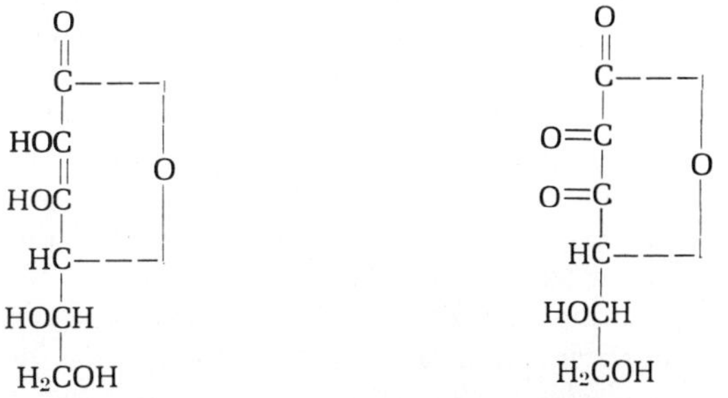

Measurement

Measured by chemical titration, the potency of ascorbic acid is expressed in milligrams. It is an active reducing agent and bleaches certain dyes rapidly. This property is used in the quantitative determination in foods and tissues.

Guinea pigs always have been the preferred experimental animals for bioassay work because of their susceptibility to a deficiency of ascorbic acid, and they are still used for demonstration of such a deficiency and for comparative assays (Fig. 7-2).

Functions

Vitamin C has a variety of roles in the life processes, but to date the specific biochemical functions of ascorbic acid are not well understood. One of its most significant roles is in the formation of *collagen*, the protein substance that cements the cells together. Collagen contains the amino acids hydroxyproline and hydroxylysine, mainly formed in the body from the amino acids proline and lysine; ascorbic acid appears to be necessary for this conversion.

It has been postulated that ascorbic acid activates the enzyme propyl hydroxylase (proline incorporated into peptide linkage) by causing the aggregation of three inactive subunits to form the active compound.[1]

Failure to synthesize collagen results in delayed healing of wounds. There is an actual increase in the amount of ascorbic acid present at the site of the wound during healing.

Because the osteoblasts fail to function properly in scurvy, bone disorganization results. Tooth dentin may also be adversely affected by vitamin C deficiency, although structural defects in the teeth rarely occur in man. Shortages of this vitamin result in weakened capillary walls, which in turn lead to hemorrhages of varying degree.

Ascorbic acid functions in the metabolism of the amino acids phenylalanine and tyrosine. In the case of tyrosine, ascorbic acid has been shown to have a role in the biosynthesis de novo of tyrosine hydroxylase.[2]

Fig. 7-1. Structural formula of ascorbic acid.

L-Ascorbic acid (reduced form)

L-Dehydroascorbic acid (oxidized form)

It is also necessary in the conversion of the inactive form of the vitamin, folic acid, to the active form, folinic acid, and in the regulation of the respiratory cycle in mitochondria and microsomes.

Ascorbic acid enhances the absorption of iron by reducing the ferric form to the more readily absorbed ferrous form.

Recent studies have suggested that ascorbic·acid may function in the process which inactivates adipose tissue lipase when energy demands have been met. This would indicate a role for ascorbic acid in phosphorylation processes.[3] Ascorbic acid may also have a role in protein deamidation reactions.[4]

Ascorbic acid sulfate (AAS) has been identified as a metabolite of ascorbic acid which may function as a sulfating agent in man. The anti-atherogenic effect of ascorbic acid, for instance, may be accounted for by the formation of cholesterol sulfate, a water soluble compound, which might serve to facilitate the removal of cholesterol from the enterohepatic circulation.[5] Equally interesting is the hypothesis that ascorbic acid functions in the conversion of cholesterol to bile acids by participating in hydroxylation reactions.[6]

Clinical observation of a number of infections accompanied by fever show a decreased blood level of ascorbic acid, indicating either increased need for this vitamin or increased destruction of it. It appears,

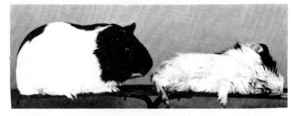

Fig. 7-2. Scurvy results from vitamin C deficiency. Guinea pigs are used for experiments in vitamin C because they need a food source of this factor, even as humans do. (*Left*) Normal guinea pig. (*Right*) Scorbutic guinea pig. (Nutrition Laboratory, Battle Creek Sanitarium)

however, that a suboptimal intake of vitamin C is not a predisposing cause of any of these diseases. It has also been observed that the normally high concentration of ascorbic acid in the adrenal cortex is depleted whenever the gland is stimulated by hormones or certain toxins. Although there is not complete agreement regarding the relationship of ascorbic acid and stress, Baker states that "there is definitely an increased requirement for ascorbic acid in all forms of stress; however, we do not, at this time, have sufficient knowledge to state an absolute or quantitative level of increased requirement."[7]

Administration of large doses of ascorbic acid appears to protect an individual exposed to very low environmental temperatures. However, the controversy involving the use of large doses of ascorbic acid to prevent and cure the common cold[8] has not been resolved. Anderson,[9] in reporting the results of a large double blind Canadian study stated that vitamin C in large amounts appeared to have some pharmacologic effects not related to its vitamin function at nutritional levels. The Food and Nutrition Board does not recommend large intakes of vitamin C.

Absorption, Storage, and Excretion

Absorption of ascorbic acid takes place in the upper part of the small intestines. It is circulated in the bloodstream to the tissues of the body. The amount of ascorbic acid in different tissues varies; adrenal and pituitary tissue, brain, pancreas, kidney, liver, and spleen have relatively high concentrations; blood cells contain more than blood serum.

Load tests which are based on the principle of tissue saturation were used to determine ascorbic acid requirements. When tissues attained their maximum concentration of the vitamin, they were said to be saturated and excess ascorbic acid was excreted in the urine. Today radioactively labeled ^{14}C-ascorbic acid is administered and, by determining

the specific radioactivity in the plasma or blood, the body pool size of ascorbic acid can be calculated. (See Table 7-1).

Human Requirement

Elaborate studies have been done to determine human requirements for ascorbic acid at different ages, under different conditions of environment, during physical exertion, in fevers, and in infections. The amount necessary to prevent frank symptoms of scurvy in humans is far less (10 mg.) than that recommended for an optimum state of health.

The National Research Council recommends 45 mg. daily for adults, 60 mg. during pregnancy, and 80 mg. during lactation. Growing children need relatively more than adults. The joint FAO/WHO Expert Committee set somewhat lower recommendations: 30 mg. for adults (males and females over 13 years), 50 mg. during pregnancy and lactation, and 20 mg. for infants and children up to 13 years old.[10]

A regular and adequate intake of ascorbic acid is emphasized because of the body's limited storage capacity and constant need.

Food Sources

It is obvious from the bar chart (Fig. 7-3) that the commonly used fruits and vegetables of Group 3 are the richest sources of ascorbic acid, with citrus fruits, strawberries, cantaloupe, and a number of raw, leafy vegetables topping the list. Canned or frozen citrus juice may be the cheapest source of vitamin C when fresh citrus fruit is scarce or expensive, and may be cheaper than tomato juice, because it takes three times as much tomato as citrus juice to supply the same amounts of vitamin C.

Many factors affect the ascorbic acid content of fruits and vegetables; variety, maturity, length of storage, part of the plant, seasonal and geographical factors are all influential. As plants mature they generally have less ascorbic acid; the sprouts of beans or grains, however, do contain vitamin C. Exposure to sunlight also tends to increase the plant's ascorbic acid content. Food value tables give average representative amounts, whereas any individual food may vary considerably from this value.[11] From analyses of the ascorbic acid content of such foods as potatoes, cabbage, and broccoli purchased during the winter in northern Vermont, the authors[12] conclude "that certain vegetables, as purchased during the winter months, provide dependable quantities of total ascorbic acid, even though they have been subjected to transportation, storage and handling."

In some countries indigenous fruits high in vitamin C are overlooked, even though they are readily

Table 7-1. Ascorbic Acid Nutritional Status in Man*

	DIETARY INTAKE	SERUM OR PLASMA CONCEN- TRATION	WHOLE BLOOD CONCEN- TRATION	BUFFY COAT CONCEN- TRATION	BODY POOL SIZE
	mg.	mg./100ml.	mg./100ml.	mcg./10⁸ cells	mg.
Well- nourished†	45	>0.60	>1.0	>16	1500
Adequate†	30-44	0.40-0.59	0.60-0.99	11-15	600-1499
Low	10-29	0.10-0.39	0.30-0.59	2-10	300-599
Deficient	<10	<0.10	<0.30	<2	0-299

*Adapted from Hodges, R. E., and Baker, E. M., Ascorbic acid, in *Modern Nutrition in Health and Disease*, ed. 5, R. S. Goodhart, and M. E. Shils. eds., Philadelphia, Lea and Febiger, 1973.

†These represent approximate ranges, not absolute values. This table is offered only as a guide to interpret current values.

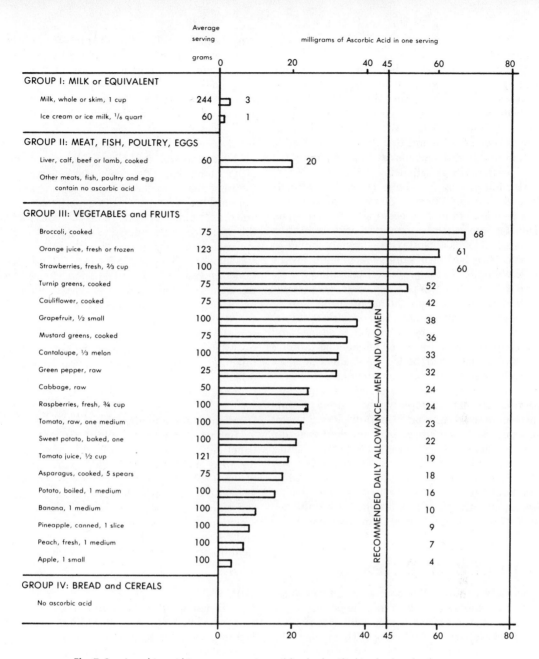

Fig. 7–3. Ascorbic acid in average servings of foods classified in the four food groups.

available. For example, in Puerto Rice the acerola (*azarole*, or West Indian cherry) has the highest ascorbic acid content of any known food.[13] Only recently has attention been called to it, and the acerola has become popular in that country. In Great Britain during World War II rosehip and black-currant syrups or jams served to supplement the meager supply of vitamin C from garden vegetables. Even before the war, in northern Russia an extract of pine needles rich

in vitamin C was being added to berry juice as a health beverage for school children. In another part of northern Europe raw turnip juice saved the lives of many infants who otherwise would have died of scurvy. Depending on diet, mother's milk may contain more ascorbic acid than average cow's milk and considerably more than is found in pasteurized milk, thus affecting the amount and the timing of additional sources needed in an infant's diet.

Stability in Foods

Of all the vitamins, ascorbic acid is the most unstable under heat, oxidation, drying, and storage, which makes it one of the most difficult nutrients to supply in adequate amounts to troops or civil populations in wartime. In World War II army rations included a lemon powder fortified with ascorbic acid; if men did not drink lemonade, as was frequently the case, their ration was deficient in vitamin C.

Alkalinity, even to a slight degree, is distinctly destructive to this vitamin; therefore, soda should never be added to food in cooking. Acid fruits and vegetables lose much less ascorbic acid on heating than nonacid foods. Vitamin C is extremely soluble in water and dissolves out of some vegetables during the first few minutes in the process of cooking.

To reduce as much as possible the loss of ascorbic acid in cooking vegetables, the use of the least possible amount of cooking water, short cooking time (water should be boiling when vegetable is added), and little chopping or cutting is recommended. Studies have shown that baked, boiled, or steamed potatoes retain a large proportion of their vitamin C if cooked whole. Fresh fruits and more especially vegetables lose vitamin C activity rapidly when stored at room temperature and somewhat less rapidly at refrigerator temperatures. Expert advice is to not shell peas, cut beans, or peel vegetables until ready to cook. Quick freezing of fruits and vegetables destroys little if any of this factor. To retain a maximum of the ascorbic acid, frozen fruits should be used promptly after thawing, and frozen vegetables should be plunged directly into boiling water for immediate cooking.

vitamin b complex

As early as 1897, Eijkman, a Dutch physician working in Indonesia, noticed that the poultry at the prison hospital showed symptoms similar to those of his patients suffering from beriberi. This malady developed in the chickens when they were fed on polished rice table scraps; recovery followed the feeding of brown rice from another prison. The results of the investigation were published in an obscure journal.

Years later great scientific significance was attached to the findings, for Eijkman had discovered that there was a deficiency in polished rice, although he had not realized its significance. Experimental work with rats, pigeons, and dogs during the early part of this century led to the recognition of a hitherto unknown food essential that came to be known as vitamin B. Animals deprived of this factor lost appetite, ceased to grow, and often developed characteristic symptoms of polyneuritis, a loss of muscular control, and partial paralysis. Many of these symptoms in animals were similar to those of beriberi in man, particularly the effects on the nervous system.

Subdivision into Separate Factors

Numerous workers began to observe a complexity of symptoms due to deficiencies among peoples with different dietary patterns. These reports were confusing until the discrepancies in experimental findings and the diversity of physiologic properties ascribed to this so-called vitamin B led to the recognition of several factors instead of one. From then on the group was known as the vitamin B complex, and each fraction received separate designation—letter, descriptive name, or chemical term—as research progressed to disclose the chemical nature of each.

At present some 12 fractions of the vitamin B complex are generally recognized, and others are postulated. Those discussed in this chapter are thiamine, riboflavin, niacin, vitamin B_6, vitamin B_{12}, folacin, pantothenic acid, and biotin, with brief comments about several others.

Distribution and Properties

Certain properties, solubility in water and distribution in many common foods, are similar for all members of the B complex. The very fact that several of the fractions occurred together in the same food gave rise to the early idea that there was only one substance. New factors identified are classified as belonging to the B complex if they are water soluble and are abundant in liver and yeast; dry yeast is the richest natural source of the B complex.

THIAMINE

The polyneuritic symptoms similar to beriberi recognized by Eijkman in his chickens resulted from lack of the vitamin B_1 fraction of the B complex. Beriberi is described in Chinese history, and some of the earliest attempts to treat it are reported from Japan and the Philippines. Recognition of its cause, and its possible cure by better diet, is a landmark in the history of nutrition. Takaki, a medical officer in the Japanese marines during the 1880s, was alarmed at the number of cases of beriberi—169 on one ship with 25 deaths. He proposed that the food must be at fault and helped plan an experiment to prove it. A special training ship was sent out on a 287-day voyage; the revised ration included more vegetables, meat, and "condensed milk," and less rice. There were only 14 cases of beriberi and no deaths on the trip; the 14 men who were sick had refused to eat the meat and the milk. According to the original report, Takaki attributed the improvement to an increase in nitrogen. The experiment, reinterpreted in view of modern knowledge, really demonstrated that foods containing more thiamine protected the men against the deficiency disease beriberi.

The pioneering work of Dr. Edward B. Vedder in the Philippines around 1910, when he cured babies dying of beriberi by feeding them a rice bran extract, and the subsequent long quest for the active principle in rice bran make a fascinating story. It is well told by Dr. R. R. Williams in his book, *Toward the Conquest of Beriberi*.[14] This account of Dr. Williams' own 26-year search for what proved to be a vitamin, its identification, and its eventual synthesis is a classic in nutrition research.

Properties

Thiamine was synthesized by R. R. Williams in 1936 as a climax to his 26 years of interest in the subject. The pure vitamin, usually sold as thiamine hydrochloride (Fig. 7-4), has a yeasty taste and odor and is water-soluble. The natural and synthetic products are identical in physiologic activity. In the dry state thiamine hydrochloride is stable and is not easily destroyed by heat or oxidation. In water solution it is less stable, but in an acid medium it is more stable than it is in a neutral or an alkaline medium.

Measurement

Thiamine content of foods may be expressed in milligrams or micrograms (1 mg. = 1000 mcg.). Human requirements and potency of synthetic compounds or concentrates are expressed more often in milligrams.

Chemical and microbiologic methods of assay have largely replaced the older bioassay methods in which rats and pigeons were used as experimental animals. Now that these rapid methods of assay are available, extensive determinations of vitamin values of foods before and after storage and cooking are possible, and tables of food values include such figures.

Functions

Thiamine, as thiamine pyrophosphate (TPP or cocarboxylase), functions as a coenzyme in at least 24 enzyme systems. In carbohydrate metabolism (Chapter 9) thiamine is necessary for the oxidative decarboxylation (removal of CO_2) of pyruvate and α-ketoglutarate which are metabolized to acetyl coenzyme A and succinyl coenzyme A respectively. In thiamine deficiency pyruvic and alpha-ketoglutaric acids tend to accumulate in the body and have been measured as a means of determining thiamine nutriture. It should be pointed out, however, that the accumulation of these two metabolites in the tissues is not necessarily the cause of the clinical symptoms of thiamine deficiency, but that they represent a biochemical abnormality which is usually related to inadequate thiamine intakes.[15]

The enzyme transketolase also requires thiamine as a coenzyme. Present in red blood cells, liver, kidney, and other tissue, transketolase is necessary for the synthesis in the body of the five-carbon sugars, such as ribose, found in DNA, RNA, and other nucleotides. The transketolase activity of the red blood cell has also been determined as a means of measuring thiamine nutriture, since it is depressed when insufficient amounts of thiamine are present in the diet.[16]

Although there is no well-defined relationship at the present time between the biochemical abnormalities and the clinical manifestations which result from thiamine deficiency, several possibilities have been suggested[17]: failure to provide sufficient energy to the cell, failure to deliver a compound essential to the heart or nerves, or an accumulation of toxic substances.

Loss of appetite, constipation, irritability and fatigue are all symptoms that have been associated with low thiamine intakes. Changes in the central nervous system affecting peripheral nerves, eye-hand coordination and mental ability are found among chronic alcoholics who have inadequate intakes of thiamine. The various forms and symptoms of beriberi are discussed in Chapter 20.

Absorption, Storage, Excretion, and Synthesis

Thiamine is absorbed from the small intestine and undergoes phosphorylation in the intestinal mucosa. It is found in cells as thiamine monophosphate or pyrophosphate. Thiamine cannot be stored to any extent in the animal body, although certain tissues—heart, brain, liver, and kidney—tend to have higher concentrations than others. These amounts decrease quickly when thiamine is not supplied, so an adequate daily intake is important. When excess thiamine is supplied, it is excreted in the urine, thus

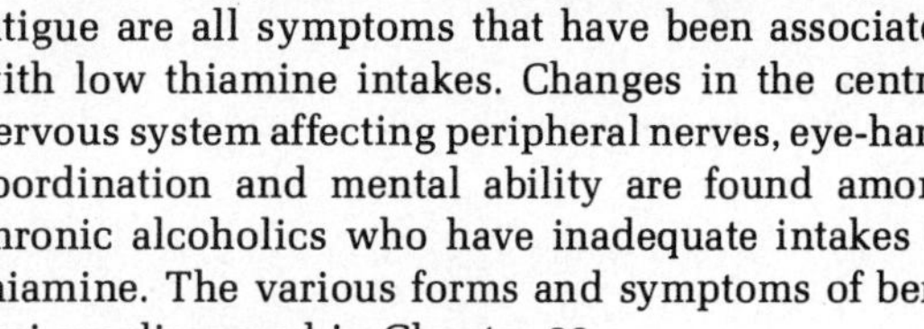

Fig. 7-4. Structural formula of thiamine.

providing another measure of the adequacy of thiamine intake.

Although some thiamine may be synthesized by bacterial action in the large intestine of humans, very little is believed to be absorbed.

Human Requirement

Since thiamine functions primarily in terms of carbohydrate metabolism, the recommended allowances suggested by both the Joint FAO/WHO Expert Committee and the National Research Council's Food and Nutrition Board are based on calorie levels. However, the FAO/WHO Expert Committee set the recommendation at 0.4 mg./1000 cal. while the Food and Nutrition Board recommends 0.5 mg./1000 cal. This latter figure indicates 1.4 mg. for the average male and 1.0 mg. for the female. An increase of 0.3 mg. over the allowance recommended for the nonpregnant woman is suggested for the pregnant woman during the last trimester and for the nursing mother. Recom-

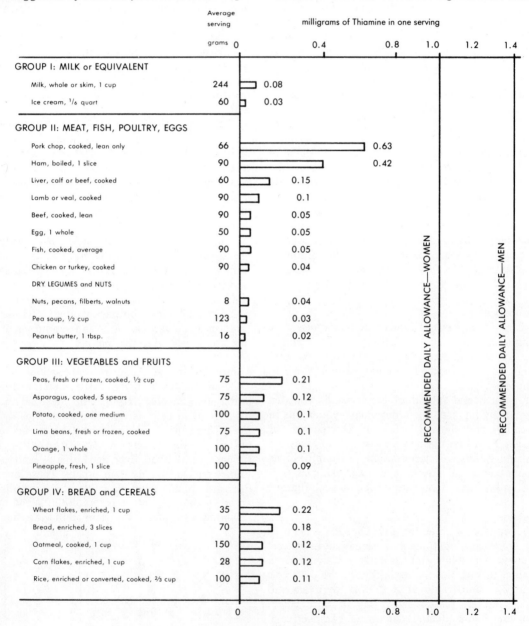

Fig. 7-5. Thiamine in average servings of foods classified in the four food groups.

mendations for infants and children are the same as for adults, 0.5 mg. of thiamine per 1000 cal. (see Chapter 10).

Food Sources

Thiamine is widely distributed in a large variety of animal and vegetable tissues, but there are few foods in which it occurs in abundance. This is strikingly emphasized in Fig. 7-5, which shows the thiamine content of average servings of some common foods. Obviously, several servings of even the better sources of thiamine are needed to meet the recommended allowance. Therefore, enrichment of bread and cereals was instigated to make it easier for the average person to meet his requirement economically. Since bread constitutes about one fifth of the calories in the average American diet, and since only a very small fraction of the bread consumed in this country is made from whole wheat, the enrichment of white flour and bread with thiamine, riboflavin, niacin, and iron was a logical step. On the basis of the average per capita consumption of flour and bread in the United States, as much as 35 percent of the daily thiamine requirement is now supplied by these foods. For more details about enriched flour and bread see Chapter 10.

Rice enrichment has been practiced for years in some of the rice-eating countries. The Rice Research Institute in the Philippines is working on the development of improved strains of rice and also on methods of enrichment, and much of the rice used in Japan is enriched.

Dry yeast and wheat germ are the richest natural sources of thiamine, but they are eaten only in relatively small amounts. Except for pork, which is outstanding, muscle meats contain less than the organs, such as liver, heart, and kidney. Fruits in general are poor sources of this vitamin.

Stability in Foods

The losses of thiamine in cooking depend on several factors, such as type of food, method of preparation, temperature, length of cooking, and the acidity or alkalinity of the cooking medium. Research indicates that on the whole fresh vegetables retain thiamine well during cooking. From a trace to 15 percent is dissolved in the cooking water, and up to 22 percent may be destroyed by cooking. If the cooking water is discarded, thiamine losses may be from 20 to 35 percent.

In acid foods this vitamin is quite stable, but its activity is destroyed rapidly by sulfite, a fact which may explain the loss of thiamine in dried fruits, such as apricots and peaches, treated with sulfur.

Thiamine is well retained in cereals, since they are generally cooked slowly and at a moderate temperature and the cooking water is used. Baked products lose about 15 percent of their original thiamine. Generally, the losses in cooking meat are greater than in cooking other foods, ranging from 25 to 50 percent of the raw value.

RIBOFLAVIN

The second member of the B complex—riboflavin—was recognized in the 1920s when it became evident that some growth-promoting properties of vitamin B were retained after heat had destroyed the antiberiberi properties. In 1932 the vitamin was identified as part of an enzyme and was synthesized in 1935.

Properties

Riboflavin (Fig. 7-6) in water solution has a yellow-green fluorescence. Although it is stable to heat, acid and oxidation, it is sensitive to alkali and in solution is easily destroyed by light. This vitamin always should be kept in dark bottles.

Measurement

The only reliable unit for riboflavin is the metric weight of the pure substance. Human requirements for this vitamin are expressed in milligrams and the amount in foods in milligrams or micrograms (1 mg. = 1000 mcg.).

Physical-chemical and microbiologic methods of assay are used for determining the riboflavin content of foods, tissues, etc.

Functions

Riboflavin functions as a part of a group of enzymes called flavoproteins which are involved in the metabolism of carbohydrates, fats and proteins. Flavin mononucleotide (FMN) and flavin adenine dinucleotide (FAD) are two important riboflavin-containing enzymes which catalyze oxidation-

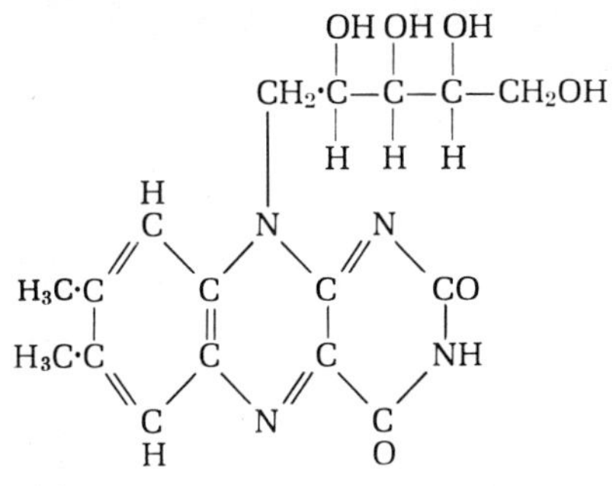

Fig. 7-6. Structural formula of riboflavin.

reduction reactions in the cells. As hydrogen carriers these enzymes transfer hydrogen from the niacin-containing enzymes to the iron-cytochrome system, after which the hydrogen is combined with oxygen to form water. Thus riboflavin is essential for the release of energy within the cell (Chapter 9.)

Since riboflavin takes part in a number of chemical reactions within the body, it is essential for normal tissue maintenance. Deficiency of riboflavin causes damage to a variety of different types of tissues. It has been demonstrated that riboflavin deficiency in man may be characterized by pallor of the mucous membrane of the lips and splitting of the lips at the angles of the mouth, a condition known as cheilosis.

Riboflavin also plays an important role in the health of the eye. Ocular symptoms appear consistently on a low riboflavin diet and may precede all other manifestations. Eye strain and fatigue, itching and burning, sensitivity to light, and frontal headaches are the most frequent complaints. Cataracts have been observed in rats, mice, chickens, and monkeys after prolonged deficiency of riboflavin. Riboflavin deficiency has also been shown to lead to adrenal cortex dysfunction in humans.[18] Recently erythrocyte glutathione reductase (EGR) activity has also been shown to be indicative of riboflavin status.[19] In man, riboflavin deficiency is apt to occur along with a deficiency of other members of the B complex.

Absorption, Storage, and Excretion

Riboflavin is absorbed through the walls of the small intestines where it is phosphorylated before entering the bloodstream. It is carried to the tissues of the body and incorporated into cellular enzymes. There is no great storage capacity in the body for this vitamin. It has been suggested that under stress the body can conserve its store of riboflavin much better than it can conserve thiamine. The excess riboflavin is excreted in the urine and urinary levels of riboflavin are used to assess riboflavin status in the body.

Human Requirement

The Food and Nutrition Board of the National Research Council has set the recommended dietary allowance for riboflavin at 0.6 mg. per 1000 cal. or 1.6 mg. for the average 23- to 50-year-old male and 1.2 mg. for the average 23- to 50-year-old female. An increment of 0.3 mg. per day for pregnancy and 0.5 mg. per day for lactation is suggested. The recommended dietary allowance for infants and children is also 0.6 mg. per 1000 cal. The actual recommendation for each age and sex group is given in Chapter 10.

The Joint FAO/WHO Expert Committee set the riboflavin recommendation at 0.55 mg. per 1000 calories for all age groups.

Food Sources

Riboflavin is widely distributed in animal and vegetable foods, but only in small amounts in most of them. Organ meats, milk, and green leafy vegetables are the outstanding food sources. This is strikingly emphasized in Fig. 7-7, which shows the riboflavin content of average servings of some common foods and the contribution they make toward the day's requirement.

The average person is not apt to get an optimum amount of riboflavin unless he consumes a generous amount of milk. The addition of riboflavin in the enrichment of flour and bread has helped to raise the average intake.

Stability in Foods

Riboflavin is stable to ordinary cooking processes but unstable in alkaline solutions. It is stable in milk—an important source—if the milk is distributed in cartons or dark bottles or otherwise protected from light. One half or more of the riboflavin in milk may be lost in two hours if exposed to light.

NIACIN

When Elvehjem reported the spectacular cure of blacktongue in dogs by means of nicotinic acid, now known as niacin, the logical supposition was that a niacin deficiency might be the cause of pellagra in humans. Later, Spies and others demonstrated that most of the classic symptoms of pellagra were relieved by the administration of niacin. However, most persons suffering from pellagra have multiple deficiencies, and it has been found that certain symptoms formerly associated with the disease are not relieved until thiamine and riboflavin are supplied along with niacin. Earlier concepts which related pellagra to a protein deficiency have been clarified by the discovery that one of the amino acids—tryptophan—is a precursor from which niacin may be synthesized in the animal body. Human pellagra is discussed fully in Chapter 20.

Properties

Nicotinic acid had long been known as a simple organic compound, but its physiologic properties were not realized until it was isolated from potent liver concentrates by Elvehjem and associates in 1937. In the dry state it is a very stable compound, and, unlike some other members of the B complex, it is even stable to alkali. Nicotinic acid is commonly called niacin to avoid confusion, because it has none of the physiologic properties of nicotine found in tobacco.

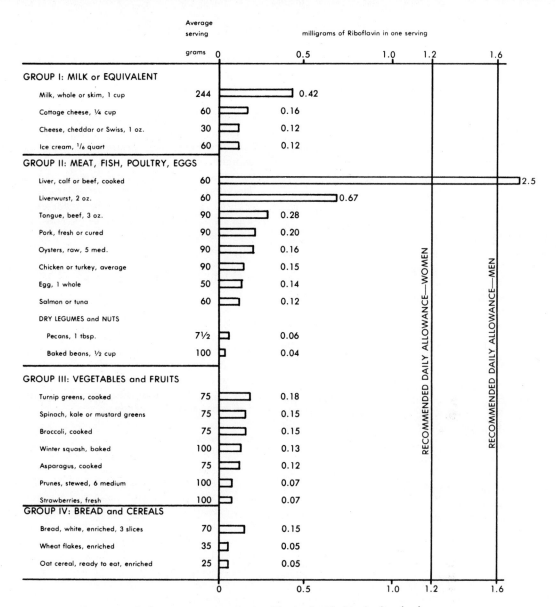

	Average serving grams	milligrams of Riboflavin in one serving

GROUP I: MILK or EQUIVALENT

Food	grams	mg
Milk, whole or skim, 1 cup	244	0.42
Cottage cheese, ¼ cup	60	0.16
Cheese, cheddar or Swiss, 1 oz.	30	0.12
Ice cream, ⅙ quart	60	0.12

GROUP II: MEAT, FISH, POULTRY, EGGS

Food	grams	mg
Liver, calf or beef, cooked	60	2.5
Liverwurst, 2 oz.	60	0.67
Tongue, beef, 3 oz.	90	0.28
Pork, fresh or cured	90	0.20
Oysters, raw, 5 med.	90	0.16
Chicken or turkey, average	90	0.15
Egg, 1 whole	50	0.14
Salmon or tuna	60	0.12
DRY LEGUMES and NUTS		
Pecans, 1 tbsp.	7½	0.06
Baked beans, ½ cup	100	0.04

GROUP III: VEGETABLES and FRUITS

Food	grams	mg
Turnip greens, cooked	75	0.18
Spinach, kale or mustard greens	75	0.15
Broccoli, cooked	75	0.15
Winter squash, baked	100	0.13
Asparagus, cooked	75	0.12
Prunes, stewed, 6 medium	100	0.07
Strawberries, fresh	100	0.07

GROUP IV: BREAD and CEREALS

Food	grams	mg
Bread, white, enriched, 3 slices	70	0.15
Wheat flakes, enriched	35	0.05
Oat cereal, ready to eat, enriched	25	0.05

RECOMMENDED DAILY ALLOWANCE—WOMEN (1.2)
RECOMMENDED DAILY ALLOWANCE—MEN (1.6)

Fig. 7-7. Riboflavin in average servings of foods classified in the four food groups.

Two forms of this vitamin—*niacin* (nicotinic acid) and *niacinamide* (nicotinamide) (Fig. 7-8)—have antipellagra activity. Therapeutic doses of nicotinic acid may cause temporary flushing or hot flashes, but niacinamide does not produce this reaction.

Measurement

Niacin in foods and niacin requirement are both expressed in milligrams of the pure chemical substance.

Chemical and microbiologic methods for niacin assay are now used generally in place of animal as-says. Dogs were the only animals with which early bio-assays could be made, and such tests were based on the blacktongue-preventing value.

Functions

Niacin, like thiamine and riboflavin, also functions as a coenzyme in energy metabolism. It is part of the enzymes NAD (nicotinamide adenine dinucleotide) and NADP (nicotinamide adenine dinucleotide phosphate), which are hydrogen carriers essential in the release of energy from carbohydrates, fats, and protein. These niacin-containing enzymes

Niacin (Nicotinic acid)   Niacinamide (Nicotinamide)

Fig. 7-8. Structural formulas of niacin and niacinamide.

transfer hydrogen from the oxidizable material (i.e., carbohydrate) to the riboflavin-containing enzymes (see Functions of Riboflavin). They are also involved in the synthesis of proteins and fats. Hence a variety of tissues, including the skin, the gastrointestinal tract, and the nervous system, are affected by niacin deficiency. (See Pellagra, Chapter 20.)

Large doses of niacin (100 to 200 times the recommended allowance) administered orally have resulted in the lowering of serum cholesterol and beta-lipoprotein levels. The mechanism of this action is not understood, and only the acid form is effective, not the amide. Undesirable effects of large doses of niacin on the metabolism of the heart muscle have been observed, however, which indicate that massive doses of this vitamin could be dangerous before prolonged physical exercise. In human subjects, intravenously administered niacin caused the depletion of cardiac muscle glycogen and endogenous lipid because the use of free fatty acids from the blood as an energy source was inhibited.[20] In addition, Winter and Boyer recently reported a case history in which large doses of nicotinamide (3 to 9 g.) taken in the treatment of schizophrenia caused liver toxicity. Thus this vitamin is not an innocuous therapeutic agent.[21]

Relationship of Tryptophan to Niacin

The amino acid tryptophan can be converted to niacin in the body. Research studies have indicated that approximately 60 mg. of tryptophan are equivalent to 1 mg. of niacin. Animal and vegetable protein contain about 1.4 percent and 1 percent of tryptophan, respectively. Table 7-2 illustrates how an approximate amount of niacin can be calculated from protein. Total niacin equals the preformed niacin

Table 7-2. Approximate Calculation of Niacin from Tryptophan

Dietary protein	60 g.
Tryptophan content 1% (approx.)	_0.01_
Tryptophan	0.60 g. or 600 mg.
60 mg. of tryptophan = 1 mg. of niacin ...	600 ÷ 60 = 10
Niacin converted from tryptophan	10 mg.

plus the niacin available from protein. A recent review [22] points out that the accepted ratio of 60:1 is not applicable under a variety of conditions, such as fasting, pregnancy, and drastically reduced intakes of niacin or tryptophan.

Recommended Dietary Allowances

Both the Food and Nutrition Board and the Joint FAO/WHO Expert Committee have established the recommended dietary allowance for niacin at 6.6 mg. per 1000 calories for all age groups. Depending on calorie intake, the 1974 NRC-RDA for adult males is from 16 to 20 mg. of niacin daily and for adult females 12 to 14 mg. daily. An increase of 2 mg. and 4 mg., respectively, above the allowance for the nonpregnant woman is recommended during pregnancy and lactation by the Food and Nutrition Board. Infants and children follow the same recommendations as adults.

Storage and Excretion

Little is known regarding the extent of storage of niacin in the body, but it is probably stored in the liver. It is eliminated in the urine largely as derivatives and, to a smaller extent, as free niacin. This diversity of end products has added to the difficulties of metabolic studies of niacin.

Food Sources

In general, meat, poultry and fish are better sources of niacin than plant products, as emphasized in Fig. 7-9, showing average servings. The use of meat drippings is recommended, because niacin is easily dissolved out of foods in cooking. Whole grain and enriched products also make a contribution. A bound form of niacin, i.e., niacytin, in wheat, corn, and rye bran is unavailable to humans.[23] Fruits and vegetables (other than mushrooms and legumes) are insignificant sources of niacin. Milk and eggs are poor sources of preformed niacin but good sources of its precursor tryptophan.

When the listed niacin content of foods in a diet fails to meet the niacin recommendations, one may calculate the approximate amount available from tryptophan (Table 7-2). In the average diet in the United States, with adequate amounts of protein, the niacin value may be increased by one third or more.

VITAMIN B₆ GROUP

Pyridoxine was identified in 1938 as a separate fraction of the B complex. Subsequently, vitamin B_6 proved to be a complex of three closely related chemical compounds—*pyridoxine, pyridoxal,* and *pyridoxamine* (Fig. 7-10)—all of which are active

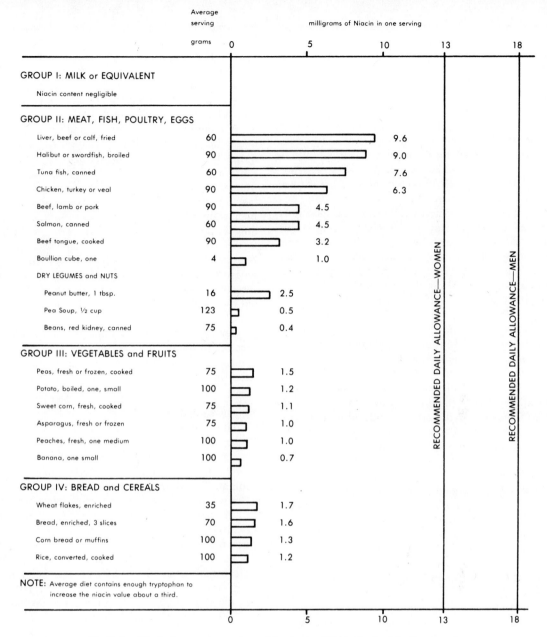

Fig. 7-9. Niacin in average servings of foods classified in the four food groups.

physiologically. The need for this factor was first demonstrated in rats, but it is now established that it is required by most animals. A deficiency is associated with a peculiar type of anemia in some species and extreme muscular weakness, dermatitis, and nervous disorders in others. Vitamin B_6 can be synthesized by intestinal organisms in the rat, but whether or not this is true in humans has not been established.

The need for and the function of vitamin B_6 in humans has been demonstrated conclusively in both adults and infants. The accidental destruction of this factor in a canned-milk formula resulted in the oc-

Fig. 7-10. Structural formulas of vitamin B_6 compounds.

currence of nervous irritability and convulsive seizures in young infants.[24] Rapid recovery followed injection of the vitamin, proving conclusively that the symptoms noted were the result of a deficiency.

Functions

The mechanism of the action of pyridoxine and its several analogues is associated closely with the synthesis and metabolism of amino acids. Pyridoxal phosphate (PALP), the coenzyme form of vitamin B_6, is necessary for transamination, the process by which the amino group (NH_2) from one amino acid is transferred to another to produce a different amino acid needed for protein synthesis. The transaminase activity (B_6-containing enzymes catalyzing transamination) of the blood can be measured as a means of assessing vitamin B_6 status.[25] Glutamic oxaloacetic acid transaminase (GOT) and glutamic pyruvic acid transaminase (GPT) are the transaminases most frequently used.

PALP-containing enzymes are also involved in decarboxylation and desulfuration (removal of CO_2 and H_2S groups) of amino acids. Chemical changes in the central nervous system, i.e., formation of serotonin from tryptophan and gamma aminobutyric acid from glutamic acid, require vitamin B_6-dependent decarboxylases. Vitamin B_6 is also essential in the synthesis of porphyrin. Certain dehydratases, racemases, transferases, hydroxylases, and synthetases also require pyridoxal-5-phosphate as a cofactor.[26]

The conversion of tryptophan to niacin requires vitamin B_6. If a large dose of tryptophan (Tryptophan Load Test) is administered to an individual with a pyridoxine deficiency, an intermediary product in the conversion—xanthurenic acid—accumulates and can be measured in the urine. When vitamin B_6 is present in adequate amounts, more nicotinic acid is formed and xanthurenic acid excretion is not increased. Folic acid metabolism is also dependent on pyridoxine-containing enzymes.

Coursin[27], in discussing several different aspects of vitamin B_6 deficiency in man, points out that in extreme cases of deficiency there have been clearcut symptoms of anemia, oxalate stone formation, or central nervous system abnormalities. In addition, consideration must be given to what appear to be suboptimal intakes by some people, as well as the increased needs of pregnant females and those taking steroid birth control pills.

An increase in the activity of inactivating enzymes (proteases) which split the peptide chains of vitamin B_6 dependent apoenzymes has been found in pyridoxine deficient rats. It has been theorized that, by reducing the level of certain apoenzymes in some tissues, the vitamin (coenzyme) is thus made available for more important enzyme functions. This finding is supported by the fact that the inactivating enzymes are found in intestine and skeletal muscle but not in heart, liver, or brain.[28]

A vitamin B_6 Dependency Syndrome of genetic origin has been identified in which the patient requires large amounts of the vitamin to prevent convulsive seizures and mental retardation. Similar deficiencies of other B_6-dependent enzymes have also been identified where only massive doses of the vitamin facilitated enzyme activity.[29] A deficiency of vitamin B_6 has been shown to influence the ability of rats to metabolize monosodium glutamate (MSG), implying that the amount of MSG required for toxicity would be decreased in pyridoxine deficiency.[30] Much research work is focusing on this vitamin at the present time and we can soon expect a better understanding of its role in nutrition.

Several antagonists function as binding agents to inactivate vitamin B_6. These include izoniazid (INH), a drug used in tuberculosis therapy, and penicillamine, used in treatment of Wilson's disease (Chapter 32).

Human Requirements

The National Research Council's Recommended Dietary Allowances for vitamin B_6 was set at 2.0 mg. per day for adults. This would provide a margin of safety and permit an intake of 100 gm. or more of protein. The allowance for pregnancy and lactation is 2.5 mg. per day. In infancy the requirement is related to the amount of protein in the milk. The ratio of vitamin B_6 to protein may be critically low in both human milk and cow's milk. Hence, the early introduction of solid foods containing vitamin B_6 is beneficial for the infant not receiving commercial formula supplemented with this vitamin. A complete list of the recommended dietary allowances for each age and sex group is given in Chapter 10.

Food Sources

Of the animal foods, pork and the glandular meats are the richest, with lamb and veal relatively better than fish or beef muscle. Considerable losses of vitamin B_6 occur during cooking. Milk and eggs are only fair sources. Of the plant foods, legumes, potatoes, oatmeal, wheat germ, and bananas are the richest, with cabbages, carrots, and other vegetables providing fair amounts. The B_6 content of foods is determined by a microbiologic method.

FOLACIN (FOLIC ACID)

Folic acid was recognized as a dietary essential for chicks in 1938 and was later shown to be a requirement of other animals. Folacin was first used clinically in 1945 by Spies, who showed it to be effective in the treatment of macrocytic anemias of pregnancy and tropical sprue, and these findings have since been confirmed.

Folic acid (pteroylglutamic acid, PGA) is not found as such in foods or in the human body (Fig. 7–11). It occurs in food chiefly as polyglutamates and as 5 methyl tetrahydrofolate (N⁵methyl THF). The body converts these to biologically active or enzyme forms of the vitamin. Folinic acid (N⁵formyl THFA) or "citrovorum factor" is one of these biologically active forms.

Functions

The major role of the enzymatically active forms of folacin is in the transfer of one-carbon units to various compounds in the synthesis of the purines and pyrimadines of DNA and RNA, and in amino acid interconversions.[31]

The amino acid histidine requires folic acid for its complete utilization. When folic acid is not available, the intermediary product, formiminoglutamic acid (FIGLU), is excreted in the urine. FIGLU excretion levels can then be used to determine folic acid nutritional status.

Folic acid deficiency in man results in megaloblastic anemia, glossitis, and gastrointestinal disturbances. Because of the interdependence of vitamins B_{12}, B_6, ascorbic acid, and folic acid, the anemia found in these deficiency diseases may be similar and may respond to treatment with one or several of these nutrients. It should be pointed out, however, that even though the anemia in pernicious anemia may be relieved by folic acid, only vitamin B_{12} cures the neurologic symptoms (see Chapter 33).

Absorption, Excretion, and Storage

Folic acid may be absorbed along the entire length of the small intestine; however, there is evidence that the jejunum is the primary site for active absorption. In addition to active energy-dependent absorption, folate also appears to be absorbed by passive diffusion. Much of the vitamin occurs in the diet in the form of polyglutamates. Before it can be absorbed excess glutamates must be removed from the side chain of the molecule by conjugases found in intestinal lumen or the cell wall.[32] The absorption of folic acid is thus controlled by the deconjugating

mechanism which may in turn be affected by conjugase inhibitors in food, i.e., yeast. The rate of absorption of conjugated folates appears to be related to the chain length.[33]

Folate, bound to a protein, is transported in the blood to bone marrow cells, reticulocytes, and perhaps other cells. Methyl-folate seems to be the chief form of the vitamin in body tissues. About half of the folic acid stored in the body is in the liver. Some folate is excreted in the bile as well as the urine. Serum levels of folacin range from 7 to 16 nanograms (1 ng. = 10^{-9} gram) per ml. of serum.

The questions of both primary (dietary) and secondary folic acid deficiency have been raised. In the case of the latter, numerous possible causes have been cited: failure to absorb dietary folate; increased urinary excretion of folic acid; increased folate destruction; interference in the synthesis or activation of enzymes necessary for folate utilization; and production of anti-folates.[34]

Human Requirement

The adult recommended dietary allowance for folacin is 400 mcg. per day. Because of the increased needs of the fetus, the allowance for pregnancy was set at 800 mcg. per day; 600 mcg. is the RDA for lactation. The infant allowance is 50 mcg. per day for the first year, at which time it is increased to 100 mcg. per day until four years of age. The recommendation for folic acid from four to six years is 200 mcg. per day; from seven to ten years it is 300 mcg. per day. The adult recommendation (400 mcg.) starts at 11 years of age and is continued throughout life for both sexes.

The Joint FAO/WHO Expert Group set 200 mcg. as the adult (over 12 years of age) allowance. It is increased to 400 mcg. for pregnancy and 300 mcg. for lactation. The recommended intake for infants 0–6 months is 40 mcg., 7–12 months 60 mcg. From one through 12 years 100 mcg. is the recommendation.[35]

Chung et al found that high-cost and low-cost diets averaged 193 and 157 mcg. of total folic acid activity respectively. A total folic acid content of 150 mcg. which should supply at least 50 mcg. of active folic acid, is considered adequate. However, the ac-

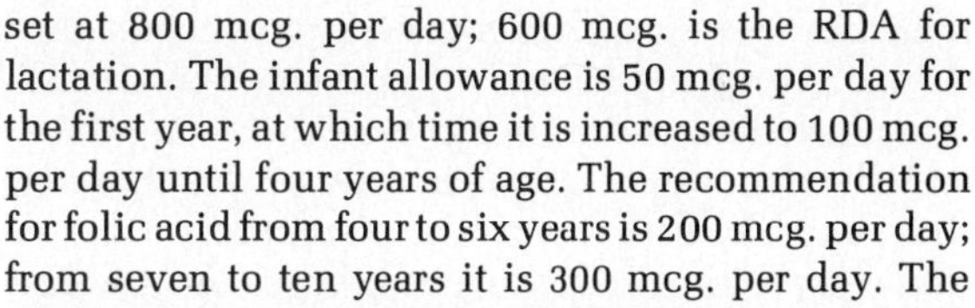

Folic acid (Pteroylglutamic acid)

Fig. 7–11. Structural formula of folacin.

tual amount of folacin in foods that is available for absorption has not been well established. (See Food Sources.) Therefore, the NRC-RDA has included a large margin of safety for this nutrient.

Because more than 100 mcg. of folic acid per day may prevent anemia but not cure the neurological symptoms of pernicious anemia, vitamin preparations which contain more than 100 mcg. of folic acid cannot be sold without prescription.

Patients receiving anticonvulsant therapy have significantly lower levels of folic acid in serum and cerebrospinal fluid than normal individuals. Administration of folic acid to these patients causes the serum level of the anticonvulsant drug to fall but does not increase the folate level in cerebrospinal fluid. Therefore, although folic acid therapy does not seem to reduce control of seizures, continued study of this therapy is important.[36] Similarly, there is no agreement regarding the reason for the folic acid deficiency reported in women using oral contraceptive agents (OCA).[37]

Food Sources

The presence of this group of factors in green leaves was the basis for the name folacin (folium, meaning leaf). In addition to their presence in green leaves, these factors are found in liver, meats and fish, nuts, legumes, and whole grains.

The availability of folacin from foodstuffs varies. In a recent study the percent of folate absorbed ranged from 92 percent for frozen lima beans to 25 percent in lettuce. Only 31 percent of the folate in orange juice was absorbed as compared with 82 percent from bananas.

Many of the folates in food are easily destroyed by storing, cooking, and other processing. Because of the destruction of folic acid activity in dried milk, it has been suggested that ascorbic acid be added as a preservative to the milk before processing.[38]

VITAMIN B_{12}

Ever since the discovery that liver is effective in the treatment of pernicious anemia, research workers have been hunting for the active principle, or "extrinsic" factor, in liver. At first it seemed that folic acid was the answer, but it proved to be ineffective in relieving many of the symptoms of the disease. In 1948 a more active substance, B_{12}, isolated from liver, was found to be effective in microgram quantites in the therapy of pernicious anemia as well as in other types of macrocytic anemias. Thus, vitamin B_{12} is probably identical with Castle's "extrinsic" factor. Its

oral effectiveness is enhanced by the "intrinsic" factor found in normal gastric juice, as was true of the active factor in liver extracts. The "intrinsic" factor is essential for the absorption of vitamin B_{12}. Pernicious anemia is discussed further in Chapter 33.

The suggestion that vitamin B_{12} may act as a growth factor for children as it does for poultry, pigs, and ruminants has not been well confirmed. The natural variation in the growth of children is so great that the relatively small effect of B_{12} is difficult to demonstrate. Furthermore, there is no evidence of a widespread deficiency of this factor among American children.

Hodgkin, the 1964 Nobel Prize winner in chemistry, and her coworkers delineated the structural formula of the vitamin (Fig. 7-12).

Properties

The structure of vitamin B_{12} was established as an extremely complex nitrogenous compound containing two major portions, the corrin nucleus (which includes cobalt) and the attached nucleotide. Active forms of this vitamin are cyanocobalamin (vitamin B_{12}), hydroxocobalamin (vitamin B_{12a}), aquacobalamin (vitamin B_{12b}), and nitritocobalamin (vitamin B_{12c}) (Fig. 7-12).

Vitamin B_{12} coenzymes are called cobamides. Cobalt, long known as a trace element essential for some animals, never before had been found in a natural organic compound.

Vitamin B_{12} is remarkably potent. It has a biologic activity 11,000 times that of a standard liver concentrate formerly used in the treatment of pernicious anemia. Thus B_{12} appears to be one of the most potent biologically active substances known. It has been administered therapeutically in doses of from 6 to 150 mcg. Comparative effects with folic acid in other types of anemia require doses of from 20,000 to 50,000 mcg.

Functions

Vitamin B_{12} functions as a coenzyme (5'-deoxyadenosyl cobalamin or methyl-cobalamin) in various chemical reactions in the cell. It is particularly important in the bone marrow where the red blood cells are formed and in nerve tissue. The synthesis of nucleic acids and hence of DNA depends on B_{12}-containing enzymes. Cobamides are thus involved in folic acid metabolism. The megaloblastic anemia which occurs in vitamin B_{12} deficiency is caused by defective cell division due to impaired DNA synthesis,[39] whereas the neurological damage appears to be related to increased levels in the nerv-

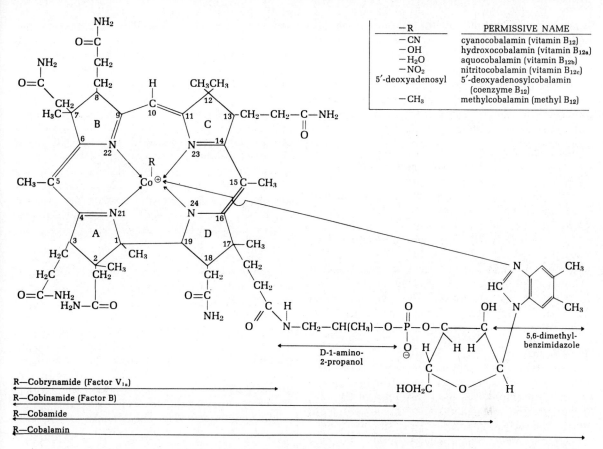

−R	PERMISSIVE NAME
− CN	cyanocobalamin (vitamin B_{12})
− OH	hydroxocobalamin (vitamin B_{12a})
− H_2O	aquocobalamin (vitamin B_{12b})
− NO_2	nitritocobalamin (vitamin B_{12c})
5′-deoxyadenosyl	5′-deoxyadenosylcobalamin (coenzyme B_{12})
− CH_3	methylcobalamin (methyl B_{12})

Fig. 7–12. Structural formula of vitamin B_{12} (cyanocobalamin). The numbering system for the corrin nucleus is made to correspond to that of the porphin nucleus by omitting the number 20. (Modified from Brown and Reynolds, Biogenesis of water-soluble vitamins. Annual Review of Biochemistry 32:419, 1963, by Herbert, V., Folic acid and vitamin B_{12}, in *Modern Nutrition in Health and Disease*, ed. 5, R.S. Goodhart and M.E. Shils, eds. Philadelphia, Lea and Febiger, 1973)

ous system of branched chain fatty acids such as methylmalonic acid and its precursor propionic acid as well as odd numbered fatty acids, C-15 and C-17.[40]

A diagnostic test for the determination of vitamin-B_{12} deficiency depends on the role of B_{12} in the metabolism of certain fatty acids. Methylmalonic acid (MMA), which requires vitamin B_{12} for its breakdown to succinic acid, is excreted in the urine of individuals deficient in vitamin B_{12} and can be measured to assess B_{12} adequacy.[41]

Absorption, Transport, and Storage

Since vitamin B_{12} has the largest and, probably, the most complicated molecule of any of the water-soluble nutrients, it is not surprising that its deficiency is caused more frequently by problems of absorption than by dietary inadequacy. Of equal interest is the fact that its active absorption requires the presence in the gastric secretions of an even larger molecule, a mucoprotein called Castle's "intrinsic factor" (IF). The B_{12}-IF complex forms in the stomach and passes through the upper part of the small intestine to the ileum, where the IF attaches itself to the epithelial cells specific to this area of the gut and thereby facilitates the transfer of vitamin B_{12} into the ileal epithelium. Calcium is also necessary for this transfer. Three hours are required for the transport of B_{12}, whereas only seconds are required for most water-soluble compounds. Since the IF is not found in lymph or plasma, it must remain in the intestinal tract.[42] Passive absorption by simple diffusion can account for a limited amount (1 to 3 percent) of absorption.

When cobalamin is released into the bloodstream, it is attached to another protein (transcobalamin II) and carried to the various tissues. Protein-bound vitamin B_{12} not immediately needed is stored in the liver, which is capable of storing relatively large amounts of this nutrient. As the quantity of the vitamin increases in the diet, the percent absorbed decreases. Serum levels of vitamin B_{12} range from 200 to 700 picograms (1 pg = 10^{-12} grams per ml.).

Although 1 to 3 percent of very large therapeutic doses of B_{12} given to pernicious anemia patients may be absorbed by simple diffusion, vitamin B_{12} usually must be administered parenterally.

Human Requirement

The Food and Nutrition Board recommends 3 mcg. vitamin B_{12} per day for adults. The allowance during pregnancy and lactation is 4 mcg. per day. (See Chapter 10 for a complete list of recommendations for each age and sex category.)

The Joint FAO/WHO Expert Group recommend 2 mcg. per day for the adult (over ten years of age). This allowance is increased to 3 mcg. for the pregnant woman and 2.5 mcg. for the nursing mother.

Pernicious anemia patients who have been treated to replenish their stores will meet their body needs with 1.5 mg. B_{12} daily, given parenterally.

Food Sources

In surveys of typical diets the remarkable difference between adequate and poor diets in the vitamin B_{12} content emphasizes the importance of the contribution made by meats and other animal products to the B_{12} intake. Dietary deficiencies of vitamin B_{12} have been found among vegans when no animal foods are consumed.

Seafoods, meats, eggs, and dairy products are all sources of vitamin B_{12}. Foods of vegetable origin do not contain vitamin B_{12} unless they are added in enrichment.

PANTOTHENIC ACID

Pantothenic acid (Fig. 7-13) is another of the vitamin B complex group first recognized as essential for rats, dogs, pigs, pigeons and chicks. The complete synthesis of pantothenic acid was accomplished in 1940. A deficiency has been reported to cause emaciation, loss of hair and graying of hair in dark animals, ulcers of the intestinal tract, and damage to several internal organs.

Functions

Pantothenic acid is a part of coenzyme A which plays a basic role in metabolism—in the release of

$$CH_2-\underset{\underset{HO}{|}}{\overset{\overset{CH_3}{|}}{C}}-CH-\overset{\overset{O}{\parallel}}{C}-NH-CH_2-CH_2-COOH$$

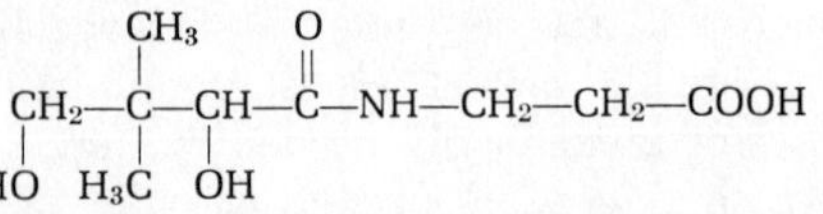

Fig. 7–13. Structural formula of pantothenic acid.

energy from carbohydrates, fats, and proteins, and also in the synthesis of amino acids, fatty acids, sterols, and steroid hormones. It is also essential for the formation of porphyrin, the pigment portion of the hemoglobin molecule.

Human Requirement

A definite dietary requirement for pantothenic acid has not been established. In a survey by Chung et al,[43] it was found that pantothenic acid activity of high-cost diets averaged 16.3 mg. per day and for the poorest diets, 6.0 mg. per day. These workers estimate that the average American diet provides from 10 to 20 mg. per day, which is liberal in terms of the estimated need of from 5 to 10 mg. per day.

Food Sources

The word *pantothenic*, meaning widespread, indicates that the distribution of this vitamin is extensive. Figures on the pantothenic acid content of foods are limited in number. Yeast, liver, kidney, heart, salmon, and eggs are the best sources. Other good sources are broccoli, mushrooms, pork, beef tongue, peanuts, wheat, rye, and soybean flour. About one half of the pantothenic acid is lost in the milling of grains, which constitute an important, if not a rich, source of this factor in the average diet. Fruits are relatively poor sources of this vitamin.

BIOTIN

Biotin (Fig. 7-14), another member of the vitamin B complex, was first isolated in 1936 as a growth essential for yeast cells. Previous to this date numerous workers had described factors called by various names but having similar antidermatitis properties in experimental animals. These several factors proved to be identical and are now known as biotin. Investigations have shown that a biotin deficiency can be produced in rats, rabbits, and monkeys by feeding them a substance called avidin found in raw egg white. Avidin inactivates biotin and is known as an antivitamin.

Biotin deficiency has been recognized in man only when diets have included large amounts of raw egg white. Intestinal synthesis of biotin is common in most animals and probably in man.

Functions

Biotin plays an essential role as a coenzyme in CO_2 fixation; fatty acid synthesis, for instance, requires a biotin-containing enzyme (acetyl-CoA carboxylase) to form malonyl coenzyme A from acetyl coenzyme A.

The role of biotin in protein and carbohydrate

metabolism is less clear, and its relationship to the synthesis of transfer RNA (Chapter 9) also needs further elucidation.

There is also some evidence that biotin is necessary for the utilization of vitamin B_{12} and that, like folic acid, it participates in one-carbon metabolism.[44]

Biotin deficiency results in lassitude, anorexia, depression, malaise, muscle pain, nausea, anemia, hypercholesterolemia, and changes in the electrocardiogram.

Human Requirement

Most American diets contain 150 to 3000 mcg. of biotin per day, which is entirely adequate for good health. Synthesis by intestinal microflora seems to provide a major source of this vitamin.

Food Sources

Few foods have been analyzed for this factor. It is abundant in liver and other organs, in mushrooms, and in peanuts. Lesser amounts occur in milk, eggs, and certain vegetables and fruits.

OTHER B-COMPLEX FACTORS

PARA-AMINOBENZOIC ACID (PABA) is a moiety of pteroylmonoglutamic acid (PGA), one of the forms of folic acid, and is no longer considered a vitamin. *INOSITOL* was first considered to be a vitamin in 1940 but there is no evidence today that humans cannot synthesize all that is needed by the body. *CHOLINE AND BETAINE.* The classification of these two nitrogenous compounds as vitamins is questioned by some. They are structural components of body cells rather than catalysts. Choline occurs in foods as well as in the body in relatively large amounts and has never been associated with a deficiency disease in man. The body can make choline from methionine, an amino acid, with the aid of vitamin B_{12} and folacin. The action of choline, betaine or methionine in the prevention of "fatty livers" is known as lipotropic (fat moving). Choline is distributed widely in plant and animal tissues, and a deficiency is not likely in the average diet. Betaine is formed by the oxidation of choline.

VITAMINS IN PATTERN DIETARY FOR ONE DAY

The contribution made by the Pattern Dietary (see Table 7-3) to the five vitamins for which we have specific recommendations and appropriate food composition tables is given in the accompanying table. Since the pattern dietary provides only 1400 calories, the foods chosen to supplement this will provide additional vitamins to bring the totals up to recommended allowances.

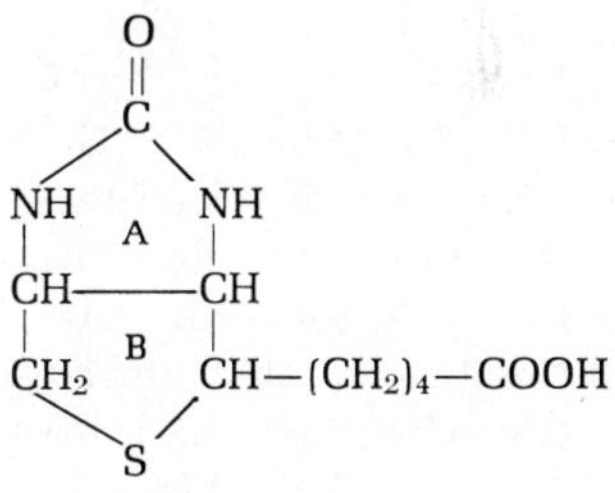

Fig. 7-14. Structural formula of biotin.

Table 7-3. Vitamins in Pattern Dietary For 1 Day*

FOOD GROUP	AMOUNT IN g.	HOUSEHOLD MEASURE	ENER-GY Kcal.	VITA-MIN A IU	THIA-MINE mg.	RIBO-FLAVIN mg.	NIACIN mg	ASCORBIC ACID mg.
Milk or equivalent	488	2 c.	320	700	.16	.84	.3	5
Meat, fish, poultry, egg	120	4 oz. cooked	376	280	.14	.23	6.1	..
Vegetables:								
Potato	100	1 medium	65	..	.09	.03	1.2	16
Green or yellow	75	1 serving	21	4700	.05	.10	.5	25
Other	75	1 serving	45	300	.08	.06	.6	12
Fruits:								
Citrus	100	1 serving	44	140	.06	.02	.3	43
Other	100	1 serving	85	365	.03	.04	.5	4
Bread, white enriched	100	4 slices	270	..	.25	.21	2.4	..
Cereal, whole grain or enriched ...	30	1 oz. dry or						
	130	⅔ c. cooked	89	..	.08	.03	.7	..
Butter or margarine.............	14	1 tbsp.	100	460	..	..	..	..
		Totals.............	1415	6945	.94	1.56	12.6	105

*For basis of calculation, see Pattern Dietary in Chapter 10.

Table 7–4. Water-Soluble Vitamins

	C	FRACTIONS OF THE VITAMIN B COMPLEX		
	Ascorbic Acid	Thiamine	Riboflavin	Niacin

Important food sources	Citrus fruits
	Strawberries
	Cantaloupe
	Tomatoes
	Sweet peppers
	Cabbage
	Potatoes
	Kale, parsley
	Turnip greens
		Pork
		Liver
		Organ meats
		Whole grains
		Enriched cereal
		  products
		Nuts
		Legumes
		Potatoes
			Liver, milk
			Meat, eggs
			Enriched cereal
			  products
			Green, leafy
			  vegetables
				Liver, poultry
				Meat, fish
				Whole grains
				Enriched cereal
				  products
				Legumes
				Mushrooms

Stability to cooking, drying, light, etc.	Unstable to heat and oxidation, except in acids Destroyed by drying and aging	Unstable to heat and oxidation	Stable to heat in cooking, to acids and oxidation Unstable to light	Stable to heat, light, and oxidation, acid and alkali
Function: Essential in	Formation of intercellular substance, cellular oxidation, and reduction	Carbohydrate metabolism, coenzyme form cocarboxylase TPP	Carbohydrate, fat and protein metabolism, coenzyme forms FMN and FAD	Carbohydrate, fat and protein metabolism, coenzyme forms NAD and NADP
Deficiency manifest as	Scurvy Sore mouth Sore and bleeding gums Weak-walled capillaries	Beriberi Poor appetite Fatigue Constipation	Eye sensitivity Cheilosis (man)	Pellagra Dermatitis Nervous depression Diarrhea
Recommended Dietary Allowance	Men and women 45 mg.	Men and women 0.5 mg./1000 cal.	Men and women 0.6 mg./1000 cal.	Men and women 6.6 mg./1000 cal.

ANTIVITAMINS OR VITAMIN ANTAGONISTS

Research in the chemical structure of vitamins has led logically to more understanding about their characteristic reactions. Some are destroyed by oxidation or light or are inactivated by reaction with other compounds. Any substance which prevents the absorption or metabolic functioning of a vitamin in the body is called an antivitamin or a vitamin antagonist; avidin is an antigonist to biotin.

One type of antagonist is a compound so similar in chemical structure that it starts to react like the true vitamin but cannot finish the reaction, thus blocking the space where the real vitamin could function. An interesting example of this type of reaction is a folic acid antagonist which has been used clinically in the treatment of malignant growths. The theory is that rapidly dividing cells may need more folic acid than normal cells, and therefore an antagonist might inhibit growth of the abnormal cells. Unfortunately, the folic acid antagonist inhibits growth in normal as well as in abnormal cells.

Antibiotics and, possibly, some of the sulfa drugs used in the treatment of infections may be vitamin antagonists. Normally, bacteria in the intestinal tract have the ability to synthesize certain vitamins. When a sulfa drug or an antibiotic is given orally, it may make some of the intestinal bacteria incapable of vitamin synthesis, thus inhibiting growth. Conversely, in other animals antibiotics seem to stimulate growth by changing the balance of the intestinal microorganisms.

STUDY QUESTIONS AND ACTIVITIES

1. From a historical point of view, which deficiency diseases were first recognized as such?
2. List properties and food sources of ascorbic acid.
3. List five functions of ascorbic acid.
4. How many fractions of the vitamin B complex are recognized today? Which ones are listed in the Recommended Dietary Allowances?
5. Which vitamins of the B complex group function in the release of energy from carbohydrates, fats, and proteins? Name the coenzyme forms of each of these vitamins.
6. Name the scientist largely responsible for isolating and synthesizing thiamine.
7. What methods may be used to assess the nutritional status of a person with respect to thiamine?
8. What single food is the best source of riboflavin in the diet? What kind of diet may result in Vitamin B_{12} deficiency?
9. Is it easy to obtain a sufficient quantity of thiamine in the diet? Which two common foods

Table 7–4. Water-Soluble Vitamins *(Continued)*

FRACTIONS OF THE VITAMIN B COMPLEX

	Vitamin B_6	Folacin	Vitamin B_{12}	Pantothenic Acid	Biotin
Important food sources	Pork Organ meats Legumes, seeds Grains Potatoes Bananas	Green leafy vegetables Liver and organ meats Milk Eggs	Liver and other organ meats, milk, eggs	Liver Organ meats Eggs, peanuts Legumes Mushrooms Salmon, whole grains	Liver Organ meats Peanuts Mushrooms
Stability to cooking, drying, light, etc.	Stable to heat, light, and oxidation	Unstable to heat and oxidation	Stable during normal cooking	Unstable to acid, alkali, heat, and certain salts	
Function: Essential in	Metabolism of amino acid—coenzyme form PALP	Blood formation Synthesis DNA, RNA, choline Amino acid metabolism	Growth, blood formation, choline synthesis, amino acid metabolism	Carbohydrate, fat and protein metabolism, coenzyme form, coenzyme A	Fatty acid synthesis carboxylation reactions
Deficiency manifest as	Convulsions Anemia Renal calculi	Megaloblastic anemia Glossitis Diarrhea	Macrocytic anemias, sprue and pernicious anemia		Lassitude Anorexia Depression Anemia
Recommended Dietary Allowance	Men and women 2 mg.	Men and women 400 mcg.	Men and women 3 mcg.	No RDA figure Probably 5-10 mg./day	No RDA figure Probably 150-300 mcg./day

are good sources? Will these supply adequate amounts? (See Table 7-3.)

10. Discuss the functions of pyridoxine in relation to protein metabolism.

11. Which vitamins are likely to be reduced in foods under the following treatment:
    (A) Bottled milk exposed to sunlight;
    (B) Cabbage kept overnight after shredding;
    (C) Vegetables to which soda has been added in cooking;
    (D) Potatoes peeled and allowed to soak 2 to 3 hours before cooking?

12. Which group of vitamins is preventive and curative of macrocytic anemias? Which one is called the "extrinsic factor" and is the one most potent in treating pernicious anemia?

13. What is meant by an antivitamin, and how is the vitamin activity destroyed or prevented?

Herbert, V.: The five possible causes of all nutrient deficiency: illustrated by deficiencies of Vitamin B_{12} and folic acid. Am. J. Clin. Nutr. 26:77, 1973.

King, C. G.: Present knowledge of ascorbic acid (Vitamin C). Nutr. Rev. 26:33, 1968.

McCormick, D. B.: Biotin. Nutr. Rev. 33:97, 1975.

————: The fate of riboflavin in the mammal. Nutr. Rev. 30:75, 1972.

Pelletier, O., and Keith, M. O.: Bioavailability of Synthetic and natural ascorbic acid. J. Am. Dietet. A. 64:271, 1974.

Review: New roles for ascorbic acid. Nutr. Rev. 32:53, 1974.

Revlin, R. S.: Riboflavin metabolism. New Eng. J. Med. 13:636, 1970.

Roe, D. A.: *A Plague of Corn. The Social History of Pellagra.* Ithaca, Cornell Univ. Press, 1973.

Schwartz, F. W.: Ascorbic acid in wound healing—a review. J. Am Dietet. A. 56:497, 1970.

For further references see Bibliography in Section 4.

SUPPLEMENTARY READING

Anderson, T. W., Reed, D. B., and Beaton, G. H.: Vitamin C and the common cold: A double blind trial. Canad. Med. Assoc. J. 107:503, 1972.

Ariaey, Nejad, M. R., et al: Thiamine metabolism in man. Am. J. Clin. Nutr. 23:764, 1970.

Darby, W. J.: Niacin. Nutr. Rev. 33:289, 1975.

Gyorgy, P.: Developments leading to the metabolic role of Vitamin B_6. Am. J. Clin. Nutr. 24:1250, 1971.

Halsted, C. H.: The small intestine in vitamin B_{12} and folate deficiency. Nutr. Rev. 33:33, 1975.

REFERENCES

1. Nutr. Rev. 31:255, 1973.
2. Nakashima, Y., et al: Arch. Biochem. Biophys. 152:515, 1972.
3. Tsai, S. C., et al: J. Biol. Chem. 248:5278, 1973.
4. Robinson, A. B., et al: Proc. Natl. Acad. Sci. U. S. 70:2122, 1973.
5. Mumma, R. O., and Verlangieri, A. J.: Fed. Proc. 30:370, 1971.
6. Genter, E., et al: Lipids 8:135, 1973.

7. Baker, E.: Am J. Clin. Nutr. 20:583, 1967.
8. Pauling, L.: *Vitamin C and the Common Cold*. San Francisco, Freeman, 1970.
9. Anderson, T. W., Reid, R. B. W., and Beaton, G. H.: Canad. Med. Assoc. J. 107:503, 1972.
10. Joint FAO/WHO Expert Committee: Requirements of Ascorbic Acid, Vitamin D, Vitamin B_{12}, Folate, and Iron. WHO Tech. Report Series 452, Geneva, 1970.
11. Merrill, A. L.: J. Am. Dietet. A. 44:264, 1964.
12. Livak, J. K., and Morse, E. H.: J. Am. Dietet. A. 41:111, 1962.
13. del Campello, A., and Asenjo, C. F.: J. Agriculture 61:161, 1957.
14. Williams, R. R.: *Toward the Conquest of Beriberi*. Cambridge, Harvard University Press, 1961.
15. Sauberlich, H. E.: Am. J. Clin. Nutr. 20:528, 1967.
16. Brin, M.: JAMA 187:762, 1964.
17. Handlin, P.: Fed. Proc. 17:31, 1958.
18. Fry, H., and Kondi, A.: Vitamins and Hormones 28:653, 1968.
19. Nutr. Rev. 30:162, 1972.
20. Lassers, B. W., et al: J. Appl. Physiol. 33:72, 1972.
21. Winter, S. L., and Barger, J. L.: N. Eng. J. Med. 289:1180, 1973.
22. Review: Nutr. Rev. 32:76, 1974.
23. Mason, J. B. Gibson, N., and Kodicek, E.: Brit. J. Nutr. 30:297, 1973.
24. Coursin, D. B.: JAMA 154:406, 1954.
25. Linkswiler, H.: Am. J. Clin. Nutr. 20:54, 1967.
26. Review: Nutr. Rev. 31:98, 1973.
27. Coursin, D. B.: Am. J. Clin. Nutr. 20:558, 1967.
28. Rose, D. P., et al: Clin. Sci. 42:465, 1972.
29. Review: Nutr. Rev. 25:72, 1967.
30. Wen, C. P., and Gershoff, S. N.: J. Nutrition 102:835, 1972.
31. Review: Nutr. Rev. 24:289, 1966.
32. Perry, J. and Chanarin, I.: Gut 13:544, 1972.
33. Review: Nutr. Rev. 30:179, 1972.
34. Review: Nutr. Rev. 24:289, 1966.
35. Chung, A.S.M., et al: Am. J. Clin. Nutr. 9:573, 1961.
36. Review: Nutr. Rev. 32:70, 1974.
37. Review: Nutr. Rev. 32:39, 1974.
38. Ghitis, J.: Am. J. Clin. Nutr. 18:452, 1966.
39. Waxman, S., Metz, J., and Herbert, V.: J. Clin. Invest. 48:284, 1969.
40. Review: Nutr. Rev. 32:204, 1974.
41. Herbert, V.: Am. J. Clin. Nutr. 20:562, 1967.
42. Wilson, T. H.: Nutr. Rev. 23:33, 1965.
43. Chung et al, op. cit.
44. Bridgers, W. F.: Nutr. Rev. 25:65, 1967.

8   energy

Energy Value of Foods
Measurement of Energy Expenditure
Rate of Energy Expenditure
Total Energy Requirements

Solar energy is the power that makes life on earth possible. However, only a fraction of all the sun's energy can be adapted or stored for future use. Even the most efficient devices presently available which are constructed for harnessing solar energy are less efficient by far than plants. In the process known as photosynthesis, plants use light energy to convert carbon dioxide and other inorganic substances into organic compounds which they need for growth and maintenance (Chapter 2). The chemical energy which either directly or indirectly drives all processes of life is held in the high-energy bonds of adenosine triphosphate (ATP), which is universal in all forms of life. Since plants can derive ATP from light energy (by a process known as photophosphorylation), they can produce and store excess carbohydrate (mostly as starch) instead of metabolizing it for energy as animals do. Thus the stored energy of plants becomes the potential energy of animals which, in turn, convert it through their metabolic processes to a usable form (ATP) to sustain their life processes.

This chapter was written by Pirkko Turkki, R.D., Ph.D., of the College for Human Development, Syracuse University.

The practice of raising animals for food is an inefficient way of utilizing plant energy. First, the animal body can capture in usable form (ATP) only about 40 percent of the total energy liberated from the oxidation of foodstuffs; the rest is released as heat. Second, a large proportion of the energy that is conserved is used for performance of work, with heat again as a by-product. Only the portions of energy utilized in the synthesis of new tissue during growth of the animal and that deposited as fat represent storage energy. A great deal of this is lost to humans when only selected parts of the carcass are used as food.

Conservation of Energy

Like inanimate matter, humans and other living creatures obey the fundamental law of conservation of energy—they can neither create nor destroy it but only transform it from one form to another. Thus, when no change is occurring in the energy stores of the body—no growth, weight gain, or weight loss—most of the energy consumed as food is accounted for as heat, either released directly in metabolic reactions or as a by-product of work performed by the body. A minor fraction is lost as unoxidized nutrients or metabolites in urine and feces, through the skin and, occasionally, the lungs (alcohol, acetone).

Energy is expended whenever work is performed by the body in the completion of any function, small or large. It does not matter whether the action is voluntary, such as walking, sitting, and the various acts involved in the performance of one's daily work, or involuntary, such as respiration, digestion, the circulation of blood, the maintenance of muscular tone, the transmission of nerve impulses, and the transport of nutrients across the membranes. Only that fraction of food energy which is captured in chemical form in the high-energy bonds of ATP can support these functions; the portion liberated as heat is useless to the body, with the exception of the small amount needed for the maintenance of body temperature.

If more energy is required for these functions than is provided for by the daily food intake, the energy reserves, primarily adipose tissue fat, are utilized. This is dramatically illustrated by the loss of body fat in starvation. Similarly, excess food intake leads to obesity (see Chapter 27).

Units of Energy

As the various forms of energy are quantitatively interchangeable, a single unit can be used to express a quantity of energy regardless of the form in which it is expended. In the past, the energy value of foods as well as the energy exchanges of the body have been expressed in terms of the calorie, which is a unit of heat. One kilocalorie, the unit used by nutritionists, is the amount of heat required to raise the temperature of 1 kg. of water 1°C. (from 15° to 16°C.). In recent years, attempts have been made to replace the calorie with the joule,* the unit for all forms of energy in the metric system and internationally accepted for use in the fields of chemistry and physics.

Adoption of the joule in place of the calorie was recommended by the VII International Congress of Nutrition in Prague (1969) and by the American Institute of Nutrition (1970). Both groups suggested that a gradual change be made in the literature, with initial inclusion of the conversion factor whenever either unit is mentioned.[1]

One kilocalorie is equivalent to 4.184 kilojoules (kJ). Since tables of food composition still list energy content of foods as kilocalories, this factor can be used when conversion is necessary or appropriate.†

Although one can anticipate that eventually completely new food composition tables will be developed with the joule as a measure of energy value, the use of the existing tables with the inclusion of both values is likely to be the next step. Both units were used in the 1969 revision of the energy allowances for the United Kingdom[2] and in the joint FAO/WHO Expert Committee Report on Energy and Protein Requirements.[3] The Food and Nutrition Board of the United States National Research Council still chose to tabulate the energy allowances as kilocalories in the 1974 revision, with the conversion factor included as a footnote.[4] A rounded value of 4.2 was recommended for practical use instead of the exact value of 4.184.

The recommended energy allowances are at best approximations and are usually rounded to the closest 50 kcal. and, with the joule, to the closest 100 kJ. For example, an allowance of 2000 kcal. equals 8368 kJ but is rounded to 8400 kJ (= 8.4 MJ [megajoule]).[5]

ENERGY VALUE OF FOODS

The total energy value of food nutrients can be determined by measuring the amount of heat produced by complete oxidation (combustion) of a known quantity of food in a *bomb calorimeter*, shown in Fig. 8-1. The apparatus is thoroughly insulated against loss of heat, and the amount of heat produced is measured by the change in temperature of a measured volume of water.

*One joule is equal to the energy expanded when 1 kg. is moved a distance of 1 meter by a force of 1 newton.
†1000 kcal. = 4184 kJ = 4.184 MJ; 1kJ = 0.239 kcal.; 1000 kJ = 1 MJ = 239 kcal.

Physiological Energy Values

The energy values of nutrients determined by the bomb calorimeter must be modified to take into account the losses in the feces and urine due to incomplete absorption and oxidation in the body. Table 8-1 shows the total and the physiological energy values of the major nutrients as determined by Atwater over 50 years ago. Whereas carbohydrate and fat are completely oxidized to CO_2 and H_2O in the body as in the calorimeter, protein metabolism is incomplete. The nitrogen of amino acids is eliminated from the body in organic forms which still contain some energy, urea being the main end product (see Fig. 9-11).

From the energy value of feces of subjects consuming typical mixed diets, Atwater estimated that, on an average, 92 percent of protein, 95 percent of fat, and 99 percent of carbohydrate is absorbed. The nitrogenous compounds excreted in urine were found to contain unused energy equivalent to 1.25 kcal per gram of protein oxidized in the body. Based on these estimates, the commonly used "Atwater factors" for protein, carbohydrate, and fat (4, 4, and 9 kcal./g., respectively) were derived. As there are slight differences in the energy contents of protein, carbohydrate, and fat from different foods, these factors are approximations only. However, they have been verified as adequate for computation of the energy content of customary American diets from the percentage composition of protein, carbohydrate, and fat.[6,7]

The energy values of foods found in tables of food composition, such as the Agriculture Handbook No. 8[8] and Home and Garden Bulletin No. 72,[9] were determined by this procedure, but more specific modified factors were employed for different types of foods on the basis of more recent information.

It should be recognized that if accurate values for energy contents of specific foods are required, the use of food composition tables is not adequate because of the wide variability in the carbohydrate, protein, and fat content of different samples of the same food, especially of animal products such as meats. Careful laboratory analysis of the composition of representative food samples is essential to calculate their energy values accurately.

Biologic Oxidation of Foodstuffs. Liberation of

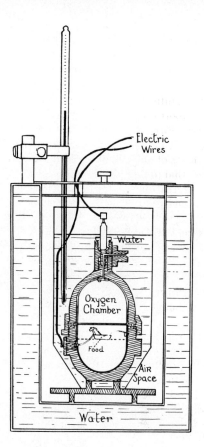

Fig. 8-1. Diagram of the parts of a bomb calorimeter. The water in the inner chamber changes in temperature when the food is burned. The water in the outer chamber acts with the intervening air space as insulation.

food energy in the body is not a process of instant combustion as in the bomb calorimeter. It is a slow, gradual redistribution of energy of the original molecules into intermediates of lower energy value with concomitant release of both heat and usable energy (as ATP) from the oxidative and other energy-yielding reactions of the metabolic pathways.

Biological oxidations include all reactions in which electrons are removed from an atom or ion which is part of the substrate; in some oxidations, the electron loss is accompanied by an addition of oxygen to or removal of hydrogen from the substance being oxidized. Oxidation of one substance (loss of electrons) always results in the reduction of another substance (gain of electrons, which may be accompanied by loss of oxygen or gain of hydrogen); oxygen is commonly referred to as an oxidizing agent or electron acceptor. Although oxygen may serve as an electron (hydrogen) acceptor in biological reactions, with

Table 8-1. Heat of Combustion and the Biologically Available Energy (kcal./g.)

	heat of combustion	loss in urine	% absorption	Atwater factor
Protein	5.6	1.25	92	4
Carbohydrate	4.1	—	99	4
Fat	9.4	—	95	9
Alcohol	7.1	trace	100	7

the formation of water (H_2O) or hydrogen peroxide (H_2O_2), most of the intermediary steps in the oxidation of foodstuffs initially involve other electron or hydrogen acceptors. The two major ones are the coenzymes nicotinamide adenine dinucleotide (NAD^+) and flavin adenine dinucleotide (FAD). Both are required for the initial breakdown of glucose, amino acids, and fatty acids as well as in the final oxidative cycle of energy production, the citric acid cycle, where the carbons of these nutrients become oxidized to CO_2 (see Chapter 9). The resulting reduced coenzymes, often referred to as "reducing equivalents" ($NADH + H^+$ and $FADH_2$), are either used in the synthesis of new compounds (in energy-requiring reductive steps) or reoxidized by the enzymes of the *respiratory chain*. Oxygen serves as the final hydrogen acceptor in this stepwise electron transfer, which is accompanied by capture of energy as ATP in the so-called *oxidative* or *respiratory chain phosphorylation*, as shown in Fig. 8–2. This oxidative phosphorylation at the respiratory chain level is the major means of ATP production in the body.

A sizeable fraction of total ATP formation takes place directly at the *substrate level*, linked to the cleavage of a high-energy bond as is seen in the conversion of 1,3-diphosphoglyceric acid to 3-phosphoglyceric acid in the glycolytic breakdown of glucose:

$$\text{1,3-diphosphoglyceric acid} \xrightarrow{\text{ADP ATP}} \text{3-phosphoglyceric acid}$$

For further discussion of energy release from protein, carbohydrate and fat, consult Chapter 9.

MEASUREMENT OF ENERGY EXPENDITURE

Though the oxidation of the energy-yielding nutrients in the body yields the same end products (CO_2, H_2O) as burning in a bomb calorimeter, the two processes are very different. In contrast to the rapid release of energy as heat in the bomb calorimeter, the slow liberation of energy in the biological oxidations allows about 40 percent of the total energy to be conserved as chemical energy of that ATP which serves as the power supply for the body's functions. However, since heat is also a by-product of all energy expended as work, production of heat can serve as a measure of energy expenditure by the body.

Direct Calorimetry

To determine the actual energy expended in a given period, a subject is placed in a chamber-calorimeter built for this purpose. It resembles a bomb calorimeter in that the heat given off by the subject is absorbed by the water in the coils surrounding the well-insulated chamber; the change in water temperature is measured. The chamber may be equipped for simultaneous determination of gas exchanges of the body. Though this method seems simple in theory, it is difficult and expensive in practice.

Indirect Calorimetry

The methods of indirect calorimetry have become widely accepted in the study of energy expenditure. They involve the measurement of oxygen consumption, with or without concurrent collection of CO_2 produced, by a subject breathing into one of several types of respiration apparatus (Fig. 8–3).

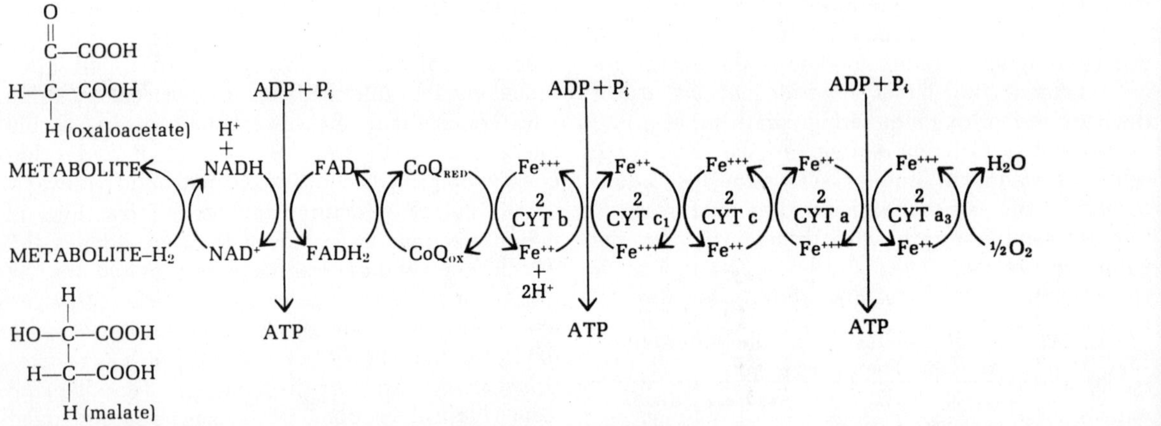

Fig. 8–2. Oxidative phosphorylation at the respiratory chain level. Consider the oxidation of malate (metabolite–H_2) to oxaloacetic acid (metabolite) in the citric acid cycle as an example. Malate dehydrogenase requires coenzyme NAD^+ which is reduced to NADH + H^+ when malate is oxidized to oxaloacetate. NADH dehydrogenase then channels the electrons from NADH to the respiratory chain, initiating a sequence of eletron transfers through the components of the chain with O_2 as the final acceptor. At certain points of the chain, the liberated energy is captured in the formation of ATP from ADP (adenosine diphosphate) and inorganic phosphate (P_i). Oxidation of some substrates is linked to the respiratory chain through the flavoprotein dehydrogenases (FAD or FMN as coenzyme) instead of the NADH dehydrogenases, resulting in two instead of three ATPs per pair of electrons.

The amount of O_2 consumed in oxidation of a food in either a calorimeter or a human body is directly related to the amount of energy liberated as heat. For example, regardless of how glucose is oxidized, the total amount of O_2 required and energy produced can be represented as follows:

$$C_6H_{12}O_2 + 6O_2 \rightarrow 6CO_2 + 6H_2O + \text{heat (664 kcal./mole)}$$

Similar equations could be used to express the oxidation of fatty acids, such as palmitic acid:

$$C_{16}H_{32}O_2 + 23O_2 \rightarrow 16CO_2 + 16H_2O + \text{heat (2340 kcal./mole)}$$

The quantity of energy produced when one liter of O_2 is consumed in the oxidation of glucose or a fatty acid can be calculated. Such values are relatively close to experimentally determined values for dietary carbohydrates and fats.

Because of the variable and unknown structure of dietary proteins, the oxidation of protein cannot be expressed by a simple equation. However, the experimentally determined energy equivalency of O_2 in oxidation of protein (4.600 kcal. per L. O_2) has been found to lie close to that of starch and fat (5.047 and 4.686 kcal. per L. O_2, respectively).[10]

Since the mixed carbohydrates and fats of the diet also differ from pure glucose or a single fatty acid, and since the body metabolizes a mixture of nutrients at the same time, an average of the three experimentally determined values (4.8 kcal. per L. O_2) is often used as a good approximation in calculations of energy expenditure from the measured O_2 consumption.

Respiratory Quotient

The amount of oxygen consumed in relation to the carbon dioxide produced in the oxidation of different foodstuffs varies with the oxygen content of the nutrient. Carbohydrates have higher oxygen content than fats (see the equations above) and, therefore, require less O_2 in the conversion to CO_2. The ratio of the volume of carbon dioxide produced to the oxygen consumed is known as the *respiratory quotient* (RQ). It is 1.0 for carbohydrate, 0.70 for fat, and about 0.8 for protein. When the mixture of the three energy-yielding nutrients is being metabolized, the value lies somewhere between 0.70 and 1.0, depending on the proportion of each. For an average mixed diet, the RQ has been found to be about 0.85. It is lowered during fasting and in uncontrolled diabetes; both are associated with decreased glucose and increased fatty acid oxidation. Insulin administration raises the RQ.

Metabolic Mixture

By measuring the urinary nitrogen excretion in addition to the O_2 consumption and the CO_2 production, one can calculate the amount of carbohydrate, fat, and protein oxidized in a given period. This is

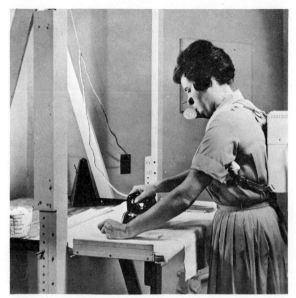

Fig. 8-3. Subject wearing respirometer to measure energy expenditure while standing to iron at a work-surface level of 36 inches from the floor. (U.S. Department of Agriculture, Office of Information)

known as the *metabolic mixture* and allows the total energy consumption to be calculated more precisely.

RATE OF ENERGY EXPENDITURE

The energy requirement of an individual consists of two major components of expenditure: (1) the energy expended for growth and maintenance and (2) the energy expended in physical activity. The total energy requirement is determined by a number of inherent and environmental factors which influence either or both components of energy expenditure and which are not totally independent variables.

Basal and Resting Metabolism

The energy expended for the maintenance of the basal activities of the body is relatively constant and includes:
1. Maintenance of muscle tone and body temperature;
2. Circulation;
3. Respiration;
4. Other glandular and cellular activities, including those related to growth.

It is customary to determine energy expenditure for these basal activities under standard conditions: the subject is lying down, awake, at complete rest; the test is taken at least 14 hours after the last meal and several hours after any vigorous exercise.

The most convenient time to comply with these conditions is in the morning before breakfast. The rate of metabolism as determined under these "standard" conditions is known as the *basal metabolic rate* (BMR). It is quite constant for individuals of the same sex, age, and body composition. Therefore, marked variations in the basal rate of metabolism are an indication of disease.

Formerly, the basal metabolism test was used extensively as a means of diagnosis, particularly in cases of hyperthyroidism, hypothyroidism, myxedema, and other endocrine disturbances which may alter the metabolic rate. Since the thyroid hormones have the greatest effect on the metabolic rate, the various thyroid function tests have gained wide acceptance in clinical diagnosis. The measurements of total serum thyroxine (T_4) or T_4-iodine and of triiodothyronine (T_3) have largely replaced the previously widely employed measurement of protein-bound iodine (PBI), which is difficult to interpret because of frequently encountered falsely high values due to iodide contamination.[11] All thyroid function tests are subject to misinterpretation unless interferences are eliminated by careful selection of appropriate methods and combinations of available tests.

Because of the specific conditions associated with the measurement of the BMR, the so-called *resting metabolic rate* (RMR) is frequently used for practical purposes. It refers to the metabolic rate at rest and under conditions of thermal neutrality. "It includes the specific dynamic action of meals, and is an average minimal metabolism for the night and the periods of the day when there is no exercise and no exposure to cold."[12]

Factors Influencing the Rate of Energy Expenditure

The maintenance component of the total energy expenditure is quite constant for an adult. There are normal variations in metabolism of different individuals, the causes of which lie within the body itself: the size, the shape, and the composition of the body, the age of the individual, and the activity of certain internal glands. It is generally accepted that a variation of from 10 to 15 percent either way from the accepted metabolic rate (all variables considered) is within normal limits.

BODY SIZE AND COMPOSITION influence the energy requirements by affecting both the resting metabolism and the amount of energy expended in the movements of the body. The resting metabolic rate is related to the proportion of actively metabolizing cell mass to the total body mass. The latter is influenced by the size of the body skeleton and the amount of adipose tissue, both of which are low in metabolic activity in comparison to that of the organ and skeletal muscle tissues. Therefore, when expressed as kcal./kg./hr., the BMR (and RMR) is quite constant for individuals with varying size but with similar proportions of these three body compartments, but varies with extreme departures from the average. Thus an athlete is likely to have a higher BMR (kcal./kg./hr.) than a sedentary individual, who in turn would have a higher rate than an obese individual. Table 8-2 shows the basal metabolic rates of adults with the recommended weights for heights.

In addition to body weight, the surface area has customarily been used as a measure of body size in studies comparing the metabolic rates of individuals or of groups of varying size, age, and sex distribution. The body surface area can be easily determined from weight and height by using nomograms developed from actual measurements of body surface areas of individuals of different heights and weights. Despite its long usage, the expression of metabolic rate in terms of surface area does not fully eliminate the variability caused by marked departures in body shape and composition. Thus grossly obese individuals tend to show lower than normal metabolic rates and women lower rates than men (who have proportionately less fat). Both differences are eliminated if the *fat-free mass** is used as the basis of expressing the metabolic rate.

* Fat-free body mass = body weight − total body fat.

Table 8-2. The Basal Metabolic Rates of Adults with Recommended Weights for Heights*

| Height | | MEN | | | WOMEN | | |
| | | Median Weight | | BMR | Median Weight | | BMR |
in.	cm.	lb.	kg.	kcal./day	lb.	kg.	kcal./day
60	152				109 ± 9	50 ± 4	1399
62	158				115 ± 9	52 ± 4	1429
64	163	133 ± 11	60 ± 5	1630	122 ± 10	56 ± 5	1487
66	168	142 ± 12	64 ± 5	1690	129 ± 10	59 ± 5	1530
68	173	151 ± 14	69 ± 6	1775	136 ± 10	62 ± 5	1572
70	178	159 ± 14	72 ± 6	1815	144 ± 11	66 ± 5	1626
72	183	167 ± 15	76 ± 7	1870	152 ± 12	69 ± 5	1666
74	188	175 ± 15	80 ± 7	1933			
76	193	182 ± 16	83 ± 7	1983			

* From Food and Nutrition Board: *Recommended Dietary Allowances,* 8th rev. Washington, D.C., National Academy of Sciences–National Research Council, 1974.

Table 8-3. Classification of Occupations According to the Extent of Physical Activity Involved*

Light Activity
Men: Office workers, most professional men (such as lawyers, doctors, accountants, teachers, architects, etc.), shop workers, unemployed men.
Women: Office workers, housewives in houses with mechanical household appliances, teachers, and most other professional women.

Moderately Active
Men: Most men in light industry, students, building workers (excluding heavy laborers), many farm workers, soldiers not on active service, fishermen.
Women: Light industry, housewives without mechanical household appliances, students, department store workers.

Very Active
Men: Some agricultural workers, unskilled laborers, forestry workers, army recruits and soldiers on active service, mine workers, steel workers.
Women: Some farm workers (especially peasant agriculture), dancers, athletes.

Exceptionally Active
Men: Lumberjacks, blacksmiths, rickshaw-pullers.
Women: Construction workers.

*From Energy and Protein Requirements. FAO Nutr. Meetings Rept. Ser. No. 52, WHO Tech. Rept. Ser. No. 522, Geneva, 1973.

With continuous improvements in the methods and standards for estimating total body fatness, fat-free body mass (sometimes referred to as lean body mass) is likely to be used more widely. This will allow more accurate assessment of the factors that alter the apparent metabolic rate but may or may not actually influence the cellular metabolic activity.

AGE AND GROWTH are responsible for normal variations in resting metabolic rate. The relative rate is highest during the first and second years of life and decreases after that, although it is still high through puberty in both boys and girls.

Although the energy requirements of children as well as of adults are usually given in terms of weight (and sex), age may be more appropriate for young children in populations where malnourishment is common, to allow for catch-up in both height and weight. For older children with irreversible stunting, energy allowances based on desirable height and weight for age could lead to obesity.

During adult life there is a steady decrease in energy expenditure. The resting metabolic rate falls due to the decrease in active cell mass and, in many instances, to the increase in total body fat. From age 40 to 60, physical activity both at work and during nonoccupational time is likely to be reduced with advancing age. Further decreases in both categories are likely after age 60, but such changes become more unpredictable due to a variable degree of disease and disabiltiy.

PHYSICAL ACTIVITY is the major determinant of variation in the rate of energy expenditure among individuals of the same sex, age, and body size and composition. Although the occupation is an important contributor to the total energy cost of physical activity, increasing leisure time or nonoccupational activities are becoming equally important, especially in the developed countries where the shortened workdays allow equal time for occupational and recreational activities.

Nevertheless, the Joint FAO/WHO Expert Committee on Energy and Protein Requirements concluded that "studies of both food intake and energy expenditure in groups of people show that by far the most important intergroup variable is the energy expenditure in the physical activity required by occupation." A rough classification of occupations into four activity categories proposed by the committee is shown in Table 8-3. It was recognized that considerable variation may occur in the amount of physical work involved in any one occupation, such as farming, due to differences in the degree of mechanization.

In the highly industrialized nations such as the United States where most occupations fall into the "light" or "moderate" activity categories, grouping of activities—both occupational and recreational—according to the estimated energy cost has provided a useful tool for estimating the total energy requirements of both groups and individuals (Table 8-4). *DISEASES* such as infections or fevers raise the BMR

Table 8-4. Examples of Daily Activities of Individuals in Light Occupations and Average Energy Expenditure in Each Category*

ACTIVITY CATEGORY	Average Energy expenditure, kcal./kg./hr.	
	Men	Women
Very Light Seated and standing activities, painting trades, auto and truck driving, laboratory work, typing, playing musical instruments, sewing, ironing	1.5	1.3
Light Walking on level, 2.5–3 mph, tailoring, pressing, garage work, electrical trades, carpentry, restaurant trades, cannery workers, washing clothes, shopping with light load, golf, sailing, table tennis, volleyball	2.9	2.6
Moderate Walking 3.5–4 mph, plastering, weeding and hoeing, loading and stacking bales, scrubbing floors, shopping with heavy load, cycling, skiing, tennis, dancing	4.3	4.1
Heavy Walking with load uphill, tree felling, work with pick and shovel, basketball, swimming, climbing, football	8.4	8.0

*Adapted from Food and Nutrition Board: *Recommended Dietary Allowances*, 8th rev., Washington, D. C., National Academy of Sciences–National Research Council, 1974.

in proportion to the elevation of the body temperature, approximately 7 percent for each degree Fahrenheit rise in temperature.

SECRETIONS OF CERTAIN ENDOCRINE GLANDS such as the thyroid, the adrenals, and the pituitary affect metabolism. The secretion of the thyroid gland has the most marked effect. Hyperthyroidism is that condition in which the metabolism is accelerated by increased production of thyroxine, while hypothyroidism is characterized by a decrease resulting in subnormal metabolism. Epinephrine (adrenalin), a secretion of the adrenal medulla, causes a temporary increase in the BMR. Those pituitary hormones which stimulate thyroid and adrenal secretions also affect the metabolic rate.

THE STATE OF NUTRITION may affect the BMR. In order to conserve energy during severe starvation or prolonged undernutrition, the body adapts by decreasing its metabolic rate, possibly by as much as 50 percent. Recent work by Rhao and Khan in India suggests that in children, malnutrition must be severe before the BMR is significantly depressed.[13]

They compared children with either kwashiorkor or marasmus with controls from the same socioeconomic group who showed no clinical signs of protein-calorie malnutrition. The BMR of the children suffering from kwashiorkor or marasmus was significantly reduced when compared to that of the controls and increased progressively with treatment. The BMR of the control group was similar to that of healthy American children, although the control group showed weight deficits ranging from 17 to 35 percent.

CLIMATE has been the subject of many studies in regard to its effect on both the resting metabolic rate and the energy expended in standard tasks. Although a lower than normal basal metabolic rate has been observed in inhabitants of some tropical communities, this finding does not seem to apply uniformly. The energy expended in standard tasks is believed to be the same within a wide temperature range, but the total energy expenditure may be increased during heavy work at high temperatures because of the additional expenditure needed for the maintenance of thermal balance in such extreme conditions.[14]

The human body has several ways of protecting itself against temperature changes. Exposure to cold initiates shivering, which consists of a series of rapid muscular contractions set up involuntarily by the body to increase heat production in order to make up for the rapid heat loss. Upon continuing exposure, nonshivering thermogenesis develops. Of course, increased heat production means increased energy expenditure.

The metabolic processes of the body under normal conditions and average daily activity produce enough heat to increase the body temperature by about 2° F. an hour if no heat were lost. However, nature has provided for a carefully controlled heat loss through perspiration, which may vary as climate and environment dictate.

Though these involuntary processes are important in the control of body temperature, they are not adequate to protect the body against extreme climatic conditions. Adjustments in clothing, housing, and level of activity are normal means of responding to changes in thermal needs.

Because of the variable and unpredictable nature of both the involuntary and voluntary adjustments to climatic changes, the Third FAO/WHO Committee on Caloric Requirements considered that "there was no quantifiable basis for correcting the resting and exercise energy requirements according to the climate."[15] They emphasized, however, the need to adjust the activity category to take into account climatic effects on the physical activity pattern and its contribution to the total energy expenditure. A similar approach was taken in the latest revision of the energy allowances for the population of the U. S. by the Food and Nutrition Board of the National Research Council.

THERMOGENIC EFFECT OF FOOD (Specific Dynamic Action). Ingestion of food is known to increase the metabolic rate above that in fasting resting conditions (BMR). This effect has been called the Specific Dynamic Action (SDA) of food, but the cause for the increased metabolic rate is still not clear. The long-held concept that the increased rate of O_2 consumption following a meal is dependent on the type of food ingested (hence "specific")—with protein having the highest effect (up to 30 percent) and carbohydrate the lowest (5 percent)—has recently been challenged. On the basis of a carefully controlled study with normal adults, Garrow and Hawes concluded that there was a similar increase in metabolic rate after a meal of a given caloric content, regardless of whether protein, carbohydrate, or fat was the source.[16]

Although the cost of increased urea synthesis resulting from oxidation of amino acids after a high-protein meal has been suggested to be responsible for the high SDA of protein,[17] Garrow and Hawes could not find any correlation between the O_2 consumption and urea production. Instead, their data seemed to support the cost of protein synthesis, as proposed by

Ashworth,[18] rather than catabolism, as the cause of the increased metabolic rate.

The magnitude of the thermic response to ingestion of food seems to be highly variable. Recent research suggests that exercise after a meal may increase the thermogenic effect of food.[19]

TOTAL ENERGY REQUIREMENTS

It should be obvious from the previous discussion that there is no single, easily quantifiable variable from which the total energy requirements can be accurately determined. Even the energy expenditure of an individual varies from day to day according to the time spent in different activities. A student studying for final exams may feel that he is working very hard, yet his energy expenditure may be considerably less than that during a regular school day when he is attending classes in different buildings on the campus and perhaps spending some time in recreational activities, such as playing tennis.

Individual variation in the amount of energy spent in a given task or activity may also be considerable. Thus energy requirements calculated from the number of hours spent in various activities are only average estimates based on a typical pattern in each activity category. For many individuals the actual energy expenditure may be higher or lower than the average.

In establishing the energy allowances for the population of the United States, the Food and Nutrition Board of the National Research Council assumed the average adult male and female to be engaged in light occupations, with a typical activity pattern consisting of 8 hours of sleeping/reclining, 12 hours of very light, 3 hours of light, and 1 hour of moderate activity. By using the energy costs shown in Table 8–4 and estimating the energy expenditure of sleep to be 90 percent of the BMR (Table 8–2), the daily allowance was established at 2700 kcal. for the reference man (70 kg.) and 2000 kcal. for the reference woman (58 kg.). Adjustments can be made for differences in body size and activity patterns by using the appropriate values from these tables. A quick estimate of the energy needs of a moderately active person may be made as follows:

Basal needs = 1 kcal./kg./hr.

Weight in kg. × 24 = BMR for 1 day;

Add 50 percent of BMR for activity to estimate the total energy need.

Although the energy allowances were established "at the lowest value thought to be consonant with good health of average persons in each age group," it was recognized that for many individuals the recommended levels are too high for a sedentary life.[20] For persons who are overweight or underweight, caloric requirements should be estimated according to the desired weight for height instead of actual weight (Table 8–2).

The energy allowances after 50 years of age were set at 90 percent of the 23- to 50- year levels on the basis of the small known decline in the BMR with age and the assumed decline in physical activity.

Although many individuals seem to be able to adjust their food intake to their energy expenditure without any special effort, this regulatory mechanism does not work as well at very low levels of energy expenditure, thus leading to obesity.[21] Instead of reduction of energy intake, the Food and Nutrition Board recommends increasing energy output through increased activity by individuals whose daily energy expenditure is below 1800 kcal. It is very difficult to maintain adequate intake of essential minerals and vitamins with low caloric intake because of the relatively low nutrient density of the average American diet, which is high in fat and sugar, providing a lot of "empty calories."

The reader should consult Chapters 17 and 18 for a discussion of energy needs of children and adolescents and Chapter 16 for those of pregnancy and lactation. Energy allowances for all age groups are shown in Table 10–1, together with the RDAs for the other nutrients.

STUDY QUESTIONS AND ACTIVITIES

1. What are the two units of energy presently used to express the energy value of foods? How can you convert one unit to the other?
2. Why are the physiological fuel values of foods different from their heat of combustion?
3. Milk has the percentage composition of 3.5 g. of protein, 4 g. of fat, and 5 g. of carbohydrate per 100 g. Calculate the caloric value of a glass of milk weighing 240 g.
4. How does the biological oxidation of the energy nutrients differ from their combustion in a bomb calorimeter?
5. Differentiate between the oxidative phosphorylation at the respiratory chain level and the substrate level phosphorylation.
6. How can the energy expenditure of an individual be estimated from the measurement of O_2 consumption?
7. What is the RQ? Why is it low during fasting?

8. What is meant by a metabolic mixture?
9. Differentiate between the BMR and RMR.
10. What are the major factors that determine the total energy requirements of an individual?
11. Estimate the energy requirements of a moderately active 50-kg. woman by the quick method. Now use Tables 8-2 and 8-4 to calculate her energy needs more carefully, using the typical activity pattern described in the text.

SUPPLEMENTARY READINGS

FAO/WHO Handbook on Human Nutritional Requirements. FAO Nutritional Studies No. 28; WHO Monograph Series No. 61, Rome, 1974.

Hegstedt, D. M.: Energy needs and energy utilization. Nutr. Rev. 32:33, 1974.

Review: Activity and energy intake in Ugandan children. Nutr. Rev. 31:84, 1973.

Review: Energy production during exercise. Nutr. Rev. 31:11, 1974.

Review: Heat production in malnourished babies. Nutr. Rev. 32:173, 1974.

Review: Thyroid function in experimental and clinical undernutrition. Nutr. Rev. 33:88, 1975.

For further references see Bibliography in Section 4.

REFERENCES

1. Ames, S. R.: J. Am. Dietet. A. 57:415, 1970.
2. Department of Health and Social Security: Recommended intakes of nutrients for the United Kingdom, reports on public health and medical subjects No. 120. London, H. M. Stationery Office, 1969.
3. FAO/WHO: *Energy and Protein Requirements.* FAO Nutr. Meetings Rept. Series No. 52, WHO Tech. Rept. Series No. 522, Geneva, 1973.
4. Food and Nutrition Board: *Recommended Dietary Allowances,* 8th rev. Washington, D.C., National Academy of Sciences–National Research Council, 1974.
5. Harper, A. H.: J. Am. Dietet. A. 57:416, 1970.
6. Bernstein, L. M., et al: U. S. Army Med. Nutrition Lab. Dept. No. 168. Denver, Fitzsimons Army Hospital, 1955.
7. Southgate, B. A. T., and Durnin, J. V. G. A.: Brit. J. Nutr. 24:517, 1970.
8. Watt, B. K., and Merrill, L. A.: *Composition of Foods: Raw, Processed, Prepared* (Agriculture Handbook No. 8). Washington, D. C., U. S. Dept. of Agr., 1963.
9. Nutritive Value of Foods. Home and Garden Bulletin No. 72, Washington, D. C., U. S. Department of Agriculture, 1970.
10. Zuntz, N.: Pflüg. Arch. Ges. Physiol. 68:191, 1897.
11. McMurry, J. F., Jr.: Postgrad. Med. 57:52, 1975.
12. Food and Nutrition Board, op. cit.
13. Rao, K. S. J., and Khan, L.: Am. J. Clin. Nutr. 27:892, 1974.
14. FAO/WHO, op. cit.
15. Ibid.
16. Garrow, J. S., and Hawes, S. F.: Brit. J. Nutr. 27:211, 1972.
17. Krebs, H. A.: in *Mammalian Protein Metabolism,* Vol. I, H. N. Munro and J. B. Allison, eds., New York, Academic Press, 1964, p. 125.
18. Ashworth, A.: Nature 223:407 (London), 1969.
19. Bray, G. A., Whipp, B. J., and Koyal, S. N.: Am. J. Clin. Nutr. 27:254, 1974.
20. Food and Nutrition Board, op. cit.
21. Ibid.

nutrient utilization: digestion, absorption, and metabolism

9

Ingestion of food initiates a multitude of physical and chemical processes which allow the body to utilize the food nutrients for maintenance of body temperature and functioning of its vital organ systems, for making new tissue for growth or repair, and for performing work. These processes are generally known as digestion, absorption, and metabolism of nutrients.

Although it is customary to study separately each of these phases of nutrient utilization, one should understand that they all go on simultaneously and are highly interdependent, although for an individual molecule they are sequen-

This chapter was written by Pirkko Turkki, R.D., Ph.D., of the College for Human Development, Syracuse University.

123

tial regarding the location and time. To illustrate, while some molecules of starch are being degraded by the digestive enzymes in the intestinal lumen, the digestion products (glucose) of other molecules ingested in the same meal are being absorbed into the epithelial cells of the mucosa. Still others are being metabolized in the mucosal cell to provide energy for continuous absorption, and some have already reached the liver and are being used to replenish the glycogen stores of this organ. Still others may have been removed from the blood by other tissues and are being oxidized to provide energy for work in the muscle or converted to fat in the adipose tissue.

digestive-absorptive processes

Because the organs and the processes of digestion and absorption may have already been studied in anatomy, physiology, and chemistry courses, this section will focus primarily on the nutrients which form the substrates, the specific enzymes involved in the hydrolysis reactions, the products that are formed by the digestive process, and the mechanisms of absorption. One should remember, however, that foods are eaten in a variety of forms and combinations; cooking and other processing methods may, there-fore, begin the breakdown of complex compounds such as starch and collagen (protein) before foods are ingested.

Although the general aspects of digestion and absorption will be discussed separately, they will be considered together for individual nutrients. It is useful to visualize the process as a whole and to focus on the transformations that take place in three sequential sites of the gastrointestinal tract: in the lumen (luminal phase), in the lipoprotein membrane of the microvilli (brushborder phase), and in the epithelial cell (intracellular phase). For a review of the structure of the gastrointestinal tract see Figs. 9–1 and 9–2.

DIGESTION

The two major and interrelated processes of digestion—i.e., the mechanical and the chemical—proceed simultaneously. In the first category are the muscular contractions of the walls of the gastrointestinal tract which move the food in solution (chyme), making contact possible between the food and the digestive enzymes. The second—chemical digestion—is the process of hydrolysis by which carbohydrates, fats, and proteins are divided into simpler units which can be absorbed through the walls of the small intestine. Table 9–1 summarizes briefly the chemical digestion of carbohydrates, fats, and proteins. They are discussed in more detail later. Each enzyme involved in the process is specific for the

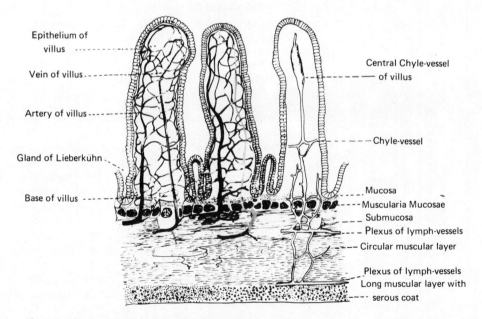

Epithelium of villus

Vein of villus

Artery of villus

Gland of Lieberkühn

Base of villus

Central Chyle-vessel of villus

Chyle-vessel

Mucosa
Muscularia Mucosae
Submucosa
Plexus of lymph-vessels
Circular muscular layer

Plexus of lymph-vessels
Long muscular layer with serous coat

Fig. 9–1. Diagrammatic drawing (after F. P. Mall) showing the great extension of absorbing surface of the intestinal lining due to projecting villi.

Table 9-1. Digestion of Carbohydrates, Fats, and Proteins

SOURCE OF ENZYME	ENZYME	+	SUBSTRATE	→	PRODUCTS
Mouth Salivary glands	Salivary amylase (ptyalin)		Starch	→	Dextrins and maltose
Stomach Gastric mucosa	Gastric protease pepsin rennin		Proteins Casein	→ →	Polypeptides Insoluble casein
	Gastric lipase		Short chain and medium chain triglycerides	→	Fatty acids and glycerol
Small Intestine Pancreas	Pancreatic proteases trypsin chymotrypsin carboxypeptidases }		Proteins and polypeptides	→	Smaller polypeptides and amino acids
	Pancreatic lipase (steapsin)		Fats	→	Mono and diglycerides fatty acids and glycerol
	Pancreatic amylase (amylopsin)		Amylose and amylopectin	→	Maltose, maltotriose and α-limit dextrins
Intestinal mucosa Brushborder	Intestinal peptidases aminopeptidases dipeptidases		Polypeptides Dipeptides	→	Smaller polypeptides and amino acids
	Intestinal saccharidases α-dextrinase (isomaltase) sucrase maltase lactase		α-limit dextrins Sucrose Maltose Lactose	→ → → →	Glucose Glucose and fructose Glucose (2 molecules) Glucose and galactose

substrate—e.g., pepsin (gastric protease) acts only on proteins and is capable of breaking them down only as far as polypeptides.

In addition to the enzymes listed in Table 9-1, there are other chemical substances which affect digestion. The stomach secretes *hydrochloric acid* (HCl) which (1) activates the gastric protease pepsinogen to pepsin, (2) creates the proper acidity for the digestion of protein, (3) acts as a bactericidal agent, and (4) increases the solubility of certain minerals such as iron and calcium. Gastric secretions also contain *mucin*, which protects the lining of the stomach from the HCl both by neutralizing the strongly acid contents and by forming a protective covering on the gastric epithelium.

Hormones, which also affect the digestive process, are produced in the mucosa of the gastrointestinal tract. Table 9-2 lists the hormones, their stimuli, and the action which they have on the secretion and motility of the gastrointestinal tract.

Bile is produced by the liver and stored in the gallbladder, which releases it into the duodenum through the common bile duct, as a result of hormonal action intitiated by the presence of fat (see Table 9-2). Bile plays an important role in the digestion and absorption of fat through emulsification, which pro-

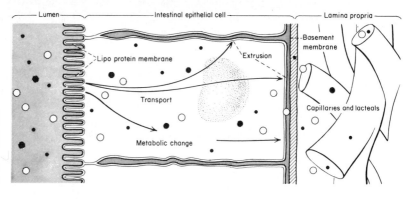

Fig. 9-2. Diagrammatic drawing, showing the process of absorption of nutrients from the lumen through the intestinal epithelial cell into the blood and lymph vessels of the lamina propria. (Ingelfinger, F. J., Gastrointestinal absorption. Nutrition Today, 2:3, 1967)

Table 9-2. Hormones of the Gastrointestinal Tract

HORMONE	STIMULUS	ACTION
Gastric mucosa		
Gastrin	Presence of protein derivatives and mechanical distension in the pyloric region.	Stimulates secretion of HCl by the gastric glands.
Small intestine mucosa		
Enterogastrone	Presence of fats, or acid chyme in the intestine.	Inhibits gastric secretion and motility.
Secretin	Presence of polypeptides and acid chyme in the duodenum.	Stimulates secretion of very alkaline enzyme-poor fluid from the pancreas.
Pancreozymin	Presence of polypeptides and acid chyme in the duodenum.	Stimulates pancreas to secrete enzyme-rich fluid.
Cholecystokinin	Presence of fat in the duodenum.	Stimulates contractions of the gallbladder, with the expulsion of bile into the duodenum.
Enterocrinin	Presence of acid chyme in the duodenum.	Stimulates secretion by glands in small intestine.

vides a larger surface for lipase action, and through solubilization of digestion products, which allows them easier access to the absorptive surface at the epithelial brushborder. These processes are performed mainly by bile salts, but the phospholipids present in bile also particpate. Bile acids (cholic and chenodeoxycholic acid) are synthesized from cholesterol and combine with the amino acids glycine or taurine in the liver to form conjugated bile acids before being secreted into the gallbladder. At the pH of the bile and intestines, they form highly soluble salts with Na^+ or K^+ and participate in the digestive process mainly as conjugated bile salts. Some deconjugation by intestinal bacteria may take place but normally this occurs in the lower part of the intestines after they have already participated in the digestion and absorption of fat (see p. 130).

Digestibility

There is strong popular conviction but not very much basic knowledge regarding the "digestibility" of specific foods and their effect on the physiology of the gastrointestinal tract. Foods are said to be "hard to digest" or, conversely, "easy to digest." They are classed as "irritating" or "gas-forming." Or they possess a quality described as "bland." Most of these terms may be traced to reported experiences of individuals who have gastrointestinal disorders, to incorrectly interpreted results of early studies of gastrointestinal function, and perhaps most frequently to long usage.

"Digestibility" of a food has been equated with the rate at which it leaves the stomach. Because fat remains longest in the stomach, it is thought to be more "difficult to digest" than protein and carbohydrate foods. Fried foods are said to be "irritating" to the gastrointestinal tract although there is little evidence to support this statement.

Some foods are also said to cause "indigestion and heartburn." Recent work by Babka and Castell[1] gives some support to this claim. They demonstrated that foods can alter the pressure of the lower esophageal sphincter (LES), which functions to prevent reflux of gastric contents into the esophagus. Of the few foods tested, diluted chocolate syrup caused an immediate and sustained decrease in LES pressure which was sufficient to cause gastric reflux in some patients. Ingestion of whole milk resulted in a slight but significant decrease and that of skim milk in an increase in the sphincter pressure. Although pure fat was found to greatly reduce the LES pressure and protein and carbohydrate to increase it, the authors pointed out that the differences found between the foods could not be explained by their protein, fat, and carbohydrate content alone.

When foods are ingested together in a meal the picture becomes even more complex. Our knowledge about the effects of individual foods on the physiology of the gastrointestinal tract when consumed in mixed diets is very scarce. It is obvious also that the factors mentioned above are not related to the true digestibility of foods. In professional usage the term digestibility refers to the proportion of the food that becomes available to the body as absorbed nutrients; the indigestible portion is excreted in the feces.

Under normal conditions the bulk of the indigestible residue consists of cellulose, pectins, and other complex carbohydrates found in foods of plant origin which cannot be degraded by the digestive enzymes in humans. The amount of bulk in the diet has received a lot of attention in recent years, as it may have a role in the development of some disorders of the colon which are common today in the Western world (see Chapters 2 and 25 for more information).

Some of the protein, fat, and carbohydrate of foods is also passed in the feces. In normal healthy individuals the average proportions of the major dietary nutrients digested (and absorbed) are: 98 percent for carbohydrate, 95 percent for fat, and 92 percent for protein. It is in this connection that the word digestibility is most meaningful and widely used by professionals. It is often expressed as a *coefficient of digestibility,* which would be 0.98, 0.95, and 0.92 for carbohydrate, fat, and protein, respectively. The coefficients of digestibility for nutrients vary with individuals and, especially with protein, with the food source. For example, the proteins of egg, milk, and meat have a coefficient of digestibility of 0.97, whereas those for plant products range from 0.89 for flour to 0.65 for most vegetables.

The amounts of nutrients lost in the feces can be greatly increased in disease states. For example, a deficiency in intestinal lactase activity results in fecal loss of milk sugar lactose and is responsible for milk intolerance in some individuals. Other disease conditions may be less specific and cause general malabsorption of nutrients. The various gastrointestinal disorders that influence digestion and absorption are discussed in Chapter 25.

ABSORPTION

Sites of Absorption

Absorption consists primarily of the transfer of nutrients from the lumen of the small intestine through the intestinal epithelium into the *lamina propria,* where the nutrients enter the blood and lymph vessels. Although limited amounts of water, alcohol, simple salts, and glucose are absorbed through the gastric mucosa, the small intestine is by far the more important organ for absorption.

Specifically, the most active absorptive area in the small intestine is the lower part of the duodenum and the first part of the jejunum (see Table 9–3). *STRUCTURE OF INTESTINAL WALL.* The inner lining, or mucosa, of the small intestine is gathered up into folds and covered by a mass of fingerlike projections (villi) which increase its surface area tremen-

Table 9-3. Sites of Absorption of Nutrients from Gastrointestinal Tract

NUTRIENT	SITE IN SMALL INTESTINE
Glucose	Lower duodenum
	Upper jejunum
Amino Acids	Lower duodenum
	Jejunum
Fats	Lower duodenum
	Upper jejunum
Iron	Duodenum
Calcium	Duodenum
Sucrose	Lower jejunum
	Ileum
Lactose	Jejunum
	Upper ileum
Maltose	Jejunum
	Upper ileum
Vitamin D	Jejunum
	Ileum
Vitamin B_{12}	Ileum

dously (Fig. 9–1). The epithelial cells which cover them have a so-called *brushborder* consisting of thousands of tiny rodlets, or *microvilli,* which further increase the surface area available for absorption.

A complex membrane made up of protein and lipid defines the outside edge of the microvilli. The exact molecular organization of this membrane is still not well understood, but it is believed to consist of a bimolecular layer of lipid in the center, covered or intermixed with protein. This membrane has a major role in the digestion and absorption of nutrients.

The single layer of epithelial cells lining the lumen rests on a connective tissue structure (lamina propria) which contains blood and lymph vessels (see schematic Fig. 9–2).

For normal absorption to occur the substrate—for instance, glucose—must enter the intestinal epithelial cell through the lipoprotein membranes, and make its way across the cell where it sometimes undergoes a chemical change. Then the substrate, glucose in this case, not only must leave on the opposite side of the cell but must pass through two additional layers of tissue before it is finally within a blood vessel. If the substrate were a fat-soluble nutrient such as a long chain monoglyceride, the process would be similar, except that it would undergo a series of changes in the mucosal cell and enter a lacteal or lymph vessel rather than a blood capillary. Fig. 9–2 schematically represents nutrients in the process of absorption.

Mechanisms of Absorption

The nutrients presented for absorption at the mucosal brushborder vary widely in regard to molecular size, solubility, and other properties. Because of the unique nature of the lipoprotein membrane of the microvilli, several mechanisms are necessary to ensure the passage into the cell of all nutrients regardless of their size and solubility characteristics. Also, as was pointed out earlier, the nutrients encounter several different barriers while passing from the luminal to the serosal side (lamina propria) of the epithelial cell and finally into the blood or lymph vessels. Therefore, more than one mechanism is likely to be involved in the total absorption process for any one nutrient.

When a solute passes "downhill" from a higher to a lower concentration, it is said to move along its concentration gradient; the process does not require expenditure of energy and is known as *passive transport*. In the same manner osmotic pressure differences and electrical gradients across the membranes also can determine the direction of movement of water and ions, respectively, by passive mechanisms.

During intestinal absorption many nutrients are transported "uphill," against the gradient; this can be accomplished only by expenditure of energy, and the process is known as *active transport*.

Several nutrients are known to be absorbed by both active and passive mechanisms. Furthermore, it is likely that in active absorption only one step, such as entrance into or exit from the mucosal cell, requires energy.

PASSIVE TRANSPORT. At least three major types of passive transport across cellular membranes are recognized:

1. *Diffusion through pores*. It is postulated that passage of water and very small water-soluble molecules takes place through *pores* or water-filled channels in the membrane. The transport by this route can proceed in either direction depending on the gradient. In addition to solubility, the size of the molecule is the major limiting factor: both monosaccharides and amino acids are too large to enter the pores.

2. *Diffusion through membrane*. Instead of molecular size, solubility within the membrane is the major limiting factor. This mechanism is believed to be of importance in the absorption of monoglycerides, fatty acids, and other substances which are lipid in nature.

3. *Carrier-mediated (facilitated) diffusion*. Water-soluble compounds which cannot pass through the pores can cross the membrane through carrier-mediated processes. These carriers, located in the lipoprotein membrane, interact with the substances to be transported and facilitate their passage, probably by rendering them temporarily membrane-soluble. Some carriers may be involved with two or more compounds such as glucose and galactose. These sugars then compete for the available carriers. The number of carriers is also probably limited, and hence carrier transport will slow down or cease as vehicles become unavailable. This passive carrier-mediated diffusion continues only until there is a balance between the solutes on both sides of the barrier.

ACTIVE TRANSPORT. In order to achieve continued absorption when there is a greater concentration in the cell or in the blood than in the lumen, a nutrient must be actively transported or pumped across the membrane barrier. These "pumps," which probably involve carriers, require energy to operate but they do permit a very large and rapid transfer into the body of such nutrients as glucose, galactose, many amino acids, sodium, and probably calcium, iron, and vitamin B_{12}.

PINOCYTOSIS. This is an amoebalike action of the epithelial cell membrane whereby a food particle or molecule is encompassed and thus brought into the cell. It may account for occasional absorption of large molecules such as those of a protein or a fat. It is unlikely that this mechanism plays an important role in the normal absorption of any nutrients.

CARBOHYDRATES

Carbohydrate (starch) digestion begins in the mouth by the action of salivary amylases which are capable of degrading starch to maltose and α-limit dextrins. The significance of salivary digestion is limited by the usually short stay and incomplete mastication of food in the mouth. By the time the food is well mixed with the gastric juice in the stomach, the action of salivary amylase is inhibited by the low pH of the medium.

The small intestine is the major site of carbohydrate digestion and absorption. In the luminal phase pancreatic amylases continue the degradation of starch where the salivary action ended, yielding maltose, maltotriose, and α-limit dextrins. No free glucose or isomaltose is formed in the lumen.[2]

The final stages of carbohydrate digestion take place by membrane-bound enzymes on the luminal side of the lipoprotein membrane of the mucosal cell (the brushborder phase). The brushborder exhibits multiple enzyme activity, most of which is believed to be of mucosal origin, but some may be due to adsorption of pancreatic enzymes from the lumen.[3] Thus digestion of starch is completed by production of glucose from α-limit dextrins by isomaltase (α-dextrinase) and from maltose and maltotriose by maltases. The common dietary disaccharides sucrose and lactose are also hydrolyzed by the mucosal disaccharidases sucrase and lactase, respectively. Figure 9–3 summarizes the major aspects of carbohydrate digestion and absorption.

Only monosaccharides can enter the mucosal cell and, subsequently, the blood. Deficient mucosal disaccharidase activity is the cause of a group of malabsorption syndromes discussed in Chapters 25 and 34.

The membrane digestion is closely integrated with the absorption of the resulting monosaccharides. Glucose and galactose are believed to share a common carrier system for transport through the mucosal cell. Although some of this transport is passive during the peak period of their production, the bulk of these sugars is absorbed by a process linked to the transport of Na^+. The exact nature of this process, including the location of the energy-requiring step, is still unsettled despite the many models that have been proposed for the system.

Fructose absorption proceeds at a slower rate than that of glucose and galactose and has been assumed to be by a passive mechanism, although the rate is relatively high when compared to passive transport of other sugars. Recent demonstration of active Na^+-dependent transport of fructose in the rat in vitro casts doubt on the interpretation of previous data in humans.[4] Existence of a separate, and possibly active, mechanism for fructose transport is also suggested by recent studies on sugar absorption in a patient with the rare defect known as glucose-galactose malabsorption[5] (see Chapter 34). An adult diagnosed as having this condition showed only minimal absorption of glucose and galactose (believed to be by passive diffusion). The rate of fructose absorption was normal, and about four times that of glucose and galactose.

After leaving the mucosal cell all monosac-

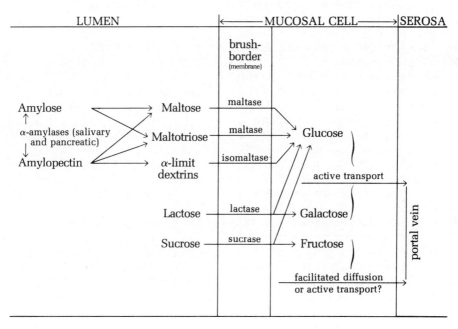

Fig. 9–3. Summary of the digestion and absorption of carbohydrates. Carbohydrate digestion in the intestinal lumen is incomplete and is finished by the membrane-bound disaccharidases. Only monosaccharides are believed to enter the mucosal cell. The action of α-amylases on starch yields maltose and maltotriose from both the amylose and amylopectin fractions; the branching points of the amylopectin molecules produce α-limit dextrins. These products, along with ingested disaccharides, lactose and sucrose, are further hydrolyzed into monosaccharides by their respective disaccharidases which are found in the membranes of the brushborder. After their passage through the mucosal cell the monosaccharides enter the capillaries of the portal venous system. (Adapted from Gray, G. M., Fed. Proc. 26:1415, 1967)

charides enter the capillaries of the portal venous system and are carried to the liver, where fructose and galactose are readily converted to glucose (see p. 139).

PROTEINS

Unlike other digestive enzymes, those with proteolytic activity are generally secreted in an inactive form. Thus the gastric initiation of protein breakdown by pepsins depends on activation of pepsinogen (the inactive form of pepsin) by HCl or by small amounts of pepsin itself. The mixture of polypeptides (known as proteoses and peptones) produced by gastric digestion is further degraded by pancreatic proteases (see Table 9–1) which principally function in the lumen of the small intestine. Trypsin, secreted as trypsinogen, is activated by intestinal enterokinase or by trypsin itself, depending on the pH of the medium. Trypsin also converts chymotrypsinogen to its active form. Both of these enzymes can degrade either intact proteins or polypeptides into smaller units, the major difference in their action being in the specificity of the peptide bonds cleaved by each. Appreciable amounts of intact protein enter the intestine daily from the intestinal secretions and desquamated epithelial cells and are digested along with the dietary proteins. Thus gastric digestion is not essential for utilization of protein in the body.

Though much of protein degradation by pancreatic proteases takes place in the lumen of the digestive tract, some polypeptide hydrolysis is also believed to occur at the brushborder by adsorbed enzymes.

The digestive process in the intestinal lumen produces a mixture of amino acids and oligopeptides which may be very complex, as one can envision from the many possible amino acid sequences that occur in proteins. Further cleavage of oligopeptides to dipeptides and amino acids is believed to result from the action of intestinal peptidases located on the brushborder.[6] Though only free amino acids are found in the portal blood after protein ingestion, a significant proportion of protein is believed to leave the lumen as small peptides which are then hydrolyzed by mucosal peptidases either in the brushborder or intracellularly.[7] Present experimental evidence favors both sites, as shown in the scheme of protein absorption proposed by Matthews (Fig. 9–4).

The transport mechanisms for amino acids, and more recently for peptides, have been the subject of intensive study. According to presently available evidence the transport of free amino acids from the lumen to the portal capillaries is accomplished by carrier-mediated processes which seem to be sodium- and energy-dependent for most amino acids. Several distinct transport mechanisms seem to exist, each of which is active with a group of amino acids with similar properties. It is also likely that individual amino acids may utilize more than one transport system.

Competition between amino acids of the same transport group has been demonstrated. This competition is avoided if the same amino acids are present as small peptides.[8] These observations suggest the existence of separate transport systems for uptake of peptides and amino acids into the epithelial cell. Other lines of evidence also support this view.

Contrary to a long-held view, the absorption of amino acids from di- and tripeptides is more rapid than from the equivalent amino acid mixtures.[9] Similarly, in some diseases involving severely impaired absorption of free amino acids due to a defective transport system (Hartnup disease, cystinuria) the same amino acids can be absorbed when they are part of small peptides.[10] The capacity to absorb peptides independently of amino acid absorption may explain the relatively good nutritional status and freedom from intestinal disturbances of patients with defective amino acid transport.

FATS AND OTHER LIPIDS

Of the dietary lipids, 90 to 95 percent are triglycerides, generally known as fats. Small amounts of di- and monoglycerides, cholesterol, and phospholipids are also ingested. Digestion, absorption, and transport of fat in the body present unique problems because of the insolubility of fat in the intestinal contents and other body fluids. Depending on the length of the carbon chain of the constituent fatty acids, there are also differences in the *solubility* of triglyceride molecules and, therefore, in the ways by which the body handles them.

The bulk of fat in a normal diet consists of so-called long chain triglycerides (LCT) with fatty acid length from 14 carbons up (including some 12 carbon fatty acids). Medium chain triglycerides (MCT, predominantly 8 to 10 carbon fatty acids) are of little significance except in therapeutic diets consumed by patients with certain malabsorption syndromes. (See Chapter 25.) Short chain triglycerides (SCT, less than 8 carbons) are utilized in a manner similar to MCT and are found mainly in milk fat.

Although differences exist in the rate of absorption of triglycerides with different fatty acid composition (chain length and saturation), it is rapid enough in normal individuals to allow 95 to 99 percent absorption with intakes up to 250 g. per day.[11]

Because of the completeness of fat absorption in

LUMEN | ←——MUCOSAL CELL——→ | SEROSA

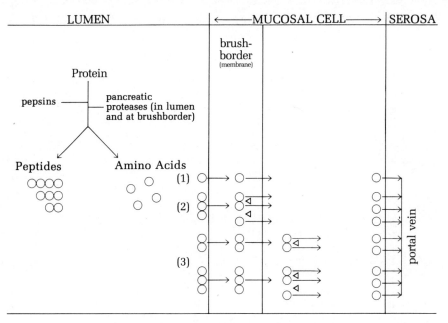

Fig. 9–4. Schematic description of protein absorption. Protein absorption may proceed by several mechanisms: (1) amino acids produced in the lumen are absorbed through the mucosal cell into the portal vein by several different mechanisms, depending on the structure of the amino acid; (2) membrane hydrolysis of small peptides upon passage into the mucosal cell; amino acids pass through the cell and enter the portal vein; (3) small peptides enter the cell and are hydrolyzed by intracellular peptidases, followed by passage through the cell and into the portal vein. The uptake of small peptides and amino acids into the mucosal cell is believed to involve separate transport systems. Although only free amino acids can enter the capillaries of the portal veinous system, their absorption from di- and tripeptides is more rapid than from the equivalent amino acid mixtures. (Adapted from Matthews, D. M., J. Clin. Path. 24 (Suppl. 5): 29, 1971)

healthy adults, comparative studies on absorption rates of dietary fats have been conducted mainly in disease states with reduced overall fat absorption, or in premature infants whose capacity to handle dietary fat is also limited. It is evident from such studies that the melting point of fat influences the rate at which it is absorbed. Thus very hard fats, those with a large proportion of completely saturated long chain fatty acids, are absorbed less readily than liquid oils with a high content of unsaturated or short chain fatty acids.[12] The effect of triglyceride composition on the overall rate of fat absorption can probably be attributed to differences both in the rate of hydrolysis and in the rate of absorption of the end products, although the mechanisms involved are not known. As was mentioned earlier, these differences are of little significance in a normal individual but may be very important in determining the extent of steatorrhea present in certain malabsorption syndromes (see Chapters 25 and 34).

Long Chain Triglycerides (LCT)

The mechanical and chemical actions of the stomach release the food fat from the protein and carbohydrate. Fat enters the duodenum in a coarse unstable emulsion. Two digestive juices essential for normal lipolysis of fat are secreted into the upper duodenum, namely bile and the pancreatic juice. The mechanical action of the intestine and the emulsifying capacity of the bile salts and phospholipids of the bile allow formation of a finely divided stable emulsion. The emulsified fat droplets consist mainly of triglycerides and of lesser amounts of diglycerides and fatty acids. They form what is known as the *oil phase,* which is dispersed in the bulk of the intestinal contents, the *water phase.*

The enzymatic hydrolysis of triglycerides takes place at the oil-water interphase by pancreatic lipase (glycerol ester hydrolase) present in the water phase. The finer the emulsion, the larger the surface area available for the enzyme action; an ample supply of lipase is normally available, making the accessibility to the substrate molecules the determining factor for the rate of lipolysis.[13]

The intestinal digestion of long chain triglycerides consists of two essential steps: hydrolysis and solubilization of the end products. The pancreatic lipase releases the fatty acids esterified at carbons 1 and 3 of the triglyceride glycerol (also known as α-positions). The resulting free fatty acids and 2-monoglycerides (remaining fatty acid in β-position) are solubilized and removed from the site of hydrolysis through formation of micelles with conjugated bile salts. Small amounts of other lipids are also found in these micelles, including cholesterol, phospholipids, and probably the fat-soluble vitamins. Though the micelles are aggregates of

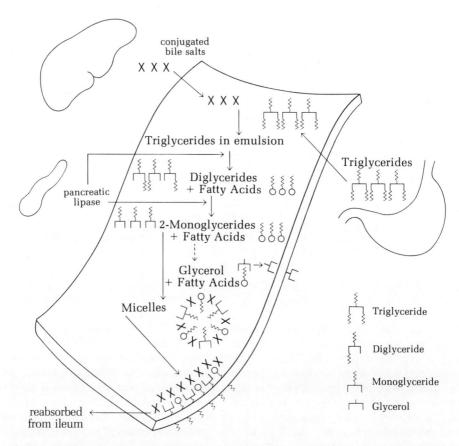

Fig. 9–5. Schematic representation of the luminal phase of digestion and absorption of long chain triglycerides (LCT). Triglycerides emulsified with conjugated bile salts are hydrolyzed into 2-monoglycerides by the pancreatic lipase. The resulting monoglycerides and fatty acids are solubilized by formation of mixed micelles with bile salts. Further hydrolysis of the micellar monoglyceride occurs but is limited. At the brushborders of the intestinal villi the micellar fatty acids and monoglycerides are absorbed into the mucosal cells whereas the bile salts pass further along the intestine until they are reabsorbed from the ileum. The absorption of fatty acids and monoglycerides is normally completed by the time the chyme reaches the midjejunum. Some of the bile salts are deconjugated by the bacteria found in the lower intestine before being reabsorbed. After passage through the mucosal cell into the portal vein, the bile salts are carried back to the liver where they are reconjugated and, along with the newly synthesized bile salts, are secreted into the gallbladder, ready to be released to the intestine again. This recycling is known as the enterohepatic circulation of bile salts. See Fig. 9–6 for the intracellular phase of LCT absorption. (Redrawn from Isselbacher, K. J., Fed. Proc. 26:1420, 1967)

molecules they are much smaller than the emulsified triglyceride droplets and they form a clear dispersion in the aqueous medium in the lumen (water phase). The major luminal events of LCT digestion and absorption are summarized in Fig. 9-5.

Micelle formation allows the monoglycerides and fatty acids to get into close contact with the absorptive surfaces of the epithelial brushborder. The minimum level of bile salts required to accomplish complete solubilization of the insoluble monoglycerides and fatty acids is known as the critical micellar concentration (CMC) of bile salts. Below this level some of the end products of hydrolysis remain in the oil phase and the entire process of digestion and absorption is slowed down.[14]

LCT are absorbed into the epithelial cell as monoglycerides, fatty acids, and glycerol. Glycerol is produced by limited hydrolysis of micellar monoglycerides, probably by intestinal lipase(s). About two thirds to three fourths of the dietary LCT are absorbed as monoglycerides.[15] The exact mechanism by which they enter the epithelial cell is not known, but the available evidence points to passive diffusion across the lipoprotein membrane. Contrary to a long-held view, some form of facilitation instead of simple diffusion may be responsible for the entrance of free fatty acids since competition among different fatty acids has been demonstrated. Recent studies suggest that fatty-acid-binding proteins in the membrane and/or inside the mucosal cell might be involved.[16]

At the site of absorption the bile salts separate from the rest of the micellar components and move farther down the intestinal lumen to the ileum where about 95 percent are reabsorbed. They pass through the mucosal cell and into the capillaries of the portal system which carries them back to the liver. If the bile salts are deconjugated in the intestine (by bacteria) before reabsorption, they are reconjugated in the liver and along with the newly synthesized bile salts are secreted into the gallbladder ready to be released once more into the duodenum as needed. The recycling is known as the *enterohepatic circulation* of bile salts.

The small fraction of bile salts lost daily in the feces is replaced by synthesis from cholesterol in the liver. This activity represents the major means of cholesterol removal from the body and can be increased by administration of certain drugs such as cholestyramine, which binds the bile salts, preventing their reabsorption and thereby increasing the conversion of cholesterol into bile acids in the liver. The net result is a reduction in blood cholesterol of hypercholesterolemic individuals (Chapter 29).[17]

The intracellular phase in the absorption of LCT is of major importance. The entering fatty acids and monoglycerides become mixed with those already present in the cell and lose their "identity." They also must undergo reconversion into triglycerides before leaving the cell.

The newly synthesized triglycerides are "packaged" into lipoprotein particles known as *chylomicrons*. The core of these particles consists of triglyceride and some cholesterol. They are covered with a protein-phospholipid "wrapping" which allows them to be dispersed in water. According to recent evidence[18] some of this dietary or exogenous triglyceride is incorporated into very low density lipoproteins (VLDL) by the epithelial cells, although this blood lipoprotein fraction is mainly known as the carrier of endogenous triglycerides synthesized in the liver (see p. 147).

Both lipoprotein particles are then released from the cells and enter the lacteals, the small vessels of the lymphatic system in the lamina propria. The contents of the lymph reach the left subclavian vein through the thoracic duct and, hence, the various sites of utilization in the body.

Medium Chain Triglycerides (MCT)

The digestion and absorption of medium chain and short chain triglycerides are similar; therefore, the discussion in this section pertains to both, although only MCT are referred to.

Gastric lipase, which has practically no activity toward LCT, can initiate the breakdown of MCT.[19] Though gastric lipolysis is considered insignificant in the digestion of fat in general, it may be important when a sizable proportion of total fat intake is in the form of MCT, as is recommended for certain therapeutic diets.

In the intestinal lumen, MCT are rapidly hydrolyzed into monoglycerides and fatty acids by the pancreatic lipase. In contrast to the long chain monoglycerides, a considerable proportion of medium chain monoglycerides normally undergoes further hydrolysis to glycerol and fatty acids before absorption.[20]

Both intact MCT and their digestion products are readily dispersed in the aqueous intestinal contents; thus, though the presence of bile salts stimulates their digestion and absorption, these processes proceed relatively rapidly even in bile-deficiency states in which ingestion of LCT causes severe steatorrhea.[21]

Uptake into the mucosal cell can also proceed at any stage of digestion; even intact MCT can enter the cell when luminal hydrolysis is incomplete, as in patients with pancreatic insufficiency. Once they are inside the mucosal cell, the hydrolysis of these glycerides (mono-, di-, and triglycerides) is completed by intracellular lipases which have little activity with long chain glycerides. This intracellular lipolysis is followed by rapid removal of the fatty acids from the cell. Unlike the LCT fatty acids, which are absorbed into the lymphatics, the MCT are directly absorbed into the portal circulation and carried to the liver, where they are readily metabolized.[22] The intracellular transformations of LCT and MCT during absorption are compared in Fig. 9-6.

Lauric acid (12 carbons), found especially in coconut oil, is usually classified as a medium chain fatty acid. In regard to the intestinal absorption, it seems to be at the borderline between the long chain and medium chain fatty acids. Although some lauric acid enters the circulation through the portal route, a considerable proportion is reesterified and enters the lymph in chylomicrons. To some extent the same is true with other fatty acids below and above lauric acid in chain length, but proportionally the portal route is the major one for fatty acids below 12 carbons and the lymphatic system for those with more than 12 carbons.

The therapeutic value of MCT preparations is based on their unique digestive-absorptive-transport behavior. Their major use is in digestive disorders (see Chapter 25) but more recently they have proven beneficial in the rare disorders of lipid transport in which chylomicron removal from the blood is defective (see Chapter 29).

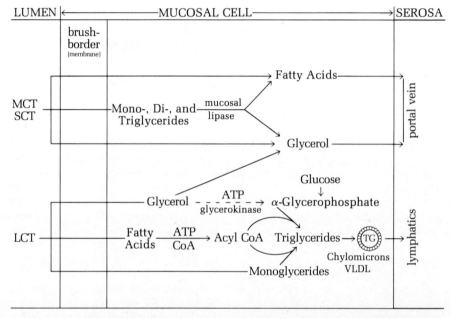

Fig. 9-6. Intracellular transformations in triglyceride absorption. Long chain triglycerides (LCT) enter the mucosal cell as monoglycerides, fatty acids, and glycerol. Monoglycerides are reconverted to triglycerides (TG) by addition of two activated fatty acids (acyl CoA). Another pathway for the reesterification of fatty acids involves addition of two acyl CoAs to "activated" glycerol, α-glycerophosphate, removal of phosphate to form a diglyceride, and addition of another acyl CoA to complete the triglyceride molecule. Metabolism of glucose provides most of the α-glycerophosphate for TG synthesis, due to limited glycerokinase activity in the mucosal cell. The newly synthesized triglycerides are "packaged" into chylomicrons, and to a lesser extent the very low-density lipoproteins (VLDL), which leave the cell and enter the lymphatics which empty to the left subclavian vein through the thoracic duct.

Medium chain and short chain triglycerides (MCT, SCT) may enter the mucosal cell intact, partially hydrolyzed (di- and monoglycerides) and as fatty acids and glycerol. The glycerides undergo intracellular lipolysis and leave the mucosal cell as fatty acids and glycerol. They enter the portal vein which carries them directly to the liver.

Thus the portal route is the major one for the transport of fatty acids with less than 12 carbons and the lymphatic system for fatty acids with more than 12 carbons. The 12 carbon fatty acid, lauric acid, is between the long chain and the medium chain fatty acids and enters the circulation through both the portal route and the lymphatic system.

Cholesterol

Cholesterol is an essential component of all animal cells and therefore is ingested in foods of animal origin. The average daily intake in a typical American diet is estimated to be 600 to 800 mg, but undoubtedly higher as well as lower intakes are common. Some cholesterol is also secreted into the intestinal tract in bile and becomes mixed with the dietary cholesterol. It exists either free or esterified with fatty acids (see Chapter 3), but the latter are cleaved in the intestine by pancreatic cholesterol ester hydrolase before absorption. The amount of cholesterol present in the intestines is small compared to the triglycerides and their digestion products, and it is easily solubilized within the bile salt-lipid micelles from which it is believed to be absorbed. It is well known that both dietary fat and bile stimulate cholesterol absorption.

Further mixing of dietary with endogenous cholesterol occurs in the mucosal cell, which actively synthesizes this compound. Some intracellular reesterification of free cholesterol also takes place, and both free and esterified cholesterol are incorporated into chylomicrons (60 to 80 percent esterified) and the VLDL.

The extent to which dietary cholesterol is absorbed in humans seems to be variable, and the information available is somewhat contradictory, especially regarding the effect of the level of dietary cholesterol on the percentage and absolute amount of cholesterol that reaches the blood. Some studies have indicated that regardless of the amount of cholesterol ingested, the daily absorption does not exeed 300 mg.,[23,24,25] whereas others have led to the conclusion that the absorptive capacity of the intestine for cholesterol is much higher.[26,27]

The results of several recent studies support the view that within the common range of cholesterol intake in American diets the amount of cholesterol absorbed is directly proportional to the dietary intake.[28,29,30] The percentage of ingested cholesterol absorbed seemed to average 40 to 50 percent of the intake. In a number of studies, cholesterol absorption in patients with diagnosed hypercholesterolemia has been found to be normal.[31,32]

It is possible that with high cholesterol intakes there is a gradual decrease in the percentage absorbed, as has been suggested by some studies.[33] More research is needed to clarify the question but, based on the presently available evidence, it seems reasonable to conclude that the amount of cholesterol absorbed is influenced by the level of cholesterol ingested.

Phospholipids

Phospholipids are found in foods of both animal and plant origin although in relatively small amounts. The main dietary phospholipid is lecithin (see Chapter 3) and, like cholesterol, it becomes mixed with endogenous lecithin both in the intestinal lumen (from bile) and inside the mucosal cell (synthesized).

Though a sizable fraction of lecithin is hydrolyzed to lysolecithin (one fatty acid removed) prior to absorption into the mucosal cell, some dietary lecithin can be absorbed intact[34] and has been found unaltered in the chylomicrons.[35] Most, however, undergoes extensive breakdown and resynthesis in the mucosal cell. Some parts of the molecule may be found in triglycerides or in other phospholipids manufactured in the cell.

metabolism

When the nutrients in the bloodstream pass through the cellular membranes of the body, they enter into the metabolic processes of the cell. Metabolism may be defined as a process by which the cells convert nutrients from food into useful energy which can be uilized for performance of work as well as for synthesis of new compounds, vital for cellular structure and function. The process by which nutrient molecules are degraded, with concurrent release of energy and subsequent elimination of waste products, is generally known as catabolism, whereas anabolism refers to the synthesis of new compounds. The anabolic processes depend on energy from the catabolic processes, both proceeding simultaneously. Some may be linked together through common intermediates. Metabolism is an ongoing process in every cell of the body, requiring a continuous supply of nutrients.

Wide variations exist among peoples and individuals in regard to daily intake of foods. Some people have meals at stated times; others cannot or do not. Fortunately, mechanisms exist which allow a steady flow of nutrients to the cells to continue for limited periods of time even though no food is ingested.

In the period immediately following ingestion of food, the levels of most nutrients in the blood rise due to absorption from the intestine. The rate of absorption varies with the nutrient, the quantity ingested, and the individual, but in general the peak level for carhobydrate (glucose) is reached in one hour and for fat (chylomicron triglycerides) in four to six hours. At the same time the uptake of nutrients by the tissues also is rapid and eventually exceeds the rate of flow from the intestine, resulting in gradual decline in the blood nutrients to fasting levels. In most individuals, fasting levels for triglycerides are attained in eight to twelve hours and for glucose in two to three hours.

The rate of protein (amino acid) absorption falls somewhere between those of carbohydrate and fat. The removal of some amino acids by the tissues is so rapid that only relatively small increases in blood levels are observed during absorption.

Upon reaching the cells, some of these nutrients enter the catabolic pathways to supply energy for immediate needs. Aside from small functional needs, the remaining nutrients are converted to various storage forms from which they can be recalled later when needed.

Glucose is converted to glycogen to replenish the tissue stores, but due to the body's limited ability to store glycogen, the remaining glucose is converted to fat and stored as triglyceride, mostly in the adipose tissue and to a lesser extent in the liver and muscle. Excess dietary fatty acids also are stored as triglyceride. Protein synthesis in the tissues is high after ingestion of a balanced mixture of amino acids; the excess is either oxidized to provide energy or first converted to glucose or fat.

The purpose of the following sections is to discuss the major metabolic pathways involved in energy production from and storage of food nutrients, and their role in the maintenance of metabolic homeostasis in the body. Though it is customary to denote certain metabolic pathways as catabolic, they may also have important anabolic functions because the intermediates may serve as substrates for biosynthetic pathways or as required intermediates for another catabolic pathway. One should then keep in mind that although the emphasis in the discussion of the various metabolic pathways is on the end products formed and on the connections between the pathways, there are numerous other directions in which some of the intermediates can be diverted, depending on the body's needs.

COMMON PATHWAYS IN ENERGY PRODUCTION

Food energy becomes available to the body cells primarily in the form of glucose, fatty acids, and amino acids carried in the blood. Though the initial catabolism of these nutrients takes place through pathways which are specific for each nutrient, only a fraction of their potential energy is released in these reactions. The end products, such as pyruvate produced from glucose, still hold the major portion of their total energy value, which becomes available only through complete oxidation into CO_2 and H_2O in the common pathways of intermediary metabolism.

Understanding the central role of the common pathways and the energy-conserving mechanism of biological oxidations is helpful for "visualizing" the role of the individual pathways in the whole metabolic process of the cell. Therefore, the common pathways are discussed first.

The common pathways involved in energy production are located in the mitochondria, which rightfully are known as the "powerhouses" of the cell. Figure 9-7 outlines the sequence of transformations through which complete oxidation of the energy-yielding nutrients is accomplished.

The Citric Acid Cycle (CAC, Krebs Cycle)

This oxidative cycle serves as a "melting pot" for the products of carbohydrate, fat, and protein metabolism after initial catabolism in separate pathways. Though it is sometimes considered as a pathway of glucose oxidation because of the carbohydrate nature of its intermediates, it does not discriminate on the basis of the origin of its substrates. Furthermore, the catabolism of several amino acids also provides intermediates for the cycle, as indicated in Fig. 9-7.

The key compound which channels the carbons of glucose, amino acids, and fatty acids into the cycle is acetyl CoA (or "active" acetate). The condensation of acetyl CoA with oxaloacetic acid initiates the series of reactions which result in the oxidation of the two acetate carbons into CO_2, with regeneration of CoA and oxaloacetic acid.

The energy generated in the oxidative steps (dehydrogenations) of the cycle is utilized in the concomitant reduction of coenzymes NAD^+ (nicotinamide adenine dinucleotide) and FAD (flavin adenine dinucleotide) and thereby conserved as "reducing equivalents" ($NADH + H^+$ and $FADH_2$). This energy can then be reclaimed by reoxidation of the coenzymes in the respiratory chain, or it may be directly used in synthetic reactions involving reductive steps specific for these coenzymes.

Electron Transport and Oxidative Phosphorylation

Reoxidation of the "reducing equivalents" is accomplished by the enzymes of the electron transport or respiratory chain, which are located in close proximity and linked to those of the citric acid cycle in the mitochondria. As discussed in Chapter 8, the oxidation-reduction steps of the respiratory chain result in transport of the "reducing equivalents" (hydrogens or electrons) from substrates to oxygen with production of H_2O. (See Fig. 8–2.) The liberated energy is "captured" for the synthesis of the high-energy bonds of adenosine triphosphate (ATP) from adenosine diphosphate (ADP) and inorganic phosphate in a process known as respiratory chain or oxidative phosphorylation.

The oxidation of each molecule of NADH yields three molecules of ATP whereas only two ATPs are recovered from each $FADH_2$ (Fig. 8–2). In addition, one high-energy bond is generated directly in the citric acid cycle by the substrate-linked phosphorylation of guanosinediphosphate (GDP) to guanosine-

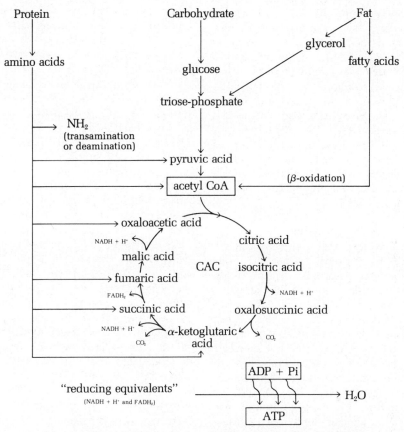

Respiratory chain linked production of ATP (oxidative phosphorylation)

Fig. 9–7. The common pathway in energy production. Carbohydrate, fat, and the carbon skeletons from some amino acids* are first converted to acetyl CoA which then channels the two-carbon units into the citric acid cycle (CAC) where they are oxidized into CO_2. Initial catabolism of other amino acids† provides several intermediates for this cycle. Oxidation of substrates in the cycle is accompanied by simultaneous reduction of coenzymes NAD (nicotinamide adenine dinucleotide) and FAD (flavin adenine dinucleotide) which then are reoxidized by the enzymes of the respiratory chain, with ultimate formation of H_2O. The energy released by the respiratory chain oxidations is "trapped" as ATP (adenosine triphosphate), three per each NADH + H$^+$ and two per each $FADH_2$ oxidized. (Pi = inorganic phosphate). In addition to the high energy bonds generated by the phosphorylation of ADP (adenosine diphosphate) to ATP (adenosine triphosphate), as shown in the illustration, another high energy bond is generated in the CAC by the substrate-linked phosphorylation of GDP (guanosine diphosphate) to GTP (guanosine triphosphate), not shown in the illustration. Thus the net yield from the oxidation of each 2-carbon unit of acetyl CoA is 12 high energy bonds.

*(alanine, cysteine, glycine, isoleucine, leucine, lysine, phenylalanine, serine, tryptophan, tyrosine)

†(arginine, aspartate, glutamate, histidine, proline, OH proline, methionine, threonine, valine, isoleucine, lysine, phenylalanine, tyrosine, tryptophan)

triphosphate (GTP). Thus the net yield from the oxidation of each 2-carbon unit of acetyl CoA is 12 high-energy bonds.

CARBOHYDRATES

Every tissue in the body is capable of removing glucose from the circulation and utilizing it for production of energy. Differences exist among tissues in regard to the essentiality of glucose as a source of energy as well as the metabolic pathways in which it is liberated. As mentioned before, the tissues of the central nervous system (CNS) and the formed elements of the blood are most dependent on a continuous supply of glucose, although adaptation to oxidation of ketone bodies (products of incomplete fatty acid oxidation) is known to take place in the CNS during long-term limited availability of glucose (prolonged fasting). Some glucose is always needed, however, and the body has means for storing it when a surplus is available and for mobilizing these stores or converting other substances to glucose when the supply is limited.

Pathways of Carbohydrate Metabolism

Uptake of glucose into the cells is the limiting step in its utilization in many tissues, including muscle, heart, and adipose tissue. Insulin is essential for glucose entrance to these tissues, whereas the process is independent of insulin in the liver and CNS.

Equally important and possibly related to glucose uptake is its phosphorylation to glucose-6-phosphate by *hexokinases* before it can enter the metabolic pathways of the cell. This reaction is practically irreversible in most tissues. Once glucose-6-phosphate is formed, it must enter the metabolic pathways and cannot be returned to the blood except from the liver and kidney, where another enzyme, *glucose-6-phosphatase*, can release free glucose. Glucose-6-phosphate serves as a link between the major pathways of glucose metabolism, which are shown in Fig. 9-8.

GLYCOLYSIS is a pathway of glucose catabolism which, under most conditions, is a necessary preliminary step for the release of all the energy biologically available in the glucose molecule. It results in the conversion of glucose-6-phosphate (either from glucose or glycogen breakdown) to two molecules of pyruvate or lactate, depending on the tissue and oxygen supply to the cell. The reactions that make up the pathway are outlined in Fig. 9-8. The energy yield of the pathway depends on the end product. Some ATP is produced directly in the pathway by substrate level phosphorylations (see Chapter 8) regardless of the

availability of oxygen. The other energy-releasing reactions involve concurrent reduction of NAD^+, which under aerobic conditions will be reoxidized, with generation of ATP.

During the periods of limited oxygen supply, such as in the muscle during vigorous exercise, pyruvate is reduced to lactate by *lactic dehydrogenase*, utilizing the reduced NAD as the coenzyme. Although this reduces the net supply of ATP, it can serve as an important source of energy for muscle by resupplying oxidized NAD for continuing breakdown of glucose and ATP production (from glycolysis), which would otherwise cease due to inability to further oxidize pyruvate and NADH.

When oxygen becomes available again, lactate can be reoxidized to pyruvate and metabolized further through the CAC. In the skeletal muscle, conversion of lactate back to pyruvate is limited. Instead, it is released into the blood and removed by the liver for reoxidation and subsequent conversion to glucose (see gluconeogenesis below). Released to the blood, this glucose becomes available to the muscle again. This recycling of glucose carbons between liver and muscle is known as the lactic acid or Cori cycle. Some pyruvate is also converted to alanine in the muscle and recycled in the same manner as lactate (both cycles are shown in Fig. 9-10).

OXIDATIVE DECARBOXYLATION OF PYRUVATE into acetyl CoA (Fig. 9-8) under aerobic conditions links carbohydrate catabolism to the common pathway (CAC) and allows releasing of the remaining energy from glucose. Decarboxylation of pyruvate involves a complex sequence of reactions in which lipoic acid and four vitamins—thiamine, pantothenic acid, riboflavin, and niacin—are required as coenzymes (TPP, CoA, FAD, NAD^+). Thiamine deficiency may be associated with elevated blood pyruvate levels due to an impairment in its conversion to acetyl CoA. The energy generated by this reaction is conserved as reduced NAD, with ultimate formation of ATP.

GLYCOGENOLYSIS results in the breakdown of glycogen and is often considered as part of glycolysis, as in many tissues the end product is pyruvate or lactate instead of glucose because of lack of glucose-6-phosphatase. In the liver, glycogenolysis releases glucose into the blood, allowing maintenance of blood glucose from glycogen stores during the postabsorptive state. In certain inherited metabolic diseases, the glycogen storage diseases, either the synthesis of glycogen or its breakdown to glucose in the liver is defective. Consequently, individuals affected with one of these conditions show a tendency to severe hypoglycemia as well as other abnormalities. By frequent feeding of small meals containing glucose (starch) these hypoglycemic periods can be prevented.

GLYCOGENESIS is an anabolic pathway which converts excess glucose-6-phosphate to glycogen, which serves as a short-term storage form of carbohydrate energy. Quantitatively, most of the body glycogen is found in the muscle, where it is stored during periods of high supply and utilized for the maintenance of metabolic intermediates when the supply of glucose

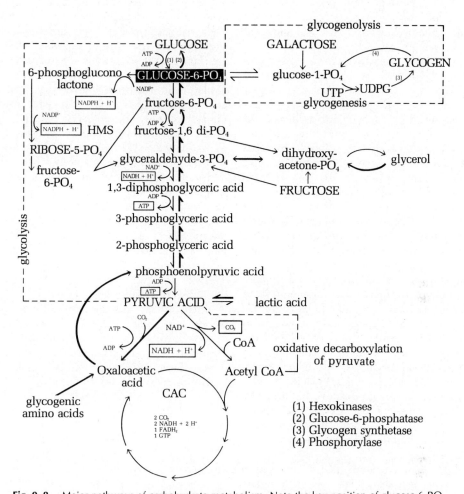

Fig. 9–8. Major pathways of carbohydrate metabolism. Note the key position of glucose-6-PO₄. Some reactions and intermediates have been deleted in order to emphasize the energy-yielding steps and the points of connection between different pathways. Heavy arrows indicate reactions involved in GLUCONEOGENESIS. Separated arrows point to individual reactions or segments of pathways where different enzymes are required for each direction. GLYCOLYSIS is the breakdown of glucose-6-phosphate to 2 molecules of pyruvate or lactate if oxygen is limited. OXIDATIVE DECARBOXYLATION of pyruvate into acetyl CoA links carbohydrate catabolism to the CAC. CAC (citric acid cycle) is the common pathway for the products of carbohydrate, fat and protein metabolism after initial catabolism in separate pathways. The condensation of acetyl CoA with oxaloacetic acid initiates the series of reactions which result in the oxidation of the 2 acetate carbons into CO₂ with regeneration of CoA and oxaloacetic acid. GLYCOGENOLYSIS is the breakdown of glycogen to glucose or, in the absence of glucose-6-phosphatase, to pyruvate or lactate. GLYCOGENESIS is the synthesis of excess glucose-6-phosphate to glycogen, mostly by the liver and muscle. GLUCONEOGENESIS is the formation of glucose or glycogen from noncarbohydrate sources in the liver or to a lesser degree in the kidneys. HMS (hexose monophosphate shunt) is an alternative pathway for the utilization of glucose-6-phosphate in certain tissues including liver, adipose, and erythrocytes.

from the blood diminishes. Liver has the highest concentration of glycogen; small amounts are found in other tissues, including adipose tissue. Though in essence the reversal of glycogenolysis, the last step in the glycogen synthesis is catalyzed by *glycogen synthetase* whereas *phosphorylase* initiates glycogen breakdown. Both of these enzymes occur in both active and inactive states and therefore are important sites of metabolic control by hormones, as noted on p. 153.

GLUCONEOGENESIS refers to the formation of glucose or glycogen from noncarbohydrate sources and takes place primarily in the liver but also to a lesser extent in the kidneys. During active gluconeogenesis (in normal fasting individuals or during periods of inadequate supply of insulin in diabetics) the substrates are amino acids and lactate, primarily from the muscle, and glycerol from the adipose tissue. Only the amino acids provide new carbons for net synthesis of glucose; lactate and glycerol are products of glucose metabolism in these tissues and represent recycling of glucose carbons between the liver and the peripheral tissues. As they cannot be further utilized in their respective tissues under the conditions of their release, gluconeogenesis from lactate and glycerol serves to clear the blood of these metabolites as well as to provide for the continuous supply of glucose for the minimal needs of the body during periods of fasting. In diabetic individuals, gluconeogenesis is high, even in the fed state, if the disease is poorly controlled, and this contributes to hyperglycemia. Because of insulin insufficiency, catabolic conditions exist in both the muscle (protein) and the adipose tissue (triglycerides), flooding the liver with gluconeogenetic substrates. Administration of insulin reverses the process by decreasing the catabolic and increasing the anabolic reactions in the extrahepatic tissues.

Essentially, gluconeogenesis is the reversal of glycolysis. As evident from Fig. 9–8, oxaloacetate plays a key role in gluconeogenesis from lactate and amino acids because the reaction from phosphoenolpyruvate to pyruvate is practically irreversible. Several other reactions or segments of glycolysis require a separate enzyme for reversal as indicated by separated arrows. Lack of one or several of these enzymes is responsible for the inability of most tissues to synthesize glucose.

HEXOSE MONOPHOSPHATE SHUNT (HMS, pentose phosphate pathway) provides an alternate pathway for the utilization of glucose-6-phosphate in some tissues, including the liver, adipose tissue, and erythrocytes. It is a complex multicyclic pathway which ultimately can achieve complete oxidation of glucose into CO_2 (3 glucose-6-PO_4 + 6 $NADP^+ \rightarrow$ 3CO_2 + 2 glucose-6-PO_4 + glyceraldehyde-3-PO_4 + 6 NADPH + 6H^+). Probably less than 10 percent of total glucose oxidation in the body takes place through this cycle, but it may play a more important role in the energy production in some tissues, such as erythrocytes. NADP (nicotinamide adenine dinucleotide phosphate) acts as a hydrogen acceptor in the dehydrogenation (oxidation) reactions of HMS, and 5-carbon sugars are produced as intermediates. Consequently, production of pentoses for nucleotide and nucleic acid synthesis and reduced NADP for fatty acid synthesis (see p. 150) are considered as two major functions of the pathway. *Transketolase*, one of the enzymes involved in the shunt, requires thiamine pyrophosphate (TPP) as the coenzyme. Measurement of erythrocyte transketolase activity with and without addition of TPP has become a useful measure in the diagnosis of thiamine deficiency.

There are other pathways which utilize glucose for the synthesis of many essential body components, but they account for a minor fraction of glucose utilization in comparison to the major pathways summarized in Fig. 9–8.

Utilization of Galactose and Fructose

Ingestion of galactose presents no problem in normal individuals. In the liver it is readily converted to uridinediphosphoglucose (UDP-glu), which can be incorporated into glycogen or converted to glucose-1-phosphate, which can then be metabolized in the pathways discussed for glucose.

1. galactose + ATP $\xrightarrow{\qquad}$
   galactokinase

   galactose-1-phosphate $\xrightarrow{\text{UDP-glu}}$
   galactose-1-phosphate
   uridyl transferase

   UDP-gal + glucose-1-phosphate

2. UDP-gal $\rightleftharpoons$ UDP-glu $\nearrow$ glycogen
   $\searrow$ glucose-1-phosphate

In a congenital disorder known as *galactosemia* (see Chapter 35) the ability to metabolize galactose is impaired due to deficiency of the enzyme *gal-1-PO_4*

uridyl transferase required for the conversion of galactose-1-phosphate to UDP-galactose. Consequently, galactose-1-phosphate accumulates in many tissues.

The major initial step in utilization of fructose in humans is considered to be its conversion to fructose-1-phosphate by *fructokinase*. Fructose-1-phosphate enters the glycolytic pathway after it is split into two 3-carbon units by an *aldolase*. Hereditary deficiency of this enzyme activity leads to a condition known as *fructose intolerance* (or fructosemia).

$$\text{fructose} + \text{ATP} \xrightarrow{\text{fructokinase}} \text{fructose-1-phosphate} \xrightarrow{\text{aldolase}}$$

glyceraldehyde + dihydroxyacetonephosphate

PROTEINS AND AMINO ACIDS
Amino Acid "Pools"

The amino acids of the circulating blood and interstitial fluid constitute an *extracellular* amino acid "pool" which is available to all cells for protein synthesis and other special needs. This "pool" represents a mixture of amino acids absorbed from the intestine and of those released from the *intracellular* "pools" of the tissues as a result of protein breakdown. Figure 9–9 depicts the interrelationships be-

tween the free amino acids and proteins in the major compartments of the body.

Except for a fluctuation observed during a 24-hour period, the average levels of individual amino acids in the plasma remain relatively constant under normal conditions. Flow of amino acids from intestinal absorption into the blood is balanced by the rapid removal by the tissues, especially by the liver. The cellular uptake of amino acids is accomplished by active transport, allowing for a rise in intracellular concentration of free amino acids, which then serve as the immediate supply for cellular needs. The intracellular free amino acid pool far exceeds in size the extracellular pool, which mainly serves a transport function. Factors that influence the cellular uptake and utilization of amino acids also regulate the extracellular amino acid pool. For example, administration of insulin, which increases amino acid uptake and protein synthesis in the tissues, causes a decrease in the plasma amino acids, whereas adrenal glucocorticoids increase protein breakdown and subsequently plasma amino acid levels.

Protein Turnover

Under the conditions of adequate protein intake, the body proteins in an adult are in a state of dynamic equilibrium with constant breakdown of the old and synthesis of the new without an appreciable change in total body protein content. The turnover (rate of renewal) of individual proteins and tissues varies

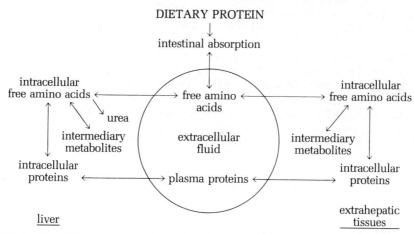

Fig. 9–9. Interrelations between amino acids and proteins in the major compartments of the body. The amino acids of the blood and interstitial fluid make up an extracellular amino acid pool which is available to all cells for protein synthesis and other special needs. Flow of amino acids from intestinal absorption into the blood is balanced by the rapid removal by the tissues, especially by the liver. The intracellular pool is much greater than the extracellular pool, which mainly serves a transport function.

widely. Thus the epithelial cells of the intestinal mucosa are renewed in less than two days, whereas the red blood cells circulate about 120 days. Of the individual proteins, serum albumin has a rapid turnover, whereas the collagen of the bone matrix is replaced very slowly. The total protein renewal in any one day represents a much higher demand for amino acids than is supplied in the diet. The balance is maintained by recycling of endogenous amino acids from the breakdown of body proteins, and synthesis of nonessential amino acids.

Protein Reserves

There are no protein stores in the body comparable to those of fat and carbohydrate; however, some body proteins are more labile than others; that is, they are called upon to supply the amino acids required for vital cellular functions when dietary supply is inadequate. Though these proteins represent functional or structural components of the cells, instead of a special storage form, they serve as body protein reserves which undergo reversible depletion and repletion, depending on the availability of and need for amino acids. The proteins of the liver are the most labile, whereas those of the brain are spared to the end. It has been estimated that individuals can lose about 25 percent of their total body protein without a serious loss of function or threat to life.

Plasma and Serum Proteins

Plasma is the liquid portion of circulating blood. The total protein content of the plasma is about 7 to 7.5 g. per 100 ml. Clotting of blood removes the plasma protein *fibrinogen*, which forms insoluble *fibrin* during the process of clot formation. All the other plasma proteins remain in the serum, a clear liquid that separates from the blood when the blood clots. Serum contains two major protein fractions, *albumins* and *globulins*, the latter being a complex mixture of simple and conjugated proteins, including glycoproteins and lipoproteins. The circulating antibodies, also known as immunoglobulins, are found in the gammaglobulin fraction.

Fibrinogen is only a minor fraction of the total plasma proteins, with a normal range of 0.2 to 0.4 g. per 100 ml. The level of plasma albumin is most susceptible to nutritional influences and is often used as a measure of protein nutrition, as is the level of total plasma proteins.

With the exception of gamma globulins, the serum proteins are synthesized in the liver and, consequently, low plasma protein levels are characteristic of chronic liver disease (cirrhosis). The cells of the reticuloendothelial system are believed to be the source of gamma globulins.

The albumin-to-globulin ratio (A/G) is altered in many disease states. Tissue destruction, inflammation, or infection is usually associated with an increase in the globulin and decrease in the albumin fraction, both of which contribute to a decrease in the A/G ratio.

Amino Acids in Intermediary Metabolism

When the protein intake is inadequate in terms of either total quantity or proportion of the essential amino acids required for protein synthesis, or if there is a deficit in the energy supply, the catabolism of amino acids exceeds their incorporation into tissue proteins and a state of negative nitrogen balance ensues (see Chapter 4). Amino acid catabolism is also a means of utilizing the energy from extra amino acids ingested in a high-protein diet.

In view of the number of different amino acids and the diversity of their structure, one can appreciate the multiplicity of metabolic pathways involved in their breakdown as well as in the synthesis of nonessential ones. Again, the catabolism of one amino acid may represent the biosynthesis of another (phenylalanine→tyrosine→further degradation) and one cannot draw a clear line between the catabolic and anabolic reactions. Discussion of the metabolism of each individual amino acid is beyond the purpose and scope of this book. Rather, the emphasis will be placed on those reactions of the amino acids which are common to most and which are essential initial steps in linking protein to the common energy-yielding pathways of intermediary metabolism. In brief, the catabolism of amino acids is essentially concerned with the separation of the amino groups from the carbon skeleton and the subsequent fate of these two components.

The carbon compounds derived from the breakdown of individual amino acids are shown in Table 9-4 (no reactions shown). Depending on the metabolic state of the body, they may be directly oxidized into CO_2 and H_2O with the production of ATP, or they may be first converted to glucose or fatty acids for later use or storage when excessive calories are ingested. Some may also be reincorporated into nonessential amino acids. The important fact is that once the amino group has been removed, the resulting carbon compounds enter the common "pool" of metabolic intermediates and are further handled as the products of carbohydrate or fat catabolism. It has become a common practice to denote as *glycogenic* those amino acids which can contribute to the net synthesis of glucose, because of the nature of the carbon compounds they yield (pyruvate or intermediates of the citric acid cycle which can be converted to glucose). Since acetyl CoA and acetoacetyl

AMINO ACID	PRODUCT OF CATABOLISM	METABOLIC FATE
Alanine	pyruvate	glycogenic
Arginine	α-ketoglutarate	glycogenic
Aspartate	fumarate	glycogenic
Cysteine	pyruvate	glycogenic
Glutamate	α-ketoglutarate	glycogenic
Glycine→serine	pyruvate	glycogenic
Histidine→glutamate	α-ketoglutarate, β-ketoglutarate	glycogenic
Proline ⎱ glutamate	α-ketoglutarate	glycogenic
OH-proline ⎰		
Methionine	succinyl CoA	glycogenic
Serine	pyruvate	glycogenic
Threonine	succinyl CoA	glycogenic
Valine	succinyl CoA	glycogenic
Isoleucine	acetyl CoA, succinyl CoA	glycogenic and ketogenic
Lysine	α-ketoglutarate, acetyl CoA, acetoacetyl CoA	glycogenic and ketogenic
Phenylalanine→tyrosine	fumarate, acetyl CoA	glycogenic and ketogenic
Tryptophan	succinyl CoA, acetyl CoA	glycogenic and ketogenic
Leucine	acetyl CoA, acetoacetate	ketogenic

CoA are precursors of ketone bodies (and fatty acids—see p. 148) but cannot supply carbons for glucose synthesis, the amino acids yielding these compounds are known as *ketogenic*. As shown in Table 9–4, only leucine is purely ketogenic and several others have both glycogenic and ketogenic potential.

The amino nitrogen is eventually excreted in the urine, mainly as urea, but small amounts are also excreted as creatinine, uric acid, and ammonia.

Deamination of Amino Acids

The first step in the degradation of most amino acids is the removal of the α-amino group. Two distinct reactions are known to occur in mammalian cells to accomplish this task. *Transamination* is the most common mechanism for amino acid deamination and involves the transfer of the amino group from one amino acid to a keto acid, with the formation of a new amino acid and a keto acid. Vitamin B_6 in the form of pyridoxal phosphate is required as the coenzyme in transaminations. *Oxidative deamination* with liberation of ammonia is another reaction for the conversion of amino acids to the corresponding keto acids.

Although most amino acids can participate in the transaminations, some play a more important role in total amino acid metabolism than others. The transaminases (amino transferases) are specific for one pair of amino and keto acids but nonspecific for the other. In the muscle, alanine-pyruvate transaminase activity seems to be especially important. When amino acids are released from the muscle, alanine accounts for a much higher proportion of the total amino acids than it represents in muscle proteins. Synthesis by transamination of pyruvate seems to be responsible.

$$\text{amino acid} + \text{pyruvate} \underset{\text{transaminase}}{\overset{\text{alanine}}{\rightleftharpoons}} \text{keto acid} + \text{alanine}$$

Alanine is removed from blood by the liver, where pyruvate is regenerated by another transamination. The pyruvate carbons are reconverted to glucose (gluconeogenesis) and released again into the circulation. This *glucose-alanine cycle* (Fig. 9–10) serves as a nontoxic carrier of nitrogen from muscle amino acid catabolism to the liver for urea synthesis.[36]

Formation of glutamate by transamination of α-ketoglutarate is another important reaction in the

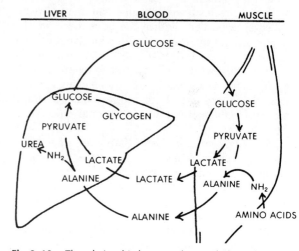

Fig. 9–10. The relationship between the metabolism of muscle and liver during gluconeogenesis. Note the parallelism of the lactic acid (Cori) cycle and the alanine cycle. The latter represents the major pathway by which the amino groups from muscle amino acids are conveyed to the liver to conversion to urea. (Redrawn from Bondy, P. K., and Felig, P., Disorders of carbohydrate metabolism in *Duncan's Diseases of Metabolism*, ed. 7, P. K. Bondy and L. E. Rosenberg, eds. Philadelphia, Saunders, 1974, p. 228)

sequence leading to final elimination of amino nitrogen from the body.

$$\text{amino acid} + \alpha\text{-ketoglutarate} \underset{}{\overset{\text{glutamate}}{\underset{\text{transaminase}}{\rightleftharpoons}}} \text{keto acid} + \text{glutamate}$$

Glutamate transaminase can use alanine as well as other amino acids as substrates. Glutamate thus formed can be oxidatively deaminated with release of ammonia.

$$\text{glutamate} \underset{}{\overset{\text{glutamate}}{\underset{\text{dehydrogenase}}{\rightleftharpoons}}} \alpha\text{-ketoglutarate} + NH_3$$

The enzyme for this deamination is very active in the liver and is believed to function in conjunction with the synthesis of carbamyl phosphate, which is the key intermediate in the conversion of ammonia to urea. Thus a series of transaminations which ultimately concentrate the amino nitrogen as glutamate prevents excessive formation of free ammonia, which is highly toxic to the central nervous system.

Deamination reactions are reversible and serve to synthesize amino acids from the corresponding keto acids and a nitrogen supply. The discovery that nitrogenous products from body protein catabolism could be utilized for this purpose has led to the introduction of new approaches to the treatment of the so-called nitrogen-accumulation diseases (chronic uremia and advanced liver desease).

It has now been well documented that in uremic patients, protein catabolism can be reduced and nitrogen balance maintained, with concurrent decline in the blood urea nitrogen (BUN) level, by limiting the dietary nitrogen intake to a mixture of essential amino acids[37] or to a small quantity of protein of high biological value.[38] Presumably, nitrogenous waste products are utilized for synthesis of nonessential amino acids (see Chapter 32).

Recent research indicates that, with the possible exceptions of lysine and threonine, even the essential amino acids could be synthesized from endogenous nitrogen when the precursor keto acids are fed.[39] By allowing further restriction of nitrogen intake to small amounts of lysine and threonine, this approach to dietary management of both renal[40] and hepatic[41] nitrogen-accumulation problems may lead to improved prognoses for patients afflicted by these serious diseases.

Urea Synthesis

Ammonia formed by the oxidative deamination of the amino acids is normally rapidly removed by conversion to less toxic excretory products, the major one

in humans being urea. Only the liver is capable of urea synthesis. The nitrogen is channeled to the cycle through carbamyl phosphate and aspartate (Fig. 9–11). Energy is required for the functioning of this cycle. It can also serve as a mechanism for synthesis of the amino acid arginine.

It should be noted that the formation of carbamyl phosphate utilizes not only ammonia but also CO_2, which is another metabolic waste product. In addition to urea synthesis, carbamyl phosphate is used for the synthesis of the pyrimidine bases which are further incorporated into nucleic acids.

When liver function is severely impaired, as in advanced cirrhosis, the urea formation is inadequate and toxic levels of ammonia accumulate in the tissues unless protein intake is restricted (see Chapter 32).

Glutamine Synthesis

Another means of detoxifying and transporting ammonia produced in the cells is by the synthesis of glutamine, as shown below.

$$\text{glutamic acid} + NH_3 \underset{\text{glutaminase}}{\overset{\text{glutamine}}{\underset{}{\overset{\text{synthetase}}{\rightleftharpoons}}}} \text{glutamine}$$

The reaction is reversible but requires a separate enzyme. Glutamine synthesis and breakdown are especially important in the kidneys where they function in the maintenance of the acid-base balance and in the conservation of cations. In metabolic acidosis glutaminase releases ammonia from glutamine. It is secreted into the tubules where it is converted to the ammonium ion (NH_4^+) and excreted in the urine as ammonium salts. In addition to removing excess H^+ from the body, excretion of the ammonium ion conserves K^+ and Na^+ which otherwise would be excreted with the acidic anions.

The fact that glutamine levels of the blood are generally high in comparison with levels of other amino acids supports its postulated role in the transport of ammonia from the tissues.

Other Uses of Amino Acids

In addition to their role in protein synthesis, energy production, and gluconeogenesis, many amino acids serve as precursors for synthesis of other biologically important compounds. *Glycine* is used for the biosynthesis of purines (nucleic acids), porphyrine (heme), creatine (p. 146), glutathione,* and conjugated bile salts (p. 126). *Phenylalanine* is

---

*A tripeptide, composed of glutamic acid, cysteine, and glycine, which serves as an activator of many enzymes.

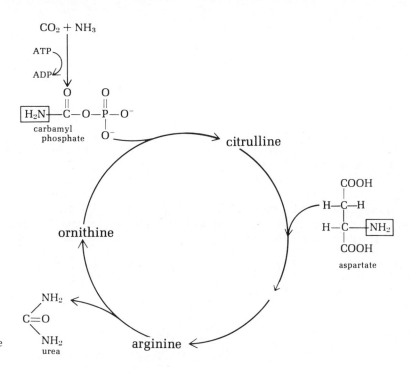

Fig. 9–11. Formation of urea by the Krebs-Henseleit cycle.

converted to *tyrosine* as a first step in its catabolism. When the enzyme phenylalanine hydroxylase, required for this conversion, is missing, a condition known as phenylketonuria results (Chapter 35). Several other enzymatic defects involving the metabolism of phenylalanine and tyrosine are also known. Tyrosine serves as a direct precursor of the hormones *epinephrine, norepinephrine,* and *thyroxine,* and of *melanin* pigment, found in the skin and hair. *Tryptophan* catabolism may involve several alternate pathways. Formation of 5-hydroxytryptophan followed by decarboxylation yields 5-hydroxytryptamine or *serotonin,* a potent vasoconstrictor and a stimulator of smooth muscle contraction. Serotonin is formed in the brain but its function in that tissue remains unknown. Tryptophan can also be converted to nicotinic acid (niacin—see Chapter 7). *Histidine* decarboxylation yields *histamine,* another physiologically active amine. Histamine stimulates the production of HCl by the gastric mucosa and is also a powerful vasodilator. It may be used in treating various allergies.

Glutamic acid decarboxylation produces *γ-amino-butyric acid* (GABA) which acts as a regulator in the tissues of the central nervous system. *Methionine* can be activated by ATP to form S-adenosyl methionine, which functions as a donor of methyl (CH_3) groups in various transmethylation reactions, including the synthesis of choline and creatine.

Protein Synthesis

The ability to produce the many different kinds of proteins needed by the body is determined by the pattern for protein synthesis which is carried in the DNA (deoxyribonucleic acid) of the cell's nucleus. Since this pattern is genetically determined, the various diseases which result from enzyme deficiencies are often referred to as "inborn errors of metabolism" (Chapter 35). For each protein a set of directions is carried on a specific segment, a gene, of the very long DNA molecule.

The DNA itself does not leave the nucleus but in a process called "transcription" its message is copied to a specific type of RNA (ribonucleic acid—messenger-RNA, or m-RNA), which carries the information to the site of protein synthesis. Each of these messenger-RNAs binds several ribosomes (particles composed of so-called ribosomal RNA and protein and located in the endoplasmic reticulum of the cell) into a polysome which then serves as a template or pattern for the assembly of amino acids into a protein.

Another type of RNA, transfer-RNA (also known as t-RNA or soluble RNA) not only recognizes a specific amino acid in the cytoplasm, but, after carrying it to the site of protein synthesis, interprets the code carried in the messenger-RNA ("translation") and delivers the amino acid to its proper place in the sequence required to form a specific protein.

Since the cells of the body are constantly manufacturing a wide variety of proteins, the need for a regular supply of the essential amino acids becomes obvious.

The general metabolic interrelations of amino acids and proteins from ingestion to excretion are summarized in Fig. 9-12.

FATS AND OTHER LIPIDS

Blood Lipids and Lipoproteins

Oxidation of fat—obtained via intestinal absorption and, during fasting, from adipose tissue—accounts for a sizable fraction of total energy production. It is no wonder then that the transport of lipids in the blood plays an important role in energy metabolism. The major forms of lipid found in normal plasma or serum are triglycerides, cholesterol, phospholipids, and free or nonesterified fatty acids (FFA, NEFA). Their origin and lipoprotein carriers are shown in Fig. 9-13 (see also Chapter 3 for composition of the different lipoproteins).

CHYLOMICRONS contain most of the triglycerides of nonfasting plasma and function to transport exogenous triglycerides and cholesterol from the intestinal mucosa, where they are formed during absorption of fat, to the other body tissues for utilization. They are the largest and least dense of the blood lipoproteins and their presence gives a milky appearance to the serum. Consequently, their removal by the tissues is often referred to as "clearing." After inges-

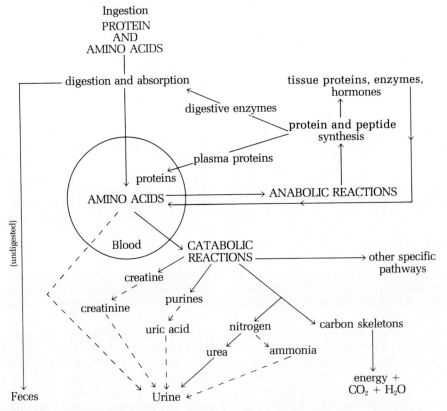

Fig. 9-12. General metabolic interrelations of amino acids and proteins. Ingested protein reaches the blood as amino acids. From this extracellular amino acid pool (including the interstitial fluid), they are actively removed by the tissues and concentrated in their intracellular pools, where they become mixed with the amino acids released from the cellular breakdown of protein. In fed state, the incorporation of amino acids into proteins is higher than their release, resulting in net increase of tissue protein. During periods of fasting or inadequate protein intake, the breakdown of protein in the tissues is high, leading to an increased release of amino acids into the extracellular pool. Under such conditions amino acid catabolism in the tissues is high. The carbon skeletons are utilized for energy production and the nitrogen is excreted in the urine, mainly as urea.

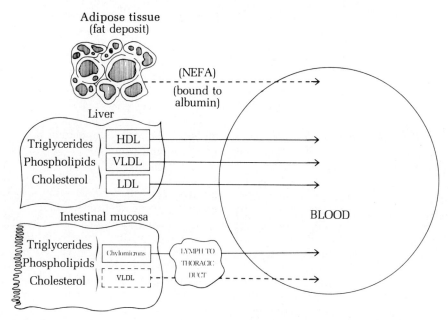

Fig. 9–13. Schematic representation of sources of plasma lipids. The major forms of lipid found in the blood are triglycerides, cholesterol, phospholipids and nonesterified fatty acids (NEFA). Their origins, adipose tissue, liver and intestinal mucosa, are shown with their lipoprotein carriers. (HDL = high-density lipoprotein or alpha lipoprotein; VLDL = very low-density lipoprotein or prebeta lipoprotein; LDL = low-density lipoprotein or beta lipoprotein) (Redrawn from *Lipids . . . in Brief*, ed. 2, with permission of Ayerst Laboratories)

tion of a fat-containing meal, the chylomicron concentration in the blood reaches its peak in about four hours and normally is cleared by eight to ten hours, depending on the individual and the amount of fat ingested. If chylomicrons are present in plasma after a twelve-hour fast, a defective clearance is suspected, as is seen in a rare familial defect known as type I hyperlipoproteinemia (see Chapter 29).

Removal of chylomicron triglycerides by the tissues involves hydrolysis into fatty acids by *lipoprotein lipase* followed by cellular uptake of the fatty acids. Lipoprotein lipase is a membrane-bound enzyme, which is believed to be present either at the cell surface or in the walls of the blood capillaries supplying the tissues. It is released and activated by administration of heparin, a natural anticoagulant found in the body. Measurement of postheparin lipolytic activity (PHLA) is a frequently used test for lipoprotein lipase activity.

Adipose tissue is the major site of chylomicron triglyceride uptake, although other tissues are known to have lipoprotein lipase activity.

THE VERY LOW-DENSITY LIPOPROTEINS (VLDL, prebeta lipoproteins) are synthesized mainly in the liver but also to a lesser extent in the intestine,

and function in the transport of endogenous triglycerides. Most of the fasting blood triglyceride is accounted for by this lipoprotein fraction. Because of the much larger amounts carried in the chylomicrons, determination of total triglycerides in nonfasting plasma has little value; the nonfasting level varies with the amount and time of fat ingestion. A high level of VLDL is usually responsible for elevation of serum triglycerides in the fasting state. The fatty acids found in the VLDL triglycerides represent two main sources: nonesterified fatty acids (NEFA) from adipose tissue triglyceride breakdown and biosynthesis in the liver from nonlipid precursors, mainly glucose.

The dietary components which most consistently influence the level of circulating VLDL are total calories and carbohydrates.[42] Weight gain is usually associated with an elevation and weight loss with a reduction in VLDL triglycerides in the blood. Ingestion of a very high carbohydrate diet (about 75 percent of total calories) causes elevation of VLDL in most individuals, whereas even normal carbohydrate intake has the same effect in so-called carbohydrate-sensitive individuals.[43] The cause for this sensitivity is not known. However, there is some evidence that the simple sugars may have a greater effect than complex carbohydrates. It should be emphasized that the populations which generally ingest a high carbohydrate (starch) diet show low average VLDL and total triglyceride levels.

The VLDL are also cleared from the blood by the action of lipoprotein lipase, as was discussed with chylomicrons.

THE LOW-DENSITY LIPOPROTEINS (LDL, beta lipoproteins) originate in the liver but may be the result of VLDL metabolism.[44] This lipoprotein fraction is a normal component of fasting plasma, accounting for about 75 percent of total serum cholesterol, and is usually elevated in individuals with hypercholesterolemia (see Chapter 29). Of the dietary factors, high cholesterol and saturated fat intake are most likely to be associated with an elevation in the level of LDL.

THE HIGH-DENSITY LIPOPROTEINS (HDL, alpha lipoproteins) consist mostly of proteins, phospholipids, and cholesterol, and their function in the body is still uncertain. There is some evidence to indicate the HDL are involved in the removal of cholesterol from the extrahepatic tissues to the liver for degradation and excretion. Occasionally an elevation of the HDL fraction is responsible for blood cholesterol elevation, especially in women taking oral contraceptives. No pathological significance is known to be associated with the elevation of HDL.[45] However, reduced levels of HDL have been reported in association with several known risk factors of cardiovascular disease, including hypercholesterolemia, hypertriglyceridemia, obesity, and diabetes mellitus. Miller and Miller have suggested that a decrease in the level of plasma HDL may accelerate the development of atherosclerosis by impairing the removal of cholesterol from the arterial wall.[46]

THE NONESTERIFIED FATTY ACIDS (NEFA) are released as a result of adipose tissue lipolysis and circulate bound to serum albumin. They constitute the metabolically most active fraction of blood lipids, although their concentration at any one time is very low. Their release from the adipose tissue is followed by a rapid uptake by other tissues, allowing a large quantity of fatty acids to pass through the blood in this form daily. Under the conditions of excessive adipose tissue lipolysis, such as in uncontrolled diabetes or after administration of lipolytic hormones (see Fig. 9-15), the uptake and utilization of fatty acids by the liver are increased. Consequent stimulation of VLDL synthesis can lead to hyperglyceridemia, which is secondary to adipose tissue fat mobilization.

BLOOD LIPID LEVELS. It is obvious that the total level of individual blood lipids represents the sum total found in the different lipoprotein fractions. In recent years their possible role in the development of cardiovascular disease has generated great interest in the blood lipid levels, not only among professionals but the public as well. Fasting levels of both cholesterol and triglyceride are relatively constant in any one individual, but wide variations exist among individuals within any population and in the average levels among populations. As is true with body weight, the average blood lipid levels tend to increase with age. The desirability of this change is being questioned. Sex differences are also evident, men generally showing higher blood lipid levels than women during the first five decades of life. One may speak about "normal" values, but these usually refer to averages or common ranges, which include a sizable proportion of the apparently healthy population. Such a range for serum triglycerides in an adult is 50 to 150 mg. per 100 ml., and for cholesterol, 150 to 250 mg. per 100 ml. Although we do not know what the optimal levels are from the standpoint of health, there is a considerable body of experimental evidence showing that a relatively small risk of cardiovascular disease is associated with cholesterol levels of 200 mg. per 100 ml. or below and with triglyceride levels of 125 mg. per 100 ml. or below. It should be emphasized that these levels do not represent cutoff points with a high risk above and a low risk below; the blood lipid levels, especially cholesterol, have a continuous relationship to the risk of cardiovascular disease (CVD). A more detailed discussion of blood lipids and CVD in relation to diet is found in Chapter 29.

Release of Energy from Fats

About 90 percent of the total energy value of fat is held in the fatty acids and the remainder in the glycerol moiety of the triglyceride molecules.

OXIDATION OF FATTY ACIDS. In order for the energy of fatty acids to be utilized, they must first be activated by formation of acyl CoA, which then can undergo a series of β-oxidations, each of which results in a release of one 2-carbon unit as acetyl CoA and acyl CoA, which is 2 carbons shorter than the original fatty acid. A schematic representation of oxidation of palmitic acid (C16:0) is shown in Fig. 9-14.

Just as was true with glycolysis in catabolism of glucose, β-oxidation releases only a small portion (about one-quarter) of total energy available in the fatty acid molecule. The remainder is held in acetyl CoA and released upon its oxidation via the CAC. Most of the common fatty acids contain an even number of carbons and yield only acetyl CoA as a

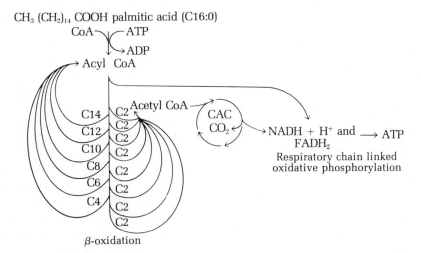

$CH_3 (CH_2)_{14} COOH$ palmitic acid (C16:0)

β-oxidation

Fig. 9–14. Schematic representation of energy production from fatty acids, using palmitic acid as an example. Palmitic acid (C:16) undergoes β-oxidation seven times, yielding 8 acetyl CoAs (two from the last cycle). Each turn of the cycle results in reduction of one FAD and one NAD which are equivalent to 5 ATPs when reoxidized. With one ATP consumed in the activation, the total yield from β-oxidation of palmitate is 34 ATPs (7 × 5 − 1 = 34). Further oxidation of each acetyl CoA in the citric acid cycle (CAC) liberates the remaining energy through the respiratory chain linked oxidative phosphorylation; 12 ATPs for each acetyl CoA, with a total production of 96 ATPs (8 × 12). The energy value of a mole of ATP is estimated to be 7.6 kcal. and the combustion of a mole of palmitate in a calorimeter yields 2340 kcal. Therefore, the efficiency of the biologic oxidation of palmitate is 42 percent. $\left(\dfrac{130 \times 7.6}{2340} \times 100 \right)$

Most fatty acids contain an even number of carbons and thus yield only acetyl CoA as a result of β-oxidation. Odd numbered fatty acids follow the same system but the final cycle (not shown) yields 1 acetyl CoA and 1 propionyl CoA. Propionyl CoA is converted to succinyl CoA and enters the CAC, thus contributing substrate to gluconeogenesis.

result of β-oxidation. Odd-numbered fatty acids can be oxidized in the same system, but the final cycle yields one acetyl CoA and one propionyl CoA. Propionyl CoA is converted to succinyl CoA, which is part of the CAC; therefore, the fatty acids with uneven carbon numbers contribute substrates to gluconeogenesis, whereas the even-numbered fatty acids do not.

FATE OF GLYCEROL. The glycerol portion of the triglyceride molecule also is glycogenic as was discussed earlier. It can also be metabolized through glycolysis without first being converted to glucose (see Fig. 9–8). The first step in the metabolism of glycerol is its conversion to α-glycerophosphate by *glycerokinase*. Because of the low activity of this enzyme in most tissues, liver is the major site of glycerol metabolism. Alpha-glycerophosphate can also be reincorporated into triglycerides, but under the conditions of high glycerol production from triglyceride breakdown, gluconeogenesis in the liver is the principal route of glycerol metabolism.

Lipid Synthesis

TRIGLYCERIDE SYNTHESIS and deposition in the adipose tissue result in the storage of excess energy in the body regardless of the form in which it is ingested.

Liver, adipose tissue, and intestinal mucosa are the major sites of triglyceride synthesis. Each can activate fatty acids to acyl CoA, from which they are esterified with glycerol, starting with α-glycerophosphate. Although adequate glycerokinase activity is present in the liver, the major source of α-glycerophosphate for triglyceride synthesis in all tissues is glucose metabolism. Triglyceride synthesis is stimulated in the fed state when availability of glucose is high. It is low during fasting, the oxidation of fatty acids for energy being favored over their incorporation into triglyceride.

DE NOVO SYNTHESIS OF FATTY ACIDS involves building the carbon chain from 2-carbon units, starting with one acetyl CoA as a primer and proceeding through successive additions via malonyl CoA, which is formed from acetyl CoA by the addition of CO_2. In the transfer of the 2-carbon units from malonyl CoA the CO_2 is released again. Because of the need for malonyl CoA as an "active" intermediate in fatty acid synthesis, the pathway is often referred to as the malonyl CoA pathway. Two B-vitamins are required in fatty acid synthesis: biotin, which participates in the formation of malonyl CoA (as well as in other carboxylations), and niacin in the form of reduced NADP, which is required in the reductions following each 2-carbon addition. The major source of acetyl CoA for fatty acid synthesis is glucose, but excess dietary amino acids may also provide it. Therefore, fatty acid synthesis from acetyl CoA is stimulated by high caloric intake, and it represents one of the major steps in the conversion of excess energy into adipose tissue triglycerides.

Chain elongation of existing fatty acids provides a means of increasing the chain length by addition of 2-carbon units until a desired length is reached. This mechanism does not produce a net increase in fatty acids, but it allows the body to alter its fatty acid composition according to its need.

Desaturation of fatty acids (formation of a double bond) is another means of altering the fatty acids available to satisfy the needs of the body. For example, the monounsaturated oleic acid (C18:1) is formed from stearic acid (C18:0). Polyunsaturated fatty acids are also synthesized from existing unsaturated fatty acids. Linoleic acid (C18:2) is converted to arachidonic acid (C20:4) by initial desaturation (removal of two hydrogens) and addition of a 2-carbon unit, followed by another desaturation. Because of the specificity of the enzyme system regarding the location at which the desaturation can take place, the structure of the unsaturated precursor determines the location of the new double bonds. Linoleic acid cannot be synthesized because no precursor is available in the body.

CHOLESTEROL SYNTHESIS. Cholesterol, a structural component in all cellular membranes, can be synthesized in all tissues. Biosynthesis from acetyl CoA in the liver and possibly in the intestine contributes to the circulating (serum) cholesterol, as does dietary intake.[47] Cholesterol ingestion exerts a negative feedback control on hepatic but not on intestinal cholesterol production.[48] Unfortunately, this mechanism is not adequate to prevent elevation of serum cholesterol induced by high influx of dietary cholesterol. With increased cholesterol intake, the maximal suppression of synthesis observed in Caucasians in the United States is about 25 percent as compared to a cholesterol free diet, whereas 36 percent suppression has been reported for Alaskan Eskimos and 50 percent for African Masai.[49] On the other hand, because of the incompleteness of this feedback mechanism, decreasing dietary cholesterol intake to below 300 mg. per day results in a fall of serum cholesterol despite the stimulation in hepatic cholesterol production.[50] As previously mentioned, the major mechanism for cholesterol degradation is through its conversion into bile acids in the liver (see p. 133).

METABOLIC INTERRELATIONSHIPS AMONG CARBOHYDRATE, PROTEIN, AND FAT IN THE MAJOR TISSUES OF THE BODY

Adipose tissue, liver, and muscle are the three major tissues which maintain the metabolic homeostasis in the body, despite the differences in their individual functions and metabolic machinery. The major factors that determine the metabolic state of these tissues are the availability of glucose and the level of insulin relative to other hormones which oppose its actions.

Adipose Tissue

Instead of being a static storage area for energy, the adipose tissue is metabolically very active and exerts a profound influence on the metabolic balance of the body. Like the proteins of muscle, the adipose tissue triglycerides are in a dynamic equilibrium, with continuous breakdown and resynthesis taking place without any appreciable change in the total fat content. During the normal course of a 24-hour day there are periods when the triglyceride synthesis exceeds the breakdown and vice versa.

In the fed state when the supply of glucose is plentiful, its utilization in all metabolic pathways in the adipose tissue is high. Under these conditions triglyceride synthesis is favored over breakdown in several ways. First, glucose oxidation in the citric acid cycle provides a large proportion of the energy needs, thereby minimizing fatty acid oxidation and directing fatty acids to triglyceride synthesis. Second, the ample supply of glucose also provides adequate amounts of α-glycerophosphate for fatty acid reesterification. Due to low glycerokinase activity, the glycerol released from triglyceride breakdown cannot be reutilized in the adipose tissue. It is released into the blood and metabolized in the liver. Third, the high rate of glucose breakdown also provides more acetyl CoA than is needed for immediate energy needs, the excess providing substrate for fatty acid synthesis. This lipogenesis serves as a means of storing carbohydrate and protein energy for the periods when intestinal absorption is not delivering nutrients to the body. The same mechanism is responsible for weight gain if more triglyceride is stored than will be mobilized to supply the daily energy needs. Finally, oxidation of glucose in the hexose monophosphate shunt yields reduced NADP (nicotinamide adenine dinucleotide phosphate) which is required for fatty acid synthesis from acetyl CoA.

In the postabsorptive state (fasting) the supply of glucose to adipose cells is low and its utilization in all pathways is reduced. Even though a high proportion of the available glucose reverts to production of α-glycerophosphate, it is not sufficient for the triglyceride synthesis to keep up with its breakdown, and fatty acids are released into the blood as NEFA. This fat mobilization is a normal mechanism for supplying the body tissues with a source of energy when blood glucose is low. Some of the NEFA is directly removed by muscle and other tissues while some is first resynthesized into VLDL triglycerides in the liver. The latter activity especially occurs when excessive mobilization of fat takes place, leading to secondary hyperglyceridemia.

Insulin has a major influence on the metabolism of adipose tissue. A high level of circulating insulin as found in the normal fed state facilitates the uptake of glucose, and secondarily favors triglyceride synthesis. Insulin also has a direct influence on the adipose tissue triglyceride storage. The first step in lipolysis (TG→DG) is catalyzed by an enzyme known as *hormone sensitive lipase*. Insulin inhibits the activity of this enzyme whereas several other hormones stimulate its lipolytic activity. Figure 9–15 shows the interrelationships of the major metabolic pathways in the adipose tissue and the hormonal influence on fat mobilization.

In the fed state the influence of insulin prevails over the lipolytic action of the opposing hormones, and fat storage takes place. When insulin activity is low (fasting), lipolysis is favored and adipose tissue fat is mobilized according to the needs of the body, in a controlled fashion. In conditions of hormonal imbalance, such as insulin insufficiency in untreated diabetes, fat mobilization continues uncontrolled. Although the blood glucose level is very high due to its inability to enter adipose and muscle cells without adequate insulin, the "message" to the adipose cell is to mobilize the energy stores. Lack of α-glycerophosphate in the cell reduces the capacity for reesterification of fatty acids and they are released into the blood.

Muscle

Both glucose and fatty acids are normally oxidized in the muscle, the proportion of each at any one time depending on the metabolic state of and nutrient supply to the body. When glucose is plentiful its uptake is high and it is converted to glycogen as well as used for energy production along with fatty acids. The amino acid uptake is also high, stimulated by the relatively high level of circulating insulin, and active protein synthesis takes place.

When blood glucose and insulin levels drop in the postabsorptive state, fatty acid uptake and oxidation increase with corresponding decrease in glucose uptake and utilization. This reciprocal relationship between glucose and fatty acid utilization in the muscle and adipose tissue has been attributed to the existence of a so-called *glucose-fatty acid cycle* proposed by Randle et al.[51] According to this concept the high levels of NEFA and their oxidation products suppress the uptake and catabolism of glucose during carbohydrate deprivation, and conversely, ingestion of carbohydrate with consequent increase in insulin level promptly reduces fatty acid release from the adipose tissue.

During the early postabsorptive period glycogenolysis provides intermediates for the citric acid cycle to allow complete oxidation of fatty acids. When fasting continues, glycogen stores become depleted and protein breakdown increases, releasing amino acids into the blood. As with fat mobilization in adipose tissue, the protein catabolism in muscle is under control and represents a normal response to provide substrates for gluconeogenesis in the liver, allowing maintenance of a blood glucose level that satisfies the minimal needs of the body. In untreated diabetes mellitus the amino acid mobilization is excessive, resulting in wasting of body tissues.

Liver

The liver plays a central role in the many homeostatic mechanisms of the body. When the flow of glucose from intestinal absorption is high, the glycogen stores of the liver are being filled, lipogenesis from glucose-derived acetyl CoA is active, and amino acids are incorporated into proteins. Glycogenolysis and gluconeogenesis are minimal. Hormonal balance again exerts a controlling influence in these metabolic events. The activity of insulin is high relative to the hormones which oppose its actions, and anabolism prevails.

When the blood glucose and insulin levels fall in the postabsorptive state, glycogenolysis increases and glucose is released into the circulation. With the reduction of glycogen stores, amino acid uptake and conversion to glucose increase. Glucose breakdown by glycolysis diminishes while the fatty acid uptake and β-oxidation accelerate. All of these adjustments

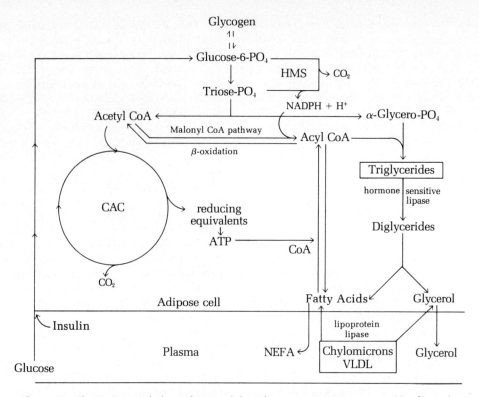

Fig. 9–15. The major metabolic pathways of the adipose tissue. Hormone sensitive lipase is activated by several hormones including epinephrine, norepinephrine, glucagon, ACTH (adrenocorticotropic hormone), and TSH (thyroid-stimulating hormone), whereas insulin inhibits it. In fed state, the uptake of fatty acids from chylomicron triglycerides by the adipose tissue is high. The level of insulin is also high, resulting in low lipolytic activity and increased uptake and utilization of glucose by the adipose tissue. Under such conditions, glucose not only provides energy, but also supplies precursors for fatty acid and triglyceride synthesis (acetyl CoA, NADPH + H+, and α-glycerophosphate). Therefore, the synthesis of triglycerides exceeds the breakdown, and storage of energy as adipose tissue triglycerides takes place. In fasting state the level of insulin and the availability of glucose and fatty acids to the adipose tissue are low. Triglyceride breakdown is stimulated by the action of the lipolytic hormones and fatty acids (as NEFA) and glycerol are released into the blood. Thus adipose tissue fat is mobilized to provide energy to the body during the periods when nutrients are not supplied by ingestion of food. (HMS = hexose monophosphate shunt; CAC = citric acid cycle; NADP = nicotinamide adenine dinucleotide phosphate; CoA = coenzyme A; ATP = adenosine triphosphate; NEFA = nonesterified fatty acids; VLDL = very low density lipoproteins)

contribute to maintenance of blood glucose levels and provide a continuous supply of glucose to the tissues that most depend on it. Figure 9–16 summarizes the balance of glucose and glucose precursors in postabsorptive man.

Ketosis

When fat mobilization from adipose tissue is high, β-oxidation of fatty aicds in the liver produces more acetyl CoA than can be oxidized in the citric acid cycle or utilized for synthetic purposes. The high concentration of fatty acids and low relative insulin activity seem to inhibit both the activity of the citric acid cycle and the conversion of acetyl CoA into fatty acids as well as the conversion of the latter to triglycerides by some mechanisms not entirely understood.

Under such conditions a high proportion of acetyl CoA is converted to acetoacetate, which is further converted to β-hydroxybutyrate and acetone, all of which are known as *ketone bodies* and are released into the blood. Ketone bodies are normal metabolites which are usually oxidized by the extrahepatic tissues at a rate comparable to their production in the liver. When the production is excessive as in prolonged fasting and in untreated diabetes, the ketone bodies accumulate in the blood (ketonemia) and spill into the urine (ketonuria), a condition known as *ketosis.* Ketoacidosis is a result of severe ketosis with concurrent loss of base from the body, leading to a drop in blood pH. Carbohydrate metabolism in the cells seems to be necessary for clearance of ketone bodies from the blood. Mild ketosis, observed when dietary carbohydrate is restricted to a very low level (as advocated for some reducing diets), is promptly reversed by increasing carbohydrate intake. Administration of insulin to a diabetic has a comparable effect. The antiketogenic effects of insulin and carbohydrate are due more to a decreased production of acetyl CoA from β-oxidation of fatty acids than to an increased utilization of ketone bodies.[52]

Hormonal Regulation of Metabolism

It is obvious from the preceding discussions that the balance between the catabolic and anabolic reactions in the body tissues is under hormonal control. Numerous hormones are known to influence nutrient metabolism in many and varied ways. Detailed discussion of the actions of individual hormones is beyond the purpose of this book. Only the major directions of such hormonal control are summarized in order to emphasize the complex integration of the many mechanisms and tissues which are involved in the maintenance of metabolic balance in the body.

Insulin is probably the only hormone which has an anabolic effect in each of its target tissues and

influences the metabolism of each of the body fuels. Table 9–5 summarizes the metabolic activity of carbohydrate, protein, and fat in normal fed and fasting states which are characterized by high and low insulin activity, respectively.

As was mentioned previously, the metabolic activity at any one time is the result of the hormonal balance rather than of the action of any one individual hormone. Thus all of the activities listed in Table 9–5 cannot be attributed to direct effects of insulin or lack of insulin. Many of the changes observed in fasting are due to the action of other hormones as well as to the decrease in insulin action. The direction of metabolic changes in diabetes mellitus is the same as in fasting, but even at the low fasting levels insulin exerts a metabolic control which is absent in diabetes.

Though many of the individual reactions which are subject to hormonal control are known, the mechanisms by which these agents act are not understood in most instances. It has become evident in recent years that the metabolic actions of several hormones are mediated by a widely distributed substance, cyclic adenosine monophosphate (cAMP), designated as a "second messenger." Hormones, the "first messengers," control the level of cAMP by influencing either its synthesis or breakdown in their target cells. Thus the "lipolytic" hormones (Fig. 9–15) elevate the level of cAMP in the adipose cells

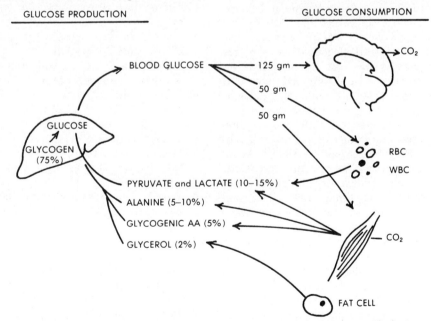

GLUCOSE PRODUCTION   **GLUCOSE CONSUMPTION**

Fig. 9–16. Balance of glucose and glucose precursors in postabsorptive man. The brain is the prime site of glucose consumption. Most of the glucose released by the liver is derived by glycogenolysis. As fasting progresses, gluconeogenesis replaces glycogenolysis as the predominant mode of glucose formation. Numbers in parentheses represent proportion of glucose output attributable to uptake of various precursors in postabsorptive state. (Redrawn from Felig, P., Metabolism 22:179, 1973. By permission)

Table 9–5. Metabolic activity of the body fuels in normal fed (high insulin) and fasting (low insulin) states

METABOLIC FUELS	METABOLIC STATE	LIVER	ADIPOSE CELL	MUSCLE
Carbohydrate	Fed	↑ glycogen synthesis ↑ glycolysis ↓ gluconeogenesis	↑ glucose uptake ↑ glucose metabolism	↑ glucose uptake ↑ glycolysis ↑ glycogen synthesis
	Fasted	↑ glycogenolysis ↓ glycolysis ↑ gluconeogenesis ↑ glucose release	↓ glucose uptake ↓ glucose metabolism	↓ glucose uptake ↓ glycolysis ↑ glycogenolysis
Fat	Fed	↑ fatty acid synthesis ↓β-oxidation ↑ triglyceride synthesis	↑ fatty acid uptake ↑ triglyceride synthesis ↑ fatty acid synthesis ↓ lipolysis	↓ fatty acid uptake ↓ fatty acid oxidation
	Fasted	↓ lipogenesis ↑ fatty acid uptake ↑β-oxidation ↑ ketogenesis	↓ triglyceride synthesis ↑ lipolysis ↑ fatty acid release	↑ fatty acid uptake ↑ fatty acid oxidation
Protein	Fed	↓ amino acid catabolism		↑ amino acid uptake ↑ protein synthesis
	Fasted	↑ amino acid uptake ↑ amino acid catabolism		↑ proteolysis ↑ amino acid release

and other tissues, whereas insulin seems to decrease its concentration in the same tissues. In the adipose tissue a high concentration of cAMP activates the hormone-sensitive lipase, thus increasing triglyceride breakdown. Conversely, lipolytic activity is reduced by low levels of cAMP.

Glucagon. In the liver the synthesis and breakdown of glycogen are controlled by cAMP. Of the hormones "antagonistic" to insulin, glucagon has probably the most powerful effect on the level of this metabolic regulator in the liver.[53] Glucagon is secreted in response to low levels of blood glucose. It increases the synthesis of cAMP, which at high levels increases glycogenolysis by activating the enzyme phosphorylase. It also inactivates glycogen synthetase, thereby preventing storage of glucose as glycogen, and stimulates gluconeogenesis. All of these actions increase the release of glucose into the blood.

Epinephrine also influences blood glucose through the cAMP-mediated mechanisms comparable to those of glucagon, but it is less potent in the liver. It is a powerful stimulus to muscle glycogenolysis, again through activation of phosphorylase by increased concentrations of cAMP. Involvement of cAMP in the regulation of protein synthesis and breakdown in muscle is likely, but the site of such control is not known for certain.

Adrenal corticosteroids are known to increase protein catabolism and interfere with protein synthesis in the peripheral tissues. They also stimulate gluconeogenesis in the liver, but the mechanism of their action remains unclear.

STUDY QUESTIONS AND ACTIVITIES

1. Identify the structural features of the intestinal mucosa which play a major role in the digestive-absorptive processes.
2. What is the main difference between active and passive absorption mechanisms?
3. Differentiate between simple and facilitated diffusion.
4. Identify the differences in the luminal phase of LCT and MCT digestion.
5. Identify the differences in the intracellular phase of digestion and absorption of LCT and MCT.
6. Describe the enterohepatic circulation of bile salts.
7. What is the role of bile salts in the digestion and absorption of LCT?
8. Describe the role of the epithelial brushborder in the digestion and absorption of carbohydrates and proteins.
9. What is the role of acetyl CoA in the production of energy in the body? In storing excess food energy?
10. What is the role of β-oxidation in the production of energy from fat?
11. List in sequence the metabolic pathways involved in the complete oxidation of glucose to produce CO_2, H_2O, and ATP.
12. Describe the roles of the Cori cycle and the glucose-alanine cycle in the skeletal muscle.
13. How is the level of blood glucose maintained in different metabolic stages (fed, fasting, and starvation)?

14. Describe how excess food energy is converted to adipose tissue fat regardless of the form in which it is ingested.
15. What are the dietary factors that most consistently influence the level of plasma VLDL? LDL? Chylomicrons?
16. Differentiate between the m-RNA, t-RNA, and ribosomal RNA as they relate to protein synthesis.
17. Compare the metabolic effects of insulin in the adipose tissue, liver, and muscle.

SUPPLEMENTARY READINGS

Biomembranes, Vol. 4A, D. H. Smyth, ed. London, Plenum Press, 1974.
  Crane, R. K.: Intestinal absorption of glucose, p. 541.
  Milne, M. D.: Hereditary disorders of intestinal absorption, p. 961.
  Wiseman, G.: Absorption of protein digestion products, p. 363.
Biomembranes, Vol. 4B, D. H. Smyth, ed. London, Plenum Press, 1974.
  Borgstrom, B.: Fat digestion and absorption, p. 555.
  Brindley, D. N.: The intracellular phase of fat absorption, p. 621.
  Jackson, M. J.: Transport of short chain fatty acids, p. 673.
Biomembranes, Vol. 7, H. Eisenberg, E. Katchaledki-Katzir, and L. A. Mason, eds. London, Plenum Press, 1975.
  Barak, Z., and Gilvarg, C.: Peptide transport, p. 167.
Connor, W. E., and Lin, D. S.: The intestinal absorption of dietary cholesterol by hypercholesterolemic (Type II) and normocholesterolemic humans. J. Clin. Invest. 53:1062, 1974.
Danielson, H., and Sjovall, J.: Bile acid metabolism. Ann. Rev. Biochem. 44:233, 1975.
Feldman, S. A., Rubenstein, A. H., Ho, K-J, Taylor, C. B., Lewis, L. A., and Mikkelson, B.: Carbohydrate and lipid metabolism in the Alaskan Arctic Eskimo. Am. J. Clin. Nutr. 28:588, 1975.
Felig, P.: Amino acid metabolism in man. Ann. Rev. Biochem. 44:933, 1975.
Kudchodkar, B. J., Sodhi, H. S., and Horlick, L.: Absorption of dietary cholesterol in man. Metabolism 22:155, 1973.
Matthews, D. M.: Intestinal absorption of amino acids and peptides. Proc. Nutr. Soc. 31:171, 1972.
Mattson, F. H., Erickson, B. A., and Kligman, A. M.: Effect of dietary cholesterol on serum cholesterol in man. Am. J. Clin. Nutr. 25:589, 1972.
Morrisett, J. D., Jackson, R. L., and Grotto, A. M. Jr.: Lipoproteins: structure and function. Ann. Rev. Biochem. 44:183, 1975.
Olsen, W. A.: Carbohydrate absorption. Med. Clin. N. Am. 58:1387, 1974.
Review: Amino acid, dipeptide and protein absorption in human beings. Nutr. Rev. 31:272, 1973.
Review: Mechanisms of carbohydrate-induced hypertriglyceridemia. Nutr. Rev. 32:74, 1974.
Review: Metabolism of alpha-keto analogues of essential amino acids. Nutr. Rev. 32:147, 1974.
Review: The role of sugars in hyperlipidemia. Nutr. Rev. 32:340, 1974.
Review: Sucrose, starch and hyperlipidemia. Nutr. Rev. 33:44, 1975.
Westergaard, H., and Dietschy, J. M.: Normal mechanisms of fat absorption and derangements induced by various gastrointestinal diseases. Med. Clin. N. Am. 58:1413, 1974.
Young, S. K., Nicholson, J. A., and Curtis, K. J.: Intestinal peptide hydrolases: Peptide and amino acid absorption. Med. Clin. N. Am. 58:1397, 1974.

For further references see Bibliography in Section 4.

REFERENCES

1. Babka, J. C., and D. O. Castell: Am. J. Digest. Dis. 18:391, 1973.
2. Gray, G. M.: Fed. Proc. 26:1415, 1967.
3. Ugolev, A. M.: Physiol. Rev. 45:555, 1965.
4. Gracey, M., Burke, V., and Oshin, A.: in Transport Across the Intestine, W. L. Burland and P. D. Samuel, eds. Baltimore, Williams and Wilkins, 1972, p. 99.
5. Phillips, S. I., and McGill, D. B.: Am. J. Digest. Dis. 18:1017, 1973.
6. Peters, T. J., Donlon, J., and Fottrell, P. F.: in Transport Across the Intestine, W. L. Burland and P. D. Samuel, eds. Baltimore, Williams and Wilkins, 1972, p. 153.
7. Matthews, D. M.: Proc. Nutr. Soc. 31:171, 1972.
8. Ibid.
9. Ibid.
10. Ibid.
11. Holt, P. R., and Clark, S. B.: Am. J. Clin. Nutr. 22:279, 1969.
12. Ibid.
13. Holt, P. R.: J. Am. Dietet. A. 60:491, 1972.
14. Ibid.
15. Ibid.
16. Marubbio, A. T. Jr., Morris, J. A., Jr., Clark, S. B., and Holt, P. R.: J. Lipid Res. 15:165, 1974.
17. McIntyre, N., and Isselbacher, K. J.: Am. J. Clin. Nutr. 26:647, 1973.
18. Ockner, R. K. F., Hughes, F. B., and Isselbacher, K. T.: J. Clin. Inv. 48:2367, 1969.
19. Cohen, M., Morgan, R. G. H., and Hofman, A. F.: Gastroenterology 60:1, 1971.
20. Ockner, Hughes, and Isselbacher, op. cit.
21. Holt, op. cit.
22. Kalser, M.: Adv. Intern. Med. 17:301, 1973.
23. Wilson, J. D., and Lindsey, C. A., Jr.: J. Clin. Invest. 44:1805, 1965.
24. Grundy, S. M., and Ahrens, E. H., Jr.: J. Lipid Res. 10:91, 1969.
25. Borgström, B., Radner, S., and Werner, B.: Scand. J. Clin. Lab. Invest. 26:227, 1970.
26. Quintao, E., Grundy, S. M., Ahrens, E. H., Jr.: J. Lipid Res. 12:233, 1971.

27. Connor, W. E., and Lin, D.: J. Lab. Clin. Med. 76:870, 1970.
28. Kudchodkar, B. J., Sodhi, H. S., and Horlick, L.: Metabolism 22:155, 1973.
29. Mattson, F. H., Erickson, B. A., and Kligman, A. M.: Am. J. Clin. Nutr. 25:589, 1972.
30. Connor, W. E., and Lin, D. S.: J. Clin. Invest. 53:1062, 1974.
31. Ibid.
32. Kudchodkar, Sodhi, and Horlick, op. cit.
33. Anon: Nutr. Rev. 29:199, 1971.
34. Blomstrand, R.: Acta Physiol. Scand. 34:147, 1955.
35. Stein, Y., and Stein, O.: Biochim. Biophys. Acta 116:95, 1966.
36. Felig, P.: Metabolism 22:179, 1973.
37. Giordano, C.: J. Lab. Clin. Med. 62:231, 1963.
38. Gioovannetti, S., and Maggiore, A.: Lancet 1:1000, 1964.
39. Close, J. H.: N. Eng. J. Med. 290:663, 1974.
40. Walser, M., Coulter, A. W., and Dighe, S.: J. Clin. Invest. 52:678, 1973.
41. Madrey, W. C., Chura, C. M., and Coulter, A. W.: Gastroenterology 5:553, 1973.
42. Albrink, M. J.: J. Am. Dietet. A. 62:626, 1973.
43. Ibid.
44. Levy, R. I., and Ernst, N.: in *Modern Nutrition in Health and Disease*, R. S. Goodhart and M. E. Shils, eds. Philadelphia, Lea and Febiger, 1973, p. 895.
45. The Dietary Management of Hyperlipoproteinemia—A Handbook for Physicians and Dietitians, Bethesda, Maryland, Natl. Heart and Lung Inst. Revised 1973.
46. Miller, G. J., and Miller, N. E.: Lancet 1:16, 1975.
47. Dietschy, J., and Wilson, J.: N. Eng. J. Med. 282:1128, 1970.
48. Ibid.
49. Ho, K-J, Mikkelson, B., Lewis, L. A., Feldman, S. A., and Taylor, C. B.: Am. J. Clin. Nutr. 25:737, 1972.
50. Levy and Ernst, op. cit.
51. Randle, P. J., Garland, P. B., Newsholme, E. A., and Hales, C. N.: Ann. N.Y. Acad. Sci. 131:324, 1965.
52. Cahill, G. F., Jr.: in *Diabetes Mellitus: Diagnosis and Treatment*, Vol. III, S. S. Fajans and K. E. Sussman, eds. New York, Am. Diabet. Assoc., 1970, p. 57.
53. Ibid.

meeting nutritional norms

10

INTERPRETATION AND USE OF RECOMMENDED DIETARY ALLOWANCES

In the discussion in preceding chapters of the various nutrients needed for health, references have frequently been made to the Recommended Dietary Allowances. These represent the establishment of a nutritional norm for planning and assessing dietary intake.

When the Food and Nutrition Board was appointed by the National Academy of Sciences–National Research Council (NAS–NRC) in 1940, it undertook as one of its most important projects the establishment of a set of figures for human needs in terms of specific nutrients. As a result of long and careful consideration, Recommended Dietary Allowances (RDA) were first published in 1943. Since then, they have been revised many times as new research data have become available. Their use has also expanded. They are used as a guide "for planning and procuring food supplies for population groups; for

157

Table 10–1. Food and Nutrition Board, National Academy of Sciences-National Research Council Recommended Daily Dietary Allowances[a] Revised 1974
Designed for the Maintenance of Good Nutrition of Practically All Healthy People in the U.S.A.

	Age (years)	Weight (kg.)	Weight (lbs.)	Height (cm.)	Height (in.)	Energy (kcal.)[b]	Protein (g)	FAT-SOLUBLE VITAMINS Vitamin A Activity (RE)[c]	(IU)	Vitamin D (IU)	Vitamin E Activity[e] (IU)	WATER-SOLUBLE VITAMINS Ascorbic Acid (mg.)	Folacin[f] (mcg.)	Niacin[g] (mg.)	Riboflavin (mg.)	Thiamin (mg.)	Vitamin B6 (mg.)	Vitamin B12 (mcg.)	MINERALS Calcium (mg.)	Phosphorus (mg.)	Iodine (mcg.)	Iron (mg.)	Magnesium (mg.)	Zinc (mg.)
Infants	0.0-0.5	6	14	60	24	kg × 117	kg × 2.2	420[d]	1,400	400	4	35	50	5	0.4	0.3	0.3	0.3	360	240	35	10	60	3
	0.5-1.0	9	20	71	28	kg × 108	kg × 2.0	400	2,000	400	5	35	50	8	0.6	0.5	0.4	0.3	540	400	45	15	70	5
Children	1-3	13	28	86	34	1,300	23	400	2,000	400	7	40	100	9	0.8	0.7	0.6	1.0	800	800	60	15	150	10
	4-6	20	44	110	44	1,800	30	500	2,500	400	9	40	200	12	1.1	0.9	0.9	1.5	800	800	80	10	200	10
	7-10	30	66	135	54	2,400	36	700	3,300	400	10	40	300	16	1.2	1.2	1.2	2.0	800	800	110	10	250	10
Males	11-14	44	97	158	63	2,800	44	1,000	5,000	400	12	45	400	18	1.5	1.4	1.6	3.0	1,200	1,200	130	18	350	15
	15-18	61	134	172	69	3,000	54	1,000	5,000	400	15	45	400	20	1.8	1.5	2.0	3.0	1,200	1,200	150	18	400	15
	19-22	67	147	172	69	3,000	54	1,000	5,000	400	15	45	400	20	1.8	1.5	2.0	3.0	800	800	140	10	350	15
	23-50	70	154	172	69	2,700	56	1,000	5,000		15	45	400	18	1.6	1.4	2.0	3.0	800	800	130	10	350	15
	51+	70	154	172	69	2,400	56	1,000	5,000		15	45	400	16	1.5	1.2	2.0	3.0	800	800	110	10	350	15
Females	11-14	44	97	155	62	2,400	44	800	4,000	400	12	45	400	16	1.3	1.2	1.6	3.0	1,200	1,200	115	18	300	15
	15-18	54	119	162	65	2,100	48	800	4,000	400	12	45	400	14	1.4	1.1	2.0	3.0	1,200	1,200	115	18	300	15
	19-22	58	128	162	65	2,100	46	800	4,000	400	12	45	400	14	1.4	1.1	2.0	3.0	800	800	100	18	300	15
	23-50	58	128	162	65	2,000	46	800	4,000		12	45	400	13	1.2	1.0	2.0	3.0	800	800	100	18	300	15
	51+	58	128	162	65	1,800	46	800	4,000		12	45	400	12	1.1	1.0	2.0	3.0	800	800	80	10	300	15
Pregnant						+300	+30	1,000	5,000	400	15	60	800	+2	+0.3	+0.3	2.5	4.0	1,200	1,200	125	18+[h]	450	20
Lactating						+500	+20	1,200	6,000	400	15	80	600	+4	+0.5	+0.3	2.5	4.0	1,200	1,200	150	18	450	25

[a] The allowances are intended to provide for individual variations among most normal persons as they live in the United States under usual environmental stresses. Diets should be based on a variety of common foods in order to provide other nutrients for which human requirements have been less well defined. From Recommended Dietary Allowances, 8th ed., Washington, D.C., NAS-NRC, 1974.

[b] Kilojoules (k J) = 4.2 × kcal.

[c] Retinol equivalents.

[d] Assumed to be all as retinol in milk during the first six months of life. All subsequent intakes are assumed to be half as retinol and half as β-carotene when calculated from international units. As retinol equivalents, three fourths are as retinol and one fourth as β-carotene.

[e] Total vitamin E activity, estimated to be 80 percent as α-tocopherol and 20 percent other tocopherols.

[f] The folacin allowances refer to dietary sources as determined by Lactobacillus casei assay. Pure forms of folacin may be effective in doses less than one fourth of the recommended dietary allowance.

[g] Although allowances are expressed as niacin, it is recognized that on the average 1 mg. of niacin is derived from each 60 mg. of dietary tryptophan.

[h] This increased requirement cannot be met by ordinary diets; therefore, the use of supplemental iron is recommended.

interpreting food consumption records; for establishing standards for public assistance programs; for evaluating the adequacy of food supplies in meeting national nutritional needs; for developing nutrition education programs; for the development of new products for industry; and for establishing guidelines for nutritional labeling of foods."[1]

Allowances vs. Requirements

Dr. Alfred E. Harper, Chairman of the Committee on Dietary Allowances, Food and Nutrition Board, in introducing the 1974 revision of the Recommended Dietary Allowances (Table 10–1) described the process and some of the problems involved in determining the allowances.

The logical starting point for estimating allowances for nutrients ... is to assemble information about estimated requirements. However, requirements differ with age and body size; among individuals of the same body size owing to differences in genetic makeup; with the physiologic state of the individual—growth rate, pregnancy, lactation; and with sex. They may also be influenced by a person's activity and by environmental conditions. Information about all these factors cannot be included in tables of allowances, although the values are presented for selected age, weight, and sex groups, as physiologic state and body size are the most important factors that influence nutritional needs.

Once the age groups have been selected, the initial problem in estimating an allowance is to establish values for average requirements. If sufficient data are available from human experiments, an average requirement can be calculated. If not, information from studies on other species or about minimum nutrient intakes of individuals in good health may have to be used.

Even when knowledge of human requirements is available, agreement about the criteria for judging when the requirement has been met may still be a problem. The requirement for a nutrient is the minimum intake that will maintain normal function and health. For infants and children, the requirement may be equated with the amount which will maintain a satisfactory rate of growth; for an adult, with the amount which will maintain body weight and prevent depletion of the nutrient from the body as judged by balance studies or the maintenance of acceptable blood and tissue concentrations. For some nutrients, the requirements may be assessed as the amount that will just prevent the development of specific deficiency signs, an amount that may differ by several fold from that required to maintain maximum body stores. A substantial element of judgment is involved in deciding where, between these extremes, the requirement has been met....

In setting allowances, it is also necessary to consider any factor that influences efficiency of utilization of the nutrient. For some nutrients, a part of the requirement may be met by a precursor which is converted to the essential nutrient within the body. In setting the allowance for vitamin A, for example, which is met in part by carotenes, consideration is given to the efficiency of conversion of carotenes to vitamin A. For some nutrients, absorption is incomplete and the allowance must reflect the proportion of the ingested nutrient that fails to gain entrance to the body. This is of major importance in setting allowances for several minerals, especially iron.

With such problems, it is perhaps not surprising that there are differences of opinion about the validity of values for requirements and allowances.[2]

The Recommended Dietary Allowances are defined in the 1974 (8th) edition as follows:

The Recommended Dietary Allowances are the levels of intake of essential nutrients considered ... to be adequate to meet the known needs of practically all healthy persons.

RDA are recommendations for the amounts of nutrients that should be consumed daily. They are estimates neither of the amounts of nutrients needed per capita in the national or local food supply, nor even in the food purchased. Thus, losses of nutrients that occur during the processing and preparation of food should be taken into consideration in planning diets based on tables of food composition.

RDA should not be confused with requirements. Differences in the nutrient requirements of individuals that derive from differences in their genetic makeup are ordinarily unknown. Therefore, as there is no way of predicting whose needs are high and whose are low, RDA (except for energy) are estimates to exceed the requirements of most individuals, and thereby ensure that the needs of nearly all are met.

RDA are intakes of nutrients that meet the needs of healthy people and do not take into account special needs arising from infections, metabolic disorders, chronic diseases or other abnormalities that require special dietary treatment. These must be considered as unique chemical problems that require individual attention.

The nutritional needs of the premature infant are also considered to fall in this category.

Continued use of certain pharmaceutical preparations such as oral contraceptives may also influence specific nutritional needs. RDA are not formulated to cover these effects. . . .

We are aware of no convincing evidence of unique health benefits accruing from consumption of a large excess of any one nutrient. Large doses of individual nutrients may have some pharmacologic action, but such effects are unrelated to nutritional function.[3]

The RDA (Table 10-1) are expressed in nutrients rather than in specific foods because these particular recommendations can be attained from a variety of different food patterns. The Committee on Dietary Allowances also points out that "to ensure that possibly unrecognized nutritional needs are met, RDA should be provided from as varied a selection of foods as is practicable."[4] One should also remember that the allowances are not minimum requirements for individuals; failure to achieve these intake levels should not be interpreted as malnutrition unless additional nutritional status information (physical, biochemical, or clinical assessment) is available and is also indicative of deficiencies.

The Dietary Standards for Canada[5] and the recommended intakes set by Joint FAO/WHO Expert Groups[6,7,8,9,10] Chapter 20, Table 20-8 also represent nutritional norms which according to Dr. J. A. Campbell of Canada are similar to RDA in "philosophy, derivation, and use of allowances. Differences in individual figures are related largely to the degree of ignorance in relating minimum requirements to recommended levels for optimal health."[11] Many other countries have also established appropriate standards in attempts to improve national dietary intakes.

Energy Allowances

The body requires food energy for metabolic processes, physical activity, growth, lactation, and maintenance of body temperature. Energy needs vary greatly with the size and activity of the individual. The energy allowances were established at the lowest level which would maintain good health. The requirements for average adults (male—70 kg., 172 cm.; female—58 kg., 162 cm.) engaged in light occupations were set for two age groups—23 to 50 years and over 50 years. They are presumed to live in an environment with a mean temperature of 20° C. (70° F.). Adjustments must be made when the characteristics of an individual or population group differ from the size, activity, or climate defined above.

The energy allowances set for infants during the first year of life are based on the general pattern of intake recorded for thriving infants. Energy allowances (kilocalories per kilogram) decrease gradually throughout infancy, childhood, and adult life. Age groups, except for the first year, are given in three- or four-year intervals up to age 23. The allowances for children are listed separately for the sexes after age 10, when differences in growth rate between boys and girls occur. Allowances are based on needs for the middle years in each age group and for light activity. Allowances for pregnancy and lactation are also included.

Although the recommended allowances are given in kilocalories, they may be converted to kilojoules as follows: 1 kilocalorie = 4.2 kilojoules.

Carbohydrate, fat, and protein provide sources of energy. Alcohol may also contribute calories to the diet. No specific recommendations were made for the proportion of calories to be derived from different sources. Attention, however, was called to the American Heart Association recommendation that energy derived from fat should not exceed 35 percent of the total, and "of that amount, less than 10 percent of total calories should come from saturated fatty acids and up to 10 percent from polyunsaturated fatty acids." Foods containing complex carbohydrate are suggested as the most appropriate replacement for fat in the diet.[12]

Warnings that surplus intake will be stored as fat and if continued will lead to obesity and be harmful to health are given in this edition, which emphasizes that the recommendations for energy are strictly estimates of average needs of population groups and not recommended intakes for individuals.[13]

Adjustment of caloric needs to size and activities, however, is not simple. Dictates of appetite and maintenance of body weight help. For extreme degrees of activity such as heavy physical work, the allowance may be increased as much as 50 percent; for sedentary people it may be reduced by 25 percent. For example, a large teen-age boy, active in athletics, may require 3600 calories, whereas his grandmother, aged 70, cannot use more than 1200 calories (one-third as many) without gaining weight.

Recommended Allowances for Other Nutrients

The specific nutrients included in the 1974 RDA and the quantities of each for the several categories of persons were based upon the consensus of authorities at the time the table was published. Since nutritional requirements differ according to age, sex, body size, physiological state, and genetic makeup, broad age-sex groups have been used for the table of RDA, while the accompanying text includes additional information for adjusting the allowances to suit unique population groups. Other nutrients not listed in the tabulation are apt to be present in adequate amounts in the usual diet, or they are trace elements or vitamins for which there are insufficient data to serve as a basis for recommendations at this time. (See Chapters 5, 6, and 7.)

Other Considerations

Intakes of some nutrients will exceed the RDA standard when the diet just provides the recommended quantities of others that are in low concentration in the food supply. For example, animal products that are naturally high in protein are important sources of several trace nutrients; to meet the allowances for some of the trace nutrients it may be necessary to exceed the allowances for protein and other nutrients.

In developing RDA, no effort was made to relate them to what, for reasons other than strictly nutritional ones, may be considered desirable intakes. For example, a diet that provided merely the recommended allowance for protein would be unacceptable to most people in countries where animal products are an important part of the diet. RDA should not be used as justification for reducing habitual intakes of nutrients.[14]

The recommended allowance values in the table are for nutrients in foods as consumed and consideration should be given to prior losses due to storage, waste, and cooking. Provision should be made for these losses in planning practical dietaries. The allowances do provide for incomplete availability or absorption of nutrients such as iron and carotene.

When the table of allowances is used to calculate the needs of population groups, the total estimate

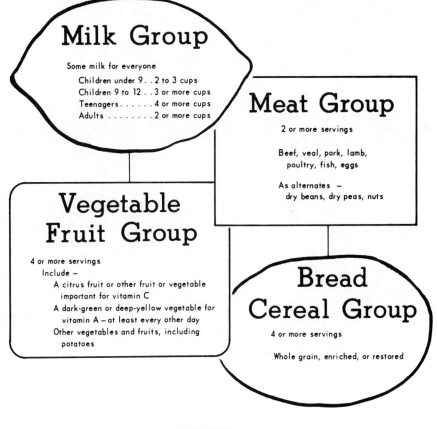

Milk Group

Some milk for everyone

Children under 9 . . 2 to 3 cups
Children 9 to 12 . . 3 or more cups
Teenagers . . . . . . 4 or more cups
Adults . . . . 2 or more cups

Meat Group

2 or more servings

Beef, veal, pork, lamb,
poultry, fish, eggs

As alternates —
dry beans, dry peas, nuts

Vegetable Fruit Group

4 or more servings
Include —
A citrus fruit or other fruit or vegetable
important for vitamin C
A dark-green or deep-yellow vegetable for
vitamin A — at least every other day
Other vegetables and fruits, including
potatoes

Bread Cereal Group

4 or more servings

Whole grain, enriched, or restored

OTHER FOODS

To round out meals and meet energy needs, most everyone will use some foods not specified in the Four Food Groups. Such foods include breads, cereals, flours; sugars, butter, margarine, other fats. These often are ingredients in a recipe or added to other foods during preparation or at table. Try to include some vegetable oils among the fats used.

Fig. 10-1. Food for Fitness: A Daily Food Guide. (Modified from Leaflet 424, U.S. Department of Agriculture, Institute of Home Economics)

Table 10–2. Evaluation of a Pattern Dietary for Its Nutritive Content[a]

Food Group	Amt. in g.	Household Measure	Energy (Kcal.)	Protein (g.)	Fat (g.)	Carbohydrate (g.)	MINERALS Calcium (mg.)	Phosphorus (mg.)	Magnesium (mg.)	Iron (mg.)	VITAMINS A (IU)	Thiamine (mg.)	Riboflavin (mg.)	Niacin (mg.)	Ascorbic Acid (mg.)
Milk or equivalent[b]	488	2 c. (1 pint)	320	17	17	24	576	452	63	.2	700	.16	.84	.3	5
Meat, fish, poultry, or egg[c]	120	4 oz., cooked	376	30	31	..	13	212	104	3.3	280	.14	.23	6.1	..
Vegetables:															
Potato, cooked	100	1 medium	65	2	..	15	6	48	22	.5	..	.09	.03	1.2	16
Deep green or yellow, cooked[d]	75	½ c.	21	2	..	6	44	28	29	.9	4700	.05	.10	.5	25
Other, raw or cooked[e]	75	½ c.	45	2	..	10	16	41	18	.9	300	.08	.06	.6	12
Fruits:															
Citrus[f]	100	1 serving	44	1	..	10	18	16	12	.3	140	.06	.02	.3	43
Other[g]	100	1 serving	85	..	..	22	10	21	16	.8	365	.03	.04	.5	4
Bread, white, enriched	100	4 slices	270	9	3	50	84	97	20	2.5	..	.25	.21	2.4	..
Cereal, whole grain or enriched[h]	130	⅔ c. cooked or 1 oz. dry	89	3	1	18	12	95	34	.9	..	.08	.03	.7	..
Butter or margarine	14	1 tbsp.	100	..	11	..	3	2	2	..	460	..	..	..	..
Totals			1415	66	63	155	782	1012	335	10.3	6945	.94	1.56	12.6[i]	105
Compare with recommended allowances[j]															
Males (70 kg., 23–50 yrs. old)			2700	56	..	..	800	800	350	10.0	5000	1.40	1.60	18	45
Females (58 kg., 23–50 yrs. old)			2000	46	..	..	800	800	300	18.0	4000	1.00	1.20	13	45

[a]Calculations from Composition of Foods. Handbook No. 8. U. S. Department of Agriculture, rev. 1963.
[b]Milk equivalents means evaporated milk and dried milk in amounts equivalent to fluid milk in nutritive content; cheese, if water-soluble minerals and vitamins have not been lost in whey; and food items made with milk.
[c]Evaluation based on the use of 700 g. of beef (chuck, cooked), 200 g. of pork (medium fat, roasted), 200 g. of chicken (roaster, cooked, roasted), and 100 g. of fish (halibut, cooked, broiled) per 10-day period, and egg occasionally.
[d]Evaluation based on figures for cooked broccoli, carrots, spinach, and squash (all varieties).
[e]Evaluation based on figures for raw tomatoes and lettuce, and cooked peas, beets, lima beans, and fresh corn.
[f]Evaluation based on figures for whole orange and grapefruit, and orange and grapefruit juices.
[g]Evaluation based on figures for banana, apple, unsweetened cooked prunes, and sweetened canned peaches.
[h]Evaluation based on figures for shredded wheat biscuit and oatmeal.
[i]The average diet in the United States, which contains a generous amount of protein, provides enough try ptophan to increase the niacin value by about one third.
[j]From the National Research Council Recommended Dietary Allowances, revised 1974.

should take into account the composition of the population, i.e., the age and sex categories. Emergency conditions may necessitate some modification in the interpretation of recommendations. It then becomes desirable to raise the food allowances of as many people as possible to maintenance levels. Rationing at such times should give special attention to the most vulnerable groups.

UNITED STATES RECOMMENDED DAILY ALLOWANCES (US-RDA)

The United States Recommended Daily Allowances (US-RDA), as distinct from the RDA established by the National Research Council are a set of standards developed by the Food and Drug Administration for use in regulating nutrition labeling (see Chapter 14). They replace the Minimum Daily Requirements (MDR) which were formerly used by the FDA for nutrient labeling. Although these new standards are derived from the NRC-RDA, they are based on a very few broad categories. The values for adults and children over the age of 4 were taken from the highest value for each nutrient given in the 1968 NRC-RDA tables for males and nonpregnant, nonlactating females 4 or more years of age except for calcium, phosphorus, biotin, pantothenic acid, copper, and zinc. Separate US-RDA values were established for infants (not more than 12 months of age), children (under 4 years old), and pregnant or lactating women. Within the next few years more and more foods should have nutrition information on the label; the US-RDA will be the reference standard for the values presented.

DAILY FOOD GUIDE

The recommended allowances for nutrients for most people can be obtained from a well chosen variety of ordinary foods including those in our markets which are commonly fortified or enriched with vitamins and minerals. The Daily Food Guide (Fig. 10–1), prepared by nutritionists in the U.S. Department of Agriculture, presents one way to select food.[15] With this aid almost anyone can get the nutrients needed from everyday foods.

Most foods contain more than one nutrient, but no single food contains all the nutrients in the amounts needed. The Daily Food Guide suggests the kinds that together supply nutrients in the amounts needed. In using the Guide one selects the main part of the diet from the four broad food groups. To this one adds other foods as desired to make meals appealing and satisfying. The additional foods should add enough calories to meet energy needs, which will vary widely for different members of the family.

Since it is possible, however, to obtain the recommended dietary allowance of nutrients in many different diet patterns because of the wide variety of foods yielding similar nutrients, anyone attempting to evaluate or teach nutrition should be conscious of this fact and avoid any tendency to use stereotyped diet yardsticks for judging individual diets.

If a patient's calcium intake is being estimated and only his milk intake is scrutinized, an entirely erroneous evaluation may be made. It is possible for some people to get enough calcium from the daily use of cheese, fish, legumes, and leafy vegetables, even though the more usual pattern would be from the use of milk. Thus, although nutrition guides such as the Four Food Groups are valuable, their limitations when applied to an individual must be recognized.

PATTERN DIETARY

The accompanying pattern dietary (Table 10–2) planned according to the Daily Food Guide provides only about 1400 calories—less than needed by an active person—but meets or approaches the recommended allowances for all nutrients for an adult male. Supplementary foods such as extra milk for children will help meet the calcium level recommended for them. In general, the foods added to meet energy needs of individuals will provide additional nutrients as well as contribute to taste and satisfaction of meals.

The iron provided in the sample dietary is low for women when compared with the 18 mg. recommended. This amount of iron is impossible to obtain unless a special effort is made to include iron-rich foods. It is suggested that perhaps women might use dried fruits for snacks instead of candy if calories permit, and try to include some type of liver in the diet at least once a week. Iron supplements may still be needed. The level of the B vitamins, which appears to be slightly low for men and boys, will be raised to RDA when calories are increased to meet their needs.

In Chapter 23 it will be noticed that hospital diets are also based upon this pattern dietary, modified as required to meet specific needs.

FOOD COMPOSITION TABLES AS A TOOL FOR ASSESSING DIETARY PRACTICES

The basic tool for the assessment of dietary practices is the knowledge of the proximate energy and nutrient composition of foods—calories, protein, fat, carbohydrate, minerals, and vitamins. The nutrients in foods are discussed in previous chapters, and an extensive table of the nutrient composition of common foods is found in Table 1, Section 4. In this section the derivation of food composition tables, commonly used tables, average servings, and the limitations of food tables are discussed.

Food Composition Tables

Food composition tables give the proximate energy, protein, fat, and carbohydrate values and the mineral and vitamin contents of a defined amount of food, usually 100 g. The household measure that approximates the gram weight may or may not be stated. Today the values for energy are given in kilocalories. However, it is possible that the joule instead of the calorie may be used in future tables. (4.2 kilojoules = 1 kilocalorie.) In all tables the values for minerals are given in milligrams with the exception of certain trace elements such as fluorine, iodine, chromium, molybdenum, and selenium, which are stated in micrograms. Calcium may be given in grams. Values are given in International Units (IU) for vitamins A, D, and E, although recently the concept of retinol equivalents has been introduced for vitamin A. (See Chapter 6.) Values for other vitamins are expressed as milligram (10^{-3} gram), microgram (10^{-6} gram), nanogram (10^{-9} gram), or picogram (10^{-12} gram). (1 mg. = 0.001 g.)

When figures from more than one food composition table are used to estimate the nutrient content of a meal or a day's food intake, care must be taken to see that the units of measurement are the same in each table. If not, it is necessary to convert the units from one table to correspond to those of the other. For example, Table 1 in Section 4 gives the thiamine values in mg., while another commonly used table gives thiamine in mcg. (1 mg. = 1000 mcg.).[16]

The term proximate analysis refers to those values in food composition tables for water, protein, lipids, carbohydrates, and ash. The term proximate is used because the figures may reflect substances which are unrelated chemically as well as the substance itself. For example: protein values are calculated from the total nitrogen in a food. Some of this nitrogen may come from nonprotein substances such as purine bases. Carbohydrate figures reflect total carbohydrate by difference: that is, the difference between the total amount of water, protein, lipid, and ash and total weight of the food. The carbohydrate figure includes pentoses and fiber in addition to mono-, di-, and polysaccharides, unless otherwise indicated. Fiber content may be determined by a routine procedure and subtracted from total carbohydrate to give an estimate of the amount of carbohydrate in foods which the body can convert to simple sugars.

In general, the figures given in food composition tables are representative values and apply to food as it is usually produced and marketed for year-round and countrywide use by the consumer. The values are derived from the research carried out in various food technology laboratories in universities, in the United States Department of Agriculture, and in industries throughout the country. The methods used for determining nutrient composition are usually those accepted by the Association of Official Agricultural Chemists. Although they are generally regarded as highly reproducible, they are not necessarily totally accurate in reflecting the amount of nutrient available. For instance, recent studies analyzing carotene values in yellow and green vegetables indicate losses of vitamin A activity of the carotenes in these vegetables when cooked or canned, which is not apparent when the usual laboratory procedures for determining this nutrient are followed.[17]

The value given for each nutrient in a food composition table represents an average (sometimes a weighted average) for the total number of samples of the particular food for which analyses were available. The figures for some nutrients were derived from the analysis of many samples, while others were derived from a limited number of analyses. In any case the actual amount of a nutrient in any specific sample of a food may vary more or less widely from the average. Average values for ascorbic acid in tomato juice ranged only from 12.5 to 16.0 mg. percent over a ten-year period, whereas, in a single year individual samples ranged from 3.2 to 21.7 mg. percent.[18] Also, averages do not tell, for example, that half the ascorbic acid in potatoes is lost after several months' storage and that an additional amount is lost in cooking and reheating.

The representative values for plant foods such as cereal grain, fruits, and vegetables reflect variability in samples due to variety (genetics), maturity, part of the plant (such as leaves, flowers, stems, or roots), seasonal or geographical differences, length and type of storage, or other factors. Also new methods or modifications of old methods of food processing may affect nutrient composition. At this time there are limited data on the mineral and vitamin contents of raw and prepared meats and poultry and on the nutrient values of baked products such as sweet rolls, doughnuts and pizza, new varieties of tomatoes which can be mechanically harvested, and a number of convenience foods.[19]

A recent statement made by research workers in the USDA when introducing a Provisional Table on the Zinc Content of Foods indicates some of the problems related to food tables.

> Values in the table . . . have been derived from data obtained by an exhaustive search of published literature and unpublished sources of information . . . . The table is called "provisional" because many of the values are derived from a limited number of analyses. It is not yet possible, from the data base available, to determine the extent to which factors such as variety, season, geographic location and fertilization may affect zinc content of some foods. The data reported here are considered by the authors to be the current best estimates for zinc content of foods as presently marketed.[20]

Commonly Used Food Composition Tables

COMPOSITION OF FOODS: RAW, PROCESSED, AND PREPARED, USDA HANDBOOK NO. 8. Since its original publication in 1950 with a revision in 1963, USDA Handbook No. 8 has been the most widely used food composition table. A new USDA food table is expected in the near future and is discussed later in this section.

Handbook No. 8 contains five tables: Table 1, Composition of Foods, 100 Grams, Edible Portion; Table 2, Nutrients in the Edible Portion of 1 Pound of Food as Purchased; Table 3, Selected Fatty Acids in Foods; Table 4, Cholesterol Content of Foods; and Table 5, Magnesium Content of Foods. Tables 1 and 2 give a description of each food item and figures for water, food energy, protein, fat, carbohydrate, ash, calcium, phosphorus, iron, sodium, potassium, vitamin A, thiamine, riboflavin, niacin, and ascorbic acid content of foods by alphabetical listing. No brand names are used to describe foods. Table 2 also gives the percentage of refuse per pound of the food as purchased. Table 3 gives the total fat, total saturated fatty acids, and the unsaturated fatty acids (oleic C18:1, linoleic C18:2) in 100 grams, edible portion, and in the edible portion of 1 pound of food as purchased. Arachidonic (C18:4) acid is not listed because very little of this fatty acid occurs naturally in foods.

The items in Tables 1, 2, and 3 have been numbered uniformly. For example, item no. 410 in all three tables refers to biscuits, baking powder, baked from home recipe. Whenever the figures in Handbook No. 8 are used to estimate the nutrient composition of a food or an intake, the item number as well as the nutrient values should be recorded on the analysis form in order to verify the figures easily.

Whenever Table 1 in Handbook No. 8 is used to identify the nutrient content of a food in other than a 100-gram portion, the appropriate calculations must be carried out. For example, the values for the 100-g. portion of milk in Table 1 will be multiplied by 2.4 to derive the figures for 240 g. (one 8-ounce cup). To derive the figures for 5 g. of butter (1 tsp.) the values for 100 g. of butter are multiplied by 0.05.

When only the household measure of a food is known, such as ½ cup string beans, this measure must be converted to grams in order to calculate its nutritive value from Table 1 in Handbook No. 8. Fabietti[21] has offered a method for converting volume to weight, or the serving of food can be weighed on a gram scale to determine its gram weight.

It is strongly recommended that anyone using Handbook No. 8 carefully study the introduction and the information in Appendices A, B, and C and have a worksheet which reflects the format of Table 1 for ease of recording the nutritive values of food intakes and for filing in patients' charts when appropriate. Table 1, Section 4, in this book is derived primarily from Handbook No. 8.

NUTRITIVE VALUE OF AMERICAN FOODS IN COMMON UNITS, USDA. This new USDA handbook is derived from Handbook No. 8 and will provide data for all constituents except fiber and ash.

> The figures, which have been calculated from the data in Agriculture Handbook No. 8, are the amounts of the nutrients in numerous specified volume measurements or units of foods. To a limited extent, values for some nutrients have been updated. In this new handbook, the weight of food in grams corresponding to the various measures or units listed will also be shown for each item. Since the problems in determining weight-volume relationships are many, a discussion of a number of practical problems has been included as an appendix.[22]

Since the fiber content of the diet is now under intensive study, it is unfortunate that this prospective publication will not contain figures for the fiber content of foods.

NUTRIENT DATA BANK. In 1973 the USDA, in cooperation with other government agencies and the food industry, initiated the establishment of a Nutrient Data Bank. Food research laboratories have been given a form for submitting food composition data. This system should make available in the future much more extensive information regarding nutrient composition of foods.

FOOD VALUES OF PORTIONS COMMONLY USED.* This food composition table, now in its twelfth edition, is commonly referred to as Bowes and Church because Anna dePlanter Bowes, a nutri-

*Church, C. F., and Church, H. N.: Food Values of Portions Commonly Used. 12th Ed. Phila., J. B. Lippincott Co., 1975.

tionist, and Dr. C. F. Church were the authors of the first edition published in 1937. The nutrient values given in this table have been derived from Agriculture Handbook No. 8, other USDA food tables, and other resources as listed in the bibliography. This publication differs from Agriculture Handbook No. 8 in that the food items are listed by groups, for example, Breads, Cereals and Cereal Products; the household measure as well as the gram weights (not necessarily 100 g.) are given; brand names are used for some items; and, in addition to total protein, the quantities of the eight essential amino acids are given when the data are available.

It contains a table of cholesterol values for a limited number of foods but no data on fatty acid composition. A valuable feature is the table on nonnutritive ingredients (additives) in foods, which gives the food additive, function, important food uses, and level of use. The chemical name is given for many but not all of the additives listed. The authors do not indicate whether or not the figures listed under level of use are levels set by the Food and Drug Administration.

NUTRITIVE VALUE OF FOODS. This food composition table, published by the USDA and also known as Home and Garden Bulletin No. 72, gives the nutritive values of 615 commonly used foods in household measures and gram weights. It was prepared as a consumer service by the Consumer and Food Economics Research Division, Agricultural Research Service. Highly motivated homemakers interested in the nutritive value of the foods they are serving to their families will find this publication useful.

FOOD INDUSTRY TABLES. Some food processors make available tables of the food composition, and in some instances, the ingredients, in their products. Some of these tables contain nutrient values derived from Agriculture Handbook No. 8, while others are figures from the analyses of the product done in the company's laboratory by food technologists. It is possible that with the institution of nutrition labeling by the U. S. Food and Drug Administration (see Chapter 14) more tables which report actual analyses of products by brand name will become available to nutrition counselors.

Average Servings

An average serving of a food is used in nutrition to describe an amount of food in a household measure by weight or volume or in a common unit which can be readily identified, such as 3 ounces of cooked meat; ½ pint or one 8-ounce cup of milk; ½ cup of cooked carrots, or one slice of bread. An average serving may or may not be a 100-g. serving. One-half cup of carrots is approximately 100 g., while 8 ounces of

milk is 240 g., almost two and one-half times 100 g. In dietetics, ½ cup refers to one-half of a standard 8-ounce measuring cup; 1 tablespoon (tbsp.) or 1 teaspoon (tsp.) refer to standard measuring spoons.

Nutrition labeling regulations (see Chapter 14) will require "serving size" to appear on each label as the basis for the nutrient content information. Recently there have been many discussions among nutritionists, food technologists, and consumer specialists as to what constitutes an average serving. Standardization, when it is finally agreed upon, should prove very helpful to the consumer as well as to the nutrition educator.

Limitations of Food Composition Tables

Since the figures in food composition tables are representative of the energy and nutrient content of a food, it must be remembered that when one calculates the nutritional value of a day's food intake, of a diet plan, or of a recipe, the results will be an *estimation* of the energy and nutrient composition, not the exact composition. If the intake of food for any period is reported accurately by an individual, or the intake is accurately observed and recorded, the analysis of energy, protein, fat, and carbohydrate in the intake, derived from commonly used food composition tables, will be reasonably accurate.

The variation of the fat composition of meat and in convenience foods may result in an overestimation or underestimation of fat in an intake, with the result that the energy composition of the actual intake may vary as much as 10 to 15 percent from the estimation. The mineral and vitamin values in any food composition table are probably the least valid figures when used to estimate intakes. These nutrients in foods vary naturally, especially in fresh fruits and vegetables, and if these foods are processed or cooked, it must be remembered that certain vitamins, and to some extent minerals, are soluble in water and that some vitamins can be destroyed by heat.

Therefore, in reports of the energy and nutrient intake of an individual for any period of time, the figures recorded should reflect the limitation of the method, that is, the use of food composition tables. For example: recording a day's energy intake for an individual calculated from a food composition table as 1832.8 kcal. connotes a degree of accuracy which cannot be achieved by this method. A more appropriate recording in this situation would be 1835 kcal., or 1825 to 1850 kcal.

This is not to imply that food composition tables are of little or no value: rather, that they must be used appropriately within the limitations inherent in the method.

SOME GENERALIZATIONS ABOUT THE NUTRIENT COMPOSITION OF FOODS

The complexity of food composition tables may "turn off" the uninitiated. The nutrition educator cannot carry a food composition table or textbook with her at all times, although she should have one readily accessible. The Daily Food Guide (Fig. 10–1) can be used to assess an individual's usual food intake, but this guide may not be adequate in all situations. Life-styles vary in our society, and food practices which differ from the Food Guide can supply adequate nutrient intakes. Some generalizations about food composition are offered in this section to assist the counselor in answering on-the-spot questions about food or in coping with the assessment of intake in the individual whose food practices are "different."

Energy

Fats and carbohydrates are the major sources of energy in the American diet today. In 1974, the USDA estimated that 3350 cal. per person per day were available for civilian consumption.[23] Eighteen percent of these calories came from fats and oils, including butter and margarine, and 17 percent from sugars and other sweeteners. Even at this level of consumption these two food groups do not contribute significantly to the intake of other nutrients such as vitamins and minerals. Thus the term "empty calories" is frequently applied to fats and sugars.

At the same time, the USDA estimated that flour and cereals represented 19 percent of the calories available for civilian consumption, and potatoes and sweet potatoes represented 3 percent. In addition to calories from carbohydrates, these two groups of food can contribute very significant amounts of protein, iron, and the B vitamins to an individual's daily nutrient intake, and, at 3 percent of the energy intake, potatoes contributed 18 percent of the 119 mg. of ascorbic acid available per capita for civilian consumption in 1974.

Fat is the nutrient which most directly affects the energy value of a food and, therefore, an individual's daily energy intake. One gram of fat yields 9 kcal. In addition to fats, oils, butter, and margarine varying amounts of fat occur naturally in foods. The variation in the amount of fat in meat is illustrated in Table 10–3. It will be noted that if one consumes 100 g. (3⅓ ounces) of broiled steak, including both the lean and fat portions, he consumes significantly more calories than if he consumes 100 g. of the cooked, lean portion only (387 vs. 200 kcal.).

The energy value of any portion of meat can be reduced by trimming off the visible fat around or between the muscle mass. However, the fat between the meat fibers of the muscle mass cannot be removed by trimming, and only partially by cooking, nor can the lipid layer of the cell membranes of meat be removed by trimming or cooking. Therefore, any portion of commonly used meats will contain some fat. Chicken, turkey, and certain lean fish (commonly classified as dry fish) have considerably less fat than muscle meat per 100 g. (see Table 10–3).

An example of the effect on the energy value of a food from which practically all the naturally occurring fat can be removed is shown in Table 10–4. Eight ounces (1 cup) of skim milk contains one-half the calories of a cup of whole milk (80 vs. 160 kcal.) while the energy value of 1 cup of partially skimmed milk reflects only a moderate reduction of total fat when compared with whole milk (145 vs. 160 kcal.).

The effect of the addition of fat to a food during preparation is illustrated in Table 10–5. Note that a potato, in and of itself, is not a "high"-calorie food, but the addition of fat during preparation markedly increases its energy value (65 kcal. for 100 g. boiled potato vs. 274 kcal. for 100 g. french-fried potato).

Gravy served with mashed potatoes may or may not be a significant source of additional calories. One cup of gravy made with 2 tbsp. flour and pan drip-

Table 10–3. Energy, Protein, and Fat in 100 Grams of Selected Meat, Fish and Poultry* (cooked without the addition of fat)

FOOD (100 g., 3½ oz.)	ENERGY (kcal.)	PROTEIN (g.)	FAT (g.)
Chicken, light meat, without skin	166	32	3
Cod, broiled	170	29	5
Beef, steak broiled			
lean and fat	387	23	32
lean	200	32	8
Pork, roast loin and shoulder			
lean and fat	373	23	31
lean	283	29	13

*See Section 4, Table 1.

Table 10–4. Energy and Fat in One Cup of Whole Milk, Skimmed Milk, and Partially Skimmed Milk*

FOOD	WEIGHT (g.)	ENERGY (kcal.)	FAT (g.)
Milk, whole[a]	244 (1 c.)	160	8.5
Milk, skim[a]	246 (1 c.)	80	Tr.
Milk, partly skimmed[b]	246 (1 c.)	145	5

*USDA Home and Garden Bulletin No. 72.
[a]See Section 4, Table 1.
[b]2% nonfat milk solids added.

Table 10-5. Energy and Fat in 100 Grams of Boiled, Mashed, and French-Fried Potatoes*

FOOD (100 g.)	ENERGY (kcal.)	FAT (g.)
Boiled[a] (½ c.)	65	Tr.
Mashed[b] (½ c.)	94	4
French-fried (20 pc.)	274	13

*See Section 4, Table 1.
[a]Pared before cooking.
[b]Milk and table fat added.

Table 10-7. Water, Energy, and Carbohydrate in 100 Grams of Selected Fruits and Vegetables*

FOOD (100 g.)	WATER (percent)	ENERGY (kcal.)	CARBO-HYDRATE (g.)
Broccoli, cooked	91	26	5
Tomatoes, raw	94	22	5
Pears, raw	83	61	15
Potato, cooked	83	65	15
Banana, raw	76	85	22
Corn, fresh, on cob	74	91	21

*See Section 4, Table 1.

pings from which *all* fat has been removed contains approximately 60 kcal., while 1 cup of gravy made with 2 tbsp. flour and pan drippings from which the fat has *not* been removed may contain as much as 500 kcal. Therefore, ¼ cup of the gravy (an average serving) *without* fat will contain 15 kcal., while ¼ cup *with* fat may contain as much as 125 kcal.

Another variation in energy value which can occur during food preparation is illustrated in Table 10-6. The two samples of veal cutlet, breaded and fried, differ in value by approximately 100 kcal. (203 vs. 294 kcal.). Standel and coworkers reported that samples A and B came from two different restaurants, and it would appear that restaurant B used more bread, which in turn absorbed more fat during the frying process as reflected in the quantity of fat and carbohydrate in sample B.[24]

The energy value of a food can vary due to the carbohydrate content. Carbohydrate yields 4 kcal. per g. The energy value of fruits and vegetables varies directly with the water and carbohydrate content, as illustrated in Table 10-7. In general certain fruits and the flowers, leaves, and stems of vegetables have a proportionately high water and low carbohydrate content, while certain fruits and seeds, tubers, and roots have less water and more carbohydrate. Fruits and vegetables, including cooked potatoes, vary from approximately 5 to 20 percent in carbohydrate content. Dry cereal grains, such as oatmeal, are approximately 8 percent water and 75 percent carbohydrate. However, since cereal grains must be hydrated in order to be digested, the average serving of cooked

cereal (½ cup or 100 g.) is approximately 83 percent water and 15 percent carbohydrate.

The addition of sugar to fruits and the addition of sugar or fats to flavor cooked vegetables increases the energy content of these foods per serving. The energy value of precooked cereals can be modified significantly by the addition of sugar during processing. For example, 1 cup of a processor's cornflakes contains approximately 80 kcal. while the same amount of flakes sugar-coated during production contains approximately 140 kcal.[25]

Sugar and fats combined with flour in desserts account for the energy value of these foods. This is illustrated in Table 10-8. Snack foods are an increasingly important source of energy in the diets of both children and adults.

The energy value of any individual's food intake is directly dependent on the size of the portions of food consumed either at a meal or as a snack. If an individual usually consumes a 200-g. serving of lean steak, not 100 g. as in Table 10-3, then the energy value of the serving will be 400, not 200, kcal. Similarly, one quarter of a 9-inch apple pie contains 615 kcal., not the 410 kcal. for one sixth of a 9-inch apple pie as in Table 10-8.

Protein

In 1974, the USDA reported that of the 101 g. of protein available per person per day for civilian consumption, 35.7 percent was provided by meat, fish, and poultry; 24.5 percent by dairy products; 19.9 percent by flours and cereals; 6.8 percent by eggs; and 5 percent by dry beans and peas, nuts, and soya flour. Approximately 67 percent of the protein available for civilian consumption was from meat, eggs, and dairy products, which provide protein of high biological value.

Meat, fish, and poultry vary from 20 to 30 percent protein (20 to 30 g. in 100 g. of food). The remainder is water (both in and around the cells), fat, undigestible connective tissue, minerals, and vitamins. Eggs are

Table 10-6. Energy, Protein, Fat, and Carbohydrate in Two Samples of Veal Cutlet Breaded and Fried*

FOOD (100 g.)	ENERGY (kcal.)	PROTEIN (g.)	FAT (g.)	CARBOHY-DRATE (g.)
Sample A	203	26.9	9.1	3.4
Sample B	294	12.9	18.8	18.4

*Standal, B. R., et al: J. Am. Dietet. A. 56:392, 1970.

Table 10-8. Energy, Fat, and Carbohydrate in Average Servings of Selected Desserts*

FOOD	WEIGHT (g.)	ENERGY (kcal.)	FAT (g.)	CARBOHYDRATE (g.)
Brownies	50 (1 bar)	242	16	25
Ice cream	100 (¾ c.)	207	13	21
Chocolate cake (with frosting)	100 (1 piece)	369	16	56
Apple pie	160 (⅙ of 9″ pie)	410	18	61

*See Section 4, Table 1.

approximately 13 percent, and milk 3.5 percent, protein.

In the United States, cereal grains, dried beans, or peas, nuts, or soya products are not considered significant sources of protein even though these foods are used widely around the world and are listed as alternates for meat in the Daily Guide published by the USDA. Cereals and dried beans or peas are usually classified as starchy (carbohydrate) foods. However, in situations where either money for food purchasing is limited or the individual prefers to use cereals and dried peas or beans, these foods can make a significant contribution to the adequacy of the intake of protein and to the intakes of iron, thiamine, riboflavin, and niacin, especially if the cereals are whole grain or enriched.

Vitamins

Milk, meat, fish and poultry, eggs, and whole or enriched grain products (cereals, breads, and flours) are the significant sources of the B vitamins. Consumed in the amounts recommended in the Daily Food Guide, these foods will supply from one half to two thirds of the recommended dietary allowances for these nutrients. The recommended servings of fruits and vegetables will supply an adequate intake of vitamin C. However, if instead of citrus fruit and tomatoes, liberal servings of fresh potatoes and other fresh vegetables and fruits are consumed daily, the diet will contain adequate amounts of vitamin C.

The fat-soluble vitamins require special attention. An adequate intake of vitamin A can be derived from dark green and deep yellow fruits and vegetables, milk fats, and fortified margarine. As a group, the fat-soluble vitamins require fat for absorption.

Minerals

The evidence presently available indicates that adequate iron intake is a problem, especially for infants 6 to 18 months of age, toddlers 1 to 3 years, adolescent girls, and women of child-bearing age. The most significant food source of iron—liver—is not a popular food and, therefore, not a widely acceptable solution to the problem. Also, since the liver is only 1.5 percent of the dressed weight of a steer, it

will probably never be available in quantities large enough to solve the problem.

In 1973, the USDA reported that approximately 18 mg. of iron per person per day was available for civilian consumption. Meat, fish and poultry, and eggs contributed 35 percent of the available iron, while flour and cereal grains contributed 29 percent due partly to the iron enrichment of flour and cereal products. Fruits, vegetables including potatoes, dry beans and peas, nuts, and soya flour contributed 25 percent of the available iron.

At present the percentage of iron absorbed from food, both that which occurs naturally and that added to enrich flour and cereal products, is not known. This problem is under intensive study and, at the same time, a higher level of iron enrichment of flour and cereal products is being proposed. In the meantime, it would appear that, if the consumption of fats, oils, and sugar and other sweeteners, which contribute only energy, was reduced, and the consumption of enriched flour and cereal products was increased, the amount of iron available for consumption would be increased without any rise in total energy consumption.

The major source of calcium in the American diet is milk and milk products, with the exceptions of butter, cream cheese, and cottage cheese. The Daily Food Guide recommends two or more cups of milk for an adult. This amount of milk contains 576 mg. of calcium—a significant contribution to the 800 mg. recommended by the National Research Council. The usual selection of foods from the other groups in the Daily Food Guide will contribute 200 to 300 mg. of calcium per day (see Table 10-2).

The addition of milk products, specifically milk solids, to bread and a variety of processed foods can contribute significantly to an individual's daily intake of calcium. The adolescent boy who eats ten slices of bread made with 4 percent nonfat dry milk will be consuming 190 mg. of calcium. Also, in areas where monocalcium phosphate baking powder is used daily to make hot breads, such as biscuits and cornbread, these foods can be significant sources of calcium.

Phosphorus is widely distributed in foods from both animal and plant sources.

Table 10–9. Nutrient Composition of Homemade and Convenience-Packaged Macaroni and Cheese*

FOOD	WEIGHT (g.)	HOUSEHOLD MEASURE	ENERGY (kcal.)	PROTEIN (g.)	FAT (g.)	CARBOHYDRATE (g.)	CALCIUM (mg.)	IRON (mg.)	VITAMIN A (IU)	THIAMINE (mg.)	RIBOFLAVIN (mg.)	NIACIN (mg.)
Homemade[a]	100	½ c.	215	8	11	20	181	0.9	430	0.10	0.20	0.9
Brand A[b]	100	½ c.	97	3.7	4.2	11.0	56	0.6	230	0.09	0.09	1.2
Brand B-1[c]	100	½ c.	179	5.8	7.1	23.0	81	NA	NA	NA	NA	NA
Brand B-2[c]	100	½ c.	170	7.8	8.4	15.5	224	NA	NA	NA	NA	NA
Brand C[d]	100	½ c.	134	5.9	6.0	13.9	127	0.4	237	0.03	0.11	0.32

*Figures courtesy Preschool Nutrition Survey.
[a]See Section 4, Table 1. Values calculated from a recipe.
[b]Canned.
[c]Same manufacturer: B-1 dry mix; B-2 frozen.
[d]Frozen.
NA—Figures not available.

Table 10–10. Nutrient Composition of Homemade and Homebaked Sugar Cookies*

FOOD	WEIGHT (g.)	HOUSEHOLD MEASURE	ENERGY (kcal.)	PROTEIN (g.)	FAT (g.)	CARBOHYDRATE (g.)	CALCIUM (mg.)	IRON (mg.)	VITAMIN A (IU)	THIAMINE (Mg.)	RIBOFLAVIN (mg.)	NIACIN (mg.)
Homemade sugar cookies[a]	20	2" diam.	89	1.2	3.3	16	15	0.3	22	.03	.03	0.2
Homebaked sugar cookies[b]	20	2" diam.	90	0.7	4.5	12	6	0.06	14	.004	.006	0.04

*Figures courtesy Preschool Nutrition Survey.
[a]Handbook No. 8 values calculated from a recipe using enriched flour.
[b]Dough, chilled unbaked, commercial, unenriched.

Convenience Foods

Convenience foods have entered the retail market in volume in the past 10 years, and the information needed to compare the nutritive values of these products with comparable products made in the home is not readily available.

Table 10-9 shows the calorie and nutrient variation in only one product—macaroni and cheese. For two of the items in the table, brand B-1 and brand B-2, all of the data are not available. Brand A is a canned product; B-1 is a dry mix; and B-2 and C are frozen products. It will be noted that the convenience-packaged products vary significantly in energy, protein, and calcium content from the product made from a commonly used home recipe.

Table 10-10 illustrates the variation in a product when enriched or unenriched flour is used. The nutrient composition of the homemade cookies was calculated from a recipe using enriched flour. From the nutrient values provided by the manufacturer for the chilled cookie dough to be baked in the home, it appears that unenriched flour is used in this convenience product. The energy values are similar.

FOODS FORTIFIED OR ENRICHED TO HELP MEET NUTRITIONAL NORMS

About 60 years ago nutritionists began to investigate how certain nutritional limitations in our food supplies could be corrected. The first large-scale experiment was the addition of iodine to salt to prevent goiter. This program was so successful that iodized salt is available in most markets today (see Chapter 5).

In the 1930's the fortification of homogenized milk with vitamin D was started in an attempt to prevent rickets in infants. Today most of the homogenized milk in our markets is fortified with 400 IU of vitamin D per quart. Much of the dry, skimmed milk is also fortified with vitamins A and D (see Chapter 6).

In the 1940's the increased use of margarines prompted the addition of vitamin A to make the content equivalent to average butter. Today all margarines in our markets are fortified with 15,000 IU of vitamin A per pound. Some margarines also have 2000 IU of vitamin D per pound added.

During World War II, the enrichment of bread and flour with iron, thiamine, riboflavin, and niacin was initiated when it was realized that repeated attempts to persuade people to use whole grains were unsuccessful. The modification of natural grains by milling had produced a more acceptable flour—whiter and with better keeping qualities, but reduced the vitamin and mineral content. Now the practice of enrichment of milled grains and breads has expanded to include not only wheat, but also corn and rice and ready-to-eat breakfast cereals. Some macaroni, spaghetti, and noodle products are also enriched. Dry infant cereals have relatively large amounts of iron as well as certain B-complex vitamins added to them. The feasibility of increased iron enrichment in flour and cereal products is presently under study, and current levels may be doubled or tripled. Enrichment of white flour and bread is now mandatory in most states and in Puerto Rico, and enrichment of cornmeal is common in southern states. Actually most of the bread and all-purpose flour sold in the United States today is enriched, although this is not mandatory in all states. However, many of the prepared foods, such as packaged mixes, frozen baked products, refrigerated doughs, and crackers are made from nonenriched flour.

Although the indiscriminate fortification of foods has been discouraged, a number of other food products have had vitamins and minerals added to them in varying amounts. Careful consideration must be given to any new proposal for fortification; for example, too enthusiastic fortification with vitamin D might be harmful for young children consuming excess amounts of this nutrient.

The 1973 Policy Statement of the Food and Nutrition Board in regard to Improvement of Nutritive Quality of Foods

> . . . endorses the addition of nutrients to foods in order to achieve enrichment or fortification when all of the following conditions are met:
>
> 1. The intake of the nutrient(s) is below the desirable level in the diets of a significant number of people;
>
> 2. The food(s) used to supply the nutrient(s) is likely to be consumed in quantities that will make a significant contribution to the diet of the population in need;
>
> 3. The addition of the nutrient(s) is not likely to create a dietary imbalance;
>
> 4. The nutrient(s) added is stable under customary conditions of storage and use;
>
> 5. The nutrient(s) is physiologically available from the food;
>
> 6. The enhanced levels attained in the total diet will not be harmfully excessive for those who may employ the foods in varying patterns of use; and
>
> 7. The additional cost is reasonable for the intended consumer.

Thus the enrichment of flour, bread, degerminated corn meal, corn grits, whole grain corn meal, white rice and certain other cereal grain products with thiamine, riboflavin, niacin and iron; the addition of vitamin D to milk, fluid skim milk and nonfat dry milk; the addition of vitamin A to margarine, fluid skim milk and nonfat dry milk; and the addition of iodine to table salt [are endorsed]. The protective action of fluoride against dental caries is recognized and the standardized addition of fluoride to water in areas in which the water supply has a low fluoride content is endorsed.[26]

STUDY QUESTIONS AND ACTIVITIES

1. The Food and Nutrition Board of the National Research Council has recommended dietary allowances for certain specific nutrients. Which ones are listed in this table (Table 10-1)?
2. These allowances are listed for different age and sex categories. For which of these are the allowances as great for young children as for a grown man? Why?
3. For which factor do the allowances vary directly with the caloric requirements?
4. Choose any dietary pattern with which you are familiar and plan a day's menu according to the Daily Food Guide (Fig. 10-1), using foods well liked by the people for whom it is intended.
5. Which nutrients are most difficult to obtain in sufficient quantities in low-cost meals in your locality at the season of the year when you are studying this chapter?
6. List the foods you ate yesterday and check to see whether all four food groups were adequately represented.
7. For what reason were the US-RDA established?
8. What are food composition tables? How are protein values calculated? What does "total carbohydrate by difference" mean? List two commonly used food composition tables and show how they differ.
9. How may preparation affect the amount of fat in a serving of pork chops? A serving of eggs? Of gravy?
10. What is meant by fortified milk? by enriched bread?

SUPPLEMENTARY READINGS

Campbell, J. A.: Approaches in revising dietary standards—Canadian, U. S. and international standards compared. J. Am. Dietet. A. 64:175, 1974.

Food and Nutrition Board: *Recommended Dietary Allowances*, 8th rev. Washington, D.C., National Academy of Sciences–National Research Council, 1974.

———: General policies in regard to improvement of nutritive quality of foods. Nutr. Rev. 31:324, 1973.

Food for the Young Family. Home and Garden Bulletin No. 85. Washington, D. C., U. S. Department of Agriculture (April) 1971.

Harper, A. E.: Recommended dietary allowances: Are they what we think they are? J. Am. Dietet. A. 64:151, 1974.

Hegsted, D. M.: Dietary Standards, J. Am. Dietet. A. 66:13, 1975.

Hertzler, A. A., and Anderson, H. L.: An historical review: Food guides in the United States. J. Am. Dietet. A. 64:19, 1974.

Leverton, R. M., Watt, B. K., Richardson, M., and Souders, H. J.: Research in agriculture and the profession of dietetics. J. Am. Dietet. A. 64:638, 1974.

Special Report: Standards of identity. Nutr. Rev. 32:29, 1974.

For further references see Bibliography in Section 4.

REFERENCES

1. Food and Nutrition Board: Recommended Dietary Allowances, 8th rev., Washington, D. C., National Academy of Sciences–National Research Council, 1974.
2. Harper, A. E.: J. Am. Dietet. A. 64:151, 1974.
3. Food and Nutrition Board, op. cit.
4. Ibid.
5. Dietary Standards for Canada. Can. Bull. Nutr. 6:No. 1, rev. 1968.
6. FAO/WHO Expert Group on Calcium Requirements. WHO Tech. Rep. Series 230, 1962.
7. Joint FAO/WHO Expert Group on Requirements of Vitamin A, Thiamine, Riboflavin, and Niacin. WHO Tech. Rep. Series 362, 1967.
8. Joint FAO/WHO Expert Group on Requirements of Ascorbic Acid, Vitamin D, Vitamin B_{12}, Folate, and Iron. WHO Tech. Rep. Series 452, 1970.
9. Joint FAO/WHO Ad Hoc Expert Committee on Energy and Protein Requirements. WHO Tech. Rep. Series 522, 1973.
10. WHO Expert Committee on Trace Elements in Human Nutrition. WHO Tech. Rep. Series 532, 1973.
11. Campbell, J. A.: J. Am. Dietet. A. 64, 1974.
12. Food and Nutrition Board, op. cit.
13. Ibid.
14. Ibid.
15. Consumer and Food Economics Research Div., Washington, D. C., Agricultural Research (rev.) 1964.
16. Church, C. F., and Church, H. N.: *Food Values of Portions Commonly Used*, ed. 12. Philadelphia, Lippincott, 1975.
17. Sweeney, J. P., and Marsh, A. C.: J. Am. Dietet. A. 59:238, 1971.
18. Farrow, R. P., et al: J. Food Sci. 38:595, 1973.
19. Watt, B. K., and Murphy, E. W.: Food Tech. 24:675, 1970.
20. Murphy, E. W., Willis, B. W., and Watt, B. K.: Abstract of Paper Presented 57th Annual Meeting, The American Dietetic Association, Philadelphia, October 8, 1974.
21. Fabietti, L. G.: J. Am. Dietet. A. 60:135, 1972.
22. Watt, B. K., et al: J. Am. Dietet. A. 64:257, 1974.
23. National Food Situation-150, USDA, November 1974.
24. Standal, B. R., et al: J. Am. Dietet. A. 56:392, 1970.
25. Brand-Name Calorie Counter, p. 8, 1969.
26. Food and Nutrition Board: General policies in regard to improvement of nutritive quality of foods, Washington, D. C., National Academy of Sciences, 1973.

11

meal management

Planning
Purchasing
Storage
Preparation
Meal Service

If mealtimes are to fulfill the nutritional needs of the various family members, as well as the many other purposes associated with such occasions in our culture, the manager, particularly the inexperienced individual, may need assistance from the nutrition educator in meal management. This chapter outlines the steps which have proven helpful in achieving successful family meals. As skill in this area is developed, some of the steps may be combined.

PLANNING

Successful meal management implies efficient use of the manager's resources—knowledge, skill, time, money, and equipment—to accomplish predetermined goals. Goals for family or group meals may differ widely depending on individual life-styles, but most managers would agree on the following three goals, although perhaps not in the order specified. Family or group meals should (1) meet the nutritional norms established for each individual member, (2) fit within the available food budget, and (3) be acceptable to each member.

Planning is the key to each step of the process, which includes the preparation of menus and shopping lists, the purchasing and storing of food,

Table 11-1. Low-Cost Food Plan: Amounts of Food for a Week[a]

FAMILY MEMBER	MILK, CHEESE, ICE CREAM[b]	MEAT, POULTRY, FISH[c]	EGGS	DRY BEANS AND PEAS, NUTS[d]	DARK-GREEN, DEEP-YELLOW VEGETABLES	CITRUS FRUIT, TOMATOES	POTATOES	OTHER VEGETABLES, FRUIT	CEREAL	FLOUR	BREAD	OTHER BAKERY PRODUCTS	FATS, OILS	SUGAR, SWEETS	ACCESSORIES[e]
	qt.	lb.	no.	lb.	lb.	lb.	lb.	lb.	lb.	lb.	lb.	lb.	lb.	lb.	lb.
Child:															
7 months to 1 year	5.70	0.56	2.1	0.15	0.35	0.42	0.06	3.43	0.71[f]	0.02	0.06	0.05	0.05	0.18	0.06
1-2 years	3.57	1.26	3.6	0.16	0.23	1.01	0.60	2.88	0.99[f]	0.27	0.76	0.33	0.12	0.36	0.68
3-5 years	3.91	1.52	2.7	0.25	0.25	1.20	0.85	2.95	0.90	0.30	0.91	0.57	0.38	0.71	1.02
6-8 years	4.74	2.03	2.9	0.39	0.31	1.58	1.10	3.67	1.11	0.45	1.27	0.84	0.52	0.90	1.43
9-11 years	5.46	2.57	3.9	0.44	0.38	2.13	1.41	4.81	1.24	0.62	1.65	1.20	0.61	1.15	1.89
Male:															
12-14 years	5.74	2.98	4.0	0.56	0.40	1.99	1.50	3.90	1.15	0.67	1.88	1.25	0.77	1.15	2.61
15-19 years	5.49	3.74	4.0	0.34	0.39	2.20	1.87	4.50	0.90	0.75	2.10	1.55	1.05	1.04	3.09
20-54 years	2.74	4.56	4.0	0.33	0.48	2.32	1.87	4.81	0.93	0.71	2.10	1.47	0.91	0.81	2.11
55 years and over	2.61	3.63	4.0	0.21	0.61	2.38	1.72	4.92	1.02	0.62	1.73	1.23	0.77	0.90	1.16
Female:															
12-19 years	5.63	2.55	4.0	0.24	0.46	2.17	1.17	4.57	0.75	0.63	1.44	1.05	0.53	0.88	2.44
20-54 years	3.02	3.21	4.0	0.19	0.55	2.34	1.40	4.17	0.71	0.55	1.31	0.94	0.59	0.72	2.13
55 years and over	3.01	2.45	4.0	0.15	0.62	2.54	1.22	4.57	0.97	0.58	1.24	0.86	0.38	0.64	1.11
Pregnant	5.25	3.68	4.0	0.29	0.67	2.80	1.65	4.99	0.95	0.66	1.52	1.06	0.55	0.78	2.56
Nursing	5.25	4.16	4.0	0.26	0.66	2.99	1.67	5.33	0.78	0.61	1.55	1.16	0.76	0.91	2.70

[a]Amounts are for food as purchased or brought into the kitchen from garden or farm. Amounts allow for a discard of about one-tenth of the *edible* food as plate waste, spoilage, etc. Amounts of foods shown to two decimal places to allow for greater accuracy, especially in estimating rations for large groups of people and for long periods of time. For general use, amounts of food groups for a family may be rounded to the nearest tenth or quarter of a pound.

[b]Fluid milk and beverage made from dry or evaporated milk. Cheese and ice cream may replace some milk. Count as equivalent to a quart of fluid milk: natural or processed cheddar-type cheese, 6 oz.; cottage cheese, 2½ lbs.; ice cream, 1½ qts.

[c]Bacon and salt pork should not exceed ⅓ pound for each 5 pounds of this group.

[d]Weight in terms of dry beans and peas, shelled nuts, and peanut butter. Count 1 pound of canned dry beans—pork and beans, kidney beans, etc.—as 0.33 pound.

[e]Includes coffee, tea, cocoa, punches, ades, soft drinks, leavenings, and seasonings. The use of iodized salt is recommended.

[f]Cereal fortified with iron is recommended.

174

and the preparation and service of meals. Since the amount of time spent in planning is most directly related to the knowledge, skill, and experience that the manager brings to the task, it decreases as these are gained. Taking time at the beginning to plan the various steps often pays dividends later on by saving time as well as money and energy when one is shopping or preparing meals.

Menu Planning

Using a guide such as the Daily Food Guide (see Fig. 10-1), the manager may plan a week's menus which take into consideration the group's preference as well as the time, energy, and money available. Since there are many food patterns that will meet the RDA (see Chapter 10), menu plans that do not conform to the Daily Food Guide should be evaluated in terms of amounts of specific nutrients and not merely food groups. Suggested changes in family menus should also be made with due consideration for the family's food pattern, rather than for stereotyped food guides. Any pattern that suits the group is a good one if it provides for regular meals and allows for a variety of foods which meet nutritional requirements.

Meal patterns in many areas of the United States have come to vary widely from the traditional three meals a day. For many Americans one or two meals plus additional minimeals appear to have become the accepted norm. This phenomenon, perhaps, offers the greatest challenge to the nutrition planner who must provide foods adequate in essential nutrients while recognizing the need to be a calorie counter. Since many of the foods included in these minimeals are so-called snack foods, the nutrient composition of these should be of great concern to the meal manager. It is expected that increased and improved nutritional labeling will assist the planner in evaluating the contribution to the diet of these foods as well as many others. Nutrition labeling when appropriately used by the planner will provide helpful information for relating serving size to calories and to amounts of essential nutrients (see Chapter 14).

Cultural preferences also determine the esthetic qualities that require consideration in menu planning. Variation in flavor, color, texture, shape, and temperature are factors which the manager should recognize in creating meals which will be acceptable to the group. Although no set rules can be applied to these elements, the manager's sensitivity to them and her creativity in dealing with them cannot be overlooked by the nutrition educator. Magazines, newspapers, and cookbooks are often helpful in these respects, especially to the inexperienced planner. Menu planning help is also available from govern-

ment publications, especially from the Home and Garden Bulletins of the USDA (see the Supplementary Readings at the end of this chapter) and the State Cooperative Extension Services, and from food trade associations such as the Cereal Institute and the National Dairy Council.

Food Plans

For more than 40 years, the USDA has published food plans as guides for determining food needs and estimating food costs of families and other population groups. Three food plans at different cost levels have recently been revised (Tables 11-1, 11-2, and 11-3). They include the low, moderate, and liberal cost food plans. The homemaker can choose the appropriate food plan according to the amount of money the family has budgeted for food costs.

As shown in the tables, there are 15 food groups in each of the food plans, and the amounts suggested in each food group vary according to age and sex of family members and the cost level of the plan selected. When properly used, the food plans will provide the recommended dietary allowances for energy, protein, calcium, vitamin A, thiamine, riboflavin, niacin, and ascorbic acid. The RDA for iodine will be met if iodized salt is used. Iron intake may be low, especially for women of child-bearing age, until the level of iron enrichment in bread and flour is increased; iron supplements for this group may be required. Iron-fortified cereal is recommended for infants and children one to two years of age. It is estimated that at least 80 percent of the RDA for vitamin B_6 and magnesium is provided and that further adjustments in the food groups may be appropriate when additional food composition data is available. Similarly, insufficient information regarding the amounts of folacin, zinc, vitamin D, and vitamin E in foods is known to make impossible reliable estimates of the levels of these nutrients provided by the plans.

Homemakers may find it more beneficial to start with the appropriate food plan rather than the Daily Food Guide, estimate the amount needed in each food group, and then prepare menus and shopping lists based on the food plan.

Table 11-4 shows the weekly quantities of food suggested according to the low-cost food plan for a family of four—mother, age 30; father, age 32; girl, age 6; and boy, age 12. The specific foods selected within each of the food groups will then depend on the availability and cost of the individual foods as well as the preferences of the family. Menus and shopping lists based on the suggested amounts of food from each of the food groups for a family of four are shown in Tables 11-5 and 11-6.

Table 11-2. Moderate-Cost Food Plan: Amounts of Food for a Week[a]

FAMILY MEMBER	MILK, CHEESE, ICE CREAM[b]	MEAT, POULTRY, FISH[c]	EGGS	DRY BEANS AND PEAS, NUTS[d]	DARK-GREEN, DEEP-YELLOW VEGETABLES	CITRUS FRUIT, TOMATOES	POTATOES	OTHER VEGETABLES, FRUIT	CEREAL	FLOUR	BREAD	OTHER BAKERY PRODUCTS	FATS, OILS	SUGAR, SWEETS	ACCESSORIES[e]
	qt.	lb.	no.	lb.	lb.	lb.	lb.	lb.	lb.	lb.	lb.	lb.	lb.	lb.	lb.
Child:															
7 months to 1 year	6.46	0.80	2.2	0.13	0.41	0.49	0.06	3.98	0.64[f]	0.02	0.06	0.05	0.05	0.19	0.08
1-2 years	4.04	1.69	4.0	0.15	0.29	1.24	0.59	3.44	1.03[f]	0.26	0.81	0.33	0.12	0.28	0.79
3-5 years	4.74	1.88	3.0	0.22	0.30	1.46	0.85	3.51	0.74	0.27	0.82	0.73	0.41	0.81	1.42
6-8 years	5.79	2.60	3.3	0.34	0.37	1.94	1.17	4.39	0.84	0.39	1.14	1.11	0.56	1.03	1.97
9-11 years	6.68	3.31	4.0	0.38	0.45	2.61	1.40	5.76	1.03	0.51	1.47	1.51	0.66	1.31	2.63
Male:															
12-14 years	7.02	3.77	4.0	0.48	0.48	2.44	1.52	4.66	0.94	0.56	1.69	1.54	0.85	1.34	3.65
15-19 years	6.65	4.65	4.0	0.29	0.47	2.73	2.00	5.45	0.80	0.67	1.98	1.82	1.05	1.15	4.41
20-54 years	3.38	5.73	4.0	0.29	0.59	2.92	1.94	5.93	0.76	0.65	1.97	1.65	0.95	0.96	2.95
55 years and over	2.97	4.64	4.0	0.19	0.70	2.91	1.69	5.88	0.89	0.53	1.58	1.45	0.87	1.05	1.50
Female:															
12-19 years	6.22	3.32	4.0	0.24	0.53	2.62	1.21	5.38	0.68	0.56	1.34	1.22	0.56	0.97	3.36
20-54 years	3.35	4.12	4.0	0.19	0.62	2.84	1.35	4.94	0.54	0.49	1.28	1.08	0.65	0.81	2.89
55 years and over	3.35	3.21	4.0	0.14	0.72	3.09	1.17	5.50	0.81	0.52	1.20	0.98	0.45	0.73	1.39
Pregnant	5.44	4.57	4.0	0.25	0.91	3.52	1.60	6.13	0.73	0.83	1.77	1.28	0.46	0.85	3.50
Nursing	5.31	5.01	4.0	0.26	0.91	3.76	1.73	6.52	0.74	0.81	1.84	1.42	0.69	1.00	3.79

[a]Amounts are for food as purchased or brought into the kitchen from garden or farm. Amounts allow for a discard of about one-sixth of the *edible* food as plate waste, spoilage, etc. Amounts of foods are shown to two decimal places to allow for greater accuracy, especially in estimating rations for large groups of people and for long periods of time. For general use, amounts of food groups for a family may be rounded to the nearest tenth or quarter of a pound.
[b]Fluid milk and beverage made from dry or evaporated milk. Cheese and ice cream may replace some milk. Count as equivalent to a quart of fluid milk: natural or processed cheddar-type cheese, 6 oz.; cottage cheese, 2½ lbs.; ice cream, 1½ qts.
[c]Bacon and salt pork should not exceed ⅓ pound for each 5 pounds of this group.
[d]Weight in terms of dry beans and peas, shelled nuts, and peanut butter. Count 1 pound of canned dry beans—pork and beans, kidney beans, etc.—as 0.33 pound.
[e]Includes coffee, tea, cocoa, punches, ades, soft drinks, leavenings, and seasonings. The use of iodized salt is recommended.
[f]Cereal fortified with iron is recommended.

Table 11–3. Liberal Food Plan: Amounts of Food for a Week[a]

FAMILY MEMBER	MILK, CHEESE, ICE CREAM[b]	MEAT, POULTRY, FISH[c]	EGGS	DRY BEANS AND PEAS, NUTS[d]	DARK-GREEN, DEEP-YELLOW VEGETABLES	CITRUS FRUIT, TOMATOES	POTATOES	OTHER VEGETABLES, FRUIT	CEREAL	FLOUR	BREAD	OTHER BAKERY PRODUCTS	FATS, OILS	SUGAR, SWEETS	ACCESSORIES[e]
	qt.	lb.	no.	lb.	lb.	lb.	lb.	lb.	lb.	lb.	lb.	lb.	lb.	lb.	lb.
Child:															
7 months to 1 year	6.94	0.97	2.3	0.14	0.43	0.60	0.06	4.71	0.64[f]	0.02	0.05	0.06	0.05	0.20	0.09
1-2 years	4.26	2.07	4.0	0.17	0.31	1.50	0.59	4.10	1.07	0.28	0.82	0.35	0.13	0.27	0.95
3-5 years	5.08	2.35	3.1	0.23	0.32	1.77	0.85	4.18	0.76	0.27	0.79	0.78	0.45	0.85	1.74
6-8 years	6.25	3.18	3.4	0.36	0.40	2.35	1.18	5.21	0.85	0.39	1.08	1.23	0.60	1.08	2.41
9-11 years	7.21	4.04	4.0	0.39	0.48	3.15	1.41	6.83	1.04	0.51	1.39	1.67	0.71	1.38	3.21
Male:															
12-14 years	7.57	4.57	4.0	0.50	0.51	2.94	1.52	5.52	0.95	0.56	1.60	1.71	0.92	1.40	4.47
15-19 years	7.18	5.59	4.0	0.31	0.50	3.29	2.01	6.45	0.84	0.69	1.92	2.05	1.07	1.20	5.36
20-54 years	3.64	6.83	4.0	0.32	0.62	3.51	1.95	6.99	0.79	0.66	1.91	1.86	0.95	1.00	3.54
55 years and over	3.24	5.54	4.0	0.19	0.76	3.52	1.68	6.97	0.89	0.54	1.49	1.57	0.94	1.09	1.82
Female:															
12-19 years	6.72	3.97	4.0	0.25	0.56	3.15	1.21	6.34	0.71	0.59	1.31	1.35	0.54	0.98	4.09
20-54 years	3.62	4.86	4.0	0.20	0.66	3.41	1.35	5.81	0.56	0.51	1.24	1.22	0.66	0.84	3.47
55 years and over	3.65	3.79	4.0	0.15	0.76	3.71	1.14	6.42	0.74	0.54	1.17	1.12	0.48	0.77	1.66
Pregnant	5.91	5.43	4.0	0.26	0.96	4.22	1.57	7.17	0.70	0.87	1.70	1.45	0.46	0.87	4.20
Nursing	5.76	5.97	4.0	0.28	0.97	4.51	1.72	7.66	0.75	0.84	1.76	1.58	0.68	1.02	4.52

[a] Amounts are for food as purchased or brought into the kitchen from garden or farm. Amounts allow for a discard of about one-fourth of the *edible* food as plate waste, spoilage, etc. Amounts of foods are shown to two decimal places to allow for greater accuracy, especially in estimating rations for large groups of people and for long periods of time. For general use, amounts of food groups for a family may be rounded to the nearest tenth or quarter of a pound.
[b] Fluid milk and beverage made from dry or evaporated milk. Cheese and ice cream may replace some milk. Count as equivalent to a quart of fluid milk: natural or processed cheddar-type cheese, 6 oz.; cottage cheese, 2½ lbs.; ice cream, 1½ qts.
[c] Bacon and salt pork should not exceed ⅓ pound for each 5 pounds of this group.
[d] Weight in terms of dry beans and peas, shelled nuts, and peanut butter. Count 1 pound of canned dry beans—pork and beans, kidney beans, etc.—as 0.33 pound.
[e] Includes coffee, tea, cocoa, punches, ades, soft drinks, leavenings, and seasonings. The use of iodized salt is recommended.
[f] Cereal fortified with iron is recommended.

Table 11-4. Weekly Quantities of Food for a Family of Four According to the Low-Cost Food Plan

	MILK, CHEESE, ICE CREAM	MEAT, POULTRY, FISH	EGGS	DRY BEANS AND PEAS, NUTS	DARK-GREEN, DEEP-YELLOW VEGE-TABLES	CITRUS FRUIT, TOMA-TOES	POTATOES	OTHER VEGE-TABLES, FRUIT	CEREAL	FLOUR	BREAD	OTHER BAKERY PROD-UCTS	FATS, OILS	SUGAR, SWEETS	ACCES-SORIES
	(qt.)	(lb.)	(no.)	(lb.)	(lb.)	(lb.)	(lb.)	(lb.)	(lb.)	(lb.)	(lb.)	(lb.)	(lb.)	(lb.)	(lb.)
Mother (30 yrs.)	3.02	3.21	4.0	0.19	0.55	2.34	1.40	4.17	0.71	0.55	1.31	0.94	0.59	0.72	2.13
Father (32 yrs.)	2.74	4.56	4.0	0.33	0.48	2.32	1.87	4.81	0.93	0.71	2.10	1.47	0.91	0.81	2.11
Girl (6 yrs.)	4.74	2.03	2.9	0.39	0.31	1.58	1.10	3.67	1.11	0.45	1.27	0.84	0.52	0.90	1.43
Boy (12 yrs.)	5.74	2.98	4.0	0.56	0.40	1.99	1.50	3.90	1.15	0.67	1.88	1.25	0.77	1.15	2.61
Total	16.24	12.78	14.9	1.47	1.74	8.23	5.87	16.55	3.90	2.38	6.56	4.50	2.79	3.58	8.28

Table 11-5. Shopping Lists for a Low-Cost Food Plan

FOOD AND QUANTITY REQUIRED (see Table 11-4)	QUANTITY PURCHASED	FOOD AND QUANTITY REQUIRED (see Table 11-4)	QUANTITY PURCHASED
Milk, Cheese, Ice Cream (16.24 qt.)		*Cereal (3.90 lb.)*	
Nonfat dry milk (2 lb.)	10 qt.	Cornflakes (1 box)	½ lb.
Homogenized milk	4 qt.	Oatmeal (1 box)	1 lb.
Swiss cheese (6 oz.)	1 qt.	Cornmeal (1 box)	1 lb.
Processed cheese (12 oz.)	2 qt.	Macaroni (1 box)	½ lb.
		Rice	1 lb.
Total	17 qt.		
Meat, Poultry, Fish (12.78 lb.)		Total	4 lb.
Hamburger	1 lb.	*Flour (2.38 lb.)*	
Frozen perch	1 lb.	White flour, all purpose	2 lb.
Stewing chicken	3-3½ lb.	*Bread (6.56 lb.)*	
Pork liver	1 lb.	White, enriched (4 loaves)	4 lb.
Canned clams (one 8-oz. can)	½ lb.	Whole wheat rolls (two 12-oz. packages)	1½ lb.
Frankfurters	1 lb.	French bread, enriched (1 loaf)	1 lb.
Tuna (one 7-oz. can)	½ lb.		
Turkey roll	2-3 lb.	Total	6½ lb.
Sausage	1 lb.	*Other Bakery Products (4.50 lb.)*	
		Graham crackers (1 box)	1 lb.
Total	12-12½ lb.	Saltines, enriched (1 box)	1 lb.
Eggs (14.9 eggs)		Chocolate Chip Cookies	1 lb.
Eggs (med.)	1½ doz.	Waffles, frozen (one 10-oz. package)	10 oz.
Dry Beans and Peas, Nuts (1.47 lb.)			
Peanut butter (1 large jar)	1 lb.	Total	3⅝ lb.
Dry beans	½ lb.	*Fats, Oils (2.79 lb.)*	
		Margarine	1 lb.
Total	1½ lb.	Cooking oil (1 pt.)	1 lb.
Dark-Green, Deep-Yellow Vegetables (1.74 lb.)		Salad dressing (½ pt.)	½ lb.
Carrots	1 lb.	Suet	¼ lb.
Squash, winter	1 lb.		
Spinach, fresh	10 oz.	Total	2¾ lb.
		Sugars, Sweets (3.58 lb.)	
Total	2⅝ lb.	Sugar	2 lb.
Citrus Fruit, Tomatoes (8.23 lb.)		Jelly (1 jar)	½ lb.
Grapefruit (2)	2 lb.	Syrup, maple-flavored (½ pt.)	½ lb.
Orange (1)	½ lb.	Molasses (½ pt.)	½ lb.
Tomato juice (one 46-oz. can)	3 lb.	Strawberry gelatin (one 4-oz. package)	¼ lb.
Frozen orange juice (two 6-oz. cans)	12 oz.		
Stewed tomatoes (one no. 2½ can)	1½ lb.	Total	3¾ lb.
Lemon juice (one 1-pt. bottle)	½ lb.	*Accessories (8.28 lb.)*	
		Coffee	1 lb.
Total	8¼ lb.	Cinnamon	1 can
Potatoes (5.87 lb.)		Salt (1 box)	1 lb.
White potatoes	5 lb.	Vinegar	1 pt.
Other Vegetables, Fruits (16.55 lb.)		Vanilla	1 bottle
Lettuce	1 lb.	Baking powder	1 can
Celery	1 lb.	Pepper	1 can
Cabbage	2 lb.	Fruit-flavored juice, enriched (one 46-oz. can)	3 lb.
Raisins	1 lb.		
Apples	4 lb.		
Pineapple	2 lb.		
Bananas	2 lb.		
Onions	½ lb.		
Cranberries	1 lb.		
Yellow beans (one no. 303 can)	1 lb.		
Green beans (one no. 303 can)	1 lb.		
Total	16½ lb.		

be priced too high for the consumer's food budget. Shopping lists are good deterrents to impulse buying in the supermarket, especially if the spouse and children accompany the shopper.

PURCHASING

Most communities offer a variety of different markets, and the wise shopper soon learns where to buy certain items. The newspaper advertisements also tell where to find specials on various foods. Usually one or two markets in close proximity to the shopper are the most appropriate choices when transportation costs are included.

If adequate refrigeration and freezer storage are available, most consumers find weekly grocery shopping most convenient. Although many stores are open seven days a week and more than 12 hours a day,

Shopping Lists

Until some experience has been gained in knowing the types and amounts of food required for various menu items, the homemaker may save time, money, and heartache by making a shopping list based on the week's menus. Most local markets usually advertise in the Wednesday or Thursday newspaper; these ads are most helpful in indicating the foods available and their prices. Substitute items should be listed for foods which may not be in the market or which may

Table 11–6. Menus for One Week of Low-Cost Meals

	BREAKFAST	LUNCH	DINNER
MONDAY	Half Grapefruit Cornflakes with Skim Milk Coffee Milk	Peanut Butter and Jelly Sandwich Carrot and Celery Sticks Apple Skim Milk	Meat Loaf Baked Potato Spinach Bread Margarine Strawberry Fluff Coffee Milk
TUESDAY	Applesauce Waffles with Syrup Coffee Milk	Tomato Soup Egg Salad Sandwich Banana Skim Milk	Broiled Perch with Lemon Baked Squash Cole Slaw Cornbread Margarine Baked Custard Coffee Milk
WEDNESDAY	Oatmeal with Raisins Coffee Milk	Macaroni and Cheese Tomato Aspic Chocolate Chip Cookies Skim Milk	Chicken with Dumplings Peas Fruit Salad Bread Margarine Rice Pudding Coffee Milk
THURSDAY	Orange Juice Cornmeal Mush Coffee Milk	Chicken Sandwich Cole Slaw Oatmeal Cookies Skim Milk	Broiled Liver with Onions Boiled Potato Yellow Beans Whole Wheat Rolls Margarine Baked Apple Coffee Milk
FRIDAY	Pineapple Slices Poached Egg on Toast Coffee Milk	Manhattan Clam Chowder Whole Wheat Rolls Indian Pudding Skim Milk	Tuna Rice Casserole Carrots Apple-Celery Salad Cheese Biscuits Margarine Lemon Pudding Cake Coffee Milk
SATURDAY	Tomato Juice Cornflakes with Skim Milk Coffee Milk	Potato Pancakes with Sausages Applesauce Coffee Milk	Baked Beans with Frankfurters Green Salad Bread Margarine Fruit Cup Coffee Milk
SUNDAY	Orange Juice French Toast with Syrup Coffee Milk	Tomato Cheese Fondue Tossed Salad Coffee Milk	Roast Turkey Mashed Potatoes Green Beans Cranberry-Orange Salad Whole Wheat Rolls Mince Pie Coffee Milk

there are frequently certain times and days when choices on various items may be limited. There may be no butcher in the meat department after 6 P.M. on weekdays or on Sunday. Many supermarkets have only leftover fresh produce on Monday. Modifications in the family menus may be made when necessary to reduce food costs. Intelligent adjustments can insure that meals are still nutritionally adequate and acceptable to the family. Unit pricing, which allows the purchaser to compare the cost per unit of different brands and different size containers, is available in supermarkets. Open dating of perishable products such as bread, milk and other dairy products, and eggs also assists the consumer by indicating how fresh a food is at the time of purchase. The date itself usually refers to the last day the product should be offered for sale in the market.

Milk and Dairy Products

Either evaporated or nonfat dry milk (fortified with vitamins A and D) is cheaper than fresh milk and is entirely satisfactory for cooking. Each product can also be used as a beverage, especially when reconstituted dry milk is mixed with equal amounts of fresh milk. It is also economical to buy dry milk in as large a package as can be stored and used without waste. Premeasured units of the nonfat dry milk cost more than the bulk form. Fresh fluid milk sold at retail food and dairy stores usually costs less than home-delivered milk or that sold at small special service stores. The ½- or 1-gallon containers, if they can be stored properly and used efficiently, usually provide some savings per quart when compared with the 1-quart container. Inexpensive cheeses are as good a source of protein as more expensive types. Processed cheeses may be cheaper than natural cheeses, especially those natural cheeses that have been aged and are labeled "sharp." Cheese foods and cheese spreads may, according to their standards of identity (see p. 222), contain more moisture than processed cheeses.

Meat, Poultry, Fish, and Eggs

One-third or more of the food dollar in the United States is spent for meat, poultry, and fish. Less expensive cuts of meat may be used when it is necessary to cut food costs. The consumer should buy meat according to grade when possible. It is important to learn to identify cuts; bones are an excellent guide for identification. A rough estimate of the cost of the edible portion of some of the apparently cheapest cuts may disclose that the cheapest cut is not always the one which has the lowest price per pound. Variety meats, such as liver, are often good buys. Fish may be cheaper than meat. Poultry today is less expensive per pound than most cuts of meat. An average 3-ounce serving of cooked meat, fish, or poultry requires 4 to 4½ ounces of fat-free and bone-free uncooked lean. The amount of meat which must be purchased to yield this depends on the amount of inedible fat and bone in a cut and on the amount of skin on poultry and fish. Table 11–7 indicates the cost of 3 ounces of cooked lean from specified meat, poultry, and fish at July 1974 prices. Today's prices may be substituted for the "retail price per pound" in column 1, and current costs (column 3) may easily be calculated by multiplying each retail price per pound by the factor in column 2, the "part of pound for 3 ounces of cooked lean."

The price-wise consumer often substitutes other kinds of main dishes for meat. Macaroni products, rice, or corn, when combined with eggs, milk, cheese, or small amounts of fish, poulty, or meat, make good alternatives for the more expensive cuts of meat. When their prices are right, dried beans, peas, or nuts may also add variety to economically planned meals. A comparison of the costs of the amounts of various

Table 11-7. Cost of 3 Ounces of Cooked Lean from Specified Meat, Poultry, and Fish at July 1974 Prices*

FOOD	RETAIL PRICE PER POUND†	PART OF POUND FOR 3 OUNCES OF COOKED LEAN	COST OF 3 OUNCES OF COOKED LEAN
Hamburger	$0.90	.26	$0.24
Beef liver	.91	.27	.24
Chicken, whole, ready-to-cook	.52	.48	.25
Chicken breasts	.75	.35	.26
Turkey, ready-to-cook	.66	.40	.26
Ocean perch, fillet, frozen	1.08	.29	.31
Ham, whole	.90	.35	.31
Pork, picnic	.72	.46	.33
Ham, canned	1.52	.25	.38
Chuck roast of beef, bone in	.95	.45	.43
Haddock, fillet, frozen	1.50	.29	.43
Pork loin roast	1.13	.50	.57
Rump roast of beef, boned	1.70	.34	.58
Round beefsteak	1.74	.34	.59
Rib roast of beef	1.52	.45	.68
Pork chops, center cut	1.54	.45	.69
Sirloin beefsteak	1.75	.43	.75
Veal cutlets	3.45	.25	.86
Lamb chops, loin	2.26	.46	1.04
Porterhouse beefsteak	2.06	.52	1.07

*From Family Economics Review, Fall 1974.
†Average retail prices in U.S. cities, U.S. Department of Labor, Bureau of Labor Statistics.

foods which supply 20 grams of protein is given in Table 11–8. In many instances, a meal will include protein from more than one of these sources; for example, 2 tbsp. (1 ounce) peanut butter (8 grams of protein); 2 slices (2 ounces) enriched bread (4 grams of protein); 1 cup (8 ounces) milk (8.5 grams of protein). Based on the prices given in the table the 20 grams of protein in this meal would cost approximately 19 cents.

Eggs of graded size show considerable variation in price—sometimes small ones are the best buy, sometimes large ones. If large eggs are 95 cents per dozen, medium eggs are a good buy if they cost less than 83 cents per dozen. Extra large eggs would be a good buy if they cost less than 12 cents more than large eggs per dozen. Grade B eggs, suitable for cakes, casseroles, and scrambling, are less expensive than Grade A.

Fruits and Vegetables

To determine the best buy in fruits and vegetables, comparisons must be made among fresh, frozen, canned, and dehydrated products in terms of the cost per serving. Table 11–9 shows the number of servings obtained from the usual purchasing unit. Count as a serving one medium-size apple, orange, banana, peach, or pear; 2 or 3 apricots, figs, or plums; ½ cup fruit with liquid.

FOOD	MARKET UNIT	PRICE PER MARKET UNIT[a]	PART OF MARKET UNIT TO GIVE 20 GRAMS OF PROTEIN[b]	COST OF 20 GRAMS OF PROTEIN
Peanut butter	12 oz.	$0.62	.23	$0.14
Eggs, large	doz.	.62	.25	.16
Bread, white enriched .	lb.	.35	.51	.18[c]
Dry beans	lb.	.78	.24	.19
Chicken breasts	lb.	.75	.25	.19
Chicken, whole, ready-to-cook	lb.	.52	.37	.19
Beef liver	lb.	.91	.24	.22
Hamburger	lb.	.90	.24	.22
Milk, whole fluid	half gal.	.78	.29	.23[d]
Turkey, ready-to-cook .	lb.	.66	.35	.23
Pork, picnic	lb.	.72	.32	.23
Bean soup, canned	11.5 oz.	.26	.96	.25
Ham, whole	lb.	.90	.29	.26
Tuna, canned	6.5 oz.	.59	.44	.26
American process cheese	8 oz.	.72	.38	.27
Ham, canned	lb.	1.52	.24	.37
Frankfurters	lb.	1.03	.36	.37
Sardines, canned	4 oz.	.40	.94	.38
Pork loin roast	lb.	1.13	.33	.38
Round beefsteak	lb.	1.74	.22	.38
Chuck roast or beef, bone in	lb.	1.09	.35	.38
Ocean perch, fillet, frozen	lb.	1.08	.36	.39
Liverwurst	8 oz.	.68	.60	.40
Salami	8 oz.	.86	.50	.43
Rump roast or beef, boned	lb.	1.70	.26	.44
Sirloin beefsteak	lb.	1.75	.28	.49
Rib roast of beef	lb.	1.52	.33	.50
Bologna	8 oz.	.71	.73	.52
Haddock, fillet, frozen .	lb.	1.50	.35	.53
Pork sausage	lb.	1.02	.52	.53
Pork chops, center cut .	lb.	1.54	.35	.53
Bacon, sliced	lb.	1.09	.52	.57
Lamb chops, loin	lb.	2.26	.31	.69
Porterhouse beefsteak .	lb.	2.06	.34	.69
Veal cutlets	lb.	3.45	.21	.74

*From Family Economic Review, Fall 1974.
[a]Average retail prices in U.S. cities, Bureau of Labor Statistics, U.S. Department of Labor.
[b]One-third of the daily amount recommended for a 20-year-old man. Assumes that all meat, including cooked fat, is eaten.
[c]Bread and other grain products, such as pasta and rice, are frequently used with a small amount of meat, poultry, fish or cheese as main dishes in economy meals. In this way the high quality protein in meat and cheese enhances the lower quality of protein in cereal products.
[d]Although milk is not used to replace meat in meals, it is an economical source of good quality protein. Protein from nonfat dry milk costs less than half as much as from whole fluid milk.

Fresh fruits and vegetables in season and when plentiful are usually cheaper than canned or frozen ones. Home frozen and canned foods are economical when the food is home-grown or purchased at the peak of the season. Help from the agents and publications of the Cooperative Extension Service is avail-

able in most communities to assist the inexperienced person with home preservation of food. Bruised or overripe soft fruits and vegetables usually involve excessive waste and hence are rarely economical to purchase. Blemishes on fruits and vegetables which may be discarded with the skin or rind, however, may influence grade and be good buys.

Prices of frozen, canned, and dehydrated fruits and vegetables vary according to brand, grade, type of process, and other added ingredients. The nutritive value of cheaper standard grades of canned fruits and vegetables is essentially the same as that of the more expensive fancy grades, and they are equally wholesome. Compare unit prices and the nutrition labeling on the can or package. The USDA publication HERR 37, *Family Food Buying: A Guide for Calculating Amounts to Buy and Comparing Costs,* * is helpful for determining the most economical buys.

Breads and Cereal Products

In general, foods prepared at home are less expensive than foods purchased ready to eat. Products made from whole or enriched grains are more nutritious than unenriched products, so it is worthwhile to check the label or ask the baker for nutrition information. Breakfast cereals cooked at home are almost always cheaper than "instant" ones. Ready-to-serve cereals in individual boxes may cost twice as much per ounce as the same cereal in a larger box. Large packages are economical for big families but not for small ones, as the contents may become stale and have to be discarded. Unsweetened cereals usually cost less per ounce than presweetened ready-to-serve cereals. Day-old bakery products may represent savings to large families who consume many loaves of bread each week. Sweet rolls, buns, and coffee cakes are expensive types of bread.

In most instances, the cost of service adds to the price of commercially prepared mixes. The convenience value of a prepared mix differs according to the experience, skill, and interest of the individual cook and must be evaluated accordingly.

STORAGE

Since many staple foods have a long storage life, large economical packages can be purchased if storage facilities are adequate. In general, these storage spaces should be away from water, drain, or heating pipes, and should be kept clean, dry, reasonably cool, and free from insects and rodents. Household chemi-

*Available from Superintendent of Documents, U. S. Government Office, Washington, D. C., 20402 at 35 cents a copy.

Table 11–9. Number of Servings of Fruits and Vegetables from Usual Purchasing Unit*

FRESH VEGETABLES	Servings per pound as purchased
Asparagus	3 or 4
Beans, lima (in pods)	2
Beans, snap	5 or 6
Beets, diced (without tops)	3 or 4
Broccoli	3 or 4
Brussels sprouts	4 or 5
Cabbage:	
Raw, shredded	9 or 10
Cooked	4 or 5
Carrots:	
Raw, diced or shredded (without tops)	5 or 6
Cooked	4
Cauliflower	3
Celery:	
Raw, chopped or diced	5 or 6
Cooked	4
Kale (untrimmed)	5 or 6
Okra	4 or 5
Onions, cooked	3 or 4
Parsnips (without tops)	4
Peas (in pods)	2
Potatoes	4
Spinach, (prepackaged)	4
Squash, summer	3 or 4
Squash, winter	2 or 3
Sweet potatoes	3 or 4
Tomatoes, raw, diced, or sliced	5

FROZEN VEGETABLES	Servings per package (9 or 10 oz.)
Asparagus	2 or 3
Beans, lima	3 or 4
Beans, snap	3 or 4
Broccoli	3
Brussels sprouts	3
Cauliflower	3
Corn, whole kernel	3
Kale	2 or 3
Peas	3
Spinach	2 or 3

CANNED VEGETABLES	Servings per can (16 oz.)
Most vegetables	3 or 4
Greens, such as kale or spinach	2 or 3

DRY VEGETABLES	Servings per pound
Dry beans	11
Dry peas, lentils	10 or 11

FRESH FRUIT	Servings per market unit as purchased
Apples	
Bananas	
Peaches	3 or 4 per pound
Pears	
Plums	
Apricots	
Cherries, sweet	5 or 6 per pound
Grapes, seedless	
Bluberries	4 or 5 per pint
Raspberries	
Strawberries	8 or 9 per quart

FROZEN FRUIT	Servings per package (10 or 12 oz.)
Blueberries	3 or 4
Peaches	2 or 3
Raspberries	2 or 3
Strawberries	2 or 3

CANNED FRUIT	Servings per can (16 oz.)
Served with liquid	4
Drained	2 or 3

DRIED FRUIT	Servings per package (8 oz.)
Apples	8
Apricots	6
Mixed fruits	6
Peaches	7
Pears	4
Prunes	4 or 5

*From *Your Money's Worth in Foods.* Home and Garden Bulletin No. 183, Washington, D. C., USDA, rev. 1974.

cals and cleaning supplies should never be stored with food.

Special attention should be paid to the storage of perishable items. Refrigerators should maintain a temperature of 45° F. or below. Fresh meat should be stored in the refrigerator loosely wrapped; all containers should be closed or covered. Many food dollars are wasted on food that spoils before it can be consumed and must be discarded. This is particularly true or frozen foods when there is not adequate freezer space in the home. A temperature of 0° F. or below is required if frozen foods are to be stored for long periods of time. Frozen concentrated orange juice can be stored for a year without losing more than 5 per-

cent of its ascorbic acid if it is kept frozen throughout the period. Fresh meats and, especially, poultry and fish require freezing if they are not cooked and consumed within a day or two of purchase.

The manner in which fresh produce is stored may alter nutritive values. Table 1 in Section 4 gives the averages values for nutrients in foods. Averages, however, do not reveal that half the vitamin C in leafy dark-green vegetables and broccoli is lost if they are stored in the refrigerator for five days or more. Raw cabbage stores well even at room temperature and storage may even increase the vitamin A value of sweet potatoes. Berries lose their ascorbic acid rapidly if they are capped or bruised.

Table 11-10. General Directions for Following a Recipe

1. Select tested recipes from reliable sources, and read them carefully.
2. Turn on the oven to the correct temperature if the product is to be baked or roasted, so that the oven will be at the desired heat when the mixture is ready for cooking.
3. Check supplies and collect the necessary ingredients in one work area.
4. Collect the needed mixing, measuring, and cooking equipment in one work area.
5. If baking or roasting, prepare the pan for the product, using the size indicated in the receipe for best results.
6. Check to see if there is anything that should be done to ingredients before adding them to the mixture, such as melting fat or chocolate, beating egg whites, or sifting dry ingredients together.
7. Use level measurements; measure exactly—dry ingredients first, then liquids, if possible, to save washing of extra utensils.
8. Combine the ingredients, following the procedure given in the recipe.
9. Bake or cook exactly as directed. Follow cooking times and temperatures given, testing for doneness as directed. Thermometers for roasting, deep-fat frying, and candymaking will be found helpful.
10. Handle finished product as directed, such as removing from pans, molding, chilling; cooling or chilling before serving; or serving at once.

PREPARATION

A reliable cookbook is a must for an inexperienced cook. Careful attention should be given to recipe amounts and instructions until the cook has developed sufficient skill to make adjustments. (See Table 11-10 for general directions for following a recipe.) It is important to realize that those ingredients which determine the shape, texture, consistency, and tenderness of a mixture are proportional; these proportions cannot be altered without changing the basic characteristics of the product. However, flavoring agents may be varied according to the preference of the family or individual. Knowledge of the terms used in recipes (Table 11-11) is important for following directions accurately.

The successful cook also selects carefully the essential equipment for food preparation.

For accurate measuring the following utensils are essential: an 8-ounce measuring cup divided into fourths and thirds or a set of measuring cups of these volumes; tablespoons and teaspoons of regulation sizes or, preferably, a set of measuring spoons.

To measure dry material by the cup, fill lightly with a spoon to brim or to indicated cup level. Do not shake the cup to level the material. This is particularly important in the case of flour sifted before measurement. Granulated sugar may be measured easily, but brown sugar should be packed firmly into the cup. Before measuring honey or syrup, rinse the cup with cold water.

Measurement of butter and margarine, when in ¼-lb. sticks, may be made by accurate division. One stick corresponds to the measurement of ½ cup. To measure bulk fat, pack firmly into cup to the desired mark of measurement. Except for that used in pastry, fat should be at room temperature. (An easy way of measuring ½ cup of shortening is to fill the cup to the one-half mark with cold water and add shortening enough to cause water to rise to the 1-cup mark. To measure ¼ cup, fill with cold water to the three-quarter mark.)

To measure dry ingredients by the tablespoon or the teapoon, fill until heaping and, with the back edge of the knife, level off all that extends above the edge of the spoon. If one-half spoonful is desired, divide the contents of the spoon lengthwise and push off one half. If one fourth is wanted, divide the remaining half crosswise and push off the portion not desired. If one eighth is desired, divide the remaining one fourth crosswise and push off the portion not needed. If one third of a spoonful is desired, divide the contents of the spoonful crosswise into thirds, pushing off the undesired portion.

To measure spoonfuls of liquid, dip the spoon into the liquid.

To measure butter or other solid fats, pack solidly into the spoon and level with a knife.

So that all the foods to be served for a meal are ready at the appointed time, the cook plans the work according to the amount of preparation and cooking time each item requires. The ability to organize a meal is one of the true tests of the cook-manager. Many beginners actually write down their work plan before they begin so that they can perform each task at the appropriate time and dovetail many steps.

Table 11-11. Terms Used in Recipes

Baste: to pour liquid over the surface of food which is being baked or roasted.

Blanch: to let food stand in hot water 3 to 5 minutes to loosen skin, remove strong flavors, or set color.

Cream: to soften shortening and to blend with sugar by rubbing with a wooden spoon or in an electric mixer.

Cut in: to blend shortening with flour with pastry blender or two knives.

Dice: to cut in small square pieces.

Fold: to add whipped cream or beaten egg whites with a careful folding motion.

Mince: to cut or to chop fine.

Pan-broil: to cook in a heated pan or on a griddle with little or no added fat.

Pan-fry: to cook in a shallow pan with just enough added fat to prevent sticking and aid browning.

Parboil: to boil in water until it is partially cooked.

Purée: to press through a sieve.

Sauté: to cook in a small amount of fat.

Scald: to heat milk until bubbles appear around the edge.

Sear: to brown quickly over direct heat or in an oven.

Shred: to cut or to tear in thin strips.

Simmer or **stew:** to cook in liquid just below boiling point.

Steep: to let stand in hot liquid below boiling point.

Milk and Dairy Products

Since at high temperatures some of the protein in milk coagulates into a film on top and a coating on the sides of the pan, milk should be heated or cooked slowly at a low temperature and not allowed to boil. It can be heated in a double boiler or with care over direct heat. Overcooking may cause off-flavors or scorching. Similarly, when baking casseroles containing a large proportion of milk it is necessary to use low oven temperatures. Cream sauces or gravies thickened with flour or cornstarch require constant stirring while cooking to prevent lumping. Care must also be taken in adding any acid foods such as tomato or lemon juice to milk because they often cause it to curdle. Add small amounts of the acid ingredient to the milk or sauce just before serving.

Evaporated milk may be substituted for fresh milk by diluting it with an equal amount of water before use. Nonfat dry milk may be sifted with the dry ingredients or reconstituted and used as a liquid.

When cheese is used in cooking, it is usually grated or finely flaked or cut into small pieces. For top-of-stove cooking, it is generally best to use a double boiler and to cook the cheese over hot water. For baked cheese dishes, a low temperature is suggested; sometimes directions call for placing the dish containing the cheese mixture in a pan of hot water. When a high temperature is used, as in toasting an open cheese sandwich under the broiler, the cooking period should be short. The texture of cheese will toughen and become stringy when it is overcooked by any method.

Meat, Poultry, Fish, and Eggs

As previously indicated, protein foods are coagulated by heat. Low-temperature cooking produces a tender product, while high temperatures tend to cause toughening. This is best illustrated in egg cookery, in that an egg cooked below the boiling point is more tender than a "boiled" egg. For baking or roasting meat, cookery experts recommend temperatures between 300° and 325° F. to get the best results for more tender meat as well as to lessen shrinkage.

MEAT. All cuts of meat, including the inexpensive ones, provide acceptable main dishes when they are properly prepared. The use of moderate temperatures and the selection of the correct method of cooking for each cut of meat are essential. Dry heat (oven roasting, oven broiling, pan broiling, and pan frying) should be used only with the tender and therefore usually the more expensive cuts of meat. Moist heat (braising, pot roasting, stewing) and the use of meat tenderizers make the less tender and less expensive cuts almost equally acceptable.

No additional moisture or fat is required for oven roasting and oven broiling. The use of low oven temperatures, checked by an oven thermometer, for roasting prevents overcooking, shrinkage in size, and loss of vitamins and of palatability that occur with high-temperature cooking. When the more tender cuts are pan fried or pan broiled, a small amount of fat is needed to guard against adherence to the frying pan. Some types of utensils are now made to be used without added fat; or a nonfat spray preparation may be used with regular utensils by the individual who is restricting fat in his diet.

In moist heat cookery such as braising, pot roasting, or stewing, the addition of an acid—either vinegar or lemon or tomato juice—to the liquid used in cooking increases the tenderizing effect of this method.

Fresh pork should be cooked until every vestige of pink coloring of the flesh has disappeared, to prevent infection with *Trichina spiralis*. Of all food animals, only pigs or hogs are susceptible to trichinosis infection, which may be passed on to humans if sufficient heat is not applied to kill any parasites present. Present methods of slaughtering and handling do not ensure against infection. Thus thorough cooking of all pork products in the home kitchen is essential.

The Meat Cookery Guide presented in Fig. 11–1 suggests the most desirable cooking methods for a variety of cuts and types of meat.

POULTRY. Chickens, the most commonly used type of poultry, are known by various terms which indicate size and, to some extent, tenderness. This is shown in the following chart:

Squab	¾-1¼ lbs.
Broiler	1¼-2½ lbs.
Fryer	2½-3½ lbs.
Roaster	3 lbs. or over
Fowl	4 lbs. or over

Proper cooking which develops and holds the delicate flavor of the meat is important in preparing chicken. Young chicken may be broiled or pan fried in a small amount of fat. Older birds should be roasted or simmered, and serve sliced, hot or cold; boiled chicken may be used for fricassee or creamed chicken. A very palatable broth can be made from the bones of roast chicken or turkey.

FISH. The general rule for cooking fish may be summed up in one sentence: Short cooking just before serving is most important. This rule is particularly applicable in the case of broiled and pan-broiled fish, which after cooking dries out quickly. The test for doneness is simple. When tried with a fork, the flesh

COOKING METHODS	BEEF CUTS	VEAL CUTS	PORK CUTS	LAMB CUTS	VARIETY MEATS
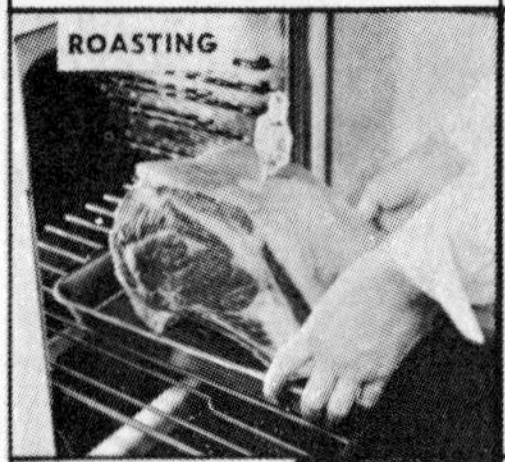 **ROASTING**	Standing Rib Rolled Rib Sirloin Chuck Ribs (high quality) Rump (high quality) Loaf	Rolled Shoulder Cushion Shoulder Arm Roast Blade Roast Rib Loin Rump Leg	Loin Rolled Shoulder Cushion Shoulder Fresh Ham (pork leg) Smoked Picnic Smoked Shoulder Butt Smoked Ham Sausages Sliced Salt Pork	Cushion Shoulder Rolled Shoulder Breast with Pocket Rolled Breast Rack Leg	Liver (beef-veal-pork-lamb)
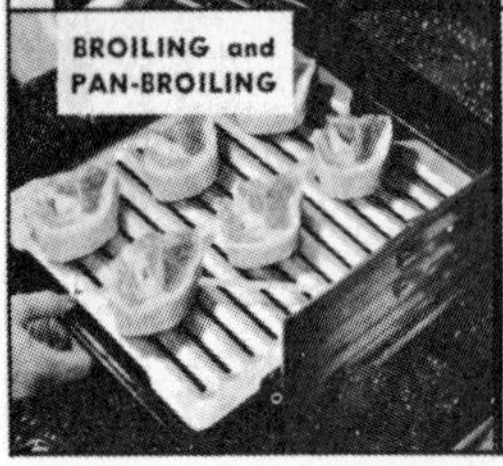 **BROILING and PAN-BROILING**	Rib Steaks Club Steaks T-Bone Steaks Porterhouse Steaks Sirloin Steaks Chuck Steaks (high quality) Rump Steaks (high quality) Patties	Veal is not broiled or pan-broiled	Fresh pork is not broiled or pan-broiled Smoked Ham Slices Sliced Bacon Sliced Canadian-style Bacon Smoked Shoulder Butt Slices	Rib Chops Loin Chops Shoulder (arm or blade) Leg Steaks Patties Choplets (from breast stuffed with ground lamb)	Liver (veal-lamb) Kidney (lamb) Sweetbreads (beef-veal-lamb)
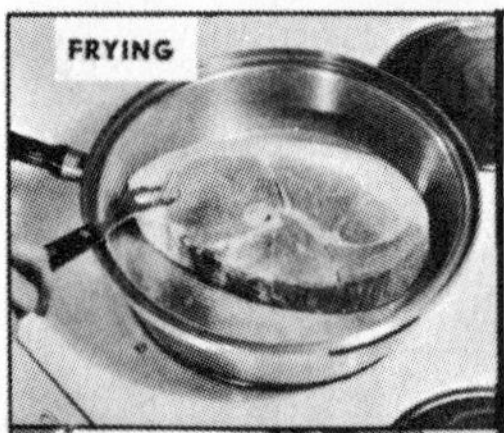 **FRYING**	Thin Steaks (tender or pounded) Patties	Chops Cutlets Steaks Patties	Sausage Sliced Salt Pork	Thin Chops or Thin Steaks	Liver (all kinds if cut thin) Tripe (after pre-cooking in water) Sweetbreads Brains
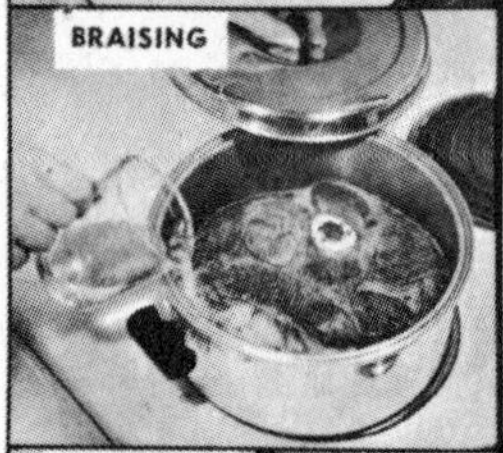 **BRAISING**	Chuck (arm or blade) Rump Round Heel of Round Brisket Plate Short Ribs Flank Shanks Ox-joints	Breast Rib Chops Loin Chops Shoulder Chops Cutlets Patties	Rib Chops Loin Chops Shoulder Chops or Steaks Fresh Ham Slices	Breast Neck Slices Shanks Riblets Shoulder (arm or blade)	Liver (beef-pork) Kidney (beef-veal-pork) Heart (beef-veal-pork-lamb) Tripe (beef) Sweetbreads (beef-veal-lamb)
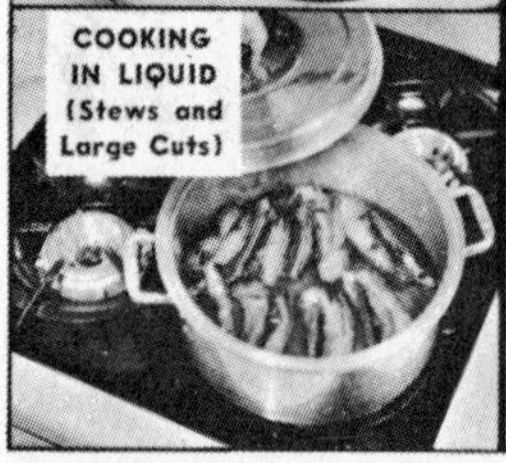 **COOKING IN LIQUID** (Stews and Large Cuts)	Neck Shank Plate Brisket Flank Heel of Round Ox-joints Corned Beef	Neck Shoulder Shanks Flank	Hocks Shanks Feet Backbones Neck Bones Spareribs Smoked Picnic Smoked Shoulder Butt Smoked Ham Shanks Smoked Spareribs Smoked Hocks	Neck Steaks Shoulder Breast	Kidney (beef-veal-pork-lamb) Heart (beef-veal-pork-lamb) Tongue (beef-veal-pork-lamb) Tripe (beef) Sweetbreads (for precooking) Brains (for pre-cooking)

Fig. 11-1. Meat cookery guide. A pressure cooker may be used for "cooking in liquid." Follow directions as given in the pressure cooker guidebook.

should flake. Sliced or quartered lemon is the chosen garnish for fish for both appearance and flavor. Suggestions for cooking fresh fish are given in Table 11–12.

EGGS. Low temperature and short cooking are also desirable for most egg dishes, as the texture will be more delicate and tender under these conditions. For this reason, soft-cooked eggs generally are coddled by being allowed to stand covered in water that has been brought to the boiling point. Hard-cooked eggs, prepared by boiling, have a firmer texture and are easier to slice or to stuff.

When they are part of a meal, eggs should be prepared just before they are to be served. Coddled eggs in their shells should be opened just before they are to be eaten.

Fruits and Vegetables

FRUITS. Most fresh fruits may be eaten raw. Fruits such as apples, pears, peaches, plums, grapes, and cherries should be washed thoroughly to remove any traces of insecticide spray residue. Berries should be washed just before serving. Strawberries should be washed before being hulled. Peaches, pears, and ap-

Table 11–12. Suggestions for Cooking Fresh Fish*

KIND OF FISH	PREPARATION AT MARKET	METHODS OF COOKING	SAUCE OR GARNISH
Bass, black	Split	Broil	Lemon
Bass, sea	Split†	Broil	Lemon
	Whole	Stuff and bake	Tomato sauce
Bluefish	Split	Broil, bake, plank	Sliced tomatoes
	Whole	Stuff and bake	Sliced pickles
			Parsley sauce
Cod, small	Whole	Stuff and bake	Anchovy sauce
large	Steaks†	Broil, bake	Melted butter
			Lemon sprinkled with paprika
Flounder	Fillets†	Bake	Lemon, parsley
Haddock, small	Whole	Stuff and bake	Mock Hollandaise sauce
large	Fillets†	Bake	
large	Steaks†	Bake, broil	Grilled tomatoes
			Tartar sauce
Halibut	Steaks†	Broil, bake, pan-fry	Cucumber sauce
	Thick slice†	Steam	Hollandaise sauce
Mackerel	Split†	Broil, bake	Sliced cucumbers
Pompano	Split	Broil, plank	Melted butter
	Fillets†	Bake	Minced parsley
			Lemon, parsley
Salmon	Steaks†	Broil	Sliced cucumbers
	Thick slice†	Steam	Egg sauce
Scrod	Split†	Broil	Melted butter
			Pepper relish
Shad	Split	Bake, plank	Lemon
			Radishes
Shad roe†		Parboil, then bake	Bacon
			Lemon
Smelts	Whole†	Broil, bake, pan-fry	Tartar sauce
Sole	Fillets†	Broil, bake	Melted butter
			Grilled tomatoes
Snapper, red	Split	Bake, broil, plank	Sliced cucumbers
Swordfish	Steaks†	Broil, pan-fry	Cucumber sauce
Trout, lake and sea	Split	Broil, bake	Melted butter
			Minced parsley
Tuna, fresh	Steak†	Bake, broil	Lemon sprinkled with paprika
	Thick piece†	Steam	Hollandaise sauce
Weakfish	Split†	Broil, bake	Sliced tomatoes
Whitefish	Split	Broil, bake, plank	Lemon
	Whole	Suff and bake	Parsley sauce

*From Heseltine, M., and Dow, U. M., *The Basic Cookbook,* ed. 5. Boston, Houghton Mifflin, 1967.
†Especially adapted to service in small family.

ples may be served whole or peeled and sliced or sectioned. They, and bananas, should be peeled or sliced just before serving or they will discolor due to oxidation. Sprinkling or dipping them in lemon juice or ascorbic acid solution or adding sugar at the time of slicing will prevent discoloration.

A melon should be tested for ripeness by feeling the "softness" of the stem end, or by the sound it makes, rather dull and thick, when slapped. Melons should be washed and chilled in the refrigerator before serving. Cantaloupe and medium-size melons are served in halves or wedges after the seeds are carefully removed. Watermelon is served in inch or 1½ inch slices or, if small, in half of a lengthwise wedge. Cut portions of leftover melon should be wrapped tightly in plastic wrap so that their aroma will not permeate other foods in the refrigerator.

Pineapple may be kept at room temperature unless it is very ripe. The easiest method of preparation is to cut the fruit in thick slices or wedges, pare each piece and remove the "eyes," then cut it into bitesize pieces.

Fresh pineapple should not be used with gelatin, as it contains a proteolytic enzyme which "digests" the gelatin and keeps it from setting. The enzyme is destroyed in canned fruit or juice.

When large oranges or grapefruit are cut in half for serving, the segments should be loosened with a curved knife made for the purpose. It should be run between the pulp and the fiber membranes, although the fiber partitions should never be cut. Oranges and grapefruit may also be served in sections by themselves or in combination with other fruits in a fruit plate or salad. They should be peeled with a sharp or serrated knife, round and round, directly into the flesh, and the sections between the membranes removed with a sharp knife.

Dried fruits should be prepared according to the directions on the package, or they may be purchased already prepared. Canned fruits, prepared with heavy or medium syrup or without added sugar, are available, and may be served in the syrup or drained for use in salads. Cooked fruits are usually stewed or baked. One should make sure that frozen fruits are thoroughly thawed before they are served.
VEGETABLES should be washed thoroughly to remove soil and traces of spray. Root vegetables should be scrubbed; asparagus, spinach, and other greens should be washed under running water to remove sand. Vegetables such as potatoes and carrots should not be pared or scraped until just before they are to be used. Peas and beans should not be shelled or corn husked until just before they are to be cooked. Outer leaves of cauliflower and cabbage should not be removed until just before they are to be used. A larger loss of vitamins occurs when vegetables are cut in small pieces. Grated carrots, for instance, lose vitamins more quickly than the sliced vegetable.

Salad greens should be separated and thoroughly washed under cold running water and allowed to drain or to be dried with a clean towel. Placing them in a plastic bag in the refrigerator will help to keep them crisp. Salads should be prepared for serving just before the meal and the dressing added at the last moment. They should be cold and crisp and attractive to the eye. They should be simple rather than elaborate and they should have a dressing which is well but moderately seasoned.

Vegetables should be cooked as short a time as possible, as long cooking destroys vitamins and changes flavor, color, and texture. The use of baking soda in the cooking of green vegetables is not recommended because an alkali such as soda hastens the destruction of the B vitamins and ascorbic acid.

Only a small amount of water should be used for boiling most vegetables. There will be little evaporation if the utensil is tightly covered and if the cooking is done over low heat. (See Table 11–13.)

Although boiling vegetables is the most common practice, other methods of preparation can be used to add interest and palatability to everyday meals. Potatoes, winter squash, onions, and tomatoes are especially attractive and flavorful when baked in the oven. Sautéing or frying such vegetables as eggplant, summer squash, parsnips, mushrooms, or peppers may add special appeal to a meal. Steaming spinach and cabbage helps to retain the natural flavor and texture as well as the nutritive value of these products. There are numerous popular vegetable combinations: two or more vegetables cooked together, or vegetables combined with protein foods such as eggs, cheese, meat, or fish, with sauces or garnishes. Imagination on the part of the homemaker will often bring about enthusiastic acceptance of vegetables where only mere tolerance existed.

For maximum retention of nutrients in canned vegetables, the liquid should be poured out and heated and the vegetables added to the liquid and heated just before serving. Directions for preparation of frozen vegetables are given on each package.

Breads and Cereal Products

Most of the bread used in the home is purchased ready-made from the supermarket. Many kinds of commercially baked breads are available to the consumer. Some are of the brown-and-serve variety, which require a short baking time before serving. Other hot breads, such as biscuits and muffins leavened with baking powder rather than yeast, are frequently prepared in the home. Enriched all-purpose flour, which forms gluten when it is mixed with liquid, gives the structure to these products. Fat and sugar tenderize and help produce the characteristic texture. Baking powder or soda is used for leavening and some salt is added for flavor. Depending on the characteristics of the product, eggs may or may not be added.

Ready-to-eat cereals require no additional prep-

Table 11-13. General Rules for Boiling Vegetables

1. Use only enough water barely to cover the vegetables. (Exceptions to this rule are noted by an asterisk.) Spinach and other tender greens need no water.

2. Bring water to boiling point and add salt before vegetable is added.

3. Cover tightly and cook over low heat only until vegetables are tender.

4. Use any remaining liquid of mild-flavored vegetables for soup or sauce.

5. Vegetables may be baked in tightly covered casseroles when the oven is being used for some other purpose. The time of cooking will be about one and a half times again as long as for boiling.

6. Variations from the general rules:
Whole artichokes, beets, the cabbage family, onions, parsnips, turnips, potatoes, and corn on the cob should be cooked in water to cover, and the water discarded. Keeping the pot tightly covered will prevent spreading the strong cooking odors of some of these vegetables through the house.
Stalks of asparagus and broccoli may be laid side by side in a skillet with one inch of water, or tied and placed upright in the top of a tall double boiler with 1 to 2 inches of water. The skillet or pot should be tightly covered.

7. When a pressure saucepan is to be used, the time chart provided with the utensils should be followed exactly for best results.

Timetable for Boiling

As vegetables differ in texture according to maturity, directions for cooking time can only be approximate.

Vegetable	Minutes	Vegetable	Minutes
Artichokes		Dandelion greens	10-20
American or Jerusalem	15-20	Eggplant	10-15
French or Globe*	20-30	Kohlrabi	20-30
Asparagus*	15-20	Mushrooms	7-10
Beans		Okra	20-25
String	15-30	Onions*	20-40
Lima	20-30	Parsnips*	30-50
Beets*	20-60	Peas	8-15
Beet greens	10-20	Potatoes*	
Broccoli*	15-25	White	20-30
Brussels sprouts*	10-20	Sweet	20-30
Cabbage*	5-10	Spinach	6-10
Carrots	15-30	Squash	
Cauliflower*	10-30	Summer	10-20
Celery	10-15	Winter	20-30
Corn*	5-10	Turnips*	15-60
Cucumbers	10-15		

*See General Rules for Cooking, No. 6, above.

aration in the home. A wide assortment is found on most grocery shelves. Milk and sugar as well as fruit may be added depending on individual choice.

When cooking porridge-type cereals such as oatmeal, farina, or cornmeal, use the proportions of ingredients shown on the package and follow the directions for cooking times.

Regular rice should not be washed before cooking. Use only the amount of water that the rice will absorb during cooking and do not rinse after cooking. Directions for cooking converted rice and instant rice are found on the package.

To make a smooth cornmeal mush, blend the cornmeal with cold water before stirring it into hot boiling water. It may be served as mush or chilled, sliced, and fried.

Macaroni products and pasta should be cooked until tender but firm. To achieve this consistency, add the pasta to rapidly boiling, salted water, and cook only until tender. The less water is used in cooking pasta, the more vitamins are retained. Thick pasta such as lasagna noodles require more water for cooking; follow directions on the package.

Variations in Food Values

Food values for prepared dishes are based on standard recipes, but people do not always use standard recipes. Obviously, cream of tomato soup made with heavy cream will have a higher calorie and fat value, and a lower calcium and protein value, than cream of tomato soup made with skim milk. Cooking methods also affect the nutritive value of food. Broiling in place of frying may greatly reduce the amount of fat and thus the calorie value of a serving of hamburger. Broiling it to the well-done stage rather than rare will further reduce the amount of fat in a serving. Water-soluble vitamins and minerals may be lost in the cooking water when vegetables or meats are cooked in liquid and the liquid is discarded.

MEAL SERVICE

The temperature and the appearance of food as it is placed before the family can be determining factors as to whether or not the meal will be consumed and enjoyed or wasted. The cook who wishes to please the group will take special pleasure in presenting attractive offerings. Children and ill people especially react to the appearance of the plate.

The type of meal service used is usually determined by the life-style of the family and may vary drastically from one meal to another. Breakfast may be an individual effort with each member preparing and serving his own food, while dinner may be served more formally to the group as a whole. In any case, responsibility for serving the meal as well as for its preparation and cleanup is frequently a shared one in today's American family. Men and women alike appear to find enjoyment in the creative aspects of meal management and also in sharing the other work involved in providing food for the family.

STUDY QUESTIONS AND ACTIVITIES

1. List your goals for family meal management.
2. What are the steps involved in providing successful family meals?
3. Using the Moderate-Cost Food Plan (Table 11–2), plan a week's menus and shopping lists for a family of four consisting of mother, age 28; father, 30; girl, 8, boy, 6. Calculate the cost of the week's food at current market prices.
4. Calculate the costs per quart of milk purchased as follows: 1-qt. homogenized milk; ½ gal. homogenized milk; 1 gal. homogenized milk; 13-ounce can evaporated milk; nonfat dry milk (bulk), one 1-lb. box; nonfat dry milk (premeasured), 1 lb.
5. Calculate the vitamin C content and the cost per serving of ½ grapefruit; ½ c. frozen orange juice reconstituted according to directions; 1 orange; ½ c. canned tomato juice; ½ c. canned grapefruit; ½ c. canned grapefruit juice.
6. What is the recommended procedure for storing fresh meats, potatoes, and bread in the home?
7. Describe the most appropriate methods for cooking tender cuts of meat and less tender cuts of meat.
8. What effect does heat have on protein foods? What precautions must be taken in cooking cheese mixtures?
9. How may cooking methods change the nutritive value of food?

SUPPLEMENTARY READINGS

Bennion, M., and Hughes, O.: *Introductory Foods*, ed. 6. New York, Macmillan, 1975.

Kinder, F.: *Meal Management*, ed. 3. New York, Macmillan, 1968.

McWilliams, M.: *Food Fundamentals*, ed. 2. New York, Wiley, 1970.

Vail, G. E., Phillips, J. A., Rust, L. O., Griswold, R. M., and Justin, M. M.: *Foods—An Introductory College Course*, ed. 6. Boston, Houghton Mifflin, 1973.

Cookbooks

General Mills: *Betty Crocker's New Good and Easy Cookbook*. New York, Golden, 1962.

———: *Betty Crocker's New Picture Cookbook*. New York, McGraw-Hill, 1961.

Heseltine, M., and Dow, V.: *The Basic Cookbook*, ed. 5. Boston, Houghton Mifflin, 1967.

Rombauer, I. S., and Becker, M. R.: *Joy of Cooking*. New York, Bobbs-Merrill, 1962.

USDA Home and Garden Bulletins

Single copies of the following publications can be obtained free from the Office of Communication, U. S. Department of Agriculture, Washington, D. C. 20250.

Freezing Combination Main Dishes . . . . HG 40
Money-Saving Main Dishes . . . . HG 43
Home Care of Purchased Frozen Foods . . . . HG 69
Storing Perishable Foods in the Home . . . . HG 78
Conserving the Nutritive Values in Foods . . . . HG 90
Family Food Budgeting . . . for Good Meals and
    Good Nutrition . . . . HG 94
Eggs in Family Meals: A Guide for Consumers . . HG 103
Vegetables in Family Meals: A Guide for
    Consumers . . . . HG 105
Poultry in Family Meals: A Guide for Consumers HG 110
Cheese in Family Meals: A Guide for Consumers HG 112
Beef and Veal in Family Meals: A Guide for
    Consumers . . . . HG 118
Lamb in Family Meals: A Guide for Consumers . . HG 124
Fruits in Family Meals: A Guide for Consumers . HG 125
Milk in Family Meals: A Guide for Consumers . . HG 127
Cereals and Pasta in Family Meals: A Guide for
    Consumers . . . . HG 150
Pork in Family Meals: A Guide for Consumers . . HG 160
Keeping Food Safe to Eat: A Guide for Homemakers HG 162
Breads, Cakes, and Pies: A Guide for Consumers . HG 186
How to Buy Nonfat Dry Milk . . . . HG 140
How to Buy Fresh Fruits . . . . HG 141
How to Buy Fresh Vegetables . . . . HG 143
How to Buy Eggs . . . . HG 144
How to Buy Beef Steaks . . . . HG 145
How to Buy Beef Roasts . . . . HG 146
How to Buy Poultry . . . . HG 157
How to Buy Meat for Your Freezer . . . . HG 166
How to Buy Canned and Frozen Vegetables . . . . . HG 167
How to Buy Beans, Peas, and Lentils . . . . HG 177
Your Money's Worth in Foods . . . . HG 183
How to Buy Cheese . . . . HG 193
How to Buy Lamb . . . . HG 195
Como Comprar Los Comestibles/How to Buy
    Food . . . A Bilingual Consumer Aid . . . . PA 976N
Food Makes the Difference: Ideas for
    Economy-Minded Families . . . . PA 934
Ideas for Leaders Working with
    Economy-Minded Families . . . . PA 937

For further references see Bibliography in Section 4.

the helping process in nutrition services

12

RESPONSIBILITY OF THE NUTRITION COUNSELOR

The chief responsibility of the health-care team is to maintain or to reestablish a positive state of well-being in the population it serves. The nutrition counselor (see Chapter 1), as a member of this team, must focus on the reinforcement or modification of food habits which promote good health. Since nutritional requirements change throughout the life-span from infancy to old age, most people will need to monitor their food practices throughout their lives. Because knowledge about nutrition is constantly increasing, most people will also need help to modify their food practices at one time or another.

The public receives nutrition information from a variety of sources other than health practitioners. Chief among these are the public communications media, which bring broad health issues to public attention and attempt via advertising to persuade consumers to change food choices. Few would

Written in cooperation with the authors by Clair Agresti Johnson, Ph.D., R.D., Assistant Professor, Medical Dietetics Division, School of Allied Medical Professions, College of Medicine, The Ohio State University.

191

argue that during the 1960s the media were chiefly responsible for changing the type of fat consumed by an entire nation. Nutrition counselors might well look to this experience as a model for implementing change. In this case, the mission of the advertising industry was to persuade the public to use one type of fat rather than another while the food industry provided an acceptable alternative.

The mission of the nutrition counselor, however, is not only to encourage the client to select among alternatives, but to discontinue one type of behavior in favor of another and to sustain this change over a lifetime. Discontinuance of smoking and curtailment of eating are examples of changes which health practitioners have historically found difficult to implement, because most people find these changes difficult to accept. Therefore, the chief responsibility of the nutrition counselor is to translate nutrition knowledge into information the client can accept and subsequently adopt.

Determining the Role of the Nutrition Counselor

Nutrition counseling is a multidisciplinary effort and, as such, counseling roles will change in relation to the context of clinical practice. Nutrition counselors can practice in a variety of settings. Some of these are: (1) the primary health-care setting, such as neighborhood health clinics, prenatal and child health clinics, and health maintenance organizations where the type of care delivered is essentially preventive in nature; (2) the secondary health-care setting, such as community hospitals and extended-care facilities where the type of care delivered is essentially crisis and rehabilitative in nature; and (3) the tertiary health-care setting, such as major medical teaching centers, where the type of care delivered is essentially complex and crisis in nature. This is not to say that preventive care cannot be delivered in a tertiary setting nor crisis care in a primary setting. The point is that before the role of the nutrition counselor can be defined it is important to know the needs of the clients served. Specifically, does the client need preventive, rehabilitative, or crisis care?

Another related consideration in role definition is the power invested in the counselor and that invested in the client. Here it becomes necessary to define power. Power is not a negative concept but rather a reality of the situation in which both the counselor and client find themselves. In other words, who is most in control? In a crisis, it is the practitioner who is most in control and has the most power to change the situation. In a rehabilitative situation, there is almost equal control and, therefore, equal power. In a preventive situation, it is the client who is in control and

who has the power to accept or reject what the counselor advocates. The counselor's role then is a dynamic one and will change as the client's needs change.

Practitioner-Managed vs. Client-Managed Care

Clients enter the health-care system at many points. Figure 12–1 demonstrates how a client can enter at one point in the system and progress or be referred to another. If, for example, a person with diabetes mellitus enters the crisis-care setting in a state of ketoacidosis, all efforts of the team are focused on the immediate treatment and care. In this situation, the care given can be said to be practitioner-managed; the primary goal at this point is to reestablish, as quickly as possible, physiological homeostasis. Once this is achieved, the health goal is the reestablishment of psychological equilibrium so that the client can begin to assume the responsibility for the continued implementation of the primary goal—a sustained positive state of well-being.

It is well to remember that during a medical crisis the client often progresses from the passive phase to the collaborative phase of his treatment and care. The nutrition counselor working in a crisis-care setting needs to be aware of these phases so that she can help the client pass through them at his own pace and with dignity. During the period of passivity the care needed can be described as essentially practitioner-managed, but as soon as the client shows an interest in the rationale of his treatment it is time for the nutrition counselor to encourage him to accept responsibility for his own management. In doing this the nutrition counselor moves from the caring role to the helping role. As this shift occurs, the client begins to move from a passive role to an active one, and true counseling begins. The counselor's objective at this time changes again and becomes one of helping the client determine his own goals and participate completely in his own care. In other words, the care delivered is client-managed.

When one compares the number of persons in crisis care or institutional settings to those in preventive care or noninstitutional settings, it is obvious that there is a greater need for clients to know how to care for themselves than for the practitioner to care for them. Yet the present health-care system is better organized to deliver crisis care than to deliver preventive care. The reason for this is understandable. In a developing nation the chief mission of health personnel is the eradication of infectious disease. As this becomes a reality, life expectancy increases, and health professions are faced with the growing problem of chronic diseases which, by their very nature, require the client to manage his own care to prevent, delay, or treat them. This type of care implies competence on the part of the client; and, if the delivery of this care is to become a reality, the counselor must see to it that the client becomes competent at caring for himself. Nutrition counselors who hope to become effective in helping the client to manage his care need to be as competent in the preventive setting as they have historically been in the crisis setting. This requires the nutrition counselor to assume the predominant role of change-agent.

As a change-agent the counselor must understand and use the helping process. In nutrition counseling the helping process can be defined as a process of intervention in which the counselor makes available to an individual the means for establishing or modifying his food practices. And, to carry out the process, the counselor must enter into a helping relationship with the client.

Nature of the Helping Relationship

A relationship refers to a connection between people, ideas, or things. A helping relationship demands a regularized pattern of interaction between counselor and client, and is built up over time. A single exchange of information does not meet these criteria. By the same token, a system involving multiple exchanges of information between the client and a variety of counselors does not lend itself to the firm establishment of the helping relationship. This has been demonstrated in research studies which suggest that patient compliance is better in private practice

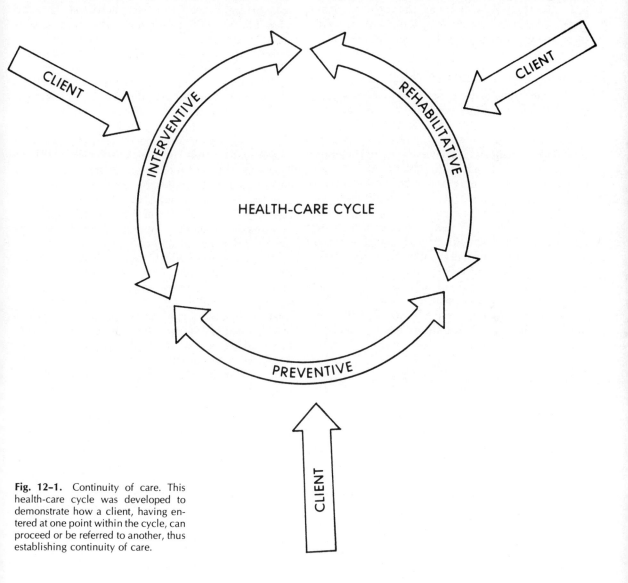

Fig. 12-1. Continuity of care. This health-care cycle was developed to demonstrate how a client, having entered at one point within the cycle, can proceed or be referred to another, thus establishing continuity of care.

than in clinics because the continuing relationship of client and practitioner is well established.[1]

The work of Rogers[2] and others has shown that the helping person must first establish a climate of trust between herself and the client. To achieve this the helping person must believe that all people can change and be able to communicate this to the client. It is important to accept *unconditionally* the client's feelings and personal meanings as the client sees them. The counselor must be warm, caring, and genuinely interested in the client. And finally, the counselor must help the client make decisions rather than have the client become dependent on her. The reason that the development of the helping relationship is so crucial to the delivery of nutritional care is that most nutritional care is implemented outside the institutional setting by the client in the context of his social environment. Therefore, the nutrition counselor is advocating a process, not a solution.

ELEMENTS OF THE HELPING PROCESS

The remainder of this chapter delineates the process of delivering client-managed nutritional care. This process is made up of several critical components (Chapter 1): *establishing and maintaining the relationship; collecting and assessing information; planning change; implementing change; and evaluating effectiveness.* It must be remembered that these components are not discrete steps toward a solution but a series of highly interrelated functions systematically planned to implement a process which has built-in evaluation criteria. Simply stated, a person who needs to lose weight must be helped to implement and evaluate a weight-reduction program. A critical step in helping the client is to determine how much weight is to be lost and at what rate. This then becomes the ultimate criterion by which both client and counselor evaluate the effectiveness of their collaboration.

Establishing the Helping Relationship

Collaboration implies that the client and counselor are working together. An important first component of the helping process is the generation of a climate conducive to the achievement of this end. This function is a continuous process in that the counselor does not simply establish the relationship and then move on to the next step. The helping relationship is one which requires constant building, and it permeates the entire process.

The first interaction with the client, however, is most critical because at this time the direction of the helping process is established. Before the nutrition counselor can do anything, she must find the answers to two important questions: What does the client expect from her and what does she expect from the client? Though one of these questions is directed to the counselor and the other to the client, it is the responsibility of the counselor to determine these answers as well as reconcile differences if any exist.

If the client seeks out the counselor's help, then the counselor's task is greatly simplified. In the case of the nutrition counselor, however, the client often enters the health-care system expecting a solution to a problem and is referred to the nutrition counselor because of a complicating factor. A classic example of this is the client who seeks medical attention because of fatigue and shortness of breath with the expectation that the health-care team will "get him well." In order to meet the client's expectations, the physician refers him to the nutrition counselor for a weight-reduction program. The nutrition counselor then finds herself in a situation where she is face-to-face with a client who came for a solution, not a process.

Here, the nutrition counselor has three major tools which can be used to help the client: force, knowledge, and client values. These can be translated into three kinds of health arguments which the counselor can use: an argument based on fear, one based on reason, and one based on trust. Health personnel have been, and continue to be, criticized for relying heavily on fear and reason, while ignoring client values. This may well be the case, but those who would advocate the third to the exclusion of the first and second are ignoring the variability of human nature as well as the reality of the clinical setting.

It is client need which should dictate the health argument used. Often, it is fear which brings the client into the health-care setting. In the preventive setting it is usually fear of losing his health; in the crisis setting, it is fear of losing his life. Both of these fears are motivating forces because they are rooted in basic values, so that in the preventive setting, the nutrition counselor might well focus on the fear motive, while in the crisis setting this is impossible. It is not, however, a question of which argument is best to employ, but which best meets the needs of a client at a particular point in time. Often, the client's self-generated fear is motive enough to establish a collaborative relationship with the counselor. When fear is not sufficient, then the counselor may try reason and, in turn, trust. It is imperative in establishing the relationship that the nutrition counselor start where the client is, not where she would like him to be.

Regardless of where the client is, he will eventually be outside the health-care setting managing his own care; and for sustained change to occur, the client's value system must be made known to the counselor. Hence the importance of developing a climate of trust so that this kind of information can be analyzed for its significance to the problem.

Collecting and Assessing Information

Collecting and assessing information provides the basis for the development of the counseling plan and, as in the establishment of the relationship, is an ongoing process. Here the nutrition counselor has two major sources: secondary and primary.

SECONDARY SOURCES: Information which can be obtained from sources other than the client or his family is described as secondary. Such sources include the client's records in any health-care setting; continuity of care or referral reports; or the information shared in health team conferences. The nutrition counselor not only uses this information but also contributes to it. She uses it to develop a nutritional care plan and contributes to it to insure continuity of care.

Analysis of the secondary information about a client and his family reveals the health problem, the objectives of care, and the resources available for the solution of the problem. Health problems are conditions or situations which obstruct the maintenance or reestablishment of a positive state of well-being. They are usually stated in a problem list and can include such conditions as poor dental hygiene or obesity. Health objectives are those goals which the health-care team wants accomplished. For example, the objectives for an obese person who has habitually practiced poor dental hygiene might be "full-mouth extraction" and "25 percent reduction in weight." The health-care team then looks to resource persons who can help meet these objectives. Health resources are those persons, departments, or agencies within or outside the health-care setting who can either solve the client's problems or help him deal with them. It is through the analysis of secondary information that the nutrition counselor can determine the health problems that will be encountered, the objectives to be achieved, and the resources to be identified for the client.

PRIMARY SOURCES: Relevant nutritional care information which is not recorded must be obtained from primary sources. These are the client himself and those persons who will help him implement his care. The nutrition counselor gathers this information in any health-care setting and must be a skilled interviewer. The counselor uses this information to develop a counseling plan as well as to keep the team informed of client progress. Analysis of primary information reveals the client's nutritional needs, problems, and resources.

Nutritional needs can be defined as that nutrient intake which best promotes or reestablishes physiological homeostasis. They can be stated as a dietary prescription or implied in the problem list. For example, the problem of obesity implies a need for a deficit in energy intake; the problem of less than adequate weight gain in an infant without organic disease implies underfeeding; a potential nutritional need may be dictated by a socioeconomic problem. In addition, nutrient monitoring may be warranted if the client is from a high-risk population, such as the pregnant teen-aged girl.

Nutritional problems, on the other hand, are reasons why the nutritional needs exist. Obesity may be the health problem but not the nutritional problem. For example, one client may be obese because he is a compulsive eater, while another may be too old to move about, have inadequate kitchen facilities, or be living on a limited budget. These clients obviously have similar nutritional needs but quite different nutritional problems related to these needs. Therefore, they will likely need different resources.

Client resources are those persons or attitudes which can assist the client in dealing with the nutritional problem, hence, in meeting the nutritional need. The person who is a compulsive eater may have strong support at home, and the person with inadequate kitchen facilities may be an active member of a church or fraternal organization. Persons too old to move about or living on inadequate funds who also have limited personal resources may need to be referred to agencies outside their primary social environment. It is through the analysis of primary and secondary information that the nutrition counselor can reconcile the differences between objectives which are defined by the health-care team and objectives which are defined by the client. Such mutually defined objectives then become the basis for the counseling plan.

Planning Change

A critical component of the helping process is the development of a plan of action. The concept of planned change implies that the change-agent knows, in advance, where she is going (objectives), how she will get there (action), and how she will know she has arrived (evaluation). In client-managed nutritional care it is important that the user of change becomes the agent of change. In other words, it is not enough to produce an attitude change in the client. To move from attitude to action, a meaningful plan is necessary. This point is extremely important. There is experimental evidence from studies of antismoking communications that both a message of threat and instructions for action are necessary to reduce or stop smoking.[3]

OBJECTIVES: Health-care objectives are directly related to the client's health problem and should reflect the common objectives of the health-care team. However, if the client is to manage his own care, then the team's objectives must be congruent, whenever possible, with the client's. For example, the health-care team in a prenatal clinic may have breast-feeding as an objective while a mother who plans to return to work four weeks after the birth of her baby may reject this objective. Equally important is the need for the nutrition counselor and the client to work together on the nutritional aspects of the health-care objectives.

Objectives are written in the client's record and will vary from client to client. There is one health-care objective, however, which is so universal that it is rarely specified. That objective is to preserve the *psychological equilibrium* of the client and his family. Viewed in this way, the importance of involving clients in the formulation of their own goals is more than an effective change strategy; it is the foundation upon which their health maintenance or recovery from disease rests.

ACTION: Once the client has developed his objectives, he must be shown how to achieve them. It is important that the nutrition counselor help the client find a way which is least disruptive to his life-style, yet conducive to health maintenance or the reestablishment of physiological homeostasis. Just as health objectives are related to health problems and client objectives to client problems, the action to be taken is related to both health and client objectives. It is at this point that the counselor must identify the specific information the client needs in order to manage his care, determine the sequence in which this will be shared with the client, and offer a variety of alternatives to the client for achieving his goals.

EVALUATION: Critical components of any plan are the evaluation criteria by which progress toward the objectives is measured. As such, evaluation criteria are directly related to the objectives. How much and what foods will the teen-aged girl eat for breakfast before going to school each morning? Is the business executive to lose one pound per week? In addition, how long should the client sustain these changes? Both client and counselor need this information. The client needs it to guide him toward his goal, and the counselor needs it to assess the client's progress. Although evaluation criteria are usually the *last* of the components mentioned in any health-care plan, they should comprise the *first* components. Objectives and evaluation criteria should be developed simultaneously so that both the health-care team and the client

know the ultimate goal, and so that the team and client can reconcile any differences.

Implementing Change

Once the change has been planned, the next step in the helping process is counseling the client in how to implement the needed change. This process is not unlike teaching children to form new ideas. But, whether teaching adults or children, the nutrition counselor is involved in a process which is commonly referred to as "adult education." Adults are free to retreat from a learning environment which they do not find satisfying. New concepts, therefore, cannot be taught in the health setting as they have traditionally been taught in the classroom. In order for the nutrition counselor to meet commonly defined objectives, she must be aware of some fundamental principles of adult education which are applicable to any learner in an open environment. These are the principles of *ego involvement* and *information need*.

Ego involvement or self-concern is pervasive in every person's actions. The nutrition counselor must continually ask what value the change being advocated has for the client. In applying the principle of ego involvement, the nutrition counselor should be sensitive to the learner's self esteem as well as her own ego involvement and goals. The self-concept of an adult affects his role as learner. A mature person perceives himself as being able to make his own decisions and to manage his own life. In fact, it is generally agreed that a person is adult when he perceives himself to be wholly self-motivating and self-directing. It is at this point that an individual experiences a deep need to be perceived by others as being self-directing. Adults, then, have a need to be treated with respect, to make their own decisions, and to be seen as unique persons. They often resent or avoid situations in which they feel they are being treated like children. Adults tend to resist learning when this is the case.

Information need is often more obvious to the counselor than to the client. However, during the process of gathering information about the client, the counselor and client jointly can often identify the information which the client needs for achieving his goals. For example, the mother of a three-month-old infant, when asked how much cereal she is feeding the baby, may respond, "Three tablespoons. Should I be feeding more?" With this response she has given the counselor a clue to what information she needs: in this case the amount, not the kind, of food.

Implementing change requires client involvement and assumes the learner is the center of the client-counselor relationship. It is recognized that this kind of teaching is time-consuming, for it involves more than handing the client a list of instructions, commonly referred to as "giving diet instructions." Giving does not imply accepting.

Evaluating Effectiveness

The effectiveness of the collaboration is tested during subsequent client-counselor encounters. At this point the nutrition counselor needs to determine whether or not the client is progressing toward his goals. If this is not being achieved, it is important for them to determine together where the relationship became ineffective.

Many nutritional care plans fail because the client's needs, problems, and resources have not been accurately identified. Some questions are so basic that they are often not asked. "Does a need exist?" is such a question. If there is evidence that the client is adequately managing his own nutritional care, it is pointless and can be disruptive to initiate a new plan of action. Some clients seen by nutrition counselors have often been counseled before. Others sustain a positive state of well-being through their own resources. Therefore, before a counseling plan is developed, it must be determined whether change is needed, as well as the nature of that change.

Weed defines a health problem as a situation which requires the health care-team to do one of three things: obtain more information, treat, or educate.[4] Many nutritional care plans are not effective because there is insufficient data to identify the client's problem. In these cases there is clearly a need for more information. On the other hand, some plans fail because the client cannot care for himself and needs to be treated or cared for by someone else. When it is determined that the client's problem is lack of information, then there is a need to educate. Also, the client's resources may not have been assessed correctly.

The client has two types of resources available to him: those within his primary social environment, or the family, and those within his extended social environment, or the community. When the client is an infant, it is obvious that the persons counseled are the parents or other caretakers. When the client is an adult, the persons counseled will vary depending on certain factors. For example, when a self-directed adult lives alone, he is the person who should be counseled. Yet, when the client is a dependent adult living with a parent, an offspring, or a spouse, counseling efforts need to be directed at both the client and his primary resource person. When the client is not in control and is being referred to an extended-care facility or a community agency, the nutritional care plan should be communicated to those persons who will care for him.

When the proper relationship has not been established, an otherwise effective care plan is doomed to failure. There are times when, despite efforts on the part of the nutrition counselor, a helping relationship cannot be established with the client. When this is the case many nutritional counselors might make a sincere attempt to proceed with the plan as best they can. Effective professional counselors, however, recognize that in these circumstances it is wiser, when possible, to refer the client to another practitioner who can better help him. Before this decision is made, the nutrition counselor should be certain that the client wants to be referred to another practitioner. She must also assure the client that she will be available at any time the client needs her. Often this open gesture of concern is enough to identify the problem obstructing the development of the helping relationship, and effective counseling can proceed.

INTERVIEWING

Interviewing is the method used by the counselor to gather primary information from a client about his usual food choices and the factors in his environment which directly affect them. Interviewing is a form of interpersonal communication which differs from social conversation in that it is guided by goals defined by either the counselor or the client and agreed upon by both. The counselor is responsible for guiding the interview to elicit the information needed to help the client.

Approaches

To elicit information not only about what a client eats but also why he eats, open-ended rather than closed questions are usually more effective. The open-ended question is one which requires the client to formulate a response, having been given a minimum of clues as to what the response should be. For example: "Do you have anything after the evening meal?" not, "Do you snack while watching TV?" The latter question not only suggests that he snacks in the evening but also watches TV, while the former asks for information without implying what the response should be.

In addition to open-ended questions, probes which elicit more detail about a response are also important. A response, "I eat cereal in the morning," should be followed by such questions as, "What kind?" "Do you put anything on it?" "How much?" "Why do you choose cereal?"

The terms breakfast, lunch, and dinner should be

avoided. A client may eat with a reasonable degree of frequency but, because the time he eats may differ significantly from what he knows are usual mealtimes for most people, he may report that he does not eat breakfast, lunch, or dinner. Or he may report a meal which he never eats to gain the counselor's approval.

One approach to gathering information when the focus is on the client is to ask him how he lives his day. With this approach the counselor can gain information about his activities as well as his food choices. When the client is a mother who is concerned about her family's meals, the counselor might start with what foods she usually buys (see Chapter 11) and then find out how she prepares food and how much each member of the family consumes.

Anxiety

Counselors use various methods to hide their anxiety. Over-ready verbal encouragement such as finishing a client's sentence for him not only reveals that the counselor is anxious but also discourages the client from giving complete information. The effective counselor learns to be comfortable with silence while the client formulates his reply. The anxious counselor can also miss the client's cues. Probing for more information when a client states, "I never eat eggs," may indicate an intolerance not discovered by other members of the health-care team, or it could indicate the client's feelings about an unfavorable experience in the past with eggs.

Clients may also be anxious. People under stress are often indirect in their communication and find it difficult to discuss some problems with an individual they have no reason to trust. Hostility is often a result of anxiety, but a client may also express hostility toward a counselor to test the counselor's acceptance of him as an individual.

Interviewing vs. Counseling

Interviewing in nutrition is the process by which the counselor gains information from the client; counseling is the process by which she imparts information to the client. In some instances the two processes may be combined. However, it is advisable to gather complete information first so that the information-giving process is carefully planned and relevant to the client's total needs.

STUDY QUESTIONS AND ACTIVITIES

1. In a prenatal clinic or a family health clinic, interview a client to obtain information about his or her usual food practices. With your instructor, formulate nutritional care objectives and observe your instructor interact with the client to validate whether or not your objectives are congruent with the client's.
2. Review a client's record and identify the nutritional component of his health-care needs. Does the information in the record indicate that the client is aware of his needs?
3. Without consulting other members, plan and implement a change in your family's usual food practices. Did your family accept or reject this change?
4. Visit a congregate meals program for the elderly and *listen* to the participants discuss the food served. Analyze the discussion with your instructor.
5. Record your own food practices for a three-day period. Analyze your record and plan and carry out *one* minor change for two weeks. Were you successful? Why or why not?

SUPPLEMENTARY READINGS

Brill, N. I.: *Working with People: The Helping Process.* Philadelphia, Lippincott, 1973.
Ginther, J. R.: Educational diagnosis in patients. J. Am. Dietet. A., 59:560, 1971.
Levanthal, H.: Changing attitudes and habits to reduce risk factors in chronic disease. Am. J. Cardiol. 31:517, 1973.
Levine, M.: The intransigent patient. Am. J. Nurs. 70:2106, 1970.
Ohlson, M. A.: The philosophy of dietary counseling. J. Am. Dietet. A. 63:13, 1973.
Slowie, L. A.: Patient learning segments from case histories. J. Am. Dietet. A. 59:563, 1971.

For further references see Bibliography in Section 4.

REFERENCES

1. Blackwell, D.: N. Eng. J. Med. 289:249, 1973.
2. Rogers, C.: Personnel and Guidance J. 37:6, 1958.
3. Levanthal, H., et al: J. Personality Soc. Psychol. 6:313, 1967.
4. Weed, L. L.: Arch. Int. Med. 127:101, 1971.

13

regional, cultural, and religious food patterns

Factors Influencing Food Habits
Food Patterns in America
Regional Food Patterns in the United States
Cultural Food Patterns
Religious Food Patterns
Unusual Dietary Practices
Food Fads

FACTORS INFLUENCING FOOD HABITS

The factors that determine individual food habits
are varied and complex. The nutrition counselor
must develop an understanding of them if she is
to fulfill her function successfully. The following
brief discussion indicates some of the influences
that help to establish food habits.

CULTURAL FACTORS. Culture may be defined as
the way of life of a group of people—usually of
one nationality or from a particular locality. Food
habits are a deeply rooted aspect of many cultures.
One culture may consider food only as a means of
satisfying hunger; another may consider eating a
duty, a virtue, or a form of pleasure; still another
may feel eating is a means of family or social
sharing.

Culture is transmitted from one generation to
another by institutions such as family, school, and
church. Over periods of time various degrees of
change occur within any given culture. The
preservation of individual cultures is an important
goal of many minority groups today. The revival of
interest in the American Indian culture, the "Black
is Beautiful" concept, and the activities of
Italian-American groups represent attempts to iden-

tify and to transmit to future generations certain aspects of a cultural identity. It is important to understand that culturally determined food practices, which vary from group to group, may nevertheless meet the basic biological needs that are similar for all peoples.

ECONOMIC FACTORS. Rising food costs and food shortages have had their impact on the food patterns of many American families. As agricultural surpluses disappeared and the world food crisis became apparent, consumers began to reexamine their buying practices and to look for alternatives for scarce and expensive foods. Although there is still a tremendous variety of foods available in supermarkets, increased prices make the selection of food for the family a real challenge.

The homemaker who has little or no concept of nutritional value bases choices on cost and on cultural and family preferences. If the food budget is unlimited so are the choices; but the homemaker who must stay within a limited budget especially needs information about nutritive values as they relate to the cost per serving of individual food items. Consumerism is rapidly developing in the United States and consumer groups are active in demanding greater honesty in the marketplace. Nutrition labeling and unit pricing are examples of recent programs introduced to assist the consumer. The nutrition counselor should help the homemaker take advantage of this information provided in the marketplace to make wise food selections.

SOCIAL FACTORS. If one recognizes that individuals belong to various social groups, the effect of group behavior cannot be overlooked when considering factors that influence food habits. The organization of society, with its many structures and accompanying value systems, plays an important part in the acceptance or rejection of food patterns.

The social groups to which one belongs—club, church, union, or fraternal organization—often have meals together, and the menus are apt to reflect the tastes of the group. For instance, union members, such as those who work in heavy industry, may be used to hearty but simple meals, either at home or in groups. On the other hand, an upper middle class club may be used to exotic foods and delicacies quite unfamiliar to the first group.

If people accept obesity or overweight as natural—in women as the accompaniment of maturity and in men as a sign of strength—it will be difficult for the nutrition counselor to persuade them to change their eating habits to accomplish weight loss. By contrast a business executive or professional person, warned of the health hazard of excess weight and too little exercise, will often seek advice and be motivated to follow it. Although socially people in such occupations may be exposed to too much or too rich food on occasion, they are able to exert self-control and to avoid overeating.

PSYCHOLOGICAL FACTORS. Food habits are an important part of human behavior. Individuals are motivated to act in terms of what they perceive as being relevant to meet their needs. Maslow[1] has defined a hierarchy of five levels of human need: (1) basic physiologic survival, (2) security, (3) belongingness, (4) self-esteem, and (5) self-actualization. Since minimum satisfaction of each level of need must be met before an individual seeks satisfaction at the next level, a thorough understanding of the person is necessary to determine effective motivation. Weight reduction for the purpose of improving self-esteem will probably not motivate the unemployed father of a large family when he is primarily concerned with his and his family's survival. Self-esteem, however, may be the motivating force for the mature woman returning to a career.

Assuming that the individual has been motivated, his or her ability to change behavior, namely food habits, will be affected by knowledge, or cognition. In this case he must have the information to select appropriate kinds and amounts of food. Thus, although a knowledge of nutrition is indispensable in affecting the desired change, information itself is useless unless the individual has accepted the need for change and is motivated to act accordingly. (See Chapter 12.)

FOOD PATTERNS IN AMERICA

Before discussing specific food patterns, it is important to consider some factors which have influenced American eating habits in general. The large number of persons of different national backgrounds living together in urban areas have made tamales, frankfurters, pizza, chow mein, sukiyaki, and many other dishes of foreign origin as American as apple pie. Just as it is difficult to define the typical American in terms of national origin, color, religion, or local region, it is equally difficult to define the "typical" American food pattern. As each national group brought its native food habits to this country and adapted them to available foods, they also dispersed them to their neighbors.

Also, because this country stretches across an entire continent, it has a variety of geographic conditions that have resulted in relatively varied regional food patterns. Fish, an important source of protein in coastal regions, is less widely used as one moves away from the sea. Soft wheat, indigenous to the South, which makes good "hot breads" but poor yeast breads, has determined regional food preferences that cannot be changed easily.

When large numbers of people of similar national origins or ethnic backgrounds settle in their own communities, they tend to be less influenced by the food habits of indigenous groups or of other cultural groups. Because of the demand for foods they are used to, their own retail stores evolve, such as the German delicatessen, the Italian fruit and vegetable market, the Chinese restaurant, and the Kosher meat market.

It may also be noted that transplanted people usually arrive poor and that it may take several generations before opportunities are available for them to achieve "middle class status." In the meantime, the frugality necessary to stretch the food dollar may develop food habits which are retained even after economic reasons for them have disappeared. French and Chinese cuisines were evolved not from unlimited food resources but rather from a set of restrictions growing out of geographic, economic, and social factors; as someone once noted, these two great national cuisines were indeed based on poverty. The evolution of "soul food" from the black culture has some of the same characteristics today.

No story of American food practices, however, is complete without mentioning the highly developed food technology which makes all foods, in a variety of forms, available in all parts of the country during all seasons of the year. Hence, the choice available to the American public is infinite, even though the individual's selection may normally derive from cultural practices.

Also, mention must be made of the effect of mass media advertising on the changing food habits of the American family. Young children especially are besieged by television commercials that advertise not only a food item but also "prizes" included in the package. Certain display techniques are used in retail stores to entice the shopper to buy an item or select a brand on the spur of the moment. Such impulse buying can increase the cost of the family's food and may at the same time reduce its nutritive value.

Mention must also be made of the increased use of alcoholic beverages and drugs among certain groups of Americans today. The high cost of such items and the physiological consequences to the people who use them excessively are well known. In cases of true alcoholism and drug addiction the appetite is reduced or perverted and cases of frank malnutrition often result.

Regional Food Patterns in the United States

Anyone who has traveled in different parts of the United States and has eaten meals typical of various regions is aware of differences in menus, food preparation, and local terms for foods or special dishes. Part of the joy of travel is in eating the traditional foods of each locality. However, national advertising in magazines and on TV has tended to popularize certain foods so that diets are not as regional in character as they once were.

People who are ill are much more likely to want familiar foods cooked in a traditional manner with familiar seasoning. Therefore, the nutrition counselor should recognize the existence of regional differences and make some adjustments in the diet so as to provide essential nutrients from familiar foods.

IN THE SOUTH, hot breads are served at nearly every meal, and baker's yeast breads are not popular. Corn and rice are common sources of carbohydrates. There is a preference for vegetables that have been cooked a long time and often with fatback. Undoubtedly some vitamins are destroyed by this process, but the common use of pot liquor conserves the nutrients which are in solution. The wide variety of greens used compensates in a measure for the low consumption of milk and cheese as sources of calcium and vitamins. The scarcity of fresh milk and refrigeration in some localitites has encouraged the use of evaporated and dry milk. Buttermilk is liked and is used when available. Because many black Americans, now living elsewhere, came from the South, their food customs reflect some of the practices of this region, as discussed later in the chapter.

IN THE SOUTHWEST, the Mexican influence is shown in the use of beans and highly seasoned dishes. Again, milk production is limited, and, while drinking fresh milk was not the custom originally, it is being introduced gradually. Mexican foods such as tortillas, tamales, enchiladas, and a wide variety of beans are popular in American homes of the Southwest as well as in Mexican families. More details of Mexican foods are given later in this chapter.

IN THE FAR WEST, the infiltration of Oriental cultures has influenced food habits. The use of a wide variety of garden produce and locally grown citrus fruits, the short-time cooking of vegetables typical of oriental cooking, and the serving of generous salads as the first course are features to be commended.

IN THE NORTH CENTRAL STATES, there is a mixed cultural background with a strong northern European and Scandinavian heritage in many localities. Homes still maintain characteristic native dishes, perhaps modified by the choice of regional ingredients. Many of these states produce and use large quantities of dairy products, especially cheeses of several varieties closely resembling European types. The so-called typical American diet is really an adaptation of much of the northern European food pattern. This is only natural since climatic conditions and crops are similar. Locally grown fruits and vegetables are used in season and preserved for winter use. This is a good custom and should be encouraged.

ON THE EAST COAST AND IN NEW ENGLAND, many traditional dishes have come down from the Pilgrim settlers. The practice of using cornmeal in Indian pudding and johnnycake was acquired from the Indians by their new neighbors. Baked beans, codfish cakes, clam or fish chowder, and turkey for festive occasions are all old New England traditions, some of which have been adopted nationally. A smaller variety of green, leafy vegetables is used in New England than in many other areas, but yellow vegetables, such as squash, turnips, and carrots, are popular.

IN ISOLATED COMMUNITIES in any part of the country, unusual food habits may be encountered. Malnutrition may result from a limited variety of foods grown locally, especially if the economic status prohibits extensive use of foods from other producing areas. Sporadic outbreaks of actual deficiency diseases have been reported occasionally. National attention has been called to such problems in Appalachia, on Indian Reservations, and among the Eskimos in Alaska. State and federal agencies are recognizing their responsibilities for these conditions quite as much as for the control of communicable disease.

IN METROPOLITAN AREAS a great variety of food patterns may be found. In large cities, there may be whole sections in which the inhabitants follow as closely as possible the food customs of the country of their origin. This influence is retained to some extent by the second generation. People who come to the city from regions of the United States where there are definite preferences for certain types of foods attempt to continue following the diet to which they have been accustomed. Usually they can be persuaded to supplement their meals with foods that are more generally available in the city than in the part of the country where their food habits were established.

Cultural Food Patterns

AMERICAN INDIAN FOOD. Over 50 percent of our present food plants originated with the Indians of South, Central, and North America. These include corn, potatoes, tomatoes, peppers, squash, pumpkins, beans, cranberries, wild rice, groundnuts, and cocoa.

The Indians also consumed a variety of wild fruits, herbs, maple sugar, small and large game, sheep and goats, wild fowl, fish, and other seafoods. The food patterns and feeding practices of various tribes differed according to their geographic location, their occupations (whether they were hunters, shepherds, fisherman, or settled agricultural groups), and their particular historical experience. "Feast or famine" is an expression which can be used to describe the quality of their early experience because they depended primarily on what was immediately available and had little provision for storing food. There are accounts of Indians fasting and gorging; however, on the whole the traditional Indian diet was probably more nutritionally adequate than many of their diets are today. Just as the trading posts introduced new items such as tea, coffee, sugar, lard, flour, and tinned milk and meat to the Indians, so did the European settlers adopt many of the Indian foods. Corn is an outstanding example of a crop developed by the American Indians and adopted and transplanted around the world by European adventurers.[2]

The Indians used open-fire cooking for their game and fish and the clambake, an Indian invention, is still popular in New England. Because of extensive food acculturation, it is difficult today to identify a typical Indian food pattern; however, dietary customs have persisted so that not only are traditional foods prepared but they are also preferred. Many of the traditional foods retain their religious and ceremonial significance and are featured on feast days. There is great interest in reviving the traditional foods and methods of preparation as part of a cultural reawakening and a desire to understand and appreciate the Indian heritage.

Since the native Indian foods are for the most part higher in nutritive value than those adopted from the European culture, it is to the nutritional advantage of the Indians to encourage the use of their traditional foods. The increased buying of expensive foods, such as soft drinks, sweets, cakes, potato chips, and crackers takes a great deal of the limited food budget of the Indians and contributes little but calories to their diets.

Soups and stews made with game or other meat and vegetables are usually well liked by Indians. They may be served with bread, especially the Indian "fry bread" (biscuit dough fried in deep fat) or cornbread. Wasna, a native dish, consists of dry berries, powdered dried meat, fat, and sugar. Fruits and vegetables which provide a source of vitamins A and C should also be encouraged rather than highly processed expensive snack foods. Wajupi is a traditional fruit pudding made from berries, sugar, and cornstarch. The practice of breast-feeding infants is a good one and should receive support from the nutrition counselor. The use of milk in children's diets after weaning rather than the carbonated beverages so popular with Indian children would be a good food habit to encourage.

Nutrition surveys on various tribes indicate mild to marked deficiencies in a number of specific nutrients. Intake of calories, calcium, riboflavin, and vitamins A and C were frequently below recommended amounts. The growth of children in all the surveys was below the norms for North American children.[3] Infant mortality rates are three times that of the general population. The incidence of disease, especially tuberculosis, still is high.[4]

THE BLACK EXPERIENCE. The food habits of the black American reflect the region of the country from which he comes. Southern blacks have the same distinctive food habits that are typical of the rest of the population in the same geographic locale. The northern black may evidence little identification with the regional patterns of the South, or on the other hand, he may have adapted many of these in his present environment. This fact was made exceptionally clear to one of the authors when planning menus with a group of paraprofessionals in a preschool center in the North. In developing a feeding program which would be supportive of the cultural backgrounds of black children, many of the "soul food" items planned and prepared by staff were new and strange to many northern blacks and whites alike, although completely familiar to blacks and whites with considerable experience of the South.

With many exceptions, the following represents what, in general, might be considered the black experience in food customs. Breakfast patterns are similar to the breakfasts of many other groups except for the very frequent use of grits in some form. If eggs and bacon, or another form of pork, are available, they are served with the grits. Hot breads, biscuits, muffins, and cornbread take the place of yeast bread at most meals.

The family usually has one main meal at a time that is determined by the activities of the family members. Greens—mustard, turnip, collard, and kale—cooked in a pot liquor with some form of pork such as fatback, salt pork, or "streak of lean," are popular. Although fresh greens are used in the South, a wide variety of frozen greens are available in northern markets. Cornbread is traditionally served with greens. Sweet potatoes, squash, lima beans, snap beans, fresh corn, and cabbage are also popular vegetables. Sweet potatoes and squash are often used in pies as the New Englander uses pumpkins. Fruits,

such as oranges, watermelon, and peaches are enjoyed when available.

Grits, rice, or potatoes provide the chief source of carbohydrate, while black-eyed peas and other dried beans may be used and contribute both carbohydrate and protein. Fried fish of all kinds, particularly that caught by members of the family in streams and lakes, are considered most acceptable. Poultry, cured and fresh pork, and some wild game, such as rabbit, woodchuck, and pheasant, are served when available. Use of meats high in bone or connective tissue with little lean tissue such as pig's ears, tails, feet, and chin bone, oxtails, neckbones, spareribs, hog maws (stomach), and chitterlings (intestines) is frequent. Frying, barbecuing, and stewing are the most popular methods of preparation even when an oven is available. Milk, milk products, and cheese are not used extensively; buttermilk, evaporated milk, and ice cream are the preferred forms. Sweets—particularly molasses, other syrups, cakes, pastries, and candy—are consumed in large quantity. Sweetened, flavored drinks often take the place of fruit juice and milk as a beverage.

"Soul food," a descriptive term for many of these dishes, connotes special feelings and emotions. It is the spirit of the provider or cook which creates an atmosphere of love and well-being for those who are to be fed. There is also the implication that from limited food resources, much happiness and enjoyment can be achieved by giving special care to the preparation of food.

Since large amounts of fat and carbohydrate are consumed, adequate or more than adequate calories are, as a rule, provided. Because relatively small amounts of meat, milk, and fish may be available the protein content of the diet of a poor southern black family is often limited. Minerals, iron, and calcium have been found inadequate in many southern black dietaries, as have vitamins A and C.[5]

DIETARY HABITS OF MEXICANS AND OTHER LATIN AMERICANS. The Mexicans freely use many varieties of beans, especially the pinto, as well as rice, potatoes, peas, and some vegetables. Chili, a variety of pepper, is also popular. The chili plant is sacred to the Mexican, who is supposed to be blessed in health if he uses it plentifully. The tomato is always prominent in Mexican cookery. Mexicans use little meat and practically always cook it with vegetables. They have a strong aversion to meat that is not perfectly fresh and slaughtered in the approved Mexican style. Chili con carne is a favorite meat dish. It consists of beef seasoned with garlic and chili peppers and cooked several hours. Tamales are also popular. They are made of corn meal and ground pork, highly seasoned, and are rolled in corn husks and steamed. Tortillas, made with ground whole corn which has been soaked in lime water and baked on a griddle, serve as a bread. Enchiladas, another favorite, are made by filling tortillas with cheese, onion and shredded lettuce. Tacos, a similar dish, is prepared by adding meat and a sauce to the tortilla. Thus some calcium is provided in tortillas and in beans in a diet which includes very little milk or cheese. The use of milk for the children should be encouraged when and if a change to the American type of bread is made. Vitamin A deficiency has been reported as the most prevalent nutritional problem among Mexican-American children.[6]

The influx of Cuban refugees into our southern states creates a need for the nutrition counselor to recognize and adjust nutrition advice and special diets to Cuban preferences. Their food pattern is similar to that of other West Indian groups where the Spanish influence predominates.

It is notable, however, that many of the more prosperous eastern South American peoples have a meat and milk consumption as high or higher than the United States. Spanish and Portuguese influences are evident in the liberal use of peppers and spices.

On the west coast of South America the situation is quite different. A few cities are prosperous, but agriculture is handicapped by desert, mountains, and jungles. The native Indian populations of the Andes in Ecuador, Peru, and Chile are short of food and especially of adequate sources of protein.

PUERTO RICAN DIETARY HABITS. The dietary pattern in Puerto Rico is similar to that of other Caribbean Islands and some Latin American countries. From the extensive work of Dr. Lydia Roberts in Puerto Rico, information is available on a typical moderate cost food supply for an adult for one day (Table 13-1). The nutrient value comes close to meeting the U. S. recommended allowances.

When Puerto Ricans migrate to the United States, as they have in great numbers, they may modify this pattern considerably according to what is available and what they can afford.

Rice, beans, and viandas (starchy root vegetables and plantains) are the staple foods, used daily. Salt codfish is used more often than fresh fish and is served with viandas, oil, and vinegar. Chicken, pork, and beef are favorite meats and are used when there is money to purchase them. Tomatoes, peppers, onions, garlic, salt pork, and seasonings (sofrito), cooked with different varieties of dried peas and beans, is a common dish. Bananas, oranges, and pineapple are popular and relatively inexpensive in Puerto Rico. Even more important are some of the native fruits which are not familiar in the North, such as mango, papaya, and the West Indian cherry, or acerola, which is now

Table 13–1. Moderate Cost Food for a Day for a Puerto Rican Adult*

FOOD	AMOUNT OF EDIBLE PORTION	WEIGHT (g.)
Rice	3 cups cooked	668
Plantain or root veg	1 serving	200
Bean, broad, kidney, or other type	1 cup	256
Onion	1 medium	110
Eggplant	1 small	100
Green Pepper	2 small	100
Tomato	1 medium	100
Mango	1 medium	200
Banana	2 medium	300
Salt Codfish	1 oz. dry	30
Goat's Milk	1 cup	244
Lard	½ cup	50
Olive Oil	2 tbsp.	28

The value of this diet is approximately:

Energy	2,506 kcal.	Vitamin A	33,500 IU
Protein	69 g.	Thiamine	1.0 mg.
Fat	77 g.	Riboflavin	1.0 mg.
Calcium	0.6 g.	Niacin	13.3 mg.
Iron	12.5 mg.	Vitamin C	195 mg.

*Adapted from information provided by Dr. Lydia Roberts, formerly of University of Puerto Rico, and Miss Ethel Robinson, formerly a teacher in rural Puerto Rico.

recognized as the richest known natural source of ascorbic acid.

Milk is not popular as a beverage except perhaps, when income permits, as café con leche, a combination of coffee and hot milk. Sweetened cocoa and chocolate made with milk are also consumed occasionally.

Puerto Ricans living in northern United States may have to adjust to different fruits in season and to canned fruits. They may well be encouraged to use more milk and cheese, and cheaper cuts of meat, to supplement the protein at meals when rice and beans are served. Acceptance of canned tomatoes in place of more expensive fresh ones out of season, margarine in place of butter, and cheaper cuts of meat would provide better nutrition for less cost.

Puerto Ricans in New York City and other urban areas are often among the lower economic groups because, having come from a more rural culture, many of them are unskilled laborers. Their poor and crowded housing may provide inadequate cooking and refrigeration facilities. Thus, they may be unable to provide their families with food as good as they had at home. Malnutrition, rickets, and tuberculosis are not uncommon among Puerto Rican children living under such conditions. The nutrition counselor can offer suggestions as to how they can improve nutrition within their budgets.

ITALIAN DIETARY HABITS. Italian-Americans, few of them today born in Italy, have adopted many food customs of the United States. Likewise, the popularity of Italian spaghetti and pizza in this country testifies to the influence that Italian food customs have had on Americans. Italians here continue to use pastas in a great variety of shapes and with many different sauces and cheeses. Similarly, bread is still an essential part of an Italian meal, although crusty white bread is now more popular than the dark breads that were a former standby.

Southern Italians may use more fish and highly seasoned foods, while northern Italians use more root vegetables and more meat. The liberal use of eggs, cheese, tomatoes, green vegetables, and fruits in the Italian cuisine is to be commended. More milk and meat might be used, both of which are popular. In general, northern Italians have better food habits than those from the south.

Italians have a strong sense of individuality. We may think of spaghetti as a typically Italian food, but not all Italians like spaghetti. They dislike foods that are not prepared to their particular tastes. They are particularly sensitive to the lack of close family ties in a hospital and therefore dread hospitalization more than one may suspect. Most Italians eat a very light breakfast: black coffee for adults and milk for children, with perhaps bread without butter. Some like the main meal at noon, others at night, but bread and cheese with coffee or wine are an acceptable light meal.

WESTERN EUROPEAN AND SCANDINAVIAN DIETARY HABITS. Most western European peoples, including Scandinavians, have food patterns not unlike those of northeastern and central North America where immigrants from these areas have settled during the past two centuries. Many American food customs of today have been derived from these countries. The lists of meats, vegetables, fruits, and grain products used by them would be a mere recital of those in our markets. To be sure, they make more frequent use of dark breads, potatoes, fish, and cheese than native Americans do. For western Europeans the differences in culinary methods, seasonings, and attitudes toward food are never serious hurdles in adjusting to American food patterns.

CENTRAL EUROPEAN DIETARY HABITS. In many of the central European countries grains and potatoes provide 60 to 70 percent of the total calories for the rural and the lower income groups. Rye and buckwheat are used, as well as wheat, for their breads. Pork and pork products, including highly seasoned sausages, are popular. Cabbage may be used raw, cooked, or as sauerkraut, and other vegetables—onions, turnips, peppers, carrots, beans, squash, and greens—are often cooked with small amounts of meat. Eggs, fresh milk, sour cream and yogurt (called by a different name in each country), cottage cheese, and other cheeses are widely used. Central Europeans bring with them many good food habits which are to be encouraged.

DIETARY HABITS OF THE MIDDLE EAST—LEBANESE, ARMENIAN, TURKISH, GREEK, AND SYRIAN. The inhabitants of the Middle East are outdoor people. Many of them are farmers: they raise their own sheep, goats, cattle, chickens, ducks, and geese; they produce their own grains and grow fruits and vegetables in abundance, wherever water is plentiful. Grains, rice or wheat, furnish the major source of energy. The whole wheat is parboiled and cracked for use as a staple starchy food at the main meal. Eggs, butter, and cheese are also produced on the farm. Lamb is the favorite meat. The food is not highly spiced but is rich in fat. The fat is cooked with the food and this takes the place of butter. Matzoon, leben, or yogurt, a sour-milk preparation, is used almost universally by these people; sweet milk is seldom used. Black coffee, heavily sweetened, in which the pulverized bean is retained—often called Turkish coffee—is the preferred beverage in many countries of the Middle East.

CHINESE DIETARY HABITS. The Chinese diet is varied, consisting of eggs, meat, fish, cereals, and a large variety of vegetables. Many plants and weeds, such as radish leaves and shepherd's purse, are used, as well as various sprouts (bean, bamboo, etc.). None of these vegetables is ever overcooked, and no cooking water is discarded; thus, nutrients are well retained. The soybean is abundant, and some 30 or more products are manufactured from it. The protein content is high and of good quality for a vegetable protein.

Rice is used freely and takes the place of American bread, particularly in southern China. In northern China, wheat, corn, and millet seed are used in abundance. The millet seed (ground or whole) is made into cakes or a thin mush, the latter being the form in which it is given to children. Noodles are widely used. Grains and, in some areas, sweet potatoes constitute the chief source of calories in the Chinese diet; grain and potato together provide from 70 to 90 percent of the total calories.

The quantity of meat eaten is small, and usually it is served with vegetables. All ingredients are cut into small pieces in conformity with an ancient law laid down by Confucius, the philosopher, specifying that food should not be eaten unless first chopped or cut into small pieces. Pork is the chief meat of the poorer classes. Lamb and goat meat and other animal foods are used when available, but beef is uncommon.

In certain parts of China, a child rarely tastes cow's milk, but water-buffalo milk is used to some extent.

Soybean milk and cheese are more common. In this country, the Chinese readily accept the use of diary products for children and adults.

The Chinese use practically every part of the animal as food (with the exception of the hair and the bones); the brain, the spinal cord, and the various internal organs, as well as the skin and the blood, are utilized. Coagulated blood is sold in the market in pieces similar to liver, and since this is one of the inexpensive foods, it is used frequently. Fish and shellfish are also in common use. They are sold alive, for the Chinese have a strong aversion to dead fish and consider them unfit for food.

Eggs, including hen, duck, and pigeon eggs, are used in abundance, when they can be afforded. The Chinese prepare what are known as fermented eggs, much relished by them, as well as other types of "preserved" eggs, which are eaten much as we in this country eat sweets.

Soy sauce, highly flavored and salted, is a frequent accompaniment to meals. It may present problems to the Chinese patient who must omit salt from his diet. This is true also of the Japanese diet.

JAPANESE DIETARY HABITS. During the past 20 years there have been spectacular changes in Japanese food habits, influenced by Western culture. Typical diets formerly included rice, bean paste soup, bean curd, vegetables and fruit, raw or cooked fish, and pickles. Now the trend is to bread as well as rice, milk, cheese, meat, and eggs. Instant foods and frozen items are available. Seafoods are served raw, smoked, fried, and, recently, as fish sausage. Japanese make a whole meal of wheat or buckwheat noodles cooked in broth and garnished with a few bits of vegetables and fish sausage and served with salty pickles. Although they are traditional tea drinkers, many of them now prefer coffee, and they like to drink milk when it is available. Many kinds of crisp salty snack foods made from rice or wheat flour, seaweed and other delicacies are popular. A Japanese or Chinese meal is complete without dessert, but at New Year's and other holidays the Japanese relish their "decoration cakes." Even the simplest one-dish meal is attractively served, and an elaborate party meal, served in 10 or 12 separate and colorful dishes of different shapes, is truly a work of art.

Religious Food Patterns

JEWISH DIETARY HABITS AND LAWS. In the United States today Jewish families differ in food habits according to whether they belong to Orthodox, Conservative, or Reform groups. Food habits may also be influenced by the country from which they or their forefathers came, as well as by Biblical and rabbinical regulations, known as the Jewish dietary laws.

According to Kaufman:

Variations in observance are due largely to differences in interpretation and importance placed on dietary laws by the three schools of thought among American Jews today. Orthodox Jews still place great value on traditional and ceremonial practices of their religion, and observe the dietary laws under all conditions. Reform Jews place much less emphasis on rules which they consider to be purely ceremonial and tend to minimize the significance of the dietary laws. Conservative Jews stand between these two groups and, while nominally adhering to dietary laws, sometimes draw the distinction between the observance of the rules in the home and outside.

Regulations include selection, preparation and service of the foods involved. The Bible gives no reason for these rules, but observant Jews feel that the rules known as Kashruth and hallowed since the time of Moses, are a positive means of self-purification and of service to their God. Although many hygienic and ethical bases have been alleged for these rules, the spiritual factors of sanctification and self-discipline are the primary motivations for those who adhere to them.[7]

Miss Kaufman also gives some definitions of Jewish terms and special foods.

A brief outline of some of the specific rules to which the Orthodox Jews conform follows:

Foods Allowed or Prohibited. Meats and Poultry. Quadrupeds with the cloven hoof that chew a cud are allowed. These include cows, sheep, goats and deer. Pork in all forms including lard and bacon is prohibited. The poultry allowed includes chicken, turkey, goose, pheasant and duck. All meats and poultry must be freshly slaughtered according to prescribed ritual and soaked in salted water to remove all trace of blood. This process is known as koshering (meaning clean), and many Jewish markets sell koshered meat and poultry. Prescribed methods of preparing meats and other foods are given in most Jewish cookbooks.
Fish. The fish prescribed in the Bible are those with fins and scales. Thus all shellfish and eels are excluded.

Food Combinations Allowed or Prohibited. The command "Thou shalt not seethe a kid in its mother's milk," repeated several times in Exodus and Deuteronomy, is the basis for never combining meat and milk in the same meal, or even cooking them in the same utensils. Eggs, fruits, vegetables, cereals and all other foods may be used without restricitions.

A striking characteristic of the Jewish diet is the richness of the food, including pastries and cakes, foods rich in fats, and preserves and conserves, as well as stewed and canned fruits. Butter, a product of milk, must not be served with meat. Most vegetables therefore are cooked with the meat. Cooked vegetables are most often served in soup. Borscht, a soup made with "sour salt" (tartaric acid) and vegetables to which sour cream is added, is a favorite dish but is not served with the meat meal. Cereals, especially barley and millet, are frequently served as a vegetable with meat or in soup.

Noodles and other egg-and-flour mixtures are used extensively as are crusty rolls.

Dried fruits, as well as fresh fruits, are popular.

Fish is served frequently, especially cod, haddock, carp, salmon, and whitefish, smoked and salted fishes—herring, salmon, and sturgeon. Gefüllte fish is a delicacy prepared in almost all Jewish homes. Chicken is considered almost an essential for the Sabbath evening meal.

Because milk in any form cannot be served with meat at the same meal, the diet of children in Jewish families that rigidly observe the dietary laws may lack the proper amount of milk. The use of more green vegetables and canned vegetables and fresh and canned fruits for the whole family, and more milk for the children should be stressed. The continued use of rye bread, legumes, coarse cereals, dried fruits, and a variety of fish which are characteristic of the Jewish diet is advantageous.

Dietary laws for the Jewish Sabbath and religious holidays are often observed by even the less orthodox groups and therefore merit comment.

Sabbath: No food may be cooked on the Sabbath. This means that all cooking for both Friday and Saturday is done on Friday. This need has led to the development of foods such as Sabbath Kugel or Sholend, Petshai, and many others.

Passover: During Passover week no leavened bread, or its product, or anything which may have touched leavened bread, may be eaten. A complete new set of dishes is used during the week. Cutlery, silver, or metal pots may be used during this holiday if properly koshered or sterilized. In actual practice this means that in every orthodox Jewish household there are four sets of dishes—the usual sets for meat and for milk foods, in addition to duplicate Passover sets.

Fast Days: Yom Kippur (the Day of Atonement); no food or drink may be taken for 24 hours. Fast of Esther: this precedes the Feast of Purim and is now observed only by the very pious. The Feast of Purim is universally observed.

ROMAN CATHOLIC. Because the Pope liberalized the dietary restrictions and fast days, customs may vary in different localities. It is well to conform to local custom with regard to foods allowed on fast days and days of abstinence.

GREEK ORTHODOX. The Orthodox laws have not changed in recent years but are interpreted somewhat more liberally. The use of meat, fish, poultry, eggs, and dairy products is still restricted on Fridays and certain Wednesdays and during the first and last weeks of the Greek Orthodox Lent.

SEVENTH DAY ADVENTISTS. Adventists in general are ovo-lacto-vegetarians; thus, they allow the use of eggs, milk and cheese as good sources of animal protein but they eat no meat, fish, or poultry. They also use nuts and legumes as sources of protein.

LATTER-DAY SAINTS. The Mormons make no food restrictions but prohibit the use of alcohol, tobacco, tea and coffee.

Understanding and Using Food Patterns

Characteristic food habits of every regional, cultural, or religious group should be respected; there are good nutritional practices in each of them and nutritional needs may be met by many different patterns of eating. Emphasis should be placed on the desirable features of the established food pattern and on methods of preparation that preserve maximum food values. Although choice of foods and methods of preparation may differ from those to which we are accustomed, it often happens that the foods used fall into the Four Food Groups and provide nutrients that meet recommended allowances.

Unfamiliar foods and methods of preparation need to be studied and possible values recognized before changes are suggested. A family may be encouraged to continue its own methods of preparation and seasoning when these are not incompatible with health, and then may gradually be helped to institute necessary changes to correct any poor practices, if these exist.

Therapeutic diets should be interpreted for the patient or the homemaker in terms of the regional, cultural, or religious food pattern. A woman of foreign birth or one from a different part of the country may have little contact outside her home and little opportunity to learn how to use foods that are new to her. The marked improvements in homes where the mother has had the opportunity to learn to adjust to local foods and customs show that instruction, as well as understanding, is an important phase of nutrition work.

In this chapter special attention is given to regional, cultural, and religious food patterns which are distinctive. A knowledge of these food preferences and attention to them may help to build the bridge of understanding between the nutrition counselor and the family in need of assistance.

Unusual Dietary Practices

More and more young American adults have adopted unusual dietary practices which are of particular concern to the nutrition counselor. Some of the more popular of these patterns will be discussed in this section.

"NATURAL" FOODS. So-called "natural" foods have become especially popular in recent years. Natural food enthusiasts use raw sugar or honey in place of refined sugar, or sea salt in place of table salt, and do not realize that the trace minerals which may be present in the impurities of such natural products are widely available in most foods. The use of olive oil in place of other fats or stone ground wheat instead of whole wheat may be taste preferences but have little nutritional significance. The question of the safety of raw milk has increased the demand for certified unpasteurized milk. This is costly and there is no absolute assurance as to its safety.

Certain vegetable juices have been credited with virtues they do not possess, such as celery juice as a treatment for rheumatism and garlic juice for high blood pressure. Juices, extracted from vegetables or fruits, have essentially similar nutritive values as the original product except for the cellulose. There is no evidence that certain vegetables or their juices have special curative properties other than as sources of nutrients.

Although it must be admitted that the number and variety of processed foods now available is often confusing, the prejudice expressed against processed foods is quite unwarranted. In general, processing is for the purpose of improving preservation, flavor, texture, nutritive value, or convenience in preparation. Seldom does such processing significantly reduce nutritive value. Moreover, as recently reported, many of the so-called natural vitamin preparations do have synthetic chemicals added. Rose hip vitamin C tablets are made from natural rose hips plus the same chemical ascorbic acid used in standard vitamin preparations; synthetic B vitamins are added to the yeast and other natural bases; and chemical solvents are used for the extraction and separation of the vegetable oils used for vitamin E preparations.[8] There is no legal definition for these "natural" products since the vitamins themselves are identical but the product may cost the consumer more. Thus, labels should be carefully read.

"ORGANIC" FOODS. The craze for "organic" foods has reached such a point that even wayside markets are advertising food grown "organically." This means that crops are grown without chemical fertilizers or pesticides and processed without the use of food chemicals or additives. People seldom realize that all organic material—compost, manure—used in growing foods "organically" must be broken down to inorganic elements before plants can absorb nutrients from the soil. Scientific tests have shown that such foods show no significant difference in nutritive value from those grown with commercial fertilizers. Salmonella contamination can result from the use of organic farming techniques.

Pesticides aid in the production of good quality foods and of increased yields, thus making larger quantities of products ever more widely available to our growing population. The use of pesticides to prevent destruction of crops by infestations of fungi, microorganisms, or insects is carefully monitored and pesticide levels well below international standards for acceptable daily intake, ADI, are reported.

Meat is considered organically grown when produced from animals raised without antibiotics or hormones and dressed without the use of chemicals. People should be aware that our regular market meats are inspected regularly; also, the constant vigilance of law-enforcing agencies regulates the use of all additives and medical agents to be sure that they are within safe limits.

The whole cult of "natural" and "organic" foods has puzzled scientific nutritionists for years, because all the evidence points to the fact that fertilizers and pesticides increase yield and that plant genetics determine the color, flavor, and nutritive value of the crop.

According to an article that appeared in the New York Times, the FDA takes the following position concerning "organic" foods:

> Organic or natural foods are not considered to be significantly different from other foods, in terms of their nutritional qualities. The FDA feels that if you want them and can afford them, they're there in the marketplace for you to buy. But they must be labeled in a manner that's neither false or misleading, and no attempt can be made in promoting these foods to suggest that they offer special health benefits. There's just no evidence to show that people living on organic or natural foods will be protected from chronic disease problems, or that they can expect better

health. Nevertheless, the interested and alert consumer can get good and nutritious food either from the so-called organic food store or the modern supermarket. The choice is and should remain open to the individual. But the main point is that we cannot hope to feed today's population with yesterday's production methods. We must use the technical advances that science and chemistry have given us if we hope to produce and preserve enough food to meet today's requirements.

The cost for organically grown groceries may be 30 percent to 100 percent more than for their nonorganic counterparts.[9]

MACROBIOTIC DIET. This diet is an outgrowth of an interpretation of Zen Buddhism introduced into the United States and Europe from Japan by Ohsawa. According to the macrobiotic system there are 10 diet plans (Diet No. -3—10% cereal, 30% vegetables, 10% soup, 30% animal products, 15% salads and fruits, and 5% desserts, to Diet No. 7—100% cereal) which may be followed to establish a healthy and happy life. In progressing from Diet No. -3 to Diet No. 7, one gradually gives up in the following order: desserts, salads and fruits, animal foods, soups, and, finally, vegetables, at the same time increasing the amount of cereal grains to be consumed. There is no scientific basis for the restrictions or recommendations of the macrobiotic system. Part of the plan for all the diets is the consumption of as little beverage as possible. Only "organically" produced fresh vegetables, fruits, or animal products are used. Foods are classified into Yang (the male principle) or Yin (the female principle), and a 5:1 balance between these is considered to be important. Because sweets and many fruits are Yin foods, the amount of these in the macrobiotic diet is small.

Most of the diet plans are low in ascorbic acid. Diet No. 7 (in which whole grain cereal, usually brown rice, is the only food consumed) is grossly inadeqate in many of the essential minerals and vitamins, as well as in good quality protein. Fortunately, not too many follow No. 7 diet plan for very long. Another danger in the macrobiotic concept is that, since the various diet plans promise to cure the body of disease and purge it of all poisons, adequate medical care may be postponed when it is needed. The American Medical Association has warned of the hazards of following this regimen.[10]

Because it is possible to have an adequate intake of nutrients on certain macrobiotic diet plans, emphasis should be placed on essential nutrients in maintaining health and well-being, and followers of this system should be counselled to select their macrobiotic foods in keeping with this principle of good nutrition. One must work within the value system or philosophy of these groups if change is to be expected. The "Hip Health Handbook" is a resource for workers in this field.[11]

VEGETARIAN DIETS. Vegetarian diets are not new. They have been followed throughout history by various groups. The Seventh Day Adventists and the Trappist monks subscribe to vegetarianism on the basis of religion. In the nineteenth century the Utopian groups advocated this dietary pattern. Among their followers were the breakfast cereal manufacturers, W.K. Kellogg and C.W. Post. Today many young people are adopting, for health, ecological, or philosophical reasons, one type of vegetarian diet or another. The practice in some instances is a belief or regulation of quasi-religious or cultist groups. Some of these groups are also natural or organic food followers or adherents of the Zen-Macrobiotic diet.[12]

Vegetarian diets usually include vegetables, fruits, cereals and breads, often whole grain, yeast, dry beans, peas and lentils, nuts and peanut butter, seeds, vegetable oils, sugars and syrups. They may also include more unusual types of food such as seaweed and bean curd, and some may permit certain animal products.

Vegans, or the **strict vegetarians,** avoid all food of animal origin including meat, poultry, fish, eggs, and dairy products such as milk, ice cream, and cheese.

Lacto-vegetarians eat dairy products but not meat, poultry, fish, or eggs.

Ovo-lacto-vegetarians include eggs and dairy products in their diets while excluding meat, poultry, and fish.

Since vitamin B_{12} is known to occur naturally only in foods of animal origin, a person following strict vegetarianism should use cereals fortified with vitamin B_{12} or a vitamin preparation which includes it. Because the chief source of calcium in our diet is milk, vegans who exclude milk products need to include daily relatively large amounts of certain dark green, leafy vegetables, such as kale, collards, mustard, turnip or dandelion greens. Soybeans, almonds, broccoli, okra, and rutabaga are also moderately good sources of calcium. Pregnant women and children especially need adequate calcium and should have milk in their diet. Similarly, pregnant women, infants and young children need to include a source of vitamin D such as homogenized milk or margarine fortified with vitamins A and D. Yeast which has been heated or cooked to inactivate it will help supply some of the riboflavin usually supplied by milk and meat. Green leafy vegetables, asparagus, broccoli, Brussels sprouts, okra, and winter squash are also good sources of riboflavin if consumed frequently in large quantity. Whole grain and enriched cereal also contribute riboflavin.[13]

If milk and eggs are included in the vegetarian diet, obtaining adequate quality and quantity of protein is not difficult. However, vegans must excercise great care in selecting and combining vegetable proteins to achieve adequate quality protein. Soybeans and chickpeas provide good quality protein, almost comparable to animal sources. Combining several kinds of vegetable sources, such as beans with corn or rice, and peanuts or peanut butter with wheat will contribute a better mixture of amino acids than either cereals or legumes alone. Meat analogs made from textured vegetable proteins (see Chapter 4) may also be used to improve the quality of proteins.[14]

The more restricted the vegetarian diet, the greater the commitment to it usually and the greater the challenge to achieve nutritional adequacy. If the nutrition counselor is to be helpful, the restrictions on food choices imposed by these dietary patterns must be accepted and the individual guided to make the best choices within the limitations. In other words, the counselor must work within the client's value system.

FOOD FADS

In this scientific age quackery still flourishes in the field of nutrition as well as in the area of drugs and medical devices. Quacks thrive by misinterpreting scientific authorities in order to sell their ideas and their products. It is estimated that some 10 million Americans spend $1 billion a year on worthless and sometimes dangerous drugs, treatments, dietary fads, and other quackery. This section focusses attention on those nutrition fads that are most widespread.

Vitamin Concentrates and Food Supplements

The promotion of vitamin and mineral supplements and special diet foods is misleading millions of people who have little need for such products. This type of deceptive advertising, which until recently appealed mainly to the "golden-agers," is now deceiving people of all ages, even teen-agers. Many people are attempting self-medication for imaginary or real illness with a multitude of irrational products. They are apt to spend much more for such products than they would for beneficial nutrients provided in an adequate diet.

Fact and Fancy

There is no magic in any specific food item. It makes little difference whether one obtains his nutrients from fluid milk or milk powder, from milk products such as cheese, yogurt, or ice cream, or whether he gets them from meat, fish or fowl, wheat germ, whole grains, or blackstrap molasses. The essential point is to get an adequate supply of each nutrient from food that tastes good.

Complicating and encouraging food fads today are the growing number of false nutritional ideas, or folklore, built up by pseudo-scientific books, pamphlets and periodicals on diets of various sorts. Some tell us that calories don't count or that arthritis can be cured by oils to lubricate joints; others tempt the unwary with a drinking-man's diet or with martinis and whipped cream. In some unreliable books there is enough of the true mixed with the false regarding food values and human needs to make it difficult for the average person to judge what is valid.

Many dietary fads may be relatively harmless but senseless. Too often they detract from the pleasure of eating, an important element of good nutrition. Variety is in itself a safeguard, and, when variety is severely limited, as it is by some fads and self-imposed restrictions, certain nutritive factors are apt to be low or absent. When fads lead to delay in seeking necessary medical advice, they can be dangerous indeed. In any event food fads may increase food costs unduly and result in the omission of foods really needed. The consequences are the same whether one is led to food faddism by the enthusiasms of the uninformed neighbor or the profit-seekers.

Hence, attention is again called to the Recommended Dietary Allowances as the nutritional norms against which any dietary pattern may be measured. If a given food plan compares favorably with the RDA, the basic nutrients for health and well-being will be supplied, and one need not be concerned with the specific dietary pattern of the individual.

STUDY QUESTIONS AND ACTIVITIES

1. Why is it essential that the nutrition counselor be able to adjust her advice on nutrition to various regional and cultural food patterns?
2. After noting the regional dietary habits in the United States, which ones in the South and in the Southwest would you recommend and encourage, and what changes would you recommend?
3. How has the transplanting of various cultures influenced the food habits of those in various regions of the United States?
4. Why is the Jewish diet one of the most difficult problems for the health worker? What are some of the dietary laws which must be respected?

5. How does the use of grains, potatoes, and animal protein vary among the different regions of Europe and Asia?
6. How can you help others to gain respect for the food habits and favorite dishes of cultural groups other than their own?
7. Which one of the unusual dietary practices mentioned in this chapter is most restrictive? Why? Is there a danger nutritional deficiencies will result from following this regimen? Explain.
8. What are the types of vegetarian diets practiced by many young people today? What nutritional problems may be found among these adherents?

SUPPLEMENTARY READINGS

American Dietetic Association Position Paper on Food and Nutrition Misinformation on Selected Topics. J. Am. Dietet. A. 66:277, 1975.

Bass, M. A., and Wakefield, L. M.: Food and nutrient intake of reservation Indians. J. Am. Dietet. A. 64:36, 1974.

Cantoni, M.: Adapting therapeutic diets to the eating patterns of Italian Americans. Am. J. Clin. Nutr. 6:548, 1958.

Chang, B.: Some dietary beliefs in Chinese folkculture. J. Am. Dietet. A. 65:436, 1974.

Dwyer, J. T., et al: The new vegetarians: The natural high? J. Am. Dietet. A. 65:529, 1974.

Fathauer, G. H.: Food habits — an anthropologist's view. J. Am. Dietet. A. 37:335, 1960.

Larson, L. B., et al: Nutritional status of Mexican-American children. J. Am. Dietet. A. 64:29, 1974.

Lowenberg, M. E.: The development of food patterns. J. Am. Dietet. A. 65:263, 1974.

Macgregor, F. C.: Uncooperative patients: Some cultural interpretations. Am. J. Nurs. 67:88, 1967.

Natow, A. B., Heslin, J., and Raven, B. C.: Integrating the Jewish dietary laws into a dietetics program. Kashruth in a dietetics curriculm. J. Am. Dietet. A. 67:13, 1975.

Nutrition Misinformation and Food Faddism — A Special Supplement. Nutr. Rev. 32: Supplement #1 (July) 1974.

Sakr, A. H.: Fasting in Islam. J. Am. Dietet. A. 67:17, 1975.

Schafer, R., and Yetley, E. A.: Social psychology of food faddism. Speculations on health food behavior. J. Am. Dietet. A. 66:129, 1975.

Todhunter, E. N.: Food is more than nutrients. Food and Nutrition News, National Livestock and Meat Board. Vol. 43, No. 6-7 (March-April) 1972.

Torres, R. M.: Dietary patterns of the Puerto Rican people. Am. J. Clin. Nutr. 7:349, 1959.

Wilson, C. S.: Food habits: A selected annotated bibliography. J. Nutr. Educa. 5: #1 Supplement 1 (January-March) 1973.

Valassi, K. V.: Food habits of Greek-Americans. Am. J. Clin. Nutr. 11:240, 1962.

For further references see Bibliography in Section 4.

REFERENCES

1. Maslow, A. H: *Motivation and Personality.* New York, Harper and Row, 1954.
2. Farr, T.: Food Management 9:45, 1974.
3. Moore, W. M., Silverberg, M. M., and Read, M. S.: Nutrition, Growth and Development of North American Indian Children. DHEW Publ. No. (NIH) 72-26, Washington, D.C., 1972.
4. Bass, M. A., and Wakefield, L. M.: J. Am. Dietet. A. 64:36, 1974.
5. Mayer, J.: Nutr. Rev. 23:161, 1965.
6. Larson, L. B., et al: J. Am. Dietet. A. 64:29, 1974.
7. Kaufman, M.: Am. J. Clin. Nutr. 5:676, 1957.
8. Kamil, A.: Nutr. Rev. 32:34, Supplement (July) 1974.
9. Review: Nutr. Rev. 32:53, Supplement (July) 1974.
10. Statement: JAMA 218 #3, 1971, reprinted, Nutr. Rev. 32:27, Supplement (July) 1974.
11. Anonymous. J. Am. Dietet. A. 61:126, 1972.
12. Dwyer, J. T., et al: J. Am. Dietet. A. 65:529, 1974.
13. Raper, N. R., and Hill, M. M.: Nutr. Rev. 32:29, Supplement (July) 1974.
14. Ibid.

14   ecology of food

The production and processing of food in the United States today is a highly developed scientific business. The 296 billion pounds of food produced each year to feed the 210 million people in this country is accomplished almost entirely by scientific farming methods using chemical fertilizers and pesticides. It would be impossible to achieve these production levels using so-called "organic farming" methods (the growing of food without the use of chemical aids) alone. In the first place, the gigantic quantities of manures and composts which would be required for our vast farm system do not exist; hence, the crop yield would be drastically reduced. Without the insecticides and herbicides, the amount of crop loss from insect and fungi infestation would increase and food shortages such as exist in the underdeveloped countries would occur.

Selective breeding of plants, another aspect of scientific farming, has developed strains of cereals, fruits, and vegetables appropriate for varying climatic and soil conditions. Other specific characteristics, such as increased resistance to certain diseases, increased amino acid content, and decreased perishability, also result from selective breeding. The nutritive value of individual foods is determined chiefly by their genetic character and not by the soil or type of fertilizer used.

Animals too have been bred for certain desired characteristics, namely the lean, meat-type hog and steer, and the tenderer, meatier chicken and turkey. Antibiotics and some hormones have been employed, in scientific feeding techniques and in the control of animal diseases, which have markedly increased the animal food production; in the United States the per capita consumption of beef has increased by approximately 70 percent and of chicken by 100 percent in the last 20 years.

Most of the food consumed in American homes today has undergone some form of commercial processing—canning, freezing, or drying (Fig. 14–1). The TV dinner is perhaps the ultimate in commercial processing, but even the fresh fruits purchased in the supermarket may have had a heat and/or chill treatment before shipping to preserve their quality. In the processing of foods to produce specific properties there may be significant changes in the characteristics and composition of the original food, such as happens in the milling of the whole wheat kernel to make white flour with good bread-making properties. Food additives may also be used as preservatives, antioxidants, stabilizers, emulsifiers, and coloring and flavoring agents.

All of these factors involved in the production and processing of food provide the American consumer with an almost limitless choice of food items throughout the year, but they also make laws and regulations essential in order to protect the safety of this food supply.

This chapter will review the factors which cause food spoilage and deterioration, the methods used for the care and preservation of food, foodborne diseases, and finally government laws and regulations which control food production and marketing.

FOOD SPOILAGE AND DETERIORATION

Any change which renders a food undesirable or unfit for human use may be called food spoilage. Although one usually thinks of spoilage as being caused by microorganisms, it can also be caused by chemical or physical changes, by enzymes, and by contamination with any foreign matter. A distinction should be made between foods *unfit* for consumption by anyone and foods which may be considered *distasteful* or *undesirable* by most Americans. For instance: snails, squid, fried grasshoppers, and fermented eggs may be delicacies in certain cultures but undesirable in others.

Microbial Food Spoilage

Food spoilage may be caused by three different groups of microorganisms: bacteria, yeasts, and molds. The stale odor of spoiled meat, the foul odor of a spoiled egg, and the souring of milk are familiar examples of bacterial spoilage. The spoilage of canned foods also is usually traced to bacterial causes.

Yeasts and molds are most familiar as causes of spoilage of fresh foods, dried foods, and foods of high sugar content. The fermentation of catsup and cider is due to yeast growth. The fuzzy growths on bread and cheese and on the surface of jams and jellies indicate mold spoilage. The spoilage of citrus fruits and other fruits and vegetables is often due to the growth of molds.

Enzymic Food Spoilage

Spoilage due to enzymic action is much more widespread than most people realize. Enzymic spoilage appears most often in loss of quality rather than as frank spoilage. The haylike flavor of frozen vegetables after long or improper storage is due to enzymic activity. Fruits and vegetables that soften or become overripe during storage may be the result of either enzymic action or mold growth. Difficulty has been encountered with some of the newer methods of food preservation, such as processing at extremely high temperatures for a very short time and preservation by irradiation with ionizing rays, since under the conditions used some enzymes are more resistant to destruction than the most resistant spoilage organisms. These enzymes can cause off odors and flavors, even though the food is perfectly sterile.

Chemical Food Spoilage

Chemical causes of spoilage include flavor changes due to oxidation; swelling of cans due to production of hydrogen by the action of food acids on the metal of the container; discoloration from the reaction of metal ions from the container with the product to produce discolored crabmeat or corn; and oxidative rancidity of fats.

Most of these situations can be prevented by using a lining in the can to protect the can and the contents; "fruit" enamel prevents the bleaching of highly colored fruits; "corn" enamel prevents corn from discoloring. Antioxidants are added to foods subject to rancidity to prevent oxidation of unsaturated fatty acids.

Physical Causes of Food Spoilage

The spoilage of foods by physical changes usually involves a change of state from a solution to a precipi-

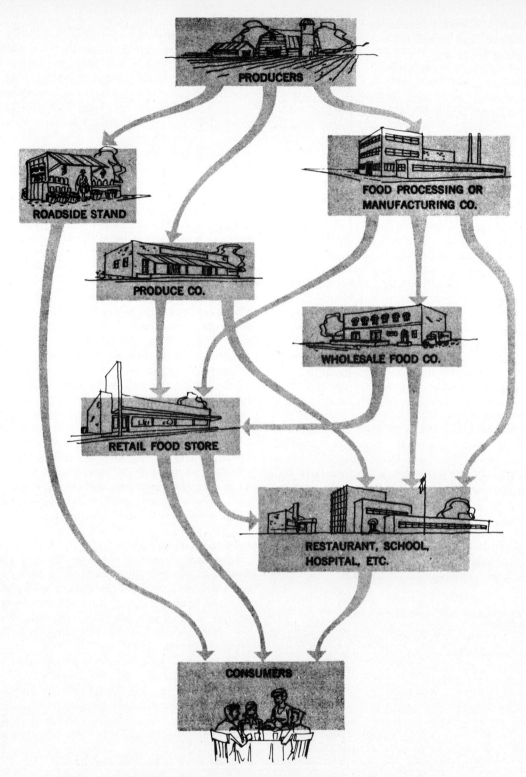

Fig. 14-1. How foods get to the consumer—the principal supply routes. (*Protecting Our Food*, Yearbook of Agriculture, U.S. Department of Agriculture, 1966, p. 239)

tate, such as is seen in sandy ice cream caused by formation of large lactose crystals during storage at fluctuating temperatures.

Exposure to light can cause spoilage in beer bottled in clear glass, with an off odor described by the industry as "skunky" beer. Sunlight can cause a tallowy off flavor in milk left too long on the doorstep and, at the same time, can destroy a high percentage of its riboflavin content.

Spoilage by Animals and Insects

One means by which the Federal Food and Drug Administration checks the sanitary conditions under which a product has been packed is to examine the product for rat hairs and droppings, insects and insect fragments, and mold hyphae. If these are present, they can confiscate an entire shipment of food and prohibit future shipments until the unsanitary conditions are corrected to the satisfaction of the Food and Drug inspector.

Often it would be chemically impossible to show any nutritional difference between a product contaminated with rat hairs and one free of contamination. However, from an esthetic viewpoint, as well as from the public health aspect—as carrier of infections —the product free of rat hairs is naturally preferred.

CARE AND PRESERVATION OF FOODS

The methods of food preservation may be divided into two general classes—bactericidal and bacteriostatic. Bactericidal methods are those which destroy the organisms. These would include cooking, canning, making jams and jellies, smoking, irradiation, and the addition of chemical preservatives. Bacteriostatic methods make conditions unsuitable for microbial growth by reducing the temperature (refrigeration and freezing), removing water (dehydration), addition of acid (pickling), or adding substances to inhibit growth (antibiotics, salt, or sugar).

Refrigeration

All perishable food products and especially those potentially hazardous foods which consist in whole or in part of milk or milk products, eggs, meat, poultry, fish, and shellfish require refrigeration. To prevent the growth of microorganisms refrigeration temperatures should be maintained at 45° F. or below if food is to be stored up to three or four days, and at 40° F. if food is to be kept longer. At temperatures between 45° F. and 140° F. (Fig. 14–2) both infectious bacteria and toxin-producing microorganisms grow rapidly. Within this range, for every 18° F. increase in temperature a tenfold increase in the rate of growth of

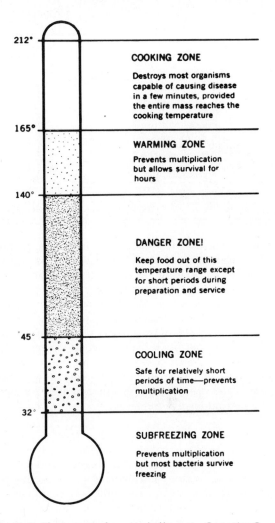

Fig. 14–2. Thermometer for control of bacteria. (*Protecting Our Food*, Yearbook of Agriculture, U.S. Department of Agriculture, 1966, p. 189)

microorganisms may occur. Food may also undergo a doubling of the bacterial growth every 15 to 30 minutes.

Almost all fresh foods sold in the U. S. have been refrigerated during part of their journey from the producer to the consumer (Fig. 14–3). If high-quality foods are to reach the consumer, the enzyme action of the fruits and the vegetables must be reduced (for these products are made up of living cells), growth of microorganisms must be inhibited, and chemical and physical changes must be prevented or slowed down.

Usually, fresh foods are stored at the lowest temperature possible at which no adverse physiological changes take place. Bananas, for example, are stored at higher temperatures during ripening (62° to 70° F.),

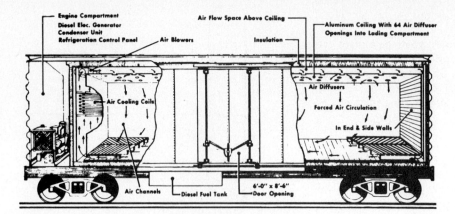

Fig. 14-3. Interior view of a modern mechanical refrigerator car. (Railway Age)

then are held at 56° to 60° F. for storage after ripening. If they are chilled below 56° F. before ripening, they develop a smoky, dull color, and if chilled after ripening the skin turns brown rapidly.

Apples and some other fruits are usually stored at 30° to 32° F. in a nitrogen atmosphere for best results. In order to maintain crispness or an attractive appearance, the humidity is usually maintained as high as possible to prevent loss of moisture, but it must also be low enough to discourage mold growth. Most fruits and vegetables are maintained at 85 percent to 90 percent relative humidity.

Freezing

Since certain varieties of fruits and vegetables have characteristics which make them better able to withstand freezing and thawing and since freezing does not improve a product that was poor quality to start with, foods for the freezer should be carefully selected for appropriate variety and quality. Vegetables are blanched before freezing to inactivate the enzymes, and fruits are either placed in a sugar syrup or treated with an antioxidant such as ascorbic acid to keep them from darkening. Some foods such as peas, beans, or shrimp may be frozen before they are packaged, but most foods are placed in cartons and then frozen rapidly at temperatures of −40° F. or below. Frozen foods should be stored at 0° F. or below.

Cooked prepared foods especially require care in preparation and sanitary handling because frequently they contain potentially hazardous mixtures (see Refrigeration) and may not be thoroughly cooked before serving. Most bacteria survive freezing, but their growth is inhibited at such low temperatures. However, Trichina, a parasite which may infect pork, is destroyed by freezing.

When foods are allowed to thaw and are kept at room temperature, spoilage actually occurs more rapidly than one might expect, since, due to a partial breakdown of cell walls and tissues, the thawed food is an excellent medium for growth of bacteria. Most foods should not be refrozen once they have thawed.

Dehydrofreezing is a process which removes about 50 percent of the water from fruits and vegetables before they are frozen. The reduction in weight and volume allows them to be shipped and stored more economically.

Cooking and Baking

Nearly all the microorganisms in a food are destroyed by proper cooking. Since this lengthens the time that a food will keep, cooking may be regarded as a method of preservation. In some cases it is a mixed blessing, as a study of food poisoning will quickly show that most cases of food poisoning are caused by consumption of a cooked food which has not been properly refrigerated. Cooking destroys the organisms that would ordinarily compete with, and hold in check, the growth of food-poisoning organisms. If inadequate cooking occurs, such as in roasting a prestuffed turkey, or if contamination of the cooked food occurs after cooking, from the hands or the nasal discharge of a food handler, the toxin-producing organisms can then grow without hindrance.

Pasteurization

The time-temperature relationship of pasteurization is based on the time at a given temperature in which all the organisms which will produce disease are destroyed. Milk as it comes from the pasteurizer is not sterile. The total bacterial count has been reduced, and all the disease-causing organisms are destroyed.

Two methods are used for milk pasteurization:

the *holding* method consists of heating milk to 63° C. (145° F.) and holding at that temperature for 30 minutes; the *high-temperature short-time* method consists of heating milk to 71.1° C. (160° F.) and holding for 17 seconds.

The reduction in bacterial count plus refrigeration increases the shelf life of many foods other than milk, such as beer, wines, etc. Mild heat treatment of concentrated citrus juices before freezing is practiced by many packers to control the enzymes which may cause clarification and/or gelation on the concentrate if it is mishandled (allowed to remain above freezing) during storage and marketing.

Canning

The canning industry has continually improved the quality and the retention of nutrients in food by increasing the rate of heating and cooling. Canned foods are sterilized by means of heating with steam under pressure (5 pounds, 227 ° F., 10 pounds, 240° F., 15 pounds, 250° F.). Agitation of the can during heating also permits faster heat penetration of the can contents and thus shortens processing time.

Originally food was preserved by boiling jars of food for hours. Now food can be sterilized in less than a second at temperatures up to 275° F. in a specially designed heat exchanger, cooled immediately, and then sealed into sterile containers aseptically. This method, known as *aseptic canning*, is now used on a small scale to process purees and baby foods, but its use is limited because of the high cost of the equipment required and the short packing periods of most canneries.

Canning has probably done more than any other discovery to help mankind maintain an adequate food supply throughout the year.

Dehydration

In the past, dehydration was looked upon as one of the least desirable methods of preservation. Technological advances during and after World War II have made possible much-improved products with special attributes of low cost, reduced weight, convenience, and keeping quality. The absence of water prevents the growth of microorganisms in dehydrated products.

The use of dehydrated foods has increased rapidly. Certain dehydrated products are used by some consumers to the exclusion of their counterparts preserved by other methods. An example of this is instant coffee, which now constitutes at least 50 percent of coffee used.

Of particular interest to the nutritionist is the availability of nonfat dried milk, which brings this excellent food to the consumer at a low price in an easily soluble form with good flavor and keeping qualities.

Certain fruits such as prunes, peaches, apricots, apples, raisins, figs, and dates are also popular consumer items. Dried legumes, onions, and parsley are available. Fish and meat may also be preserved by drying.

Other items in this multimillion-dollar business include cake, muffin, cornbread, pancake, and roll mixes (which are mixtures of dehydrated ingredients); instant potato, fruit-flavored juices and dessert mixes; precooked dehydrated cereals, rice, and tapioca; soups; and dried active yeast. Dried stabilized eggs (whole eggs, egg yolk, or egg white) are used widely in bakery products but have not as yet reached wide distribution on a retail scale.

Freeze-Drying

This process consists of first freezing the food and then removing the water under a vacuum. The food is packaged in the presence of an inert gas such as nitrogen. Freeze-dried foods rehydrate very readily and retain their original shape and volume. The most widely used freeze-dried product today is coffee, although seafoods, meats, poultry, fruits, and vegetables have been tested and found acceptable.

Chemicals as Preservatives

Chemical preservatives are among the oldest forms of food preservation—salt, sugar, vinegar are the most familiar ones. Other types of chemical preservatives are also used. Some are effective for a particular type of food or against a particular spoilage organism. They are called antioxidants, inhibitors, fungicides, and sequestrants. Ascorbic acid is frequently used as an antioxidant in commercial canning and freezing to prevent the enzymatic browning of fruits and vegetables. Sorbic acid is used to prevent mold growth on cheese, and sodium benzoate is used to preserve cider from yeast fermentation and margarine from spoilage by mold. Sodium propionate, calcium propionate, or sodium diacetate are used in bread to prevent mold growth. In general, however, chemical preservatives have had a long hard fight to stay in foods, due to adverse public opinion about their use and strict regulation by the Food and Drug Administration. When a food can be preserved satisfactorily without chemicals, chemical preservatives are not allowed. For example, catsup will keep because of the preservative effects of acids, sugars, and spices, and for that reason sodium benzoate which for years had been added to catsup may no longer be used. (See section on Food Additives.)

Antibiotics

Various antibiotics have some limited usefulness in food preservation. Growth of spoilage organisms can be inhibited by antibiotics but cannot be completely prevented. These substances are of value in extending the periods for which foods can be kept fresh during processing and storage. For instance, the addition of oxytetracycline (Terramycin) or chlortetracycline (Aureomycin) to the ice slush in which poultry is cooled after dressing can extend the shelf life of the poultry 7 to 10 days. This is allowed in the United States in the processing of poultry if the residue is no more than 7 parts per million. At this level practically all of the antibiotic is destroyed by cooking.

Because antibiotics are drugs, their use in processing and their presence in foods is carefully regulated by the Food and Drug Administration. For use in food processing they must be heat labile and, therefore, destroyed by cooking. It must be demonstrated that residues left in foods will not sensitize individuals and cause allergic reactions. Not only would this create health problems for individuals but would limit the therapeutic value of the antibiotics. Also, tolerance levels for specific antibiotics in specific foods must be established by the Food and Drug Administration before they may be used in processing. Equal care must be taken to ensure that antibiotic residues are not left in animal food products from the treatment of farm animals during their lives.

Radiation

The newest method of food preservation is still in the experimental stage. The Armed Forces Food and Container Institute at Natick, Mass., has been doing extensive research on food irradiation in one of the best equipped laboratories in the world for this purpose. They are testing various types of foods in different designs of containers to determine levels of irradiation which will safeguard the food without changing its flavor. Obviously, food does not become radioactive in the process. F. P. Mehrlich, Technical Director, explains:

The radiation preservation process involves exposing food to electrons so the food itself is not cooked in the process. Raw foods remain raw. Different effects are obtained, depending on the level of irradiation provided.

At the lowest levels, in the order of 7,500 rads, sprouting of potatoes and onions is inhibited, extending their postharvest storage life well into

the next harvest. At slightly higher levels, human pathogens like trichinosis-causing worms and liver flukes are destroyed, making infested pork and fish safe for human consumption. At still higher levels, insect larvae and eggs are destroyed, eliminating insect damage in packaged cereal and permitting previously infested fruits across quarantine barriers.

At even higher levels, pathogenic bacteria like Salmonella are inactivated. At the same time so are most of the bacteria present, thereby extending the refrigerated shelf life and marketing radius of fresh foods.

Finally, at the highest levels, in the order of 4.5 million rads, all bacteria are killed and prepackaged food can be kept without bacterial spoilage, in the absence of refrigeration. The military and civilian advantages of such a process are readily apparent.[1]

A *rad* is a unit of absorbed ionizing radiation. It corresponds to an energy absorption of 100 ergs per gram of material. A lethal dose for man is between 500 and 600 rads.

Since many foods become unacceptable at radiation levels above 500,000 rads due to off flavor and odor, it is probable that research will develop a combination of heat, radiation, and refrigeration to retain the highest quality of certain foods. Heat destroys enzymes which are resistant to destruction by radiation.

EFFECTS OF FOOD PROCESSING ON NUTRIENT COMPOSITION
Canning

Properly canned fruits and vegetables have approximately the same nutrient composition as fresh ones. It is possible that the canned products might be better than the fresh if the latter are not protected in shipment from farm to market or are stored incorrectly and cooked by the homemaker. Some nutritive loss, especially of the heat-labile water-soluble vitamins, ascorbic acid, thiamine, vitamin B_6, and pantothenic acid, occurs during the canning process. Additional losses occur during storage depending on the temperature at which canned goods are stored. Canned fruits and vegetables stored for a year at 65° F. or below lose much less ascorbic acid and thiamine than if stored at 80° F. The use of the liquid from canned fruits and vegetables also reduces the loss of water-soluble nutrients.

The calorie value of most canned fruits is greater than fresh due to the addition of sugar during processing. The majority of canned vegetables will differ in sodium composition compared with fresh ones because salt (NaCl) is added during processing.

Losses of heat-labile water-soluble vitamins, such as thiamine and vitamin B_6, also occur in the canning and storage of meat, poultry, and fish products. However, since the cooking of fresh meat, fish, and poultry in the home also results in similar losses, these products have approximately the same nutritive composition. Salt (NaCl) is usually added to these foods in processing.

Freezing

Frozen vegetables and fruits may also lose small amounts of the water-soluble vitamins during the blanching and freezing process; however, this loss is similar to the loss from fresh foods prepared in the home. The temperature at which frozen foods are stored also affects nutrient losses. Freezers should be maintained at 0° F. or below if food is to be stored for more than a few days.

Frozen fruits, vegetables, meat, fish, and poultry will be comparable in nutrient composition to the fresh products if other food items are not added. Plain frozen vegetables, without the addition of butter or sauces for seasoning, are equal to fresh or canned ones. Salt, and in some instances monosodium glutamate, may be added to plain frozen vegetables. When salt is added it is listed on the label. Frozen fruits may or may not have sugar added during processing. Frozen orange juice concentrate does not have sugar added, but most of the orange-flavored breakfast drinks do have sugar added. The calorie value of frozen meat, fish, or poultry can be greater than fresh if a gravy or sauce has been added or if the product is breaded and fried before freezing, such as frozen fish sticks.

Dehydration

Drying and storing of protein foods, such as milk, fish, meat, and legumes, may result in some loss of biological value or a reduction in the protein efficiency ratio (PER). Nutrition labeling information will have to consider these data although it is probably of limited concern to high-protein consuming Americans.[2]

Ascorbic acid losses in dehydrated fruits and vegetables are considerable. Thiamine levels may also be decreased in dehydrated products. Some loss of fat-soluble vitamins A and E have been reported in dehydrated foods.[3]

FOODBORNE DISEASES AND TOXINS

Foods may be contaminated by a variety of pathogenic organisms. These contaminants may be various worms, molds, bacteria, viruses, and other organisms or the toxins produced by them. The appearance, taste, and smell of the food so infected may show no change and thus give no warning to the consumer.

These infections may be present in the food at its source, such as animals infected with tuberculosis, brucellosis, salmonellosis, tularemia, tapeworms, or trichinae, and may be carried to the consumer if the food is undercooked.

Food may also be infected by food handlers who are convalescent from infectious diseases. They may be in apparent good health but still carry infectious organisms. The organisms may be distributed on food by hands soiled with urine or feces or by spray of oral and nasal secretions by coughing and sneezing over the food being prepared. Contamination may also come from the butcher block or from the handling of an infected animal before working with the food in question.

Dust falling on uncovered foods and the feces and the bodies of insects may also convey pathogenic organisms to a food supply. Covering of cooked foods and refrigeration can do much to cut down on the number of pathogenic organisms in foods. Cooked foods should be cooled as quickly as possible by pouring or sorting into flat pans and promptly refrigerating rather than by allowing them to cool at room temperature. Often the period required for cooling in a warm kitchen is sufficient for bacteria to grow rapidly.

Bacterial Contamination of Food and Water

SALMONELLA infection is a term used to cover a large group of infections caused by several species of the Salmonella organism and common to man and several animals and birds. Salmonellosis is an infection of the intestinal tract, and symptoms begin to appear from 8 to 48 hours after contaminated food has been eaten. Symptoms typically are headache, vomiting, diarrhea, fever, and cramps. An attack may last a few hours or several days. Infants and debilitated older people may be most seriously affected and death may result. Antibiotics do little to relieve an attack; fluids and a bland diet are the usual treatment.

The Center for Disease Control in Atlanta, Georgia, reported that salmonellosis has become a major national problem, whereas a generation ago it was seldom recognized as such. Even today cases go unreported because they are mistaken for "24-hour flu" or "stomach upset." They state that some 20,000 cases of salmonella infection are reported each year but that the actual incidence is probably 2 million cases per year. In this decade salmonella have been traced to well water, frozen turkey, fresh chicken, eggs, smoked fish, ground beef, and a contaminated batch of powdered milk.

Many varieties of salmonella may be carried by contaminated foods. Because these bacteria grow easily in moist foods of low acidity and may continue to be viable even in some dry foods, strict control of food sanitation and cooking procedures at home and in institutions, especially, is essential. The usual path of infection is from animals or animal products to man. Precautions in regard to utensils, dishwashing, and food handling are outlined by Werrin and Kronick.[4] Salmonella are readily destroyed by usual cooking procedures and by pasteurization but not by freezing. Note the incident of turkeyborne multiple infection below.

THE TYPHOID BACILLUS is another species of salmonella and may be carried by contaminated water or shellfish. In the United States, however, an outbreak of typhoid fever can usually be traced to a food handler who is a "carrier" of the organism. Fortunately, the disease responds to an antibiotic, and the course is not as serious as it once was.

SHIGELLOSIS is closely related to salmonellosis. Shigella also are enteric bacteria and are the etiologic agents of bacillary dysentery in man. Young children and newborn animals are most seriously affected.

CLOSTRIDIUM PERFRINGENS. Perfringens poisoning, which results in gastrointestinal disturbances, is caused by certain strains of Clostridium perfringens, a spore-forming bacteria that grows in the absence of oxygen. The spores are resistant to heat, ordinary cooking, drying, freezing, curing of meats, and to irradiation. To prevent their growth, meats should be cooked rapidly and refrigerated promptly below 40° F.

The symptoms of Cl. perfringens food infection are mild gastroenteritis, abdominal cramps, and diarrhea 8 to 16 hours after eating infected food, and may be accompanied by nausea and headache. The illness is usually mild and of short duration, with recovery within 24 hours.

A report of three consecutive outbreaks of foodborne disease in one week was recently investigated and traced to turkey infected with both salmonella and Cl. perfringens. The turkey prepared ahead and served at three banquets in one week caused food poisoning in 23 percent of the persons present at the first, in 35 percent of those at the second, and in 69 percent of those at the third banquet. The 20- to 22-pound turkeys had been purchased frozen, thawed at room temperature, boiled for 4 hours and allowed to cool in water overnight. They were stored in a refrigerator but were probably at room temperature for

some time during preparation and prior to reheating before service at each banquet. This is an example of poor food handling, if not poor sanitation.[5]

STREPTOCOCCAL INFECTIONS. Hemolytic streptococcus is the type most commonly carried by food. Food and utensils may be contaminated by a carrier, from nasal discharge or skin infection. Strep sore throat, strep ear infections, and scarlet fever are all caused by strains of hemolytic streptococci.

TULAREMIA, sometimes called rabbit fever, is caused by infection with Pasteurella tularensis. It is transmitted from rodents by flies, fleas, and ticks and may be acquired by man from the handling of infected animals. It is characterized by an ulcer at the site of inoculation, followed by inflammation of the lymph glands and by headache, chills, and fever. It is recommended that hunters use rubber gloves when dressing wild game.

Toxins Produced by Bacteria and Molds

The bacteria that produce exotoxins in foods are of two types quite different in growth habits and in the clinical symptoms of poisoning.

STAPHYLOCOCCUS FOOD POISONING. Staphylococcus bacteria are responsible for many cases of food posioning. Most people are sensitive to the exotoxins produced by these bacteria, and serious illness can result if enough of the toxin is present in the food. The toxin affects only the gastrointestinal tract, and the onset of symptoms occurs within one to eight hours after infected food is eaten. The symptoms are severe nausea, vomiting, and abdominal cramps. This kind of food poisoning is rarely fatal.

Most outbreaks of this type of food poisoning have been caused by the bacteria in prepared or unheated foods such as custard-filled pastries, cream pies, salads, precooked meats such as ham, sandwiches, and creamed dishes. The bacteria get into food from boils, infected cuts, coughing, and sneezing by food handlers followed by improper storage and inadequate reheating of foods before service. The flavor and appearance of the food may not change. Control of this type of food poisoning is largely a matter of education of food handlers.

BOTULISM. Botulism is a rare form of food poisoning. It occurs when foods have been underprocessed. Botulin (the toxin) may also be found in some meat products such as sausage (the Latin word for sausage is botulus). Since Cl. botulinum is a strict anaerobe, it can grow only under conditions in which air is excluded, such as in a can or deep inside a product.

In recent years commercially processed foods have been relatively free of any poisoning caused by

Cl. botulinum. However, in 1963 two instances of cases were caused by canned tuna fish and one by smoked fish frozen in polyethylene bags.

In 1971, two cases were reported as the result of the use of canned soup and resulted in a massive recall of all soups and sauces processed by that particular company.

The *toxin* produced is one of the most deadly biological poisons known. On average, mortality is about 25 percent for the diagnosed and reported cases. Occasionally, entire families are killed by botulism. An antitoxin, trivalent "A, B, E," is widely available across the U.S. through the Public Health Service.

Home-canned foods account for the vast majority of the 10 to 20 botulism outbreaks which occur each year. Low-acid foods should be preserved only by means of a pressure cooker process. Boiling canned foods for 10 minutes will also destroy the toxin.

The toxin is absorbed directly from the stomach and the intestinal tract. In about 8 to 72 hours it affects the nervous system, causing double vision, difficulty in swallowing, loss of speech and, when lethal, respiratory failure in from 3 to 6 days.

TOXINS FROM MOLDS (MYCOTOXINS). Aflatoxin, a toxin produced by *Aspergillus flavus,* a fungus found in peanuts (groundnuts) which have been improperly dried, has been found to be carcinogenic in rats. No acute illness is caused in man from eating foods contaminated by these toxins, but it is wise to destroy any moldy foods in which the mold was not deliberately introduced. Although certain mycotoxins "have been proven to cause cancer in animals the question remains open concerning human health."[6] The fungus itself can cause serious infection of the respiratory tract, sinuses, eyes, and ears. It is difficult to diagnose, which is especially important if it is to be treated with specific drugs.

Research in India and other Asian countries is aimed at prevention of the damaging mold on peanuts. Commercial peanut products designed for human consumption in the United States are toxin-free, even if produced from contaminated nuts, because any trace of aflotoxin is removed in the refining process.

Naturally Occurring Toxins

It is well known that many varieties of mushrooms are poisonous and have been mistaken for edible types with disastrous results. There is no simple test which will identify edible types other than botanical characteristics.

A few plants used as foods are safe at one time and not at another. The young white shoots of pokeweed frequently are eaten with safety as greens in the early spring, but the later green shoots may cause severe illness. The green leaves of rhubarb may contain enough oxalic acid to cause illness, but the succulent leaf stems are eaten without any untoward effects. Clams and mussels on the Pacific coast may build up toxins during the summer due to an infection from certain plankton (red tide).

Viral Infections

INFECTIOUS HEPATITIS is the most common of viral infections spread by contaminated food. It may be spread by the consumption of contaminated water, milk, or other food or by the blood of persons carrying the hepatitis virus. A food handler who is a carrier may cut his finger and thus contaminate food; this may not be discovered for some time. The incubation period is from 10 to 50 days and the virus may be in the blood 2 to 3 weeks before the onset of the disease.

Parasitic Infections

Parasitic infections are not confined to the tropics as is sometimes thought. They may be transmitted by food or drink, often by infected fish, shellfish, or crustacea.

TRICHINOSIS is the parasitic disease most likely to be encountered in the United States and is caused by improperly cooked pork from pigs that were infected with *Trichinella spiralis.* Symptoms of the infection in man include fever, muscle pain, sweating, chills, vomiting, and swollen eyelids. Outbreaks have been reported from homemade sausage and other pork products improperly cured. Trichinosis can be avoided if pork is well cooked (internal temperature of at least 137° F.) or properly cured.

Protozoan Infections

AMEBIC DYSENTERY, caused by *Entamoeba histolytica,* is another infection that may be carried by food and food handlers. It is common in the tropics. Once it is acquired, the organism remains in the tissues of the intestinal tract and causes intermittent attacks until the individual is treated. Abscesses of the liver may be a complication.

SAFEGUARDING THE FOOD SUPPLY

The food industry is the nation's largest industry and depends upon the work of thousands of scientists and experts to predict needs and regulate food production and processing in the United States. People in general do not have the means or the skills to examine how meats are handled, to check fruits and vegetables for residues of pesticides or processed foods for harmful preservatives or accidental contaminants or packaged goods for insect infestation. Through Congress, however, laws have been passed making certain federal agencies responsible for protecting the safety of our food supplies. Such agencies as the Food and Drug Administration, the Federal Trade Commission, and the Department of Agriculture have extensive programs for safeguarding our foods.

U.S. Department of Health, Education and Welfare — Food and Drug Administration

FEDERAL FOOD, DRUG AND COSMETIC ACT. Under the Food, Drug and Cosmetic Act, the Food and Drug Administration (FDA) of the Department of Health, Education and Welfare (DHEW) has jurisdiction over the safety of foods shipped interstate or manufactured in a territory of the United States or the

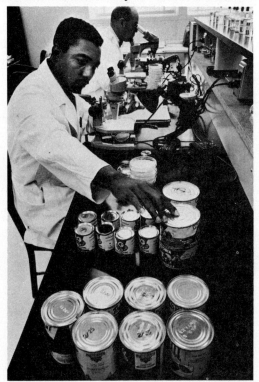

Fig. 14-4. FDA'S enforcement effort for foods is mainly concerned with food plant sanitation and the wholesomeness of ingredients and finished products. The Federal Food, Drug, and Cosmetic Act (1938) makes it illegal to ship in interstate commerce a food that comes from unsanitary premises. To enforce this section of the Act, FDA inspects food processors to insure that the factories are sanitary. FDA is responsible for establishing safety standards for additives in foods. (FDA Publ. No. 1. U.S. Department HEW, Washington, D.C.)

District of Columbia. Federal regulations also control imported and exported foods. Foods manufactured and sold within a state's boundaries are not subject to federal regulation but are controlled by the food regulations of the state in which they are produced (Fig. 14-4).

Adulteration of Foods. A food is considered to be adulterated if it is filthy, putrid, or decomposed, if noncertified colors are used, if the container is made of a substance injurious to health (e.g., lead), if there is dilution or substitution, or if there is omission of a valuable ingredient. Food is also considered to be adulterated if it contains meat from a diseased animal or one that died by means other than slaughter.

Standards. Standards of identity, quality, and fill have been established under federal regulations. A **standard of identity** defines what a food product is. It determines what ingredients must be included, the minimum and maximum amounts of each, and additional ingredients that are optional. Standards of identity have been set for such products as milk and cream; cheese and cheese products; eggs and egg products; margarine; mayonnaise, French dressing, and salad dressing; frozen desserts; flours; macaroni and noodle products; jellies and preserves; canned fruit and fruit juices; vegetables and vegetable products. Only the optional ingredients used in these products must appear on the label. Hence, the nutrition educator needs to know that even though salt may not appear in the list of ingredients on the label of the catsup bottle, it is included in the standard of identity; therefore, catsup is a food to be avoided on a sodium-restricted diet.

Standards of quality have been established chiefly for canned fruits, vegetables, and meats. Foods that do not meet the minimum standards for quality must be labeled substandard. These foods are not usually sold on the retail market.

Standards of fill are specifications for the amount of food that must be in a container. They were established to prevent the use of deceptive containers and to provide guidelines for foods such as cereals and crackers that tend to "shake down" after being packaged.

Pesticide Control. An amendment to the Food, Drug and Cosmetic Act of 1938 was passed in 1954 to establish safe limits of pesticide chemical residues on fresh fruits and vegetables. The chemical pesticide sprays range in toxicity to man from virtually harmless to extremely toxic and dangerous poisons. To control their use the FDA has published a list of more than 2000 tolerance levels for pesticide chemicals and has established a zero tolerance for certain pesticides such as cyanides, mercury-containing compounds, and selenium-containing compounds, which are extremely dangerous.

To protect the consumer, foods which are shipped in violation of FDA regulations are subject to seizure. The manufacturers may be fined and/or imprisoned, depending on the circumstances.

Food Additives. The Food Additives Amendment of 1958 and the Color Additive Amendment of 1960 govern the use of intentional and incidental food additives. These amendments are designed to protect the public from the presence in foods of any substance not demonstrated to be safe under the recommended conditions of use as judged by competent experts.

Food additives are prohibited specifically by the Food, Drug and Cosmetic Act where they are used to mask faulty processing and handling techniques, to deceive the consumer, and to aid processing at the expense of a substantial reduction of the nutrition value of the product, and where good manufacturing practices do not require the use of an additive to produce a food item economically.

Intentional food additives include preservatives, antioxidants, stabilizers, emulsifiers, and coloring and flavoring agents. Well over 1000 such additives are being used in food processing today, and these are continually being investigated by the Food and Drug Administration.

The GRAS list, published by the FDA, is a list of 675 substances used in food which are *Generally Recognized As Safe.* Other approved food additives not on the GRAS list are known as regulated food additives. All GRAS list items are currently under review to determine their usage rates in the American food supply and their relative safety in terms of amounts consumed.

Saccharin has been removed from the GRAS list to an "interim regulated additives" list and will remain on that list until the National Academy of Sciences reports on the evaluation of research to determine if saccharin can cause cancer. Glycine and brominated vegetable oil have also been transferred to the interim list until further study on their toxicity is complete. Those GRAS list additives which have now been placed on the regulated additives list with the reasons for this action are as follows:

> Carrageenan, a vegetable gum—to allow the FDA to define permissible sources for the substance;
> Carob bean gum and probably all natural gums—to establish permissible levels for their use;
> Amino acids—to establish permissible levels.

In addition, four additives, the sweeteners mannitol and sorbitol and the preservatives methylparaben and propylparaben, have been proposed by the FDA as the first substances for the FDA-affirmed GRAS list.

The manufacturer has the burden of proof for the usefulness and safety of a proposed additive. Usually, judgment of safety is based on the result of experiments on three or more types of animals to determine acute toxicity and chronic toxicity at levels far above those intended for use in foods. The maximum level of consumption of an additive in a day's food must be determined or estimated. The minimum level which will produce deviations from normal in animals is studied carefully to determine what effects may be expected in humans, and an adequate margin of safety must be established to reduce to a minimum any hazard to the health of people of varying ages and physiological states. Any additive shown to be a carcinogen in any experimental animal is automatically not approved. The removal of cyclamates from the approved list of additives was based on this regulations.

Although safety of food additives is a problem of extreme importance, it is practically impossible to demonstrate absolute proof of safety of an additive for all people in a population which may include a few very sensitive individuals and others in poor physiological condition, as well as those suffering from a disease of one sort or another.

The use of nitrites and nitrates in cured meats is under serious consideration at the present time. Since their presence in food may result in the formation of nitrosamines, some of which have been shown to be carcinogenic under certain conditions, their use continues only because nitrite acts to prevent the spore formation from *Cl. botulinum* in these meat products.[7]

The incidental additives, usually undesirable, which may appear in food products include:
1. Pesticides (used for plant and animal pest control);
2. Fertilizers (utilized by plants);
3. Feed adjuvants and drugs (antibiotics, hormones, tranquilizers, and enzymes);
4. Chemicals used in packaging materials (may migrate into the food).

These regulations are monitored by FDA officials, and the public is protected when foods which do not conform to them are found.

POLLUTION. The hazards of environmental pollution to our food supply have become a national concern. The rapid increase in the contamination of air, water, and soil as a result of increased population and technological advances requires diligent monitoring by those persons responsible for safeguarding the nation's health.

Of special concern is the possible presence of

radioactive materials in food. For example, the milk supply requires constant radiation surveillance because of the possible presence of strontium-90 or iodine-131, two potentially harmful substances, especially in infants and children. Although most of the Sr-90 is excreted from the body, small amounts may be deposited in bones. Larger amounts of I-131 are absorbed and have a carcinogenic effect on the thyroid gland. Currently the amounts of radioactive fallout in our food supply are well below danger levels.

Another problem of environmental contaminants involves the toxic metals (see Chapter 5) including mercury, lead, and cadmium. The FDA alerted the public to the excessive amounts of mercury in certain types of fish. Swordfish, in particular, has been identified as containing potentially harmful levels and was removed from the market. Although the presence of mercury has been detected in tuna fish, these amounts were not as alarming and tuna fish may still be purchased. In fact, most of the fresh tuna fish is now examined before it is canned and only that fish which is below guideline levels is canned for the consumer market.

The pollution of inland lakes and streams and coastal waters from industrial wastes and sewage has not only reduced the available supply of fish from these sources but also has increased the health hazard from the consumption of that supply which remains.

FAIR PACKAGING AND LABELING ACT. The Fair Packaging and Labeling Act of 1966, known as the "truth in packaging" law, provides for more informative and more prominent labeling of packaged foods. The regulations concerning labeling include the following requirements: (1) the common name of the food with appropriate descriptions, such as whole, sliced, diced, or chopped, must appear in bold type on the principal display panel; (2) the name and address of the manufacturer, packer, and distributor must be conspicuous on the package; (3) the net contents of the package must be stated in terms of standard measure and the number and size of servings (no misleading statements such as "giant quart" or "jumbo pound" may be used); (4) the common names of ingredients must be listed in legible type in decreasing order of their prominence in the food.

Nutrition Labeling

All prepared and packaged foods shipped in interstate commerce after July 1975 in which label or advertising claims are made must carry nutrition labeling. The objectives of this labeling program are to provide consumers with nutrition information about packaged foods; to assist in the nutrition educa-

tion of the consumer; to encourage improvement of the nutritional content of foods; and to safeguard the nutritional value of the food supply.

Although nutrition labeling for most foods is voluntary, it must be used for all fortified and enriched foods, such as fortified milk and enriched flour. If, however, enriched flour is one of many ingredients in a product, nutrition labeling is not mandatory. The sodium content of a food may appear on the label without full nutrient disclosure.

Formats for the nutrition label, exemplified in Table 14–1, have been standardized and must include the following:

Serving size;
Servings per container;
Calorie content per serving;
Protein content per serving—grams;
Carbohydrate content per serving—grams;
Fat content per serving—grams;
Percentages per serving of the US-RDA of protein, vitamin A, vitamin C, thiamine, riboflavin, niacin, calcium, and iron.

Other optional nutrients may be included— vitamin D, vitamin E, vitamin B_6, folic acid, vitamin B_{12}, phosphorus, iodine, magnesium, zinc, copper,

Table 14–1. Example of Nutrition Information on Cereal Package*

NUTRITION INFORMATION
PER SERVING

SERVING SIZE: One ounce (1 1/3 cups) corn flakes alone and in combination with ½ cup vitamin D fortified whole milk.
SERVINGS PER CONTAINER: 12

	Corn Flakes	
	1 oz.	with ½ cup whole milk
CALORIES	110	190
POTEIN	2 g.	6 g.
CARBOHYDRATES	24 g.	30 g.
FAT	0 g.	4 g.

PERCENTAGE OF U.S. RECOMMENDED
DAILY ALLOWANCE (US-RDA)

	Corn Flakes	
	1 oz.	with ½ cup whole milk
PROTEIN	2	10
VITAMIN A	25	25
VITAMIN C	25	25
THIAMINE	25	25
RIBOFLAVIN	25	35
NIACIN	25	25
CALCIUM	†	15
IRON	10	10
VITAMIN D	10	25
VITAMIN B_6	25	25
FOLIC ACID	25	25
PHOSPHORUS	†	10
MAGNESIUM	†	4

*(Cereal Institute, Inc.)
†Contains less than 2 percent of the US-RDA of these nutrients.

biotin, and pantothenic acid. The fatty acid composition and/or cholesterol content of a food may also appear on the label.

Several types of foods may be presented with two sets of figures. Foods such as bread for which there is reliable data that they are consumed more than once a day, may carry an additional set of figures which show the nutrients in a day's intake. A product which requires preparation in the home may carry a second column of figures showing the nutrient value of the finished product provided the directions for its preparation are given on the package.

The FDA has also proposed that certain claims be prohibited from appearing on the label. These would include any statements which suggest or imply:

That the food can prevent, cure, mitigate, or treat any disease or symptom;

That a balanced diet of ordinary foods cannot supply adequate nutrients;

That the lack of optimum nutritive quality of a food, by reason of the soil in which food was grown, is or may be responsible for an inadequacy or deficiency in the quality of the daily diet;

That the storage, transportation, processing, or cooking of a food is or may be responsible for an inadequacy or deficiency in the quality of diets;

That the food has nutritional properties when

such properties are actually of no significant value or need in human nutrition; and

That a natural vitamin in a food is superior to an added vitamin, or that there is any difference between natural and synthetic vitamins.

The US-RDA (see Chapter 10) was adopted as the standard reference for all nutrition labeling. As shown in Table 14–2, these standards recognize differences in protein quality by establishing two levels of recommended intakes. One recommended intake level is for protein with a protein-efficiency ratio (PER—a biological index of protein quality) less than casein; a lower recommended intake level is given for food protein sources with a PER value equal to or greater than casein. For products whose protein quality is less than 20 percent that of casein, the statement "not a significant source of protein" must be inserted in place of grams per serving.

Nutrition labeling promises to be a most valuable consumer program; however, it must be recognized that the costs of implementing, sustaining, and regulating the program will be in the millions of dollars. An estimate of one cent per case of product has been suggested, and this cost will have to be shared by the consumer. Thus, if the consumer is to get her money's worth from nutrition labeling, a large-scale educational program will have to be introduced. All nutrition educators will have to share responsibility for

Table 14–2.   U.S. Recommended Daily Allowances (US-RDAs) for Essential Nutrients

	INFANTS BIRTH TO 12 MONTHS (TENTATIVE)	CHILDREN UNDER 4 YEARS OF AGE	ADULTS AND CHILDREN 4 OR MORE YEARS OF AGE	PREGNANT OR LACTATING WOMEN
*Nutrients which MUST be declared on the label**				
Protein, "low quality protein" (g.)	28	65	65	65
Protein, "high quality protein" (g.)	20	45	45	45
Protein, "proteins in general" (g.)	28	65	65	65
Vitamin A (IU)	1500	2500	5000	8000
Vitamin C (ascorbic acid) (mg.)	35	40	60	60
Thiamine (vitamin B_1) (mg.)	0.5	0.7	1.5	1.7
Riboflavin (vitamin B_2) (mg.)	0.6	0.8	1.7	2.0
Niacin (mg.)	8	9	20	20
Calcium (g.)	0.6	0.8	1.0	1.3
Iron (mg.)	15	10	18	18
Nutrients which MAY be declared on the label				
Vitamin D (IU)	400	400	400	400
Vitamin E (IU)	5	10	30	30
Vitamin B_6 (mg.)	0.4	0.7	2.0	2.5
Folic acid (Folacin) (mg.)	0.1	0.2	0.4	0.8
Vitamin B_{12} (mcg.)	2	3	6	8
Phosphorus (g.)	0.5	0.8	1.0	1.3
Iodine (mcg.)	45	70	150	150
Magnesium (mg.)	70	200	400	450
Zinc (mg.)	5	8	15	15
Copper (mg.)	0.6	1	2	2
Biotin (mg.)	0.05	0.15	0.3	0.3
Pantothenic acid (mg.)	3	5	10	10

*Whenever nutrition labeling is required.

assisting the consumer in understanding and using the information provided. At the present time many fresh foods will not contain nutrition labeling so that an equal amount of emphasis by the nutrition educator will have to be placed on the nutritive values of these foods if the homemaker is to select an adequate diet for herself and her family.

DIETARY SUPPLEMENT AND DRUG PROPOSAL. According to a recent FDA proposal, any food product to which one or more nutrients is added in amounts equal to 50 percent or more of the US-RDA per serving must be labeled "dietary supplement." If this proposal becomes effective, it would make the consumer aware of the fact that she is getting a large amount of a specific nutrient or nutrients; the decision to select such a food could be based on the need for the nutrient.

In addition, any food or pill which has a nutrient or nutrients added in amounts over 150 percent of the US-RDA would be classified as a drug and subject to the laws governing drugs. There has been considerable controversy over this proposal, and the nutrition educator should be alert to the final action taken.

Nutritional Guidelines for Classes of Food

At the present time the FDA is in the process of deciding the various classes of food for which nutritional guidelines will be determined. The first guidelines established were for frozen "heat-and-serve" dinners. In order to state on the label that it "provides nutrients in amounts appropriate for this class of food as determined by the U.S. Government" a dinner must contain at least the following items:

1. One or more sources of protein derived from meat, poultry, fish, cheese, or eggs. These sources, excluding their sauces, gravies, etc., must provide at least 70 percent of the total protein in the frozen dinner.
2. One or more vegetables or vegetable mixtures other than potatoes, rice, or cereal-based product.

Table 14-3. FDA Guidelines for Nutrients in Frozen "Heat-and-Serve" Dinners

NUTRIENT	FOR EACH 100 CAL. OF THE TOTAL COMPONENTS	FOR THE TOTAL COMPONENTS
Protein, g.	4.60	16.0
Vitamin A, IU	150.00	520.0
Thiamine, mg.	0.05	0.2
Riboflavin, mg.	0.06	0.2
Niacin, mg.	0.99	3.4
Pantothenic acid, mg.	0.32	1.1
Vitamin B_6, mcg.	0.15	0.5
Vitamin B_{12}, mcg.	0.33	1.1
Iron, mg.	0.62	2.2

3. Potatoes, rice, or cereal-based product (other than bread or rolls).

Frozen dinners that comply must provide at least the quantities of nutrients in Table 14-3 for each 100 calories or for the total of the three major components, whichever is greater.

Other Laws Administered by the Food and Drug Administration

THE RADIATION CONTROL FOR HEALTH AND SAFETY ACT protects the public from unnecessary exposure to radiation from medical x-ray and electronic products such as microwave ovens.

THE PUBLIC HEALTH SERVICE ACT regulates the sanitary practices of interstate carriers, and provides for a sanitation program to control public health problems associated with the production, processing, and distribution of products by the food service, milk, and shellfish industry.

THE TEA IMPORTATION ACT regulates the quality of imported tea.

THE MILK IMPORT ACT demands certification that imported milk products meet U.S. requirements.

U.S. Public Health Service

Standards have been established for the chemical quality of drinking water by the U.S. Public Health Service.[8] The toxic or other physiological effects from ingestion of excessive quantities of given substances are outlined, and limits for their permissible concentration in drinking water are indicated. The chemicals listed include alkyl benzene sulfonate (detergent), arsenic, barium, cadmium, carbon-chloroform extract, chloride, chromium, copper, cyanide, fluoride, iron, lead, manganese, nitrate, phenols, selenium, silver, sulfate, zinc, and total dissolved solids.[9]

Traces of these chemicals and others can get into food in dangerous amounts through ignorance or accident in the home: antimony, cadmium, mercury, insecticides, detergents, kerosene, lye, washing soda, and silver polish, to name the more obvious. The swallowing of poisons is a common cause of death among children in the United States. It is imperative that poisonous chemicals be plainly marked and kept as far as possible from food supplies.

Federal Trade Commission

False advertising of foods, drugs, and cosmetics through media such as television and radio is under the jurisdiction not of the FDA but of the Federal Trade Commission.

U.S. Department of Agriculture

FEDERAL MEAT INSPECTION ACT. Through the Bureau of Animal Industry (BAI), the Secretary of Agriculture administers regulations concerning the meat industry. Formerly, laws provided for the inspection of all cattle, sheep, swine, and goats slaughtered for transportation or sale as articles of interstate or foreign commerce. A law passed in late 1967 provides for similar inspection and regulation of all meats sold for human consumption anywhere in the United States. The carcasses and parts of all such animals found to be sound, healthful, wholesome, and fit for human food are stamped "Inspected and Passed." Animals found to be unfit for human food are separated and stamped "Inspected and Condemned." Carcasses which have been condemned for food purposes must be destroyed under the supervision of a federal inspector.

The Secretary of Agriculture also enforces the regulations concerning imported and exported meat and meat products, as well as those concerning the labeling of horsemeat. Horsemeat may be used for human food, but strict labeling is required to prevent its use as a substitute for beef.

A law passed in 1957 provides for compulsory inspection of poultry and poultry products and is similar in nature to the Meat Inspection Act.

USDA GRADE STANDARDS AND INSPECTION SERVICE FOR PROCESSED FOODS. The Fruit and Vegetable Division of the Agricultural Marketing Service, United States Department of Agriculture, develops grade standards for processed foods and supplies an inspection service for processed fruits, vegetables, and related foods.

The federal grading of foods aids in informing processors, sellers, brokers, distributors, and buyers concerning the class, the quality, and the condition of the product. The grades serve as a basis for arriving at a value of the product for purposes of securing a loan, payment of damages, or sale of the product.

State Regulations

It is the responsibility of the states to regulate food production and processing of certain products which do not leave the state. The state also controls such things as pasteurization of milk, inspection of cattle and goats for brucellosis and tuberculosis, and regulations concerning the sale of margarine. Many state food regulations are similar to the federal regulations, but others may prohibit some things which are allowed by federal law. Food processors must satisfy the regulations of the state in which they operate and the states in which the food is sold, as well as the

federal regulations. Oregon is the first state to adopt regulations defining organic foods. In New York, mandatory unit pricing of most food items sold in large-volume retail stores began in 1975.

Local municipal sanitary codes may also regulate food production and processing to the extent that they may be more restrictive than state or federal codes, but not less so.

STUDY QUESTIONS AND ACTIVITIES

1. List three techniques that are used in scientific farming to increase food production. How is the safety of these methods regulated to protect the consumer?
2. Which foodborne bacteria, carried most often in eggs or poultry, have been responsible for recent outbreaks of gastrointestinal disease?
3. What disease carried by water, milk, or food is due to a virus? How long after exposure may it take to develop?
4. Name some of the activities of the FDA stemming from the Federal Food, Drug and Cosmetic Act.
5. What is meant by standards of identity? What implications are there for the nutrition counselor in relation to labeling and standards of identity?
6. What types of food additives may be considered "intentional"? Why are they used and how are they controlled?
7. How would you answer someone who questioned the safety of the many additives foods contain today? Of the use of pesticides and the danger of traces of these being present in food?
8. What labeling procedures must be followed as a result of the "truth in packaging" law?
9. What is nutrition labeling? What is the standard reference for nutrition labeling?

SUPPLEMENTARY READINGS

Beloian, A.: Nutrition labels: A great leap forward. FDA Consumer, Sept. 1974.

Coon, J. M.: Natural food toxicants—a perspective. Nutr. Rev. 32:321, 1974.

Eyl, T. B.: Alkyl mercury contamination of foods. JAMA 215:287, 1971.

Food and Drug Administration: Fact Sheets (available from FDA consumer representative). U.S. Department HEW, Washington, D.C.

Hodges, R. E.: The toxicity of pesticides and their residues in food. Nutr. Rev. 23:225, 1965.

Moore, J. L., and Wendt, P. F.: Nutrition labeling—a summary and evaluation. J. Nutr. Educa. 5:121, 1973.

Public Health Service, U.S. Department HEW: You Can Prevent Foodborne Illness. Folder, 1967. Hot Tips on Food Protection. Folder, 1966. Government Printing Office, Washington, D.C. 20201.

Pyke, M.: Food technology and society. Nutr. Rev. 28:31, 1970.

Scientific Status Summary by the Institute of Food Technologists' Expert Panel on Food Safety and Nutrition. Chicago. Botulism, 1972; Mercury in food, 1973; Nitrites, nitrates and nitrosamines in food—a dilemma, 1972; Nutrition labeling, 1973.

For further references see Bibliography in Section 4.

REFERENCES

1. Mehrlich, F. P.: *Protecting Our Food.* Yearbook of Agriculture, Washington, D.C., U.S. Department of Agriculture, 1966, p. 204.
2. Labuza, T. P.: Food Tech. 27:20, 1973.
3. Ibid.
4. Werrin, M., and Kronick, D.: Am. J. Nurs. 65:528, 1965.
5. Note. Nutr. Rev. 25:94, 1967.
6. Keenan, J.: FDA consumer (Nov.) 1974, p. 18.
7. IFT Expert Panel on Food Safety and Nutrition: *Nitrites, Nitrates and Nitrosamines in Food—a Dilemma.* Chicago, Institute of Food Technologists, 1972.
8. U.S. Public Health Service: J. Am. Water Works A. 53:935, 1961.
9. Wright, C. V.: Public Health Rep. 77:628, 1962.

application of nutrition
to critical periods
throughout the life span

15

growth and development

Relationship of Nutrition to the Growth Process
The Growth Cycle
Nutrition in Brain Development and Behavior

RELATIONSHIP OF NUTRITION TO THE GROWTH PROCESS

The terms "growth" and "development" imply all the complex physiological changes which take place during conception (when a single-celled ovum is fertilized by a single sperm), during embryogenesis (as cells divide and differentiate to form the structures of the fetus), and during fetal life (as growth and maturation of the fetus occur). These terms also apply to the complex physiological, psychological, and sociological changes which take place during infancy, throughout childhood and adolescence, and into young adulthood.

Growth and development depend on both the genetic or hereditary background of the individual and the physical and cultural environment into which he is born. The food which provides the nutrients required for physical growth is one environmental factor essential for growth and development, while the feeding process itself, at least during infancy and childhood, is an integral part of psychosocial development. A poor environment—for example, one providing inadequate nutrition—can prevent an individual from reaching his full genetic potential not only in terms of physical size and strength but also, according to all indications of contemporary research, in terms of cognitive development as well.

Growth

Growth occurs continuously from conception to full maturity, but it is not a uniform process. It consists of two periods of rapid growth separated by a period of more or less uniform but slower increase in size. The first period of rapid growth occurs in fetal life and early infancy, the second during adolescence.

Physical growth may be defined as an increase in the size of an individual as measured by changes in weight and/or height. It is an exceedingly complicated process brought about by an increase in the number of cells as a result of cell division and by the enlarging of the size of cells from increases in their protein content. Winick discusses four phases of normal growth:

1. Hyperplasia: rapid cell division with cell size remaining constant. The cell number is determined by measuring the total amount of DNA in an organ and dividing it by the DNA content per diploid cell for the particular species (6.0 picograms (pg) in the human).

2. Hypertrophy: an increase in cell size accompanied by a slowing down of cell division. Cell size increases due to an increase in protein content. The average weight per cell or protein content per cell is determined by weighing the organ or by determining its total protein content and then dividing by the number of cells.

3. Cessation of cell division while individual cells continue to grow from increased protein content.

4. Cessation of growth (maturity) as protein synthesis and degradation come into equilibrium.[1]

Both animal research and limited studies of humans have shown that different organs are at various phases of growth at different times. However, during prenatal life and for variable periods into postnatal life, all organs are undergoing cell division. Growth by cell division in the human brain begins to slow down at birth but continues until about 10 months of age. Hypertrophy, increase in size of cells, continues after hyperplasia ceases. (The relationship of nutrition to mental development will be discussed later in this chapter.) Nerve and lymphoid tissue grow most rapidly in the early years, the body as a whole more slowly; genital tissues remain almost dormant until puberty. Figure 15–1 shows the different rates of growth for various body tissues.

Obesity in adults may well be related to these phases of growth. There is evidence that infants who are overnourished at the stage when adipose tissue cells are rapidly increasing accumulate more fat cells in their bodies than infants whose weight gain is more carefully controlled. It is believed that this excess of adipose tissue cells persists throughout life with, of course, persistent problems of overweight.[2,3] Infant feeding is discussed in Chapter 17.

Thus the nutrition counselor should recognize, when working with mothers, that undernutrition or overnutrition during the critical phases of growth for an organ can affect the ultimate number of cells in that organ and this in turn may have permanent effects on its function. If undernutrition or overnutrition occurs at a later phase of growth, the size of the organ may be temporarily smaller or larger but returns to normal when the nutritional needs of the individual are met. The degree of recovery seems to depend on when the damage occurred during the growth process; how long it lasted; and how severe it was. Therefore, malnutrition has the most lasting effects when it occurs early in life, persists over a long period of time, and is severe enough to suggest or require hospitalization.

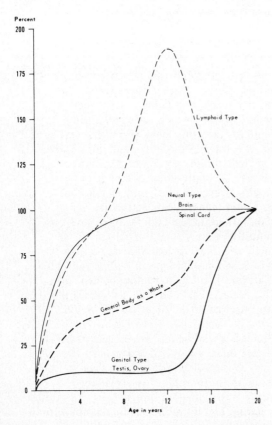

Fig. 15–1. Growth of various body tissues. (Scammon, R. E., *The Measurement of Man*. Minneapolis, University of Minnesota Press)

Development

Development or maturation refers to the progressive increase in the capacity to function both physically and mentally and is closely associated with growth. The growth process or growth cycle as it is used in this chapter refers also to development.

THE GROWTH CYCLE
Fetal Growth During Pregnancy

During the first two months of pregnancy when the cells for the various organs and for the arms, legs, eyes, and ears are differentiating, the growth rate is relatively slow and the quantitative nutritional demands are small. *Qualitatively,* however, they are extremely important. Animal research indicates that severe malnutrition during embryonic development can produce spontaneous abortions or congenital abnormalities in the newborn. Although these findings have not been proven in humans, there remains the implication that, since this critical period occurs at an earlier stage in pregnancy than most women seek medical advice, it is most desirable for young women to acquire good dietary habits before pregnancy.

The next seven months of pregnancy are often referred to as the growth period because the weight of the fetus increases 500-fold, from about 6 g. at 9 weeks to approximately 3500 g. at birth. Skeletal development begins during the second month of intrauterine life and will continue after birth until the end of puberty. Fatty tissue begins to build up by the sixth month. A maternal weight gain of about one-half pound per week is normal during the last two months of gestation. Inadequate nutrition of the fetus during this time may result in stillbirths, prematurity, or "small-for-date" babies. This period of growth, because of its greater nutritional demands, is more sensitive to *quantitative* nutritional inadequacies than the earlier period of differentiation.[4]

Throughout the course of pregnancy there is also growth of the maternal tissue. About half of the weight gained during a normal pregnancy represents increases in the mother's tissues—growth of tissues in the uterus and in the breasts, and the development of the placenta. Nutritional needs during pregnancy are discussed in Chapter 16.

Infancy—Growth and Development During the First Year

Rapid cell division continues into the postnatal period for varying amounts of time for different organs. During the early months of life growth is more rapid than at any other time. Infants will double their birth weight in about five to six months. After that the weekly gain is slower—four to five ounces—for the rest of the year, and they will usually triple the birth weight by the end of the first year.

The infant will grow in length, from 20 to 22 inches at birth to 30 to 32 inches by the end of a year. At birth the head is large in proportion to the rest of the body and will continue to grow. This is the time when the brain and nervous system are developing rapidly, and during this period a supply of essential nutrients is crucial for normal mental development.

The gastrointestinal system of a full-term infant can digest protein, emulsified fats, and simple carbohydrates.

The body of the newborn infant contains a higher proportion of water than that of older children. The muscles are poorly developed and the amount of subcutaneous fat is limited but will increase during the first year. The skeleton is not fully calcified, and there is a high percentage of cartilage. Girls have a greater skeletal maturity at birth than boys by about one month. A full-term infant has a store of iron and a high hemoglobin level—nature's way of providing for the early months on milk which is low in iron. The iron stores are gradually depleted, however, unless either the milk is supplemented with iron in some form or iron-rich foods are added two or three months after birth (see Chapter 17).

Preschool and School Age Growth (One to Nine Years)

Growth during the second year of life slows down, and a weight gain of 8 to 10 pounds is considered average. Thus infants who tripled their weight during the first year will be approximately four times their birth weight at the end of two years. From about two to nine years the average annual weight gain is approximately five pounds.

Annual increments in height gradually decrease from birth to maturity except for the period of the adolescent growth spurt. Birth length is usually doubled by four years. The average gain is about two and one-half inches per year until adolescence.

Body composition changes during childhood; baby fat disappears at the same time that muscles increase in size and bones harden. Body proportions also become more like the adult form as legs lengthen at a rapid rate while head growth decelerates. Motor coordination progresses at a fast rate, as does intellectual development.

The Adolescent Growth Spurt

It is during adolescence that the second very rapid growth period occurs. This is usually between the ages of 10½ and 13 for girls and 13 and 16 for boys, although it may be sooner for early-maturing children and somewhat later for late-maturing children. Girls grow approximately three inches per year, while boys may grow as much as four inches per year during the growth spurt. From ages 13 to 16 years girls continue to grow but at a much slower rate. In contrast, boys' growth rate declines less rapidly and they continue to grow until the late teens.

The growth spurts occur in all directions—in length and weight of bones, in muscle mass, in the laying down of body fat in the soft tissues, in the widening of the shoulders in boys and the broadening of the hips in girls, and in the accelerated growth of genital tissue. Hands and feet are usually the first to grow, followed by hips, chest, and shoulders. By age 10 girls will have undergone a fivefold increase in muscle cell number; further increase in either number or size will be small. Boys, in contrast, at age 18 will have 14 times as many muscle cells as at birth, and they may continue to increase in size for another five years.[5] Girls will have increasingly greater proportions of fat. Increases in height due to lengthening of the long bones, particularly the femur and tibia, occur until the epiphyses of the bones close at the end of puberty.

When the nutrients supplied by the blood stream are inadequate to permit optimum growth of these long bones, merely shorter stature may be found without obvious signs of malnutrition. Protein is essential for the formation of the new cartilage cells in the epiphysis of the long bones which later become calcified to form bone. Evidence that the adolescent growth spurt may be slowed down by nutrient and especially protein limitation has been reported by Mitchell.[6] The changes in stature over 65 years of Japanese youth show a remarkable parallelism with the food limitations during the war years and subsequent increase in consumption of animal protein, which has more than doubled during prosperous years. Fig. 15-2, showing the changes in stature in Japanese boys over a period of 65 years (including World War II and later), seems to show that teenagers were more susceptible than younger children to limitations and more responsive to postwar improvements in food. The response of girls was similar but not quite as striking. The commonly accepted association of calcium with bone growth needs to be supplemented by the concept of the need for good quality protein for the lengthening of bone before calcification occurs.

Biological age at this period is a much better guide to growth and development than is chronological age. The total period of rapid adolescent growth seldom lasts more than two or three years, when adult build and stature are reached. However, growth in skeletal muscle mass continues. A further "lengthening out" may occur in both males and females up to age 30. Garn and Wagner point out that, "In a growth sense, adolescence does not terminate with college entrance but continues well beyond, to age 25 to 30 for muscle mass, to age 30 for stature, to age 30 to 40 for skeletal mass and life long for skeletal volume."[7]

Physical growth is usually measured by changes in height and weight with age. Stature is the more

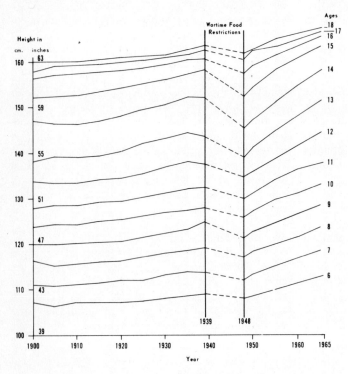

Fig. 15-2. Secular changes in the height of Japanese boys of school age, 1900-1965. (Data from the Japanese Ministry of Education Report for 1965. Tokyo)

significant criterion because variations in build and the amount of adipose tissue may cause wide variations in weight. However, Cheek et al report that the growth of adipose tissue in normal children is so predictable and uniform that weight can be a good measure of "metabolic size" in boys and girls from 5 to 17 years.[8] Development other than physical growth is more difficult to measure: it deals with muscle strength and coordination, with mental health, and with adaptations and attitudes.

NUTRITION IN BRAIN DEVELOPMENT AND BEHAVIOR

One of the most interesting and dramatic aspects of nutrition today is its relationship to brain development in young children. Evidence clearly indicates a close association between severe protein-calorie malnutrition and impaired brain and behavioral development,[9,10,11] but the degree to which malnutrition alone is the cause of depressed cognitive development has not been clearly defined.

The brain and central nervous system grow rapidly during fetal life and early infancy, and by approximately 10 months of age, the total number of cells in the brain has reached its maximum. Different regions of the brain, each made up of their characteristic cell types and each controlling different functions, show their own specific cell division growth patterns. This is followed by myelination of nerve fibers and the establishment of synaptic connections which extend into the third year of life.[12] By the time a child is four years old, some 90 percent of the brain has been formed. Along with the increase in size there is a continuous complex evolution of the anatomy, biochemistry, and physiology of the brain. The formation and functioning of the brain and nerve fibers and the laying down of the myelin sheaths demand that adequate nutrients of the right type be available at this critical period.[13]

During the early formative years as the brain acquires each new specific function it integrates the process into its total pattern of performance and experience. Experimental evidence suggests that the timing of this overall procedure is of utmost importance. Each new function seems to make its appearance chronologically at a critical period of development. Therefore, any disruption of the normal sequence may result in limitation of the capacity of the brain in some specific ability. This damage may not be evident immediately but may show up at a later age.

Studies of the brains of young children who have died of malnutrition and others who died accidentally indicate that severe malnutrition during early life can result in reduced numbers of brain cells in malnourished infants as compared with normal children.[14]

Winick suggests three different effects of malnutrition on brain growth depending on when it occurs:
1. Marked reduction in brain cell number when fetal malnutrition (low-birth-weight infants) and severe malnutrition during the first year of life occur.
2. Moderate reduction in brain cell numbers as a result of severe malnutrition during the first year in normal-birth-weight infants.
3. No reduction in brain cell numbers when malnutrition occurs after the first year, but possible reduction in cell size.[15]

Early malnutrition has also been found to reduce or alter numerous biochemical features as well as the rate of myelin formation.

The significance of the various brain abnormalities and their effects on brain function are not clearly understood. A recent report of the National Research Council summarizes the "possible modes of interference with learning and behavior by malnutrition" as follows:

First, abnormalities of morphologic, biochemical, and/or physiological characteristics may so alter normal brain function as to reduce learning abilities. Secondly, the developmental process may be impaired by decreased exposure and responsiveness to environmental stimuli during critical periods when essential sequences of experience must be acquired to provide for continued orderly development. Third, the learning process may be disrupted by adverse changes in personality, emotionality, and behavior of the child. These changes may interfere with the interpersonal relationships that are necessary for learning experience. Furthermore, malnutrition among the persons in social contact with the child may militate against their providing adequate learning experience.[16]

Thus, the relationship between malnutrition and mental development in humans is extremely complicated because the environment of poverty in which we find severe malnutrition is almost always lacking in those other characteristics which are also important for an individual to reach full mental potential. The disadvantaged child is therefore at high risk not only in terms of limited physical growth but also in regard to psychosocial and cognitive development.

At present, it is impossible to say whether malnutrition, *per se*, contributes more or less to the depressed cognitive development of previously malnourished children than do unfortunate social and environmental conditions. No investigation has completely addressed the question of the relative importance of malnutrition versus social environmental factors in cognitive development; the findings have consistently been that both are significant.[17]

The immediate program of action seems clear. "Every child born alive is entitled to the normal development of his or her physical and mental potentials."[18] Thus Dr. György prefaced his recommendation that a crash program for better nutrition in early childhood be followed by a long-term educational program toward this same goal. As more and more types of intervention programs for the young child are initiated, particularly in infant and child care centers, it is important that the total growth process of the child be considered by those responsible for program planning.[19] Equal emphasis and attention must be given to the physical, emotional, social, and intellectual development of the infant and child. All who are involved in the physical care of infants should understand the intimate relationship between the various components of the developmental process. Cuddling, smiling, and talking to the baby while he is being fed a nutritionally adequate diet all contribute to his total development. Good mothering with the *wrong* diet is just as devastating as poor mothering with the *right* diet. The goal is good mothering with the right diet.

STUDY QUESTIONS AND ACTIVITIES

1. What is meant by physical growth? How is it accomplished?
2. What are the phases of growth? How do these relate to brain size? to obesity?
3. When do the two periods of most rapid growth occur? At what age does muscle mass growth cease?
4. What are the differences in nutritional demands during the two stages of pregnancy: differentiation and growth? What are the effects if these demands are not met?
5. What effect does severe malnutrition during infancy have on brain growth?
6. What kinds of growth occur during adolescence?

SUPPLEMENTARY READINGS

Birch, H. A., and Gussow, J. D.: *Disadvantaged Children— Health, Nutrition and School Failure.* New York, Harcourt Brace Jovanovich, 1970.
Chase, H. P., and Martin, H. P.: Undernutrition and Child Development. N. Eng. J. Med. 282:933, 1970.
Cravioto, J., and DeLicardie, E. R.: The long-term consequences of protein-calorie malnutrition. Nutr. Rev. 29:107, 1971.
Dayton, D. H.: Early malnutrition and human development. Children 16:210 (Nov.-Dec.) 1969.

Dobbing, J., and Sands, J.: Quantitative growth and development of human brain. Arch. Dis. Child. 48:757, 1973.
Food and Nutrition Board: The relationship of nutrition to Brain development and behavior. Washington D.C., National Academy of Sciences—National Research Council, 1973.
Martin, H. P.: Nutrition: Its relationship to children's physical, mental, and emotional development. Am. J. Clin. Nutr. 26:766, 1973.
Nutrition and Cell Growth. Dairy Council Digest, Vol. 41, No. 6 (Nov.-Dec.) 1970.
Review: Growth of the human brain: Some further insights. Nutr. Rev. 33:6, 1975.
Symposium: Nutrition, Growth and Mental Development. Am. J. Dis. Child., 120:395, 1970.
Winick, M.: *Malnutrition and Brain Development.* New York, Oxford University Press, 1976.

For further references see Bibliography in Section 4.

REFERENCES

1. Winick, M.: Food and Nutrition News, Vol. 40, No. 7, (April) 1969.
2. Hirsch, J., and Knittle, J. L.: Fed. Proc. 29:1516, 1970.
3. Eid, E. E.: Brit. Med. J. 2:74, 1970.
4. Giroud, A.: *The Nutrition of the Embryo.* Springfield, Ill., Thomas, 1970.
5. How Children Grow. NIH-PHS DHEW Publ. No. (NIH) 73-166, Washington D.C., 1973.
6. Mitchell, H. S.: J. Am. Dietet. A. 44:165, 1964.
7. Garn, S. M., and Wagner, B.: The adolescent growth of the skeletal mass and its implications to mineral requirements. Chap. 11 in *Adolescent Nutrition and Growth*, F. Heald, ed. New York, Appleton-Century Crofts, 1969.
8. Cheek, D. B. et al: Body composition: anthropometric growth and heat production. Chap. 12 in *Adolescent Nutrition and Growth*, F. Heald, ed. New York, Appleton-Century Crofts, 1969.
9. Cravioto, J., and DeLicardie, E.: Am. J. Dis. Child. 120:404, 1970.
10. Chase, H. P., and Martin H. P.: N. Eng. J. Med. 282:933, 1970.
11. Yatkin, U. S., and McLaren, D. S.: J. Ment. Defic. Res. 14:25, 1970.
12. Nutr. Rev. 33:6, 1975.
13. Coursin, D. B.: Undernutrition and brain function. Borden's Rev. Nutr. Res. 26:1, 1965.
14. Rosso, P., Hormazabal, J., and Winick, M.: Am. J. Clin. Nutr. 23:1275, 1970.
15. Winick, M.: Med. Clin. N. Am. 17:69, 1970.
16. Food and Nutrition Board: The relationship of nutrition to brain development and behavior. Washington, D.C., National Academy of Sciences—National Research Council, 1973.
17. Ibid.
18. György, P.: Am. J. Clin. Nutr. 14:65, 1964.
19. Dibble, M. V., and Lally, J. R.: J. Nutr. Ed. 5:200, 1973.

nutrition in pregnancy and lactation

16

NUTRITIONAL DEMANDS OF PREGNANCY

Pregnancy makes many demands on the prospective mother, not the least of which are her nutritional needs and those of the unborn infant. Although an undernourished mother may produce a healthy child, studies of nutrition of women during pregnancy have shown a definite relationship between the diet of the mother and the condition of the baby at birth. These studies have also shown that some of the complications of pregnancy, such as anemia, toxemia, and premature delivery, may result from a diet inadequate for the nutritional needs of the mother and the baby. Moreover, if the mother has always eaten a diet adequate in all essentials and is in good health, she has a much better chance of bearing a healthy baby than does the mother who has consistently had a poor food intake.

The Teen-Age Mother

In the United States there are approximately 200,000 babies born each year to teen-age mothers 17 years of age and younger. These young mothers represent a high-risk population because there are more cases of toxemia and an increased number of

237

premature deliveries and low-birth-weight infants in this age group. It has been found that preeclampsia and essential hypertension occur more often in the white teen-age patients than in patients between 21 and 25 years of age. Weight gain over 25 pounds is more common in the young black girls and anemia and essential hypertension are frequent complications in this group.

The percentage of low-birth-weight babies (under 2500 g.) born to young teen-age mothers is considerably higher than those born to more mature mothers. The highest percentage of low-birth-weight infants were born to nonwhite mothers under 15 years of age. Infant mortality rates are also higher for infants born to young mothers, particularly to young girls who have had repeated pregnancies.

Many of these teen-age pregnancies occur out of wedlock. Society has imposed certain stigmas upon them and has developed punitive attitudes toward them. The pregnant teen-ager often has to drop out of school; she may be shunned by her family and may find medical care difficult to obtain. Hence, many young people do not have the guidance of a physician or a prenatal clinic early in their pregnancy, and adequate counseling often comes too late for the prevention of complications. To help solve these problems many communities have introduced health and education programs to meet the particular needs of the pregnant adolescent. The Consortium on Early Childbearing and Childrearing, a federally funded project under the auspices of the Child Welfare League of America, provides through its publication "Sharing" information about these programs and related research.

Nutritional requirements for the adolescent during pregnancy vary widely, depending on the rate of growth and stage of maturation of the expectant mother. Early-maturing girls who reach menarche at the peak of their growth spurt may conceive before their skeletal, including pelvic, maturation has been completed. Because calorie requirements parallel the growth curve (Figs. 18–3 and 18–4), these girls have high caloric needs. Protein and calcium requirements are also high. Calorie restrictions imposed on these teen-agers may not only affect the birth weight of their infants but their own adult stature. Approximately 10 to 12 percent of pregnant teen-agers are overweight and an equal number are underweight. Even for the obese teen-ager who must meet her own nutritional demands as well as those of the fetus, some weight gain should be allowed during pregnancy.[1] The special care that should be given to the diet plans for these young girls is discussed later in this chapter.

Nutrition Studies in Pregnancy

The effect of food intake on the condition of the newborn is best illustrated by the now classic studies of Burke and her coworkers at the Harvard School of

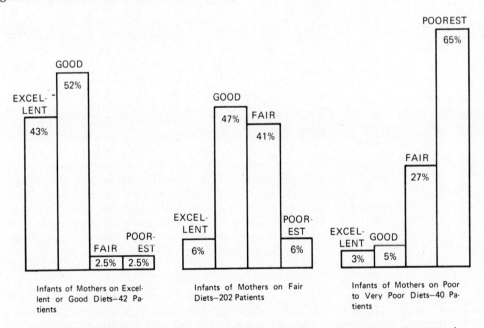

Fig. 16–1. Condition of infants at birth in relation to the prenatal diet of the mother. Note the decrease in excellent and good ratings for infants and the increase in fair and poorest infants as the diet goes from good to poor. (Adapted from Burke, B. S., et al, J. Nutrition 38:453, 1949)

Public Health and the Boston Lying-In Hospital.[2] Figure 16–1 shows the relationship of the mother's diet to the health of the baby. In a study of 284 women, it was found that those on good or excellent diets (42 mothers) had babies in good or excellent condition at birth, with only two exceptions. The mothers on fair diets (202 patients) had babies rated largely as good or fair. Those mothers on poor to very poor diets (40 patients) had babies rated as fair or poorest, with only three exceptions. The poorest infants were those who were stillborn or born prematurely, who died within three days of birth, who had congenital defects, or who were functionally immature.

The question sometimes is asked, What is meant by a "poor" diet? Such a diet is usually low in most necessary food nutrients; there may even be one food group, such as milk, entirely missing. An example is that of a young, pregnant woman, living in a housing development, whose husband leaves for work early. Usually she gets up and joins him in a cup of coffee and a piece of Danish pastry for breakfast. In the morning and again in the afternoon she visits her neighbors, at which time more pastry and coffee are consumed. Often she is not hungry at lunch, nor does she enjoy preparing food only for herself, so that frequently lunch either is skipped or takes the form of a piece of fruit. Fortunately, she may have a good dinner when her husband returns in the evening, but this is not sufficient to meet her nutritional needs, except perhaps for calories. Another person drank up to 15 cups of tea daily, each with 2 teaspoonfuls of sugar, and consequently was seldom hungry for other food.

It will be seen from the foregoing that the importance of nutrition in pregnancy is poorly recognized by a large section of the population, and that nutrition counselors, as well as many others in the medical field, must assume more responsibility for teaching this group better nutrition.

Nutritional Requirements

Table 16–1 shows the Recommended Dietary Allowances for girls and women at various ages with added allowances for pregnancy. The RDA will vary with the weight, the age, and the activity of the woman and should be used only as a guide.

CALORIES. If the physical activity of the woman remains the same during the second and third trimesters of pregnancy, an additional 300 calories daily is suggested to meet the gross energy cost of 80,000 kcal.

Table 16–1. Recommended Daily Dietary Allowances for Girls and Women at Various Ages, with Added Allowances for Pregnancy*

	RECOMMENDED DAILY ALLOWANCES FOR NONPREGNANT WOMEN				RECOMMENDED DAILY ALLOWANCES ADDED FOR PREGNANCY
	11-14[a] years old	15-18[b] years old	19-22[c] years old	23-50[d] years old	
Calories (kcal.)	2400	2100	2100	2000	300
Protein (g.)	44	48	46	46	30
Vitamin A (IU)	4000	4000	4000	4000	1000
(RE)	800	800	800	800	200
Vitamin D (IU)	400	400	400		e
Vitamin E (IU)	12	12	12	12	3
Ascorbic acid (mg.)	45	45	45	45	15
Folacin (mcg.)	400	400	400	400	400[f]
Niacin (mg.)	16	14	14	13	2
Riboflavin (mg.)	1.3	1.4	1.4	1.2	0.3
Thiamine (mg.)	1.2	1.1	1.1	1.0	0.3
Vitamin B_6 (mg.)	1.6	2.0	2.0	2.0	0.5
Vitamin B_{12} (mcg.)	3	3	3	3	1
Calcium (mg.)	1200	1200	800	800	400
Phosphorus (mg.)	1200	1200	800	800	400
Iodine (mcg.)	115	115	100	100	g
Iron (mg.)	18	18	18	18	h
Magnesium (mg.)	300	300	300	300	150
Zinc (mg.)	15	15	15	15	5

*Adapted from Food and Nutrition Board: Recommended Dietary Allowances. Washington, D.C., National Academy of Sciences — National Research Council, 1974.

[a] Weight, 44 kg.; height, 155 cm.
[b] Weight, 54 kg.; height, 162 cm.
[c] Weight, 58 kg.; height, 162 cm.
[d] Weight, 58 kg.; height, 162 cm.
[e] 400 IU of vitamin D is recommended for the pregnant adult woman.
[f] The diet may be supplemented with 200 to 400 mcg. of folacin daily.
[g] 125 mcg. of iodine per day is recommended for pregnancy.
[h] It is recommended that the diet be supplemented with 30 to 60 mg. of iron per day.

for a nine-month pregnancy. The building of new tissue in the woman, the placenta, and the fetus, an increased work load associated with the activity of the woman, and an increased basal metabolic rate contribute to increased energy needs. However, decreased physical activity, particularly during the third trimester, may more than compensate, to the point that no additional calories may be needed. Blackburn and Calloway state:

> If a pregnant woman's occupation involves externally paced work, such as on an assembly line or with a production quota, her energy expenditure will increase according to the increment in body weight. Left to her own inclination a pregnant woman will slow her pace so that she works at a comfortable rate; her daily energy expenditure will be greater, equal to, or less than her non-pregnant level according to the use to which she puts the excess time left after performing a fixed number of tasks.[3]

Although the pregnant adolescents in this study were extremely sedentary, many pregnant women today are employed in strenuous occupations, in addition to their household work. Many are also actively involved in the care of small children. The physician, by carefully observing weight changes, is best able to recommend necessary calorie modifications. For adequate protein utilization, energy intake should not go below 36 kcal./kg. of pregnant body weight. In any case the calorie increase is small, and food must be carefully chosen if the other nutrient increases are to be met while keeping the total calories within the recommended allowance. Table 16–2 shows a suggested dietary pattern during pregnancy.

PROTEIN REQUIREMENT. The protein intake must be increased in pregnancy because of its specific contributions to growth and because, as a rule, a diet low in protein is lacking in other nutrients.

Studies indicate that approximately 925 g. of protein are deposited in the fetus and accessory tissues of the woman. The amount increases throughout successive quarters of pregnancy as follows: 0.6, 1.8, 4.8, and 6.1 g. per day.[4] There is also evidence that during early pregnancy protein may be stored in maternal tissue and used later when the needs for growth of the fetus are greatest. An additional allowance of 30 g. of protein is therefore recommended to provide the protein which is accumulated by the fetus and accessory tissues during pregnancy.

Extra protein in the diet will be supplied by additional milk, meat, poultry, fish, and eggs (Table 16–2). Skim milk, liquid or dried, can be used to increase protein without adding considerably to the total calorie intake. Inexpensive dried skim milk can be used in creamed soups and casserole dishes; 1 or 2 tablespoons can also be added to regular milk to increase the protein content. Sample menus which meet the recommended dietary allowances for pregnancy are shown in Table 16–3.

CALCIUM AND PHOSPHORUS REQUIREMENTS. The pregnant woman must be supplied with calcium and phosphorus in quantities large enough for her own needs and those of the bony framework of the body of the growing fetus and for the formation of its teeth. Approximately 25 g. of calcium are found in the full-term infant, most of which (200 to 300 mg. daily) is deposited during the last trimester. In addition, the mother may store calcium in her own body as a reserve for the high demands of lactation. An additional allowance of 0.4 g. of calcium and phosphorus per day is recommended at this time. Again, a quart of milk a day will supply a large proportion of the needed calcium and phosphorus, as well as a good proportion of the necessary protein.

MAGNESIUM REQUIREMENT. The NRC-RDA recommends an additional 150 mg. of magnesium per day during pregnancy. The additional milk, plus the meat, whole-grain cereals, vegetables, and fruit will supply the extra amount.

IRON REQUIREMENT. An adequate iron supply during pregnancy is no less important than that of calcium. Besides the woman's need for iron, the developing fetus is building its own blood supply. When the baby is born its blood has a hemoglobin content of from 20 to 22 g. per 100 ml. This high level is needed in fetal life for oxygen uptake at the placenta, where oxygen is at lower pressures than it is in the lungs. Soon after birth some of the hemoglobin begins to break down until a normal level of 13 to 14 g.

Table 16–2. Suggested Dietary Pattern During Pregnancy

Whole or skimmed milk: 1 qt. (1 oz. of cheddar cheese is equivalent to 8 oz. milk).

Lean meat, fish, poultry, eggs, dried peas, beans, and nuts: One liberal or two small servings (4 oz.) of meat, fish, or poultry; liver is desirable at least once each week. One egg equals approximately one-half of a small serving. Dried peas, beans, or nuts may be used as meat substitutes.

Fruit: Two or more servings (1 cup, 200 g.) each day. One serving should be citrus fruit or other good source of ascorbic acid.

Vegetables: Two or more servings of cooked or raw vegetables (1-1½ cups, 200-300 g.) each day; these should include dark green leafy or deep yellow vegetables; in addition, a medium potato (150 g.) should be eaten daily.

Bread and cereal: Whole-grain or enriched bread, at least 4 slices daily (½ cup of cereal is equivalent to 1 slice of bread).

Butter or margarine: One to 2 tablespoons.

Additional foods: Consisting of either more of the foods already listed or other foods of one's own choice adjusted to individual energy needs and in relation to desired weight gain.

Vitamin D: Some form of vitamin D to supply 400 IU such as 1 qt. of milk would supply.

Table 16–3. Sample Menus for Pregnancy

FOR PREGNANT WOMEN OF NORMAL WEIGHT	FOR PREGNANT ADOLESCENT GIRLS OF NORMAL WEIGHT
Breakfast	**Breakfast**
Orange juice—4 oz.	Orange juice—4 oz.
Scrambled egg	Cornflakes or grits
Toast—1 slice	Scrambled egg
Butter or margarine	Toast—1 slice
Coffee	Milk—½ pint
Midmorning	**Midmorning**
Milk—½ pint	Milk—½ pint
Lunch	**Lunch**
Meat, cheese, or peanut butter sandwich	Hamburger on a bun
Carrot sticks	Cole slaw
Oatmeal cookies	Oatmeal cookies
Milk—½ pint	Milk—½ pint
Midafternoon	**Midafternoon**
Milk—½ pint	Frankfurter on a bun
	Milkshake or fruit juice—½ pint
Dinner	**Dinner**
Roasted or broiled beef, pork, liver, or fish	Roasted or broiled beef, pork, liver, or fish
Broccoli or greens	Broccoli or greens
Baked potato	Baked or french-fried potatoes
Butter or margarine	Butter or margarine
Green salad with French dressing	Green salad with French dressing
Fresh or canned fruit	Fruit
Coffee, tea, or milk	Milk—½ pint
Bedtime	**Bedtime**
Milk or cocoa—½ pint	Fruit juice or cocoa—½ pint

per 100 ml. of blood is reached. The iron from the hemoglobin breakdown is stored in the infant's liver to serve as a supply during the first few months of life when the diet of milk provides little iron. If the woman's intake of iron is low, this will reflect itself in the level of her own hemoglobin and, eventually, in the level of hemoglobin and iron available for storage in the infant.

Foods especially high in iron, such as livers of beef, chicken, and pork, should be included frequently in the pregnant woman's diet. Other good sources are heart, kidney, tongue, all lean meats, chicken, eggs, most green, leafy vegetables, potatoes, whole-grain or enriched bread, dried fruits, and dried peas and beans. It is not always easy to include sufficient iron in the daily diet, especially in the low-income group. The physician may prescribe some type of supplementary source of iron. Because of the difficulty of obtaining a sufficient intake of iron from food alone, the National Reseach Council's Committee on Maternal Nutrition recommends that the diet of the pregnant woman be supplemented with 30 to 60 mg. of iron per day as medication.

IODINE REQUIREMENT. Iodine is also an important element in the diet of the pregnant woman. An additional 25 mcg. of iodine per day is recommended for a woman over 18 during pregnancy. A deficiency of this element during pregnancy may cause goiter in the child or in the woman. The use of iodized salt is suggested for those who live in areas in which the soil and the drinking water are known to be deficient in iodine.

ZINC REQUIREMENT. An additional 5 mg. of zinc per day is recommended during pregnancy to meet the needs of the fetus and maternal tissue. Meat, poultry, dry beans, eggs, and milk are good sources of zinc.

VITAMIN REQUIREMENTS. All vitamins are essential for the metabolism of living tissue, and doubly so in growth.

Foods rich in vitamins are those which have been discussed as essential for other nutrients: milk and milk products, eggs, meat, fish and poultry, and especially liver, whole-grain and enriched breads, green and yellow vegetables, citrus fruits, tomatoes, cabbage, and potatoes. All these must be supplied liberally in the diet of the pregnant woman if she is to meet her own nutritional needs as well as those of the growing fetus.

The proper utilization of calcium and phosphorus depends on the inclusion of a certain amount of vitamin D in the diet. Most areas today offer both whole and skim fluid milk to which 400 IU of vitamin D per quart has been added. Some physicians order vitamin D for their patients as a medication, although not all obstetricians subscribe to this practice. Because of recent evidence indicating a relationship between abnormal calcium deposition in infants and excessive vitamin D intakes during pregnancy, the pregnant woman should be cautioned against overdosage with supplements.

Mineral oil in any form interferes with the absorption of the fat-soluble vitamins and should be avoided.

In addition to increased amounts of vitamin A,

vitamin E, thiamine, riboflavin, niacin, vitamins B_6 and B_{12}, and ascorbic acid (Table 16-1), the pregnant woman may require a daily supplement of 0.2 to 0.4 mg. of folacin to protect the fetus and provide for the maternal organism.

The use of vitamin supplements (except for folic acid and possibly vitamin D) is not necessary unless, because of illness or other problems, the woman is unable to eat an adequate diet. The physician is best able to determine whether or not supplements are needed.

FOOD SELECTION IN PREGNANCY

Table 16-2 lists the foods and the quantities of each that, if consumed daily by the pregnant woman, will meet the Recommended Dietary Allowances except for iron and folic acid. Such a food intake represents the so-called excellent diet found by investigators to be most likely to produce a superior infant and to maintain the woman's health at an optimum. Routine salt restriction or too rigid weight control should not be necessary if the pregnancy is proceeding normally.

Two menus based on the foregoing table, one for adult pregnant women and one for pregnant adolescent girls, are presented in Table 16-3. It is assumed that both groups are of normal weight. Note that calories and calcium have been increased in the menu for pregnant adolescent girls to provide for their own growth needs and those of the fetus.

Adaptations for Cost and Food Habit Patterns

It may be difficult for the woman to follow the suggested diet pattern if she has a strong dislike for a food such as milk or liver, if her food habits are culturally very different, or, most frequent of all, if the cost of the diet is higher than she can afford. However, some adaptations can be made without impairing the nutritive value of the diet too greatly. The use of dried skim milk for part or all of the whole milk will lower the cost substantially. The use of chocolate and coffee flavor, a dash of vanilla extract or of cinnamon or nutmeg may change the taste of milk sufficiently so that the woman will drink it. Some women who do not like whole milk because it makes them "sick" may be able to drink buttermilk. Milk, either fluid or dried, may be used in desserts, creamed soups, and scalloped dishes. As has already been indicated, a 1-ounce slice of cheddar (hard) cheese has approximately the same protein and calcium content as an 8-ounce glass of milk. This may be an acceptable substitute for those who use cheese somewhat more

readily than large quantities of milk. Liver, another food sometimes heartily disliked, may be eaten as liverwurst or as a liver spread in a sandwich, or it may be disguised in a variety of ways in cooked dishes.

In general, meat and eggs are expensive foods. Dried beans and peas, used by many groups in the United States as well as in many other countries, serve as a partial substitute at lower cost. However, they must not replace the use of animal protein to too great a degree, for the legumes do not supply as good a quality of protein. Fish and eggs are excellent meat substitutes in areas and at times of year when they are cheap.

Fruits and vegetables, bought fresh in season, are usually least expensive. However, the frozen fruit juices, especially orange and grapefruit juice, and canned tomato juice are comparatively inexpensive sources of vitamin C all year round. In the Southeastern section of the United States, the frequent use of greens with their accompanying "pot liquor" provides a considerable source of calcium and vitamin C in the diet. Carrot sticks and celery strips, stored in the refrigerator, will provide a low-calorie snack to satisfy the craving for nibbling and at the same time help to meet the vegetable requirements.

Desserts made from milk, eggs, and fruit, unsweetened or flavored with noncaloric sweetening, give a psychological "lift" to the pregnancy woman.

Pica

An abnormal craving for nonfood substances (pica), such as starch and clay, has been reported by certain women during pregnancy. This practice appears to be most prevalent among black women, particularly in the South, where it is often a traditional practice accepted within the immediate community. A study by Edwards and associates in Alabama showed that the caloric intake of pregnant women who consumed starch and clay was reduced when these substances were omitted from the diet, indicating that they were either appetite stimulators or that deprivation of them was so emotionally upsetting as to reduce appetite.[5] In general, the diets of these women tended to be low in protein, iron, and calcium. Although the birth weight and length of the infants born to these mothers were similar to those of the control groups' infants, fewer babies born to the starch- and clay-eating mothers were rated in good condition at birth.

Nutrition Education

The needs of pregnant girls or women for nutrition information will vary. The mother having her second or third baby who feeds her family with good judgment will probably do the same for herself. All she may need is a review of dietary essentials with perhaps some suggestions for the less costly foods if her income is limited. On the other hand, a mother with a large family and a low income may need considerable guidance in wise spending. National and cultural dietary patterns will influence the choice of foods in many families and need to be reckoned with. Chapters 10 and 13 will be of help in this matter.

The most urgent nutritional problem is that of the very young pregnant woman. It has been said that "nutrition for pregnancy begins before conception," and, above all, this is true of the mother under 20. The diet of many teen-age girls is low in calcium and vitamin C. There is also a tendency to an inadequate iron intake.

The nurse, the dietitian, and the physician will have to use patience, imagination, and persistence in persuading women who are not doing so to follow an adequate diet. The woman who asks for calcium pills because she does not like milk needs to be taught that milk is a rich source of other needed nutrients besides calcium and to be encouraged to use a variety of methods for including it in her diet. On the other hand she may be allergic to milk or lactase deficient and will require calcium pills. The young girl needs help in understanding her body's new needs, and possibly the help of the social worker or community agency in providing a good diet. The use of the attractive health literature available may aid the woman in following an improved diet, both for herself and for her family.[6] It is very possible that the foundation for good nutrition for the whole family may be laid in the obstetrician's office or the prenatal clinic.

COMPLICATIONS OF PREGNANCY INVOLVING DIET

Vomiting

During the first trimester of pregnancy the mother-to-be may be troubled with nausea. Certain foods which previously have been eaten without difficulty now may cause distress. Fats are a common cause of upset. Fluids taken with meals may also precipitate vomiting. Dry toast or a few unsalted crackers eaten before arising may be of help. Fluids should be drunk between meals, not with the meal. Skim milk may be tolerated better than whole milk. Often the nausea disappears by the middle of the day, and the woman can make up her dietary needs by increasing her food intake in the late afternoon, at dinner, and before bedtime.

Vomiting, if it persists and becomes pernicious, should be treated by a physician.

Overweight in Pregnancy

Pregnancy usually is a time of well-being and often is accompanied by an excellent appetite. Most doctors guard against excessive weight gain as being detrimental to both the woman and the fetus. The average weight gain during pregnancy of 24 (20 to 25) pounds includes the following:

Full-term baby	7.7 pounds
Placenta	1.4 pounds
Amniotic and body fluids	1.8 pounds
Enlarged uterus	2.0 pounds
Enlarged breasts	0.9 pounds
Blood volume increase	4.0 pounds
Interstitial body fluids	2.7 pounds
Maternal storage—fat	3.5 pounds

Although a maternal weight gain of 20 to 25 pounds is normal and desirable, especially if the mother is to nurse her infant, if additional weight is gained it usually accrues to the mother's total weight gain and is undesirable except for those women who were underweight before pregnancy. Figure 16-2 shows a pattern of normal prenatal gain in weight. Certain factors contribute to some variability in weight gain. Teen-age mothers tend to slightly higher gains than more mature women; thin women gain more than obese women. Women having their first pregnancy gain more than women having second, third, or fourth babies.

The Committee on Maternal Nutrition has stated the following in relation to nutrition and weight gain during pregnancy:

> An average weight gain during pregnancy of 24 lb. (range 20-25 lb.) is commensurate with a better than average course of pregnancy. This would be a gain of 1.5 to 3.0 lb. during the first trimester and a gain of 0.8 lb. per week during the remainder of pregnancy. There is no scientific justification for routine limitation of weight gain to lesser amounts. . . .

> The pattern of weight gain is of greater importance than the total amount—a sudden sharp increase after about the 20th week of pregnancy may indicate water retention and the possible onset of pre-eclampsia. There is no evidence that the total amount of gain during pregnancy has, per se, any causal relationship to pre-eclampsia.

> Severe caloric restriction, which has been very commonly recommended, is potentially harmful to the developing fetus and to the mother, and almost inevitably restricts other nutrients essential for growth processes. Weight-reduction regimes, if needed, should be instituted only after pregnancy has terminated.[7]

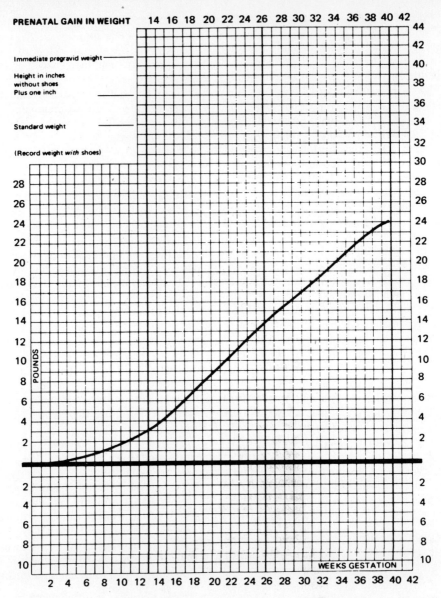

PRENATAL GAIN IN WEIGHT

Immediate pregravid weight ———

Height in inches
without shoes
Plus one inch   ———

Standard weight   ———

(Record weight *with* shoes)

POUNDS

WEEKS GESTATION

Fig. 16-2. Gain in weight grid. Pattern of normal prenatal gain in weight. (U.S. Department HEW, Social and Rehabilitation Service, Children's Bureau)

Care must be taken that any calorie-restricted diet in pregnancy is not so low in calories that the protein in the diet is used partly for energy instead of for growth. Oldham has shown that this occurs when the diet is below 1500 calories, even when the protein of the diet is adequate.[8] Probably no diet in pregnancy should fall below 1500 calories, and it may be more realistic to allow an 1800-calorie diet. If the woman adheres to this, there should be no impairment of her health or the infant's, and her weight gain should remain at a minimum.

If there is a tendency to gain too much weight, such foods as sugar, candy, jelly and other sweets, salad dressings, fried foods, fatty meats, cake, pie, and desserts, and carbonated beverages should be limited or omitted entirely. It may be necessary to limit bread and potatoes; and skim milk may be substituted for whole milk (see Chapter 27).

A problem arises with the person who believes that milk is "fattening" and reduces or omits it in her diet. As explained earlier, the substitution of calcium pills for milk markedly lowers the protein and the vitamin content of the diet and should be discouraged.

Table 16–4. Diets for Pregnancy Varying in Caloric Content*

FOOD	2300 CALORIES	1800 CALORIES	1500 CALORIES
Milk	1 qt. whole	1 qt. whole	1 qt. skimmed
Meat, fish, and poultry	4 oz.	4 oz. lean	4 oz. lean
Eggs	1	1	1
Fruit	1 serving citrus, 1 other	1 serving citrus, 1 other	1 serving citrus, 1 other
Vegetables	4 servings, including potato and dark green leafy or yellow vegetable	4 servings, including potato and dark green leafy or yellow vegetable	4 servings, including potato and dark green leafy or yellow vegetable
Bread and cereals	4 servings whole-grain or enriched	4 servings whole-grain or enriched	4 servings whole-grain or enriched
Butter or margarine	3 teaspoons	3 teaspoons	3 teaspoons
Other foods	Sugar, desserts, fat for cooking; other foods to meet caloric needs	None	None

These diets may be restricted in sodium as follows (see Chapter 30 for details of food restriction):
1. *Moderate sodium restriction*—1000 to 1500 mg. sodium. Prepare all food without salt: do not add salt at table; omit all salted foods such as salted butter and bacon.
2. *Severe sodium restriction*—300 to 400 mg. sodium. Prepare all food without salt; do not add salt at table; omit all salted foods such as salted butter and bacon. Use only low sodium milk. Use only fruit for dessert.

*Adapted from the Woman's Clinic of The New York Hospital. The above diets meet the Recommended Dietary Allowances of the National Research Council for pregnancy with the exception of calories for the 1800- and the 1500-calorie diets and iron in all diets.

Table 16–4 shows a comparison of the recommended diet for pregnancy for a woman of normal weight, containing approximately 2300 calories, and the restrictions necessary to bring this down to 1800 and 1500 calories. All these meet the Recommended Dietary Allowances for specific nutrients, except for calories (in the 1800 and the 1500 calorie diets) and iron. The physician may wish to prescribe folacin and iron supplementation as a precaution against the anemias of pregnancy.

Underweight in Pregnancy

The severely underweight woman and the woman who does not gain normally during her pregnancy are of as great concern as the obese woman. The reason for the underweight may be economic; this may often be discovered by the nutrition worker, who will direct the client to a community agency for help. Supplementary foods for pregnant and lactating women and children under four are available through many health agencies as part of a federally sponsored program for women, infants, and children (WIC). If the cause is psychological—such as a severe depression—or physical, the physician will take the appropriate measures.

Anemias of Pregnancy

In the latter months of pregnancy there may be a slight lowering of the hemoglobin content of the woman's blood due to physiological adjustments. By this time her total blood volume has increased considerably to provide for the placental circulation. This may not be accompanied by a corresponding increase in red blood cells; consequently, a degree of hemodilution occurs. However, it is of slight degree and usually is not mistaken for anemia of pregnancy.

True anemia occurring during pregnancy is due most often to an iron deficiency. Even healthy American women usually do not have iron stores large enough to meet the demands of pregnancy. Iron supplementation will aid greatly in maintaining the hemoglobin at normal levels in these patients. During the second and third trimester of pregnancy, an oral iron supplement of 30 to 60 mg. of ferrous salts is recommended. It is also essential, however, that the woman be urged to include foods rich in iron and protein in her diet, or other deficiencies may appear.

As explained earlier in this chapter, the infant's level of hemoglobin at birth and the supply of iron available for storage for use in the first few months of life are curtailed when the mother's iron intake is inadequate. The result is anemia of infancy, which is not an uncommon finding.

Megaloblastic anemia of pregnancy may be due to poor food intake, vomiting, or the fetal demands for folacin. It is characterized by an extremely low red blood cell count and an equally low hemoglobin and has some other findings associated with pernicious anemia, with which it may be confused. The administration of folic acid causes an immediate and dramatic rise in red blood cells and hemoglobin, and in appetite. Studies indicate that the folic acid requirement during pregnancy is greatly increased as compared with the minimum adult requirement.[9] The Committee on Maternal Nutrition suggests a supplement of 400 mcg. of folacin per day. If the woman does not receive treatment before the birth of the infant, the infant also will show some of the symptoms of megaloblastic anemia. It may be treated with folic acid, or, if the mother is being treated while nursing, the infant will receive enough folic acid from its mother's milk to restore its blood components to normal.

Toxemia of Pregnancy

The cause of toxemia of pregnancy is not known. It is characterized by an elevation in blood pressure, proteinuria, and rapid weight gain due to edema. In the eclamptic stage there may be convulsions and coma. There is considerable controversy over the influence of nutrition on the development of toxemia. Toxemia occurs more frequently in pregnant women on poor diets, and particularly on low protein intakes, than in corresponding groups on good diets. Epidemiologic studies show a direct relationship between the incidence of toxemia and an individual state's per capita income. The poorer the state the greater the number of cases of toxemia reported.[10]

Findings of Burke and Kirkwood show that 44 percent of the women on poor or very poor diets, 8 percent on fair diets, and none on good or excellent diets developed symptoms of toxemia.[11] Tompkins

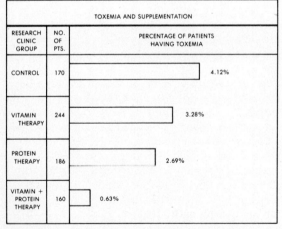

Fig. 16–3. Toxemia and supplementation. (Tompkins, W. T., and Wiehl, D. G., Nutritional deficiencies as a causal factor in toxemia and premature labor. Am. J. Obst. & Gynec. 62:898, 1951)

and Wiehl have shown that supplementation of the diet with protein and vitamins greatly reduced the incidence of toxemia in their patients (see Fig. 16–3).[12] Although McGanity and his group in Nashville, Tenn., were not able to relate nutritional status to health during pregnancy as clearly as other investigators, they do report an increased incidence of toxemia in mothers who ate less than 1500 calories and 50 g. of protein per day during the last trimester.[13] All these findings reinforce what was said earlier in this chapter; we have not so far provided adequate medical care, including nutrition education, for all those requiring such help during pregnancy.

In the past few years a question has arisen about the relation of salt intake to toxemia. Robinson,[14] studying over 2000 pregnant women, advised half to increase their salt intake and half to lower it. He found a lower incidence of toxemia in those having the higher salt intake. Mengert placed 48 patients with proven toxemia either on a high salt intake or on a very low one. No difference in the progress of the disease was noted between the two groups of women in this study.[15] The Committee on Maternal Nutrition discourages the routine use of salt restriction and diuretics during pregnancy.

Cardiac Disease and Pregnancy

It should be remembered that the nutritional requirements of the pregnant woman with cardiac disease are the same as those of the noncardiac pregnant woman. If it is necessary to limit the salt intake, note the suggestions for moderate sodium restriction in the notes given in Table 16–4. The very low sodium diet probably should be reserved for patients being cared for in the hospital.

Diabetes and Pregnancy

Again the diabetic woman's diet must be increased to meet her larger needs and those of the growing fetus. The insulin dosage will have to be augmented accordingly. For further discussion of pregnancy and diabetes see Chapter 28.

DIET DURING LABOR

During the early part of labor, if feeding by mouth is permitted by the physician, the diet should consist mainly of carbohydrates, as they leave the stomach quickly. Protein and fat tend to remain in the stomach considerably longer, which may result in aspiration if anesthesia is given. The diet may be soft or liquid and may include white-bread toast with jelly, soda crackers, canned or cooked fruits, gelatin, fruit juices, ginger ale, broth, and tea or coffee with sugar but no milk or cream. By the time the patient is in active labor, most obstetricians prefer that no food be given by mouth so as to prevent the possibility of vomiting and of aspiration of food into the trachea. Intravenous fluids are given to maintain water balance if labor is prolonged.

DIET FOLLOWING DELIVERY

A liquid diet usually is given for the first meal after delivery. After that, there is a return to the normal diet. If the mother nurses the infant, there must be an even greater allowance of food than there was during pregnancy.

DIET IN LACTATION

Lactation makes even greater demands in some respects on the maternal organism than does pregnancy. After birth the child still may be fed from the mother's body, the food now being produced by the mammary glands instead of being supplied through the bloodstream, as before birth. As the infant gains in weight and becomes increasingly active, the food supply from the mother must increase.

Supply of Mother's Milk

A normal infant will consume daily 2½ ounces of mother's milk for each pound of its weight. An 8-pound infant will consume approximately 20 ounces, while a 15-pound one will consume about 35 ounces. Since human milk has a caloric value of 20 calories per ounce, it will be seen readily that a nursing mother must have several hundred additional calories per day to supply food for the infant.

Dietary Requirements

The recommended dietary allowance for energy for the nursing mother producing 850 ml. of milk daily is 500 additional calories above her normal needs for the first three months of lactation. This recommendation is based on the 80 percent efficiency with which maternal dietary energy is converted into energy in milk. The production of 100 ml. of milk

Table 16–5. Recommended Dietary Allowances for the Lactating Woman 23 to 50 Years, 58 kg., 162 cm.

NUTRIENT	AMOUNT
Energy (kcal.)	2500
Protein	66 g.
Vitamin A	6000 IU (1200 RE)
Vitamin D	400 IU
Vitamin E	15 IU
Ascorbic acid	80 mg.
Folacin	600 mcg.
Niacin	17 mg.
Riboflavin	1.7 mg.
Thiamine	1.3 mg.
Vitamin B_6	2.5 mg.
Vitamin B_{12}	4 mcg.
Calcium	1.2 g.
Phosphorus	1.2 g.
Iodine	150 mcg.
Iron	18 mg.
Magnesium	450 mg.
Zinc	25 mg.

requires approximately 90 kcal. It also takes into account the calories available (200 to 300 per day for 100 days) from the 3.5 pounds of fat stored by the mother who gained 24 pounds during pregnancy. Thus the allowance provides for the production of milk as well as for the readjustment of maternal body fat stores following pregnancy. If lactation continues beyond three months or if the mother's weight falls below ideal weight for height, the mother's energy allowance should be increased.[16]

Besides the increase in energy requirements, there are also increases in the requirements for protein, minerals, and vitamins. To cover the needs of milk production and to allow for 70 percent efficiency of protein utilization, an additional 20 g. of protein is recommended. Increasing maternal protein intake in very poorly nourished mothers has been shown to increase the volume of breast milk produced, while the proximate amount of protein in human milk remains relatively constant.[17] Similarly, vitamins and minerals which will be used in milk production must be supplied in adequate amounts or the mother's own tissues may become depleted. Supplements of vita-

Table 16–6. Sample Menu for a Day for a Lactating Mother

BREAKFAST	LUNCH	DINNER
Orange juice	Vegetable soup	Green salad
Oatmeal or grits with milk	Cottage cheese with fruit salad	Baked ham
Poached egg on toast	Biscuit with butter or margarine	Scalloped potatoes
Milk. Coffee if desired	Gingerbread with topping	Green beans
	Milk. Coffee if desired	Bread with butter or margarine
		Sliced peaches
		Milk. Coffee if desired
Midmorning	Midafternoon	Bedtime
Milk	Fruit juice	Milk

min A, vitamin C, thiamine, and riboflavin given to malnourished mothers have resulted in increased amounts of these nutrients in the milk.[18] Low levels of vitamin B_{12} have been found in the breast milk of Indian women who were lacto-vegetarians.[19] Table 16–5 shows the recommended dietary allowances for the lactating woman.

Between-meal feedings often are advisable during lactation. Plenty of fluids should be taken to replace the water secreted in the milk. A typical sample menu for a day is shown in Table 16–6.

It should be remembered that the mother must return to a normal food intake when she weans the infant or she will gain excess weight.

STUDY QUESTIONS AND ACTIVITIES

1. Even the normal healthy woman who has been eating an adequate diet will require more dietary essentials during pregnancy. Review the Recommended Dietary Allowances for women in various conditions. Which allowances increase in ratio to the energy allowance? What other essentials should be increased during pregnancy?
2. What do nutrition studies show concerning the adequacy of diets in pregnancy of large groups of women in the United States?
3. Give several reasons why the adolescent may have serious nutrition problems in pregnancy. Name some of the ways in which these can be met.
4. Why is the nutrition of the woman previous to pregnancy so important?
5. Discuss the results of an inadequate intake of protein in pregnancy. In what forms may extra protein be added to the diet?
6. The mineral requirement is naturally larger during pregnancy. How may the calcium and the phosphorus requirements be fulfilled? What are the food sources of iron? How may the iodine requirements be met?
7. What danger to the infant may result from nutritional anemia in the mother? Explain.
8. List the foods and the quantity of each that must be included daily in the diet of the pregnant woman.
9. Plan a menu for a day for a healthy pregnant woman of average weight with a limited income.
10. Using Chapter 13 as a guide, write a menu for a day for a pregnant woman with a food pattern not typically American. Be sure that it is adequate for the needs of pregnancy.
11. During the first trimester there may be trouble with nausea. How may the menu be modified to relieve this?
12. If for any reason the quota of fluid milk cannot be taken each day, how may milk be used otherwise in the diet? Suggest appetizing, easily digested dishes which may be used in the menu.
13. During the third trimester toxemia may appear. Is there anything to indicate that diet may act as a preventive? If so, state the evidence.
14. How may the diet in pregnancy be restricted in sodium? Should salt be restricted routinely in pregnancy?
15. Lactation makes greater demands upon the mother than does pregnancy. What food increases should be made to provide for the supply of milk? Plan a menu differing in content from the sample menu in Table 16–6, but equivalent to it in other respects.
16. What would you say to the woman who asks about substituting calcium pills for milk?

SUPPLEMENTARY READINGS

Blackburn, M. L., and Calloway, D. H.: Energy expenditure of pregnant adolescents. J. Am. Dietet. A. 65:24, 1974.

Chopra, J. G.: Effect of steroid contraceptives on lactation. Am. J. Clin. Nutr. 25:1202, 1972.

Jacobson, H. N.: Nutrition and pregnancy. J. Am. Dietet. A. 60:26, 1972.

Lindheimer, M. D., and Katz, A. I.: Sodium and diuretics in pregnancy. N. Engl. J. Med. 288:891, 1973.

Medical News: Malnutrition during pregnancy. JAMA 212:44, 1970.

Prenatal Care. Children's Bureau Publication No. 4. Washington, D.C., U.S. Department HEW, 1973.

Semmens, J. P.: Implications of teenage pregnancy. Obstet. Gynec. 26:77, 1965.

Thompson, M. F., et al: Nutrient intake of pregnant women receiving vitamin-mineral supplements. J. Am. Dietet. A. 64:382, 1974.

For further references see Bibliography in Section 4.

REFERENCES

1. Committee on Maternal Nutrition—Food and Nutrition Board: Maternal nutrition and the course of pregnancy. Washington, D.C., National Academy of Sciences—National Research Council, Summary Report, 1970.
2. Burke, B. S., et al: J. Nutrition 38:453, 1949.
3. Blackburn, M. L., and Calloway, D. H.: J. Am. Dietet. A. 65:24, 1974.
4. Hytten, F. E., and Leitch, I.: The Physiology of Human Pregnancy, ed. 2. Philadelphia, Davis., 1971.

5. Edwards, C. H., et al: J. Am. Dietet. A. 44:109, 1964.
6. Good examples are *Prenatal Care*, Children's Bureau Publication No. 4, 1973, and *When Your Baby Is on the Way*, Children's Bureau Publication No. 391, 1961, U.S. Department of Health, Education and Welfare. Local and state health departments also have good material available.
7. Committee on Maternal Nutrition—Food and Nutrition Board, op. cit., p. 13
8. Oldham, H.: Bull. Matern. Welf. 4:10, 1957.
9. Alperin, J. B., et al: Arch. Int. Med. 117:681, 1966; Willoughby, M. L. N., and Jewell, F. J.: Brit. Med. J., 5529:1568, 1966.
10. Committee on Maternal Nutrition—Food and Nutrition Board, op. cit., p. 163.
11. Burke, B. S., and Kirkwood, B. B.: Am. J. Publ. Health 40:960, 1950.
12. Tompkins, W. T., and Wiehl, D. G.: Am. J. Obst. & Gynec. 62:898, 1951.
13. McGanity, W. J., et al: Am. J. Obst. & Gynec. 67:501, 1954.
14. Robinson, M.: Am. J. Obst. & Gynec. 76:1, 1958.
15. Mengert, W. F.: Am. J. Obst. & Gynec. 81:601, 1961.
16. Food and Nutrition Board: *Recommended Dietary Allowances*. Washington, D.C., National Academy of Sciences—National Research Council, 1974.
17. Jelliffe, D. B., Gurney, M., and Jelliffe, E. F. P.: Cajanus 6:156, 1973.
18. Belavady, B.: Indian J. Med. Res. 57:63, 1969.
19. Jathar, V. S., et al: Arch. Dis. Child. 45:236, 1970.

17

nutrition during infancy and early childhood —from birth to three years

Nutritional Requirements of Infants
Breast Feeding vs. Formula Feeding
Formulas—Types and Sources
Feeding Difficulties in Infants
Introduction of Solid Foods
Other Considerations in Infant Feeding
The Toddler

Because of the rapid rate of growth during the first year, infancy is one of the most critical periods in the life cycle as far as food is concerned. Nutrient needs in relationship to size are high, and optimal nutrition at this time is very important to health and vigor throughout life. Many mothers with their first babies feel insecure and are concerned about what and how to feed the infant. The nutrition counselor should be able to advise and help the mother develop skills in this area.

NUTRITIONAL REQUIREMENTS OF INFANTS

THE ENERGY REQUIREMENT of infants is much greater per unit of body weight than that of older children or adults. During the first year energy allowances range from 120 kcal/kg. at birth to 100 kcal/kg. at the end of the year. The RDA for energy is, therefore, stated as 117 kcal/kg. for the first six months and 108 kcal/kg. for the second half of the first year (see Table 17-1). This is from 3½ to 2½ times the adult requirement per unit of weight.

There are several reasons for this difference in requirements. The infant is growing rapidly, but is doing so at a decreasing rate, which is reflected by the reduction in kcal/kg. during the first year.

He has a greater surface area in proportion to his weight than the adult and, consequently, a greater heat loss. Additional calories are also needed for increased activity. The accompanying table (Table 17-2) shows the approximate distribution of the caloric needs of the infant at the 120 kcal./kg. level.

Both breast milk and infant formulas (normal dilution) supply approximately 20 calories per ounce (67 calories per 100 ml.); thus 24 ounces of human milk or formula will supply about 480 calories or 120 calories per kilogram for the 4 kg. infant (120 cal. × 4 kg. = 480 cal.).

THE FLUID REQUIREMENT for normal healthy infants is about 150 ml. (5 ounces) per kilogram of body weight in 24 hours. This amount is usually consumed in the formula or from the breast. If extra water is lost from the skin, lungs or gastrointestinal tract, such as in hot weather, fever, or diarrhea, additional water should be given. When solid foods replace formula or breast milk in the infant's diet, some extra fluids may also be necessary. This is especially true if the solid food is high in protein, sodium chloride, or potassium.[1] (See Chapters 5 and 34 for a discussion of fluid and electrolyte balance in the normal and in the sick child.)

THE PROTEIN REQUIREMENT in the first year of life is greater per unit of body weight than at any other time of life. It gradually decreases from 2.2 gm. per

Table 17-2. Distribution of the Energy Needs of the Infant

	CALORIES/KG. OF BODY WEIGHT/24 HRS.
Basal metabolism	60
Activity	25
Growth	30
Loss in stools	5
Total	120

kilogram during the first six months to 2.0 gm. per kilogram for the second half of the first year. The RDA for protein during infancy (Table 17-1) is based on the "amount of protein provided by the quantity of milk required to ensure a satisfactory rate of growth."[2] The protein content of the body increases during the first year from 11 to 14.6 percent while there is a 7 kg. increase in body weight.

Most of the infants in the U. S. today who are not breast fed receive a modified cow's milk formula which closely simulates human milk. Because protein provides from 9 to 11 percent of the total calories in the usual infant formulas, 1 ounce of formula will supply approximately 0.5 g. of protein. Thus the 4 kg. infant receiving 24 ounces of formula (20 calories per ounce) will get approximately 12 g. of protein per day. (RDA = 8.8 g.)

FAT REQUIREMENT. No specific requirement for fat can be stated, but the caloric value of fat is essential during the early months of life when energy requirements per unit of body weight are high. Human milk provides 48 to 54 percent of its calories as fat, cow's milk—46 to 50 percent. Most commercial formulas

Table 17-1. Recommended Dietary Allowances for Infants During the First Year*

	0-6 MONTHS 6 kg. - 60 cm.	6-12 MONTHS 9 kg. - 71 cm.
Energy (kcal)	117 kcal/kg. (702)	108 kcal/kg. (972)
Protein (g.)	2.2 g./kg. (13.2)	2.0 g./kg. (18)
Vitamin A (RE)	420†	400
(IU)	1400	2000
Vitamin D (IU)	400	400
Vitamin E (IU)	4	5
Ascorbic Acid (mg.)	35	35
Folacin (mcg.)	50	50
Niacin (mg.)	5	8
Riboflavin (mg.)	0.4	0.6
Thiamin (mg.)	0.3	0.5
Vitamin B_6 (mg.)	0.3	0.4
Vitamin B_{12} (mcg.)	0.3	0.3
Calcium (mg.)	360	540
Phosphorus (mg.)	240	400
Iodine (mcg.)	35	45
Iron (mg.)	10	15
Magnesium (mg.)	60	70
Zinc (mg.)	3	5

*Adapted from Recommended Dietary Allowances. National Academy of Sciences—National Research Council. Washington, D.C., 1974.
†Assumed to be all as retinol in milk during the first six months of life. All subsequent intakes are assumed to be half as retinol and half as beta-carotene when calculated from international units. As retinol equivalents, three-fourths are as retinol and one-fourth as beta-carotene.

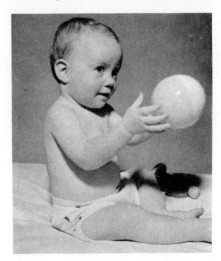

Fig. 17-1. Signs of good nutrition. Note the straight back, well-developed body, alertness, and good coordination of this child. (The New York Hospital)

provide 35 to 50 percent of the calories as fat. In order for infants to acquire adequate calories from the limited amount of formula they are able to consume, at least 15 percent of the calories provided must come from fat. The fat must be in an easily digestible form, preferably emulsified. Fomon[3] points out that loss of fat in the stools may be excessive if whole or evaporated milk without added carbohydrate is fed to the infant and suggests that the change from formula to whole milk be delayed until the infant is taking two jars of carbohydrate-rich commercially prepared strained food or the equivalent in table food.

Fat is also a carrier of fat-soluble vitamins. As described in Chapter 3, the infant requires small amounts of the essential fatty acid EFA—linoleic acid. Human milk is an excellent source of EFA, providing 6 to 9 percent of total calories as linoleate, whereas cow's milk provides 1 to 2 percent, which is the minimum recommended level. Commercial formulas, by using a combination of vegetable oils, usually contain at least 3 percent.

Carbohydrates in Infant Feeding.

Thirty-seven percent of the calories in human milk are from carbohydrate, while 29 percent in cow's milk, and approximately 42 percent in commercially prepared infant formula are from carbohydrate.

Lactose, the natural carbohydrate of mammalian milks, has many advantages. It provides calories in nonirritating and easily available form. Its slow breakdown and absorption probably have a beneficial effect on calcium absorption in the intestinal tract. Most commercial formulas use lactose as the preferred carbohydrate, although a variety of other carbohydrates which modify the flavor (sucrose, corn syrup solids, dextrose, dextrins, maltose,) or consistency (arrowroot starch, cornstarch, modified cornstarch and tapioca starch, banana powder, carrageenan) may be added to commercially prepared formulas. For economy and for the convenience of the mother preparing a formula at home, cane sugar (sucrose), or corn syrup can be used, the amount calculated according to the caloric need.

Minerals
CALCIUM–PHOSPHORUS–MAGNESIUM. The recommended dietary allowances for calcium, phosphorus, and magnesium during the first year of life apply to bottle-fed infants. These recommendations are given in Table 17–1. To prevent hypocalcemic tetany during the first week of life, a calcium-phosphorus ratio similar to that of human milk (2:1) is more desirable for the newborn than the Ca:P ratio

(1.2:1) found in cow's milk. The NRC's recommendation for a Ca:P ratio of at least 1.5:1 for the first weeks of life is found in several commercial formulas. For later infancy, the cow's milk Ca:P ratio is suggested. The approximate amounts of these minerals supplied by human milk and by cow's milk are shown in Table 17–3.

IRON. Although the normal-term infant is born with a store of iron, this is depleted by 6 months of age and hemoglobin levels fall below normal by 1 year unless an adequate source of iron is provided in the infant's diet. The RDA for infants is based on 1.5 mg. of iron per kilogram per day during the first year of life. This is a difficult recommendation to meet without the use of a supplement.

Because both human and cow's milk are poor sources of iron, breast-fed infants and those receiving whole cow's milk formulas need the early introduction of a good source of iron in their diets. Commercial infant formulas fortified with iron are available and supply about 8 to 12 mg. of iron per quart. They are prescribed by many physicians as the chief source of iron during the first 6 months when the RDA is 10 mg. per day.

Table 17–3. Comparative Nutritive Value of Human Milk and Cow's Milk
(Nutrients per 100 g. of fluid milk)

	HUMAN	COW'S
Energy (kcal.)	77	65
Protein (g.)	1.1	3.5
Fat (g.)	4.0	3.5
Carbohydrate (g.)	9.5	4.9
Water (g.)	85.2	87.9
Total ash (g.)	0.2	0.7
Calcium (mg.)	33	118
Phosphorus (mg.)	14	93
Magnesium (mg.)*	4	12
Sodium (mg.)	16	50
Potassium (mg.)	51	114
Iodine (mcg.)	3	4.7
Iron (mg.)	0.1	0.5
Zinc (mg.)	0.3-0.5	0.3-0.5
Vitamin A (IU)	240	140
Vitamin E (IU)†	0.2-0.5	0.02-0.25
Vitamin D (IU)*	2.1	1.3
Vitamin K (mcg.)*	1.5	6.0
Ascorbic acid (mg.)	4.3	1.1
Thiamin (mg.)	0.01	0.03
Riboflavin (mg.)	0.04	0.17
Niacin (mg.)	0.2	0.1
Folacin (mcg.)	5.2	5.5
Vitamin B_6 (mg.)*	0.01	0.064
Vitamin B_{12} (mcg.)*	0.03	0.4

Figures adapted from Watt, B.K., and Merrill, A.L., Composition of foods, raw, processed, prepared. Agr. Handbook No. 8. U.S.D.A., 1963 except as noted.
*Fomon, S. J.: Infant Nutrition. Ed. 2. Philadelphia, W. B. Saunders, 1974.
†Recommended Dietary Allowances. National Academy of Sciences—National Research Council Publ. No. 1964. Washington, D.C., 1968.

Infant (dry) cereals, also fortified with iron, may be introduced by the second or third month. Because many of these supply approximately 1 mg. of iron per tablespoon, they provide the additional iron recommended for the 6 to 12 month old infant (15 mg. of iron for a 9 kg. infant), assuming the iron-fortified formula is continued.

If the 6- to 12-month-old infant is to get 15 mg. of iron as specified in the RDA, both the iron fortified formula and infant cereal must be continued throughout the first 18 months rather than making a change at 4 to 6 months to whole cow's milk and using other forms of cereal as is the current practice. Approximately 5 to 6 mg. of iron will be supplied by the fortified formula, 5 to 6 mg. by the fortified cereal, and 4 to 5 mg. by the addition of meat, egg, and vegetables and fruits carefully selected for their iron content.

IODINE. Table 17–1 gives the recommended dietary allowance for iodine during the first year. Although the amount of iodine in human milk and cow's milk varies depending on the quantity that has been consumed in food and water, the breast-fed infant of an adequately nourished mother is assumed to receive at least the recommended amounts. In regions of the United States where the soil is low in iodine, feeding practices in dairies may increase the amount of iodine in cow's milk. The early introduction of strained foods to the infant's diet may also be a source of iodine depending on the nature of the soil in which they were grown. In addition, at least one of the major manufacturers (Gerber) of commercially prepared strained foods uses iodized salt in processing.

ZINC. Human and cow's milk contains approximately the same amount of zinc. Low zinc concentrations in hair have been found in infants with a history of poor appetite and growth retardation.[4]

FLUORINE. In technically advanced countries the magnitude of the dental caries problem exceeds that of all other nutritional diseases. It has been dramatically demonstrated that six-year-old children born after fluoridation started in one community had significantly fewer cavities than 10- or 11-year-old children using the same water supply but born before fluoridation started.[5] These differences suggest that fluoride prophylaxis during infancy is desirable. The advisable intake proposed by Fomon,[6] 0.5 mg. per day, is approximately the amount which would be ingested by infants fed formulas diluted with equal parts of water fluoridated at the usual level of 1 ppm.

Other trace elements—copper, chromium, cobalt, manganese, molybdenum and selenium—are assumed to be essential for the infant in extremely small amounts which are supplied by the usual diet.

VITAMINS. The recommended dietary allowances for the vitamins (Table 17–1) may be met by breast milk or cow's milk formulas consumed at a rate of approximately 800 ml. per day with the following exceptions:

Vitamin D. The breast-fed infant should receive a supplement of 400 I.U. of vitamin D per day after about 5 days of age. If the infant is bottle-fed with a commercial formula already fortified providing this amount of vitamin D, no further supplement is necessary.

Vitamin E. Human milk is higher in vitamin E content (2 to 5 I.U. of α tocopherol per liter) and will meet the infant's requirement, whereas cow's milk is relatively low (only about 1/10 to 1/2 of the amount in human milk) in vitamin E content and will not meet the RDA. Most of the commercial infant formulas have had vitamin E added to them and supply approximately 5 I.U. per quart. Some vitamin preparations for infants also include vitamin E.

Vitamin K. The Committee on Nutrition of the American Academy of Pediatrics[7] recommends that every newborn infant receive a single parenteral dose of 0.5 to 1.0 mg. of phytylmenaquinone (vitamin K) soon after birth. This is especially important for breast-fed infants since human milk (15 mcg./liter) provides much less vitamin K than cow's milk (60 mcg./liter) and thus vitamin K deficiency in the newborn period is more common in breast-fed infants.[8]

Precautions are necessary in the use of the fat-soluble vitamins, which should be given in the amounts recommended but not in excess of them, because an excess of these factors can be toxic (see Chapter 6).

Ascorbic Acid. Ascorbic acid is a limiting factor for bottle-fed infants whose formulas are subjected to high heat processing. Infants should receive a supplementary source of ascorbic acid by the tenth day of life. A synthetic source of this vitamin rather than orange juice is frequently recommended for small infants because it minimizes any sensitizing reaction. Most commercially prepared infant formulas have had ascorbic acid added to them, and since these require no further heat processing, the vitamin C is available. When used according to the directions on the label, 1 quart of prepared formula supplies approximately 50 mg. of ascorbic acid.

Folacin. The recommended dietary allowance for folacin during the first year is supplied by either human milk or cow's milk, both of which are relatively good sources of this nutrient. Folic acid has been added to several of the prepared commercial formulas in amounts to supply 30 to 50 mcg. of folacin per quart formula.

BREAST FEEDING VS. FORMULA FEEDING

There is much evidence that the earliest experiences of the newborn infant are of great importance to his total growth and development. This is particularly true of the way he obtains his food. Even at this early stage, he will react to the emotions of the mother, and this is of more importance than whether he is breast- or formula-fed. If the mother is relaxed and confident, the infant will respond to her and, through her, to the world about him with trust and confidence. Conversely, if the mother is tense and overanxious, or if the feeding is hurried, the infant becomes aware of discomfort. In response, he may be fretful or cry, which could prevent his taking the food he needs.

Certain psychological advantages have been attributed to breast-feeding. Many mothers derive satisfaction from feeling they are the source of their infant's nutriment. Also, breast-feeding permits early establishment of an intimacy with the child that bodes well for the mother-child relationship.

A mother should be encouraged to breast-feed her infant, but she should not be made to feel guilty if she prefers to bottle-feed him. If he is cuddled and made comfortable when he is being fed, whether by breast or by bottle, his feelings will be warmth and comfort.

Human milk from a well-nourished mother, when consumed in amounts sufficient to fulfill caloric needs, will meet the recommended intakes for all nutrients and there is no need for supplementation except for vitamin D, iron, and fluoride.

While breast-feeding is nature's way to feed the baby, relatively few young mothers in the U. S. today nurse their infants for more than a few days and many do not do so at all. In poor areas or where medical aid is not available, breast milk may be safer than a poor formula or one unhygienically prepared. Breast milk also has the advantage of freedom from contamination and of requiring no preparation. The bifidus factor in human milk is often referred to as the "intestinal guardian" because it appears to inhibit growth of certain pathogenic organisms by creating an acid environment in the gastrointestinal tract. The lysozyme content of human milk, which is much higher than cow's milk, may also have a bactericidal effect. Lactoferrin, an iron-binding protein in milk, has been shown to inhibit the growth of bacteria by denying them iron. Human milk also contains antibodies important in immunizing the infant against certain infectious diseases. Moreover, human milk is less likely to cause allergic reactions.

The lactating woman will find, however, that she needs more food than a non-lactating woman of her age and size and it may cost her more per week to feed herself during the time that she is sharing her nutriment with her infant.

Since certain drugs may pass from the mother's blood to her milk, Catz and Giacoia[9] have advised that the nursing mother not receive medications such as: antimetabolites, most cathartics, radioactive drugs, anticoagulants, atropine, and thiouracil. In addition, they recommend that certain other drugs such as oral contraceptives, barbiturates, and cough medicines with codeine be given only under careful medical supervision.

The decision of whether to breast-feed or bottle-feed the infant should be made during pregnancy. If the mother decides to breast-feed, instructions for the preparation of her breasts prior to delivery should be given by the nurse. Some young mothers will breast-feed their infants if careful teaching and psychological as well as physical preparation is instigated early in pregnancy. Moreover, the nursing mother must be sure to have the proper diet (see Chapter 16) and get sufficient sleep and relaxation; otherwise she will not produce enough milk.

Table 17–4 shows the approximate quantity of milk consumed by an average infant under normal conditions, proving that the mother must eat properly if she is to produce this quantity of milk.

The thick, yellowish fluid which appears the first few days of nursing (colostrum) will nourish the baby until the milk comes a few days later. The infant should be laid beside the mother with his cheek close to her breast. He will turn his head toward the breast trying to find the nipple (rooting reflex), and the mother can help him by holding the breast so that he can get the nipple into his mouth. To express the milk and prevent nipple irritation, most of the areola should be in the infant's mouth and not just the tip of the nipple.

Nursing the baby will in itself increase the milk supply of the mother, and she will be able to satisfy

Table 17–4. Approximate Quantities of Milk Consumed by an Average Infant During the First Six Months of Life

	G.	Oz.
1st day	10	1/3
2d day	90	3
3d day	190	6 1/3
4th day	310	10
5th day	350	11 1/2
6th day	390	13
7th day	470	15 2/3
3d week	500	16
4th week	600	20
8th week	800	26 1/2
12th week	900	30
24th week	1,000	33

his needs with an ever-increasing supply as he keeps growing. At first the infant may be satisfied after he has emptied only one breast, but if he does not give signs that he is full, he should be given the other breast. He should be started on this breast at his next feeding to be sure it is emptied.

If the infant is not getting enough to satisfy his hunger from the breast feeding, the doctor may prescribe an additional formula for him, to be given after he has been at the breast, or solid food such as cereal may be introduced. For one reason or another, the mother may wish to skip a breast feeding occasionally, and in such a case a formula feeding may be substituted. Beal[10] points out that in the United States today, the whole concept of breast feeding has changed not only because of the tendency to supplement with formula but also because semisolid foods are introduced early in infancy. Very few infants receive only breast milk even for the first two months of life.

FORMULAS—TYPES AND SOURCES

The physician usually determines the type of feeding for the newborn infant. Various factors, such as availability, ease of preparation, cost, and (most important) the infant's needs, should be considered in recommending the type and amount of feeding to be given.

FRESH COW'S MILK. Although there is a tendency toward the earlier introduction of undiluted fresh, whole homogenized, or skim milk, this is rarely the form prescribed for the newborn. (See Chapter 34.)

Because whole cow's milk contains more protein and mineral salts and less milk sugar than human milk, it is usually modified for the newborn by dilution with water and the addition of some form of sugar. Most homogenized milk is fortified with 400 I.U. of vitamin D per quart.

EVAPORATED WHOLE MILK has much to recommend it for use in infants' formulas but it is less used than it formerly was. Because evaporated milk is already sterilized, it is easy to prepare. The heat processing and homogenizing it undergoes results in both a soft, easily digested curd and well-distributed digestible fat. Evaporated milk contains 400 I.U. of vitamin D per reconstituted quart and is less expensive than commercial formula. It is available in two different size cans: 5½-ounce and 13-ounce.

CONDENSED COW'S MILK with its high sugar content is considered undesirable for infant feeding.

SKIM MILK, deficient in calories as well as in essential fatty acids, is not recommended for infant feeding.

PREPARED COMMERCIAL FORMULAS are by far the most popular type of infant feeding for the newborn. They are available in a variety of forms: powdered, concentrated-liquid, ready-to-use, and in feeding bottles, ready-to-feed. Their cost is related to their ease of use. Currently, the two most popular forms are the concentrated-liquid, $0.02 per ounce (normal dilution) and the ready-to-use at approximately $0.025 per ounce. Several brands are marketed, with and without added iron. A variety of vitamins have been added to each different brand. Almost all of them contain supplements of vitamins A and D, ascorbic acid and vitamin B_6, whereas others may also contain vitamin E, folic acid, vitamin B_{12}, and other B complex vitamins.

Commercial formulas may also have been modified in one or more of the following ways:

Butterfat is removed and a vegetable oil or oils are added to increase the amount of unsaturated fatty acid, particularly the essential fatty acid, linoleic acid. This makes the cow's milk formula more like breast milk in essential fatty acid content, and fat in this form is better tolerated by the infant.

The protein is treated to produce a softer, more flocculent curd which is more easily digested by the infant.

The milk is diluted to reduce the calcium and, to make up for this dilution in terms of calories, sugar—usually lactose or corn syrup solids—is added. Both of these modifications make the formula more like breast milk.

Dialysis may be used to reduce the sodium content of cow's milk.

Examples of commercially prepared formulas are given in Table 17–5.

Only by carefully reading the labels on the individual brands can one be sure of the exact nutritive content of the formula. The nutrition counselor should urge the mothers to follow the specific directions for the form she is using. Dilution of a ready-to-use can of formula will reduce the infant's nutritive intake, whereas failure to dilute the concentrated-liquid form may result in too strong a formula which the infant may vomit. Care should also be taken to sterilize the bottles, nipples, and can opener, and water, if it is to be added.

If facilities for sterilizing bottles or refrigeration are unavailable, for instance, in a home emergency or when traveling, the individual 4-, 6-, or 8-ounce bottles called nursettes may be an excellent way to ensure a safe supply of milk for the infant.

Table 17–6 gives a comparison of the costs of infant formulas made from different forms of cow's milk.

Table 17-5. Examples of Commercially Prepared Milk-Based Formulas Marketed in the United States[a]

Components			
Protein	Nonfat cow milk	Demineralized whey and nonfat cow milk	Nonfat cow milk and soy-protein isolate
Fat	Vegetable oils	Vegetable oils and oleo oil	Corn oil
Added carbohydrate	Lactose or corn syrup solids	Lactose	Sucrose
Examples	Enfamil[b] (Mead) Similac[c] (Ross)	SMA[d] (Wyeth)	Similac Advance (Ross)[f]
Major constituents (g./100 ml.)			
Protein	1.5-1.6	1.5	3.6
Fat	3.6-3.7	3.6	1.6
Carbohydrate	7.0-7.1	7.2	6.6
Minerals	0.3-0.4	0.3	0.7
Caloric distribution (% of calories)			
Protein	9	9	26
Fat	48-50	48	27
Carbohydrate	41-43	43	47
Minerals per liter			
Calcium (mg.)	550-600	445	1000
Phosphorus (mg.)	440-455	330	800
Sodium (meq.)	11-17	7	17
Potassium (meq.)	16-28	14	32
Chloride (meq.)	12-24	10	29
Magnesium (mg.)	40-48	53	85
Sulfur (mg.)	130-160	145	310
Copper (mg.)	0.4-0.6	0.4	1
Zinc (mg.)	2.0-4.2	3.2	4
Iodine (mcg.)	40-69	69	100
Iron (mg.)	trace-1.5[e]	12.7	18
Vitamins per liter			
Vitamin A (I.U.)	1700-2500	2650	3000
Thiamin (mcg.)	400-650	710	750
Riboflavin (mcg.)	600-1000	1060	900
Niacin (mg.)	7-8.5	7	10
Pyridoxine (mcg.)	320-400	423	700
Pantothenate (mg.)	2.1-3.2	2.1	5
Folacin (mcg.)	50-100	32	100
Vitamin B_{12} (mcg.)	1.5-2.0	1.1	2.5
Vitamin C (mg.)	55	58	50
Vitamin D (I.U.)	400-423	423	400
Vitamin E (I.U.)	8.5-12.7	9.5	6.3

[a]Some are marketed in other countries as well.
[b]Enfalac in Canada.
[c]Multival in some European countries.
[d]S-26 in other countries. Product marketed as SMA in other countries has different composition.
[e]Products also available with 12 to 13 mg. iron per liter.
[f]Older infant formula.
From Fomon, S. J.: *Infant Nutrition*, ed. 2, Philadelphia, W. B. Saunders, 1974.

GOAT MILK, seldom used today in the United States for infant feeding, is still used in many parts of the world. Experience shows that it is nutritionally adequate in most respects, except for folacin. Infants receiving goat milk as their major source of calories should receive folacin supplements. Goat milk was formerly used to feed infants who had an allergy to cow's milk; it is still used occasionally today and is available in drug and grocery stores. Goat-milk fat differs from fat in cow's milk in that it contains more essential fatty acids and has a greater percentage of medium- and short-chain fatty acids. These differences suggest that the fat of goat milk may be more readily digested than that of cow's milk.

MILK SUBSTITUTES. Certain infants are born with a sensitivity to the proteins of all milks. This may be mild enough to cause irritability only, or it may be severe enough to cause violent illness and even death. Several preparations have been devised as formulas to approximate human milk in carbohydrate, protein, fat, mineral, and vitamin content. These contain no milk at all. Soybean preparations are used most commonly.[11] Usually, the protein in the soybean can be taken by infants allergic to the proteins of milk. A milk substitute having meat protein as a base,[12] with added vitamins and minerals, has also proved to be adequate nutritionally for such infants. (See Table 34-4, Chapter 34.)

Table 17-6. Comparison of Costs of 1 Quart of Infant Formula Made from Different Forms of Cow's Milk

Homogenized milk	
22 oz. milk—10 oz. water	$ .22
1 oz. sugar	.03
1 ml. multivitamins with iron	.10
	.35
Evaporated milk	
11 oz. milk—21 oz. water	.22
1 oz. sugar	.03
1 ml. multivitamins with iron	.10
	.35
Commercial Formulas	
(vitamins and iron added)	
Powdered form (normal dilution)	.53
Liquid-concentrate (normal dilution)	.64
Ready-to-feed	.83
Nursettes—5$^1/_3$ 6-oz. bottles	1.98

If these milk substitutes are properly supplemented, infants do as well on them as on other formula feedings. A discussion of the nutritive adequacy of milk substitutes and a table of composition have been prepared by the Committee on Nutrition of the American Academy of Pediatrics.[13]

Galactosemia and lactose intolerance in infants and children are discussed in Chapters 34 and 35.

TEMPERATURE FOR FEEDING. The formula may be given at room temperature or warmed to body temperature if desired. If the formula has been stored in the refrigerator, it should be allowed to stand long enough to reach room temperature, or the bottle may be placed in warm water until it reaches the desired temperature.

The temperature of milk should be tested by shaking a few drops on the inside of the wrist. The older infant may tolerate his formula straight from the refrigerator.

HOW OFTEN TO FEED. Much has been said in recent years about so-called "self-demand schedules of feeding." For many years infants were fed by the clock, regardless of whether they were hungry earlier or later than the scheduled time. Today we recognize that the time to feed an infant is when he is hungry, whether the interval is 2, 3, 4, or even 5 hours. The inexperienced mother may need help in recognizing the difference between a hunger cry and a cry for something else.

A newborn infant may wake up to be fed eight to ten times in 24 hours. By the time he is a month old, there may be three hours between feedings. Most infants establish themselves on a schedule of four-hourly feedings by the time they are between two and three months old. During this time, too, the infant will begin to sleep through the night after a late evening feeding. The nutrition counselor should also recognize that the frequency of feeding will be influenced by the attitude of the mother as well as by other demands on her time.

"BURPING" THE INFANT. Once or twice during a feeding, the infant should be given a chance to bring up any swallowed air. Holding him up so that his stomach is against the mother's shoulder and gently patting him on the back will help to eliminate the air. An even better way is to hold the infant in a sitting position on the mother's knee, with his chin held in the palm of her hand. By leaning the infant forward and gently stroking or patting his back, swallowed air is released.

PSYCHOSOCIAL ASPECTS OF INFANT FEEDING. If the mother is feeding her infant by bottle, she should hold him as though she were breast-feeding him, cradled in her arm, in order to give him the same sense of nearness and companionship. It is important that she feel relaxed and unhurried and that she enjoys this time with her infant. It is particularly important that the bottle-fed infant not be overfed. Since the mother cannot tell how much the breast-fed infant has consumed she is inclined to assume that the infant is satisfied when he stops sucking, whereas, the mother who is bottle-feeding may urge the infant to completely finish the bottle. This early training may be the beginning of overfeeding and one of the causes of obesity in later life.

Moreover, the infant should not be allowed to eat by himself by means of propping the bottle up beside him. In this way his nutritional needs may be met but not his need for love and contact.

By feeding "on demand," the mother also eliminates the infant's frustration of hunger and helps him develop trust and security in the feeder. Talking and repeating sounds to the infant while he is being fed is a valuable learning experience and may be an important aspect of his later intellectual development.

FEEDING DIFFICULTIES IN INFANTS

VOMITING AND REGURGITATION. Vomiting may result from a number of causes and may or may not be a serious symptom. In regurgitation only small amounts of food are lost, while in vomiting the contractions are sufficiently strong to empty the stomach. Regurgitation may be avoided by "burping" the infant once or twice during a feeding. Occasional vomiting is usually caused by overdistention of the stomach due to the ingestion of too large or too frequent feedings or to the swallowing of air. It may also be caused by an imbalance of the food constituents,

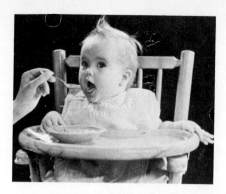

Fig. 17-2. The right start for the baby. Liking comes through learning to like. Teach the flavor of a variety of foods early. (Gesell A., and Ilg, F. L., *Behavior of Infants*. Philadelphia, Lippincott)

especially an oversupply of fat, which delays emptying of the stomach. Persistent vomiting may be a symptom of infection, obstruction, or other serious ailment and should be referred promptly to the physician. The cause should be determined and the feedings adjusted accordingly.

COLIC. An infant who has hard crying spells shortly after eating is said to be "colicky." The colic, or severe abdominal cramping pain, may be caused by distention due to the swallowing of air; to gas formed by bacterial fermentation of undigested food; to overfeeding or underfeeding; to cold, excitement, or only to being tired. The infant may have to be "burped" again. Making sure he is warm may help. Mothers are apt to think that his feeding is wrong, but changing the feeding usually does not help. Spock[14] says that these babies seem to grow and gain weight better than most, and that generally, the condition disappears at the age of three to four months.

DIARRHEA. Loose stools may be serious, and the doctor should be consulted at once. See Chapter 34 for diseases in which diarrhea is a symptom.

CONSTIPATION. Constipation in infancy is not infrequent. Many mothers are concerned when the infant has only one bowel movement per day or on alternate days. The number of movements per day is not of so much importance as is the consistency of the stools. If the feces are hard and expelled with difficulty, then the child may be said to be constipated and should be treated accordingly.[15] Increasing the amount of fruit in the diet and giving additional water usually relieves constipation. If it persists, the doctor should be consulted.

INTRODUCTION OF SOLID FOODS

Fomon[16] has introduced the German word "Beikost": other than milk or formula, to describe the semi-solid foods used in infant feeding. Since this term may be unfamiliar to the readers of this text, the authors will continue to refer to such foods as solids or semi-solids.

The time for the addition of supplementary foods to the diet of the breast- or formula-fed infant has undergone marked changes in the past 20 years. Whereas earlier, no solid foods were introduced until the end of the first year, the pendulum has swung all the way to the opposite extreme of offering the infant semi-solids during the first month of life. Beal[17] has found that the average infant's willing acceptance of cereal occurs at two and one-half to three months, of vegetables at four to four and one-half months, of meat and meat soups at five and one-half to six months, and of fruit at two and one-half to three months. Earlier introduction of solid foods tended to meet with resistance by the infant. Beal also has shown that the age of transition from infant foods to the family diet has decreased from approximately two years to 13 months.

Later studies, however, indicate that most infants are fed some semi-solid foods before they are two months old and that they begin to eat foods from the family diet before the end of the first year. In the following paragraphs, the authors have indicated approximate ages for the introduction of new foods.

CEREALS. Cereals are usually added to the infant's diet before he is two months of age. Dry, precooked cereal preparations are fortified with iron, whereas the "wet-packed" jars of cereal may or may not be iron-fortified.

Dry, precooked cereals must be mixed with warm formula or whole milk, while others may only need to be warmed. The cooked cereals eaten generally by the family may be prepared according to package directions and given to the infant. Coarse cereals must be strained, and all of them should be thinner than those prepared for the family—thin enough to drop from a spoon. Only a small amount of cereal should be used at first, and this is generally given with the midmorning feeding. The original small amount may be increased gradually, and in a few months it may be of a thicker consistency. By the fourth or the sixth month, the infant will be taking from ¼ to ½ cup twice during the day.

FRUITS. Cooked, strained fruits and ripe banana may be added to the infant's diet when he is between two and three months old. Like cereals, these may be purchased in cans or jars, all ready for infant use, or they may be prepared at home. Cooked fruits should be put through a puree sieve or strainer. Strained apple sauce, prunes, peaches, pears, and apricots are suitable. Ripe mashed banana may also be given.

Starting with a teaspoonful once or twice a day, the infant will soon take 2 to 3 tablespoonfuls. Most infants like fruit and take it readily. This helps them to accept other solid foods, the taste of which may not appeal to them quite as much.

VEGETABLES. By the third or fourth month, or even earlier, strained vegetables are usually introduced. Those added first are peas, string beans, spinach, carrots, beets, and squash. Fresh, frozen, or canned vegetables are suitable. If prepared at home, they should be cooked in a small amount of water, as would be done for the family meal, and the infant's portion put through a puree sieve or a strainer. Again, these and other varieties of vegetables are available in cans or jars in most grocery stores, prepared and ready for serving after they are warmed. Starting with a teaspoonful at one feeding—and, later, as part of lunch—the infant will soon be taking 2 to 3 rounded tablespoonfuls. Potatoes, both sweet and white, may be added a little later, but potatoes in any form are one of the last vegetables to be accepted by most infants.

EGG YOLK. Egg yolk is a good source of iron, but since other infant foods are now fortified with iron, eggs can be deferred until other foods have been started. Eggs may cause an allergic reaction, the white more than the yolk, which is the reason the yolk is given first. The egg may be cooked hard by placing it in boiling water, turning off the heat and letting it stand, covered, for 20 minutes. Cooking changes the protein to make it less allergenic.

Egg yolks should be crumbled and given by spoon or mixed with cereal or vegetables at first. A fourth of a yolk is a good quantity with which to start. If the infant accepts it well and there are no signs of allergy, the quantity may be increased until he is taking a whole yolk, usually at the breakfast feeding. Whole egg may be given by the time he is a year old.

Prepared egg yolk is now available in jars ready to serve, as are other infant foods.

MEAT. Meats may be added as early as three to four months or as late as six months, depending on the doctor's judgment of the infant's need for them. The most convenient way of serving meat to the infant is by canned, strained beef, beef heart, liver, lamb, chicken, veal, and pork preparations available in cans and jars at most grocery stores. To prepare meat for the infant at home, the mother should buy a lean cut of beef, pork, lamb, veal, or poultry. It may be simmered or pan broiled and then put in a blender with sufficient water to achieve the desired consistency. Liver may be prepared in the same way. If a blender is not available, a fork or dull knife may be used to scrape meat off fibers from the surface of a cooked or cleaned raw piece of meat. If raw meat is used, the resulting meat pulp may be heated until it is brown in a custard cup set in a small pan of water over heat.

Meats add protein, iron, and some of the B complex vitamins to the infant's diet. Again, it is best to begin slowly with a teaspoonful or less at the evening feeding, increasing the quantity as the infant grows older.

Widening Variety in the Infant Diet

By the time they are six months old, most babies will be eating some foods from each of the four food groups. They may also be starting to take some milk or fruit juice from a cup. In addition to milk, a good meal plan for an infant of this age is to give him cereal and egg yolk at breakfast, vegetable and meat for lunch, and cereal and fruit for supper. The quantities will depend on his appetite. If there is a tendency toward constipation, giving fruit at breakfast as well as at supper may help.

ADDITIONAL FOODS, 6 TO 12 MONTHS. The infant will welcome a piece of dried bread, toast, or an infant teething biscuit to hold in his hands and chew on, particularly if his teeth are beginning to appear. If potato has not already been given, it can be added at this time, mashed fine. Puddings made mainly with milk, such as junket, cornstarch, tapioca, and rice pudding, may also be added occasionally for variety. A small piece of a white, nonoily fish, such as flounder, haddock, or halibut, may be substituted for meat now and then. It should be poached gently in water to cover until it flakes, and all bones carefully removed.

By the time he is nine months old, it is time to try serving some of the junior foods, or foods mashed with a fork, instead of strained foods. The change should be made gradually and should not be forced. Vegetables and fruits may be tried this way first. Meat is better served strained until after the first year, because it is so much more difficult to swallow.

A piece of crisp bacon or a bit of raw, peeled apple is also often enjoyed by babies, when they are allowed to hold it in their hands and suck on it.

Mixed dishes, either junior foods or appropriate ones from the family table, may also be added. These include spaghetti with meat sauce, macaroni and cheese, and tuna fish and noodles.

As the infant becomes acquainted with a variety of things, including his food, he will want to explore it with such tools as he has at his command. To quote Rabinovitch:[18] "In the second half of the first year, the baby will begin to mess with food, to feel its texture and consistency, to finger-feed himself as he recognizes his growing dexterity. Such experimentation, often difficult for the cleanliness-and-germ-conscious mother, is essential for the child as he

Table 17-7.   Proximate Composition of Selected Commercially Prepared Baby Foods and Home-Prepared Foods of the Same Name[a]

PRODUCT	Energy Kcal./100 G.	PROXIMATE ANALYSIS (G./100 G.)					
		Water	Protein	Fat	Carbohydrate Total	Carbohydrate Fiber	Ash
Chicken and noodles, cooked from home recipe[b]	153	71.1	9.3	7.7	10.7	trace	1.2
Strained chicken noodle dinner[c]	46	88.5	2.0	1.0	7.1	0.3	1.1
Spaghetti with meatballs in tomato sauce cooked from home recipe[d]	134	70.0	7.5	4.7	15.3	0.3	2.2
Junior spaghetti, tomato sauce, and meat[c]	70	82.9	2.7	1.7	11.0	0.3	1.4

[a]Adapted from Anderson, T. A., and Fomon, S. J.: Commercially prepared strained and junior foods for infants. J. Amer. Diet. Ass. 58:520, 1971.
[b]From Watt and Merrill, 1963, item 752.
[c]Mean calculated from data in Table 16-2.
[d]From Watt and Merrill, 1963, item 2165.

learns to relate to food by messing, smelling and pouring. That a high degree of parental fortitude is necessary to allow for these developmental realities goes without saying."

WEANING. The weaning of an infant from sucking from a nipple to taking milk from a cup is not an abrupt transition as infants are fed today. As soon as the infant is introduced to the supplementary foods discussed earlier, he is on the way to being weaned. He will have learned to drink from a cup by the time he is seven to nine months old. If he still shows a desire to suck, he may have a bottle once a day. He may be drinking homogenized milk and eating a variety of foods. The proportion of calories derived from milk will decrease gradually as he obtains more of his nutrients from other foods—junior foods for a time and then simple foods from the family table.

OTHER CONSIDERATIONS IN INFANT FEEDING

COMMERCIAL BABY FOODS. The widespread use of commercial baby foods by mothers in the U. S. today makes knowledge of these foods especially important. Anderson and Fomon[19,20] have discussed the many factors which must be considered in using them, such as the differences and similarities between various groups of infant foods. See Section 4, Table 1, Baby Foods—Cereals, Fruits, Meats, Poultry and Eggs, and Vegetables, for the nutritive values of these foods. Table 17-7 shows a comparison of the proximate composition of the commercially prepared infant foods and similar home-prepared foods. Note the much lower calorie, protein, and fat content of the commercially prepared foods, due to the higher water content, as compared with home-prepared items.

SALT IN COMMERCIAL BABY FOODS. The amount of salt added to baby foods by the manufacturer has been a matter of recent concern. In the report from the subcommittee of the Food and Nutrition Board dealing with food protection, it is noted that the current levels of salt in baby food, although substantially more than what is required by the infant, are neither harmful nor beneficial to the infant. "There is no valid scientific evidence in support of the contention that addition of salt to infant foods contributes to development of hypertension or other disease states in adult life, nor is there valid evidence that the practice is not harmful, or that salt levels now consumed by infants in the U. S. overburdens excretory mechanisms."[21] Because salt is added more for the mother's taste than the infant's, it was recommended that the amount of salt in all foods be limited to 0.25 percent, and that no additional salt be added to foods such as fruits, currently prepared without it.

SATIETY, the mechanism by which the infant is made aware that he has had enough, varies widely in infants. In some, the reaction is sharp and they actively resist further feeding attempts. In others, satiety is less sharply defined and interest in eating wanes gradually after a period of playfulness. Still others do not seem to know when they have had enough and will vomit what they cannot handle. Remember, overfeeding in infancy may establish an undesirable food pattern for later life.

CRITERIA FOR JUDGING NUTRITIONAL ADEQUACY. The criteria for judging adequate nutrition in an infant are: a steady gain in weight; a moderate increase in subcutaneous fat; the development of firm muscles; good elimination; and an infant who is happy, sleeps well, and shows normal curiosity about his surroundings.

OVERNUTRITION. The nutrition counselor should be particularly aware of the hazards of overnutrition. She must be able to relate these to the mother who may look upon a fat baby as a healthy, happy baby and sees no cause for alarm.

Infants who show an excessive weight gain from overfeeding even as early as six weeks of age are reported to have a greater tendency toward overweight and obesity later in childhood.[22] As previously discussed in Chapter 15, there may also be an increase in the total number of fat cells in the body of

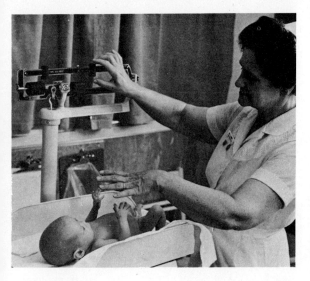

Fig. 17-3. The rate at which a child gains weight is dependent on many factors. As long as he gains weight and length steadily, and exhibits the other signs of good nutrition, there is no cause for worry. (Broadribb, V., *Foundations of Pediatric Nursing*, ed. 2. Philadelphia, Lippincott, 1972)

an infant who is overnourished during the phase of rapid fat-cell division and this condition persists throughout his life. Although the reasons are not clear, a recent study gives evidence that obese infants also have a higher incidence of respiratory infections than those of normal weight.[23]

THE TODDLER
Nutritional Requirements of Early Childhood
The recommended dietary allowances for one- to three-year-olds are shown in Table 17–8.

CALORIES. The calorie needs from one to three years are relatively low (Table 17–8) and hence, in order to ensure a diet adequate in other nutrients, careful selection of the toddler's food is essential.

PROTEIN. Protein needs for growth of muscles and other tissue are relatively high during this period. They are easily met, however, if the toddler consumes a pint of milk and 1 to 2 ounces of meat each day.

MINERALS. Calcium, phosphorus, and magnesium recommendations also depend on the inclusion each day of 1 pint of milk and 1 to 2 ounces of meat.

The recommended dietary allowance for iron, 15 mg., is not easily met with the usual diet at this age and a supplement may be necessary until increased levels of enrichment are achieved.

In areas where iodine in the soil is limited, a small amount of iodized salt in cooking and seasoning adequately provides for the recommended amounts of iodine.

VITAMINS. A varied menu such as that shown in Table 17–9 will provide an adequate intake of vitamins if the toddler's appetite permits its consumption. Foods high in ascorbic acid and vitamin A should be served each day. If fortified milk is not used, a vitamin D supplement is necessary.

Feeding the Toddler
The one-year-old begins to show a decided change in appetite and interest in food. Beal[24] has shown that, on the average, girls at six months and boys at nine months decrease their milk intake markedly. For girls this persists until two to three years of age and then slowly milk intake begins to rise. In contrast, boys have a somewhat steeper decrease in milk intake than girls but recover more rapidly and by two and one-half years have reached a higher level than girls. Other foods, too, are not taken as eagerly as formerly, and some may be refused altogether. This should not be interpreted as a "poor" appetite but rather, the normal appetite for that age.

All this is due in large measure to a decrease in growth rate and, therefore, to the quantitative need for food. Also, at this age, the young child is becoming increasingly intrigued by his surroundings—parents, sisters and brothers, and the paraphernalia of the home, all of which vie for his attention. He wants to play with his food to feel its texture, and he tries to feed himself with his hands, refusing the same food when it is offered on a spoon.

This can become an anxious time for the inexperienced mother, accustomed to the voracious appetite of infancy (or to the busy nurse facing a ward full of

Table 17–8. Recommended Dietary Allowances for the 1- to 3-Year-Old*

	1-3 Years (13 kg.)
Energy (kcal.)	1300
Protein (g.)	23
Vitamin A (I.U.)	2000
(R.E.)	400
Vitamin D (I.U.)	400
Vitamin E (I.U.)	7
Ascorbic acid (mg.)	40
Folacin (mcg.)	100
Niacin (mg.)	9
Riboflavin (mg.)	0.8
Thiamine (mg.)	0.7
Vitamin B_6 (mg.)	0.6
Vitamin B_{12} (mcg.)	1.0
Calcium (mg.)	800
Phosphorus (mg.)	800
Iodine (mcg.)	60
Iron (mg.)	15
Magnesium (mg.)	150
Zinc (mg.)	10

*From Recommended Dietary Allowances. National Academy of Sciences—National Research Council Publ. Washington, D.C., 1974.

Table 17–9. Suggested Meal Plan for the 1- to 3-Year-Old*

BREAKFAST
Fruit or juice
Cereal with milk
Toast
Butter or margarine
Milk

LUNCH OR SUPPER
Main dish—mainly meat, eggs, fish, poultry, dried
 beans or peas, cheese, peanut butter
Vegetable or salad
Bread
Butter or margarine
Dessert or fruit
Milk

DINNER
Meat, poultry or fish
Vegetable
Relish or salad
Bread
Butter or margarine
Fruit or pudding
Milk

SNACKS BETWEEN MEALS
Dry cereal, with milk or out of the box
Simple cookie or cracker
Raw vegetables
Canned, fresh or dried fruit
Cheese wedge
Fruit sherbet or ice cream
Toast, plain or cinnamon
Fruit juice
Fruit drinks made with milk and juice

*From *Your Child from 1 to 3*, Children's Bureau, U.S. Dept. H.E.W., 1966. Revised 1967; reprinted 1969.

restive children). Unless the mother is guided correctly, food and eating may become a battleground between her and the child and may lay the groundwork for the anorexia and emotional upsets related to food and eating which so often occur in the preschool years. It is important for her to understand that changes in food acceptance and the need for exploration are a part of the normal growth pattern and that all children go through this process.

Physically, the child is learning motor mastery of his body—eye, hand, and mouth coordination, chewing, swallowing, the use of mouth and throat muscles. He "puts everything into his mouth." From his earliest days his mouth has served him as a sensory organ. He now uses it to explore whatever is within reach. Moreover, from the very beginning his feedings establish his primary relationships with other people. If the mother is helped to understand and is able to enjoy her baby's developing skills and interests even when she is frustrated by the spilled milk, the dropped spoons, and the gleeful contrariness, she is less likely to worry him over the food which he does or does not eat.

THE DIET OF THE ONE-YEAR-OLD differs only slightly from that described. It includes not much more than a pint of milk a day plus foods from each of the other four food groups. His vegetables and fruits are mashed or chopped instead of strained, and he has started on "finger foods." He is introduced to the family meal schedule with a midmorning and a midafternoon snack of fruit juice or milk. The cup largely supplants the bottle, and he may start to try feeding himself with a spoon.

DURING THE SECOND YEAR more solid foods are added, such as chopped or sliced fruits and vegetables; ready-to-eat cereals as well as hot cereals; chopped liver, lean meat, fish, and poultry instead of the strained variety. Whole egg replaces egg yolk. Cottage cheese and other mild cheeses may be used. Butter or fortified margarine is used with toast. The two-year-old also enjoys custard and puddings.

FOOD FROM THE FAMILY TABLE. By the time the infant reaches his first birthday his usual food is often from the family table. It is important that the family-food fed to the toddler is appropriate both in nutritive value and in consistency. Because caloric intake is limited, the one-year-old cannot afford calories that do not contribute equal amounts of other nutrients. Soft drinks, candy, many types of cookies, pastries and cakes supply too many calories and not enough protein, vitamins, or minerals for the toddler. The nutrition counselor should discourage mothers from feeding the toddler these foods except, perhaps, on special occasions.

When the toddler's meat comes from the family table it should be tender and cut into small pieces. Rich gravies and sauces are not appropriate for this age. Except for finger items, other foods should be cut into bite-size pieces.

Very small portions (1 to 2 tablespoonfuls) seem to encourage the toddler to eat. He should have the option of refusing certain foods as well as having additional servings of those he likes.

MAKING FOODS EASY TO EAT for beginners helps them to develop independence in feeding themselves and will prevent accidents. Small plastic cups or tumblers are easier to handle than glass or china. If they are not filled too full, there will be less spilling.

OVERUSE OF MILK. Earlier in this chapter it was stated that most children decrease their milk intake in favor of other foods sometime during the first year. Because milk has been the center of the diet in infancy, there is a tendency to think that it must continue to be so. When milk continues to provide the largest part of the one- to two-year-old's diet, nutritional anemia may result. The one- to two-year-old may cut his milk intake down to a pint or even less a day and, instead, eat a variety of other foods, many of which help supply his need for iron. He slowly resumes milk drinking, but it will be some years before he is able to consume a full quart and still eat a variety of other foods.

ABNORMAL CRAVINGS – PICA. Pica is a craving for unnatural foods or for nonfood substances such as clay or chalk. It is most apt to occur in children between the ages of 18 and 24 months of age. Lourie et al[25] found no correlation between the occurrence of pica and nutritional deficiencies. Gutelius et al[26] supplemented the diet of some pica children with vitamins and minerals but failed to reduce the incidence of this craving among their subjects. These workers agree that pica is a complicated environmental, cultural, and psychological problem most apt to occur among children of mothers who also practice pica themselves.

STUDY QUESTIONS AND ACTIVITIES

1. Why is breast feeding considered to be highly desirable for both mother and infant?
2. What should the mother's attitude be if she bottle-feeds the infant?
3. What foods in what quantity should be included in the mother's diet if she is nursing her infant? (See Chapter 16.)
4. How much iron should a four-month-old infant get per day? How can this be supplied by food?
5. Is there evidence that fluoride in an infant's diet has any prophylactic effect during later childhood?
6. Which nutrients are most apt to be the limiting factors in breast-fed infants?
7. Formerly there were problems in weaning an infant from formula. Why and how has this situation changed with recent methods of infant feeding?
8. Prepared commercial formulas are used generally in artificial feeding. How do they compare in composition with human milk? How do they compare in cost with either whole or evaporated cow's milk formulas?
9. Supplementary foods are introduced into the infant's diet gradually. What is the first supplement generally advised and in what amount? In what order are other foods introduced?
10. Why are we concerned today about overnutrition in infants?
11. What changes take place in the small child's food habits at about one year of age? Why does this occur?
12. Why do later emotional problems with food and appetite often have their origin at this period?
13. How can the nutrition counselor help to allay the mother's anxiety and sense of frustration about her child's food habits at ages one to three years?
14. How much milk is the one- to two-year-old likely to be willing to drink? What may happen if he is forced to drink a quart of milk daily?

SUPPLEMENTARY READINGS

Anderson, T. A., and Fomon, S. J.: Commercially prepared, strained, and junior foods for infants: Nutritional considerations. J. Am. Dietet. A. 58:520, 1971.
————: Commercially prepared infant cereals: Nutritional considerations. J. Pediat. 78:788, 1971.
Brown, R. E.: Breast feeding in modern times. Am. J. Clin. Nutr. 26:556, 1973.
Children's Bureau: U.S. Dept. H.E.W., Washington, D.C. Breast Feeding Your Baby. C.B. No. 8, 1965; Your Baby's First Year. C.B. No. 400, 1962; Infant Care. 1973; Your Child From 1-3. 1966.
Committee on Nutrition, American Academy of Pediatrics: Vitamin D intake and the hypercalcemia syndrome. Pediatrics, 35:1022, 1965. Iron balance and requirements in infancy. Pediatrics 43:134, 1969.
Cowell, C., et al: Survey of infant feeding practices. Am. J. Publ. Health 63:138, 1973.
Economy in Nutrition and Feeding of Infants. Am. J. Public Health 56:1756, 1966.
Editor's Column: Prop the baby, not the bottle. J. Pediat., 79:348, 1971.
Fomon, S. J.: Infant Nutrition, ed. 2. Philadelphia, Saunders, 1974.
————: Prevention of Iron-Deficiency Anemia in Infants and Children of Preschool Age. Public Health Service Publ. No. 2085. DHEW, Washington, D.C., 1970.
————: Skim milk in infant feeding, JAMA 63:156, 1973.
————: What are infants fed in the United States? Pediatrics 56:350, 1975.
————, and Anderson, T. A.: Practices of low-income families in feeding infants and small children with particular attention to cultural subgroups. DHEW Publ. No. (HSM) 72:5605, Washington D.C., 1972.
Maternal Child Health Service: Nutrition and feeding of infants and children under three in group day care. DHEW Publ. No. (HSM) 72-5606, Washington, D.C., 1971.
O'Grady, R.: Feeding behavior in infants. Am. J. Nurs. 71:736, 1971.
Review: Overfeeding in the first year of life. Nutr. Rev. 31:116, 1973.
Schmitt, M. H.: Superiority of breast-feeding—fact or fancy. Am. J. Nurs. 70:1488, 1970.

For further references see Bibliography in Section 4.

REFERENCES

1. Fomon, S. J.: *Infant Nutrition*, p. 261. Philadelphia, W. B. Saunders, 1974.
2. Food and Nutrition Board: Recommended Dietary Allowances. National Research Council–National Academy of Sciences, Washington, D. C., 1974.
3. Fomon, S. J., op. cit. p. 166.
4. Hambridge, M., et al: Pediatric Res. 6:868, 1972.
5. Dunning, J. M.: N. Eng. J. Med. 272:30, 1965.
6. Fomon, S. J.: op. cit., p. 350.
7. Committee on Nutrition. American Academy, Pediatrics 28:501, 1961; 48:483, 1971.
8. Keenan, W. J., et al: Amer. J. Dis. Child. 121, 271, 1971.
9. Catz, C. S., and Giacoia, G. P.: Drugs and metabolites in human milk. In Galli, C. et al: *Dietary Lipids and Postnatal Development*, New York, Raven Press, 1973, p. 247.
10. Beal, V. A.: J. Am. Dietet. A., 55:31, 1969.
11. Two such products are ProSobee, made by Mead Johnson and Co.; and Mull-Soy, made by Syntex Laboratories.
12. Meat Base Formula, Gerber Products Co.
13. Pediatrics 31:329, 1963.
14. Spock, B.: *Baby and Child Care*, rev. ed. New York, Hawthorn Books, 1968.
15. Your Baby's First Year. Children's Bureau, DHEW Publ. No. 400. Washington, D. C., 1962.
16. Fomon, S. J., op. cit., p. 408.
17. Beal, V. A.: Pediatrics 20:448, 1957.
18. Rabinovitch, R. D., and Fischoff, J.: J. Am. Dietet. A. 28:614, 1952.
19. Anderson, T. A., and Fomon, S. J.: J. Am. Dietet. A. 58:520, 1971.
20. Anderson, T. A., and Fomon, S. J.: J. Pediat. 78:788, 1971.
21. Filer, L. J.: Nutr. Rev. 28:184, 1970.
22. Nutr. Rev. 28:184, 1970.
23. Tracey, V. V., et al: Brit. Med. J. 1:16, 1971.
24. Beal, V. A.: J. Nutrition 53:499, 1954.
25. Lourie, R. S., et al: Children 10:143, 1963.
26. Gutelius, M. F., et al: Am. J. Clin. Nutr. 12:388, 1963.

18

nutrition for children and youth

Nutritional Requirements of Children and Youth
Food Habits and Eating Practices
Child Nutrition Programs

Children and youth comprise approximately 35 percent of the total population of the United States today. The youth-oriented society of the 1970s has increasingly focused attention on the needs of young people. New and innovative programs dealing with all aspects of childhood and adolescence, from comprehensive medical care projects for children and youth to coordinated health and educational centers for teen-age mothers and their infants, are developing in many communities. Of particular concern in all of these are the needs of the disadvantaged child and the opportunities available to him. Nutritional assessments, dietary counseling, and nutrition education should be an integral part of all programs for children and youth.

This chapter will examine nutritional requirements of various age groups through adolescence and food habits and eating practices as related to nutritional requirements and developmental levels. The role and influence of child nutrition programs is also discussed.

NUTRITIONAL REQUIREMENTS OF CHILDREN AND YOUTH

The Recommended Dietary Allowances, Table 18–1, for children from four through ten years are the same for boys and girls. There is a gradual increase in

265

Table 18-1. Recommended Dietary Allowances for Children and Youth*

Age (Years)	MALES AND FEMALES		MALES		FEMALES	
	4–6	7–10	11–12	15–18	11–14	15–18
Energy (kcal.)	1,800	2,400	2,800	3,000	2,400	2,100
Protein (g.)	30	36	44	54	44	48
Vitamin A (I.U.)	2,500	3,300	5,000	5,000	4,000	4,000
(R.E.)	500	700	1,000	1,000	800	800
Vitamin D (I.U.)	400	400	400	400	400	400
Vitamin E (I.U.)	9	10	12	15	12	12
Ascorbic Acid (mg.)	40	40	45	45	45	45
Folacin (mcg.)	200	300	400	400	400	400
Niacin (mg.)	12	16	18	20	16	14
Riboflavin (mg.)	1.1	1.2	1.5	1.8	1.3	1.4
Thiamine (mg.)	0.9	1.2	1.4	1.5	1.2	1.1
Vitamin B_6 (mg.)	0.9	1.2	1.6	2.0	1.6	2.0
Vitamin B_{12} (mcg.)	1.5	2.0	3.0	3.0	3.0	3.0
Calcium (mg.)	800	800	1,200	1,200	1,200	1,200
Phosphorus (mg.)	800	800	1,200	1,200	1,200	1,200
Iodine (mcg.)	80	110	130	150	115	115
Iron (mg.)	10	10	18	18	18	18
Magnesium (mg.)	200	250	350	400	300	300
Zinc (mg.)	10	10	15	15	15	15

*From Food and Nutrition Board: Recommended Dietary Allowances. National Academy of Sciences–National Research Council, Washington, D.C., 1974.

Table 18-2. A Daily Guide to Foods Needed by Children and Their Families*

TYPE OF FOOD	EACH DAY

Milk Group
Milk, whole or skim
Children under 11 ....2 to 3 cups
Children 11–18 ....3 or more cups

Dairy products such as:
Cheddar cheese, cottage cheese, and ice cream .... May be used sometimes in place of milk

Vegetable-Fruit Group .... 4 or more servings
Include—
A fruit or vegetable that contains a high amount of vitamin C: Grapefruit, oranges, and tomatoes (whole or in juice), raw cabbage, green or sweet red pepper, broccoli, and fresh strawberries.

A dark green or deep yellow vegetable or fruit for vitamin A: You can judge fairly well by color—dark green and deep yellow: broccoli, spinach, greens, cantaloupe, apricots, carrots, pumpkin, sweet potatoes, winter squash.

Other vegetables and fruits, including potatoes.

Meat and Meat Substitutes .... 2 or more servings
Include—
Meat, poultry, fish, or eggs.
Dried beans or peas, peanut butter, and nuts can be used as meat substitutes.

Breads and Cereals .... 4 or more servings
Whole grain, enriched, or restored bread and cereals or other grain products such as cornmeal, grits, macaroni, spaghetti, and rice.

Plus Other Foods
To round out meals and to satisfy the appetite, many children will eat more of these foods, and other foods not specified will be used, such as butter, margarine, other fats, oils, sugars, and unenriched refined grain products. These "other" foods are frequently combined with the suggested foods in mixed dishes, baked goods, desserts, and other recipe dishes. They are a part of daily meals, even though they are not stressed in the food plan.

*Adapted from Your Child from 6 to 12. Children's Bureau, U.S. Dept. HEW, Publ. No. 324. Washington, D.C., 1966.

growth and therefore, in the recommended amounts for most nutrients throughout childhood. However, because the adolescent growth spurt is markedly different for boys than it is for girls, separate recommendations are given for each starting at age 11.

If the Daily Guide to Foods Needed by Children and Their Families (Table 18–2) is followed, using appropriate servings for different age groups, plus other foods suggested in the guide, the recommended dietary allowances for children and youth will be met.

CALORIES. The RDA for calories during childhood, four through ten years, is based on an allowance of 80 calories per kilogram of body weight. After age ten there is a decrease in the calories per kilogram for both boys (45 calories per kilogram) and girls (38 calories per kilogram).

It is important to understand, however, that these recommendations represent average amounts for groups of children. An individual child may require more or less calories than the RDA, depending on his size, activity, and rate of growth.

Adequate calories must be supplied if growth is to proceed normally. When caloric intake is below the requirement, protein foods will be used for energy instead of for tissue building. Macy and Hunscher[1] have shown that "a difference in intake of as few as ten calories per kilogram of body weight per day (or approximately four calories per pound) may make the difference between progress and failure in satisfactory growth."

Figs. 18–1 and 18–2, which compare differences in increments of height and calorie intake between early- and late-maturing boys and girls, are good illustrations of why food intake of individual children must be adjusted to specific needs.

If a *growth chart* such as Fig. 18–3 is used for recording height and weight, deviations from normal patterns can readily be seen. The chart shown is for boys from age two to 13. Similar charts have been constructed for girls of this age, for infants, for both boys and girls, and for adolescent boys and girls. They are based on careful measurements of a selected group of children followed for the years specified and, as can be seen, show a wide range of variation.

The 50th percentile in both height and weight curves represents the median of all children measured. A child of stocky build is below the median for height and may be slightly above the median for weight. On the other hand, the tall, rangy child is well above the median for height and may or may not be below the median for weight.

The height and the weight recorded on such a chart at six-month or yearly intervals show graphically how a child is progressing within his particular growth pattern. For example, a drop to a lower percentile in weight from one measuring period to the next may indicate inadequate energy intake, particularly if the height trend is in the same direction. The nutrition counselor will wish to determine the reason for this deviation. Likewise, a shift in weight to a higher percentile, if not accompanied by a similar height increase, may signal overnutrition.

The basic foods listed in Table 18–2 need to be supplemented by varying amounts of butter or mar-

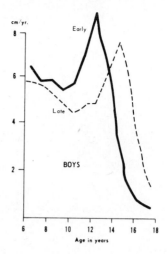

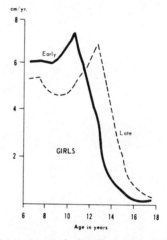

Fig. 18–1. Increments in the height of early and late maturing boys and girls (means of 20 in each group). (Mitchell, H. S., et al, The adolescent growth spurt and nutrient intake. Presented at the International Congress of Nutrition, Hamburg, Germany, August 8, 1966)

garine, salad dressings, jams, jellies, desserts, and, occasionally, other sweets to meet the energy needs of different age groups.

PROTEIN. Protein needs to be increased with growth, and protein intake should rise as calories are increased if there is a variety of foods in the diet. The milk and meat groups, including fish, eggs, cheese and peanut butter, meet protein needs adequately. However, if calories are obtained largely from carbohydrates, including candy and soft drinks in excess, both the quantity and the quality of the protein intake suffers.

MINERALS. Milk in the amounts recommended is the main source of *calcium* and *phosphorus* and, together with meat, contributes significant amounts of magnesium and zinc. Iron needs for children can be

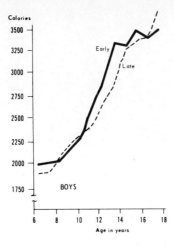

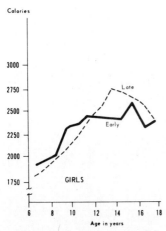

Fig. 18-2. Total caloric intakes of early and late maturing boys and girls (means of 20 in each group). (Mitchell, H. S., et al.: The adolescent growth spurt and nutrient intake, Presented at the International Congress of Nutrition, Hamburg, Germany, August 8, 1966)

met by an adequate intake of meat, eggs, green leafy vegetables, whole grain and enriched breads, and cereals and potatoes. Dried beans, peas, and peanut butter contribute a share of iron if these products are a staple of the diet. Adolescent boys may be able to meet the RDA for iron if they consume large quantities of foods to meet energy needs. The adolescent girl, however, probably needs an iron supplement, particularly after menstruation begins and iron is lost from the body. The necessary *iodine* is supplied by the use of iodized salt in cooking or as seasoning.

VITAMINS. Vitamin needs are more likely to be met when a variety of foods is included in the diet. Milk, butter, fortified margarine, and green and yellow vegetables and fruits will provide vitamin A. Milk fortified with vitamin D will ensure a sufficient intake of this vitamin. The B-complex vitamins will be in-cluded if good quality protein foods, as well as enriched bread and cereals, appear frequently in the diet. Children and adolescents who consume strictly vegetarian diets (vegans) may not receive adequate amounts of vitamin B_{12}. In Southern states, where cornmeal rather than wheat flour is frequently used, it is important to obtain enriched cornmeal when possible. In at least one Southern state, rice must be enriched by law.

Vitamin C needs are not met as easily as other nutritional requirements. Poor children especially do not always receive adequate amounts of ascorbic acid. Citrus fruits and tomatoes may be expensive items when not in season. Many of the fruit-flavored juices which are popular drinks with children do supply significant amounts of ascorbic acid in the amounts consumed. If these are used to replace citrus juices, their vitamin C content should be investigated. Raw potatoes are a good source of this vitamin but lose a large percentage of it in commercial processing, and the processed form of potato is the one most frequently found in the diets of children and adolescents. Cabbage and other leafy vegetables, raw especially, contribute some of this vitamin to the diet.

FOOD HABITS AND EATING PRACTICES
The Preschool Child—3 to 5 years

The daily food guide (Table 18-2) serves as the basis of the diet for the three- to five-year-old child, although size of servings is about half the average size used for older children and adults. A good estimate for size of a serving at meals is approximately 3 table-spoons for the three-year-old and 4 tablespoons for the four-year-old. The three- to five-year-old should be encouraged to drink 1 to 1½ pints of milk (regular or skim) a day. Some of this milk requirement may be provided in creamed soups and custards or other desserts included in his meals. Helping prepare and serve "instant puddings" is real fun for the preschooler and is also an excellent way to increase milk consumption in this age group.

Whole fruits and vegetables, both cooked and raw, should begin to appear in his menu. Meat should be cut in small pieces rather than ground. Remember that often at this age, a child will gladly eat such foods as raw carrots and lettuce with his fingers but refuse them if he has to use a fork or a spoon, because it is too difficult to manage the food with them.

It is usually desirable for the preschool child to have a midmorning, midafternoon, and bedtime snack in addition to his regular meals. Some pediatricians feel that there is room for further study and research on the question of the number of meals best suited to the needs of the preschool child. Stitt[2] won-

BOYS

NAME   BIRTH DATE   NO.

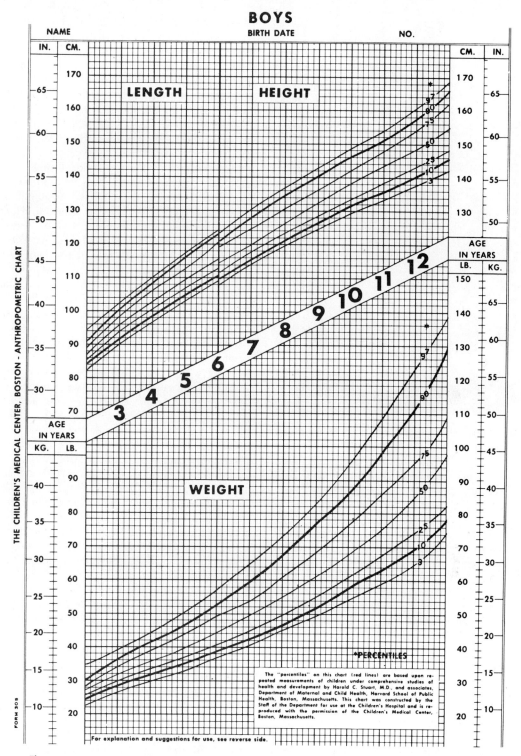

Fig. 18-3. Anthropometric height—weight chart for boys. For explanation of use see text. The break in height at the 6 year level occurs because up to that time the length of the child has been measured as he lay recumbent, while after this age the standing height is measured. The 50th percentile is the median range. Most children will fall somewhere between the 10th and 90th percentiles. (Children's Medical Center, Boston, Mass.)

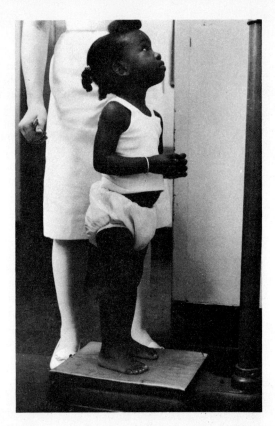

Fig. 18-4. A healthy child at the Pediatric Clinic, The New York Hospital. Note sturdy build, straight back, and alert interest in being weighed. (Children's Bureau photograph)

ders "whether good nutrients distributed fairly evenly over the waking hours may not be what many children seem to reach toward." Milk, if not consumed at a regular meal, or fruit juice accompanied by bread, crackers, or plain cookies, may form a good light meal or snack. Desserts, to be appropriate for the three- to five-year-old child, should furnish essential protein, minerals, and vitamins as well as calories. They should not be given as rewards for finishing a meal or withheld as punishment for not doing so, but perhaps even offered with the meal if the child prefers.

Children differ greatly in their natural preferences for food, but some patterns emerge clearly. "Finicky" food habits and food jags are characteristic of this age group. They may want to eat nothing except peanut butter sandwiches and fruit juice, or two to three hard cooked eggs at a sitting, but these patterns usually do not persist for very long, and soon they will settle down again to normal meals. The overall pattern of food intake from week to week and month to month is more important than the occasional food binge or refusal.

Project Head Start, serving children aged three to five, has offered an opportunity of studying the food preferences of children from low income families. These children usually lack experience with a wide variety of foods. Thus any program for the disadvantaged child should include a variety of new foods as well as culturally familiar foods.

PRESCHOOL DAY CARE CENTERS. As a result of the intensive demand for adequate child-care facilities, more and more day care centers are opening in our communities. The Child Development Center, a term currently being used for some of these, indicates their focus on the total development of the child—physical, psychosocial, and intellectual. Many of these centers not only serve meals as part of the physical care of the child but also use food and mealtimes as an integral part of the learning and socializing processes. They afford excellent opportunities for developing good food habits in children.

The breakfast and/or lunch served in the day care center provides an opportunity to introduce children to fruit juices, fruits in season, and raw vegetables. Children are pretty sure to like the familiar and simple main dishes, bread and butter, and milk. Eating in company with other children, perhaps for the first time, often encourages the less venturesome to try something new. A story about a new food and a small sample served attractively may make the difference between rejection and acceptance. Parent involvement in the programs of the center provides a chance for nutrition education for the entire family.

A professionally qualified nutrition consultant should be available to group day-care programs on a regular basis. The consultant should participate in developing and implementing written policies for the nutritional care of the children. These should include guidelines for planning, buying, storing, preparing, and serving food to meet nutritional needs, training of food service workers, and nutrition education programs for staff, children, and parents. A nutritional assessment, including dietary practices, should be made at the time each child enters the program and, if necessary, an individualized nutritional care plan should be established. The child's growth progress, food pattern, and mealtime behavior should be recorded and included in regular staff and parent conferences. Opportunities should be provided for parents to visit the center and to participate in mealtime activities. Menus should be posted in appropriate places in the center and made available to parents to facilitate planning of meals served in the home.[3] See Special Food Service Program for Children on p. 275.

The School Age Child—5 to 10 years

The basic food plan (Table 18–2) is the same for the school age child as it is for the preschooler, except that serving sizes increase until they are equal to or greater than the average adult serving.

The meal patterns for the school age child may vary depending on what the school provides and to what extent these services are used by the family. In any case, the mother needs to plan the family's meals around the school situation.

Breakfast for the child going off to school is an important meal. Because many mothers today have a variety of responsibilities, the preparation of this meal is often shared with the whole family. The school age child with a minimum of help can prepare a simple breakfast. Many schools in low-income areas have introduced a breakfast program to provide disadvantaged children with a good start for the school day.

Under certain circumstances, especially if the school does not have a school lunch program, a bag lunch has to be carried from home. The bag lunch should be planned to supplement breakfast and dinner in terms of foods selected from the food guide. Many children still need and enjoy snacks during this period. The after-school snack particularly is important and should be planned so as not to interfere with the evening meal.

Children's food habits develop along with other aspects of their growth. The five- to seven-year-olds prefer plain foods such as meat, potatoes, raw vegetables, milk, and fruits. Although most casserole dishes, mixtures of all kinds, fat meats, and gravies are not liked, spaghetti and meat sauce, pizza, and macaroni and cheese are notable exceptions. By six or seven, they are willing to try new foods and to accept foods previously disliked. By eight, there is a ravenous appetite with few refusals but strong preferences. Food may be judged by odor or color, and food served attractively makes an impression. By nine, the child usually has a keen interest in food, likes to help prepare it, and is positive in his likes and dislikes. Some eat everything at this age, but plain foods are still preferred.

One of the best methods for developing good food habits in children is for the whole family to eat wisely. If the mother and father, knowing that they can expect variations in acceptance of foods by their children, maintain a reasonably firm stand about overall behavior, mealtime can and should be one of the pleasant times of day for the whole family.

Children are great imitators. Although they may object to being asked to conform, they may, on the other hand, be heard to say proudly to some friend, "My mother won't let me eat that."

ROLE OF THE ELEMENTARY SCHOOL. For many children, elementary school is an introduction to group feeding. This can be difficult if the school does not make special provisions for the first and, perhaps, second graders. The hurry and confusion of most school cafeterias does not provide a conducive atmosphere for the average six-year-old to eat and enjoy his lunch. A smaller group in a quieter place, such as the classroom, is a more satisfactory arrangement for this age. This arrangement also affords an opportunity to use the luncheon meal as an educational tool to develop the child's interest in food.

The nutritional contributions of the school lunch are particularly important to those children who do not receive adequate food at home. However, all children can share the social aspects of group feeding, and this in itself may be enough incentive for a child to try an unfamiliar food or to drink his milk because the other children do. The National School Lunch Program is discussed on p. 273.

The Challenges of Youth—10 to 18 years

Because the growth spurts of girls and boys usually occur at different ages (11 to 13 or 14 years for girls and 12 to 15 years for boys), their nutritional requirements during adolescence also vary. Before the spurt, the recommendations are only slightly higher than for seven- to ten-year-olds and after the growth spurt taper off to the adult level.

All the foods included in the Daily Guide to Foods Needed by Children and Their Families (Table 18–2) are essential in the diet of the adolescent but in markedly increased quanitites. A rapidly growing boy will need a quart of milk or its equivalent each day to meet his calcium requirement, and girls during their period of rapid growth also need a quart of milk daily. Skim milk may be substituted for whole milk if excess weight, real or imaginary, is a factor. The increased milk intake will provide good-quality protein for growth as well as calcium. All the other foods listed, eaten in sufficient quantity, will provide for the greatly increased physiologic needs during this period of growth and stabilization.

In addition to adequate calcium, protein, and calories, girls need an iron supplement when menses begin. An adequate amount of foods high in iron, such as lean meats, liver, eggs, green leafy vegetables, enriched breads, and cereals and potatoes, should also be included in the daily food intake. This is a period when the young girl, who may be looking forward to marriage and motherhood, should be helped to realize that good nutrition is an important factor in the bearing of healthy babies.

During the period of rapid physical growth and sexual development, there is a concurrent maturing of the whole personality, with its attendant strains and stresses. The identity crisis of the teen-ager results in a drive for independence from parental restriction, coupled with an increased need for guidance and reassurance. There is a tremendous need for peer group approval, and fads in food habits are prevalent. The adolescent must be given the opportunity to make his own decisions, and parents should be understanding of this urge for independence, yet they should also be willing to help when needed.

Because boys and girls differ in their response to this growth period, they are discussed separately.
BOYS. As shown in Fig. 18-5, the diets of adolescent boys at all ages were generally found to be adequate for protein, vitamin A, riboflavin, and ascorbic acid; however, iron, calcium, and thiamine were low in the diets of certain age groups.

The adolescent spurt stimulates appetite, as is well recognized. The energy and nutrient requirement for this spurt in any one boy is not known. If the increments of height gained as shown in Fig. 18-1 are compared with the caloric intake for the same boys (Fig. 18-2), it is not surprising that the early maturers experienced an earlier increase in food intake than the late maturers.[4]

That serious undernutrition in boys still exists is known from the number of army recruits rejected as being physically unfit; but, on the whole, the nutritional outlook for boys is good.
GIRLS. With many girls the story is different. Despite the abundance of food in the United States and the inclusion of nutrition education in most elementary and high schools, the USDA Food Consumption Survey (Fig. 18-5) shows that teen-age girls, at all ages, comprise one of the most poorly fed groups in our population. The most serious deficits are in iron and calcium, with smaller numbers deficient in vitamin A and thiamine. This finding is particularly critical in view of today's early marriage and childbearing ages (see Chapter 16), because of the additional nutritional demands being made on the young mother's body.

The caloric intake of adolescent girls shows quite a different picture from that of boys (see Figs. 18-1 and 18-2). One can almost read into these graphs the psychology of the early-maturing girls who are concerned about their rapid growth and increase in height ahead of boys their age. Thus, they curtail their total food and often choose unwisely with respect to essential nutrients. The late-maturing girls do not make as drastic a reduction in caloric intake until much later.

The concern of teen-age girls often centers on weight reduction, whether necessary or not. There is probably no great harm in this, if the essential foods to meet nutritional needs are included in the diet. However, if soft drinks, candy and other sweets are substituted for milk, fruits, and vegetables, as is often the case, there may be a reduction in essential minerals and vitamins though not in calories.

ADOLESCENT OBESITY. A word of warning concerning adolescent obesity is necessary in any discussion of nutritional needs of this age group. Although the basic cause of juvenile-onset obesity is not well-understood, the fact that most fat children remain fat adults indicates an urgent need to prevent the development of obesity when possible and to treat it promptly when it occurs.

A minority of boys and girls have the habit of consuming more calories than they can use for energy and growth and thus become overweight for their height and age. Whether this is due to underactivity, to overeating, or to a combination of the two, adolescent obesity presents a real problem to the teen-ager's social and emotional adjustment as well as to future health. Obese adolescents are discriminated against in many ways. They are rejected by their peer group, harassed by their parents, set apart from the average by the fashion industry, laughed at in movies and on television, and generally excluded from the mainstream of teen-age life.[5]

Improving the poor self-image that the obese adolescent frequently has is usually the first step in his treatment. As his self-confidence is developed, his determination to effect change can often be depended on to motivate him through the long and difficult struggle with weight control. Although adolescent weight control is more successful with parental understanding and cooperation, the teen-ager must be the one responsible for his food intake. Weight control is discussed in Chapter 27.

CHILD NUTRITION PROGRAMS

The Food and Nutrition Service of the U.S. Department of Agriculture is responsible for the Child Nutrition Programs which were authorized either by the National School Lunch Act of 1946 or the Child Nutrition Act of 1966. The purpose of these programs is to safeguard the health and well-being of the nation's children. The Child Nutrition Programs include 1) the National School Lunch Program, 2) the School Breakfast Program, 3) the Special Milk Pro-

Sex—Age (Years)	Protein	Calcium	Iron	Vitamin A Value	Thiamine	Ribo-flavin	Ascorbic Acid
Male and Female:							
Under 1			x x x x				
1-2			x x x x				
3-5			x x				
6-8							
Male:							
9-11		x					
12-14		x x	x x x		x		
15-17		x	x				
18-19							
20-34							
35-54		x					
55-64		x x					
65-74		x x					
75 & over		x x x		x		x x	x
Female:							
9-11		x x x	x x x x		x		
12-14		x x x	x x x x	x	x		
15-17		x x x x	x x x x		x x		
18-19		x x x	x x x x	x	x		
20-34		x x x	x x x x		x	x	
35-54		x x x x	x x x x		x	x x	
55-64		x x x x			x	x	
65-74		x x x x	x	x	x x	x x	
75 & over		x x x x	x	x x	x x	x x x	

x—1 through 10%   xx—11 through 20%   xxx—21 through 29%   xxxx—30% or more

Fig. 18–5. Nutrients less than the recommended dietary allowances. (National Academy of Sciences—National Research Council, 1968) (From Food Intake and Nutritive Value of Diets of Men, Women and Children in the U.S., Spring, 1965. U.S. Department of Agriculture, Agricultural Research Service.)

gram, and 4) the Special Food Service Program for Children.

In order to participate in Child Nutrition Programs, schools and child-care institutions must agree to the following regulations:

1. To operate the food service on a nonprofit basis for all children without regard to race, color or national origin;

2. To provide free or reduced-price meals to children unable to pay the full price. These children must not be identified nor discriminated against in any way; and

3. To serve meals that meet the minimum nutritional requirements established by the Secretary of Ag-

riculture. This does not apply to schools and institutions that participate only in the special milk program.

Generally, these programs are administered through the State Education Departments; however, in those states where the law and other restrictions prohibit agencies from administering programs in private schools and child-care institutions, the Food and Nutrition Service, USDA, directly administers the program.

The *National School Lunch Program* assists schools in providing nutritionally adequate lunches to children by making available direct financial aid, donated foods, nonfood assistance, and technical guidance. The lunches served must meet the requirements for the "Type A lunch pattern." This pattern has been designed to provide approximately one-third of the RDA for children and includes as a minimum:

1. One-half pint of fluid milk as a beverage. Recent regulations define this to mean "fluid types of unflavored whole milk or lowfat milk or skim milk or cultured buttermilk which meet State and local standards for such types of milk and flavored milk made from such types of milk which meet such standards."

2. Two ounces (edible portion as served) of lean meat, poultry, or fish; or 2 ounces of cheese; or one egg; or one-half cup of cooked dry beans or peas; or four tablespoons of peanut butter; or an equivalent combination of these foods. To be counted in meeting these requirements these foods must be served in a main dish or in a main dish and one other menu item. When an egg or one-half cup of cooked dry peas or beans is served, it is nutritionally desirable to have an additional source of protein such as meat, cheese, or peanut butter.

3. A three-fourths cup serving that consists of two or more vegetables or fruits or both. Full strength vegetable or fruit juice may be counted to meet not more than one-fourth cup of this requirement.

4. One slice of whole grain or enriched bread; or a serving of cornbread, biscuits, rolls, or muffins made of whole-grain or enriched meal or flour.

5. One teaspoon of butter or fortified margarine.

The number of children participating in the school lunch program has steadily risen, although recently the need to increase the price of lunches has resulted in decreased pupil participation. Future changes in the program will probably aim at increasing the participation of children from low-income families and of teenagers. There is also a movement underway—although not likely to be implemented in the near future—for a universal school lunch program which would guarantee each child at least one nutritionally adequate free meal each day. Bettelheim,[6] in support of such a concept, discusses the ways in which food and the manner of its delivery may influence present and future behavior of children:

> . . . in order to make going to school attractive, and learning feasible, I would suggest that we first concentrate on feeding all children there. And by this I do not mean something akin to existing food programs which provide food as food, and not as an essential part of the educational enterprise. Instead I suggest centering the school experience around satiation of the children's needs, building the school day around meals, beginning with breakfast in the morning,

a snack at midmorning, lunch at noon, and another snack at the end of the school day. Money spent on such programs would pay off much better than that spent on practically any other expense, be it textbooks, teaching machines, etc. I would give it priority even over school buildings. But this program would have to be entirely different from the mass feedings that is characteristic of most of our food programs. The meals I have in mind are not just filling of the stomach, but an enrichment of the total personality around a common meal—which requires that only a small group should eat together, and eat with those who are supposed to educate not only their minds, but nurture their total personalities.

Many innovative changes have already occurred in school feeding programs and these as well as future ones will require careful evaluation in terms of the goals of the program. Satellite feeding systems have been used whereby those schools which do not have adequate kitchens are served from other schools where kitchen facilities are available. Similarly, some school systems have established central kitchens not located in school buildings, which provide food for the entire school system. Commercially prepared convenience foods both canned and frozen in individual-sized containers have been introduced to meet the needs of schools where facilities are inadequate. Food service management companies and caterers also provide the food for some schools under the National School Lunch Program. To increase flexibility without reducing standards, menu planning techniques designed to meet predetermined nutrient requirements are being developed and tested as an option to the Type A pattern. Alternate or engineered foods have also been introduced. These include enriched macaroni with fortified protein and textured vegetable protein products. (Chapter 4) One of the changes which caused great concern among nutritionists was that permitting the sale of competitive foods, generally from vending machines, at the same time and place as the school lunch.[7] Hallahan[8] has suggested that the choice of competitive foods "be under the supervision of the person or persons responsible for the total food operation who are concerned with the establishment and maintenance of the highest standards of good nutrition."

There is a continuing concern for the development of effective nutrition education programs in the schools. The Department of Agriculture is currently supporting the preparation and evaluation of curriculum materials in this area and some states have mandated nutrition education as part of the school curriculum.

THE SCHOOL BREAKFAST PROGRAM was established in 1966 to assist schools in providing breakfasts to pupils from low-income families or to children who had to travel long distances to school. It is available today to all schools.

According to the regulations, the breakfast pattern must include as a minimum each of the following:

1. One-half pint of fluid milk served as a beverage, or on cereal, or used in part for each purpose.
2. A one-half cup serving of fruit or full-strength fruit or vegetable juice.
3. One slice of whole-grain or enriched bread or an equivalent serving of cornbread, biscuits, rolls, muffins, etc. made of whole-grain or enriched meal or flour; three-fourths cup serving of whole-grain or enriched or fortified cereal; or an equivalent quantity of any combination of these foods.

To improve the nutrition of participating children, school breakfasts should also include as often as practicable: one egg; or a one-ounce serving (edible portion as served) of meat, fish, or poultry; or one ounce of cheese; or two tablespoons of peanut butter; or an equivalent quantity of any combination of any of these foods. Additional foods may be served with breakfast as desired.

An "alternate breakfast" consisting of a formulated grain-fruit product called fortified breakfast cake has been approved for use in breakfast programs especially in those schools without kitchen facilities. These products when served with one-half pint of milk will provide, with the exception of calories, approximately one-fourth the US–RDA for children. Critics of this program have been concerned not only about encouraging the use of cake for breakfast but also about giving credence to the idea that all cakes would be equally nutritious.

All pupils in participating schools can buy breakfast at a reasonable price. Children from low-income families are eligible for free- or reduced-price breakfasts under the same guidelines established for the school lunch program.

THE SPECIAL MILK PROGRAM'S purpose is to encourage the consumption of milk by children. All public and private schools and child-care institutions are eligible to participate. Under this program schools and other institutions are reimbursed in part for all the milk sold to children at reduced cost.

THE SPECIAL FOOD SERVICE PROGRAM FOR CHILDREN assists all public and nonprofit child care institutions in providing nutritionally adequate meals—breakfast, lunch, dinner, and between meal supplements. Guidelines for participation in this program are similar to those of the school lunch program and must include specific types of foods in minimum amounts according to the ages of the children.

Breakfast: Milk, fruit or juice, and bread or cereal;

Lunch or Supper: Milk, meat or alternate, two or more vegetables or fruits, bread and butter or margarine; and

Between Meals: Milk or fruit or vegetable or juice, and bread or cereal.

Institutions may receive assistance in the form of donated commodities, cash reimbursements, or financial help to buy food service equipment and technical guidance to establish and operate the food service program.

STUDY QUESTIONS AND ACTIVITIES

1. What are some food preferences and prejudices of children at various ages?
2. What is the probable effect of a poor breakfast on the total food intake? Why do American families so often eat an inadequate breakfast?
3. Why do you think adolescent girls eat so much more poorly than boys in the same age group? Have you had experience with this problem yourself?
4. What are the food needs of the teen-ager? Do girls have additional nutritional needs as compared with boys? What are these, why do they occur, and how may they be met?
5. How is the Daily Guide to Foods Needed by Children and Their Families adapted to meet the nutritional needs of the various age groups?
6. Why is adolescent obesity of particular concern to the nutrition counselor?
7. Observe a preschool child during mealtime either in the hospital or at a day-care center. What was the menu served to the child? What were the portion sizes? Approximately how much of the various items did the child eat? Describe his eating skills. Were there any opportunities for socializing during the meal?
8. Describe four programs included in the Child Nutrition Programs. What is the Type A pattern lunch? Plan a week's menus for lunch which meets the Type A pattern for elementary school children.
9. What forms of assistance are available to day-care centers through the Special Food Service Program for Children? Discuss the role of the nutrition consultant to group day-care programs.

SUPPLEMENTARY READINGS

Beal, V. A.: Dietary intake of individuals followed through infancy and childhood. Am. J. Public Health 51:1107, 1961.

————: Iron nutriture from infancy to adolescence. Am. J. Public Health 60:666, 1970.

Bettelheim, B: Food to Nurture the Mind. The Children's Foundation, 1026 17th St., N.W. Washington, D.C., 1970.

Children's Bureau: Your Child from 6 to 12. 1966. Moving into Adolescence. 1966. Washington, D.C., U.S. Department of Health, Education, and Welfare.

Dibble, M. V., and Lally, J. R.: Nutrition in a family-oriented child development program. J. Nutr. Educa. 5:200, 1973.

Gussow, J. D.: Improving the American diet. J. Home Econ. 65:6, 1973.

Hammar, S. L.: The role of the nutritionist in an adolescent clinic. Children, 13:217, (November-December) 1966.

Hueneman, R. L.: A review of teen-age nutrition. Health Service Reports 87:823, 1973.

Lukaczer, M.: The national school lunch program in 1973. Some accomplishments and failures. Nutr. Rev. 31:385, 1973.

Owen, G. M., et al: A study of nutrition status of preschool children in the United States, 1968–70. Pediatrics 53: No. 4, Part II, Supplement (April) 1974.

Read, M. S.: Malnutrition, hunger and behavior II. J. Am. Dietet. A. 63:386, 1973.

Sulby, A. B., Diodate, A., and Karsch, B. B.: Family day care: The nutritional component. Children Today 2:12 (May-June) 1973.

Thomas, J. A., and Call, D. L: Eating between meals—a nutrition problem among teen-agers? Nutr. Rev. 31:137, 1973.

Review: What is USDA doing about nutrition education? School Food Service J. 27:31, 1973.

For further references see Bibliography in Section 4.

REFERENCES

1. Macy, I. G., and Hunscher, H. A.: J. Nutrition 45:189, 1951.
2. Stitt, P. G.: Nutrition Education Conf., Washington, D.C., Jan. 29, 1962.
3. Dibble, M. V., and Lally, J. R.: J. Nutr. Educa. 5:200, 1973.
4. Mitchell, H. S., et al: Proc. VII, Int. Cong. Nutrition, 1967.
5. Peckos, P. S.: Food and Nutrition News (December-January) 1970-71.
6. Bettelheim, B.: Food to Nurture the Mind. The Children's Foundation, 1026 17th Street, N.W., Washington, D.C., 1970.
7. Review: Child Nutrition Programs. Dairy Council Digest 45: No. 1, (January-February) 1974. National Dairy Council, Chicago.
8. Hallahan, I. A.: J. Am. Dietet. A. 62:652, 1973.

PLATE 1

(*Top, left*) Dermatitis of hands and neck in a case of pellagra. (New York)

(*Top, right*) Beefy red glossitis in a patient with multiple B complex deficiency. This is characteristic of pellagra or sprue. (New York)

(*Center, left*) Late chronic glossitis with complete papillary atrophy, probably resulting from prolonged B complex deficiency. (Newfoundland)

(*Center, right*) Angular stomatitis and dermatitis, probably due to a riboflavin deficiency. (Grace A. Goldsmith, M.D., Tulane University)

(*Bottom, left*) Advanced gingivitis: marked swelling of papillae with loss of tissue and retraction of gums (Newfoundland). Nutritional factors most apt to be associated with such a condition in Newfoundland are ascorbic acid and some of the B vitamins.

(*Bottom, right*) "Granulated" eyelids, or conjunctival follicular hypertrophy, is common in malnourished children. It begins with reddening and thickening of the lower lid. (Florida)

(Plate 1 from Jolliffe, Norman, Tisdall, F. F., and Cannon, Paul R.: Clinical Nutrition, New York, Hoeber.)

PLATE 1

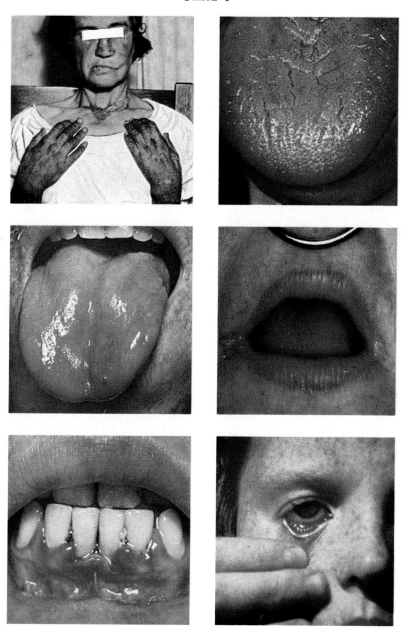

19

geriatric nutrition

Nutrition of Older People
Food Requirements Change With Age
Planning Meals For Older People
Community Food and Nutrition Programs
  For the Older Age Adult

Nutritional requirements for the mature person and the older adult are not fundamentally different from those of the young adult. However, because the aging process gives each age group unique characteristics, geriatric nutrition is worthy of special consideration.

The difference between the terms *aged* and *aging* should be clearly defined: the aged are people; aging is a continuous process. Aging begins at conception and terminates at death. Thus, birth, growth, maturation, and senescence are all part of the normal aging process. Aging proceeds more rapidly during the growing years because change is more rapid at that time. In the adult, the aging process slows down and the rate of this change may be further retarded; the active period of life may be extended by good health practices. Thus, since there are persons who, in terms of chronological age, may be considered old but are in fact young in appearance, attitude, and/or stage of the biological aging process, the term aged is not appropriate when referring to a chronological age group. Consequently, the term aging, which is both relative and multidimensional, is more generally descriptive of the older adult population.[1]

277

The population figure of 20 million persons over 65 years of age in the United States in 1971 is about double the number for that age group in 1940. Of this number, over 60 percent are widowed or unmarried, and many live alone. One-half of the women and one-third of the men over 65 years living alone had annual incomes under $1000. Medical science, which is largely responsible for the increase in the number of senior citizens alive today, is also challenged to learn more about the degenerative and chronic diseases common in this group. The social sciences also have a responsibility to help make later years of life worthwhile.

Besides the obvious changes of aging, there are invisible changes within the body that may develop as gradually as greying hair. Therefore, authorities emphasize that an adult's nutrition must be considered in terms of the past, the present, and the future. The nutritional state of a person at 70 or 80 reflects not only his current food practices but all of his previous dietary history as well. This can be observed by anyone with a long close association with older persons. As Dr. Swanson[2] comments:

> The older a person grows, the longer and more complex is his dietary history. The variations in nutritional status and dietary needs of a group of adults thus are bound to be greater than corresponding variations in a group of young people. Recommendations for the food needs of this age group must be pointed especially to the needs of individuals.

> The same nutritional principles that describe adequate diets for earlier periods of life apply to the diets of adults. Even though the adult has grown up—matured—his basic food supply still must provide all the nutrients necessary for maintaining body structure and for operating its machinery.

Good nutrition is only one of the habits which help to maintain strength and vigor, and it can be practiced three times a day—but it is abused more frequently than any other.

It has been demonstrated repeatedly that older people can adjust to different circumstances, learn new skills, and adopt new food habits. We cite a few examples: the 80-year-old man who learned to eat salads when a thoughtful housekeeper chopped them to make them easier to eat yet kept them colorful and attractive; the two women in Fig. 19–1 serving as hospital volunteers, feeling useful and adapting themselves to needed tasks; the elderly homemaker still trying new gadgets and ready-prepared foods to make work easier and also add interest and variety to meals for two. "Never too old to learn" is a far truer adage than "You can't teach an old dog new tricks."

None of us is too young to begin thinking about improving our health prospects for later years. People buy annuities and life insurance for the future; why shouldn't they consider other steps which may give even greater security and comfort?

NUTRITION OF OLDER PEOPLE

Food Habits and the Consequences

Food habits of older people do not always coincide with their food needs. Several surveys of the food choices of older people have been made in different localities; all report much the same trends. In a Boston

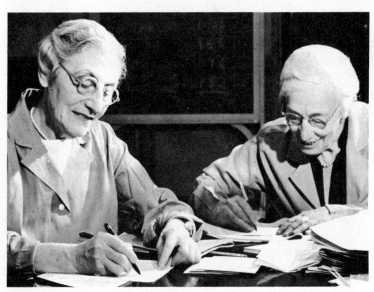

Fig. 19–1. Two long-faithful volunteers happy doing a needed job. (The New York Hospital)

survey of 104 geriatric patients, most of them over 70, Davidson[3] found a marked decrease in consumption of meat and milk and an increased use of eggs, but no caloric deficit. In fact, 84 percent of the men and 71 percent of the women were above desirable weight. He observed factors that seemed to affect the food habits of these elderly retired people: social situation (over half of them lived alone), reduced income, limited cooking and refrigeration facilities, marketing difficulties, condition of the teeth, sense of smell, problems of swallowing, food faddism, and long-standing misconceptions about good nutrition.

When 24-hour diet recall tests were administered to approximately 4000 participants entering congregate meal programs sponsored by the Administration on Aging, only 3 percent were found to have "good diets." In other words, only this small number met 100 percent of the Recommended Dietary Allowances (1968) for protein, calcium, iron, vitamin A, thiamine, riboflavin, and vitamin C. Eleven percent met 2/3 of the RDA for these nutrients and were classified as having "fair diets," while 86 percent were below 2/3 of the RDA for one or more nutrients and were classified as having "poor diets." Many of the older people did not consume any milk products, or fruits and vegetables, and a large number reported having fewer than three meals each day.[4]

SUSCEPTIBILITY TO FADS. Unfortunately, many adults in late middle age, or older, are misled in their search for "eternal youth" or relief from their aches and pains. They hear and believe the TV and radio promotions of various panaceas—elixirs or multivitamin and mineral mixtures claimed to be remedies for all sorts of ills. They read and believe the fad health books, especially those that have been flooding the book market during the past decade. It is well-known that food and nutrition quackery thrives in areas where middle income retired people congregate. So-called health food stores may carry many desirable food items, but they also stock a variety of items ("health foods") promoted by the faddists. The cost of fad foods may divert money from other food items or from other needs. Indiscriminate use of vitamin and mineral supplements may also cost the older individual money that could more appropriately be used to purchase a better quality diet, one more generally beneficial to health.

FOOD REQUIREMENTS CHANGE WITH AGE. The dietary requirements of later life are influenced by a number of factors such as general health; degree of physical activity; changes in ability to chew, digest, and absorb food; efficiency in the use of nutrients by the tissues; alteration in the endocrine system; emotional state; and mental health. The nutrient and calorie allowances that maintain one person in optimum health may be inadequate or more than adequate to meet the needs of another, apparently similar, individual. Dr. Swanson's comment is especially pertinent:[5]

A person at 70 is an historical record of all that has happened to him—his injuries, infections, nutritional imbalances, fatigues, and emotional upsets. Old people, therefore, differ from each other much more than do younger folk. All this needs to be considered in food planning for any old person. Each one is an individual, quite unlike anyone else.

Calorie Needs

The major physiologic change occurring with age is a decrease in the number of functioning cells, which results in a slowing down of metabolic processes. This, together with a decrease in physical activity, may reduce the energy needs of the older adult. For example, a woman over 50 years of age weighing 128 pounds may need only 1800 calories whereas she needed 2000 or more at age 23. If she does not reduce her caloric intake to conform to her needs, she will store the excess as fat—which is so common in older people, particularly women.

WHEN CALORIES NEED TO BE REDUCED. The food sources of reduced calories must be chosen with care to include all essential factors, in higher proportion than that needed in former years because the total food consumed is less. There is an obvious need for foods which carry a full quota of proteins, minerals, and vitamins. It is essential to reduce comsumption of empty calories—sugar, rich desserts, cakes, candies, fats, and alcohol.

Reduction in total calories involves a most difficult task of alteration of food habits. For the majority of persons, habit is perhaps one of the greatest obstacles in the path to an optimal diet. The longer the habits are continued, the more fixed they become. The food habits of older people are apt to be so fixed that it is difficult to change them unless the way is made easy.

Whoever is planning or preparing the meals for overweight persons—the homemaker herself, a health aide or housekeeper—can eliminate some calories behind the scenes (if necessary) while still keeping meals attractive and in the familiar pattern. If people do not see the high calorie foods, one psychological barrier has been overcome. By substituting for rich cakes and pastries such items as puddings and custards made with skim milk, angel food cake and more fruit desserts, gelatins, whips, etc., calories are saved without sacrificing flavor. Also, low-calorie salad dressings, less butter or margarine on vegetables, and gravies made with a minimum of fat are devices for the cook to use before the food reaches the table.

When appropriate, the nutrition counselor concerned with the continuing education of the patient may make specific suggestions along this line in keeping with the socioeconomic status of the patient and his cultural pattern of eating.

Surplus calories are not the only reason for curtailing carbohydrates and fats in the diets of older people. Impaired glucose tolerance associated with a delayed insulin response is a fairly common occurrence in older people, especially women. When this is found, a reduction in the total amount of carbohydrate, but especially in the amount of sugar in the diet, is advisable.

Fats are the most concentrated source of calories and often the invisible component of common foods. For those who eat out, foods fried in deep fat are apt to be popular, since fats give flavor and satiety value to meals. However, since the ability to digest and absorb fat appears to decrease with advancing years, too much fat may result in indigestion or discomfort for some older adults.

The most serious problem for the middle aged and past middle aged group concerns the type and amount of fat in the diet and their relation to the blood cholesterol level and to the incidence of atherosclerosis. There are still many uncertainties and misconceptions concering this problem, which is discussed in Chapters 3 and 29.

WHEN CALORIES NEED TO BE INCREASED. Quite another problem exists for the really elderly, or the disabled and shut-in who may not get enough food to meet energy or other nutritional requirements. If they live alone or have poor cooking facilities, they may have little incentive or opportunity to market and cook for themselves.

Sometimes appetite fails to tempt the very elderly to eat enough food or the right kind of food. The reduced calories in such cases seldom carry enough of the essential nutrients.

The undernutrition which may occur can be relieved by attention to foods with low bulk and concentrated calories that are high in protein, vitamins, and minerals and are prepared in a tasty way. This may not be easy for the person living alone to achieve; even for someone living with a large family, attention to the younger members of the family may seem more important to the homemaker than tempting the appetite of an elderly grandmother. For others the same problem may stem from the necessity of eating in hotels or restaurants where food does not appeal to the appetite or may be too expensive.

Protein Requirements

Apparently, protein needs are not reduced appreciably with age, and yet many older people eat less protein than they did when younger. This is most likely to happen where marketing is difficult, cooking facilities are poor, or the money for food is limited. It can also happen among those with a better economic status when denture troubles, lack of appetite, or too little energy prevent the preparing or the eating of meats or other protein foods.

Some good-quality protein is essential at each meal regardless of age. The Recommended Dietary Allowances (0.8 g./kg. body weight) suggest no reduction in protein with age, as they do in calories. Thus, the proportion of protein making up the total calories is increased.

The requirement for certain amino acids may even be increased to meet changes in body function with age. Bigwood[6] found the methionine and lysine requirements of six male subjects 50 to 70 years of age to be substantially greater than that of younger males.

Special attention may need to be given to meeting the protein requirements of the older person if he is sharing in the family meals planned to meet the higher caloric food habits of younger members of the family. An extra glass of skim milk at meals or between meals may be consumed to supplement smaller servings of meat, fish, or other high protein main dishes. If the person lives alone, milk, cheese, and eggs are often used as alternates for meat, fish, or poultry because of ease in preparation. Adequate calories tend to spare protein, so that the total food intake should always be taken into account.

Mineral Requirements

The calcium needs of older people seem to be as great as the needs of younger adults.

Inadequate calcium intake along with some endocrine disturbance may cause the loss of calcium from the bones and lead to osteoporosis and resulting fragility, so frequently responsible for fractures. Lowered gastric acidity and hepatic and pancreatic insufficiency may contribute by impairing calcium absorption. Increased excretion of calcium due to impaired kidney function or to reduced physical activity may also play a role in osteoporosis. Dr. Swanson's comments are pertinent.[7]

We cannot consider bony tissue in the adult as static material. It is a dynamic substance, which constantly remodels itself. Formation of new bone and destruction of old bone go on simultaneously. These processes approximately balance each other in the healthy adult .... As a person grows older, however, the process of bone destruction may overbalance that of bone building. That this occurs is suggested by observations that the average weight of the skeleton decreases gradually after age 35. The extent to which such decalcification may proceed without injury is not known. We do know that it does not always occur in all individuals.

But we cannot ignore the fact that osteoporosis, or deficient bone substance, certainly is not uncommon in later life . . . . It is commoner among older women than among men. Persons with marked osteoporosis tend to eat food poor in a number of nutrients, including calcium. They also tend to improve in health and to store calcium when the diet is improved.

Osteoporosis is prevalent among older people around the world. The reason for poor calcium absorption or utilization in older people is still subject to speculation. There is a possibility that traces of fluorine in drinking water may improve calcium utilization and thus decrease the incidence of osteoporosis. A survey of people living in high and low fluoride areas of North Dakota[8] showed osteoporosis more common in the low fluoride areas than in the higher fluoride areas. This finding served to confirm earlier suggestions of the benefit of fluoride for older people.

At present the best suggestion is to provide liberal amounts of milk and milk products. These may be used in cooking, creamed soups, milk desserts, and other such foods. The use of nonfat dry milk is to be encouraged in cooking as an inexpensive source of good protein and calcium. Present evidence favors about 0.8 g. of calcium per day.

Needs for other minerals for the elderly are apparently similar to those for all adults, as discussed in Chapter 5.

Vitamin Requirements

Unfortunately, little is known regarding the vitamin requirements of older people and whether there is a change associated with age or with chronic disease. However, there is no evidence that vitamin requirements are reduced with advancing years, and it is safe to assume that older people need all the vitamins they did in earlier years.

If there has been merely a marginal supply of any vitamin in the diet for many years, a reduction in total food eaten may be sufficient to precipitate minor nutritional deficiencies. The time factor of advancing age may permit cumulative effects to show up.

PLANNING MEALS FOR OLDER PEOPLE

The planning of menus to meet the needs of the older age group presents problems which are as varied as the circumstances in which such people live. They may be living alone, or with one or two other older people, and marketing and preparing meals for themselves; they may be the older member in a younger family; they may be cared for by a practical nurse or a housekeeper. Whoever is responsible for planning and preparing their food should be aware of

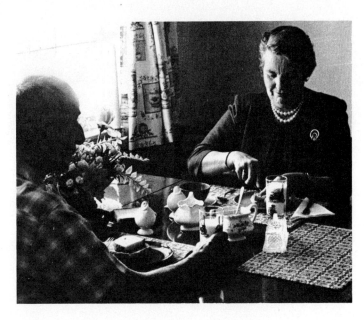

Fig. 19–2. Good food and a pleasant environment enliven the day for this retired couple. (U.S. Department HEW, Administration on Aging)

individual likes and dislikes, and special needs and limitations. There are numerous factors, such as ignorance of nutritional facts, food prejudices, fear of new foods, lack of money, limited cooking facilities, poor dentition, and poor appetite, which should be considered. The Daily Food Guide described in Chapter 10 is as important for meeting the nutritional needs of older people as for younger ones. The nutrition counselor may be able to advise or help with the planning where such problems seem to interfere with adequate nutrition.

The elderly person, too often a forgotten member of the household, may require some special foods or food preparation, but so far as possible he or she should be a member of the family at mealtime and eat foods prepared for the family. If digestive ability is limited, the family meals should be planned so that the older person may avoid fried foods, rich sauces, pastries, and other foods that disagree with him. When lack of mealtime appetite makes an adequate food intake difficult, a midmorning and a midafternoon snack such as hot malted milk or orange juice, may be offered. A hot drink at bedtime may be welcomed by an older person and may help to induce sleep.

The older handicapped person, living alone, may encounter real difficulties in preparing meals for himself. Homemaking for the Handicapped offers many suggestions to those with physical limitations to assist them in acquiring homemaking skills.[9]

When groups of older people are confined in institutions or nursing homes, they sometimes become depressed. Volpe and Kastenbaum[10] reported on a ward of 34 confused and debilitated older men who were agitated and hostile and had poor appetites. They were transferred to a larger ward where a record player was installed and games provided and where there were large tables for meals. They dressed in white shirts and ties and had an afternoon snack of beer, crackers, and cheese. Within a month the atmosphere changed and behavior improved.

Bulletins and pamphlets published by national and state agencies and by insurance companies give simple information about food for older people.

Making simple food attractive and appropriate to the specific needs of an elderly person may be appreciated far out of proportion to the effort involved. This is particularly important when an event in their honor is celebrated such as a birthday, anniversary, or other special occasion. By considering the texture and consistency of various menu items as well as their relationship to any diet modification, appropriate meals that will be enjoyed by all can be planned.

COMMUNITY FOOD AND NUTRITION PROGRAMS FOR THE OLDER-AGE ADULT

Many communities have programs which provide services especially appropriate for the older-age adult. The following discussion indicates the variety of opportunities which may be available to the senior citizen in his community. The nutrition counselor should become knowledgeable about the resources in her local area.

FOOD STAMPS AND DONATED COMMODITIES. The local community may have a food stamp or donated commodities program to aid all low income persons in obtaining an adequate diet. Many older age adults, living on very limited incomes, are eligible for assistance from a program which the local community provides. The welfare department determines eligibility, depending on the size and income of the family unit.

In the food stamp program, those eligible to participate must purchase food stamps at a bank or other authorized agency. The actual purchasing power of these stamps is greater than the amount which the consumer pays for them. The stamps or coupons may be used to buy food in any cooperating retail store. Although food stamps represent a real saving in terms of food dollars, many older citizens with very little cash to spend hesitate to make the proportionately large monthly or semimonthly investment which is necessary to purchase the coupons. This aspect of food budgeting is an area where the nutrition counselor may be able to help the older client understand the long term advantages of such a program.

The local welfare department also certifies eligibility for donated commodities depending on the family size and income. In this program, certain donated foods are made available for pickup by eligible recipients at specific times and places. This system, although supplying a variety of different kinds of foods at no cost to the recipient, is often difficult for the elderly person: the place and time may be inconvenient as far as transportation is concerned; the packaging may be too large for the one- or two-member family; or the food processing may not be appropriate for modified diets, as in the case of sodium restriction. Foods may also be included that are unfamiliar to the older person. By understanding various aspects of the problem, the nutrition counselor may be able to assist the senior citizen to plan for the economical use of donated foods.

HOME HEALTH OR NEIGHBORHOOD AIDES. For the person capable of remaining in the home where assistance in meal management can be furnished, home health or neighborhood aides have been made available by certain community agencies. These aides are trained to go into homes to "provide advice, nutrition counseling, education, information services, and moral support on such matters as marketing, food preparation, handling and storage, uses of equipment, and budgeting."[11] Nurses together with other members of the home care team such as dietitians, nutritionists, or home economists, help train and supervise home health aides. The provision of these services enables an elderly person to continue to maintain himself for longer periods of time in his own home than could be possible otherwise.

PORTABLE MEALS PROGRAMS. Often referred to as meals-on-wheels, portable meals programs have been initiated in many cities by various community groups. They are for the home-bound person who cannot prepare his own meals. They often provide two meals a day (one hot and one cold) for five days a week. Because breakfasts and weekend meals are usually not included, participants in these programs must have some additional resource for providing meals in the home.

COMMUNITY GROUP FEEDING PROGRAMS. In recent years a variety of group-feeding projects have been started in communities to provide the older adult with good nutrition in a sociable atmosphere. Federal grants have helped sponsor many of these in different locations throughout the country. All sorts of facilities have been used, from churches and schools to housing projects and senior citizen day care centers. For the older person who is able to go to the center and is interested in meeting people, these programs offer recreational as well as nutritional benefits. Many of these centers also include nutrition or consumer education programs.

In 1972, a new Title VII of the Older Americans Act of 1965 established the Nutrition Programs for the Elderly. Since the goal of this program is to provide older Americans, particularly those with low incomes, with low cost, nutritionally sound meals served in strategically located centers, such as schools, churches, community centers, senior citizen centers, and other public and private facilities where they can obtain other social and rehabilitative services, many of the community congregate meal programs are now supported in large measure by federal funds granted under this legislation. Besides promoting better health among the older segment of the population through improved nutrition, these programs are aimed at reducing the social isolation of old age, offering older Americans an opportunity to live with dignity and companionship. No one aged 60 or over or his or her spouse can be denied participation in a Nutrition Program for the Elderly by virtue of economic status. Thus, those able to afford to contribute are expected to do so in accordance with schedules developed by local projects.

Guidelines for Nutrition Programs for the Elderly require that the following meal pattern be adopted, which should provide at least one-third of the RDA for the participants in the program:

> meat or alternate—three ounces cooked edible portion of meat or meat alternate
> vegetables and fruits—two one-half cup servings
> enriched or whole bread or alternate—one serving
> butter or margarine—one teaspoon
> dessert—one-half cup
> milk—one-half pint
> optional beverages—as desired.

Menus must be posted in a conspicuous location in each congregate meal site. Special menus where feasible and appropriate should be available to individuals in the programs. The delivery of food and supportive services may be made also to homebound participants.

If the Project Director is not a Registered Dietitian or Nutritionist, one should be employed by the project to review and advise on policy decisions regarding the nutrition component, to plan, review, and approve all menus, to coordinate special diet menus with general menus, to plan and implement nutrition education for staff and participants, and to provide diet counseling.

An important feature of the Nutrition Programs is the Outreach service. Outreach tries to seek out and identify the maximum number of hard-to-reach, isolated, and withdrawn eligible individuals and then provide them with the opportunity to participate in the program.

The senior citizen is often hesitant about searching for and requesting help; so it is especially important for the nutrition counselor to know the opportunities available and how to take advantage of them.

STUDY QUESTIONS AND ACTIVITIES

1. Surveys have shown that older people are apt to omit certain foods from their diets. Which ones are these and which nutrients are deficient as a result?
2. Why is the caloric requirement of older people reduced? How much reduction in caloric intake is recommended between ages 23 and 51?

3. What advice would you give an older person who should reduce his calorie intake? How may calories be increased for the underweight older person?
4. What disease in older people may result from failure to absorb or utilize calcium? What suggestions are offered that may help to improve calcium utilization?
5. If an elderly person shares the family fare but eats less of everything than younger members, which nutrients may be lower than recommended? How can this be remedied?
6. In what circumstances may the use of vitamin concentrates be justified?
7. If an older person with whom you are associated is a food faddist, how would you attempt to correct his false ideas? What reliable sources of information would you recommend?
8. What nutrition services for older people are available in your community?

SUPPLEMENTARY READINGS

Alvarez, W. C.: Osteoporosis, a disease that attacks millions. Geriatrics 25:77, 1970.
Berman, P. M., and Kersner, J. B.: The aging gut 2. Diseases of the colon, pancreas, liver and gallbladder, functional bowel disease and iatrogenic disease. Geriatrics 27:117, 1972.
Current Comment: Nutrition and eating problems of the elderly. J. Am. Dietet. A. 58:43, 1971.
Exton-Smith, A. N.: Physiological aspects of aging: relationship to nutrition. Am. J. Clin. Nutr. 25:853, 1972.
Greenberg, B.: Reaction time in the elderly. Am. J. Nursing 73:2056, 1973.
Gress, L. D.: Sensitizing students to the aged. Am. J. Nursing 71:1968, 1971.
Luhrs, C. E.: Feeding the elderly. Am. J. Clin. Nutr. 26:1150, 1973.
Pelcovits, J.: Nutrition for older Americans. J. Am. Dietet. A. 58:17, 1971.

Schlenker, E. D., et al: Nutrition and health of older people. Am. J. Clin. Nutr. 26:1111, 1973.
Sherman, E. M. and Brittan, M. R.: Contemporary food gatherers: a study of food shopping habits of an elderly urban population. The Gerontologist 13:358, 1973.
Sherwood, S.: Sociology of food and eating: implications for action for the elderly. Am. J. Clin. Nutr. 26:1108, 1973.
Shock, N. W.: Physiologic aspects of aging. J. Am. Dietet. A. 56:491, 1970.
Turner, T. B.: Beer and wine for geriatric patients. Editorial. JAMA 226:779, 1973.
Wells, C. E.: Nutrition programs under the Older Americans Act. Am. J. Clin. Nutr. 26:1127, 1973.

REFERENCES

1. Beattie, W. M.: Matching services to individual needs of the aging in Working With Older People: A Guide to Practice. III The Aging Person: Needs and Services. DHEW—PHS—HSMHA #1459, Washington, D.C., 1970.
2. Swanson, P.: Nutrition Needs, After 25. Food. The Yearbook of Agriculture. Chap. 28. USDA, Washington, D.C., 1959.
3. Davidson, C. S.: Am. J. Clin. Nutr. 10:181, 1962.
4. Bechill, W. D., and Wolgamot, I.: Nutrition for the Elderly. DHEW Publ. No. 73:20236, Washington, D.C., 1973.
5. Swanson, P.: op. cit.
6. Bigwood, E. J.: Nutritio et Dieta 8:226, 1966.
7. Swanson, P.: op. cit.
8. Bernstein, D. S.: JAMA 198:499, 1966.
9. May, E. E., Waggoner, N. R., and Boettke, E. M.: Homemaking for the Handicapped. New York, Dodd, Mead, 1966.
10. Volpe, A., and Kastenbaum, R.: Am. J. Nurs. 67:100, 1967.
11. Howell, S. C., and Loeb, M. B.: Nutrition and aging—a monograph for practitioners. The Gerontologist 9:77 (Autumn) 1969.

For further references see Bibliography in Section 4.

20

malnutrition—
a world problem

NUTRITION PLANNING:
A PRIORITY IN NATIONAL DEVELOPMENT

Estimates indicate that there are a billion and a
half women, men, and children in the world today
suffering from severe, moderate, or mild
malnutrition.[1] Most of these people live in
developing countries. The capacity of
malnourished adults for work may be significantly
reduced and their potential as family providers and
as bearers of children may be equally affected.
Some children will die from malnutrition; larger
numbers will suffer physical, and possibly mental,
retardation and will be more susceptible to
infectious diseases.[2] Due to the synergistic effect of
the combination of malnutrition and infection,
malnourished children are not only more apt to
contract infectious diseases such as diarrhea, upper
respiratory infections, bronchitis, and measles, but
are also less able to withstand the effects of such
diseases than children who are adequately

nourished. The high mortality rate from infectious disease among children in developing countries is a reflection of the nutritional status of these children.

Recent findings of a five-year study, The Inter-American Investigation of Mortality in Children, identified nutritional deficiency as the most important factor contributing to the very high childhood mortality in Latin America. Low birth weight or malnutrition was either a primary or secondary cause of death in more than half of the 35,000 deaths of children under the age of five years.[3] Because of improved medical care in the last thirty years, more children may survive severe episodes of illness during early life, but at school age these survivors show signs of physical underdevelopment and appear to be withdrawn and uninterested in their environment.[4]

Consequently, the degree to which long term effects of malnutrition may relate to the socioeconomic development of a nation is becoming of increasing concern to government planners in developing countries. Low productivity, poor quality of life, increased expenditures for health and medical care, and low returns from educational investments are some costs that accrue to a nation which is not concerned with improving the nutritional status of its poor. Thus, for economic as well as for humanitarian reasons, nutrition should have a high priority in national development plans. Nutrition intervention programs can be planned in terms of cost effectiveness—an important consideration as they compete for the limited resources available for development in poorer countries. Moreover, government decision makers must realize that expanding employment opportunities and larger incomes would increase consumption among low income groups.

Since FAO's Agricultural Commodity Projections for 1970-1980, based on national food balance sheet data submitted by member countries, indicate that there are adequate levels of food supplies available for human consumption, the major problem remains one of distribution—among nations, among rich and poor within a nation, and even among individual family members. Government decisions regarding food policies will largely determine whether individual nations and the world as a whole will have a surplus or a deficit of food in the future. These complex issues must be examined by nutritionists, agricultural specialists, food technologists, economists, bankers, and development planners before political decisions on policy can be made and implemented by individual nations. The present world food crisis (Chapter 1) suggests an immediate urgency for such action.

INTERNATIONAL PLANNING TO CONTROL FAMINE

The World Food Conference and the follow-up meeting held in Rome in 1974 (Chapter 1) are examples of international planning aimed at preventing future famines such as those that occurred in Bangladesh and Biafra. Of the many recommendations made at the meetings, four are considered to be the most significant. They are: (1) the establishment of a World Food Council to oversee international activities for improving the food situation, (2) a consultative group to coordinate investments in agricultural development, (3) an early warning system to detect impending famines, and (4) a world food reserve to be distributed in time of famine. Considerable progress has been made in implementing the first two suggestions while the latter two proposals have lagged.

The World Food Council, with 36 member countries, is funded by the United Nations Secretariat budget and is responsible to the General Assembly. It coordinates the activities of existing agencies such as the Food and Agricultural Organization as well as any new agencies which develop. It first met in 1975. The Consultative Group on Food Production and Investment in Developing Countries was established under the auspices of the World Bank to identify places and projects around the world where major financial investment is needed to improve food production. It helps donor countries and agencies to funnel aid money into useful projects.

In order to detect famines the early warning system must have access to up-to-date information on weather, crop forecasts, and production figures from all large countries. China and the Soviet Union have in the past been reluctant to provide such data and their future responses are not predictable. There are also many problems in establishing a world food reserve, since it would require keeping quantities of grain out of normal market channels to be available for famine prevention. The U.S. Department of Agriculture is presently reluctant to buy and store grain. It prefers that grain stocks be held by the private sector, so that grain could be sold on the world market instead of being stored for famine relief. It is thus obvious that, although major steps have been taken to prevent famines, the problem is still far from being resolved. Since famines are dramatic causes of severe malnutrition which attract world attention, and they are so far from being dealt with effectively, it is feared that even less will be done to alleviate unpublicized food shortages which exist among smaller segments of population groups.

IDENTIFICATION OF NUTRITION PROBLEMS

The extent of malnutrition in the world today is difficult to determine because specific deficiency diseases with obvious clinical signs are not encountered as frequently as they were a half-century ago. Instead, the presence of more moderate and less clearly identified forms of malnutrition are foremost in terms of public health. Health workers are challenged not only to identify and treat nutritional deficiencies but also to understand and prevent the causes of malnutrition before children and adults are handicapped by its effects.

The medical history which includes a dietary history, combined with a physical examination and appropriate laboratory tests, remain the most important tools in diagnosing individual nutritional problems. Morbidity and mortality statistics can give helpful information regarding the prevalence of malnutri-

tion. Physical growth data may also be used as an indicator of the status of a community in regard to nutrition. The causes of malnutrition are multiple and frequently overlap in a given situation. They include problems related to the physical environment, social structure, family development and child rearing patterns, agricultural practices, or natural disasters. An understanding of how these various factors interrelate in specific communities is important for all health personnel. The encouragement of breast feeding at the same time that more emphasis is placed on immunization programs could, in many instances, improve the nutritional status of large numbers of young children.

Nutritional problems may be classified into three main groups according to their geographical range and prevalence. First, those which are common to most of the developing countries: protein-calorie malnutrition (PCM), nutritional anemia, endemic

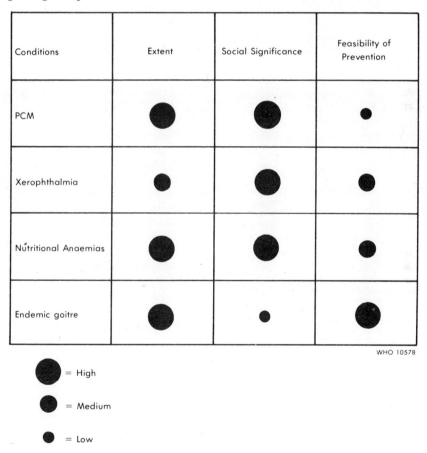

Fig. 20–1. Priorities among nutritional conditions. (Bengoa, J. M., in *Nutrition, National Development and Planning,* A. Berg, N. S. Scrimshaw, and D. L. Call, eds. Cambridge, MIT Press, 1973)

goiter, ariboflavinosis, and dental problems; secondly, those found in certain areas of developing countries: xerophthalmia and rickets; and lastly, those limited to very specific areas: pellegra, beriberi, and scurvy.[5]

According to Bengoa[6] there are four conditions which, because of their prevalence, social significance, and feasible prevention (Fig. 20-1), should have the highest priority from an international point of view:

1. Protein-calorie malnutrition, which has a high prevalence, a high mortality rate and can produce irreversible physical and mental damage in those who survive. Although the feasibility of eradicating PCM at the present time is recognizably low, the consequences of this problem are so extreme that it must be given first priority.
2. Xerophthalmia, which is less prevalent but more easily prevented than PCM. This disease not only contributes to childhood mortality but also causes irreversible blindness in its victims.
3. Nutritional anemias, which, like PCM, have high prevalence and contribute to mortality from many other conditions also have negative effects on an individual's working capacity. The feasibility of prevention is similar to that of xerophthalmia.
4. Endemic goiter, which has less social significance than the first three conditions, but is as prevalent as PCM and the nutritional anemias and much more feasible to prevent.

PROTEIN-CALORIE MALNUTRITION (PCM)

The term, protein-calorie malnutrition (PCM), is used to identify a complex group of related nutritional problems, as shown in Table 20-1. Since energy intake is regarded by many authorities to be the more important problem in childhood malnutrition today, the term energy-protein malnutrition (EPM) is also used to describe these conditions.[7] Children with PCM are always retarded in their growth and development but other clinical symptoms vary with the age and condition of the child and the intensity of the causal factors. A severe deficiency of both calories and protein results in nutritional marasmus; whereas a severe protein deficiency with more adequate energy intake may result in kwashiorkor. Both of these are severe, the latter, an acute disease from which the child either dies quickly or, with suitable medical care, recovers quickly. Nutritional marasmus may also terminate in death if not treated. Some children present symptoms of an intermediate or mixed form of PCM showing clinical signs of both marasmus and kwashiorkor. Most of the children suffering from PCM present a moderate form of the disease and many may go unrecognized unless an infectious disease, famine, or some other factor precipitates a more severe form. In community studies made between 1963 and 1972 in Latin America, Africa, and Asia, it was estimated that 100 million children between birth and four years of age were suffering from severe or moderate protein-calorie malnutrition. In addition, the number of children in these areas who show signs of nutritional dwarfing is unknown.[8]

Nutritional Marasmus

The age of a child is an important factor in determining whether severe protein-calorie malnutrition will appear as nutritional marasmus or kwashiorkor. Marasmus is more likely to develop in children under one year of age when breastfeeding fails or is not carried on for a sufficient length of time and suitable foods for weaning either are not available or feeding practices discourage their use. The decreased incidence of breastfeeding among mothers in developing countries contributes greatly to the high proportion of deaths due to nutritional deficiency and diarrheal disease. Records of hospital admissions in many countries indicate that the number of cases of marasmus is increasing while kwashiorkor is becoming less frequent.

As indicated in Table 20-1, the infant with marasmus is more than 40 percent below standard body weight. There is an absence of subcutaneous fat, muscle wasting, and diminution of height or length. (See Undernutrition, Chapter 34.) Edema is not noticeable.[9] The marasmic infant looks like a little old man, whith a big head and huge eyes, wrinkled face, and tiny body. Such infants are particularly susceptible to infectious disease and their mortality rate is high.

Table 20-1. Simplified Classification of PCM*

CATEGORIES	BODY WEIGHT % OF STANDARD	BODY HEIGHT	EDEMA	DEFICIT OF WEIGHT FOR HEIGHT
Kwashiorkor	80-60	Affected	+	+ +
Marasmus	<60	Affected	0	+ +
Mixed forms (marasmic kwashiorkor)	<60	Affected	+	+ +
Underweight child (moderate PCM)	80-60	Affected	0	Minimal
Nutritional dwarfing	<60	Pronounced deficit	0	Minimal

* Reprinted from Bengoa, J. M., *Nutrition, National Development and Planning*, A. Berg, N. S. Scrimshaw, and D. L. Call (eds.), 1973, by permission of the MIT Press, Cambridge, Mass.

Kwashiorkor

In 1933, Dr. Cicely Williams, a British pediatrician working in West Africa, first described this disease in children from one to four years of age. She called it by its local name, "kwashiorkor," and found that milk could cure it. The name means: the disease the deposed baby gets when the next one is born.[10] The picture of a mother from Uganda (Fig. 20-2) is a striking example: the healthy infant in arms and the "deposed" one by her side.

Although kwashiorkor was first described and named in Africa, it has also been recognized to exist in Latin America and Asia. Severe protein-calorie malnutrition tends to appear as kwashiorkor rather than marasmus when the child is over one year old. The presence of edema is its most distinguishing characteristic, Table 20-1. Invariably, growth is retarded although the presence of edema may conceal the degree of emaciation. Kwashiorkor is caused by severe protein deficiency relative to energy intake, although it may be superimposed on any degree of marasmus and is frequently precipitated by the occurrence of an infectious disease. Kwashiorkor is an acute condition of short duration in which recovery or death occurs relatively rapidly. The mortality rate even among hospitalized children is high. The child is apathetic and miserable. There may also be disorders of pigmentation of the skin and hair and some liver enlargement.

Kwashiorkor is found in areas where starchy roots or tubers are the staple food, or less commonly, where cereals are the staple food. Although cereal grains are better sources of protein than starchy roots or tubers,

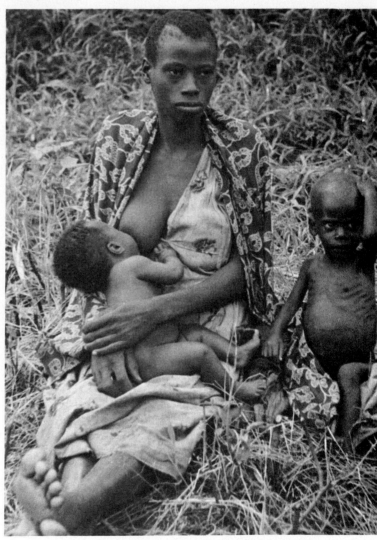

Fig. 20-2. The older child in this picture shows the protein calorie deprivation and the malnutrition that occurred when he was "deposed" or replaced at the mother's breast by the new baby. He is subsisting on starchy foods and a few vegetables. (From Dr. John Bennett, Nutrition Unit, Ministry of Health, Kampala, Uganda)

many cereal grains do not have sufficient good quality protein relative to their bulk and energy value to serve as appropriate weaning foods for young children when milk is not available.[11]

MIXED FORMS OF SEVERE PROTEIN–CALORIE MALNUTRITION. As shown in Table 20-1, some children show clinical signs of both marasmus and kwashiorkor. They present a weight deficit of more than 40 percent of standard weight which is indicative of nutritional marasmus; in addition, they have edema and other symptoms of kwashiorkor. It has been recognized that an infant with marasmus may develop kwashiorkor as a result of protein losses incurred during acute infection. Similarly, an infant in whom kwashiorkor has been diagnosed may, when edema disappears during treatment, appear marasmic.[12]

MODERATE FORM OF PROTEIN–CALORIE MALNUTRITION. More children suffer from the moderate form of PCM than the severe form. Although there is not total uniformity in the diagnosis of this form, a weight deficit of 25 to 40 percent below standard is the general criterion used to determine it. Children with moderate PCM may become severely malnourished as a result of diarrhea or other infectious diseases. The practice of feeding the sick child a very limited diet consisting primarily of carbohydrate can precipitate acute malnutrition in the preschool age group.

NUTRITIONAL DWARFING. Children who have survived PCM and a series of infectious diseases during infancy and the toddler and preschool periods often show signs of nutritional dwarfing when they reach school age. It is difficult to distinguish between the child who has suffered permanent growth retardation and the one who could "catch up" if his marginal subsistence diet were improved. The distinguishing characteristic of nutritional dwarfing is the pronounced deficit in body height as compared to standard heights. Children with this condition are often thought to be years younger than their actual chronological age, although their facial expressions may be more mature.

Inadequate diets, particularly in terms of protein, among teen-agers may also result in retarded growth during the adolescent spurt. This situation seems to have occurred in Japan from 1939 to 1948, resulting in shorter stature, especially of teen-agers, at the end of the war than before.[13]

PREVENTION AND TREATMENT OF PROTEIN–CALORIE MALNUTRITION. Since PCM has been found to occur in early infancy in developing countries where the practice of breast feeding is no longer common, mothers should be encouraged to breast feed their infants as long as they can.[14] They should also be encouraged to add other appropriate foods to the infant's diet at about four or five months of age. These foods should be of a consistency suitable for the infant and should be free of contamination with harmful pathogens. Mixtures of cereals and legumes, such as rice and red peas, made into a porridge and rubbed through a strainer, may be used in combination with fruits and vegetables, such as mashed bananas and sweet potatoes. By the time the infant is six months old, he may be fed many of the same foods the rest of the family consumes provided that they are soft or tender, not too highly seasoned, and that he continues to be breast fed.[15] Table 20-2 shows the FAO/WHO recommended daily intakes for calories and protein.

The feeding of the sick child is also an important factor in the prevention of PCM. It is the cultural practice in many areas to feed the child with diarrhea or other infectious disease a very limited diet, often consisting of a thin gruel such as rice or barley water. Since these illnesses tend to be frequent and severe among children living in poverty with poor housing and unsanitary conditions, the dietary treatment is extremely important and mothers need to be made aware of the increased nutritional needs during these periods. If possible, the infant should be fed his usual diet of breast milk and other soft bland foods. Since loss of body fluids during diarrhea may be the most critical factor, he should be given additional water which has been boiled, with perhaps barley or rice to make a very thin gruel.

In the absence of adequate amounts of animal milk, the availabilty of appropriate "weaning food," those foods which will replace breast milk, is critical to the prevention of malnutrition in the toddler and the preschool child. Cereal and legume mixtures are relatively bulky foods in terms of calories and proteins and young children may not be able to consume large enough quantities of them to meet their needs if other sources of calories and proteins are not also included in the diet. Because of the bulk of these foods and the small capacity of the child's stomach, frequent feeding is an important aspect of nutritional care. Four or five meals per day for the child rather than one or two, which may be the common adult practice, is advisable.[16] Moreover, additional, more concentrated sources of both calories and proteins should be added. Starches, tubers and roots, other vegetables, and fruits can contribute additional calories as well as essential vitamins and minerals. Small amounts of eggs, meat, fish (including fish protein concentrate), unfortunately considered by some cultures to be inappropriate foods for children, would add good quality protein to the child's diet. Peanuts (ground nuts) and soy bean products can also provide good sources of high quality protein. Of course, if milk is available and tolerated, the young child should receive generous amounts of it. Since fresh milk is easily contaminated with harmful bacteria which grow readily in it, it should be pasteurized or boiled for the young child. Dry skim milk (DSM) has been widely distributed by various international agencies such as UNICEF, Catholic Relief Services, and Church World Service, and can be added to other foods to increase their protein content.

In some developing countries, especially in urban areas, a processed "weaning food" protein-rich mixture is available as a substitute for milk. The problem, however, is that although this food may cost less than milk or meat, it does usually cost more than the cereals it replaces and thus, it is often more expensive than the lowest income groups can afford to purchase in sufficient quantities for child feeding. One of the first of these was prepared at the Institute of Nutrition of Central America and Panama (INCAP) in Guatemala City. This mixture, called Incaparina, consists of either a cornmeal or a rice base with soy and cottonseed flour and is available in several Central American countries. Dr. Behar of INCAP is shown in Fig. 20–3 examining a child with kwashiorkor who shows the typical lesions, edema, sparse hair, and apathetic expression. The second picture (Fig. 20–4) shows the same child after being fed Incaparina for six weeks.

Other mixtures of vegetable proteins which have been developed include Pronutro in South Africa, Faffa in Ethiopia, Laubina in Lebanon, Saci in Brazil, and Bal Ahar and Bal Amul in India. A corn-soy milk (CSM) and a wheat-soy blend (WSB) have been commercially produced in the United States for distribution throughout the world. Vitasoy is an example of a protein-rich beverage bottled and marketed in Hong Kong which accounts for 25 percent of the soft drink sales.

Since generous amounts of good quality protein are required for the treatment of kwashiorkor, milk or a protein-rich milk substitute is essential. Specific dietary treatment depends on the severity of the disease and other deficiency symptoms which may be present. The child may be too sick in the beginning to consume more than small, frequent feedings of relatively dilute mixtures of milk or other formula. As his condition improves, he will be able to take larger quantities of more concentrated mixtures.

VITAMIN DEFICIENCIES
Vitamin A Deficiency—Xerophthalmia

The prevention of xerophthalmia has been given the second highest priority by J. M. Bengoa, Chief Medical Officer of the Nutrition Division of the World

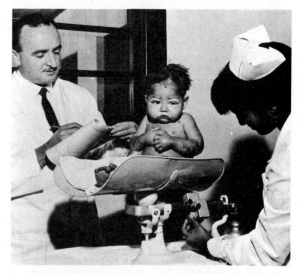

Fig. 20–3. Dr. Moises Behar of INCAP examines a child suffering from kwashiorkor, showing edema, skin lesions, and lethargic expression. (UNICEF photo)

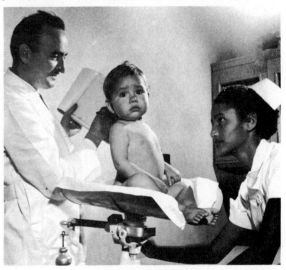

Fig. 20–4. The same child being examined at INCAP in Guatemala, after being fed Incaparina for six weeks. (UNICEF photo)

Health Organization.[17] It is not unusual for protein-calorie malnutrition and vitamin A deficiency to occur together, with severe consequences. When xerophthalmia accompanies PCM, the mortality may be as high as 80 percent, whereas it is about 15 percent in a group which is equally malnourished but not deficient in vitamin A.

The signs of vitamin A deficiency are predominantly ocular and the preschool child (30 to 36 months is the age of peak incidence) is especially vulnerable to the severe forms that cause blindness.

Xerophthalmia due to vitamin A deficiency is the most important single cause of blindness in many developing countries. It has been widely reported in various parts of the world including especially Southeast Asia, India, the Middle East, parts of Africa, and Latin America. One must recognize that in terms of human suffering and economic loss, the cost of blindness is incalculable. In comparison, the cost of prevention is almost negligible.[18]

CLASSIFICATION OF STAGES OF XEROPHTHAL-MIA. The ocular signs of vitamin A deficiency include night blindness, conjunctival xerosis, Bitot's spots, corneal xerosis, and keratomalacia. The stages of xerophthalmia are on a continuum from one stage to the next and have been classified as follows:[19]

X0—only night blindness present;

X1—xerosis of the conjunctiva, with or without night blindness and with or without Bitot's spots;

X2—xerosis of the cornea, superficial reversible, changes of the corneal epithelium;

X3—irreversible corneal changes, involving the corneal stroma, leading to loss of substance and perforation and possibly keratomalacia (softening of the cornea);

X4—scars presenting as corneal opacity (nebula), a total or partial milk white opacity (leucoma), a protrusion of the cornea (staphyloma) or shrinkage and wasting of the eye (phthisis bulbi).

Stage X0, or night blindness, indicates a functional impairment of the retina and is difficult to diagnose in the young child (one to four years) unless the mother is aware that the child cannot see well at night. For screening purposes, the child may be asked to walk into a darkened room.

The first sign of xerophthalmia is xerosis of the conjunctiva (stage X1). This dryness and dullness associated with the stability of the pre-corneal film is considered complete alteration of the reflection of light from the conjunctiva. Night blindness and Bitot's spots (accumulation of debris and fatty material near the edge of the eye) are frequently present at this stage. At stage X2, when there is xerosis of the cornea itself, the pre-corneal film fails to cover the cornea which now appears dry and opaque. Small erosions or perforations begin to occur if treatment with massive doses of vitamin A is not provided within two or three days of inception, and irreversible damage will soon result. However, if treated the corneal xerosis will clear up within a short period of time.

Irreversible damage occurs once deeper layers of the cornea are involved, as in stage X3. The cornea may liquefy and melt away resulting in large perforations and extrusion of the iris, the lens, and the vitreous. The permanent scarring effects (stage X4) may differ depending on whether or not intraocular pressure was restored at stage X3. It is essential that medical and paramedical personnel be alert to the signs of xerophthalmia and that, in order to prevent blindness, treatment be instituted immediately when symptoms are recognized.

ETIOLOGY OF XEROPHTHALMIA. The development of xerophthalmia is complex and often involves dietary as well as nondietary factors. It frequently results from deficiencies of protein and calories as well as vitamin A and its onset is often precipitated by infectious disease.

The reduction in serum proteins found in kwashiorkor includes a reduction in the amount of retinol-binding protein and thus also a decrease in the amount of vitamin A or retinol in the blood. When increased levels of protein are fed without additional vitamin A the concentration of vitamin A in the blood increases due apparently to utilization of previously available stores. In marasmus, however, xerophthalmia is not associated with low levels of serum protein but rather with a lack of vitamin A. Thus, in the case of xerophthalmia and marasmus, only administration of vitamin A at the proper time will cure the xerophthalmia.[20]

Breast feeding protects the infant from xerophthalmia so that the greatest incidence occurs in children over one year old. There is also a seasonal variation in the incidence which appears to relate both to seasonal availability of food sources of carotene and vitamin A and to the occurrence of infectious diseases.

TREATMENT AND PREVENTION OF XEROPHTHALMIA. Because of the extremely serious consequences of vitamin A deficiency and the high cost of identifying specific cases, two stages of prevention have been suggested; one as a short term measure and the other as a long range goal.[21] Presently, the most practical and immediate way to control vitamin A deficiency in high risk areas appears to be the periodic (usually at six-month intervals) oral administration of large doses (200,000 I.U.) of retinol to preschool children, 1 to 5 years of age. This may be done as part of routine procedures in child health programs. India, Indonesia, Bangladesh, and certain other areas have mass campaigns employing special mobile units participating in the project. Since vitamin A can be stored in the liver, children treated by this method maintain enhanced serum levels of vitamin A for 4 to 6 months. Moreover, in areas where large doses of vitamin A have been given to children, the incidence of xerophthalmia has been greatly reduced. It is important, however, that all health personnel working in the programs are aware of the risks of overdosage and are supervised by medically qualified personnel.[22]

The long term goal, however, should be to improve the child's diet so as to insure adequate intake of vitamin A. The success of this method will depend on the effectiveness of nutrition education. Good dietary sources of vitamin A are available in most countries with high rates of xerophthalmia but these foods are not fed to children in adequate amounts. Consequently, there is great need to identify those green leafy and yellow vegetables which in terms of their carotene content will satisfy the vitamin A requirements of children. (See Table 20-2.) Another good source of carotene is the red palm oil available in certain parts of Africa. Ultimately, in order to increase the amount of vitamin A in young children's diets, the nutrition educators will have to face the difficult task of modifying culturally determined child feeding practices.

Fortification of a staple foodstuff is also a possibility provided there is a food regularly consumed by children in sufficient quantity. The enrichment of sugar with vitamin A currently being assessed in Central America should be carefully evaluated in terms of its overall nutritional effect on children.

Night Blindness (Nyctalopia) and Glare Blindness (Hemeralopia)

INCIDENCE. Mild deficiencies of vitamin A with a variety of manifestations still occur in more prosperous areas of the world. One of the early signs long associated with this deficiency is night blindness. In Labrador and Newfoundland, where the condition has been recognized for generations, the popular remedy is fish liver, which the people rarely eat as food but will take as medicine. Varying degrees of night blindness are discovered among children and adults in the U. S. when instruments for detecting and measuring adjustment to dull light are used for routine examinations of large groups. In general, it tends to be more prevalent among low-income groups, but some cases are found in almost any group.

Glare blindness (hemeralopia), closely related and essentially similar to night blindness, was recognized when automobile drivers complained of being unable to drive at night because of the glare of headlights (Fig. 20-5). During World War II pilots were examined especially for this condition, and a liberal intake of vitamin A was recommended as a preventive.

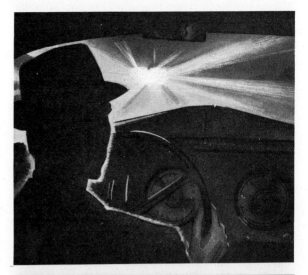

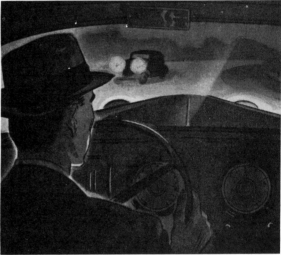

Fig. 20-5. (Top) "Glare blindness" often is a symptom of vitamin A deficiency. Headlights dazzle the eyes and cause discomfort. The driver is blinded temporarily by oncoming headlights, and the edge of the road is seen with difficulty. (Bottom) An adequate intake of vitamin A protects against "glare blindness" or remedies it. Properly focused headlights no longer dazzle so blindingly, and the road edge can be seen almost immediately after the headlight glare has passed.

ETIOLOGY AND PATHOLOGY. Both nyctalopia and hemeralopia are functional disorders resulting from the slowed regeneration of visual purple in the retina of the eye. The difficulty is usually due to an insufficient supply of vitamin A to function with the protein of the retina for the regeneration of visual purple, which is bleached to visual yellow under the influence of bright light. Regeneration of visual purple takes place in the dark, but replenishment of vitamin

A from the bloodstream is essential to continue the reaction, i.e., to permit the adaptation in the shortest possible time (see Chapter 6).

SYMPTOMS AND DIAGNOSIS. A person may have a mild degree of either night or glare blindness and not be aware of it unless his attention is drawn to it by some circumstance or special test. One person may be slower than another in adjusting to the dull light of a movie theater, but neither is aware of a difference. This is not a condition which causes sufficient discomfort to prompt one to seek medical advice unless it reaches an advanced stage.

TREATMENT. A daily intake of 5000 I.U. of vitamin A is more than enough to prevent night blindness or any related condition.

Other Conditions Due to Vitamin A Deficiency

CUTANEOUS LESIONS may appear early in adults and have a characteristic appearance. Papules tend to form around hair follicles on outer surfaces of arms, legs, shoulders, and lower abdomen, and are described as having a "gooseflesh" appearance. They usually disappear when an adequate food source of vitamin A is provided.

EPITHELIAL TISSUE CHANGES may occur as a result of vitamin A deficiency; normal secretory epithelium is replaced by dry, keratinized epithelium which is more susceptible to invasion by infectious organisms.

GENITOURINARY-TRACT CHANGES also may occur as a result of vitamin A deficiency. In the female, the epithelial cells in the vagina undergo changes which interfere with the normal estrus cycle, and in the male atrophic changes in the testes may occur, resulting in permanent damage.

For food sources of vitamin A and further discussion of the subject see Chapter 6 and Table 1, Section 4.

Thiamine Deficiency

INCIDENCE. Mild or chronic thiamine deficiency is more often part of a depletion of the whole group of B complex vitamins. Such a chronic multiple deficiency may be a contributing factor in malnutrition in children. It also should be recalled that the thiamine allowance is related to total calorie intake (see Chapter 7).

Beriberi

The frank deficiency disease known as beriberi is of special significance among the rice eaters of the Orient, where it still occurs, although less frequently than formerly.

Beriberi is described in Chinese history, and some of the earliest attempts to treat it are reported from Japan and the Philippines. The recognition of its cause and of its possible cure by better diet is one of the landmarks in the history of nutrition. The story is well told by Dr. R. R. Williams in his book entitled, Toward the Conquest of Beriberi.[23] This account of Dr. Williams's own 26-year search for what proved to be a vitamin, of its identification and eventual synthesis, is a classic in nutrition research. Dr. Williams prior to his death in 1965 had been the moving spirit behind the practical use of thiamine and other factors of the B complex for the enrichment of rice in the Philippines and some other oriental countries. This has resulted in a marked reduction in the incidence of beriberi. In fact, beriberi has almost disappeared from Japan where the prophylactic use of thiamine and enrichment of rice are common.

"In Thailand, Malaysia, and Vietnam, however, beriberi has increased in recent years as more efficient small mechanical mills replace hand pounding, which left some of the germ and hull. Moreover, most of the increase has been in infantile beriberi, with its recognized high mortality."[24]

According to Scrimshaw:

... infantile beriberi is one of the most dramatic deficiencies, for a child may be apparently well and die from this condition in a few hours. It is due to low thiamine levels in breast milk. Recovery is equally dramatic when the mother is given thiamine. [The initial stage is characterized by] vomiting, restlessness, pallor, anorexia and insomnia.... In the subacute form further vomiting, puffiness of the face and extremities, oliguria, abdominal pain, dysphasia, aphonia and convulsions may appear. This type may go on to a fatal episode or may become chronic.

There need be no signs of beriberi in the mothers of infants affected.[25]

SYMPTOMS AND PATHOLOGY. Beriberi in adults and older children is of three main types: the chronic dry, atrophic type generally found only in older adults, often associated with prolonged consumption of alcohol; the fulminating acute type which is more serious and dramatic but occurs rarely; and the mild subacute form which is most common. This third type

has characteristic nervous manifestations, including alterations in tendon reflexes. Paresthesia is common.... Sensations of fullness and tightening of the muscles and muscle cramps are common at night. Cardiovascular signs and symptoms range from breathlessness on exertion and palpitation to tachycardia, cardiac dilation and some degree of congestive heart failure. Coexisting deficiencies of ascorbic acid, riboflavin, niacin and vitamin A are common.[26]

TREATMENT. Adequate food sources of thiamine are sufficient to prevent any of the deficiency conditions described, but, when the pathologic symptoms appear, more concentrated sources of thiamine usually are necessary for prompt recovery. Anorexia and nausea are often so severe as to preclude an adequate food intake until symptoms have been relieved by the administration of concentrates.

Since most of the cases diagnosed as beriberi in regions where it is prevalent are suffering from multiple deficiencies, it is customary for the physician to prescribe B-complex concentrates rather than pure thiamine and to seek improvement in the diet. The dosage for therapeutic purposes is often several times the recommended allowance of thiamine with other factors in proportion. (See Table 20-2 for recommended allowances of vitamins for different age and sex categories. See Chapter 7 for rich food sources of thiamine and other fractions of the B complex.)

BERIBERI HEART DISEASE. Beriberi heart disease is described as a distinct clinical entity by Gubbay.[27] The pathology includes right heart failure, edema, and peripheral vasodilation. Beriberi heart disease is due to a deficiency and is curable if the deficiency is corrected in time.

Nutritional Disorders of the Central Nervous System

Several acute disorders of the central nervous system have been associated with alcoholism. Similar disturbances may also occur in the absence of alcoholism when there is a prolonged deficiency of food intake, as in gastric carcinoma or when anorexia is a complication of other conditions such as pregnancy.

Experimental work in pigeons in 1938 first demonstrated that a severe thiamine deficiency could produce brain lesions. In 1942 British prisoners-of-war developed nervous disorders which disappeared with small doses of thiamine.

Subsequent clinical research has identified the lesion in man as polioencephalitis, an inflammatory disease of the gray substance of the brain. This is due in most, if not all, cases to a thiamine deficiency.

POLYNEUROPATHY is defined as a disease which involves many nerves and affects the peripheral nerves. The symptoms are remarkably similar to those of classical beriberi and are usually relieved by thiamine or vitamin-B-complex therapy. Under some circumstances a deficiency of pyridoxine or pantothenic acid may give rise to similar symptoms. The chief ones are weakness, numbness, partial paralysis and pain in the legs. The legs are affected earlier than the arms. Motor, reflex and sensory reactions are lost in most cases. Recovery is a slow process involving weeks or months, and a year may pass before a patient is able to walk unaided.

WERNICKE'S DISEASE is closely associated with Korsakoff's psychosis, and the combination is often referred to as the Wernicke-Korsakoff syndrome. The specific nutritional factor mostly concerned is thiamine. This syndrome may occur apart from alcoholism but is most frequently encountered in chronic alcoholics (see Chapter 32). The chief symptoms are ophthalmoplegia (paralysis of the eye muscles), nystagmus (involuntary rapid movement of the eyeballs), and ataxia (failure of muscular coordination). The ophthalmoplegia is relieved promptly after a few adequate meals; the other symptoms respond more slowly to thiamine therapy, indicating, perhaps, some structural damage to the nerve tissue. Wernicke's disease is a medical emergency and massive doses of thiamine (as much as 250 mg. per day) may be prescribed. Mental symptoms such as apathy, drowsiness, inattentiveness, and inability to concentrate or sustain a conversation seem to clear up upon thiamine administration.

THE KORSAKOFF SYNDROME is characterized by memory defect and confabulation (a form of mental confusion consisting of giving answers and reciting experiences without regard to truth). These symptoms may not respond to thiamine therapy as do the other mental symptoms mentioned in the preceding paragraph. There is evidence that the damage to the nervous system in the Korsakoff syndrome may be structural rather than biochemical, and that thiamine deficiency of long standing may be responsible.

THE AMBLYOPIA (dim vision) accompanying alcoholism and formerly attributed to the toxic effects of alcohol and tobacco is probably of nutritional origin.[28] Clinical experiments have demonstrated recovery following improved nutrition, with vitamin B complex—and, more specifically, thiamine—the important factor.

Riboflavin Deficiency

INCIDENCE. No well-defined deficiency syndrome or disease with a long history, such as scurvy or beriberi, is associated with a lack of riboflavin. However, dietary and clinical evidence of riboflavin deficiency or borderline intake has been reported from Taiwan, Korea, the Philippines, East Pakistan, and Turkey.[29] Riboflavin deficiency was the deficiency most commonly reported from these countries, which are predominantly rice-eating. Ariboflavinosis as it exists today is seldom fatal, but it is a serious handicap. It must be remembered that a person with a riboflavin deficiency is likely to have associated deficiencies of thiamine and niacin.

Table 20-2. Recommended Intakes of Nutrients (FAO/WHO)

AGE	BODY WEIGHT (kilograms)	ENERGY (1) kilocalories	ENERGY (1) megajoules	PROTEIN (1, 2) grams	VITAMIN A (3, 4) micrograms	VITAMIN D (5, 6) micrograms	THIAMINE (3) milligrams	RIBOFLAVIN (3) milligrams	NIACIN (3) milligrams	FOLIC ACID (5) micrograms	VITAMIN B$_{12}$ (5) micrograms	ASCORBIC ACID (5) milligrams	CALCIUM (7) grams	IRON (5, 8) milligrams
Children														
<1	7.3	820	3.4	14	300	10.0	0.3	0.5	5.4	60	0.3	20	0.5-0.6	5-10
1-3	13.4	1360	5.7	16	250	10.0	0.5	0.8	9.0	100	0.9	20	0.4-0.5	5-10
4-6	20.2	1830	7.6	20	300	10.0	0.7	1.1	12.1	100	1.5	20	0.4-0.5	5-10
7-9	28.1	2190	9.2	25	400	2.5	0.9	1.3	14.5	100	1.5	20	0.4-0.5	5-10
Male adolescents														
10-12	36.9	2600	10.9	30	575	2.5	1.0	1.6	17.2	100	2.0	20	0.6-0.7	5-10
13-15	51.3	2900	12.1	37	725	2.5	1.2	1.7	19.1	200	2.0	30	0.6-0.7	9-18
16-19	62.9	3070	12.8	38	750	2.5	1.2	1.8	20.3	200	2.0	30	0.5-0.6	5-9
Female adolescents														
10-12	38.0	2350	9.8	29	575	2.5	0.9	1.4	15.5	100	2.0	20	0.6-0.7	5-10
13-15	49.9	2490	10.4	31	725	2.5	1.0	1.5	16.4	200	2.0	30	0.6-0.7	12-24
16-19	54.4	2310	9.7	30	750	2.5	0.9	1.4	15.2	200	2.0	30	0.5-0.6	14-28
Adult man (moderately active)	65.0	3000	12.6	37	750	2.5	1.2	1.8	19.8	200	2.0	30	0.4-0.5	5-9
Adult woman (moderately active)	55.0	2200	9.2	29	750	2.5	0.9	1.3	14.5	200	2.0	30	0.4-0.5	14-28
Pregnancy (later half)		+350	+1.5	38	750	10.0	+0.1	+0.2	+2.3	400	3.0	30	1.0-1.2	(9)
Lactation (first 6 months)		+550	+2.3	46	1200	10.0	+0.2	+0.4	+3.7	300	2.5	30	1.0-1.2	(9)

[1]Energy and Protein Requirements. Report of a Joint FAO/WHO Expert Group, FAO, Rome, 1972.—[2]As egg or milk protein.—[3]Requirements of Vitamin A, Thiamine, Riboflavin and Niacin. Report of a Joint FAO/WHO Expert Group, FAO, Rome, 1965.—[4]As retinol.—[5]Requirements of Ascorbic Acid, Vitamin D, Vitamin B$_{12}$, Folate and Iron. Report of a Joint FAO/WHO Expert Group, FAO, Rome, 1970.—[6]As cholecalciferol.—[7]Calcium Requirements. Report of a FAO/WHO Expert Group, FAO, Rome, 1961.—[8]On each line the lower value applies when over 25 percent of calories in the diet come from animal foods, and the higher value when animal foods represent less than 10 percent of calories.—[9]For women whose iron intake throughout life has been at the level recommended in this table, the daily intake of iron during pregnancy and lactation should be the same as that recommended for nonpregnant, nonlactating women of childbearing age. For women whose iron status is not satisfactory at the beginning of pregnancy, the requirement is increased, and in the extreme situation of women with no iron stores, the requirement can probably not be met without supplementation.

SYMPTOMS AND PATHOLOGY. Before any true clinical symptoms appear, a mild riboflavin deficiency may be responsible for a type of light sensitivity and dimness of vision, followed later by itching, burning, and eyestrain. Later clinical manifestations are a shiny red mucosa of the lips with cracking at the corners of the mouth, known as cheilosis, a beefy red tongue, and roughened skin around the mouth and the nose, often accompanied by sebaceous exudate.

TREATMENT AND PREVENTION. Common food sources of riboflavin are listed in Chapter 7. Milk and organ meats are the richest natural sources. Enriched bread is also a good economical source.

Niacin and Tryptophan Deficiency—Pellagra

INCIDENCE. Pellagra is still found in India, South Africa, and Egypt where there are large numbers of poor peasants living on maize or, sometimes, on millet. It has become rare in recent years in Yugoslavia and Romania where wheat has replaced some of the maize in the diets of these Eastern Europeans. The enrichment of bread and other cereal grains resulted in the disappearance of pellagra in the United States and Western Europe.[30] There is also a low incidence of pellagra in those areas of the world, e.g., Mexico and Central America, where maize is treated with lime, which apparently makes the niacin content more available.[31]

Isolated cases of pellagra may occur in any area in persons confined to a restricted diet low in protein and niacin. This can happen in older people with self-imposed restrictions or in someone with allergies to a number of protein foods. Alcoholic pellagra is essentially identical with endemic pellagra. It is caused by the substitution of alcohol for food.

SYMPTOMS AND PATHOLOGY. On exposure to sun, persons whose diets supply inadequate tryptophan and are deficient in niacin acquire a scaly, pigmented dermatitis over the exposed areas. Depending on type of clothing and extent of exposed skin, the areas most affected are face, neck, back of hands, elbows, knees, and ankles. The classic "three D's" *dermatitis, diarrhea,* and *dementia* may still describe the symptoms, although dementia is rare. Anemias are frequent, probably owing to associated deficiencies. Glossitis (sore tongue) suggests a relationship to the disease blacktongue in dogs.

TREATMENT AND PREVENTION. Large doses of niacin usually in the form of niacinamide are used in the treatment of pellagra. The addition of milk, eggs, meat, nuts, and certain vegetables (see Chapter 7) would supply the factors missing in the typical pellagra-producing diet.

The best form of prevention of pellagra has been the improvement of the socioeconomic status of people living chiefly on maize or corn diets. When a more varied diet is introduced, perhaps where individuals have gained some land of their own to raise additional foods or money with which to purchase what are usually the more expensive items in the diet, endemic pellagra disappears. Roe summarizes the situation as follows:

> It is not, however, the opportunity for social, economic and agricultural progress that determines the decline of pellagra but rather the extension of the benefits of progress to all members of society. The current situation in India, South Africa and Egypt points up the fact that pellagra will be with us until the dispossessed achieve their right to freedom from want and can choose to eat the foods that prevent the disease.[32]

Ascorbic Acid Deficiency and Scurvy

HISTORY AND INCIDENCE. Scurvy is probably the oldest recognized deficiency disease. Although its specific relationship to ascorbic acid was not recognized until the 20th century, its prevention by the use of fresh foods was practiced much earlier. Prevalent in Europe during the 19th century and earlier, for centuries scurvy was attributed to a limited food supply. On the long voyages which followed the discovery of America, sailors were often obliged to subsist for long periods on salt fish and meats, hardtack, or other breadstuffs, entirely deprived of any fresh food. The outbreaks of scurvy on such voyages were frequently so severe that there was scarcely enough of the crew left to man the vessel. In 1772, however, Captain Cook commanded a voyage which lasted three years, during which not one man was lost because of scurvy. This fact he attributed to the use of a "sweet wort" made from barley and sauerkraut. Subsequently, limes or lemons were included in the supplies, since they had been found to be antiscorbutic, i.e., scurvy preventive.

Scurvy probably was responsible for most of the deaths among the pilgrims in the Massachusetts Bay Colony during that first hard winter. There was an outbreak of mild scurvy in northern Maine during the depression years, the early 1930s. Outbreaks of the disease have also been associated with famine or war areas, when the food supply was limited. Historically, its occurrence was reported during polar expeditions or other circumstances in which supplies of fresh food were unavailable. Expert dietetic advice was sought in planning the food supplies for the more recent polar expeditions in order to avoid the possibility of a vitamin-C shortage, because scurvy is greatly dreaded by explorers.

Eskimos seldom have scurvy on their native diets but are susceptible to it when they adopt the "white man's diet." On their native diets they may include organ meats and mosses that supply ascorbic acid. It is also reported that some groups eat meat raw or undercooked, thus retaining the slight amount of ascorbic acid that may be present.

The only cases of scurvy in adults reported in this country are in men living alone and preparing inadequate meals or in psychoneurotic individuals on bizarre diets. During the 1960s an increased number of cases of infantile scurvy had been reported in the medical literature from such areas as Canada, Newfoundland, and Australia. A survey in Canada during 1961-1963 found 87 cases of infantile scurvy.[33] These cases occurred mostly in small communities where there was ignorance, poverty, and poor health supervision. As a result of these findings, Canada has enacted a regulation permitting the addition of ascorbic acid to evaporated milk, commonly used in infant feeding.

Scurvy is relatively rare in the underdeveloped areas of the world. Many of these countries are in the tropical and subtropical zones where fruits and vegetables are plentiful and widely consumed.

Frank scurvy is so rare in the U. S. today that medical students seldom have a chance to observe the disease. Yet the history of this disease and its prevention is worthy of note.

SYMPTOMS AND PATHOLOGY. The principal symptoms of scurvy are restlessness, loss of appetite, general soreness to touch, sore mouth and gums with bleeding and loosening of the teeth, petechial skin hemorrhages, and swelling of the legs with special tenderness about the knee joints (see Fig. 20-6). Anemia may occur as a result of the loss of blood.

Marginal symptoms of this disease are sallow skin, muddy complexion, lack of energy, and fleeting pains in limbs and joints. Irritability, retarded growth, and tooth defects may also accompany this dietary deficiency.

Mild manifestations of ascorbic acid deficiency in adults may easily be overlooked or ignored. Tendency to bruise easily, slow healing of minor wounds, and pin-point hemorrhages may be indications of tissue depletion of this factor.

TREATMENT. An adequate supply of ascorbic acid is the obvious treatment for all these conditions, but what is an adequate supply? This problem is reflected in the differences between the Recommended Dietary Allowances of the National Research Council, Table 10-1, and the FAO/WHO Recommended Intake of Nutrients, Table 20-2. For rich food sources of ascorbic acid and for a discussion of its properties and losses in cooking, see Chapter 7. Ascorbic acid in tablet form is stable and relatively inexpensive. It is useful when fresh foods are not available or must be omitted from the diet for any reason. This synthetic form has been used to promote wound healing and to act as a food supplement in emergency rations.

Vitamin D Deficiency—Rickets

"The disappearance of rickets" is the title of an article[34] reviewing the history and prevention of vitamin-D-deficient rickets as a triumph of medicine and nutrition. As late as 1940 rickets was still a common disease of early childhood in northern climates.

One cannot be complacent, however, about the overall decrease in rickets since, in the 1960s, a survey by the Committee on Nutrition of the American Academy of Pediatrics[35] reported 843 cases of rickets in five years among hospital pediatric admissions. It would seem that the general use of antirachitic supplements in infant feeding would have precluded the possibility of this deficiency still being a public health problem. Of course, the widespread use of vitamin D supplements in infant feeding has reduced the incidence in northern climates. Although it is rare in tropical countries in general, where children spend more time out of doors and expose more of their skin to the sun, a 1967 survey in North Africa reported that 45 to 60 percent of the children examined showed

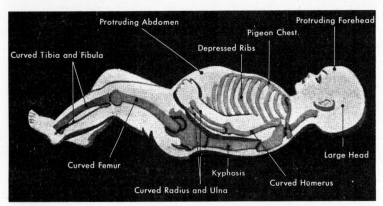

Fig. 20-6. The symptoms of rickets. (Abbott Laboratories)

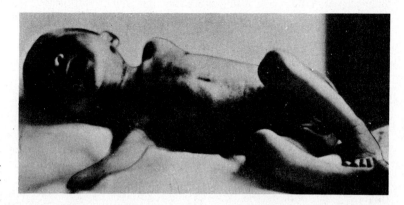

Fig. 20-7. Infantile scurvy. Typical contractions of extremities from pain. (Hoffmann-La Roche, Inc.)

some signs of rickets.[36] Children of dark-skinned races living in northern climates are even more susceptible to rickets than children of the white race.

SYMPTOMS AND PATHOLOGY. Rickets is a disease of infancy and early childhood in which the bones do not calcify properly as they grow. They become pliable, malformed, and distorted, which results in such evident deformities as pigeon chest, enlarged wrists and ankles, and bowed legs or knock knees when the leg bones are not strong enough to support the child learning to walk. All these symptoms are shown in the schematic drawing of a child with rickets (Fig. 20-7). The enlargement or beading of the ribs, frequently called "the rachitic rosary," may be less evident in a plump infant than in an emaciated one, but it is characteristic. Profuse sweating and restlessness are early symptoms of rickets in infants. Growth may not be retarded at first, since nature seems to allow the bones to increase in length to keep up with growth in soft tissues if other nutrients are adequate. Prolonged and severe cases usually show stunted growth.

TREATMENT AND PREVENTION. The major factors involved in the prevention of rickets—calcium, phosphorus, and vitamin D—have been discussed in Chapters 5 and 6. Since the geographic incidence of rickets and practical experience indicate that it is more often a deficiency of vitamin D which causes rickets in children, attention is directed to the problem of adequate and reliable sources of this factor in regions where sunshine cannot act as the natural preventive agent. Obviously, when children can be exposed to an adequate source of ultraviolet light (sunshine or ultraviolet lamp), sufficient vitamin D may be synthesized to regulate the utilization of minerals for bone building. Vitamin preparations containing vitamins A and C in addition to vitamin D are readily available for infants in the U. S.

Vitamin D milk is a convenient and reliable antirachitic agent. Since milk contains the minerals calcium and phosphorus and is a natural food for children, it seems to be the most suitable carrier for added vitamin D. Fortified evaporated milk is especially convenient for use in vicinities where fresh vitamin D milk is not available. Dry skim milk may also be fortified with vitamin D.

PRECAUTIONS. It is wise to caution mothers against the simultaneous use of several supplementary sources of vitamin D because it is possible to give too much (see Chapter 6).

OSTEOMALACIA. Incidence and Pathology. Prolonged deficiency of dietary calcium and vitamin D or sunlight may result in osteomalacia, sometimes called adult rickets. This condition is characterized by poor calcification of the bones with increasing softness, so that they become flexible, leading to deformities of limbs, spine, thorax, or pelvis. These bone changes may be accompanied by rheumatic pains and exhaustion.

Osteomalacia is rare in Western countries but still occurs in the Middle East and the Orient, especially among women following several pregnancies and when they nurse their infants for extended periods of time. The high incidence of osteomalacia among women in certain parts of India where the rite of purdah is still practiced and among Bedouin Arab women who wear long black garments and live in dark tents testifies indirectly to the protective action of sunshine on exposed skin. In many of these same areas the diet consists largely of cereals and root vegetables low in calcium.

Osteomalacia is often confused with osteoporosis, which may occur in older women in any country, even the most prosperous. The etiology of osteoporosis is not well understood but is more likely due to a metabolic or endocrine disturbance than to a deficiency (see Chapter 33).

Prevention and Treatment. Prevention of osteomalacia, like rickets, is entirely possible by means of a diet adequate in calcium and phosphorus and with a supply of vitamin D or exposure to sunlight.

The diet of patients suffering from osteomalacia should be adequate in all respects but especially in calcium and vitamin D. In countries where milk is not readily available other food sources of calcium and the protective vitamin should be supplied.

MINERAL DEFICIENCIES
Nutritional Anemia

As a world problem nutritional anemias, particularly iron-deficiency anemia, are widespread and generally more serious than has previously been recognized. They are responsible for considerable ill health and some mortality in most areas of the world including the more developed countries. The most vulnerable groups in terms of iron deficiency anemia are pregnant women, infants, and young children. It is estimated that 20 percent of the United States population, and between 10 to 25 percent of European women, are affected by iron deficiency anemia. In Africa, 6 to 17 percent of the adult men, 15 to 50 percent of the adult women, and 30 to 60 percent of the children under 15 years of age suffer from iron deficiency anemia. Similar figures are also reported for Asia where it is estimated that as high as 92 percent of the children under two years of age are affected. Reports from the Middle East indicate that 20 to 25 percent of pregnant women and 25 to 70 percent of the children are anemic. Mortality as high as 10, 20 and 40 per 100,000 population are reported in some South American countries.[37]

Chapter 33 includes a discussion on the etiology and dietary treatment of anemias. See Chapter 5 for information on iron requirements and dietary sources.

To increase the amounts of iron in the diets of children and women during child bearing years iron enrichment of wheat and other grains has been adopted in many developed countries. An increase in the level of enrichment is currently under consideration in the U.S. More information on the availability of iron in various foods and in supplements used for fortification is important. Although the general practice of enrichment of staple foods should be recommended in countries where the food iron content of the diet is less than 6 mg. per 1000 calories, the extent and level should be determined by the individual countries, depending on the general composition of the national diet.

Endemic Goiter and Cretinism—Iodine Deficiency—Incidence

The cause of simple goiter is failure of the thyroid gland to obtain a supply of iodine sufficient to maintain its normal structure and function. The lack of iodine is usually a result of an environmental deficiency of iodine.

Since iodine in surface soil shows a very uneven distribution and plants absorb iodine from the soil, the iodine content of foodstuffs varies with the locality in which they are grown. Thus we find simple goiter most common in those parts of the world where the surface soil is low in iodine and where salt water fish are not commonly eaten. Due to increased facilities for food distribution in the United States today, city people are less confined to food grown in one locality and the incidence of simple goiter seems to be decreasing.

Iodized salt, which is on the market in most areas of the United States, has proved to be beneficial in reducing the incidence of goiter, as evidenced by examination of schoolchildren. In one state in which goiter was almost eliminated, it again became prevalent when the emphasis on the use of iodized salt was relaxed. If the spectacular decrease in the incidence of goiter which resulted from the use of iodized salt in the United States is to continue, effective nutrition education must support its use.

Similar programs using iodized salt have been successful in sharply reducing the incidence of endemic goiter in Argentina, Czechoslovakia, France, Guatemala, New Zealand, Switzerland, and Yugoslavia. Injection of iodized oil has also been used successfully as a prophylactic agent in such areas as New Guinea and Zaire. There are, however, many parts of the world where endemic goiter continues to be an important medical problem. They include the Middle East, Southeast Asia, the Himalaya region, most of Central Africa and many of the Latin American countries (Fig. 20–8). It should be recognized that where the incidence of moderately severe and severe endemic goiter is high, endemic cretinism and deaf mutism are also found among the population. Stanbury et al[38] suggest that in certain areas of Zaire, the Andes, New Guinea, and Southeast Asia 5 percent of all surviving persons are significantly retarded. The implications of this finding are serious in terms of economic and social development in these countries. *SYMPTOMS AND PATHOLOGY.* Many criteria have been suggested for identifying the prevalence of simple goiter. Enlargement of the thyroid may exist in 5 to 10 percent of the adolescent or preadolescent population even when ample iodine is available in their diets. Thus guidelines are essential to determine the scope of the problem. The following scheme of classifying thyroid conditions has been suggested:[39]

Grade Oa: Thyroid not palpable, or if palpable not larger than normal.

Grade Ob: Thyroid distinctly palpable but usu-

ally not visible with the head in a
normal or raised position; considered to be definitely larger than
normal, i.e., at least as large as the
distal phalanx of the subject's
thumb.

Grade I: Thyroid easily palpable and visible
with the head in a normal or a raised
position. The presence of a discrete
nodule qualifies a patient for inclusion in this grade.

Grade II: Thyroid easily visible with the head
in a normal position.

Grade III: Goiter visible at a distance.

Grade IV: Monstrous goiter.

The thyroid, as a result of iodine deficiency, becomes enlarged and, with chronic stimulation over
time, becomes nodular. Hypothyroidism may also result if the deficiency is sufficiently severe. In the
female, endemic goiter appears to persist throughout
the life span, whereas it decreases in the male following adolescence. In addition to iodine deficiency,
dietary goitrogens, and perhaps genetic factors may
influence the severity of the disease.

Endemic goiter may be said to exist in a community when more than 5 percent of the adolescents or
preadolescents have Grade I goiter, or when more
than 30 percent are assigned to Grade Ob or above.
Urinary excretion of iodine may be used to confirm
this finding. If large numbers of the sample population excrete less than 50 mcg. of iodine every 24 hours
(or per gram of creatinine) the conclusion of endemic
goiter due to iodine deficiency would be reinforced.[40]

Where the incidence of endemic goiter, as defined
by Grade I or above thyroid enlargement, is greater
than 20 percent of the population, endemic cretinism
can also be diagnosed. The symptoms of endemic
cretinism may include all or a combination of the
following: mental retardation, deafness, deaf mutism,
retarded growth, neurological abnormalities, and
hypothyroidism. Cretins are usually deaf-mute but it
is not certain whether deaf mutism without mental
retardation can be the result of endemic cretinism.
Thus it is difficult in field surveys to trace and identify cretins. It is believed that cretinism results when
the fetus receives insufficient iodine. Although proof
is still lacking, cretinism may also be the result of low
levels of thyroid hormone in the maternal blood.[41]

PREVENTION. Both endemic goiter and cretinism
can be prevented by supplying adequate amounts of
iodine. The most successful programs have been
those where sodium or potassium iodide have been
added to table salt. Various countries have found different concentrations to be beneficial. In the U.S., one

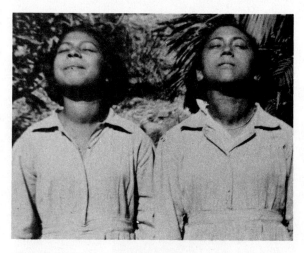

Fig. 20-8. Goiter is so common among youth of mountainous
regions of South America that a child without goiter is ridiculed
as a "bottleneck." (Photo FAO, Rome)

part of iodide is added to 10,000 parts of salt, in
Finland, one part of iodide is added to 25,000 parts of
salt, and in India, the concentration used is one part
iodide to every 40,000 parts salt. Iodide may be lost
during storage of salt which is high in moisture or
other impurities.

In remote areas of the world where the distribution of iodized salt is not practicable, intramuscular
injection of iodized oil has proved effective. It has
been administered to females up to the age of 45
and to males up to 20 years of age. Amounts currently
used in this program require new injections approximately every three years.

Iodine prophylactic programs should be carefully
monitored by health personnel. Surveillance of the
target population is particularly important after administration of iodized oil because of the large initial
dose. Persons over the age of 40 especially should be
examined after three to six months so that any cases of
thyrotoxicosis can be diagnosed and treated. Surveys
by trained personnel every two or three years should
be carried out to evaluate the effectiveness of the
iodized salt or oil program in reducing the incidence
of endemic goiter and cretinism.

GOITROGENS. The availability of dietary iodine
may be affected by goitrogenic substances which
interfere with iodine utilization. These are found in a
number of plant species, among them cabbage, Brussels sprouts, soy beans, and peanuts. They are of significance only when the intake of iodine is borderline, and their effect can be compensated for by an
adequate intake of iodine.

DENTAL CARIES
Incidence

Dental caries is probably the most common disease that affects human beings. Authorities estimate that only about 2 percent of the people of the United States have escaped having at least one dental cavity. Contrary to the regional and the endemic incidence of some other deficiencies, dental caries is so common that nearly everyone has experienced it. Few adults in western civilization have absolutely perfect teeth. Figures on incidence of caries among population groups vary according to locality and race. The prevalence among blacks is lower than among whites of comparable age in the same locality. In the underdeveloped countries, primitive peoples as a rule show a lower incidence than do civilized populations. However, as soon as primitive populations are touched by civilization, and native foods are replaced by processed foods, an increase in dental caries follows.

Etiology

Dental caries has been variously attributed to inheritance, metabolic disturbances, specific or multiple food deficiencies, conditions in the mouth, including composition of saliva, and lack of fluorine in the water supply. None of these entirely explains the high incidence or varying degree of susceptibility to caries encountered among children of the same family with similar dietary and mouth hygiene habits.

Extensive research has been conducted in an attempt to understand carious changes in teeth and thus be better able to prevent or inhibit them. It is now generally agreed that dental caries is unquestionably of bacterial origin with certain other contributing factors. Bacterial metabolism and growth in the mouth lead to destruction of both tooth enamel and dentin. Carbohydrates must be present in the crevices of the teeth for caries-producing organisms to grow. Heredity and nutrition during the period of tooth development will affect the resistance to decay at a later date. Saliva is protective, but much is yet to be learned about hereditary, nutritional, endocrine, and other variables that determine the physical consistency, the chemical composition, and the rate of flow of saliva. It is now also recognized that teeth are more resistant to caries when the fluoride ion is incorporated in the crystal lattice of the enamel and the dentin.

The inverse relationship between incidence of dental caries and the fluorine content of drinking water has given impetus to the use of fluorine as a prophylactic agent. A review of caries control in the U.S.[42] indicated that controlled fluoridation had reduced the incidence of caries by 50 to 70 percent among young people whose teeth were formed during the period of fluoridation.

Prevention

It is generally agreed that fluorine is the only known agent ordinarily included in food and water that is capable of exercising mass control of dental caries. It is effective during the period of calcification of the crown of the tooth and through the period of eruption.

Among the authorities who have studied the problem, it is agreed that the simplest, cheapest, and most far-reaching method of ensuring adequate fluoride is through the fluoridation of drinking water. This procedure will supplement, but not supplant, other dental health measures.

The level of fluorine which seems to be protective without being harmful is 1.0 part per million (ppm.) of drinking water. Mottled enamel (dental fluorosis) is apt to occur when fluorine in the water supply exceeds 2 ppm., as it does naturally in communities in several Western states. Indeed, it was the absence of caries in persons with mottled enamel that first called attention to the protective action of fluorine.

Consideration has been given to media other than water as possible means of administering fluorides to children where the community water supply is not fluoridated. Rusoff and coworkers[43] tried milk as a vehicle for fluoride administration in the school lunch program. The amount added was such that ½ pint of milk supplied 1 mg. of fluoride. This was tried on 171 children over a period of 3½ years and resulted in a 70 percent reduction in caries incidence in teeth erupting after the initiation of the experiment.

Calcium, phosphorus, or vitamin D deficiencies during and preceding the eruption of teeth undoubtedly account for some faults in structure. The teeth, once fully developed, are not as apt to be influenced by diet later.

EARLY DIAGNOSIS AND TREATMENT OF NUTRITIONAL FAILURE

The insidious development and delayed clinical evidence of malnutrition make the problem particularly serious. This subject is of great concern to nutritionists, public health nurses, physicians, and others who are frequently in close contact with children and with families living on low incomes and an inadequate food supply. There is ample room for further study and observation of these marginal deficiencies among all groups of the population, but especially among lower income groups, in which the vicious circle of malnutrition, lack of strength and possibilities for self-improvement, and continued low income offers little opportunity for real positive change.

Before clinical signs of nutritional deficiencies appear, there must be biochemical abnormality. Although specific biochemical lesions are difficult to detect, low levels of certain nutrients in blood and/or urine can be determined by laboratory tests and are indicative of probable deficiency states. (Table 10, Section 4, gives the current guidelines for criteria of nutritional status for laboratory evaluation.) These low levels may persist for varying periods of time before clinical symptoms of a deficiency manifest themselves, Table 20–3. The pattern for the development of nutritional deficiencies is shown in Fig. 20–9.

Table 20–3. Physical Signs Indicative or Suggestive of Malnutrition*

BODY AREA	NORMAL APPEARANCE	SIGNS ASSOCIATED WITH MALNUTRITION
Hair	Shiny; firm; not easily plucked	Lack of natural shine; hair dull and dry, thin and sparse; hair fine, silky, and straight; color changes (flag sign); can be easily plucked
Face	Skin color uniform; smooth, pink, healthy appearance; not swollen	Skin color loss (depigmentation); skin dark over cheeks and under eyes (malar and supra-orbital pigmentation); lumpiness or flakiness of skin of nose and mouth; swollen face; enlarged parotid glands; scaling of skin around nostrils (nasolabial seborrhea)
Eyes	Bright, clear, shiny; no sores at corners of eyelids; membranes a healthy pink and are moist. No prominent blood vessels or mound of tissue or sclera	Eye membranes are pale (pale conjunctivae); redness of membranes (conjunctival injection); Bitot's spots; redness and fissuring of eyelid corners (angular palpebritis); dryness of eye membranes (conjunctival xerosis); cornea has dull appearance (corneal xerosis); cornea is soft (keratomalacia); scar on cornea; ring of fine blood vessels around corner (circumcorneal injection)
Lips	Smooth, not chapped or swollen	Redness and swelling of mouth or lips (cheilosis); especially at corners of mouth (angular fissures and scars)
Tongue	Deep red in appearance; not swollen or smooth	Swelling; scarlet and raw tongue; magenta (purplish color) of tongue; smooth tongue; swollen sores; hyperemic and hypertrophic papillae; and atrophic papillae
Teeth	No cavities; no pain; bright	May be missing or erupting abnormally; gray or black spots (fluorosis); cavities (caries)
Gums	Healthy; red; do not bleed; not swollen	"Spongy" and bleed easily; recession of gums
Glands	Face not swollen	Thyroid enlargement (front of neck); parotid enlargement (cheeks become swollen)
Skin	No signs of rashes, swellings, dark or light spots	Dryness of skin (xerosis); sandpaper feel of skin (follicular hyperkeratosis); flakiness of skin; skin swollen and dark; red swollen pigmentation of exposed areas (pellagrous dermatosis); excessive lightness or darkness of skin (dyspigmentation); black and blue marks due to skin bleeding (petechiae); lack of fat under skin.
Nails	Firm, pink	Nails are spoon-shape (koilonychia); brittle, ridged nails
Muscular and skeletal systems	Good muscle tone; some fat under skin; can walk or run without pain	Muscles have "wasted" appearance; baby's skull bones are thin and soft (craniotabes); round swelling of front and side of head (frontal and parietal bossing); swelling of ends of bones (epiphyseal enlargement); small bumps on both sides of chest wall (on ribs)—beading of ribs; baby's soft spot on head does not harden at proper time (persistently open anterior fontanelle); knock-knees or bow-legs; bleeding into muscle (musculo-skeletal hemorrhages); person cannot get up or walk properly
Internal Systems:		
Cardiovascular	Normal heart rate and rhythm; no murmurs or abnormal rhythms; normal blood pressure for age	Rapid heart rate (above 100 Tachycardia); enlarged heart; abnormal rhythm; elevated blood pressure
Gastrointestinal	No palpable organs or masses (in children, however, liver edge may be palpable)	Liver enlargement; enlargement of spleen (usually indicates other associated diseases)
Nervous	Psychological stability; normal reflexes	Mental irritability and confusion; burning and tingling of hands and feet (paresthesia); loss of position and vibratory sense; weakness and tenderness of muscles (may result in inability to walk); decrease and loss of ankle and knee reflexes

*From Christakis, G., ed.: Nutritional Assessment in Health Programs, American J. Public Health, 63:Supplement (November) 1973.

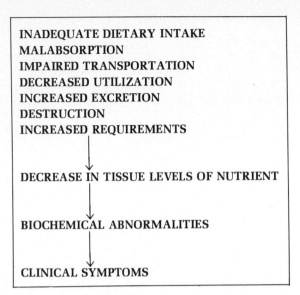

INADEQUATE DIETARY INTAKE
MALABSORPTION
IMPAIRED TRANSPORTATION
DECREASED UTILIZATION
INCREASED EXCRETION
DESTRUCTION
INCREASED REQUIREMENTS

↓

DECREASE IN TISSUE LEVELS OF NUTRIENT

↓

BIOCHEMICAL ABNORMALITIES

↓

CLINICAL SYMPTOMS

Fig. 20–9. Pattern for development of nutritional deficiencies.

STUDY QUESTIONS AND ACTIVITIES

1. What are the relationships between malnutrition and infectious diseases? Explain nutritional dwarfing.
2. What are the four most significant recommendations from the 1974 World Food Conference?
3. What are the most prevalent nutritional deficiencies in the world today?
4. What age group is most susceptible to marasmus? Why?
5. What are the most likely symptoms of kwashiorkor? What is the meaning of the word kwashiorkor and where did it come from?
6. What contributions has INCAP made in the control and treatment of PCM or kwashiorkor? What do the letters INCAP stand for?
7. What other deficiency may complicate the picture in PCM?
8. Which vitamin deficiency is most widespread and most serious in the world today? What are the consequences?
9. What diseases other than beriberi may result from a thiamine deficiency? What is a common complication?
10. Why is pellagra not as serious a problem in the U.S. today as it was formerly? Is it found elsewhere in the world? What food pattern is most apt to be found associated with pellagra?
11. Which deficiency disease is widespread in the developed countries? What means have been used to combat its incidence in the U.S.?
12. What progress is being made in the control of dental caries? What stands in the way of greater success in this area?
13. What is the world distribution of common goiter? Is there a proved method of control and how successful has it been?
14. What steps might be or are being taken toward earlier diagnosis or detection of mild forms of nutritional failure?

SUPPLEMENTARY READINGS

Berg, A: *The Nutrition Factor: Its Role in National Development.* Washington, D.C., The Brookings Institution, 1973.

Berg, A., Scrimshaw, N. S., and Call, D. L., eds.: *Nutrition, National Development and Planning.* Cambridge, MIT Press, 1973.

FAO/WHO: Handbook on Human Nutritional Requirements. Rome, FAO Nutritional Studies No. 28; WHO Monograph Series No. 61, 1974.

McClure, F. J.: Water Fluoridation. Bethesda, DHEW, National Institutes of Health, National Institute of Dental Research, 1970.

Olson, R. E., ed.: *Protein-Calorie Malnutrition.* New York, Academic Press, 1975.

Oomen, H. A. P. C.: Vitamin A deficiency, xerophthalmia and blindness. Nutr. Rev. 33:161, 1974.

Roe, D. A.: *A Plague of Corn: The Social History of Pellagra.* Ithaca, Cornell University Press, 1973.

Stansbury, J. B., et al: Endemic goiter and cretinism: public health significance and prevention. WHO Chronicle, 28:220, 1974.

REFERENCES

1. Berg, A.: *The Nutrition Factor: Its Role in National Development.* The Brookings Institution, Washington, D.C., 1973.
2. Bengoa, J. M.: WHO Chronicle 28:3, 1974.
3. Pan American Health Organization: *Patterns of mortality in childhood.* Scientific Publication No. 262, Washington, D.C., 1973.
4. Bengoa, J. M.: in Nutrition, National Development and Planning. Ch. 12. A. Berg, N. S. Scrimshaw, D. L. Call, eds. Cambridge, MIT Press, 1973.
5. Ibid.
6. Ibid.
7. McLaren, D. S.: Lancet 2:93, 1974.
8. Bengoa, J. M. (1973): op. cit.
9. Ibid.
10. Williams, C. D.: Lancet 2:1151, 1935.
11. WHO Chronicle 27:487, 1973.
12. Bengoa, J. M. (1973) op. cit.

13. Mitchell, H. S.: J. Am. Dietet. A. 44:165, 1964.
14. WHO Chronicle 28:276, 1974.
15. Williams, C.: Cajanus 7:37, (February), 1974.
16. Bengoa, J. M. (1973): op. cit.
17. Ibid.
18. WHO Chronicle, 27:28, 1973.
19. Oomen, H. A. P. C.: Nutr. Rev. 32:161, 1974.
20. Zaklama, M. S., et al: Am. J. Clin. Nutr. 26:1202, 1973.
21. Oomen, H. A. P. C.: op. cit.
22. WHO Chronicle 27:28, 1973.
23. Williams, R. R.: *Toward the Conquest of Beriberi*. Cambridge, Harvard University Press, 1961.
24. Scrimshaw, N. S.: N. Eng. J. Med. 272:137, 1965.
25. Ibid.
26. Ibid.
27. Gubbay, E. R.: Canad. M.A.J. 95:21, 1966.
28. Victor, M., and Adams, R. D.: Am. J. Clin. Nutr. 9:379, 1961.
29. Williams, R. R.: J. Am. Dietet. A. 36:31, 1960.
30. Roe, D. A.: *A Plague of Corn: The Social History of Pellagra*. Ithaca, Cornell University Press, 1973.
31. Joint FAO/WHO Expert Committee: Requirements of Vitamin A, Thiamine, Riboflavin and Niacin. Geneva, WHO Tech. Report Series No. 363, 1967.
32. Roe, D. A., op. cit.
33. Demers, P., et al: Canad. M.A.J. 93:573, 1965.
34. Harrison, H. E.: Am. J. Public Health 56:734, 1966.
35. Report: Pediatrics 29:646, 1962.
36. Joint FAO/WHO Expert Committee on Nutrition—Seventh Report. Geneva, WHO Tech. Report Series No. 377, 1967.
37. Bengoa, J. M. (1974): op. cit.
38. Stanbury, J. B., et al: WHO Chronicle 28:220, 1974.
39. Perez, C., et al: Technique of Endemic Goiter Surveys In: Endemic Goitre. Geneva, WHO Monograph Series No. 44, 1960.
40. Stanbury, J. B.: op. cit.
41. Dunning, J. M.: N. Eng. J. Med. 272:30, 84, 1965.
42. Ibid.
43. Rusoff, L. L., et al: Am. J. Clin. Nutr. 11:94, 1962.

For further references see Bibliography in Section 4.

section three
diet in disease

21 introduction to diet in disease

Diet Therapy
Classification of Dietary Modifications
The Therapeutic Dietitian
Assessment of Patient Needs

DIET THERAPY

Diet therapy is that component of the treatment of an individual with an acute or chronic disease which involves the modification of food intake. It may be the primary mode of therapy, such as the energy-restricted diet used to treat uncomplicated obesity. It may be used in conjunction with therapeutic agents, such as diet combined with insulin to treat diabetes. Or, diet therapy may be supportive of other modes of treatment, such as the progression from a liquid to a regular diet following surgery.

Traditionally therapeutic diets have been classified according to the disease being treated: for example, diabetic diet, cardiac diet, ulcer diet, or renal diet. These labels indicate a patient's diagnosis but do not indicate the nutritional problem associated with the disease process or the modification in food and/or nutrient intake required in the treatment of the disease. At the same time these labels do not indicate the nutritional problems which may be common to a number of diseases. The patient with the renal complications which may occur in long-standing diabetes, the patient with the renal complications of severe cardiac failure, and the patient with primary renal disease all have similar problems

309

with the excretion of the end products of protein metabolism and with fluid and electrolyte balance. All of these patients will require some modification of their protein, fluid, sodium, and, in many situations, potassium intake.

The patient's diagnosis will continue to be the primary focus of the physician's medical plan of care although those physicians who are using the problem-oriented patient record may also identify the nutritional problem.[1] For example: hyperglycemia is often one of the problems listed in the physician's progress notes for the patient with diabetes. With this trend of identification of the nutritional problem by physicians, the labeling of therapeutic diets today and in the future should reflect the modifications of food and/or nutrient intake required to treat the problem, not the disease per se. Although the chapter headings in this section appear to contradict this statement, the food and/or nutrient modifications required to treat the nutritional problems associated with the disease are presented at the beginning of each chapter.

CLASSIFICATION OF DIETARY MODIFICATIONS

Therapeutic diets may be modified in consistency or bulk, in energy content, or in the kinds and amounts of nutrients, such as protein, fat, carbohydrate, minerals, vitamins, and/or fluids and electrolytes.

Consistency or Bulk

Foods are modified in consistency or bulk for patients with chewing and swallowing difficulties and with diseases of the gastrointestinal tract, such as peptic ulcer, diarrhea, or constipation. Modification in consistency may vary from a liquid diet administered by nasogastric tube to a diet of well-cooked food. Modification in bulk may vary from a diet totally devoid of fiber to a diet high in fiber (nondigestible residue).

Energy

The energy content of a diet is modified for overweight (overfat) and underweight patients. The obese individual requires a diet restricted in calories but adequate in all other nutrients. The underweight individual requires an increase in calorie intake with a reasonable distribution of protein, fat, and carbohydrate and adequate amounts of minerals and vitamins. In many complex situations the calorie content of the diet pattern must be given the same consideration as other nutrients. For example, in chronic renal failure the basal energy needs must be met. Otherwise amino acids will be deaminized to provide carbon

units for the Citric Acid Cycle and the nitrogen from such amino acids will contribute to the amount of urea the kidney has to excrete (see Chapter 9).

The chronically ill older person living alone or the disturbed individual admitted to psychiatric often requires total nutritional rehabilitation including an increased calorie intake. These individuals may also be dehydrated as well as underfed and will require rehydration as well as a diet adequate in calories and all nutrients.

Modification in calorie intake is also used as a preventive measure. Any adult who reduces his energy expenditure for any reason requires a decrease in calorie intake. For most adult patients hospitalization reduces energy expenditure.

Kinds and Amounts of Nutrients

The kinds and amounts of nutrients are modified when problems of nutrient utilization occur. Problems involving the digestive-absorptive process occur frequently. Interference with the flow of bile into the duodenum usually requires a modification in the amount, and in some situations the kind, of fat intake. Total fat intake may be reduced, or medium chain triglycerides may be substituted for long chain ones. Patients who have an insufficient amount, or a total lack, of the digestive enzyme lactase require a diet reduced in the amount, or totally devoid, of the disaccharide lactose.

Problems of nutrient utilization in intermediary metabolism require a variety of modifications. In the diet of the patient with diabetes mellitus the amount of protein and the amount and kinds of fat and carbohydrate are modified to achieve a reasonable level of blood glucose and lipids. For the infant with phenylketonuria, the amount of the essential amino acid phenylalanine is restricted just to meet the need for this essential nutrient. Such an infant is unable to metabolize excessive amounts of phenylalanine through the tyrosine pathway due to a lack of the enzyme phenylalanine hydroxylase.

Problems in the utilization of lipids also occur. The polyunsaturated fatty acid composition of a diet may be increased and saturated fatty acid decreased either to prevent or to treat patients with atherosclerosis, and the amount of cholesterol in a diet is reduced in the treatment of a patient with familial hypercholesterolemia.

Problems also occur in fluid and electrolyte balance and in the excretion of the end products of metabolism. The patient in chronic renal failure faces both problems. He requires a diet restricted in fluid, electrolytes, and protein. However, the food selected to supply the limited amount of protein must contain protein of high biological value to provide the essential amino acids needed by the patient and, at the same time, limit the nonessential amino acids to reduce the amount of nitrogen to be excreted by the kidneys.

Whatever the modification, care must be taken to ensure the nutritional adequacy of the therapeutic diet. When such a diet cannot for any reason provide an adequate intake of vitamins and minerals, the physician should be informed so that he can supplement the diet with vitamin and mineral preparations.

THE THERAPEUTIC DIETITIAN

The therapeutic dietitian is the primary nutrition counselor in the health-care team. She is prepared to enter into the helping relationship (see Chapter 12) with a patient to assist him in modifying his usual food choices as part of the treatment of his medical problem. The therapeutic dietitian may interact with patients in the in- or outpatient facilities of a hospital, in a health maintenance organization, in a neighborhood health center, or in any other medical care setting. She may share her *functions* with, or delegate them to, another member of the health-care team, such as the physician, nurse, nurse practitioner, social worker, dietetic technician or aide, or the home health aide. However, the therapeutic dietitian is never privileged to delegate her *responsibility* for the quality of nutritional care of any patient to another member of the team.

In 1971 the American Dietetic Association described the therapeutic dietitian as the clinical nutrition specialist:

A person with expertise in nutritional care. One who can evaluate the nutritional status of a person, plan his nutritional care, and direct implementation of the plan. Such a specialist would work with other members of the health-care team, but would accept responsibility for the diet prescription and the patient's nutritional care.[2]

The phrase "can evaluate the nutritional status" might more appropriately read "can evaluate the nutritional needs." The data required to evaluate a patient's nutritional status are rarely available to the therapeutic dietitian or any other member of the health-care team. A complete evaluation of a patient's nutritional status requires a series of complex, and at present, not well-validated biochemical tests; these tests are not done routinely in the hospital to evaluate nutritional status (see Chapter 1). With the biomedical data which are available and the assessment of psychosocial needs, the therapeutic dietitian today can identify a patient's nutritional needs.

ASSESSMENT OF PATIENT NEEDS

In the medical setting the assessment activity (see Chapter 12) takes on additional significance. The needs of the hospitalized patient whose diet is modified as part of the treatment of his acute or chronic disease may differ significantly from the needs of clients who are well. Together with all the factors in the patient's situation of which the dietitian must be aware, she must seek to discover his reaction to hospitalization and to understand his behavior in, for most people, an unfamiliar and anxiety-producing situation.

Hospitalization most often disrupts the life-style of a patient and forces him to interact with numerous unfamiliar individuals—physicians, nurses, dietitians, technicians—and, perhaps for the first time in his life, to share a room with a stranger. At the same time a patient may have very little time to think about and accept the diagnosis. For instance, between his noon and evening meal he may find he must change his food habits because the physician may have discovered after completing the glucose tolerance test that morning that the patient has diabetes mellitus.

As one seeks to help a patient accept a therapeutic modification of his food practices as part of the treatment of his disease, it must be kept in mind that his food habits are part of his social and cultural heritage. In addition certain psychological factors and his physical condition will influence his acceptance of food during his illness. Some of the factors which one needs to consider in assessing a patient's needs are discussed in the following paragraphs.

Cultural Factors

Cultural heritage, family background and status, religious customs, family methods of food preparation and service, emotional attitudes toward food, as well as exposure to nutrition education, food fads, and superstitions all contribute to an individual's food habits and acceptance of food during hospitalization. A variety of ethnic food patterns may be encountered (see Chapter 13). The Orthodox Jewish, the Puerto Rican, the Mexican, the Polish, and the Italian patient may have food habits different from one another and from those of other Americans. At the same time, care must be taken to avoid cultural patronage; for example, a patient whose surname identifies him as a member of an ethnic group may represent the third or fourth generation of his family. He may have been born and lived his whole life in the United States, and his food habits may be typically American.

In the United States, food patterns may vary widely by region although modern transportation and communications media have modified these patterns to some extent. However, even today, a patient from the South who finds himself in a Northern hospital may feel that, because of the way vegetables are cooked, they are insipid and uninteresting, and he may refuse to eat them.

Most people live in families and eat their meals with others. To eat in bed and by oneself may accentuate the illness in the patient's mind. Some hospitals try to meet this problem by having as many patients eat together as possible, and here a room for four or six patients may actually be a better setting than a single room with its lone private patient. Even a sodium-restricted diet may be accepted when its restrictions are shared with a fellow patient.

Psychological Influences

Illness may change a person's psychological orientation to everyday occurrences and personal relationships; the need for the familiar and the customary is immeasurably increased. Because what, how, and with whom we eat is an everyday occurrence, illness, which interrupts this pattern, may have serious psychological repercussions. The fear, the worry, the insecurity, and the frustration that possess the patient as he changes from an independent, healthy individual to one dependent on others in illness is often expressed through regressive behavior. Fussiness, anorexia, or demands for extra attention are traits that may be exhibited by the worried patient. Babcock says that "it is easier to show discouragement through anorexia than it is to explain that one is feeling inadequate and depressed in the presence of a frightening disease or a disheartening experience."[3]

The apparent apathy or uncooperativeness of a patient may mean not that he does not want to eat, but that the food offered to him is unacceptable because of its emotional connotations. His food habits have developed slowly through the years and have become a personal and guarded part of himself, so that many foods may be associated with specific feelings and emotions separate from their nutritional significance. Such foods as milk, cocoa, custards, junket, creamed and strained foods, first met with in infancy, become associated with the dependency and the security of that period. Some adults will refuse such foods despite their apparent nutritional value simply because they resent the dependency of illness. Because of the sense of security they convey, others may cling to using these same foods, even though they may not be desirable nutritionally or psychologically.

Desserts, sweets, and delicacies have become re-ward foods to many people because they first were received as a reward for cleaning one's plate or being a good child. It is not surprising that adolescents, and older people too, indulge in excessive intake of such foods when they are under stress and in need of psychological reward.

In the United States some foods have gained special status. Steaks, chops, green salads, and butter are four examples of these foods. Patients may resent suggestions to reduce the cost of food by substituting ground meat for steaks and chops, or margarine for butter. On the other hand the homemaker who is well aware of the cost of food uses ground meat and margarine.

Tea, coffee, and alcoholic beverages may be thought of as adult foods by some patients because they were forbidden to them as children. Excessive use of these beverages, to the exclusion of milk, may be an expression of a desire to seem mature. On the other hand, some cultural groups use tea, coffee, and alcoholic beverages regularly as part of the daily diet for the whole family, including the children.

It must not be forgotten that the appearance of the food and the tray also will produce a psychological effect which may determine acceptance or rejection of the meal. Hot food must be served *hot* and cold food *cold*. A pot of *hot* coffee or tea may make the remainder of a restricted diet acceptable. It tells the patient, as no words can, that those about him really care about him and are making every effort to make his food as palatable as possible.

The therapeutic diet itself may have meaning for the patient that is not evident to the professional staff. Everyone rejoices with the patient who progresses from a liquid diet to one containing solid food as concrete evidence that he is getting better. But, should that patient ask if he must follow a sodium-restricted diet for the rest of his life, are we aware that he may be inquiring in reality if he is going to have cardiac disease permanently, with all that this implies? The therapeutic diet which must be of long duration may give the patient a real sense of deprivation, with depressing overtones that are difficult to resolve.

All those concerned with nutrition need to be cognizant of what food means to people under various circumstances. Attempts to change long-established and deeply ingrained patterns may be met with resistance. The overzealous nutrition counselor who is trying to teach a patient "what is good for him, nutritionally," may interpret the patient's response as "ignorance" or "lack of cooperation." Pumpian-Mindlin writes: "To accomplish the prime purpose of regulating and guiding what goes into a patient's mouth, one must learn to listen carefully to what first comes out of the same mouth. . . . Otherwise one may find himself in the position of having more than mere words thrown back in one's face."[4] We must be able to interpret what the patient says or does not say about food, what he does with food, and how he reacts to food service in the light of his emotional as well as his metabolic needs. Whatever dietary changes may be necessary for his therapy must be made within this framework if they are to be successful.

Physical Condition

Through observation, the physical characteristics of the patient which may influence his acceptance of food or ability to feed himself may be identified. Older patients may have lost some of their teeth, making chewing difficult if they are placed on a general house diet. Some individuals will use poor fitting dentures for cosmetic reasons and remove them at mealtime. The adolescent boy with a fractured jaw may complain bitterly of hunger because his liquid house diet has not been modified sufficiently in calorie content or frequency of feeding to satisfy his needs. Patients recovering from oral surgery will not appreciate the effects of citrus juices on a sore mouth. Assessment of the ability to swallow is critical for certain patients if aspiration and its adverse effects are to be avoided.

Patients with emphysema and other respiratory difficulties may be forced to eat and drink slowly and, therefore, may need their trays for a longer period of time than other patients. Providing adequate nutrients and fluids for these individuals may require four or five meals per day.

Many individuals with sight problems, including the blind, can and prefer to feed themselves. They will need to be oriented to the placement of dishes and other articles on their trays. They may need help in pouring beverages, in opening milk cartons, and in removing protective coverings from foods. Individuals with poor manipulative skills such as the arthritic or the multiple sclerosis patient may need the same kind of assistance. Assessing the ability of any handicapped individual and providing the proper assistance not only will reduce his frustrations and promote his independence but also may help him to achieve a reasonable nutrient intake.

Every patient does not require the same size serving of food. "Appetite poor" recorded on the dietitian's Kardex after meal rounds may really mean that the patient was served too much food not, as this note is usually interpreted, that the patient did not eat enough food. A high-calorie diet for an 82-year-old, 5-foot 1-inch chronically ill woman may be 2000 calories and for a 27-year-old, 6-foot 2-inch man after a hemorrhoidectomy, 3500 calories.

The long-term or chronically ill patient presents a special challenge to both the dietitian and the nurse. Cycle menus which repeat the same menus every two to four weeks are used in many hospitals. The long-term or chronically ill patient may experience two or three periods of a cycle menu plan; this may be a problem, even though the menu items are familiar and acceptable to him. Family members or friends can often be helpful when a patient becomes bored with the hospital's food by occasionally providing a favorite dish from home, although they will need direction from the dietitian so that their contribution will fit his diet plan.

Interval nourishments for the chronically ill patient need to be carefully planned. A 400-calorie milkshake at 10:30 A.M. may result in the patient's refusal of an 800-calorie meal at 12:00 noon. Four meals, with the last one served at 8:00 or 9:00 P.M., may be a more effective plan for providing for his nutrient needs, especially if he is accustomed to an evening snack at home.

The scheduling of treatments, diagnostic tests, and nursing care are often critical factors in obtaining a proper food intake. The best meal of the day for some of these patients is breakfast because they are rested or, for some of the older patients, because breakfast has always been an important meal. As the day progresses they may become increasingly tired and tend to eat less. Therefore, treatments should be planned so that the patient may rest before the noon and evening meals. Some of these patients may require only minimal assistance at breakfast and considerably more at the evening meal.

The patient restricted to prolonged bed rest benefits from nursing care procedures which promote the maximum movement by, or of, himself. Research has shown that immobilization, even with adequate food intake, promotes negative nitrogen and calcium balance which may result in progressive muscular weakness. Turning and positioning the patient as ordered by the physician and providing passive exercise during personal care will help to prevent the adverse metabolic effects of immobility (see Chapter 24).

Nutritional Status

There are very limited data on the nutritional status of patients admitted to general hospitals. Even the limited data available in practically every hospitalized patient's chart—height and weight by age and sex and hemoglobin and hematocrit—have not been collected and analyzed to indicate the status of the average patient. With the computerization of patient data it is possible that this information will be available in the future.

Recently, Bollet and Owens reported the frequency of protein and certain vitamin deficiencies (vitamins A, C, and E) in 315 medical service patients.[5] The patients were selected by diagnostic category, not because of any indication of nutritional deficiencies. The authors state that their data reflect the frequency with which nutritional deficiency can occur in the average patient but did not measure the true frequency of the occurrence.

They observed the best nutritional status in those patients with the diagnosis of diabetes mellitus. There was a greater frequency of low body weight in this group as compared to their other study subjects, which they attributed to nutrition counseling and the patients' attention to diet. The patients with the poorest overall nutritional status were those with liver disease due to alcoholism; those with the next lowest nutritional status were patients with hyperthyroidism, a hypermetabolic state.

A significant number of patients with peptic ulcer disease (42 percent) and those with rheumatoid arthritis (37 percent) had low blood ascorbic acid levels. In patients with peptic ulcer disease, this was attributed to dietary practices; without supplements of vitamin C, the usual diet used to treat patients with peptic ulcer can be low in ascorbic acid. The frequency of low ascorbic acid levels in patients with rheumatoid arthritis is well known although poorly understood. It has been suggested to be the result of drugs used to treat this disease.

Although the data are limited, the work of Bollet and Owens provides some clues to the nutritional status of patients admitted to the medical services of a general hospital.

Potential for Learning

As early as possible in her interaction with a patient, the dietitian will attempt to discover through observing, listening, and interviewing what he knows about nutrition and diet; his attitudes toward his diet and illness; and his readiness for learning, when necessary, how to manage his diet.

Studies tell us that, as our nutrition education programs in elementary and secondary schools have been improved, we have a better educated young adult population today than in the past. If we are to avoid boring patients by giving them nutrition information they already have, we need to find out what they know and how they use their knowledge. In this way we can discover the problem, if any, and focus our teaching on the patient's real need (see Chapter 12).

As we listen to the patient, his vocabulary will give us numerous clues as to the words and kinds of explanations we will need to use in teaching him. For example, if the patient is a newly diagnosed diabetic who is an organic chemist, he may expect the nutrition counselor to use the word "carbohydrate"; whereas, the mother of six children who reads and understands at the sixth-grade level will need to be approached quite differently. In helping her to understand diabetes and her diet we would more likely use the word "sugar."

With the increasing use of programmed instruction, any member of the health-care team will want to watch for clues as to whether or not a patient is literate, in English or any other language. We have not always been aware of this in the past as we used printed instructions, since children, friends, or other patients may have interpreted such instructions for the patient.

The dietitian, who begins diet instruction as early as possible during the patient's hospitalization, can use the trays served each day to demonstrate the kinds and amounts of food he will be eating at home. At the same time, she can involve him or a member of his family in the planning of his daily menu. The wife of a patient who will require a sodium-restricted diet for the years ahead may demonstrate her understanding of the dietitian's instructions and her skill in adjusting her methods of food preparation by bringing her husband the "fruits" of her labors. At the same time she may feel a certain satisfaction from participating in her husband's care. This approach to patient education not only prepares the individual and his family for his discharge but also, in many instances, stimulates the patient's interest in learning about his diet.

STUDY QUESTIONS AND ACTIVITIES

1. Select a patient who has been identified as a "feeding problem." With the assistance of your clinical instructor, determine what the patient's problem really is and with her guidance attempt to work toward a solution to the problem.

2. In the supine position with only one pillow to elevate your head, have someone feed you ½ cup of hot broth, two crackers and ½ cup of pudding or clear gelatin. Record the time it took you to consume all the food and fluids and your reaction to this experience. Write an outline of what you would use when instructing an individual responsible for feeding a hospitalized patient in the same position.

3. With your clinical instructor select a patient whose name identifies him as a member of some ethnic group. Interview this patient to find out what foods he commonly eats. Was his name a valid or an invalid clue to his usual food practices? In conference discuss this clinical encounter with your classmates.

SUPPLEMENTARY READINGS

ADA position paper on education for the profession of dietetics. J. Am. Dietet. A. 59:372, 1971.

Butterworth, C. E., Jr.: Editorial: Malnutrition in the hospital. JAMA 230:879, 1974.

Davies, G. J., et al: Special diets in hospitals: Discrepancy between what is prescribed and what is eaten. Brit. Med. J. 1:200, 1975.

Kocher, R. E.: Monitoring nutritional care of the long-term patient. I. Policies and systems that support the ongoing evalution of care. J. Am. Dietet. A. 67:45, 1975.

Natow, A. B., et al: Integrating the Jewish Dietary Laws into a dietetics program. J. Am. Dietet. A. 67:13, 1975.

Ohlson, M. A.: The philosophy of dietary counseling. J. Am. Dietet. A. 63:13, 1973.

Spangler, A. A., et al: Physicians' attitudes on dietitians' contributions to health team care. J. Am. Dietet. A. 65:647, 1974.

Walters, F. M., et al: Nutritional needs of the outpatient—an overview. J. Am. Dietet. A. 61:170, 1972.

For further references see Bibliography in Section 4.

REFERENCES

1. Weed, L. L.: N. Eng. J. Med. 278:593-600, 652-657, 1968.
2. ADA position paper on education for the profession of dietetics. J. Am. Dietet. A. 59:372, 1971.
3. Babcock, C. G.: J. Am. Dietet. A. 28:222, 1952.
4. Pumpian-Mindlin, E. J.: J. Am. Dietet. A. 30:576, 1954.
5. Bollet, A. J., and Owens, S.: Am. J. Clin. Nutr. 26:931, 1973.

22

feeding the hospitalized patient

Background Data
Management of Patient Food Service
Progressive Hospital Diets
Fluid Intake

The community general hospital is viewed today not only as a medical care facility but also as a community center for health education. Therefore, the food served to patients in the hospital should exemplify proper meal planning for the community as well as provide for the nutritional needs of each patient. At the same time, well-prepared and attractively served food acceptable to the majority of patients enhances the hospital's image in the community.

BACKGROUND DATA
The Diet Order
A patient's diet prescription is ordered by his physician, and will be found in the orders written by him at the time the patient is admitted to the hospital. The order which the physician writes will depend on the patient's condition and may vary from nothing-by-mouth (N.P.O., *nil per oris*) to a normal or regular diet. The diet order is changed as the patient's condition changes. If he is known to have a disease which requires the modification of his diet as a part of his treatment, or if diagnostic procedures during hospitalization indicate a disease which can be treated by diet therapy, a therapeutic diet will be ordered.

In most but not all instances, the patient with a prescription for a therapeutic diet will require counseling prior to discharge from the hospital so that he can manage this aspect of his treatment at home. To avoid inadequate initial counseling, those who are working with the patient must anticipate his discharge and consult with the physician regarding his plans for the patient. Some physicians will anticipate discharge when they write the therapeutic diet prescription, for example, "diabetic diet and instruct for discharge." In any situation, counseling begins with the interpretation of the diet prescription to the patient when the physician writes the order.

The physician is legally responsible for the patient's medical care plan, including the diet order. He may delegate the formulation of the diet order to the therapeutic dietitian or he may formulate the prescription in consultation with her. However, he cannot delegate his ultimate responsibility for the order to the dietitian or to any other member of the team. If the therapeutic dietitian is to participate in the formulation of the diet order, she is responsible for familiarizing herself with the patient's medical problem before making any decisions or recommendations about the order. At the same time the dietitian is responsible for keeping up-to-date in both the theory and practice of therapeutic dietetics.

The Diet Manual

The diet manual is a compilation of routine and therapeutic diet plans and includes an explanation of the rationale for each plan. It is used for ease of communication by the members of the health-care team. The manual serves as a guide to the kinds and amounts of foods and beverages the dietary department provides to fulfill the patient's diet order. A copy of the manual used by a hospital is usually available in each clinical unit for the convenience of doctors and nurses. Under Medicare, in the Conditions of Participation for Hospitals, the dietary department is required to have an up-to-date manual which has been approved jointly by the medical and dietary staffs.[1]

In teaching hospitals and in many large hospitals, physicians, dietitians and other members of the health-care team working together in committee frequently compile a diet manual for use in their institutions. In some communities a committee of physicians and dietitians representing all the hospitals will compile a manual for community-wide use. Many of these diet manuals are available for purchase. Diet manuals have also been compiled by state or district dietetic associations or by state health or welfare agencies for use by small hospitals, extended-care facilities, and nursing homes. (See partial list of diet manuals at the end of this chapter.)

As a general rule the first section of a manual will describe routine diet plans for infants, children, and adults, including soft and liquid diet plans. Subsequent sections will describe a variety of therapeutic diets used in the treatment of disease, test diets required by certain diagnostic procedures, and food composition tables. Diet manuals often differ in terms used to describe diets and in the recommendations for the foods used in a diet plan. These differences reflect variations in interpretation of theory relating to therapeutic dietetics or regional or cultural variations in food acceptance.

The Patient's Medical Record

A record or chart for each hospitalized patient is available in the clinical unit. These charts have been standardized by the American Hospital Association and include demographic data obtained on admission—the patient's name, address, sex, age, physician, admitting or provisional diagnosis, etc.; graphic data—temperature, pulse, respiration, and fluid intake and output; nursing notes—reports of treatment procedures, food acceptance, and any expression of psychosocial problems either observed by the nurse or verbally communicated to her by the patient or his relatives and friends; the medical history elicited by the physician, the diagnosis, and the physician's daily progress notes; laboratory data and x-ray reports; reports of any operative procedures; and consultants' comments and progress notes. The patient's orders may be a part of his chart during hospitalization, or the orders for all patients in a clinical unit may be kept in one folder or notebook in the unit office. The patient's record is available and used by all qualified professional personnel working with the patient; all personnel are equally responsible for sharing information and *protecting the confidentiality* of this information.

It is the policy in some but not all hospitals that the dietitian records her findings in the patient's chart on a page usually identified as dietitian's notes. These should include the patient's diet history, acceptance or rejection of food, food intolerances, diet order and any therapeutic diet plan, progress, and counseling notes. If the physician is using the problem-oriented system in his daily progress notes, it is advisable for the dietitian to use the same problem identification in labeling her notes.[2] Guidelines for the therapeutic dietitian in making notations in the medical record are available.[3] Any notes written in a patient's record should be *legible*, in the *third* person, *concise*, and *factual*, with no expression of opinion or judgment of the patient's behavior. For example, noting that the patient "cheats on his diet" reflects a judgment. A more appropriate recording is: "The patient is unable to manage his diet because . . . ," followed by an identification of the reason for his behavior, such as "he cannot afford to purchase food required" or "he does not understand reason for therapeutic diet."

The dietitian's notes are used to communicate with the other members of the busy health-care team just as she uses their notes to keep up with a patient's progress. The dietitian's notes should be a part of the patient's permanent record so that she can review them before subsequent contact with the patient, or so that they are available for use by another dietitian who may have contact with the patient at a later date.

The following sections in this chapter discuss the management of patient food service, the general principles used in establishing the routine diet plans—sometimes referred to as house diets or progressive diets—and meeting the fluid needs of patients. The brief discussion of the management of food service is presented for members of the health-care team other than dietitians.

MANAGEMENT OF PATIENT FOOD SERVICE

The Administrator of Dietetic Services

In large hospitals in the United States menu planning, food purchasing and preparation, and the delivery of meals to the clinical units are directed by a qualified administrative dietitian. The administrator of dietetic services is described by the American Dietetic Association as:

> A person competent in the management of complex food service operations using a systems approach and integrating nutrition principles; an executive who participates in defining objectives, formulating policies, and who employs all the tools of business management, automation, creative planning, and delegation.[4]

With the knowledge explosion in both management science and in food, nutrition, and related biomedical sciences, the nutritional care of patients in large hospitals today requires the expertise of both the administrator of dietetic services and the therapeutic dietitian. Together these two members of the dietetics profession plan and implement the nutritional care of patients. At the same time all the members of the health-care team, including dietitians, must coordinate their services for the comfort and satisfaction of the patient. For example, interrupting a four-year-old child's lunch to draw blood can be as hazardous to his nutritional care as serving an inadequate diet; or serving breakfast trays one-half hour later than scheduled can disrupt a variety of treatment schedules for many of the patients in a clinical unit. Communication and cooperation among patient-care services are achieved most effectively by a patient nutritional care committee, having responsibility for establishing routines which best serve the patient.

Food Service Management Systems

Two management systems are used in hospitals today. Under one system the hospital administers all aspects of the dietary department, including both the nutritional care of patients and employee food service. All the members of the dietary department staff are employees of the hospital, and the director of the department is directly responsible to the hospital administrator or one of his assistants.

Under a second system the hospital contracts with a food service or catering company to manage all aspects of the dietary department. In many situations all employees of the dietary department including the dietitians are employees of the food service company. However, it would seem advisable for the therapeutic dietitian to be an employee of the hospital, since her counseling services to patients are not in all instances directly related to daily food service: for example, the dietitian giving service in the ambulatory care clinics of the hospital, or the one who is a member of the team in a clinical research center. Either system, properly managed, can provide quality food service to patients and employees and expert dietary counseling to both inpatients and outpatients.

In small hospitals and skilled nursing homes the food service may be managed by a food service director who is not prepared to plan diets, normal or therapeutic, or to counsel patients. A consultant dietitian is employed by these institutions to assess the nutritional needs of the patients and to plan their nutritional care. She is also responsible for assisting the food service employees to implement these plans, and for counseling the patients.

Food Service Delivery Systems

Two types of food delivery systems, centralized and decentralized, are used to deliver food to the patient area. In centralized service, a patient's tray is completely assembled in or near the food production area and delivered to the patient area in a specially designed cart or by a conveyor system or dumbwaiter. The tray is delivered to the patient directly from the cart or from a service pantry.

Decentralized service refers to the method by which bulk food is transported from the production area to a service kitchen in the patient area. The patient's tray is assembled in the service kitchen and delivered to the bedside. Either system requires that nursing and dietary departments carefully coordinate their schedules so that patients receive palatable, attractive food.

Cost analysis of these two systems has generally shown that the centralized one is the most economical method for serving adult patients. However, decentralized service is to be preferred in pediatric units caring for children ages 2 to 12. Portion size varies by age and appetite in this group to such an extent that tray service in or close to the patient area is desirable in order to avoid overwhelming children with more food than they can eat. The needs of the adolescent can be met, where necessary, with double adult size servings.

In some hospitals the patient's tray is delivered to the bedside by a dietary department employee, in others by an employee of the nursing service. In either situation the individual who delivers the tray needs to know of any recent change in the patient's status, and must be informed about meals to be delayed or omitted for tests and treatments. Errors of this type in the delivery of trays can add to the discomfort of the patient and the cost of medical care by increasing the time the patient is required to stay in the hospital. At the same time any personnel responsible for the delivery of the tray to the patient must be trained to help the patient and to protect both himself and the patient from infection.

Meal Service Schedules

Traditionally hospital dietary departments have served patients three meals a day—morning, noon, and night. When necessary, beverages and snacks have been available between meals. This schedule is used by many hospitals and appears to reflect the habits of the patients they serve.

Recently, due to labor costs and problems of staffing in the dietary department, new meal service schedules have been adopted. In some hospitals food is served four times a day: a continental breakfast, usually coffee and a roll, at 7:00 A.M.; brunch or lunch at 10:30 A.M.; dinner at 3:30 or 4:00 P.M.; and a snack, usually a sandwich and beverage, at 8:00 or 8:30 P.M. The continental breakfast and the evening snack are frequently served on disposable materials and, with the exception of coffee, prepared by the food service workers at low work-load periods during the day. Within an eight-hour workday one group of highly skilled cooks can prepare both the brunch and the dinner. Some hospitals use a five- rather than a four-

meal plan, which includes the brunch and dinner meals plus three snack-type meals.

Certain patients in the general hospital requiring therapeutic diets cannot participate in a four- or five-meal service schedule. The labile diabetic will need meals served on his usual schedule, usually three well-spaced meals with a bedtime (h. s., *hour of sleep*) snack. An 800-calorie diet for an obese patient cannot be distributed in four or five meals. If one were to attempt this the patient would be correct when he said, "I am eating like a bird."

Where patient acceptance of the four-meal plan has been evaluated it has been discovered that patients like the plan. Nursing personnel have also accepted this revised meal schedule. They point out that on busy medical units fewer patients miss a major meal due to delayed breakfasts for tests or treatments, and the patients enjoy the snack served in the evening at the end of visiting hours. The four- or five-meal plan has been successful in those extended-care facilities and nursing homes which serve geriatric patients who may often need frequent, small meals.

Selective Menus

The hospital patient is offered a daily menu from which he can select his meals. Two or more items in each section of the menu are usually offered; for example, at dinner there may be a choice of roast beef or fried chicken, mashed or baked potato, etc. The printed menus are marked by the patient each day usually for service the next day. In some hospitals menu items for soft and liquid diets may also be included on the regular diet menu. (See the following section, Progressive Hospital Diets.)

Selective menus, even when alternatives are limited, have improved patient food acceptance. Patients with poor vision or who cannot read need assistance. All selective menus need to be evaluated daily to insure adequate nutrient intake by the patient. The individual who consistently selects a less than adequate diet needs professional guidance.

In some but not all hospitals, the patient requiring a therapeutic diet is also offered a selective menu. This patient must be guided by the dietitian so that his menu selections will fulfill his diet plan. This system provides the dietitian with the opportunity to guide the patient early in his hospital stay to become familiar with his therapeutic diet and to counsel the patient appropriately. The selective menu can serve as a "paper and pencil test" of a patient's knowledge of his therapeutic diet and serve to identify for the dietitian, as counseling progresses, areas where reinforcement is needed.

Table 22-1. Evaluation of a Pattern Dietary for Its Nutritive Content[a]

Food Group	Amt. In g.	Household Measure	Energy (Kcal.)	Protein (g.)	Fat (g.)	Carbo-hydrate (g.)	MINERALS Cal-cium (mg.)	Phos-phorus (mg.)	Magne-sium (mg.)	Iron (mg.)	VITAMINS A (IU)	Thia-mine (mg.)	Ribo-flavin (mg.)	Niacin (mg.)	Ascorbic acid (mg.)
Milk or equivalent[b]	488	2 c. (1 pint)	320	17	17	24	576	452	63	.2	700	.16	.84	.3	5
Meat, fish, poultry or egg[c]	120	4 oz., cooked	376	30	31	..	13	212	104	3.3	280	.14	.23	6.1	..
Vegetables:															
Potato, cooked	100	1 medium	65	2	..	15	6	48	22	.5	..	.09	.03	1.2	16
Deep green or yellow, cooked[d]	75	½ c.	21	2	..	6	44	28	29	.9	4700	.05	.10	.5	25
Other, raw or cooked[e]	75	½ c.	45	2	..	10	16	41	18	.9	300	.08	.06	.6	12
Fruits:															
Citrus[f]	100	1 serving	44	1	..	10	18	16	12	.3	140	.06	.02	.3	43
Other[g]	100	1 serving	85	..	..	22	10	21	16	.8	365	.03	.04	.5	4
Bread, white, enriched	100	4 slices	280	9	3	50	84	97	20	2.5	..	.25	.21	2.4	..
Cereal, whole grain or enriched[h]	130 30	⅔ c. cooked or 1 oz. dry	89	3	1	18	12	95	34	.9	..	.08	.03	.7	..
Butter or margarine	14	1 tbsp.	100	..	11	..	3	2	2	..	460	..	..	..	..
Totals			1415	66	63	155	782	1012	335	10.3	6945	.94	1.56	12.6[i]	105
Compare with recommended allowances[j]															
Males (70 kg., 23-50 yrs. old)			2700	56	..	..	800	800	350	10.0	5000	1.40	1.60	18	45
Females (58 kg., 23-50 yrs. old)			2000	46	..	..	800	800	300	18.0	4000	1.00	1.20	13	45

[a]Calculations from Composition of Foods, Handbook No. 8. U. S. Department of Agriculture, rev. 1963 or Table 1, Section 4.
[b]Milk equivalents means evaporated milk and dried milk in amounts equivalent to fluid milk in nutritive content; cheese, if water-soluble minerals and vitamins have not been lost in whey; and food items made with milk.
[c]Evaluation based on the use of 700 g. of beef (chuck, cooked), 200 g. of pork (medium fat, roasted), 200 g. of chicken (roaster, cooked, roasted), and 100 g. of fish (halibut, cooked, broiled) per 10-day period and egg occasionally.
[d]Evaluation based on figures for cooked broccoli, carrots, spinach, and squash (all varieties).
[e]Evaluation based on figures for raw tomatoes and lettuce, and cooked peas, beets, lima beans, and fresh corn.
[f]Evaluation based on figures for whole orange and grapefruit, and orange and grapefruit juices.
[g]Evaluation based on figures for banana, apple, unsweetened cooked prunes, and sweetened canned peaches.
[h]Evaluation based on figures for shredded wheat biscuit and oatmeal.
[i]The average diet in the United States, which contains a generous amount of protein, provides enough tryptophan to increase the niacin value by about one third.
[j]From the National Research Council Recommended Dietary Allowances, revised 1974.

PROGRESSIVE HOSPITAL DIETS

Regular, Standard, General Diet

Various terms are in current use to describe the normal hospital diet which will provide a patient with the energy and nutrients he needs. It is intended for the patient whose condition does not require a therapeutic diet. The pattern dietary, Table 22-1, reproduced here for the convenience of the reader (see Chapter 10), illustrates the basic pattern used to plan the regular hospital diet. This pattern furnishes the nutrients needed to meet the NAS-NRC Recommended Dietary Allowances for an adult, with the exception of calories and iron.

It is expected that additional items will be chosen from the selective menu to meet a patient's needs for calories. A limited number of items, such as milk and sugar for coffee and a cookie served with canned fruit for dessert, will need to be added to this 1400-calorie diet plan by an older patient who requires 1600 to 1700 calories per day. On the other hand, a patient requiring 2400 calories per day may select more bread or rolls and butter, a simple dessert, and a larger serving of meat to meet his calorie needs. In any situation it is well to remember that some patients may require fewer calories than usual, since even ambulatory patients are less active during hospitalization than they are at home or at work.

The nutritional adequacy of a regular diet depends not only on the patient's selection of foods and the amount served but also on the protection of the nutrients in food during preparation and cooking, including the time and temperature of these processes (see Chapter 11). The foods chosen for the regular diet will reflect the preferences characteristic of the cultural background and the economic status of the majority of those served by the institution. For example, two hospitals may serve the same cut of beef, one as pot roast and the other as sauerbraten. The choice of food will further be determined by its suitability for quality and quantity of preparation, its availability, and current market costs and conditions.

The regular diet may be modified in selection and methods of preparation and in consistency for patients who cannot tolerate a regular diet but do not require a therapeutic diet. These modifications of the regular diet are the light or convalescent diet; the soft diet, including the surgical soft, medical soft, and dental soft diets; and the full liquid and clear liquid diets. Table 22-2, Foods Used in Progressive Hospital Diets, illustrates the types of food used in planning regular, light, soft, and full liquid diets; and Table 22-3, Typical Menus for Progressive Hospital Diets, illustrates how these foods are used in menu plans.

Light or Convalescent Diet

A light, or convalescent, diet is intended for convalescent patients not yet able to tolerate the regular diet and for those with minor illnesses. It must be appetizing and readily digested. The chief difference between this diet and the regular diet is the method of preparation. The foods are cooked simply, and fried foods and rich pastries are omitted. Other fat-rich foods, such as nuts, avocado and salad dressing, are avoided. Bran and strong or gas-forming vegetables are to be avoided, as well as most raw vegetables and fruits. All foods included in the soft and the liquid diets may be served on the light diet. In some hospitals this classification is omitted.

Soft Diet

The soft diet is soft in texture and consists of liquids and semisolid foods. It is an intermediate step between the liquid and the light or regular diets. It is indicated in certain postoperative cases, in acute infections, and in some gastrointestinal conditions; also, it may be ordered for the debilitated patient for ease of eating.

It is low in residue and is readily digested. Few or no spices or condiments are used in the preparation. It is somewhat more restricted than the light diet in fruit, meat, and vegetables.

The foods used in the medical soft diet are generally the same as those used in the soft diet in Table 22-2. In the surgical soft diet less tender meats and certain vegetables and fruits may be puréed or blenderized.

Dental or Mechanical Soft Diet

The regular diet may need modification for patients with poor teeth or none, or with dentures which they are unable or unwilling to wear. Additional cooked vegetables or juices should be substituted for salads, and no whole meats should be served, unless the physician approves of the patient's eating whole tender meats. Otherwise the diet should follow the foods used in the light diet.

Full Liquid Diet

Liquid diets are usually prescribed for the postoperative patient, or the patient acutely ill with an infection, gastrointestinal tract disturbances, or a myocardial infarction. See Table 22-2 for the kinds of fluids used and Table 22-3 for a suggested menu.

Clear Liquid Diet

If the patient's condition requires it, only clear fluids may be offered him. In addition to water, clear broth, fruit juices, thin gruels made with water, plain

Table 22-2. Foods Used in Progressive Hospital Diets

TYPE OF FOOD	REGULAR DIET	LIGHT DIET	SOFT DIET	FULL LIQUID DIET
Fruits	All	All cooked and canned fruits, citrus fruits, bananas	Fruit juices, cooked and canned fruits (without seeds, coarse skins or fiber), bananas	Fruit juices, strained
Cereals and cereal products	All	Cereals: dry or well-cooked, spaghetti and macaroni, not highly seasoned	Same as light diet	Gruels, strained or blended
Breads	All	Enriched and whole-wheat bread, crackers	Same as light diet	
Soups and broths	All	All	Broth, strained cream soups	Same as soft diet, or blended
Meat, fish, and poultry	All	Tender steaks and chops, lamb, veal, ground or tender beef, pork, chicken, sweetbreads, liver, fish	Tender chicken, fish and sweetbreads, beef, lamb, and pork	
Eggs	Eggs cooked all ways	Soft-cooked eggs	Same as light diet	Eggnog*
Dairy products	Milk or buttermilk; cream; butter; cheese, all kinds	Milk or buttermilk; cream, butter; cottage and cream cheese, cheddar cheese used in cooking	Same as light diet	Milk or buttermilk, cream
Vegetables	All, including salads	Cooked vegetables: asparagus, peas, string beans, spinach, carrots, beets, squash Salads: tomato and lettuce Potatoes: boiled, mashed, creamed, scalloped, baked	Cooked vegetables: same as light diet Salads: none Potatoes: same as light diet	Vegetable juices
Desserts	All	Ices, ice cream, junket, cereal puddings, custard, gelatin, simple cakes, plain cookies	Same as light diet	Ices, ice cream, gelatin, junket and custard
Beverages	All	Tea, coffee, cocoa; coffee substitutes; milk and milk beverages; carbonated beverages	Same as light diet	Same as light diet

*Because of the danger of salmonella infection when raw egg is used, a pasteurized commercial eggnog preparation is recommended.

gelatin, and tea and coffee are generally used. Carbonated beverages may or may not be used, depending on the policy set by the physicians and dietitians. In some hospitals simple solids such as plain crackers or dry toast are served with the clear liquid diet.

SPECIAL PROBLEMS WITH LIQUID DIET. Both the clear and the full liquid diets are low in nutritive value. The clear liquid diet is used for only limited periods of time, usually no longer than 24 to 36 hours. When the full liquid diet must be used for a period of time, special attention must be given to improving its

nutritive value. Skim milk powder, protein supplements, cream, and sugars may be used to increase its protein and calorie content.

Patients receiving liquid diets will require a feeding every two to three hours during the day and evening. When it is not possible for the dietary department personnel to serve these patients other than at regularly scheduled mealtimes, nurses have found it helpful to remind themselves of a patient's need for an interval feeding by noting this at the proper time interval in the nursing care plan. Also, when the dietitian or nurse observes that a patient is ready for

Table 22-3. Typical Menus for Progressive Hospital Diets

REGULAR DIET	LIGHT DIET	SOFT DIET	FULL LIQUID DIET
		Breakfast	
Fresh pear	Orange	Orange juice	Orange juice, strained
Oatmeal with milk or cream	Oatmeal with milk or cream	Oatmeal with milk or cream	Strained oatmeal gruel with milk or cream
Scrambled eggs	Soft scrambled eggs	Soft scrambled eggs	Coffee with cream and sugar
Buttered whole-wheat toast	Buttered whole-wheat toast	Buttered whole-wheat or white toast	
Coffee with cream and sugar	Coffee with cream and sugar	Coffee with cream and sugar	10 A. M.
			Eggnog*
		Dinner	
Vegetable soup	Vegetable soup	Strained vegetable soup	Broth
Roast veal	Roast veal	Ground veal	Ginger ale with ice cream
Mashed potato	Mashed potato	Mashed potato	Coffee with cream and sugar
Buttered carrots	Buttered carrots	Buttered carrots	
Tomato salad with French dressing	Tomato salad with French dressing	Bread: whole-wheat or white	
Bread: whole-wheat, rye, or white	Bread: whole-wheat, rye or white	Butter	
Butter	Butter	Vanilla ice cream with chocolate sauce	
Peppermint stick ice cream	Peppermint stick ice cream		3 P. M.
Milk	Milk	Milk	Malted milk or buttermilk
		Supper	
Cream of pea soup with crackers	Cream of pea soup with crackers	Cream of pea soup with crackers	Strained cream of pea soup
Macaroni au gratin	Macaroni au gratin	Macaroni au gratin	Plain gelatin with whipped topping
Head lettuce salad with Russian dressing	Head lettuce salad with French dressing	Buttered beets	Tea with cream and sugar
Bread	Bread	Bread	
Butter	Butter	Butter	
Fruit gelatin	Fruit gelatin	Plain gelatin with whipped topping	9 P. M.
Tea with cream and sugar	Tea with cream and sugar	Tea with cream and sugar	Hot cocoa

*See note, Table 22-2

more than a liquid diet, either one can tactfully suggest this to the physician so that he will revise the patient's diet order.

FLUID INTAKE

Fluids are essential to all body functions and must be provided by foods and beverages each day (see Chapter 5). Unless the physician prescribes otherwise, adult patients should drink 1000 to 1500 ml. of fluid per day as beverages served with meals and water available in the patient's unit. Some patients will need to be reminded to drink this quantity because their usual routines—coffee breaks, stopping for a drink each time they pass a water fountain, having a glass of beer or carbonated beverage at bedtime—have been interrupted by hospitalization.

In situations where fluid intake is critical and the daily amount of oral fluid intake is defined in the physician's orders for a patient, close communication between dietary and nursing services is required to carry out the order for fluids and, at the same time, satisfy the patient. Water is not a popular beverage in our society today and the order to force fluids to 3000 ml. per day may be difficult to achieve without the use of coffee, tea, fruit juices, or carbonated beverages between meals, in addition to fluids served with meals. The problem is even more critical for the patient in chronic renal failure when fluid intake is limited to 500 or 800 ml. per day. This patient will usually want as much fluid with his meals as possible within the limitations of any concurrent sodium and potassium restrictions, while nursing service will need some water to give medications. In this situation the dietitian and the nurse will work together with the patient to carry out the order for fluids and to satisfy the patient. Where applicable, critical problems of fluid intake, other than infection, are discussed in succeeding chapters.

Infection

In patients with acute infection, excessive fluid loss may occur through the skin and lungs and through the gastrointestinal tract (diarrhea) which, without the replacement of fluid, can result in dehydration. Electrolyte depletion or retention can also occur. Severe dehydration with electrolyte imbalance can lead to death. Asiatic cholera is a dramatic exam-

feeding the hospitalized patient   323

ple: this infection produces a sudden, massive diarrhea which within a few hours leads to shock (hypovolemia) and death. A recent example was the outbreak of cholera in India.

Severe dehydration due to infection is usually treated by intravenous fluids (dextrose and water and/or electrolyte solutions). At this stage many individuals will not tolerate fluids by mouth. When oral fluids are tolerated, not only water but broth, tea, coffee, carbonated beverages, fruit and vegetable juices, and milk should be offered. These beverages, in addition to adding variety, also contribute to the patient's electrolyte intake. (100 g. canned tomato juice contains approximately 200 mg. sodium and 227 mg. potassium; see Table 4, Section 4). Most of these fluids will also contribute to the patient's carbohydrate intake.

In addition to fluid and electrolyte loss, an elevation in body temperature is always accompanied by an increase in metabolism. In most febrile conditions (acute or chronic) the basal metabolic rate is increased 7 percent for each degree Fahrenheit rise in temperature (12 percent for each degree Centigrade). As a result, the carbohydrate stores are quickly exhausted, and body protein and fat are used for energy if insufficient food is eaten. As soon as the patient with an infection can tolerate food as well as fluids, he should be assisted in selecting food which will meet his energy and other nutrient needs.

STUDY QUESTIONS AND ACTIVITIES

1. Compare the menu selections of a group of patients on regular diets with the pattern dietary in Table 22–1. Will the selections of each patient provide adequately for his energy and nutrient needs?
2. Using the selective menu for a regular diet from any hospital in your community, check to determine whether or not any combination of meal selections for a day will provide an adequate nutrient intake for a twenty-five-year-old postpartum mother who is breast-feeding her newborn infant.
3. Compare the soft diet in the diet manual your hospital uses with the soft diet in Table 22–2. Are there any major differences in the foods used in the two plans? With the help of your clinical instructor, identify the reasons for these differences.
4. With the assistance of your clinical instructor, ob-

tain the diet history of a patient and record your findings in his record. Did you use any judgmental words or phrases? Was your writing legible? Was your spelling correct?
5. Obtain a record of the 24-hour intake of a patient on a clear liquid diet. Using the food composition tables in Section 4, estimate his calorie and nutrient intake. How adequate was this diet for him?

SUPPLEMENTARY READINGS

DeMarco, M. R., and Lovell, J. O.: Centralized food service. Hospitals 47:109, June 1, 1973.
Ohlson, M. A.: Use of dietary manual to promote communication. J. Am. Dietet. A. 62:534, 1973.
Reed, R. M.: Conventional system may be best. Hospitals 47:161, July 16, 1973.
Robinson, C. H.: Updating clinical dietetics: Terminology. J. Am. Dietet. A. 62:645, 1973.
Worthington, B. S.: Effect of nutritional status on immune phenomena. J. Am. Dietet. A. 65:123, 1974.
Zolber, K.: Producing meals without meat. Hospitals 49:81, June 16, 1975.

For further references see Bibliography in Section 4.

DIET MANUALS

Knoxville Area Diet Manual. Committee of the Knoxville District Dietetic Association and the Knoxville Academy of Medicine, 1973.
Manual of Applied Nutrition. Baltimore, Md., Nutrition Department, Johns Hopkins Hospital, 1973.
Mayo Clinic Diet Manual, ed. 4. Philadelphia, Saunders, 1971.
Mike, E. M.: Diet Manual. New York City, The Babies Hospital, The Presbyterian Hospital, 1972.
Ohlson, M. A.: Experimental and Therapeutic Dietetics, ed. 2. Minneapolis, Burgess, 1972.
St. Luke's Hospital Diet Manual. Cleveland, Ohio, Department of Dietetics, 1973.
Turner, D.: Handbook of Diet Therapy, ed. 5. Chicago, University of Chicago Press, 1971.

REFERENCES

1. Conditions of Participation for Hospitals. Soc. Sec. Adm., HIR-10, 1968.
2. Weed, L. L.: N. Eng. J. Med. 278:593-600, 652-657, 1968.
3. Guidelines for Therapeutic Dietitians on Recording in Patients' Medical Records. Chicago, Am. Hospital Assoc., 1966 (in revision, 1974).
4. J. Am. Dietet. A. 59:372, 1971.

food composition— a basic tool of diet therapy

23

The dietary modifications prescribed for any patient must be translated into the foods and serving sizes he is familiar with, and into a meal pattern similar to that of his family. This insures a greater probability that the diet will be accepted and used and, thus, be successful in terms of therapeutic goals. At the same time, one may encounter a patient whose usual food practices require drastic changes, not just modification, because of the complexity of his problem. Such a patient will need special support and understanding as he struggles to change his food practices (see Chapter 12).

To be able to design simple or complex therapeutic diet plans, the nutrition counselor must have extensive knowledge of both the kinds and amounts of nutrients in food (see Chapter 10). She must be familiar with the effect of food processing on the nutrient composition of foods and, with today's increasingly complex manipulation of nutrient intake in the treatment of certain diseases, she needs to know the composition of specially formulated foods and supplementary feedings used to implement various therapeutic diet plans. She should be an expert in food preparation and know how the adjustment of ingredients in a recipe may modify the dish.

Most nutritional misinformation among members of the health care team today is due to a lack of quantitative, not qualitative, knowledge of the energy and nutrient composition of food. For example, a physician may order a 1500-calorie diet but complain strenuously when his patient has two slices of toast for breakfast although the patient, perhaps a farmer, has been used to a substantial breakfast. Within the limits of his diet order the patient chose two slices of toast for his breakfast meal plan. When questioned the physician said, "Bread is fattening." He did not realize that one slice of bread contains approximately 70 calories and that two slices (140 calories) could be included in the breakfast plan for this patient's 1500-calorie diet. Many lay people share the same lack of information, such as the banker who says, "Potatoes and bread are fattening," while munching a glazed doughnut with his midmorning coffee.

The therapeutic dietitian, or any other nutrition counselor, may use the Daily Food Guide (Chapter 10) as a standard for assessing the adequacy of an individual's nutritional intake. However, this standard may not be adequate in all situations. Life-styles vary in our society and food practices which differ from the Food Guide can supply adequate intakes of nutrients. The diet of an adolescent boy who will not eat dark green or deep yellow vegetables in any form can still supply adequate vitamin A because of the amount of fortified skim milk he is drinking each day.

In addition, the therapeutic dietitian responsible for the calculation of therapeutic diets cannot approach the nutrient content of foods in the traditional way such as, milk for calcium, meat for protein, liver for iron. She must be aware of the significance of the total energy and nutrient content of a food. For example, one pint of milk (16 oz.) contributes approximately 1/3 of the protein, 3/4 of the calcium, and 1/2 of the riboflavin recommended daily by the NRC for the 23 to 50 year-old-man, while 3½ ounces of broiled hamburger contributes approximately 1/2 of the protein, 1/3 of the iron, and 1/3 of the niacin for the same individual. Together the pint of milk and 3½ ounces of broiled hamburger contribute almost 1/4 of this man's daily energy needs when whole milk is used; or less, if he drinks skim milk.

At the same time the therapeutic dietitian must be prepared to answer on-the-spot questions from other members of the health-care team regarding both the qualitative and quantitative nutrient composition of foods. On rounds in the clinical setting with the renologist and his coworkers, the therapeutic dietitian

can expect to be asked, "Is there potassium in tomato juice?" or, "How much potassium is in 100 ml. of tomato juice?"

The therapeutic dietitian cannot be a "walking" food composition table. However, with a knowledge of general nutritional composition she can readily answer questions about the qualitative aspects of foods. With the repeated use of the nutrient values of common foods, she can evaluate the nutrient content of a food with a reasonable degree of accuracy without constant reference to food composition tables. The knowledge of qualitative and quantitative nutrient composition of foods is the dietitian's unique contribution to the health-care team and she cannot expect the other members of the team to develop expertise in this area comparable with hers.

This chapter presents special resources for planning and a system for the calculation of diet patterns for therapeutic diets. The reader is urged to review at this point the discussions on food composition tables and the general information about the nutrient composition of foods in Chapter 10, Meeting Nutritional Norms. Additional information pertinent to planning modified diets is given in this chapter.

FOOD COMPOSITION AND THERAPEUTIC DIETS
Basic Food Composition Tables

The food composition tables discussed in Chapter 10 and Tables 1 to 6 in Section 4 of this book are the primary resources for calculating the majority of modified diet patterns. Frequently additional resources are required for more extensive information than is included in the tables in Section 4 and for calculating some of the more complex diet patterns; e.g., values for the naturally occurring simple sugars in fruits and vegetables. A discussion of these special resources follows.

Special Food Composition Tables

SUGARS. Only limited data on the mono-, di-, and poly-saccharide content of foods are available because no standardized analytical method has been formulated until recently. Also, the free sugar content of fruits and vegetables will vary by variety and stage of maturity; e.g., a partially ripe vs. a ripe banana. A partially ripe banana will contain significantly more starch than a ripe one (8.8 gm. vs. 1.2 gm. per 100 gm. edible portion).[1]

The most readily available information about the sugar which occurs in foods has been published by Hardinge and coworkers.[2] Table 1 in Hardinge's work is a tabulation of the data in the literature prior to 1965 and gives values for the sugars in fruits, vegetables, legumes, milk and milk products, and nuts and nut products. Table 2 gives limited data on less common sugars such as arabinose, raffinose, stachyose, and sorbitol. In 1970 Yee, Shallenbarger, and Vittum[3] published the results of their own analyses of free sugars in fruits, vegetables, and legumes. They give values for glucose, fructose, sucrose, raffinose, and stachyose.

The figures for sugars in foods are used to calculate diets limited in simple sugars for the treatment of carbohydrate induced hyperlipidemia and to identify foods to be avoided in lactose intolerance or other disaccharide malabsorption problems, and in galactosemia, fructosuria, or any other condition where the intake of a specific sugar must be avoided or limited.

AMINO ACIDS. Table 3 in Section 4 of this book was derived from Amino Acid Content of Foods, USDA Home Economics Research Report, No. 4. Unfortunately, values for the amino acid composition of all commonly used foods are not available in Research Report No. 4 or any other publication. It can be anticipated that this handbook, published in 1957, will be revised in the near future, since the method for analyzing the amino acid composition of foods has been modified in recent years. In 1968 the USDA published an updated report on two amino acids, phenylalanine and tyrosine, in fruits and vegetables.[4]

The amino acid composition of diets may be modified for individuals with inborn errors of intermediary metabolism. When the error occurs in the metabolism of an essential amino acid such as phenylalanine or the branched chain amino acids, leucine, isoleucine, and valine, the intake is monitored to provide the individual's needs for these essential nutrients without an excess. In planning diets for patients in renal failure or in impending hepatic coma, it is necessary to calculate amino acid values so that adequate essential amino acids and limited amounts of nonessential amino acids are provided.

LIPIDS. The fatty acid values in Table 2 of Section 4 were derived from USDA Handbook No. 8 and the cholesterol figures from the recent findings of Feeley, Criner, and Watt.[5] Some manufacturers of soft margarine give the amounts in grams of the saturated and polyunsaturated fatty acids and cholesterol found in a specified quantity of their product. Recent articles on the fatty acid composition of foods are listed in the Supplementary Readings at the end of this chapter.

The values for the fatty acid and cholesterol contents of foods are used to calculate diet patterns for patients with hyperlipidemias and/or elevated blood cholesterol levels.

ELECTROLYTES. Table 5, Section 4, gives figures for the sodium, potassium, and magnesium content of foods. Values for a limited number of foods may also be found in recent issues of professional journals.

In addition to food, drinking water may, or may not be a significant source of sodium. This depends on the geological characteristics of an area and on the method used to treat water supplies. In some areas of the United States, local water supplies contain a significant amount of naturally occurring sodium (more than 2 mg. per 100 ml.). In some instances the equipment used to soften home water supplies adds sodium to the water.

Convenience Foods

Uncertainty about the energy, protein, fat, and carbohydrate contents of convenience foods, as well as their sodium and potassium content, make these foods unusable in therapeutic diet plans requiring complex manipulation of energy and nutrient content, e.g., energy restricted, protein, and/or electrolyte restricted, or gluten restricted diets. The administrator of dietetic services in the general hospital is faced with the same dilemma. Convenience food items served to patients on regular diets are rarely appropriate for therapeutic diets unless the suppliers of the foods will prepare them according to rigid specifications set by the dietitian.

Dietetic Foods

Foods for special dietary use have been on the market in the U.S. for many years. The most commonly available ones have been fruits canned without the addition of sugar; bread made without salt, vegetables canned without sodium; and artificially sweetened pudding mixes, gelatin dessert powders, cookies, jellies, candy, gum, and carbonated beverages. The labels of these products state the energy and nutritive value of a specified serving of the contents of the container as required by the Food and Drug Administration regulations. It has recently been proposed that the U.S. Congress modify these regulations as part of the Nutrition Labeling Legislation (see Chapter 14).

ARTIFICIAL SWEETENERS. Prior to 1969 when the Food and Drug Administration prohibited the use of cyclamate because research showed it to cause bladder tumors in rats, it was the most widely used nonnutritive sweetener. Before the ban went into effect, approximately half of the carbonated beverages sold in the United States were artificially sweetened with cyclamate or a combination of cyclamate and saccharin. Today sodium or calcium saccharin and sorbitol are the most widely used nonnutritive sweeteners but the products in which they are used do not have the same taste acceptance as those sweetened with cyclamate. The safety of both cyclamate and saccharin as food additives is under intensive study at present.

There are a variety of sweeteners on the market which contain saccharin combined with small amounts of mono- or disaccharides and, therefore, cannot be classified as nonnutritive. Each product must be evaluated before use, especially if the diet is restricted not only in calories but also in simple sugars.

DIET BREADS AND MARGARINES. Both of these products contain fewer calories per serving than the regular products. One slice of diet bread weighing approximately 18 gm. contains approximately 45 to 50 kcal., while one slice of regular bread weighing approximately 23 gm. contains 70 kcal. Three teaspoons of the diet margarines contain approximately the same number of calories as one teaspoon of regular margarine. The energy content of diet margarines vary by brand; the nutrition label of a brand should be checked for energy content per serving.

Before recommending any dietetic products, the energy and nutrient content per serving must be estimated and the quantities to be used carefully defined to avoid serious errors. Two slices of diet bread (90 to 100 kcal.) cannot be substituted for one slice of regular bread (70 kcal.). Also, many patients are confused about dietetic foods. They think that any food labeled dietetic may or must be used on their diets. For example, a woman who was restricting her energy intake because she was obese used canned vegetables without sodium added even though she did not have to restrict her sodium (salt) intake. The vegetables were labeled "dietetic," therefore, she thought she must use them in her low calorie diet.

MEDIUM-CHAIN TRIGLYCERIDES (MCT). Fat in the ordinary diet contains mainly the long-chain fatty acids, palmitic (C16:0), stearic (C18:0), and oleic (C18:1). The products of absorption of these fats are transported by the lymphatic system as chylomicrons to the thoracic duct and into the general circulation (see Chapters 8 and 9). Digestion and absorption are dependent on the availability of bile salts and pancreatic lipase. In several malabsorption syndromes (see Chapter 25) it is the long-chain fatty acids which are frequently not absorbed and are excreted in the feces.

About five percent of naturally occurring fat contains short- and medium-chain fatty acids, C6:0 to C12:0. Hashim et al[6] showed that these are hydrolyzed to glycerol and fatty acids by the mucosal enzymes and are absorbed directly from the villi into the capillary bed without reesterification; they are then transported via the portal vein to the liver.

The synthesis of a fat containing only medium-chain fatty acids was accomplished by the hydrolysis of coconut oil and the distillation of the fatty acids. The short- and medium-chain fatty acids, C6:0 to C12:0, being the lightest, came off first. They were reesterified with glycerol to form a fat (an oil) which can replace regular fat in the diet. This product, containing almost entirely caprylic (C8:0) and capric (C10:0) fatty acids, is called medium-chain triglyceride or MCT.

Greenberger and Skillman[7] reviewed the use of MCT in the treatment of malabsorption syndromes and point out that it is effective as a substitute for ordinary dietary fats in reducing steatorrhea and the loss of sodium, potassium, and calcium in the feces in cystic fibrosis, celiac disease, intestinal lymphangiectasia, chylothorax, and small bowel resection. It has not proved effective in inflammatory bowel disease, massive bowel resection, or impending hepatic coma.

Medium-chain triglycerides yield 8.2 to 8.4 kcal. per gram and are available as MCT oil* or in a powdered-formula diet (Portagen)*. MCT oil can be substituted for regular cooking oils. Schizas and coworkers[8] and Howard and Morse[9] have published recipes using MCT oil. The powdered-formula diet is used in infant feeding and as a beverage by adults.

PROTEIN-FREE WHEAT STARCH PRODUCTS. These products are essentially free of protein and are used as a source of energy in protein-restricted diets used in the treatment of renal and hepatic disease. They are also gluten-free and can be used in the treatment of gluten-induced enteropathy. Their use and the problems encountered with them in food preparation are discussed in detail in Chapter 25, Diet in Gastrointestinal Disease and Chapter 31, Renal Disease.

Food Supplements

There are a variety of products available which can be used to supplement energy or energy and protein intakes. These products vary widely in availability, energy and nutrient density, acceptability, and cost. Some of them are used as beverages while others may be added to reinforce commonly used beverages and foods. The food and nutrient contents are supplied by the producer and should be carefully evaluated for the individual patient before using because in some instances the ingredients or electrolyte content may not be appropriate.

EXCHANGE SYSTEM OF DIET CALCULATION

Therapeutic diet orders which prescribe a quantitative modification in nutritive intake require the

*Mead Johnson Laboratories, Evansville, Ind.

Table 23-1. Daily Food Guide Compared with Exchange System

DAILY FOOD GUIDE	EXCHANGE SYSTEM
Milk Group	Milk Exchange
Meat Group	Meat Exchange
Vegetable Fruit Group	Vegetable Exchanges
	Group A
	Group B
	Fruit Exchanges
Bread Cereal Group	Bread Exchanges
	Fat Exchanges

calculation of a dietary pattern for the patient's use in selecting food each day. These dietary patterns may be calculated from food composition tables, by a system using composite figures for food groups (the Exchange System), or by programming the computer properly.

By the 1940s, dietitians and physicians were aware that food composition tables used to calculate therapeutic diets, especially diets for the diabetic patient, were cumbersome, time consuming, and needlessly precise, and that an individual does not have the time or inclination to calculate for each day the energy and nutrient composition of the food required to fulfill his dietary prescription.

After careful study, a committee of the American Dietetic Association, working cooperatively with the Committee on Education of the American Diabetes Association and representatives of the Diabetes Branch of the United States Public Health Service, published a simplified system of diet calculation for diabetic patients known today as the Exchange System.[10] Although originally planned for the calculation of dietary patterns for patients with diabetes, this Exchange System, or modifications of it, are widely used to calculate other therapeutic diets: for example, energy-restricted or fat-restricted diets.

The term "exchange" reflects the problems that a patient with diabetes encountered in the management of his diet prior to 1950. Frequently his instructions focused on menus, not dietary patterns. A breakfast menu might be ½ cup of orange juice, ½ cup of cooked oatmeal, one cup of milk, one slice of toast, and one teaspoon of butter. After two or three weeks of this meal he would ask, "Can't I have something in place of orange juice?" He would be offered ½ cup of grapefruit juice in "exchange" for ½ cup of orange juice. As a solution to this problem, foods of similar nutritive composition were grouped together for "exchanges" and formalized into the Exchange System.

The groups are: milk, whole, skim, and evaporated; meat, including fish and poultry and such meat alternates as eggs and cheese; fruits; vegetables; bread, including cereals and cereal products, legumes and certain vegetables; and fats, including seed oils, margarine, and butter.

The food groups in the Exchange System are similar to, yet differ to some extent from, the groups in the Daily Food Guide. Table 23-1 illustrates the similarities and differences in these two classifications. The milk, meat, and bread-cereal groups of the Daily Food Guide are also in the Exchange System. The vegetable-fruit group of the Daily Guide becomes two items in the Exchange System, vegetable exchanges, and fruit exchanges. The vegetable exchanges are subdivided further into two groups, group A and group B. Fat exchanges are included in the Exchange System but not in the Daily Food Guide.

Table 23-2 gives the average protein, fat, carbohydrate, and energy values for each exchange. These values are averages of the nutrient values of the foods in a group weighted by frequency of use. Table 23-3 is adapted from the original committee report to illustrate how the carbohydrate value (7 gm. per ½ cup) for the vegetables in group B was derived from weightings based on the usual rate of consumption.

Table 23-4 gives the lists of the foods included in each exchange group. With the exception of the meat serving, which is one ounce, the serving sizes of the items within each exchange are average servings. The average serving of meat for an adult is approximately 3 or 4 ounces or three or four times the protein, fat, and energy values given in Table 23-2 for a meat exchange. Whenever the term "cup" is used to define a serving in dietetics it will be remembered that it

Table 23-2. Nutrient Composition of Food Exchanges*

GROUP†	AMOUNT	WEIGHT (g.)	PROTEIN (g.)	FAT (g.)	CARBOHYDRATE (g.)	ENERGY (kcal.)
Milk, whole	½ pt. (8 oz.)	240	8	10	12	170
Vegetables, Group A	as desired	..	..	..	..	..
Vegetables, Group B	½ cup	100	2	..	7	35
Fruit Exchanges	varies	..	..	..	10	40
Bread Exchanges	varies	..	2	..	15	70
Meat Exchanges	1 oz.	30	7	5	..	75
Fat Exchanges	1 tsp.	5	..	5	..	45

*Tables, 23-2 and 23-4 modified from Caso, E. K.: J. Am. Dietet. A., 26:575, 1950.
†For lists of foods in each exchange, see Table 23-4.

food composition—a basic tool of diet therapy 329

Table 23–3. Data Used to Calculate the Composition of Vegetables—Group B

FOOD	CARBOHYDRATE CONTENT (Starch and sugar) g./100 g.	WEIGHTINGS (Based on usual rate of Consumption)
Beets	8.0	3
Carrots	7.5	4
Onions	7.2	1
Peas, green (medium)	9.0	4
Pumpkin	5.1	—
Rutabaga	6.7	½
Squash, winter	4.9	2
Turnip	4.6	1
Weighted Average	7.0	

means the standard eight-ounce measuring cup, and a teaspoon or tablespoon refers to standard measuring spoons.

Each list of foods in Table 23–4 should be studied carefully and any special directions should be noted, for instance: that when skim milk is substituted for the whole milk calculated in the diet pattern, two fat exchanges should be added to replace the fat in the whole milk; or, that vegetable exchanges in group A are not assigned any energy or carbohydrate values in Table 23–2. The nutrient values of each exchange apply only to the serving size of the food as described, not for example, to fruits canned or frozen with sugar added, or cooked meat served with gravy. It will also

Table 23–4. Exchange Lists

(Adapted from Meal Planning with Exchange Lists, The American Dietetic Association, 430 N. Michigan Ave., Chicago, Ill. 60611)

FOODS THAT NEED NOT BE MEASURED
(Insignificant carbohydrate or calories)

Coffee	Cranberries (unsweetened)
Tea	Mustard (dry)
Clear broth	Pickle (unsweetened)
Bouillon (fat free)	Saccharin
Lemon	Pepper and other spices
Gelatin (unsweetened)	Vinegar
Rennet tablets	Seasonings

Chopped parsley, mint, garlic, onion, celery salt, nutmeg, mustard, cinnamon, pepper and other spices, lemon, saccharin, and vinegar may be used freely.

LIST 1. MILK EXCHANGES

One exchange of milk contains 8 gm. of protein, 10 gm. of fat, 12 gm. of carbohydrate, and 170 calories.

This list shows the different types of milk to use for one exchange:

Type of Milk	Amount to Use
Whole milk (plain or homogenized)	1 c.
*Skim milk	1 c.
Evaporated milk	½ c.
Powdered whole milk	¼ c.
*Powdered skim milk (nonfat dried milk)	¼ c.
Buttermilk (made from whole milk)	1 c.
*Buttermilk (made from skim milk)	1 c.

One type of milk may be used instead of another, for example, ½ cup of evaporated milk in place of 1 cup of whole milk.

*Skim milk and buttermilk have the same food values as whole milk, except that they contain less fat. Two fat exchanges are added when 1 cup of skim milk or buttermilk made from skim milk is used in place of whole milk calculated in a diet pattern.

LIST 2. VEGETABLE EXCHANGES: GROUP A

Group A contains little protein, carbohydrate, or calories. 1 cup at a time may be used without counting it.

Asparagus	Cauliflower
*Broccoli	Celery
Brussels sprouts	*Chicory
Cabbage	Cucumbers
*Escarole	Lettuce
Eggplant	Mushrooms
*Beet greens	Okra

LIST 2. VEGETABLE EXCHANGES: GROUP A (Continued)

*Chard	*Pepper
*Collard	Radishes
*Dandelion greens	Sauerkraut
*Kale	String beans, young
*Mustard	Summer squash
*Spinach	*Tomatoes
*Turnip greens	*Watercress

*These vegetables contain a lot of vitamin A.

LIST 2. VEGETABLE EXCHANGES: GROUP B

Each exchange contains 2 gm. of protein , 7 gm. of carbohydrate, and 35 calories.

½ cup of vegetable equals 1 exchange:

Beets	Pumpkin
*Carrots	Rutabagas
Onions	*Squash, winter
Peas, green	Turnip

*These vegetables contain a lot of vitamin A.

LIST 3. FRUIT EXCHANGES

One exchange of fruit contains 10 gm. of carbohydrate and 40 calories. This list shows the different amounts of fruits to use for one fruit exchange:

Fruit	Amount to Use
Apple (2" diam.)	1 small
Applesauce	½ c.
Apricots, fresh	2 medium
Apricots, dried	4 halves
Banana	½ small
Blackberries	1 c.
Raspberries	1 c.
*Strawberries	1 c.
Blueberries	⅔ c.
*Cantaloupe (6" diam.)	¼
Cherries	10 large
Dates	2
Figs, fresh	2 large
Figs, dried	1 small
*Grapefruit	½ small
*Grapefruit juice	½ c.
Grapes	12

Table 23–4.   (Continued)

LIST 3. FRUIT EXCHANGES (Cont.)

Fruit	Amount to Use
Grape juice	¼ c.
Honeydew melon	⅛ medium
Mango	½ small
*Orange	1 small
*Orange juice	½ c.
Papaya	⅓ medium
Peach	1 medium
Pear	1 small
Pineapple	½ c.
Pineapple juice	⅓ c.
Plums	2 medium
Prunes, dried	2 medium
Raisins	2 tbsp.
*Tangerine	1 large
Watermelon	1 c.

*These fruits are rich sources of vitamin C.

LIST 4. BREAD EXCHANGES

One exchange contains 2 gm. of protein, 15 gm. of carbohydrate, and 70 calories.

This list shows the different amounts of foods to use for one bread exchange:

Bread, Cereal, Etc.:	Amount to Use
Bread	1 slice
Biscuit, roll (2″ diam.)	1
Muffin (2″ diam.)	1
Cornbread (1½″ cube)	1
Cereals, cooked	½ c.
Dry, flake, and puff types	¾ c.
Rice, grits, cooked	½ c.
Spaghetti, noodles, cooked	½ c.
Macaroni, etc., cooked	½ c.
Crackers, graham (2½″ sq.)	2
Oyster (½ c.)	20
Saltines (2″ sq.)	5
Soda (2½″ sq.)	3
Round, thin (1½″)	6
Flour	2½ tbsp.
Vegetables:	
Beans and peas, dried, cooked	½ c.
(Lima, navy, split pea, cowpeas, etc.)	
Baked beans, no pork	¼ c.
Corn	⅓ c.
Popcorn	1 c.
Parsnips	⅔ c.
Potatoes, white	1 small
Potatoes, white, mashed	½ c.

LIST 4. BREAD EXCHANGES (Cont.)

Bread, Cereal, Etc.:	Amount to Use
Potatoes, sweet, or yams	¼ c.
Sponge cake, plain (1½″ cube)	1
Ice cream (omit 2 fat exchanges)	½ c.

These foods are measured carefully because they contain significant amounts of carbohydrate.

LIST 5. MEAT EXCHANGES

One meat exchange contains 7 gm. of protein, 5 gm. of fat, and 75 calories.

This list shows the different amounts of foods to use for one meat exchange:

Meat	Amount to Use
Meat and poultry (medium fat)	1 oz. cooked
beef, lamb, pork, liver, chicken, etc.	
Cold cuts (4½″ x ⅛″)	1 slice
salami, minced ham, bologna, liver- wurst, luncheon loaf	
Frankfurter (8-9 per lb.)	1
Egg	1
Fish: haddock, etc.	1 oz.
Salmon, tuna, crab, lobster	¼ c.
Shrimp, clams, oysters, etc.	5 small
Sardines	3 medium
Cheese: Cheddar type	1 oz.
Cottage	¼ c.
*Peanut butter	2 tbsp.

*Peanut butter is limited to 1 exchange a day unless the carbohydrate in it is allowed for in the calculated diet pattern.

LIST 6. FAT EXCHANGES

One fat exchange contains 5 gm. of fat and 45 calories.

This list shows the different foods to use for one fat exchange:

Fat	Amount to Use
Butter or margarine	1 tsp.
Bacon, crisp	1 slice
Cream, light	2 tbsp.
Cream, heavy	1 tbsp.
Cream cheese	1 tbsp.
Avocado (4″ diam.)	⅛
French dressing	1 tbsp.
Mayonnaise	1 tsp.
Oil or cooking fat	1 tsp.
Nuts	6 small
Olives	5 small

be noted that certain vegetables are listed with the bread exchanges. These contain 15 gm. of carbohydrate per serving as listed, such as ¹/₃ cup of corn. The items in the fruit exchanges are listed by serving size that yields 10 gm. of carbohydrate. Bacon and nuts are listed in the fat exchanges, not in the meat exchanges, as might be expected. Their primary contribution to the diet in this system is fat rather than protein.

Average values for minerals and vitamins have not been calculated for the Exchange System because of the wide variations within each exchange. For example, whole milk contains vitamin A, while skim milk, unless fortified with vitamin A, does not. Therefore, giving a vitamin A value to a milk exchange would imply that all items listed in the exchange contain vitamin A. When a diet pattern is calculated by the Exchange System, care must be taken to insure proper mineral and vitamin composition.

The dietitian uses the Exchange System to calculate a diet pattern which translates the physician's diet order into the kinds and number of servings of food (exchanges) to be consumed by the patient each

food composition—a basic tool of diet therapy   331

day. She uses the nutrient values in Table 23–2 to calculate this pattern. The patient then selects the specific foods he wants to eat at each meal using the foods listed in Table 23–4. Examples of the use of the Exchange System to calculate dietary patterns are found in subsequent chapters, e.g., a 1500-calorie diabetic dietary pattern Chapter 28.

Dietitians have modified the nutrient composition of the food exchanges to reflect the changes in the food supply since 1950. For example Ohlson[11] has adjusted the meat exchange values to 8 gm. protein, 3 gm. fat, and 60 calories to reflect the use of leaner meats and an increasing use of poultry and fish. A dietitian can calculate an Exchange System for an individual patient using the food composition tables and the frequency of food usage within each group and thereby satisfy the patient's usual food choices. In other words the nutrient composition of the Exchange System can be adjusted to the food likes and dislikes of an individual within the constraints set by his diet order.

Although this Exchange System and any other reflect average and not specific energy and nutrient values, the therapeutic successes that result when the values are used to calculate diet patterns demonstrate that the method is accurate enough to serve this purpose. The only method for determining the actual energy and/or nutrient intake of an individual is the laboratory analysis of an aliquot of the foods actually consumed by him. This technique is used in metabolic studies and requires a highly skilled research team including the dietitian. In this setting she plans the diet described in the research protocol, prepares the aliquots for laboratory analyses, and closely monitors the serving and the patient's consumption of food and beverages.

STUDY QUESTIONS AND ACTIVITIES

1. Weigh one level standard tablespoon of each food on a gram scale: granulated sugar, powdered sugar, corn syrup, instant potatoes, dry skim milk powder, infant cereal, and margarine. Is there a difference in the weights?
2. Weigh ½ standard measuring cup of each food on a gram scale: cooked carrots, cooked string beans, applesauce, orange juice, milk, and ginger ale. Are there differences in weight? What does this tell you about the accuracy of using volume as a measure of food composition?
3. Select what you think is a 3-ounce serving of each one of the foods listed below and then weigh it on a

gram scale: American cheese, cottage cheese, sliced bologna, hamburger patty, frankfurter, lettuce, raw carrot strips, potato chips, and jelly beans.
4. Using the data in Table 1, Section 4, calculate the gram weight of each item in the fruit exchanges which contains 15 gm. carbohydrate. Translate the gram weight for each item into portion size (volume).
5. Using the information obtained from a patient about the frequency with which he consumes the items in the meat exchanges, calculate the weighted values for protein, fat, and energy of his usual choices. Are these values similar to or different from those in Table 23–2? Would you use the values in Table 23–2 or those which reflect his food choices in calculating a diet pattern for him?

SUPPLEMENTARY READINGS

Adams, C. F.: Nutritive Value of American Foods in Common Units. USDA Agricultural Research Service, Agricultural Handbook No. 456. Washington, D.C., (November) 1975.
Anderson, B. A., et al: Comprehensive evaluation of fatty acids in food. II. Beef products. J. Am. Dietet. A. 67:35, 1975.
Fabietti, L. G.: Method for converting food volume to weight. J. Am. Dietet. A. 60:135-137, 1972.
Feeley, R. M., et al: Major fatty acids and proximate composition of dairy products. J. Am. Dietet. A. 66:140, 1975.
Koch, R.: Safety of aspartame as a sweetener. N. Eng. J. Med. 292:596, 1975.
Posati, L. P., et. al: Comprehensive evaluation of fatty acids in foods. I. Dairy products. J. Am. Dietet. A. 66:482, 1975.
———: Comprehensive evaluation of fatty acids in foods. III. Eggs and egg products. J. Am. Dietet. A. 67:111, 1975.
Special Report: The effects of food processing on nutritional values. Nutr. Rev. 33:123, 1975.
Watt, B. K., et al: Food composition tables for the 70's. J. Am. Dietet. A. 64:257, 1974.

For further references see Bibliography in Section 4.

SPECIAL FOOD TABLES

Goddard, V. R., and Goodall, L.: Fatty Acids in Food Fats. Home Economics Research Report No. 7, U.S. Dept. of Agriculture, 1957.
Orr, M. L., and Watt, B. K.: Amino Acid Content of Foods. Home Economics Report No. 4, U.S. Dept. of Agriculture (December) 1957.
Orr, M. L.: Pantothenic Acid, Vitamin B_6, and Vitamin B_{12} in Foods. Home Economics Research Report No. 36, U.S. Dept. of Agriculture (August) 1969.

REFERENCES

1. Hardinge, M. E., et al: J. Am. Dietet. A. 46:197, 1965.
2. Ibid.
3. Yee, C. Y., et al: Free sugars in fruits and vegetables. Ithaca, N. Y. Food and Life Sciences Bulletin, No. 1, 1970.
4. McCarthy, M. A., Orr, M. L., and Watt, B. K.: J. Am. Dietet. A. 52:130, 1968.
5. Feeley, R. M., et al: J. Am. Dietet. A. 61:134, 1972.
6. Hashim, S. A., et al: J. Clin. Invest. 43:1238, 1964.
7. Greenberger, N. J., and Skillman, T. C.: N. Eng. J. Med. 280:1045, 1969.
8. Schizas, A. A., et al: J. Am. Dietet. A. 51:228, 1967.
9. Howard, B. D., and Morse, E. B.: J. Am. Dietet. A. 62:51, 1973.
10. Caso, E. K., et al: J. Am. Dietet. A. 26:575, 1950.
11. Ohlson, M. A.: Experimental and Therapeutic Dietetics, ed. 2. Minneapolis, Burgess Publishing Co., 1972.

24

handicapping problems—self-feeding, chewing, swallowing

Skills Necessary for Self-Feeding
Motor Performance Problems
Special Nutritional Care Problems
Special Programs

Patients with physical handicaps may have difficulty achieving an adequate nutrient intake because they may be unable to feed themselves; or they may be limited in their ability or be unable to suck, bite, chew, or swallow fluids and/or foods. Severe arthritis may affect the joints of the fingers, the elbow and the shoulder to such an extent that the adult patient cannot feed himself; or affect the jaw so that he may even have difficulty biting and chewing. Some patients after a cerebral vascular accident (stroke) may be unable to swallow clear liquids but may be able to swallow semisolids such as "soupy" mashed potatoes or soft ice cream.

Infants and children with neuromuscular defects such as cerebral palsy may present numerous problems that require carefully planned and consistently implemented feeding training programs in order to achieve their potential for self-feeding. Until a cleft palate with or without a cleft lip is repaired surgically an infant with this congenital anomaly has special feeding problems.

This chapter was written in cooperation with Nancy D. Herrick,*
M.S., M.P.H., Chief of Nutrition, and Marian F. Chase, M.S., L.P.T.,
Chief of Physical Therapy, Nisonger Center, The Ohio State University Affiliated Center for Mental Retardation and Developmental Defects.
*Deceased.

334

Table 24–1. Progressive Levels of Motor Skills Necessary for Self-Feeding

Sucking
Sitting and head balance
Upper extremity control sufficient to bring hand to mouth
Cup and utensil grasp
Ability to sip and take liquids from cup
Ability to take food from spoon with lips
Ability to bite, chew and swallow with a minimum of drooling

It is necessary to assess the individual needs of each handicapped patient when determining the method of feeding and/or feeding training to be used to assist him in achieving his potential. There are two major aspects of this assessment: (1) the individual's nutritional needs; and (2) his physical capacity. To assess nutritional needs, the patient's age, height, weight, activity level, and any disease requiring diet modification must be identified. His physical capacity must be evaluated to set reasonable goals for his self-feeding or feeding training program. In certain situations special attention must be given to the consistency of food required to overcome the difficulty.

The skills necessary for self-feeding: coping with problems of positioning, sucking, biting, chewing, and swallowing; adaptive equipment; selected nutritional care problems; and special programs for the handicapped are discussed in the following sections of this chapter. The nutritional needs of infants, children, and adults are presented in other chapters and are not repeated here.

SKILLS NECESSARY FOR SELF-FEEDING

Table 24–1 lists the progressive levels of motor performance necessary for self-feeding. Although it is not necessary that all skills at each level be completely mastered before progressing to the next one, some evidence of skill or readiness is necessary at all levels if self-feeding is to be achieved. These are the developmental tasks the normal infant and young child goes through in achieving the ability to feed himself, and the skills the normal individual uses throughout life. The neurologically handicapped infant may present problems in progressing to one or more levels in sequence, while the recently handicapped adult may lose his ability to perform at one or more levels.

MOTOR PERFORMANCE PROBLEMS
Positioning

The normal feeding position for humans is upright and requires the ability to sit up and control the balance of the head. Proper positioning of the hand-icapped patient should be based on the assessment of his ability to hold himself upright. Aspiration of fluids or food into the bronchi can be hazardous to the individual who cannot maintain head balance.

Patients with limited ability to support the trunk may be helped to sit at the table by stabilizing the trunk with a binder or strap secured at the pelvis. The patient is also more stable if his feet are firmly positioned flat on the floor or on a footstool. Figure 24–1 illustrates this method. If the patient is in a wheelchair, the footrest is used. This method permits the patient to concentrate on his food rather than worrying about falling off his chair. It also eliminates constricting the chest or "hanging" which happens frequently when a binder is placed under the arms.

If the patient is seated in an armchair, pillows at each side and a headrest may be used for stabilization. A lapboard, or an over-bed table adjusted to the appropriate height, is useful to the patient in a wheelchair or armchair. When a lapboard is used, it is advisable to have it equipped with a raised edge so that the patient with poor motor skills is not frustrated by having dishes and other equipment slide off the board onto the floor. For the small child, a highchair is often appropriate because of the protection it offers on all four sides. For the larger child it is helpful to use a cutout table with a strap placed across the back of the chair to hold him close to the table.

Sucking—Straw Drinking

The problems encountered in the neurologically handicapped infant may include limitation in the ability to suck. Initially the mother is taught to stroke

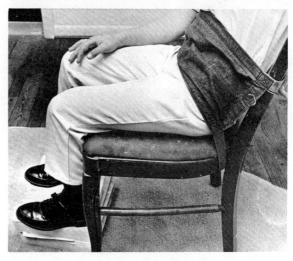

Fig. 24–1. A child with poor trunk control stabilized by a binder at the pelvis and feet supported. (Note use of telephone directories as a footstool.)

often helpful because it prevents crushing the straw (Fig. 24-3). As the patient progresses in his ability to suck through the straw the length and diameter may be increased. This allows him to take thicker fluids that usually contain more energy and nutrients than thinner fluids.

Biting, Chewing, and Swallowing

The patient who has the ability to bite and chew, or who can reestablish this ability, can be offered food of various textures and, therefore, a more acceptable diet. Patients with neurological diseases who have difficulty biting and chewing and, at the same time, can take food without choking, should be encouraged to bite off small amounts of soft or semisolid foods; for example: a small amount of mashed potato or a small bite of a well-cooked carrot strip. The food should be directed to alternate sides of the mouth and the patient encouraged to use his tongue to move the food in his mouth. The patient should chew and swallow each bite before he takes more food. Food may become lodged between the teeth and inside of the cheeks in patients with facial paralysis or a very high palate,

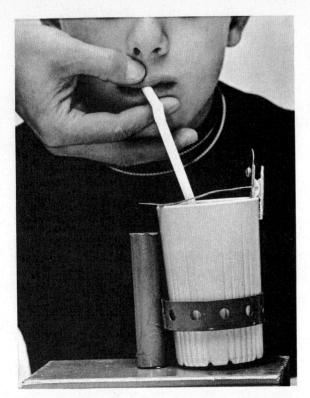

Fig. 24-2. Applying light pressure to lips to help patient develop ability to drink through straw. Note adaptive cup holder and straw holder.

the infant's cheek and stimulate the oral area to elicit the sucking reflex. However, the infant may need to be tube fed during the first months to insure adequate fluid, electrolyte, and nutrient intake (see Chapter 34). Stimulation and some oral feeding may be done even though tube feeding is necessary.

Straw drinking, a form of sucking, may be used with the neurologically handicapped child or handicapped adult. It aids in the development of the facial and oral musculature and with breath control—an important aspect of speech development. Also, many severely involved patients are helped to obtain an adequate fluid intake through straw drinking.

Initially a short straw with a small diameter should be used. The patient should be instructed to take one sip at a time until he is able to suck continuously. If he has difficulty holding his lips closed around the straw, light pressure may be applied with the fingers. Figure 24-2 illustrates this method in the feeding training program for a child. Flex straws (Fig. 24-2) may be helpful in some situations. For the severely involved patient a plastic straw with an inch or two of rubber tubing attached to the mouth end is

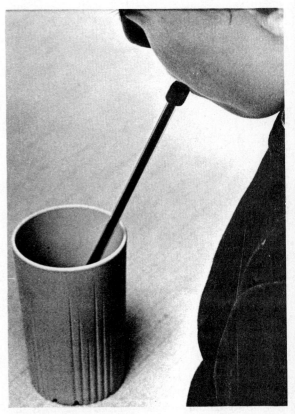

Fig. 24-3. Plastic straw with rubber tip to prevent crushing end of straw.

and it may become necessary to use a finger to dislodge it.

It is obvious that any patient who is unable to swallow cannot be offered fluids or foods by mouth and must be tube fed (see Chapter 26). On the other hand, these patients need to be evaluated continuously so that if there is any indication that the ability to swallow is developing or has been reestablished, they are offered fluids and food by mouth. One indication of this would be the ability to swallow the saliva.

Adaptive Equipment

Adaptive equipment may be used in the beginning of any feeding training program. However, the objective is to move from adaptive equipment to independent skill as soon as possible if the situation permits. For the quadraplegic adult or the neurologically handicapped child, adaptive equipment may be a part of his life if he is to achieve and maintain some degree of self-feeding skills. Figure 24–4 shows the device a neurologically handicapped child might need to help him feed himself.

There are many adaptive devices on the market today to help those who need them. However, many of these can be constructed easily in the hospital or home to fit the needs of the individual. The basic areas in which adaptive devices are most often required are difficulty in sucking (discussed previ-

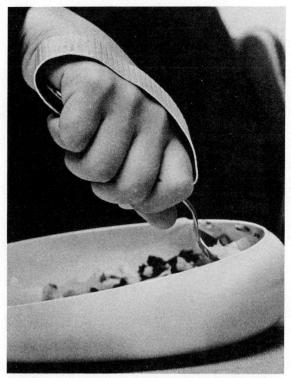

Fig. 24–5. Spoon with loop handle and scoop guard plate.

ously), poor grasp, poor upper extremity strength, and poor coordination of hand-to-mouth movements.

Poor grasp may be aided by the use of a "loop handle" on a spoon or fork (Fig. 24–5). The use of the fork is encouraged, especially if hand-to-mouth coordination is good, because it is often easier to "spear" bits of food than get them on a spoon. Handles that are built up with tape, sponge or foam rubber, wood, or other materials to fit the patient's needs are effective and relatively inexpensive to replace when they become soiled. Cups with handles on both sides (bouillon cups) or small, lightweight cups can be more easily grasped with both hands (Figs. 24–5, 24–6).

A patient with poor upper extremity strength may be helped by raising the height of the table. Swivel feeders as shown in Fig. 24–4 may be used with patients who have very weak upper extremities.

The scoop plate (Fig. 24–5) or the plate with a guard attached to one side can be used with the patient with poor coordination in the upper extremities. A piece of wet foam rubber under the plate, or a hole in a lapboard cut to fit a plate, keeps the dish from sliding. Plates with suction cups attached to the underside are also available. As illustrated in Fig. 24–2, cup holders and straw holders stabilize these items.

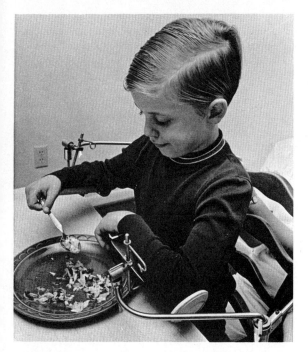

Fig. 24–4. Swivel feeder for child with very weak upper extremities.

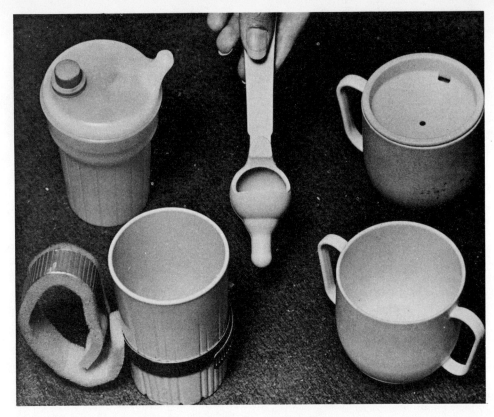

Fig. 24–6. Devices used to facilitate drinking.

Table 24–2 lists the most common handicapping conditions and the feeding disabilities most frequently encountered by these patients.

SPECIAL NUTRITIONAL CARE PROBLEMS
Fluid Intake

Handicapped patients, especially those who can take only sips of fluids slowly by mouth, present a special problem. Care must be taken that they do not become dehydrated or overhydrated if they are also receiving intravenous fluids. Accurate records of fluid intake and output are a very important part of the nutritional care plan. If the patient cannot help himself, he must be offered fluids frequently. If he can manage himself, care must be taken that his glass, cup, or an adapted drinking device is conveniently placed within his reach. Adequate fluid intake is important in the prevention of urinary tract infection and, for some patients, the prevention of nephrolithiasis (see Chapter 31).

Activity and Nutrient Utilization

Immobility even in healthy individuals with adequate energy and protein intakes promotes a nega-tive nitrogen balance. The loss of nitrogen is primarily from the muscle mass. Immobility in healthy individuals also promotes a negative calcium balance with calcium loss primarily from the long bones. Negative nitrogen and calcium balances also occur in immobilized patients; for example, a patient immobilized by the application of a cast, or one immobilized after a cerebral vascular accident. Muscular activity combined, whenever possible, with weight bearing on the long bones reverses the negative balances in both the healthy and the sick individual. Therefore the physically handicapped individual requires a daily activity program for the effective utilization of his nutrient intake.

Consistency of Food

Two concerns should be kept in mind regarding the consistency of food offered the handicapped patient: (1) its nutritional value and (2) the progression from semiliquid to more solid foods as the patient progresses.

Generally, it is difficult to keep a reasonable proportion of protein, fat, and carbohydrate in semiliquid diets (see tube feeding in Chapter 26). Also, if milk is used extensively as a beverage, with

Table 24-2. Handicapping Conditions and Feeding Disabilities

HANDICAPPING CONDITIONS	FEEDING DISABILITIES				
	Inability to suck, close lips	Inability to bite, chew, swallow	Poor grasp	Poor hand-mouth coordination	Poor trunk and upper extremities control
Cerebral Vascular Accident					
with facial paralysis	+	+		+	
with hemiplegia on dominant side	+	+	+	+	+
Cerebral Palsy					
athetoid type	+	+	+	+	+
ataxic type			+−	+	+
spastic type				+−	+
Traumatic Spinal Cord Injury					
paraplegia					
quadraplegia			+	+	+
Muscular Dystrophy					
Duchenne's			+	+	+
fascio-scapular-humeral	++	+	+	+	+
Multiple Sclerosis	+	+	+	+	+
Parkinson's Disease	+	+	+	+	+
Myasthenia Gravis			+	+	+
Rheumatoid Arthritis			+	+	+−
Severe and Profound Mental Retardation	+	+	+	+	+

+Moderate
++Severe
+−Varies

mashed potatoes and cereals, and in other foods, the daily calcium intake may be excessive while the iron intake may be inadequate. At this time the relationship of calcium intake to the formation of kidney stones in the relatively immobile patient is not well understood, but it is probably advisable that daily calcium intake not exceed the NRC's Recommended Dietary Allowance (see Chapter 10).

Continuous evaluation of a patient's progress is necessary if he is to be helped to progress from semisolid to solid foods. It has been observed that individuals may not progress because they are not encouraged and assisted to try more solid foods.

Weight Control

Weight control is a very important aspect of the nutritional care of the handicapped patient. Persons with paralysis or other motor dysfunctions that permanently limit physical activity require fewer calories to meet their energy needs. In these situations the diet pattern must be carefully planned so that adequate nutrients, without excessive calories, are consumed each day. The patient who is obese when he acquires his handicapping condition should be helped to lose weight for his own benefit and for the benefit of those who give him physical care. Special care must be taken to avoid obesity in the infant and young child (see Chapter 34).

Constipation

Persons with paralysis or hypotonia often become constipated due to immobility and a diet low in roughage. Regular bowel movements may be encouraged through promoting as much physical movement as possible and a diet with adequate roughage (see Chapter 25).

SPECIAL PROGRAMS
Feeding Training of the Neurologically Handicapped Infant

In a number of centers in the United States, intensive study of the training of the neurologically handicapped infant and child is in progress to assist these children in developing their fullest potential for participation in the activities of daily living. The feeding training aspect of this program is concerned not only with the nutritional needs of these children but also with the development of self-feeding skills, so they may eat with their families at home and with others when away from home.

Careful study of each stage in the self-feeding process is being done. For example, the elements of feeding oneself with a spoon include grasping the spoon; getting food onto it; lifting the spoon to the mouth; placing the spoon in the mouth; taking the food from the spoon with the lips; removing the spoon from the mouth; returning it to the plate; and chewing and swallowing the food.

It has been observed that using the fingers is the best way to begin the program. Having peanut butter, pudding, or mashed potatoes on the fingers often encourages hand-to-mouth action. When spoon feeding is introduced, foods which stick to the spoon, such as cooked cereal, mashed potatoes or mashed carrots, and thick puddings, are used.

The staffs of these centers recognize that the key to success in the feeding training programs are repeating the activity, giving gentle yet consistent encouragement, giving only the required amount of help, and knowing when the child does not need assistance.

When the neurologically handicapped child who has been carefully trained to achieve his potential for self-feeding is admitted to a pediatric unit for an acute illness, the personnel should seek the help of the mother so that he can maintain the skills he has acquired and not regress.

The Handicapped Homemaker

The homemaker who is handicapped can often perform her usual activities of meal preparation by using specialized equipment and methods. These activities can be programmed by an occupational therapist or through use of manuals such as the *Mealtime Manual for the Aged and Handicapped* by Klinger *et al* (New York, Simon & Schuster, 1970) or *Homemaking for the Handicapped* by May *et al* (New York, Dodd, Mead, 1966).

STUDY QUESTIONS AND ACTIVITIES

1. Have a classmate or friend feed you liquids and solids while you are lying on your back without your head raised. What difficulties did you encounter with sipping, chewing, and swallowing?
2. Feed or observe the feeding of a patient recovering from a stroke. How long did it take? Did the individual consume a reasonable energy and nutrient intake at this meal (one quarter to one half of his daily needs)?
3. Once a day for a week observe a skilled therapist work on developing self-feeding skills in a handicapped child. Did the child make any progress?
4. Analyze one day's energy and nutrient intake of a handicapped person in a hospital or skilled nursing facility. Was the intake adequate to meet this individual's needs?

SUPPLEMENTARY READINGS

Cornelius, M. S.: Feeding handicapped patients. J. Am. Dietet. A. 67:136, 1975.

Gaffney, T. W., and Campbell, R. P.: Feeding techniques for dysphagic patients. Am. J. Nurs. 74:2194, 1974.

Gresham, G. E.: Residual disability in stroke survivors—the Framingham study. N. Eng. J. Med. 293:954, 1975.

Manning, A. M., and Means, J. G.: A self-feeding program for geriatric patients in a skilled nursing facility. J. Am. Dietet. A. 66:275, 1975.

Nutrition and Feeding Techniques for Handicapped Children. Developmental Disabilities Program, California Dept. of Health, Sacramento, Ca., 95814, 1974.

Ogg, H. L.: Oral-pharyngeal development and evaluation. Physical Therapy 55:235, 1975.

Weber, B.: Eating with a trach. Am J. Nurs. 74:1439, 1974.

Zickefoose, M.: Feeding the child with a cleft palate. J. Am. Dietet. A. 36:129, 1960.

For further references see Bibliography in Section 4.

diet in gastrointestinal disease

25

Diet therapy in gastrointestinal disease is concerned with problems which may occur in the esophagus, at the lower esophageal sphincter, and in the stomach; in the small bowel, including the duodenum, jejunum, and ileum; in the large bowel (the colon), including the rectum and anus; and in the appendages to the tract—the liver, gallbladder, and pancreas. There is good evidence that dietary modifications are effective in the treatment of a number of malabsorption problems due to: (1) the lack of or inadequate amounts of specific pancreatic or intestinal enzymes required to hydrolyze certain constituents of food; (2) the lack of conjugated bile salts from the liver to form a microemulsion of fat to facilitate its absorption in the small intestine; or (3) a structural or functional defect of the villi of the small intestine, particularly in the distal duodenum, proximal jejunum, and terminal ileum, which interferes with the hydrolysis and/or transport of nutrients.

There is also good evidence that certain chemical constituents of beverages such as the caffeine in coffee; theobromine in tea and chocolate; and alcohol enhance the secretion of hydrochloric acid by the parietal cells in the antrum of the stomach.

341

Otherwise the significance of diet therapy in the treatment of a variety of gastrointestinal diseases such as peptic ulcer and ulcerative colitis is not clear. There are limited data on the effects of the chemical and physical characteristics of the nutrients in foods as consumed in meals on the structure and functions of the gastrointestinal tract. At the same time there is no consensus as to the definition of the term "bland diet," a diet widely used in the treatment of peptic ulcer.

This confusion in diet therapy in peptic ulcer disease reflects to some extent the confusion at present regarding its etiology. The problems met in working with physicians treating patients with peptic ulcer are best described by Fein's observation that "opinion regarding diagnosis and treatment of stomach disease may vary from locality to locality and from gastroenterologist to gastroenterologist."[1]

Also, the lay public has many misconceptions. Foods are said to be "hard to digest," which is equated with the rate at which food leaves the stomach. Or, foods may be classified as "irritating" or "gas forming" (see later in this chapter). There is no question that certain foods may cause gastrointestinal discomfort in some individuals. This may be due to a specific substance in food such as the lactose in milk in a lactase-deficient patient, or it may be an allergic response to a food protein.

Since food carries many emotional overtones, it is to be expected that the emotional state of an individual will affect his digestion. The layperson often attributes his "indigestion" or diarrhea to anger or anxiety; and in a three- or four-year-old child the excitement of a birthday party or the anticipation of a trip to a favorite relative can initiate vomiting. Likewise, many neuroses and even psychoses may give rise to gastrointestinal symptoms.

Symptoms ascribed to disorders in the gastrointestinal tract may be due to pathologic conditions in other systems of the body. For example, severe congestive heart failure, chronic renal disease, space-occupying lesions in the central nervous system such as brain tumors, and infections such as pneumonia, bacteremia, and pulmonary tuberculosis are often accompanied by symptoms of gastrointestinal distress.

Succeeding sections of this chapter present diet therapy in diseases of the esophagus and stomach, the small intestine, and the colon. The reader is advised to review the anatomy of the gastrointestinal tract and its appendages and to review in this book Chapter 9, Nutrient Utilization, and Chapter 24, Handicapping Problems, particularly the sections on chewing and swallowing. Malabsorption caused by cystic fibrosis and certain disaccharides which occurs primarily in infants and children is discussed in Chapter 34; the surgical removal of sections of the intestines or the colon presents problems in diet therapy which are discussed in Chapter 26. Liver disease is discussed in Chapter 32.

DIAGNOSTIC PROCEDURES IN GASTROINTESTINAL DISEASE

Five common procedures used in the diagnosis of gastrointestinal disease are: (1) indirect visualization of the gastrointestinal tract by fluoroscopy or x-ray photographs after a barium meal has been ingested; (2) direct visualization of the esophagus, stomach, and duodenum by an endoscope; (3) analysis of gastric secretions for the quantity of hydrochloric acid being produced; (4) examination of intestinal tract tissue obtained by peroral suction biopsy; and (5) absorptive function tests.

Roentgenography

Roentgenography of the gastrointestinal tract is an important diagnostic procedure. It may be done by x-ray photography or by direct examination with a fluoroscope, or, usually, by both. By this means the progress of an opaque "meal" of barium sulfate may be followed through the entire upper digestive tract, and motility (including peristalsis), emptying time, general tonus, defects of outline indicative of ulcer or carcinoma, and other signs of abnormalities can be studied in detail. The barium meal is given in the morning, or at least 12 hours after the taking of food or drink. This test is known as an upper gastrointestinal series (UGI).

A barium enema (BE) is used to visualize the large bowel. The patient is prepared by enemas, or by a clear liquid diet for 48 to 72 hours and enemas, so that the bowel is free of fecal material. This procedure is used when cancer, diverticula, ulcerative colitis, or aganglionic megacolon is suspected.

Endoscopy

The mucosa of the esophagus, stomach, and duodenum can be visualized directly by an endoscope, a flexible tube with a light at the end which is inserted through the mouth and esophagus into the stomach. It has an eyepiece through which the physician can examine the area.

Gastric Analysis

This test is carried out in the morning, before the patient has received any food. A tube is passed from the mouth into the stomach, and any gastric secretion present is withdrawn. The patient may then be given an injection of histamine, a drug that stimulates gastric secretion. The gastric contents are withdrawn at intervals, for an hour or longer. All samples, including the fasting one, are examined for the presence of undigested food, bile, and blood, and tested for the quantity of free and total hydrochloric acid each contains.

In the normal individual no remnants of a previous meal or of blood should be present. A small amount of bile is sometimes regurgitated from the duodenum. The amount of acid present in the fasting specimen in a normal individual is 2.0 ± 1.8 mEq. per hour for females and 3.0 ± 2.0 mEq. per hour for males. After histamine stimulation the commonly accepted normal values are 16 ± 5 mEq. of acid per hour for females and 23 ± 5 mEq. of acid for males.

If a higher range of acid is found, the condition is called *hyperchlorhydria* and may indicate the presence of an ulcer in the stomach or the duodenum. If the range is much below normal, it is termed *hypochlorhydria*. It may indicate gastric disease in the presence of other findings. *Achlorhydria* denotes that no hydrochloric acid is present. It may occur in gastric disease, and is often found in patients with pernicious anemia.

Peroral Suction Biopsy

The peroral biopsy tube is used to obtain tissue specimens from the duodenum, jejunum, and ileum. These specimens can be analyzed for structural defects such as the flattened villi in gluten-induced enteropathy, or functional defects such as the level of disaccharidases in suspected deficiency.

Absorptive Tests

Various absorption tests are used to diagnose small bowel problems, such as the quantitative fecal fat test, the d-xylose absorption-excretion test, the lactose tolerance test, and the vitamin B_{12} absorption test. During the collection of stool for the quantitative fecal fat test the adult patient must consume a diet of 100 g. of fat per day. The absorption of less than 95 percent of the ingested fat is indicative of malabsorption. The other absorptive tests are well described in Todd-Sanford's Clinical Diagnosis by Laboratory Methods, edited by Davidsohn and Henry.[2]

THE UPPER GASTROINTESTINAL TRACT—
PEPTIC ULCER
Terminology

The term gastric ulcer denotes an eroded lesion in the stomach, usually occurring along the lesser curvature or near the pylorus. A duodenal ulcer is the same type of lesion, but is found in the first part of the duodenum. It is much more common than a gastric ulcer. Whether an ulcer occurs in the stomach or in the duodenum, the treatment is similar. They will be considered together here under the term peptic ulcer. Peptic ulcer disease may be acute with bleeding and other complications, or chronic with periodic recurrences of the acute phase.

The diagnosis of ulcer is commonly made by gastric analysis and by fluoroscopy and x-ray findings. Hyperacidity and hypersecretion of gastric juice are usually found in examination of the stomach contents, and the ulcer crater is often plainly visible on the roentgenogram.

Symptoms

PAIN. Pain in the epigastrium, occurring more or less regularly from one to three hours after meals, is characteristic of peptic ulcer. It is usually of a burning or gnawing type and is relieved by food or nonabsorbable antacids. The pain complained of by the peptic ulcer patient when the stomach is empty is due to the action of the highly acidic gastric juice on the open lesion, since no food or antacid is present to neutralize the gastric acid.

HEMORRHAGE AND PERFORATION. Sometimes hemorrhage is the first indication of the presence of an ulcer; or, hemorrhage may occur if the ulcer goes untreated. Sudden weakness and tarry stools, the latter due to the presence of blood, are the outstanding symptoms, and the patient is usually hospitalized at once. If perforation of the gastric or the duodenal wall accompanies the hemorrhage, the situation is extremely serious and the patient is subjected to emergency surgery.

Etiology

The etiology of peptic ulcer is presently under intensive investigation. It is not clear whether both types of ulcers, duodenal and gastric, are caused by similar or different problems. However, there is general agreement that there are three factors involved in the development of all peptic ulcers. These are: (1) the presence of gastric acid and pepsin, usually but not always, in amounts greater than normal; (2) decreased mucosal resistance to the action of gastric acid and pepsin; and (3) a higher degree of reaction to emotional stress and a higher level of anxiety in patients with peptic ulcer compared to people who do not develop ulcers.[3]

Gastric acid and pepsin must be present for the development of a peptic ulcer. It has been observed that in the absence of gastric acid and pepsin ulcers do not develop. However, the converse is not true, i.e., that in the presence of elevated levels of gastric acid and pepsin, ulcers will occur. A small percentage of hypersecretors do not develop peptic ulcers. Also, not all individuals who develop ulcers have elevated levels of gastric acid and pepsin. Although the mechanism(s) are not well understood, the lesion in peptic ulcer appears to be caused by a combination of two factors, the presence of gastric acid and pepsin and decreased mucosal resistance to the action of acid and pepsin.

The role of emotional stress is also not well understood. It is possible that stress may stimulate gastric acid and pepsin secretion or may reduce mucosal resistance in some way.

Principles of Diet Therapy

The goal of the medical treatment of peptic ulcer is to reduce the secretion of gastric acid and pepsin and to neutralize the gastric acid which is secreted, to protect the ulcerated area from irritation and to promote healing. Anticholinergic drugs are used to reduce secretions, and nonabsorbable antacids are used to neutralize gastric acid. For many years, dietary programs have been an integral part of the medical treatment of peptic ulcer. These programs have varied from a severely restricted milk and cream regimen to a bland diet regimen or a liberal regimen of frequent feedings of those foods the patient tolerates. Numerous clinical research studies have been conducted in an attempt to identify the best therapeutic diet plan for the treatment of peptic ulcer, but as yet there is no firm evidence for one specific approach to diet therapy in ulcer disease. In the following discussion an attempt is made to analyze and summarize the major controversies of diet in peptic ulcer disease.

PROTEIN. When any food is ingested, it distends the antrum of the stomach. This process initiates the release of the hormone *gastrin*, which in turn stimulates gastric acid secretion. As it enters the antrum, the protein in food buffers the gastric acid. Later, the products of the gastric digestion of protein and other gastric secretagogues (see later) are major stimulators of gastric acid secretion.[4] In normal individuals when the pH of the contents in the pyloric area drops to approximately 2.0 or less, gastrin release is inhibited. In the patient with active peptic ulcer disease the early buffering of gastric acid by protein relieves the pain, while the later drop in pH due to stimulation by the products of gastric protein digestion causes the pain which many ulcer patients experience one to three hours after meals. To neutralize the gastric acid, the patient with an active ulcer takes an antacid one hour after a meal. However, if the pH of the gastric contents does not drop to 2.0 or less, gastrin release is

not inhibited and gastric acid secretion continues. Therefore, anticholinergic drugs are included in the therapeutic plan to reduce the vagal stimulation of gastrin release.

Although the protein in all foods stimulates gastric acid secretion, there is some evidence that the protein in milk may be a less potent stimulant than the protein in meat. This could be related to the fat in milk. However, the excessive use of milk is not recommended. (See discussion on fat in this section.)

Even though the products of protein digestion are major stimulators of gastric acid secretion, protein is included in the diet of the patient with peptic ulcer disease. The daily diet should provide at least 0.8 g. per kg. of body weight. If extensive blood loss has occurred, it is advisable to include 1 to 1.5 g. per kg. to support red blood cell synthesis and maturation.

GASTRIC SECRETAGOGUES. In addition to the products of gastric protein digestion, it has been demonstrated that the methyl xanthines, caffeine and theobromine, cause an increase in gastric acid secretion. Alcohol is a mild stimulant of acid secretion but also is damaging to the mucosal barrier. Although not a secretagogue, aspirin (salicylic acid) damages the mucosal barrier.

Alcohol and beverages containing caffeine and/or theobromine, such as coffee, tea, chocolate, and cola beverages, are omitted from the diets of patients with ulcer disease. Meat extractives in meat-based soups and in meat drippings used to make gravies are also classified as gastric secretagogues and, therefore, are omitted from the diet.

FAT AND CARBOHYDRATES. Fat inhibits gastric secretion while carbohydrates neither stimulate nor inhibit it. Partly because fat inhibits gastric secretion, hourly feedings of a mixture of milk and cream have been used in the early phase of treatment of acute peptic ulcer disease. The hourly feedings of approximately 3 to 4 ounces of the milk and cream mixture are combined with between-feeding doses of antacid to neutralize the gastric acid stimulated by the products of the digestion of the protein in the milk. This regimen was designed by Sippy in 1915 and became known as the Sippy diet. The milk and cream mixture was commonly referred to as "gastric mixture." Between-meal feedings of milk and cream were continued during the convalescent phase.

This regimen is still used occasionally in the early treatment of the acute phase of peptic ulcer disease. However, with increasing knowledge of the relationship of the type of dietary fat to the level of serum cholesterol and development of atherosclerosis (see Chapter 29) the effects of a diet high in milk fat have been questioned. Sandweiss, in a study of 180 ulcer patients, found the mortality from heart disease 14 percent higher than in the general population.[5] Recently, when the Sippy regimen is ordered, whole or skim milk is used in place of milk and cream.

It is generally agreed that the diet for the treatment of peptic ulcer disease should be moderate in fat, 80 to 100 g. per day, and contain sufficient carbohydrate to provide an adequate energy intake.

ROUGHAGE. Raw fruits and vegetables, especially those with skins and small seeds such as strawberries and tomatoes, and unrefined cereals and flours have been excluded from diets for peptic ulcer because of their fiber content, commonly referred to as roughage. From limited research it was suggested that the roughage in these foods is mechanically irritating to the ulcer in acute peptic ulcer. More research is needed to document whether or not roughage does irritate the ulcer crater.

pH OF BEVERAGES. There has been considerable controversy about citrus juices and other beverages with a pH of 4.0 or less. Some diet programs have included them while others have excluded them. Further research by Castell and colleagues (see Reflux Esophagitis) may demonstrate that orange juice may be contraindicated in the diets of those patients with peptic ulcer who report distress after drinking it.

SPICY FOODS. Spices are often excluded from diet programs for peptic ulcer. One group of investigators has shown that the use of considerable amounts of cinnamon, allspice, thyme, sage, paprika, clove, and other spices produced no increase in gastric secretions in patients with gastric ulcers. In five out of fifty patients in this study, some difficulty was encountered with chili, black pepper, mustard seed, and nutmeg.[6] This work and the more recent work of Castell and colleagues suggests that spices may be tolerated, although there may be some individual differences.

SIZE OF MEALS. Distention of the antrum stimulates gastric acid secretion. Therefore, in acute peptic ulcer, feedings of small to moderate volume may be used in an attempt to avoid excessive distention of the antrum. In such cases, frequent feedings are required to achieve a reasonable energy and nutrient intake. For the patient with a healed ulcer, Fordtran suggests that frequent small meals are contraindicated because of the repeated stimulus by food to gastric secretion, especially in duodenal ulcer patients who are hypersecretors.[7]

SUMMARY. The diet for the patient with peptic ulcer should meet the individual's energy needs and provide adequate amounts of protein and moderate

Table 25–1. American Dietetic Association Position Paper on Bland Diet in the Treatment of Chronic Duodenal Ulcer Disease*

I. [The ADA] recognizes that the rationale (chemically and mechanically non-irritating) for the bland diet is not sufficiently supported by scientific evidence.

  A. Spices, condiments, and highly seasoned foods are usually omitted on the basis that they irritate the gastric mucosa. However, experiments have indicated that no significant irritation occurs, even when most condiments are applied directly on the gastric mucosa. Exceptions are those items which do cause gastric irritation, including black pepper, chili powder, caffeine, coffee, tea, cocoa, alcohol, and drugs.

  B. Milk has been the basis of diets for duodenal ulcer for many years. One of the primary aims in dietary management of duodenal ulcer disease is to reduce acid secretion and neutralize the acid present. While milk does relieve duodenal ulcer pain, the acid neutralizing effect is slight. Its buffering action could be overweighed by its ability to stimulate acid production. Most foods stimulate acid secretion to some extent; protein provides the greatest buffering action and is also the most powerful stimulus to acid secretion. The use of milk therapy has been greatly reduced over the past decade, owing to a better knowledge of its side effects and allergic reactions. The controversy regarding the use of milk still continues. There are those who still advocate the regular use of milk, primarily during the active stage of acute duodenal ulcer; however, strict insistence on its use during remission is unwarranted.

  C. Roughage, or coarse food, has been excluded from the diet on the basis that it aggravates the inflamed mucosal area. There is no evidence that such foods as fruit skins, lettuce, nuts, and celery, when they are well masticated and mixed with saliva, will scrape or irritate the duodenal ulcer. Grinding or puréeing of foods is necessary only when the teeth are in poor condition or missing.

  D. The effect of a bland diet on the healing of duodenal ulcer has been studied extensively. Investigations have compared various bland diets with regular or free-choice diets. The results indicate that a bland diet made no significant difference in healing the ulcer. One such study demonstrated that the acidity of the gastric contents was frequently lower when a free-choice diet was taken. Many foods have been incriminated as the cause of gastric discomfort and are subsequently eliminated from a patient's diet. Studies done on patients with and without documented gastrointestinal disease indicate that those with gastrointestinal disease cannot be distinguished by food intolerance. Symptoms of intolerance were more related to individual response than to intake of specific food or the presence of disease.

II. Believes that scientific investigation supports the validity of frequent, small feedings in the management of patients with duodenal ulcer disease. These have been found to offer the most comfort to the patient; additionally, acidity of the gastric contents is lower with small-volume, frequent feedings. It must also be recognized that rest, preferably in bed, rapidly reduces duodenal ulcer symptoms. This is a specially important factor in the healing of the ulcer.

III. Believes the following points should be of major consideration in developing a dietary plan for duodenal ulcer patients.
  A. Individualization of the dietary plan, since patients differ as to specific food intolerances, living patterns, life styles, work hours, and education.
  B. Utilization of small volume, frequent feedings.
  C. Provision of educational materials relative to dietary support.

IV. Advocates the continued pursuit of current research and recommends that valid information be utilized in up-dating dietary regimens.

V. Suggests that dietetic practitioners be cognizant of the possible harmful effects of a milk-rich bland diet in patients who have a tendency towards hypercalcemia and/or atherosclerosis.

*Approved by the Executive Board, May 21, 1971, as Position Paper Number 0000H. J. Am. Dietet. A. 59:243, 1971.

Table 25-2. Progressive Peptic Ulcer Routine—Acute Phase

Milk and cream, half and half, or milk, or skim milk 3 oz. every hour alternating with nonabsorbable antacid on the half hour

Supplements (given in 3 small meals, adding 2 or 3 foods each day as tolerated, in addition to hourly milk feedings):

Eggs
Soft cooked or poached

Cereal
Refined, cooked cereals only

Toast and crackers
White, refined bread and crackers

Cottage and cream cheese
May be substituted for an egg

Strained cream soup
Made of bland, low residue vegetables such as asparagus, corn (cream), peas, spinach, and strained before serving

Baked or soft custard, gelatin, junket

Purée fruits and vegetables
Those available as infant foods are suitable

---

amounts of fat. Because blood loss may occur, special attention must be given to foods which are high in iron. If necessary, an iron supplement is prescribed. Future research may demonstrate more clearly whether or not there are individual intolerances to citrus juices and "spicy" foods. If citrus fruits and juices are not tolerated, a vitamin C supplement can be prescribed.

Today there is firm evidence that gastric secretagogues, commonly referred to as gastric stimulants, should be avoided by the patient with peptic ulcer. There is limited evidence and considerable controversy about the effectiveness of frequent "bland" meals in the treatment of ulcer disease. Because of this controversy the American Dietetic Association published the association's position paper on the bland diet in the treatment of chronic duodenal ulcer disease, given in Table 25-1.[8] Section III of this paper states the generally, but not completely, accepted guidelines for planning diets for patients with peptic ulcer.

Diet Plans

In this section the traditional diet plans and the liberal plan for the treatment of peptic ulcer are presented for the reader's convenience. The bland diet is frequently used in the treatment of gastrointestinal diseases other than peptic ulcer. These may be patients receiving certain medications such as steroids, patients with hiatus hernia, or patients recovering from acute gastritis.

PROGRESSIVE PEPTIC ULCER ROUTINE—ACUTE PHASE. The diet plan for the acute phase of peptic ulcer disease is given in Table 25-2 and is a modification of the original Sippy regimen, which restricted the acutely ill patient to hourly servings of milk and cream for 21 days. Then limited servings of refined cereals, eggs, and custard were added. Later this plan was reduced to 14 days with the addition of other simple foods such as toast, cottage cheese, and milk-based soups. It is used today by some physicians for a short period of time in the early treatment of the patient who is bleeding on admission to the hospital.

PROGRESSIVE PEPTIC ULCER ROUTINE—CONVALESCENT PHASE. The convalescent peptic ulcer diet plan in Table 25-3 is a further modification of the Sippy regimen using bland foods and restricting roughage and condiments. As the patient progresses from the acute to the convalescent stage, the hourly feedings of milk are discontinued and six small meals or three meals with between-meal feedings are served. Table 25-4 shows a menu of three meals and three between-meal feedings for a convalescent peptic ulcer patient.

BLAND DIET. Table 25-5 lists the foods included in a bland diet that may be used by some physicians as soon as the acutely ill patient with a peptic ulcer has improved. The convalescent ulcer diet plan in Table 25-3 is then omitted. The bland diet plan, which is somewhat less restrictive than the convalescent diet plan, may also be used after discharge from the hospital. Table 25-6 gives a typical day's menu using a bland diet. Most convalescent ulcer patients are advised to distribute this food into three small meals and three between-meal feedings to avoid gastric distention (see Table 25-4). For example, the canned pears and the bread and butter in the noon meal menu may be eaten at 3:00 P.M.

LIBERAL DIET. Some clinicians advocate a liberal diet in the treatment of peptic ulcer. The diet plan is usually based on the patient's usual dietary practices provided that his food choices provide an adequate nutrient intake. He should be counseled to omit any food that has regularly caused gastric distress. He may be advised to eat frequently—midmorning, midafternoon, and before retiring, together with three small meals—and to avoid excessive use of alcoholic beverages, tea, and coffee.[9] Other clinicians are of the opinion that the bedtime feeding should be omitted because it might result in an excessive secretion of gastric acid and, therefore, gastric distress in the early morning hours.[10]

The total calories in the diet of the patient of normal weight should be that required to maintain weight. The obese patient should be assisted to lose weight.

Table 25-3. Progressive Peptic Ulcer Routine—Convalescent Phase

FOODS USED

Milk
Milk, cream, buttermilk

Cheese
Cottage, cream; other mild, soft cheeses. Cheddar cheese may be added later.

Fats
Butter or margarine

Eggs
Soft or hard cooked, poached, scrambled

Meats
Tender beef, lamb, veal; sliced chicken; liver; fish, poached, broiled or baked; crisp bacon; smooth peanut butter

Soups
Cream soups, using only vegetables listed below

Vegetables
Well-cooked or canned: asparagus, beets, carrots, peas, green or wax beans, spinach; mashed squash or pumpkin; mashed or baked white and sweet potato (no skins)

Fruits
Applesauce, baked apples without skin, ripe or baked bananas, diluted fruit juices, stewed or canned pears, peaches and peeled apricots, purée of all dried fruits except figs
It is advisable to take citrus fruit juices after eating some of the other foods of the meal, or to dilute them half and half with water.

Breads, cereals, macaroni products
Enriched white bread, fine whole wheat or light rye bread; refined cereals; all ready-to-eat cereals except those containing bran; oatmeal; macaroni, spaghetti, noodles

Desserts
Ice cream, plain; custard; simple puddings of rice, cornstarch, tapioca or bread without fruit or nuts; gelatin desserts (with fruit as permitted above); sponge and other plain cakes, sugar cookies

Beverages
Milk, cream, buttermilk. Postum, and decaffeinated coffee if allowed by physician

Condiments
Moderate amounts of sugar, jelly and salt; others if permitted by physician

FOODS TO BE AVOIDED

Fats
All fried foods

Meats and fish
Smoked and preserved meats and fish; pork; meat gravies

Soups
All meat soups; all canned soups

Vegetables
All raw vegetables; all gas-forming vegetables, including cabbage, cauliflower, brussels sprouts, broccoli, cucumbers, onions, turnips, radishes

Fruits
All raw fruits except orange juice and ripe banana

Breads and cereal
Coarse breads and cereals; hot breads

Desserts
Pastries, nuts, raisins, currants, and candies

Beverages
Coffee, tea, alcoholic, and carbonated beverages

Condiments
All condiments except salt, unless permitted by physician

Table 25-4. Menu for Progressive Peptic Ulcer Routine—Convalescent Phase

Breakfast	Dinner	Supper
Orange juice	Chicken, sliced	Cream of spinach soup
Eggs, scrambled	Baked potato (no skin)	Cottage cheese
White toast	String beans purée	White-bread toast
Butter or margarine	White bread	Butter or margarine
Jelly	Butter or margarine	Milk
Milk	Milk	
10 A.M.	**3 P.M.**	**9 P.M.**
Cornflakes with milk	Canned peaches	Applesauce
Milk	Plain cookies	Milk
	Milk	

Counseling the Patient

The physician's diet order determines the approach to dietary counseling. The personality of the patient may be a factor in the diet the physician chooses. A patient with an ulcer often expects some dietary restrictions.[11] If he is a worrisome, overanxious individual, he may find a carefully controlled regimen such as a bland diet more to his liking than to be told he can eat what he wants. On the other hand, the patient who is able to take his diagnosis in stride or who finds dietary restrictions irksome may do very well on a liberal dietary regimen.

Patients who are employed may need some suggestions about what to eat at coffee break time or at noontime in a cafeteria or restaurant; or what to include in a bag lunch. The homemaker responsible for preparing a bland diet may need some assistance in modifying food preparation methods.

diet in gastrointestinal disease 347

Table 25-5. Bland Diet

PRINCIPLES

1. Low in fiber and connective tissue
2. Little or no condiments or spices, except salt in small amounts
3. No highly acid foods
4. Foods simply prepared

FOODS USED

Milk
Milk, cream, buttermilk, yogurt

Cheese
Cream, cottage and other soft, mild cheeses

Fats
Butter and margarine

Eggs
Boiled, poached, scrambled in Teflon pan or top of double boiler

Meat, fish, fowl
Roast beef and lamb; broiled steak, lamb or veal chops; stewed, broiled or roast chicken; fresh tongue; liver; sweetbreads; baked, poached or broiled fish

Soups
With milk or cream-sauce foundation

Vegetables
Potatoes, peas, squash, asparagus tips, carrots, tender string beans, beets, spinach. (In severe cases these vegetables are puréed.)

Fruits
Orange juice, ripe bananas, avocados, baked apple (without skin), applesauce, canned peaches, pears, apricots, white cherries, stewed prunes

Bread, cereals, macaroni products
White bread and rolls, crackers, all refined cereals; macaroni, spaghetti, noodles

Desserts
Custard, junket, ice cream, tapioca, rice, bread or cornstarch pudding, gelatin desserts, junket, sponge cake, plain cookies, prune, apricot or peach whip

Beverages
Milk, buttermilk, cocoa, malted milk, fruit juices (if tolerated), coffee or tea (if allowed)

FOODS TO BE AVOIDED

Fats
Fried or fatty foods

Meat, fish
Smoked and preserved meat and fish; pork

Vegetables
All raw; all cooked except those listed above

Fruits
All except those listed above

Desserts, sweets
Pastries, preserves, candies

Beverages
Alcoholic beverages; carbonated drinks unless prescribed by the doctor

Condiments
Pepper, other spices, vinegar, ketchup, horseradish, relishes, gravies, mustard, pickles

Table 25-6. Typical Menu for Bland Diet

Breakfast	Noon Meal	Evening Meal
Banana, ripe	Roast lamb	Cream of potato soup
Farina with milk	Mashed potatoes	Cheese Soufflé
1 egg, poached	Peas	Fresh spinach
White-bread toast	White bread	White bread
Butter or margarine	Butter or margarine	Butter or margarine
Coffee or substitute	Canned pears	Applesauce with sugar cookies
Cream	Tea or milk	Milk
	Cream	Small glass orange juice*
	Small glass tomato juice*	

*If tolerated.

Surgical Treatment

Peptic ulcer tends to be recurrent. If the ulcer proves to be resistant to medical treatment, or if it recurs fairly frequently, surgery is usually necessary. (For the dietary regimen following surgery for peptic ulcer, see Chapter 26.)

OTHER DISORDERS OF THE UPPER GASTRO-INTESTINAL TRACT

Achalasia

Achalasia or cardiospasm is a motor disorder of the esophagus in which the lower esophageal sphincter (LES) is constricted and impedes the flow of food and fluid into the stomach. At the same time the normal peristaltic action of the upper part of the esophagus is inadequate. Difficulty in swallowing (dysphagia) is the most common symptom. As the problem progresses, food and fluid do not pass from the esophagus into the stomach and are regurgitated. As a result weight loss occurs. Dilatation of the upper part of the esophagus and inflammation of the lower end of the esophagus may also result.

The patient may be treated by a series of mechanical dilations of the stricture of the lower esophageal sphincter or, if necessary, by surgery. When the patient has recovered from the dilation procedure clear liquids are offered and, if the patient does not experience dysphagia, a regular or bland diet is ordered. Frequent small feedings may be better tolerated than three regular meals. Daily food intake should be closely monitored, especially in those patients who have experienced significant weight loss prior to treatment, or who may be apprehensive about their ability to swallow food.

Reflux Esophagitis

Esophagitis occurs when the gastric contents reflux into the lower esophagus. The condition may be mild, or it may be severe enough to cause bleeding and ultimately esophageal stenosis. It is often complicated by the presence of hiatus hernia. The primary function of the lower esophageal sphincter is to prevent the reflux of gastric contents into the esophagus, and it is generally agreed that reflux esophagitis is caused by a hypotensive and, therefore, incompetent lower esophageal sphincter. The most common clinical symptom is "heartburn" (pain high under the sternum). Regurgitation of gastric contents into the mouth, usually during the night or when bending over, also occurs.

Esophagitis is treated by vigorous antacid therapy and by the prevention of reflux by gravity. The patient is advised to remain in an upright position after eating meals and to elevate the head of the bed to reduce reflux during sleep. A bland diet, excluding coffee, tea, and alcohol, in combination with antacid therapy has been used to treat reflux esophagitis. Also a regular diet, excluding coffee, tea, and alcohol and limited in fat, has been recommended with meals equal in size and moderate in quantity to minimize gastric distention.

Recent research indicates that in normal subjects a test meal of fat significantly decreases esophageal sphincter pressure; carbohydrate increases pressure only slightly.[12] Further research demonstrates that slight but significant decreases in lower esophageal sphincter pressure occurred with whole milk in contrast to a significant increase in pressure with skim milk.[13] A chocolate syrup with only 1.25 percent fat also lowered sphincter pressure. The investigators attribute these results to the caffeine and theobromine in chocolate. A tomato mixture representing "spicy" foods and orange juice produced considerable variation in pressure and frequent secondary esophageal contractions. The investigators suggest the use of skim milk in the treatment of "heartburn" from gastric reflux and the avoidance of spicy foods, orange juice, and chocolate. Because of the caffeine content of coffee and of theobromine in tea, these beverages should also be excluded.

Although the evidence is limited, it would seem advisable that patients with reflux esophagitis eat regular meals of equal size and avoid coffee, tea, alcohol, chocolate, citrus juices, and "spicy" foods and limit the quantity of fat at each meal. Although the mechanism is not well understood, reflux esophagitis frequently occurs in the obese individual and improves with weight reduction. Therefore, the diet may also be restricted in energy content. If both tomato and orange juices are omitted from the diet, a vitamin C supplement should be prescribed to insure an adequate intake.

Hiatus Hernia

The term hiatus or diaphragmatic hernia refers to herniation of the cardiac portion of the stomach into the thoracic cavity. The esophagogastric junction slides up and down through the herniation depending on body posture, abdominal distention, and gastric filling. Hiatus hernias are usually asymptomatic. However, when the lower esophageal sphincter is incompetent, gastric reflux occurs and the patient develops reflux esophagitis (see previous discussion).

If bleeding occurs in hiatus hernia, the clinician may order a bland or convalescent ulcer diet, described earlier in this chapter. However, excessive fat intake should be avoided. In severe cases which do not respond to medical therapy, surgery may be advised.

Hemorrhagic Gastritis

Hemorrhagic gastritis is essentially an inflammation, which may be localized or diffuse, of the gastric mucosa. It is characterized by bleeding from superficial lesions as compared with the deeper, localized lesions of peptic ulcer. The glands which secrete gastric acid and pepsin are not involved. It may follow the ingestion of aspirin, alcohol, or toxic substances; be associated with staphylococcal food poisoning or with infection; or be the terminal event in the uremia of renal disease.

The treatment will vary with the cause. For example, if toxic substances have been ingested in an attempt to commit suicide, gastric lavage is used; or if aspirin or alcohol has caused the bleeding, ingestion of these is eliminated. When the bleeding is controlled, vigorous antacid therapy is used to neutralize the gastric acid in order to protect the gastric mucosa.

When tolerated, a full liquid diet (see Chapter 22) with frequent small feedings is usually offered. Depending on the problem, solid foods such as dry toast, crackers, cooked cereals, and soft-cooked eggs may be added to the diet. The patient may progress to a bland or regular diet as tolerated.

Atrophic Gastritis

Compared with hemorrhagic gastritis, in which the gastric glands are not involved, atrophy of the gastric glands in atrophic gastritis leads to the hyposecretion of gastric acid (hypochlorhydria). Most patients are asymptomatic, while some complain of indigestion. Atrophic gastritis may accompany organic diseases such as cancer, pernicious anemia, iron deficiency anemia, and chronic infection such as syphilis. There is also evidence that bile reflux from the duodenum into the stomach may cause chronic gastritis. The treatment consists of discovering and treating the underlying cause.

Indigestion

Indigestion, characterized by "heartburn," regurgitation of gastric contents, frequent belching, and a sense of fullness, is symptomatic of various gastric and other organic diseases. When no organic disease is found, the indigestion is said to be functional. Functional indigestion may be due to poor food habits and hurried and irregular meals; to food idiosyncrasies and possible allergies; or to tension and anxiety.

Individuals who live for much of the day on doughnuts and pastries accompanied by frequent cups of coffee or carbonated beverages, with a proper meal only in the evening, are good candidates for indigestion. Overeating, especially of very sweet and fatty foods, may be the cause of indigestion. Rapid eating, particularly when under pressure, resulting in "bolting" of food cannot help causing gastric discomfort. For all these, the treatment consists of finding time for rest and relaxation and adopting more moderate food habits. These patients may have to be persuaded of the necessity for such changes and reassured that it is their food habits and not organic disease which has caused their discomfort.

Certain foods have been labeled as difficult to digest, although the reason is not always clear. Such foods as lobster, crab, sardines, peanuts and nuts, raw apples, garlic, and pickles are in this group. The gas-forming vegetables and fruits may cause discomfort, either because of coarse cellulose or their volatile oils. Common gas-forming foods are cabbage and its relatives—brussels sprouts, broccoli and cauliflower, dried peas and beans, onions, turnips, green peppers, radishes, cucumbers, and melons. If any of these foods are known to be troublesome, they should be omitted from the diet. True food allergies are discussed in Chapter 33.

Disturbed or anxious patients whose gastric distress is an outcome of their emotional problems are in need of medical guidance and help. They should be given sympathetic support and reassurance. A bland diet may be found to be of help in treatment.

Cancer of the Stomach

DELAYED DIAGNOSIS. Because the onset usually is very gradual and there are no distressing symptoms in the early stages of cancer of the stomach, it is frequently overlooked until too late to effect a cure. For this reason, any continued abdominal discomfort should be investigated, even though seemingly inconsequential.

SYMPTOMS AND DIAGNOSIS. Lack of appetite over a considerable period of time with loss of weight and strength are symptoms suggestive of carcinoma. Vomiting, particularly of food eaten many hours before, may occur and sometimes newly acquired constipation is a symptom. The absence of free hydrochloric acid in the gastric contents is suggestive, although in the earlier stages it may be increased. Occult blood is frequently present in the stools. The most important methods used in diagnosis are roentgenography and endoscopy. The early discovery of this condition, when surgical intervention is more likely to be successful, is of utmost importance.

DIETARY ADAPTATIONS. When either a subtotal or a total resection of the stomach has been performed, the diet should follow that outlined in the chapter on preoperative and postoperative diets for peptic ulcer surgery (see Chapter 26).

Often in inoperable carcinoma of the stomach, patients feel that if only they could eat they would get well; therefore, the diet is difficult to prescribe. A bland or a convalescent ulcer diet is indicated, or even a liquid diet, particularly if there is obstruction or bleeding. However, the patient's morale may be benefited most by serving a regular house diet as long as possible and letting him choose from his tray what appeals to him.

DISORDERS OF THE SMALL INTESTINE
Malabsorption

Intestinal malabsorption is any state in which there is a disturbance in the net absorption of any constituent in the gastrointestinal tract—fluid, electrolytes, or nutrients—across the intestinal mucosa, from the mucosal to the serosal. There may also be excessive secretion of fluids and electrolytes into the lumen of the tract from the serosal to the mucosal side.[14] In practice the term also encompasses the problem of maldigestion of food nutrients as well as their absorption.

The final digestion (hydrolysis) and absorption of nutrients takes place primarily in the cells of the distal duodenum and the jejunum and to a lesser extent in the ileum. Maldigestion results when there are insufficient amounts of pancreatic enzymes and fluids entering the duodenum, an inadequate flow of bile from the liver to emulsify fats, or insufficient amounts or a deficiency of the digestive enzymes in the cells of the villi of the small intestine. Maldigestion can also occur when there are structural defects in the small intestine such as flattened villi or when there is increased peristaltic activity (peristaltic rushes). Maldigestion results in a decrease in net absorption of protein, fat, and carbohydrate because they have not been hydrolyzed to the substances which can be absorbed—hexoses, amino acids, fatty acids, and monoglycerides. The undigested nutrients, modified to some extent by intestinal bacteria, are excreted by the large bowel.

Malabsorption may be primary, such as lactose malabsorption due to a hereditary lack of lactase, or secondary, such as lactose malabsorption due to lactase deficiency following gastrointestinal infection.[15] The common symptoms of malabsorption are weight loss in adults or growth retardation in infants and children, abdominal distention and cramping, and diarrhea or steatorrhea.

DIARRHEA. In diarrhea the stools are fluid or semifluid and increased in number. In addition to water, the stool also contains sodium and potassium and frequently undigested food. With significant fluid and electrolyte losses dehydration and weight loss result. In infants and children the fluid and electrolyte losses may be critical.

STEATORRHEA. Steatorrhea means excessive fat in the stools. With massive maldigestion of fats the stools are frothy, large, foul smelling, and shiny in appearance. The number of stools per day is increased; they also contain significant amounts of water and electrolytes.

Disaccharide Problems—
Lactose Intolerance

Intolerance to lactose, the sugar of mammalian milk, is due to a deficiency or insufficiency of the enzyme lactase, the greatest quantity of which is found in the proximal jejunum. Lactose intolerance is characterized by intestinal distention, cramps, and diarrhea. The lactose tolerance test, and in some instances peroral suction biopsy, are used to confirm the suspected diagnosis.

Congenital lactase deficiency is a rare disease occurring in infants. Diarrhea following the ingestion of breast milk or cow's milk is severe and life threatening. A lactose-free infant formula relieves the symptoms immediately (see Table 34-4, Chapter 34, p. 484). As the infant grows the dietary restrictions discussed under dietary treatment should be observed.

Acquired lactose intolerance, which occurs in children after age six and in adults, is more frequent in people whose heritage derives from countries in Asia and Africa. In these areas milk, and therefore lactose, are not consumed postweaning. The implications of the cultural heritage are not known at present. In some individuals with acquired lactose intolerance there is an insufficiency rather than a deficiency of lactase. Often the patient has recognized his intolerance to milk and has excluded it from his diet.

Secondary lactase deficiency can occur as a result of damage to the intestinal villi by infection.[16] Infants are often intolerant of lactose during and for a period following gastrointestinal infection. Lactose intolerance has also been reported in celiac-sprue, tropical sprue, cystic fibrosis, ileitis, colitis, and kwashiorkor. This intolerance is due, in part, to mucosal damage in the jejunum.

Severe milk intolerance may also occur following subtotal gastrectomy with a gastrojejunostomy in patients who were able to drink milk without symptoms prior to the operation. This problem may result from the reduction in the amount of jejunal surface containing lactase.

DIETARY TREATMENT. In lactase deficiency all sources of lactose are excluded from the diet. This includes milk and cheese and foods containing milk such as ice cream, milk chocolate, cream soups, other creamed dishes, and breads made with milk. The list of ingredients on the labels of all food packages must be read carefully since milk in some form is widely used in convenience foods and in numerous other products including baby foods. Also, lactose is an ingredient of some medications.

Individuals with an insufficiency, but not a total lack, of lactase tolerate small amounts of milk as a beverage with meals or in food such as bread. This should be encouraged for the calcium it contributes to the diet. Also, it has been reported that fermented dairy products such as buttermilk, cottage cheese, and yogurt are tolerated by some lactose intolerant individuals.[17] This is possibly due to the modification of the lactose in these products by bacterial fermentation during processing.

To date no studies of lactose intolerant individuals report the supplementation of the diet with calcium medication. However, without supplementation, the calcium intake will be inadequate, since milk is the most significant dietary source of calcium.

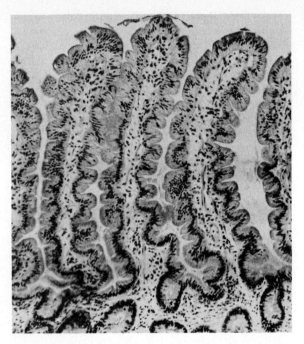

Fig. 25-1. Jejunal biopsy. Normal jejunum. The villi are slender and of uniform size. The epithelial cells are intact in all areas. (Benson, G. D., Kowlessar, O. D., and Sleisenger, M. H., Adult celiac disease with emphasis upon response to the gluten-free diet. Medicine 43:1, 1964)

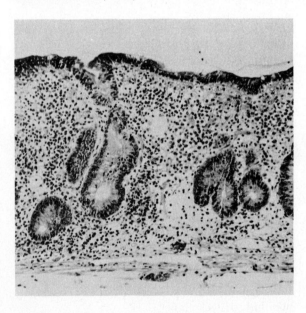

Fig. 25-2. Jejunal biopsy. Adult celiac disease. Pretreatment biopsy showing severe changes. There is complete absence of villi, thinning of the mucosal surface, and disorganization of the epithelial cells. (Benson, G. D., Kowlessar, O. D., and Sleisenger, M. H.; Adult celiac disease with emphasis upon reponse to the gluten-free diet. Medicine 43:1, 1964)

Celiac-Sprue (Gluten-Induced Enteropathy, Celiac Disease, Nontropical Sprue)

Although the term celiac disease was originally applied only to children who exhibited this malabsorption syndrome, it is generally accepted today that what formerly was called nontropical sprue is in reality adult celiac disease and may be referred to as celiac-sprue. It has been observed that a number of patients who developed celiac disease in adult life had a history of the disease in childhood. With the discovery that the gluten in cereal grains is the toxic agent, the syndrome is now also known as gluten-induced enteropathy.

SYMPTOMS. Celiac-sprue is characterized by steatorrhea, with the passing of at least two to three stools a day. These are described as bulky, foamy, light colored, and foul smelling. They contain a high percentage of fat, fatty acids, and calcium soaps, resulting from incomplete digestion and absorption in the intestinal tract.

Due to the loss of fat and other nutrients in the stool a whole complex of symptoms results. There is often marked weight loss, muscle wasting, anorexia, and debilitation; in infants and sometimes in adults there is a typical "pot belly"; there is anemia due to poor absorption of iron and folic acid; there may be tetany, bone pain, and fractures resulting from the poor absorption of calcium and vitamin D; and hypoprothrombinemia and roughening of the skin may be present because fat-soluble vitamins K and A are not absorbed. Occasionally patients have glossitis and peripheral neuritis, possibly due to an inadequate absorption of the B vitamins. More recent findings suggest that there may also be a deficiency of vitamin E due to faulty fat absorption, and of vitamin B_6.

DIAGNOSIS. The finding of unabsorbed fat and fatty acids in the feces and the history and appearance of the patient give the first clue to the diagnosis. A jejunal biopsy, viewed under the electron microscope, reveals marked changes in the jejunal mucosa. Instead of the fingerlike projections of the villi with their brushborder, the mucosa is flat and thickened and appears to have varying degrees of epithelial cell atrophy, now recognized as characteristic of celiac disease (see Figs. 25-1 and 25-2). It is suspected that an immunological reaction in the tissues of the villi causes the changes in the jejunal mucosa.

In 1953 three Dutch investigators Dicke, Weijers, and van de Kamer reported that wheat, rye, and oat cereals were responsible for the steatorrhea and other symptoms of celiac disease in children.[18] When they excluded these cereals from the diets of their patients there was prompt and marked improvement. In a subsequent report these same authors showed that the two major components of wheat protein, glutenin and gliadin, which are also present in rye protein and, to a lesser extent, in oat protein, were the offending substances.[19] They indicated that the specific substance in the cereal gluten is the amino acid glutamine when it is bound in a peptide (a partial breakdown product of protein digestion). When they tested their treated patients with bound glutamine the symptoms recurred. This did not happen when they tested these same patients with glutamine alone. The more recent work of Cornell and Townley supports these findings.[20]

Glutamine, the amide of glutamic acid, occurs widely in all food proteins but the greatest concentration is found in the gluten of wheat, rye, barley, and, to a lesser extent, in oats. Although rice and corn also contain glutamine—but in smaller amounts than the other cereals—they are well tolerated in patients with celiac-sprue.

DIETARY TREATMENT. From the work of the Dutch investigators with children, and of others with adults with nontropical sprue, a "gluten-free" diet which excluded the use of wheat, rye, barley, and oats was begun and soon proved to be successful in controlling the disease. Foods used in the gluten-free diet are presented in Table 25-7. In the patient with severe diarrhea, the diet may be restricted in residue until the diarrhea is controlled.

Table 25-7. Gluten-Free Diet

CHARACTERISTICS

1. All forms of wheat, rye, oatmeal, buckwheat, and barley are omitted, except gluten-free wheat starch.
2. All other foods are permitted freely, including fats and starches.
3. The diet should be high in protein and calories. Mineral and vitamin supplements may be needed if malnutrition is present. After that, the diet should be sufficient to maintain normal growth and development in children, and normal weight in adults.

FOODS USED

Milk
2 glasses or more. Flavored if desired. More for children

Cheese
As desired. Cottage and pot cheese only for very young children

Fats
Butter and other fats as desired. (Note restrictions under "Foods To Be Avoided.")

Eggs
1 to 2 a day

Meat, fish, fowl
1 or 2 servings daily (not breaded, creamed or served with thickened gravy; no bread dressings). Otherwise prepared as desired

Soups
All clear and vegetable soups; cream soups thickened with cream, cornstarch, or potato flour only

Vegetables
As desired, except creamed. Include 2 servings of green or yellow vegetables and at least 1 raw vegetable daily. (The last may be omitted for very young children.) Rice may be substituted occasionally for potato.

Fruits
As desired; 2 or 3 servings daily. Include citrus fruit once a day.

Bread and cereals
Bread made from rice, corn, or soybean flour and gluten-free wheat starch only
Cornflakes, corn meal, hominy, rice, Rice Krispies, Puffed Rice, precooked rice cereals

Desserts
Any of the following: Jello, fruit Jello, ice or sherbet, homemade ice cream, custard, junket, rice pudding, or cornstarch pudding (homemade)

Beverages
Milk, fruit juices, ginger ale, cocoa. (Read label to see that no wheat flour has been added to cocoa or cocoa syrup.) Coffee (made from ground coffee), tea, carbonated beverages

Condiments and sweets
Salt; sugar, white or brown; molasses; jellies and jams; honey; corn syrup

FOODS TO BE AVOIDED

Fats
Cream sauces made with wheat flour; commercial salad dressings except pure mayonnaise. (Read labels.)

Meat, fish, fowl
Meat patties or meat, fish, or chicken loaf and pies made with bread or bread crumbs; croquettes; breaded meat, fish, or chicken. Chili con carne and other canned meat dishes. Cold cuts unless guaranteed pure meat. Bread stuffings
All gravies or cream sauces thickened with wheat flour

Soups
All canned soups except clear broth. All cream soups unless thickened with cream, cornstarch, or potato flour

Vegetables
Any prepared with cream sauce or breaded

Bread, cereals, macaroni products
All bread, rolls, crackers, cake and cookies made from wheat or rye; Ry-Krisp; muffins, biscuits, waffles, pancake flour and other prepared mixes; rusks, Zwieback, pretzels; any product containing oatmeal, barley, or buckwheat
Breaded foods, bread crumbs
All wheat and rye cereals; wheat germ, barley, oatmeal, buckwheat, kasha
Macaroni, spaghetti, noodles, dumplings

Desserts
Cakes, cookies, pastry; commercial ice cream and ice cream cones; prepared mixes, puddings. All homemade puddings thickened with wheat flour

Beverages
Postum, malted milk, Ovaltine. For adults: beer, ale

Sweets
Commercial candies containing cereal products. (Read labels.)

WARNING: *Read labels on all packaged and prepared foods.*

The exclusion of all cereal grains except corn and rice from the diet may seem to be an easier matter than it actually is. Wheat flour and wheat-bread products are used in such a variety of ways in food preparation that their elimination poses many problems. Not only must all wheat bread and rolls be omitted, both white and whole wheat, but all breaded products, bread stuffing, gravies and cream sauces thickened with wheat flour, macaroni, spaghetti, noodles, biscuits, crackers, cakes, and cookies made from wheat flour. Rye grain, with the exception of rye breads, pretzels, and Ry-Krisp, is less commonly used and, therefore, is omitted more easily. Oatmeal is excluded, as it caused a recurrence of symptoms when reintroduced into the diet. Barley and buckwheat are also excluded, as their effect in the intestinal tract in this disease is not known. For adults, beer and ale must be omitted, since they may contain cereal grain residues.[21]

In place of the cereals which must be excluded, bread, biscuits, and cookies made from rice, corn, and soy flour, and wheat starch are used. (See Chapter 31 for wheat starch products.) Cornflakes, corn meal, hominy, rice, Rice Krispies, Puffed Rice, and pre-cooked rice cereals may be used. Cornstarch and potato flour can be used to thicken gravies and cream sauces. Because wheat flour is in such common usage, it is well to check the labels on commercially prepared foods for content before using them on this diet to be sure that no wheat flour or modified wheat starch has been used in their preparation. Postum, malted milk, and Ovaltine are examples of commercial products made from or containing cereal grains. Where such content is not included in the label, the food had better be omitted if there is a question.

When the individual has a concurrent lactase deficiency, milk in all forms will also be excluded from the diet.

The physician may augment the diet with mineral and vitamin supplements to correct deficiencies and hasten recovery. Although fat excretion persists to some extent, fat is well tolerated and there is no need to limit it in the diet.

Results and Prognosis. The response of the patient with celiac disease to the elimination of the offending cereal grains is often dramatic, and may occur within 24 hours to a week. The appetite returns, the patient begins to regain lost weight, the stools become less fatty and less frequent, and a sense of well-being is quickly apparent.

The long-term effects of adherence to the gluten-free diet are equally striking. Benson et al, reporting on 32 patients with adult celiac disease followed for a number of years, found that there was improvement in every diagnostic finding, including in most cases a return to normal mucosal structure.[22] The degree of improvement was in direct proportion to the careful adherence to the diet. That the diet does not cure the disease is shown by the fact that symptoms recur if the patient consumes food containing gluten.

Other Findings. Weser and Sleisenger and others have reported that lactase deficiency and the absorption of undigested lactose occurred in some patients in whom celiac disease was untreated or who did not follow their diets carefully.[23] Symptoms were abdominal cramps, distention, and diarrhea, and were relieved when lactose and gluten were omitted from the diet. That this is not a permanent defect is shown by the fact that patients who had maintained a strict gluten-free diet for two years or more had no symptoms of lactase deficiency.

Tropical Sprue

Tropical sprue, another malabsorption syndrome, is endemic in the native populations of some tropical and subtropical areas in the world, notably Puerto Rico and Southeast Asia. Military personnel as well as other residents from temperate countries who are stationed in these areas also may develop tropical sprue, either during their stay in the host country or on their return home.

The symptoms are diarrhea, with loss of nutrients, especially fat, weight loss, and macrocytic anemia. If the disease is of long standing, there will be severe malnutrition, megaloblastic bone marrow changes, and villous atrophy of the jejunal mucosa, eventually leading to the typical flat mucosa of celiac disease.

The syndrome responds dramatically to the administration of folic acid and antibiotics. In some patients, despite continuance of therapy, the megaloblastic anemia recurs due to deficient absorption of vitamin B_{12}. There is prompt response to vitamin B_{12} therapy. The response to a gluten-free diet is minimal, and an ordinary, nutritionally adequate diet, increased in calories and protein to counteract malnutrition and weight loss, is sufficient. With treatment, patients become asymptomatic and eventually the intestinal mucosa returns to normal.

The etiology of tropical sprue is still in doubt. It has been thought to be due to a diet deficient in folic acid or to an interference with its absorption, but there is no basis for this hypothesis other than the response to treatment with folic acid. There is some evidence of the presence of an infective agent, because of the response to antibiotic therapy, but no pathogens have been demonstrated.

Pancreatitis

ETIOLOGY. Pancreatitis, or inflammation of the pancreas, may be acute or chronic; the acute form may or may not progress to the chronic one. The etiology of pancreatitis is poorly understood at present. Three hypotheses are proposed to explain the disease: (1) obstruction of the pancreatic duct; (2) regurgitation of bile from the common duct up the pancreatic duct; and (3) the reflux of duodenal contents into the pancreatic duct. The role of pancreatic enzymes in the pathogenesis of pancreatitis is also under investigation.

It has been observed that pancreatitis is associated with other diseases. Acute pancreatitis may occur with biliary tract disease, infection, alcohol ingestion, and hyperlipoproteinemia Types 1, 4, or 5. Chronic pancreatitis is associated with chronic alcoholism, untreated biliary tract disease, and familial abnormalities of the sphincter of Oddi.

The most common symptom of pancreatic disease is abdominal pain. Nausea, vomiting, and steatorrhea due to a deficiency of pancreatic lipase also occur. Hypovolemia, leading to circulatory failure, and paralytic ileus frequently accompany severe, acute pancreatitis.

DIETARY TREATMENT. The presence in the duodenum of dilute hydrochloric acid and the products of protein digestion normally stimulate the flow of pancreatic juices and enzymes, while the presence of fat stimulates the flow of bile. The dietary treatment of pancreatitis is derived from these principles.

In severe acute pancreatitis intravenous feedings of fluid, electrolytes, and dextrose (see Chapter 26) are given. When oral feedings are tolerated, liquids containing primarily carbohydrate are offered because it is the nutrient which has the least effect on pancreatic exocrine excretion. During recovery, and with milder attacks, frequent small feedings containing carbohydrate and protein and limited in fat are given. Antacid therapy is used to neutralize gastric acid secretion. The diet is limited in fat because pancreatic lipase is deficient and with concurrent biliary disease bile may also be deficient. If hyperlipoproteinemia is present, the diet may be modified to treat this problem (see Chapter 29).

Chronic pancreatitis may be treated by a regular or bland diet limited in fat. When necessary, pancreatic extracts are given orally and are taken with each meal and snack. Medium chain triglycerides can be used as a source of energy because they do not appear to require pancreatic lipase or bile for digestion (see discussion of MCT oil in Chapter 23). If glucose intolerance develops due to lack of insulin, the diet may be restricted in carbohydrate (see Chapter 27).

Providing an adequate energy and nutrient intake for the patient with pancreatitis is difficult. The diet tends to be low in energy due to the fat restriction, and the patient's food intake is poor because of constant pain. Supplementary vitamins may be required. Every effort should be made to give the patient the foods that he can tolerate, and in such quantity that his nutritional needs continue to be met. In all cases of pancreatitis alcohol is prohibited.

Gallbladder Disease

ETIOLOGY. The most common form of gallbladder disease is cholelithiasis (gallstones) complicated by cholecystitis (inflammation of the gallbladder) and occurs more frequently in women over 40 years of age than in any other group. The largest proportion of stones are composed of cholesterol. It is suspected that the cholesterol in bile precipitates to form cholesterol stones when the amount of bile salts and lecithin in bile is inadequate to keep the cholesterol in solution.[24]

SYMPTOMS. The major symptom of gallbladder disease is acute or intermittent epigastric pain. Indigestion, intolerance to fatty and spicy foods, and nausea and vomiting may also occur. If the flow of bile into the duodenum is decreased or the cystic duct is obstructed, jaundice and steatorrhea can occur. A survey of hospitalized patients by Koch and Donaldson indicates that some patients with gallbladder disease have pain when they eat fat while others do not.[25]

DIETARY TREATMENT. Gallbladder disease is treated primarily by surgery. Prior to surgery the diet is restricted in fat to reduce the contractions of the gallbladder and, therefore, avoid pain. If the individual is grossly obese, surgery is delayed whenever possible until there is an appropriate weight loss.

Table 25–8 shows the foods containing significant amounts of fat, which must be used in limited quantities, and foods high in fat, which must be omitted. If the patient reports gastric distress from eggs, they

Table 25–8. Restrictions and Omissions on a Low Fat Diet

FOODS LIMITED

Milk to 1 pint daily
Eggs to 1 daily
Butter or margarine to ½ tablespoon daily
Lean meat, fish or fowl to 1 serving daily
    (If skim milk is used, meat may be increased to 2 servings without altering the fat limitation.)

FOODS OMITTED

Cream; cheese other than pot or cottage cheese
All fried foods
Salad oils; salad dressings; gravies
All meat high in fat, such as pork, bacon, ham, goose, duck, fatty fish
Pastry; cake; cookies; ice cream
Nuts, olives, avocados

should be omitted. Table 25-9 gives a low fat bland diet menu. A fat-restricted bland diet is usually well tolerated. If the individual is obese, the fat-restricted diet may need to be further restricted in total calories to achieve weight loss. This is achieved by restricting carbohydrate (see Chapter 27).

Regional Ileitis (Crohn's Disease)

ETIOLOGY. Regional ileitis is a chronic, progressive disease of the ileum of unknown etiology. It may first involve the terminal segment of the ileum proximal to the ileocecal valve, but, eventually, it will spread along the ileum and may involve the jejunum. For this reason the disease is sometimes called regional enteritis. The term regional refers to the fact that healthy areas of the bowel may alternate with diseased ones. Despite occasional remissions, the disease is progressive.

SYMPTOMS. The condition is characterized by hyperplasia (enlargement due to cell increase) of the lymphatics, which eventually interferes with the blood supply of the mucosa of that section of the intestinal tract which is affected. This in turn gives rise to edema and ulceration, scarring of the mucosa, thickening of the intestinal wall with narrowing of the lumen of the bowel, and obstruction. The most common symptoms are persistent diarrhea and pain.[26]

Because of the persistent diarrhea, there may be marked malnutrition. If the disease is extensive, there will be poor absorption of food nutrients, further accentuating the poor nutrition. A chronically ill patient may be markedly underweight and show signs of protein depletion. Anemia may be present due to blood loss and to poor absorption of iron and vitamin B_{12}. There may be insufficient absorption of fat-soluble vitamins as evidenced by hypoprothrombinemia and roughened skin. If medical treatment fails to restore the patient's nutritional status, or if there is obstruction, surgery may be indicated. See Chapter 26 for dietary care in the latter case.

DIETARY TREATMENT. The diet in regional ileitis should be high in protein and calories, and low in residue, as described in the next section of this chapter. The patient may eat better when the diet is divided into six meals during the day and evening, and if he is given some choice. Seasonings and cold fluids are not well tolerated and should be omitted. Vitamin supplements should be given as additions to the diet. Vitamins K and B_{12} and, possibly, iron should be given as parenteral medications, since they are not sufficiently absorbed from the intestinal tract.

Chalfin and Holt report lactose intolerance in three out of five patients with ileitis.[27] Two of these had a history of milk intolerance previous to the disease. The restrictions for lactase deficiency discussed earlier in the chapter should be observed in cases where the diagnosis has been established.

DISORDERS OF THE LARGE BOWEL
Dietary Residue

Patients with problems in the terminal ileum and large bowel may require a low residue diet. These patients may have regional ileitis, ulcerative colitis, malignant or nonmalignant lesions of the colon or rectum, or hemorrhoids. Regional ileitis and ulcerative colitis are generally treated medically. Progression of the disease may lead to surgery: ileostomy in regional ileitis, and colostomy or ileostomy in ulcerative colitis. In all situations the low residue diet is generally used as part of medical treatment or in preparation for surgical treatment of the patient.

RESIDUE IN FOODS. The foods used in the residue-restricted diets are low in vegetable fiber to decrease the volume of fecal material. The elastin fibers of meat are restricted for the same reason. Fiber is that portion of food (cellulose, hemicellulose, and lignin) that is not enzymatically digested in the digestive tract. Fruits, vegetables, nuts, and whole grains are the major contributors of fiber. The term "roughage" is also used to refer to fiber.

It is generally agreed that meats free of elastin fibers, fats such as butter and margarine, and highly refined carbohydrates such as flour, spaghetti, maca-

---

Table 25–9. Very Low Fat, Bland Diet Menu in 6 Meals *

Breakfast	Lunch	Dinner
Stewed prunes	Cottage cheese	Sliced chicken
Cream of Wheat	Toast, slightly buttered, 2 slices	Baked potato
Milk, whole, ½ cup	Jelly or honey	Soft-cooked string beans
Postum	Applesauce	Canned apricots
Sugar	Tea, sugar	Tea, sugar
10 A.M.	**3 P.M.**	**8 P.M.**
Toast, slightly buttered, 2 slices	Junket made with skim milk	Crackers
Jelly or honey	Crackers	Jelly or honey
Skim milk, 1 glass	Jelly or honey	Skim milk, 1 glass

*This diet will contain approximately 70 g. of protein, 25 g. of fat, 325 g. of carbohydrate and 1750 calories.

Table 25-10. Diets Varying in Residue

FOODS	RESIDUE-RESTRICTED DIET	MODERATE RESIDUE DIET	MINIMAL RESIDUE DIET
Milk*	Milk, buttermilk, yogurt, cream	Same	Same
Cheese	Cottage, cream*, Cheddar	Same	Cottage, cream only*
Fat	Butter, margarine	Same	Same
Eggs	Cooked, poached, scrambled in double boiler	Same	Same
Meat, fish, fowl	Tender chicken, fish, sweetbreads, ground beef and lamb	Same	Ground, tender meat; minced chicken and fish
Soups and Broths	Broth, strained meat-base soups	Same	Broth only
Vegetables	Cooked vegetables: asparagus, peas, string beans, spinach, carrots, beets, squash; potatoes—boiled, baked	Vegetable juice; vegetable purée, cooked asparagus tips, carrots, potatoes—boiled, mashed, baked	Unseasoned vegetable juices in limited amounts*
Fruits	Fruit juices, cooked and canned fruits (without skins, seeds or fiber), bananas	Fruit juice, fruit purée, ripe bananas, cooked, peeled apples, apricots, peaches, pears, plums	Fruit juices, preferably citrus in limited amounts*
Bread, cereals	Refined, enriched bread and cereals; macaroni, spaghetti, noodles, rice, crackers	Refined, enriched bread and cereals only, macaroni, spaghetti, noodles, rice, white crackers	As in moderately low residue
Desserts	Ices, ice cream*, junket*, cereal puddings*, custard*, gelatin, plain cake and cookies; all without fruit and nuts	Same	Same
Beverages	Tea, coffee, carbonated beverages	Same	Tea, coffee as permitted
Condiments	Salt, moderate amounts of pepper, other mild spices, sugar	Salt and sugar	Salt and sugar

*If tolerated

roni, noodles, rice, and sugar add minimal residue to the fecal contents of the large bowel. Bananas and potatoes, which are low in residue, are exceptions in classifying fruits and vegetables as high in residue.

Limited evidence exists which indicates that milk may add residue to the fecal contents. As a result there is controversy about the use of milk in residue-restricted diet plans. It has been observed that some adult ulcerative colitis patients have insufficient amounts of lactase and respond favorably to a moderate lactose restriction.[28] (See discussion of lactose intolerance earlier in this chapter.)

Tea, coffee, meat extractives, condiments, spices, and carbonated beverages are usually not excluded from the residue-restricted diet. Fruit and vegetable juices may be excluded in some situations, not because of residue, but because the organic acids in these beverages may stimulate peristaltic action.

RESIDUE-RESTRICTED DIETS. Residue-restricted diets may be ordered at various levels of restriction. Table 25-10, Diets Varying in Residue, presents one example of levels of residue-restricted diets.

The Minimal Residue Diet in Table 25-10 may be used to prepare a patient for bowel surgery or immediately after surgery. It is seen that the foods used in this diet are limited and that this diet can be inadequate in calcium and vitamins A and C. If used for any period of time, it should be supplemented with mineral and vitamin preparations.

The Moderate Residue Diet in Table 25-10 may be used as the patient progresses after bowel surgery, in the early medical treatment of regional ileitis or ulcerative colitis, or for the symptomatic control of diarrhea. The Residue-Restricted Diet in Table 25-10 is usually the one used over a period of time by individuals with regional ileitis or ulcerative colitis.

Ulcerative Colitis
ETIOLOGY. Ulcerative colitis is an inflammatory disease of the colon, encountered in all age groups from very young children to the elderly. The etiology is unknown. No organism has been isolated as a cause of the disease. It has been ascribed to allergy, especially to milk, wheat, and eggs. In addition, there are indications that colitis may occur on an emotional basis, since these patients are often very painstaking and meticulous and seem to have more than an ordinary dependence on others.[29]

SYMPTOMS. The disease is characterized by friability and hyperemia of the mucosa, leading to many small areas of bleeding ulceration. This may involve only a part of the rectum or the colon, but in advanced stages of the disease it usually involves the entire area of the large bowel. The stools, which may be as frequent as 15 to 20 a day, are semiliquid and contain blood and mucus. The patient suffers from the discomfort of the frequent stools and the accompanying cramps, and he is usually malnourished, often to an extreme degree. Anemia may be present due to blood loss, and the patient may be severely underweight. The disease is usually treated conservatively by medical means, but in advanced cases surgery may be resorted to and a colostomy or ileostomy performed. See Chapter 26 for dietary care in the latter case.

DIETARY TREATMENT. Dietary treatment in colitis is supportive rather than curative. A patient previously well controlled by diet and medication may have diarrhea when emotionally upset, even though he is adhering to his prescribed diet.

The frequency of the stools, the degree of bleeding and ulceration of the colon, and the general malnutrition present in all patients with severe colitis demand the use of a diet low in residue and as high in protein and calories as the patient can tolerate. The omission of roughage will prevent irritation of the inflamed colon, and the high protein, high caloric diet will help to restore the patient to a better nutritional status. Vitamin and iron supplements should be given.

Either the moderate residue diet or the minimal residue diet listed in Table 25–10 is suitable for the very ill colitis patient. It should be served in six small meals at first. Unfortunately the diet is not very palatable or colorful, and care must be taken to serve the food as attractively as possible. As his condition improves, the patient progresses to a residue-restricted diet.

Lactose intolerance may further complicate the dietary treatment of the patient with ulcerative colitis. Chalfin and Holt report improvement of symptoms when lactose was withdrawn in four patients with colitis who had flat lactose tolerance curves.[30] One of these had had milk intolerance for many years prior to the onset of colitis. Buttermilk or yogurt may be tried, but if they are not tolerated even these dairy products should be omitted.

Since colitis seems to have strong emotional components, a self-selected diet may be used to help the patient to achieve some degree of independence. The doctor may allow him to choose his own diet and encourage him to try whatever food appeals to him, even those which would seem to be contraindicated, such as foods high in residue. All members of the health-care team must be supportive as well as permissive, giving the patient confidence and encouraging him to make his own decisions. As the patient's feeling of security increases, he will eat larger and more nutritious meals, with the subsequent healing of the colon and a gain in weight and strength.

FOOD ACCEPTANCE. Patients with colitis are fussy about their food and often extremely hard to please. They wish others to make choices for them, yet refuse to eat the food when it appears on the tray. They have the irritability of the badly nourished patient and need much understanding and encouragement. Fortunately, most patients recover, at least for a time, and can return to a more or less normal diet.

Diverticulosis

Diverticulosis occurs primarily in the sigmoid colon and is characterized by an increase in both intraluminal pressure and segmentation and by luminal narrowing. The greatest prevalence of the disease occurs in individuals over 50 years of age living in Western societies. Epidemiological and experimental evidence suggests that diverticulosis is due to Western diets from which the natural fiber or roughage has been removed by food processing. As a result, diets without natural roughage lead to a reduction in the fecal bulk entering the sigmoid colon, and the low fecal bulk produces luminal narrowing, increased segmentation, increased pressure, and possibly hypertrophy of the colonic muscles. Many patients with diverticulosis have no symptoms, while others may experience moderate to severe discomfort characterized by lower abdominal pain and distention. In some situations diverticulosis may be complicated by diverticulitis.

DIETARY TREATMENT. Traditionally diverticulosis has been treated with a residue-restricted diet. Recently it has been demonstrated that a high fiber diet which increases fecal bulk is a more effective treatment. In one study the symptoms of diverticulosis were relieved in 71 percent of the subjects by the use at each meal of special wheat bran wafers. The wafers increased each subject's daily intake of dietary fiber.[31]

The most significant food sources of fiber are unprocessed wheat bran, unrefined breakfast cereals, and whole wheat and rye flours. Raw and dried fruits, raw vegetables, and legumes are also important sources. However, it appears that the fiber in wheat bran is more effective than that in raw fruits and vegetables in increasing fecal bulk. Significant, but not excessive, amounts of wheat bran must be used; the quantity that has been generally effective is 6 teaspoons daily.

During an acute attack of diverticulitis with bleeding from the mucosa of the colon, a moderate or minimal residue restricted diet is used.

Cancer of the Bowel

In all cases of constipation, or of constipation alternating with diarrhea, particularly if these symptoms are of short duration and in the face of otherwise normal living habits, there is the possibility of neoplastic growth of some section of the colon or the rectum. If this diagnosis is established by the use of proctoscopic and roentgenographic examinations, the patient is subjected to surgery. See Chapter 26 for postoperative diets.

Constipation

A common disturbance of the digestive tract is constipation. However, there is considerable confusion as to what is meant by this term. Although a daily bowel movement has been stressed as desirable, there are many people for whom an evacuation every other day or even every third day is normal. Moreover, evacuation may occur regularly until an emotional upset occurs, in which case there may either be an increased number of bowel movements, almost diarrhea, or retention of the feces for a day or two, resembling constipation. The matter usually straightens itself out when the strain is relieved. However, if the person becomes anxious when no daily bowel movement occurs and begins to resort to cathartics or enemas, a vicious pattern is set up, and it may be difficult to effect a return to normal habits.

Chronic constipation may be due to the individual's dietary and living habits. Insufficient rest, hurried, irregular meals, a food intake which does not meet the nutritional needs of the body, and too sedentary a life all may contribute to poor bowel function. The problem here is to help the patient to accept a more regular mode of living, including a diet that meets all his nutritive requirements and a reasonable amount of exercise.

Elderly patients may suffer from constipation because muscle tone is relaxed, the dietary intake is inadequate for nutritional needs, and activity is diminished.

DIETARY TREATMENT. In most cases of so-called constipation, a normal diet (see Chapter 10) containing roughage in the form of fresh and cooked fruit and vegetables and including whole-grain bread and cereals will provide sufficient bulk to maintain regular bowel evacuation. Where such regularity needs to be reestablished—for instance, following an illness in which the mobility of the patient has been greatly limited—the addition of stewed fruit and of fruit juices to the ordinary diet will be found helpful. Prune juice, particularly, taken at bedtime or the first thing in the morning, is usually effective.

Elderly patients should not use foods with a high bran content for fear of impaction. Cooked fruits and vegetables are often better tolerated by the older patient than raw ones, except for bananas.

LAXATIVE ABUSE. The abuse of laxatives can lead to structural changes in the terminal ileum and colon.

On roentgenography the terminal ileum appears tubelike in structure and the ileocecal sphincter becomes wide and gaping. The colon becomes dilated and loses its normal mucosal pattern. Hypokalemia (low blood potassium) also occurs with laxative abuse.[32] Laxative abuse, like any substance-abuse problem such as alcohol or drugs, can result in long-term chronic ill health. Individuals who take excessive amounts of laxatives need continuous help to accept and use corrective diet therapy.

STUDY QUESTIONS AND ACTIVITIES

1. Which component of gastric juice is thought to be responsible for the development of a peptic ulcer? What are some possible causes for its increase in gastric juice?
2. Of what symptoms does the patient with peptic ulcer usually complain?
3. Explain the principles underlying the dietary treatment of peptic ulcer. What is the purpose of the antacid medication?
4. Is the Sippy diet in the early stages adequate for normal nutritional needs? What nutrients are likely to be low?
5. Why may the Sippy regimen contribute to the development of atherosclerosis?
6. Write out the dietary instructions for a secretary with achalasia who has been placed on a bland diet.
7. Name some of the causes of gastritis. Plan a menu for a day for a patient with hemorrhagic gastritis. Is it adequate for normal nutritional needs?
8. What are some of the causes of "indigestion" that are not due to an organic lesion? Write a diet for a homemaker who complains of heartburn and gastric discomfort. What are some of the questions you would ask her before giving her instruction?
9. What does the term "malabsorption syndrome" mean?
10. Which two tests are most frequently done to determine disaccharidase deficiency?
11. Name six foods or food groups which must be omitted in lactose intolerance.
12. What is the older term for adult celiac disease?
13. What are the symptoms of celiac-sprue? What does the term "steatorrhea" mean? What pathologic changes are found in the jejunal mucosa?
14. Why is the so-called gluten-free diet used in celiac-sprue? Which cereals must be omitted?
15. Plan a diet for an adult patient with celiac-sprue who eats at home; for a secretary with this disease who eats her lunch at a drugstore counter.

16. What is the difference between celiac-sprue and tropical sprue? How is the latter treated?

17. What is a medium chain triglyceride? Why may it be used effectively in some diseases of the small intestine?

18. Why does a patient with gallbladder disease have pain on the ingestion of fat?

19. Which foods should be avoided, which limited, on a low-fat diet?

20. Write a low-fat general diet for a patient with gallbladder disease who is 20 pounds overweight. Use Chapter 27.

21. Why may a low-fat bland diet be ordered for a patient with pancreatitis? Which foods must be omitted? Which severely restricted?

22. Why should a patient with ileitis have a residue-restricted diet? Can such a diet meet all the patient's nutritional requirements? How may additional calories and proteins be included?

23. Why may hospitalized patients develop constipation? Which groups are especially vulnerable? Name some simple remedies by which the problem may be corrected without the aid of cathartics.

24. Plan a diet for a working man with diverticulosis, using a diet high in fiber.

SUPPLEMENTARY READINGS

PEPTIC ULCER

Donaldson, R. M. Jr.: The muddle of diets for gastrointestinal disorders. JAMA 225:1243, 1973.

Freidman, G. D., et al: Cigarettes, alcohol, coffee and peptic ulcer. N. Eng. J. Med. 290:469, 1974.

Isenberg, J. I.: Peptic ulcer disease. Postgrad. Med. 57:163, 1975.

McKegney, F. P.: Psychosomatic aspects of gastrointestinal disease. Postgrad. Med. 57:43, 1975.

Morrissey, J. F., and Barreras, R. F.: Antacid therapy. N. Eng. J. Med. 290:550, 1974.

OTHER UPPER GASTROINTESTINAL DISORDERS

Behar, J., et al: Medical and surgical management of reflux esophagitis: A 38-month report of a prospective trial. N. Eng. J. Med. 293:263, 1975.

Cohen, S.: Recent advances in management of gastroesophageal reflux. Postgrad. Med. 57:97, 1975.

Ivey, K. J.: Gastritis. Med. Clin. N. Am. 58:1289, 1974.

Ingelfinger, F. J.: How to swallow, belch and cope with heartburn. Nutrition Today 8:4, 1973.

Lasser, R. B., et al: The role of intestinal gas in functional abdominal pain. N. Eng. J. Med. 293:525, 1975.

MALABSORPTION

Ament, M. E.: Malabsorption syndromes in infancy and childhood. J. Pediat. 81: Part I, 685, Part II, 867, 1972.

Gray, G. M.: Carbohydrate digestion and absorption: Role of the small intestine. N. Eng. J. Med. 292:1225, 1975.

DISACCHARIDE PROBLEMS

Bayless, T. M., et al: Lactose and milk intolerance: Clinical implications. N. Eng. J. Med. 292:1156, 1975.

Lebenthal, E., et al: Correlation of lactose activity, lactose intolerance and milk consumption in different age groups. Am. J. Clin. Nutr. 28:595, 1975.

Rayfield, E. J., et al: Impaired carbohydrate metabolism during a mild viral illness. N. Eng. J. Med. 289:618, 1973.

CELIAC-SPRUE

Ferguson, A., et al: Cell-mediated immunity to gliadin within the small-intestinal mucosa in coeliac disease. Lancet 1:895, 1975.

Patey, A. L.: Gliadin: The protein mixture toxic to coeliac patients. Lancet 1:722, 1974.

TROPICAL SPRUE

Klipstein, F. A., and Corcino, J. J.: Malabsorption of essential amino acids in tropical sprue. Gastroenterology 68:239, 1975.

Viteri, F. E., and Schneider, R. E.: Gastrointestinal alterations in protein-calorie malnutrition. Med. Clin. N. Am. 58:1487, 1974.

PANCREATITIS

Cameron, J. L., et al: Acute pancreatitis with hyperlipemia: Incidence of lipid abnormalities in acute pancreatitis. Ann. Surg. 177:483, 1973.

Sarles, H., and Tiscornia, O.: Ethanol and chronic calcifying pancreatitis. Med. Clin. N. Am. 58:1333, 1974.

Taubin, H. L., and Spiro, H. M.: Nutritional aspects of chronic pancreatitis. Am. J. Clin. Nutr. 26:367, 1973.

GALLBLADDER DISEASE

Coyne, M. J., and Schoenfield, L. J.: Gallstone disease. Postgrad. Med. 57:153, 1975.

Swell, L., et al: Current concepts of the pathogenesis of cholesterol gallstones. Med. Clin. N. Am. 58:1449, 1974.

Shaffer, E. A., et al: Bile composition at and after surgery in normal persons and patients with gallstones: Influence of cholecystectomy. N. Eng. J. Med. 287:1317, 1972.

THE LARGE BOWEL

Ament, M. E.: Inflammatory disease of the colon: Ulcerative colitis and Crohn's colitis. J. Pediat. 86:322, 1975.

Benson, J. A.: Simple chronic constipation: Pathophysiology and management. Postgrad. Med. 57:55, 1975.

Findlay, J. M., et al: Effects of unprocessed bran on colon function in normal subjects and in diverticular disease. Lancet 1:146, 1974.

Kirwan, W. O.: Action of different bran preparations on colonic function. Brit. Med. J. 4:187, 1974.

Plumley, P. F., and Francis, B.: Dietary management of diverticular disease. J. Am. Dietet. A. 63:527, 1973.

Scala, J.: Fiber—the forgotten nutrient. Food Tech. 28:34, 1974.

Walker, A. R. P.: Dietary fiber and the pattern of diseases. Ann. Int. Med. 80:663, 1974.

For further references see Bibliography in Section 4.

PATIENT RESOURCES

Celiac Disease Recipes. Hospital for Sick Children, 555 University, Toronto 5, Ontario, Canada.

Low Gluten Diet with Tested Recipes. 3rd rev. Gastrointestinal Section, Univ. of Michigan Medical Center, Ann Arbor, Michigan, 1964.

Sheedy, C. B., and Keifetz, N.: Cooking for Your Celiac Child. New York, Dial, 1969.

Wood, M. N.: Delicious and Easy Rice Flour Recipes. Springfield, Ill., Thomas, 1972.

Wood, M. N.: Gourmet Food on a Wheat Free Diet. Springfield, Ill., Thomas, 1972.

REFERENCES

1. Fein, H. D.: in *Modern Nutrition in Health and Disease*, ed. 5, R. S. Goodhart and M. E. Shils, eds. Philadelphia, Lea and Febiger, 1973, p. 770.
2. Davidsohn, I., and Henry, J. B., eds.: *Todd-Sanford's Clinical Diagnosis by Laboratory Methods*, ed. 14. Philadelphia, Saunders, 1969.
3. Fordtran, J. S.: in *Gastrointestinal Disease*, M. H. Sleisenger and J. S. Fordtran, eds. Philadelphia, Saunders, 1973, Chapter 51.
4. Davenport, H. W.: *Physiology of the Digestive Tract*, ed. 3. Chicago, Medical Year Book, 1971.
5. Sandweiss, D. J.: Am. J. Digest. Dis. 6:929, 1961.
6. Schneider, M. A., et al: Am. J. Gastroent. 26:722, 1956.
7. Fordtran, op. cit.
8. J. Am. Dietet. A. 59:243, 1971.
9. Spiro, H. M.: *Clinical Gastroenterology*. New York, Macmillan, 1970.
10. Fordtran, op. cit.
11. Caron, H. S., and Roth, H. P.: J. Am. Dietet. A. 60:306, 1972.
12. Nebel, O. T., and Castell, D. O.: Gastroenterology 61:778, 1972.
13. Babka, J. C., and Castell, D. O.: Am. J. Digest. Dis. 18:391, 1973.
14. Jefferies, G. H., et al: Gastroenterology 46:438, 1964.
15. Rayfield, E. J., et al: N. Eng. J. Med. 289:618, 1973.
16. Ibid.
17. Gallagher, C. R., et al: J. Am. Dietet. A. 65:418, 1974.
18. Dick, W. K., et al: Acta paediat. 42:34, 1953.
19. van de Kamer, J. H., et al: Acta paediat. 42:223, 1953.
20. Cornell, H. J., and Townley, R. R. W.: Gut 15:862, 1974.
21. Sleisenger, M. H., et al: J. Am Dietet. A. 33:1137, 1957.
22. Benson, G. D., et al: Medicine 43:1, 1964.
23. Weser, E., and Sleisenger, M. H.: Gastroenterology 48:571, 1965.
24. Swell, L., et al: Med. Clin. N. Am. 58:1449, 1974.
25. Koch, J. P., and Donaldson, R. M., Jr.: N. Eng. J. Med. 271:657, 1964.
26. Crohn, B. B.: JAMA 166:1479, 1958.
27. Chalfin, D., and Holt, P. R.: Am. J. Digest. Dis. 12:81, 1967.
28. Spiro, op. cit.
29. Kirsner, J. B.: JAMA 169:433, 1959; Rider, J. A., and Moeller, H. C.: Am. J. Gastroent. 37:487, 1962; Fullerton, D. T., et al: JAMA 181:463, 1962.
30. Chalfin and Holt, op. cit.
31. Plumley, P. F., and Francis, B.: J. Am. Dietet. A. 63:527, 1973.
32. Cummings, J. H.: Gut 15: 758, 1974.

nutritional care—surgical and burn therapy

26

Principles of Nutritional Care
Tube Feedings
Diet Therapy After Gastrointestinal Surgery
Nutrition Following Burns

Good nutritional status is an asset for patients who are to undergo surgery. This is relatively easy for those undergoing elective surgery for problems that do not interfere with eating an adequate diet, such as gynecological or orthopedic surgery or surgery for uncomplicated cholelithiasis, hernia, thyroid disease, and tonsillitis. Patients who are to undergo cardiac surgery or kidney transplantation need the appropriate dietary treatment prior to surgery to reduce operative risks (see Chapters 30 and 31).

The obese surgical patient is a particular risk, especially for the anesthesiologist, because inhalant anesthesias may be sequestered in the fat depots and impede normal recovery from anesthesia postoperatively. When possible the obese patient should be counseled to lose weight prior to surgery (see Chapter 27).

Patients with cancer of the oral cavity, esophagus, larynx, stomach, small intestine, or colon may come to surgery in a nutritionally debilitated state. The nutritional rehabilitation of these and certain other patients cannot be done until after surgery, because these conditions may interfere with chewing and swallowing or with digestion, absorption, and excretion.

The key factors of postoperative nutritional care

362

are: (1) maintenance of energy, fluid, and electrolyte balance; (2) adequate energy-protein intake; and (3) adequate total nutrient intake to promote wound healing and resumption of normal activities.

Principles of postoperative nutritional care, postoperative oral feeding routines, tube feedings, diet therapy used after surgery of the gastrointestinal tract, and the nutritional care of the severely burned patient are discussed in this chapter.

PRINCIPLES OF NUTRITIONAL CARE
Metabolic Responses to Surgery and Trauma

Surgical intervention or acute trauma due to accidents or burns elicit the same sequence of metabolic responses. These responses can be categorized as the catabolic phase, the anabolic phase, and the fat gain phase.

CATABOLIC PHASE. Surgery or trauma activates the neuroendocrine system, particularly the pituitary and adrenal glands, promoting a hypermetabolic state. This phase is also referred to as the stress reaction. During the catabolic phase there is loss of body cell mass, primarily in muscle tissue, which results in a negative nitrogen and potassium balance; retention of extracellular fluid with the retention of sodium; change in energy source from glucose to fat; and alteration in the pH of the blood. After serious traumas such as burns or after most surgery the peristaltic and absorptive functions of the gastrointestinal tract are reduced.

ANABOLIC PHASE. The anabolic phase is characterized by positive nitrogen balance until the nitrogen lost during the catabolic phase is restored; sodium and water excretion and potassium retention; return of peristalsis to normal; and slow weight gain. The anabolic phase begins five to seven days or earlier after most surgery. With extensive burns or complex surgery it may be delayed for much longer.

FAT GAIN PHASE. This final metabolic phase, during which the fat lost during the catabolic phase is regained, may last for two or three months.

Nutritional Needs

ENERGY. For the majority of patients in the immediate postoperative period, the needs for energy, fluids, and electrolytes are supplied by intravenous solutions of 5 percent dextrose, combined if necessary with electrolytes and water-soluble vitamins. It is estimated that after trauma an adult requires 40 to 70 kcal. per kg.[1] (2800 to 4900 kcal. for a 70-kg. man). There are 170 kcal. in each 1000 ml. of 5 percent dextrose, and no more than 2500 to 3000 ml. (415 to 510 kcal.) can be administered safely in 24 hours.

Therefore, the total energy needs of an adult cannot be met by a 5 percent dextrose solution. More concentrated solutions of dextrose cannot be used since they cause thrombosis in peripheral veins. During this period stores of body fat serve as the primary energy supply, and the dextrose administered intravenously spares body proteins to some extent.

In general the average patient will be able to take food and fluid orally in one to three or four days after surgery. For some patients it may be necessary at this point to supply energy, nutrients, and fluids by nasogastric, gastric, or jejunal tube. As soon as the patient can tolerate fluids and foods, he is offered a diet adequate in energy and nutrients to meet his needs to insure proper wound healing and a return to his normal activities. (See the discussion about monitoring food acceptance in this section.)

When the gastrointestinal tract cannot be used for any extensive period of time after surgery, e.g., after massive bowel resection after a mesenteric infarct, hyperalimentation through a catheter inserted into the superior vena cava during surgery is used.[2] The *hyperalimentation* solution contains fluids, electrolytes, minerals, vitamins, dextrose, and a source of nitrogen and is prepared under sterile conditions in the pharmacy; its administration is monitored by the physician.

PROTEIN. The loss of cell body mass accompanied by a negative nitrogen balance during the catabolic phase is poorly understood. In severe trauma as much as 30 grams of nitrogen, equivalent to 2 pounds of muscle tissue, can be lost in one day.[3] Significant losses of protein can also occur as a result of blood losses during surgery or trauma and because of atrophy of bone and muscle in the immobilized patient.

The negative nitrogen balance of the catabolic phase is generally attributed to the breakdown of amino acids to supply substrate for the gluconeogenic pathway with the urinary excretion of nitrogen as urea and ammonia. However, the recent work of O'Keefe and Sender suggests that the reaction to moderate stress involves a decrease in the rate of cellular protein synthesis without an acute rise in the rate of protein breakdown.[4]

Protein metabolism during the catabolic phase of the metabolic reactions to surgery and trauma is presently under intensive study. The focus of this research is on whether or not intravenous solutions of amino acids, alone or in combination with dextrose, administered in the immediate postoperative period are effective in reversing the negative nitrogen balance of the stress reaction.[5] However, Moore writes that an early intravenous source of amino acids is not required for wound healing in the catabolic phase.[6]

The critical factor is the return to adequate oral alimentation in a reasonable period of time postoperatively. On the other hand, a prolonged period of time postoperatively without adequate energy and nutrient intake (starvation) does have adverse effects on all aspects of recovery from surgery or trauma. Therefore, the postoperative patient must be monitored carefully by the medical team for his readiness for, and his acceptance of, oral fluids and foods to support a positive nitrogen balance during the anabolic phase.

MINERALS AND VITAMINS. Wound healing requires adequate supplies of minerals, trace elements, and vitamins as well as energy and amino acids. For example, the synthesis of collagen, which is a basic process of wound healing, requires vitamin C. Protein synthesis, in general, requires a variety of trace elements and vitamins as well as amino acids. (See Chapter 7, Water-Soluble Vitamins, and Chapter 9, Nutrient Utilization.)

Monitoring Nutritional Care and Food Acceptance

PREOPERATIVE ROUTINES. Whenever possible a careful and extensive diet history and the specific food and fluid likes and dislikes of the patient should be obtained prior to surgery. The diet history is an important component of the assessment of nutritional status before surgery, and the patient's likes and dislikes can be used in menu planning postoperatively.

POSTOPERATIVE ROUTINES. After the return of normal peristalsis, the first oral feeding offered is a clear liquid diet. Clear liquids such as broth and gelatin are used to test the patient's tolerance for fluids by mouth. Clear liquids are also less hazardous if vomiting with aspiration occurs. If clear liquids are well tolerated, the patient may progress to a full liquid diet and then to a soft and finally a regular diet. (See Chapter 22 for a description of these diets.) For some patients the progression is directly from clear liquids to a regular diet.

It must be remembered that the clear liquid diet is nutritionally inadequate in calories, protein, and other nutrients; therefore, such patients should be observed carefully so that they may progress to an adequate diet as soon as it is tolerated. Because of cultural expectations of food for illness, an older patient who could be offered a regular diet after clear liquids may accept a soft diet more readily before progressing to a regular diet. Patients with a concurrent disease such as diabetes mellitus or heart disease should be returned to their appropriate therapeutic regimen. Serious postoperative complications can occur if the appropriate diet is not offered. (See also the section in this chapter on diet therapy after gastrointestinal surgery.)

The acceptance of food and fluid by the postoperative patient must be monitored at each feeding to insure that he achieves an adequate intake of energy and all nutrients to support his metabolic needs in order to avoid postoperative malnutrition and its sequelae.[7] Whenever necessary, an estimate of the patient's energy and nutrient intake for the previous 24 hours should be recorded in his medical record each morning. This information should be available as part of the assessment of the patient's progress toward recovery.

In some instances the nutritional needs of a patient may be met by a combination of oral feedings and hyperalimentation. This regimen is used in preparation for discontinuing hyperalimentation. The kinds and amounts of fluids and foods to be offered to the patient are planned jointly by the physician and dietitian; the physician is responsible for determining the amount of hyperalimentation solution given each day. When this occurs the energy and nutrient intake by mouth must be recorded daily (preferably at each feeding) to avoid an imbalance in the intake of energy, nitrogen, and electrolytes. Therefore, the electrolytes, as well as the energy and nutrients provided by the oral feedings, must be estimated and recorded.

PREPARATION FOR DISCHARGE. Before discharge it should be ascertained that the postoperative patient is selecting and consuming a diet totally adequate to promote full recovery; and he should be counseled to continue these practices at home without gaining excessive weight during the fat gain phase.

Because many patients become fatigued easily for a period after surgery, attention should be given to the home situation. Special care should be taken to identify the mother with a large family or the individual who lives alone. Such individuals may need assistance after discharge with food buying and preparation at home. Otherwise their recovery may be delayed. If relatives or friends are not available to assist them, a home health aide can be requested to help two or three times a week, or daily if required. For the patient over 65 this service is provided by Medicare. Some of these individuals may need to transfer to an extended-care facility before returning to their own homes. The social worker can assist the nurse and the dietitian in these situations.

TUBE FEEDINGS

Feeding by nasogastric, gastric, or jejunal tube is used when it is not possible for the patient to take food otherwise. This may occur when there is an obstruction in the esophagus or after surgery for oral or esophageal cancer; when the esophagus and, in some cases, the stomach has been injured by strong alkali solutions; after gastrectomy for cancer; or when the patient is recovering from trauma to the head or a cerebral vascular accident (stroke). The tube feeding must be liquid, yet contain reasonable proportions of all the nutrients essential for adequate nutrition, especially if it is to be used permanently or over a considerable period of time.

There are three general types of tube feedings: (1) primarily a milk-base solution; (2) a milk-base solution with suspended solids from strained or blenderized foods; and (3) low residue and elemental tube feedings. Commercial preparations of all types are generally available and used by hospitals.

Nutrient Composition of Tube Feedings

CALORIES. Standard tube feedings, prepared in the hospital or obtained from commercial sources, contain approximately 1 calorie per milliliter. Therefore, 1500 ml. of standard tube feeding contain 1500 calories, and 2000 ml. contain 2000 calories. Tube feedings can be prepared which contain ½ calorie per milliliter or 1½ calories per milliliter. The more dilute feeding (½ calorie per milliliter) is generally used as the first feeding to test tolerance. The more concentrated feeding (1½ calorie per milliliter) is used to rehabilitate the nutritionally debilitated patient.
PROTEIN, FAT, AND CARBOHYDRATE. Tube feedings should contain reasonable proportions of protein, fat, and carbohydrate. Whole milk, which contains approximately ⅔ calorie per milliliter, evaporated milk, nonfat dry milk solids, pasteurized powdered egg, liquefied meats (baby foods), and various carbohydrates are used to provide the protein, fat, and carbohydrate in standard nasogastric and gastric tube feedings.

Table 26-1 gives the ingredients and nutrient analyses of 1000 ml. of an inexpensive, standard tube feeding containing one calorie per ml., 100 calories per 100 ml., or 1000 calories per 1000 ml. (1 quart). This feeding contains 42 g. of protein, 55 g. of fat, and 94 g. of carbohydrate per 1000 ml. Two thousand ml. of this feeding contains 2000 calories, 84 g. of protein, 110 g. of fat and 188 g. of carbohydrate.

Table 26-2 gives the ingredients and nutrient analysis of a blenderized tube feeding containing 1 calorie per ml., 100 calories per 100 ml., or 1000 calories per 1000 ml. (1 quart). This feeding contains 50 g. of protein, 46 g. of fat and 106 g. of carbohydrate per 1000 ml. It has been observed that blenderized tube feedings are better tolerated than the standard, milk-based, solution.
MINERALS AND VITAMINS. Both the standard and the blenderized tube feedings require supplementation with thiamine. The standard formula requires supplementation with vitamin C and iron if a liquefied meat other than liver is used. In some hospitals the vitamins are added during the preparation of the tube feeding; in others, the vitamins are ordered and given to the patient as medication.

Commercial Tube Feedings

Table 26-3 gives the composition of energy and selected nutrients per 100 ml. of commercial products representative of the types of tube feedings available in 1974. (These values will not apply if the product is modified in the future.) The energy and nutrient values were calculated for 100 ml. from the producers' information because tube feedings are commonly administered in 100-ml. units, e.g., 300 to 400 ml. per feeding. Therefore, the 100-ml. unit can be used to estimate the nutritional value of one feeding or of the total amount administered in a 24-hour period. If estimates of other electrolytes, trace minerals, and other vitamins are required, these values can be calculated from the product label.

Table 26-4 lists the basic ingredients, exclusive of the minerals and vitamins, in each product in Table 26-3. It will be noted that two standard tube feedings, Ensure and Isocal, are lactose-free. These products are used to avoid diarrhea and other gastrointestinal tract disturbances in patients with a history of milk intolerance or lactase deficiency. Vivonex Standard and High Nitrogen are elemental diets containing nutrients in a readily absorbable form—highly purified amino acids, essential fatty acid, glucose, and glucose oligosaccharides. These two products are used when a major portion of the gastrointestinal tract has been removed during surgery (short bowel syndrome), or when an excessive amount of protein has been lost, such as in extensive second- and third-degree burns.

With the exception of Vivonex High Nitrogen, the feedings listed in Table 26-3 are also useful beverages as nutritional supplements to a regular diet. The strong taste of the purified amino acids in Vivonex High Nitrogen, which is difficult to mask with flavorings, makes this product unacceptable as a beverage. The smaller quantity of amino acids and the flavorings in Vivonex Standard make this a more palatable beverage.

Special Considerations

FIRST FEEDING. To avoid adverse reactions to tube feeding, such as gastric distention and diarrhea, the first feeding should be dilute—½ to ⅔ calorie per milliliter. The standard tube feeding can be diluted with water to ½ calorie per milliliter; or whole milk, if tolerated, at ⅔ calorie per milliliter can be used for the first feeding.

The volume of the first feeding should be re-

Table 26-1. Standard Tube Feeding (1 calorie per milliliter)

FOOD	WEIGHT IN G.	HOUSE-HOLD MEASURE	ENERGY (Calories)	PROTEIN (g.)	FAT (g.)	CARBO-HYDRATE (g.)	CALCIUM (g.)	IRON (mg.)	VITAMIN A (IU)	THIA-MINE (mg.)	RIBO-FLAVIN (mg.)	NIACIN (mg.)	VITAMIN C (mg.)
Evaporated milk	400	1 can	548	28.0	31.6	38.6	1.000	0.4	1,280	0.16	1.36	0.8	4.0
Corn syrup	70	¼ c.	200	..	..	52.5	0.030	2.7	..	..	..	..	..
Puréed liver*†	100	1 jar	94	14.0	3.1	2.4	0.006	6.8	25,655	0.057	2.25	9.4	27.4
Corn oil	20	1½ tbsp.	177	..	20.0	..	..	..	..	..	..	..	..
Water—add to make 1000 ml.													
Totals per 1000 ml.			1,019	42.0	54.7	93.5	1.036	9.9	26,935	0.217	3.61	10.2	31.4
Totals per 100 ml.			102	4.2	5.5	9.4	0.104	1.0	2,694	0.022	0.36	1.0	3.1

*Strained baby food.
†Other baby meats can be used, but there is a decrease in mineral and vitamin content.
DIRECTIONS: Place all ingredients in a mechanical blender and mix 10 minutes. Place in sterile containers, label and refrigerate immediately. Shake well before pouring.

Table 26-2. Blenderized Tube Feeding

FOOD	WEIGHT IN G.	HOUSEHOLD MEASURE	ENERGY (Calories)	PROTEIN (g.)	FAT (g.)	CARBOHYDRATE (g.)	CALCIUM (g.)	IRON (mg.)	VITAMIN A (IU)	THIAMINE (mg.)	RIBOFLAVIN (mg.)	NIACIN (mg.)	VITAMIN C (mg.)
Milk, whole	244	1 c	160	8.5	8.5	12	0.288	0.2	350	0.08	0.42	0.2	2
Dry skim milk (instant)	16	2 tbsp.	58	6.0	..	8	0.206	0.2	..	0.06	0.62	0.2	2
Cream, 20%	100	½ c.	211	3.0	21.0	4	0.102	..	840	0.03	0.15	0.1	1
Egg, pasteurized powder*	30	4 tbsp.	163	13.0	12.0	1	0.054	2.3	1,180	0.11	0.30	0.1	..
Corn syrup	70	½ c.	200	..	..	52.5	0.030	2.7	..	..	..	..	..
Strained pears†	70	½ jar	48	0.2	..	11.5	0.007	0.2	26	0.09	0.10	0.3	..
Strained peas†	70	½ jar	38	2.8	..	6.3	0.007	0.8	350	0.05	0.06	0.7	7
Strained beef	100	6 tbsp.	99	15.0	4.0	..	0.008	2.0	..	0.01	0.16	3.5	..
Orange juice	100	½ c.	45	1.0	..	11.0	0.009	0.1	200	0.09	0.01	0.3	45
Water, add to make 1000 ml.													
Totals per 1000 ml.			1,022	49.5‡	45.5	106.3	0.711	8.5	2,946	0.52	1.82	5.4	57
Totals per 100 ml.			102	5.0	4.6	10.6	0.07	0.85	295	0.052	0.18	0.5	5.7

*Pasteurized powdered egg is used to avoid salmonella. Fifteen g. is equivalent to one egg.
†Strained baby foods. These can be changed daily. This alters nutrient composition somewhat.
‡Can be increased, if necessary, by addition of protein supplement.

DIRECTIONS: Place all ingredients in a mechanical blender and mix 10 minutes. Strain, place in sterile containers, label and refrigerate immediately. Shake well before pouring.

Table 26-3. Energy and Nutrient Composition of 100 ml. Commercial Tube Feeding* Compared with 100 ml. Whole Milk

Energy and Nutrients	Whole Milk	MILK-BASED FEEDINGS			LACTOSE-FREE FEEDINGS		BLENDERIZED FEEDINGS		LOW-RESIDUE FEEDINGS			MCT OIL LACTOSE-FREE	AVAILABLE NITROGEN FROM AMINO ACIDS	
		Meritene Liquid	Nutri-1000	Susta-cal	Ensure	Isocal	Compleat-B	Formula 2	Flexical	Precision LR	Precision High Nitrogen	Portagen	Vivonex Standard	Vivonex High Nitrogen
Energy (kcal.)	65	100	100	100	106	104	100	100	100	131.9	125	100	100	100
Protein (g.)	3.5	6	3.25	6.0	3.7	3.37	4.0	3.75	2.2	2.9	5.2	3.5	0.33†	0.66†
Fat (g.)	3.5	3.3	5.5	2.3	3.7	4.37	4.0	4.0	3.4	0.1	0.06	4.5	0.145	0.07
Cho (g.)	5.0	11.5	10.6	13.8	14.5	13.0	12.0	12.1	15.5	29.8	29.9	11.4	22.1	21.0
Calcium (mg.)	118.0	141.7	115.0	100.0	42.0	63.0	62.0	130.0	50.0	55.0	33.0	100.0	44.0	26.6
Iron (mg.)	tr.	1.7	0.6	1.6	0.95	0.94	1.1	1.5	0.5	1.25	0.75	1.8	0.55	0.33
Sodium (mg.)	50.0	91.7	50.0	92.5	74.0	50.0	137.5	45.0	35.0	83.0	116.6	60.0	86.0	77.1
Potassium (mg.)	140.0	166.7	140.0	205.5	127.0	130.0	143.5	210.0	150.0	104.0	108.3	150.0	116.9	70.2
Vitamin A (IU)	140.0	415	250.0	464.0	265.0	260.0	312.0	50.0‡	250.0	340.0	208.0	400.0	277.0	166.0
Thiamine (mcg.)**	30.0	166	100.0	139.0	170.0	200.0	87.5	70.0	70.0	139.0	83.0	150.0	66.6	40.0
Riboflavin (mcg.)	170.0	166	100.0	166.0	180.0	225.0	106.0	120.0	85.0	139.0	83.0	180.0	66.6	40.0
Niacin (mg.)	0.1	0.8	0.75	2.0	2.1	2.6	0.62	1.0	0.9	1.3	0.42	1.8	0.74	0.44
Ascorbic A. (mg.)	1.0	8.0	5.0	5.5	16.0	15.6	4.0	5.0	5.0	5.0	2.5	8.0	3.8	2.3

*Calculated from producers' information.
†Available nitrogen in form of highly purified amino acids.
‡Preformed vitamin A only. Adequate carotene present.
**1 mcg. = 0.001 mg.

Table 26-4. Major Ingredients in Tube Feedings Listed in Table 26-3

PRODUCT	PRODUCER	MAJOR INGREDIENTS
Meritene Liquid	Doyle Pharmaceutical Co., Minneapolis, Minn. 94710	Concentrated sweet skim milk, corn syrup solids, vegetable oil, sodium caseinate, sucrose . . . salt . . . Chocolate flavor also includes cocoa, cellulose flour . . .
Nutri-1000	Syntex Laboratories, Inc., Palo Alto, Ca. 94304	Skim milk, corn oil, sucrose, corn syrup solids . . .
Sustacal Liquid	Mead Johnson Laboratories, Mead Johnson & Co., Evansville, Ind. 47721	Concentrated sweet skim milk, sugar, partially hydrogenated soy oils, sodium caseinate, corn syrup solids . . . salt . . .
Ensure	Ross Laboratories, Division of Abbott Laboratories, Columbus, Oh. 43216	Water, corn syrup solids, sucrose, corn oil, sodium and calcium caseinate, soy protein isolate . . .
Isocal	Mead Johnson Laboratories	Corn syrup solids, soy oil, sodium caseinate, MCT oil, soy protein isolate . . .
Compleat-B	Doyle Pharmaceutical Co.	Deionized water, maltodextrin, beef purée, green bean purée, pea purée, nonfat dry milk, corn oil, sucrose, peach purée, reconstituted orange juice . . .
Formula 2	Cutter Laboratories Inc., Berkeley, Ca. 94710	Water, nonfat dry milk, beef, sucrose, carrots, corn oil, orange juice concentrate, egg yolks, green beans, farina . . .
Flexical	Mead Johnson Laboratories	Sucrose, corn syrup solids, enzymatically hydrolyzed casein, soy oil, tapioca starch, MCT oil . . .
Precision LR	Doyle Pharmaceutical Co.	Maltodextrin, pasteurized egg white solids, sugar . . . vegetable oil . . .
Precision High Nitrogen	Doyle Pharmaceutical Co.	Maltodextrin, pasteurized egg white solids, sugar . . . vegetable oil . . .
Portagen	Mead Johnson Laboratories	Corn syrup solids, sugar, MCT oil, sodium caseinate, corn oil . . .
Vivonex Standard	Eaton Laboratories, Division of Morton-Norwich Products, Inc., Norwich, N. Y. 13815	Purified amino acids, linoleic acid, glucose, glucose oligo-saccharides . . .
Vivonex High Nitrogen	Eaton Laboratories	Purified amino acids, linoleic acid, glucose, glucose oligo-saccharides . . .

stricted to 40 to 60 ml. administered in one hour. A drip meter attached to the feeding tube is used to control the flow. Most patients tolerate tube feedings best when the feeding has been warmed to room temperature. If the first feeding is well tolerated, the next feedings can be increased by 50 to 100 ml. increments up to the volume per feeding—usually 300 to 400 ml. every three to four hours.

The dilute feeding should be continued for approximately 24 hours. If the patient tolerates the dilute feeding without gastric distress or diarrhea, feedings containing 1 calorie per milliliter can be used. However, if diarrhea occurs with the more concentrated feedings, the dilute feeding should be continued. For the comfort of the patient and to avoid adverse reactions, all feedings by tube should be given slowly.

RECORDING INTAKE. After the feeding is given, the amount and type should be recorded separately from the water used to test the patency of the tube or to give medications. Only when this is done can the adequacy of the calorie and nutrient intake of a patient be appraised with any degree of accuracy.

HAZARDS OF TUBE FEEDING. There are three major hazards of tube feeding: (1) contamination of the feeding leading to gastrointestinal infection; (2) too concentrated a feeding (hypertonic), particularly in protein and sodium, leading to diarrhea and dehydration and an elevated blood urea nitrogen level; and (3) diarrhea and other gastrointestinal problems due to lactose intolerance.

To avoid contamination, the tube feeding made by the dietary department should be prepared daily under clean conditions and delivered to the refrigerator in the patient area in sterile containers. To open commercial tube feedings that are packaged in cans, a sterile opener must be used. After the appropriate amount for a feeding has been measured out, the supply of feeding should immediately be refrigerated. With the exception of an unopened can of a commercial product, all tube feedings that have been in the refrigerator for 24 hours are discarded.

An excessive intake of protein and sodium without adequate fluid intake can lead to dehydration with hypernatremia and an elevated blood urea nitrogen (BUN) level. This is particularly hazardous for older patients with impaired renal function.[8] Therefore, when a tube feeding for an older patient provides more than 1½ to 2 g. of protein per kilogram of body weight per day, the fluid intake and output should be carefully measured and recorded daily, and the intake of protein in grams per kilogram of body weight should also be recorded daily in the patient's chart. Too concentrated a feeding can also result if the commercial products which come in powdered or concentrated form are not reconstituted according to the producers' directions.

If watery diarrhea occurs in a patient receiving a tube feeding that has been administered correctly, it may be due to the carbohydrate content. Excessive amounts of milk and, therefore, lactose may cause diarrhea in some patients. In this case a feeding which is lactose-free should be used. A careful diet history prior to surgery will often identify these individuals so that this problem can be avoided with the first feeding.

DIET THERAPY AFTER GASTROINTESTINAL SURGERY
Diet After Gastric and Duodenal Surgery

The patient whose gastric or duodenal ulcer does not respond to medical treatment is the most common candidate for gastric surgery. He may have a vagotomy and pyloroplasty or partial gastrectomy and vagotomy.

PRINCIPLES OF POSTOPERATIVE DIET THERAPY. There are various approaches to the feeding of patients after gastric surgery. Two principles appear to apply to all routines: (1) the restriction of the total volume of any feeding during the immediate postoperative period, with gradual increases as tolerated; and (2) the restriction of concentrated carbohydrate, particularly excessive amounts of sucrose, and in some situations, lactose.

After peristalsis has returned and the patient has tolerated clear fluids by mouth—beginning with 30 ml. per feeding on the first day and increasing to 60 ml. on the second day—the patient is offered six to eight small feedings of soft or solid foods, neither very hot nor very cold.[9] A small feeding in this situation may be limited to 3 or 4 ounces increasing gradually to 8 to 10 ounces. For example, one poached egg and one slice of buttered toast is approximately 3 ounces of food.

Fluids including milk may or may not be included in the small frequent feedings. After gastric surgery the contents of the stomach may pass into the small intestine before it is in proper solution and cause distention of the jejunum. When this happens the patient complains of nausea, cramps, diarrhea, lightheadedness, and extreme weakness. This occurs 15 to 30 minutes after meals and is known as early dumping syndrome. It has been observed that this occurs less frequently if the patient avoids too much fluid with his meals.[10]

It has also been observed that excessive amounts of carbohydrate, especially sucrose and in some patients lactose, cause the early dumping syndrome. Therefore, sucrose is usually restricted in the diet of the patient immediately after gastric surgery. Candies, jams, jellies, frosted cakes, and beverages sweetened with sucrose are not used. After recovery from gastric surgery many patients tolerate moderate amounts of sugar.

Some but not all individuals, after gastric surgery, develop lactose intolerance; therefore, some clinicians exclude milk after surgery.[11] However, other clinicians exclude milk only after the patient has experienced distention and diarrhea that are relieved by the exclusion of milk.

Nutritional Care of the Patient After Gastric Surgery

Table 26-5 lists the foods used after gastric surgery. These foods can be used in six to eight small meals. If any of the foods listed were not well toler-

Table 26-5. Foods Used After Gastric Surgery

Milk*

Eggs and Cheese
  Eggs—boiled, poached, scrambled, or omelets
  Cottage cheese

Meat, Fish, Poultry
  Any type—baked, broiled, boiled, or in simple mixed dishes

Potato, Rice, Macaroni, Spaghetti, Noodles
  Plain or in simple mixed dishes

Bread, Crackers
  Enriched white bread and rolls toasted or plain in sandwiches
  Saltines and other plain crackers

Vegetables†
  Soft cooked vegetables

Fruits
  Cooked or well-drained canned fruit

Fat
  Butter, margarine, mayonnaise, bacon, and cream cheese

Desserts
  Cooked or well-drained canned fruit
  Baked custard or plain vanilla pudding*

---

*If tolerated.
†Avoid gas-forming vegetables. These are cabbage, cauliflower, brussels sprouts, broccoli, cucumbers, onions, turnips, and radishes.

ated by the patient before surgery, it is advisable to avoid them in the postoperative period.

Patients should be observed closely to check their food acceptance so that the volume of food in a meal can be increased as tolerated. Most patients after recovery from gastric surgery eventually eat normal amounts of food at a meal, but they should be advised to increase the amount of food at each meal slowly after discharge. As the volume consumed at each meal increases, the number of meals can be decreased from 6-8 to 4-5.

One dietitian who works closely with patients after gastric surgery tests each one's tolerance for concentrated carbohydrate before discharge.[12] She serves a sweet such as cake, ice cream, or jelly with toast at one meal and observes the patient's tolerance carefully.

Late Dumping Syndrome or
Postgastrectomy Hypoglycemia

A few patients develop severe dumping syndrome after gastric surgery. After taking sugar by mouth they have an elevated blood glucose level (hyperglycemia). This is followed by a precipitous drop of blood glucose to below normal levels (hypoglycemia) at which time the patient is dizzy, feels faint, and is nauseated. These patients usually have diarrhea and lose weight. They find it difficult to maintain a normal weight status.

A high-protein, high-fat, low-carbohydrate diet is usually well tolerated by these patients. One diet plan that has been used successfully contains 20 meat exchanges, 20 fat exchanges, 4 bread exchanges, 3 fruit exchanges, and 2 vegetable exchanges[13] (see Chapter 23). The food is served in six meals without fluids. One cup of coffee or tea with 40 percent cream is served one hour before breakfast, lunch, and dinner. If possible, medications requiring water should also be given one hour before meals.

The dietitian plans the diet with these patients daily and the nurse should report to her any symptoms of the dumping syndrome the patient may have.

After the severe symptoms of the syndrome are controlled, individual patients may tolerate an increase in complex carbohydrate such as bread, potatoes, and other starches but may need to avoid using sugar in any form. These individuals may also be lactose-intolerant and need to exclude all milk from their diets.

Bowel Surgery

Many patients require surgery in other sections of the gastrointestinal tract. This may be small or large bowel resection, hemorrhoidectomy, or ileostomy or colostomy.

POSTOPERATIVE NUTRITIONAL CARE. Postoperatively, after testing with clear liquids, these patients are usually given a residue-restricted diet. They progress from a minimal to a moderate residue diet. (See the residue-restricted diet plans in Table 25-10.)

Most patients with colostomies are able before long to return to their regular food practices, provided that these are adequate for their nutritional needs. They should omit foods that were not well tolerated before surgery, but no food is contraindicated once the patient has recovered from the operation.

The ileostomy patient may present a special problem. If a significant portion of the terminal ileum has been removed, there is a decrease in vitamin B_{12} absorption because it is absorbed in the terminal ileum. In this case it may be necessary to give vitamin B_{12} parenterally. After recovery from surgery, the ileostomy patient is able to tolerate a regular diet, although he may be advised to avoid excessive roughage which has in some patients obstructed the stoma.

SHORT BOWEL SYNDROME. In some situations a large portion of the ileum may be removed at surgery. Because of a decrease in the amount of absorptive surface, these individuals often have difficulty maintaining a reasonable nutritional status. Depending on the extent of the bowel surgery the nutritional needs of these patients may be met postoperatively by venous hyperalimentation or by an elemental tube feeding (Vivonex Standard or High Nitrogen). An elemental tube feeding is used for oral alimentation because the nutrients in these feedings are absorbed primarily in the terminal duodenum and the proximal jejunum. Dilute feedings administered with a drip meter are used first, followed by an increase in concentration as tolerated by the individual patient (see section on tube feedings).

It has been observed in some patients with extensive small bowel resection that, with time, there is hypertrophy of the remaining mucosa of the small intestine resulting in a larger absorptive surface. At this point these patients may respond to a diet of *small* frequent feedings high in protein and carbohydrate and relatively low (60 to 80 g.) in fat. Medium chain triglycerides* have been used in such diets to supply energy, but in general the results have not been satisfactory.

NUTRITION FOLLOWING BURNS

Patients with extensive burns present nutritional problems much more far-reaching even than those

*MCT Oil, Mead Johnson Laboratories, Evansville, Ind.

who have undergone major surgery. As a result of the stress reaction there is massive loss of fluids and electrolytes, and serum proteins are lost by exudation from the burned areas. There is extensive tissue breakdown, lasting for periods of weeks as evidenced by tremendous losses of nitrogen and potassium in the urine. Such nitrogen losses continue for the first 30 days, then gradually diminish as healing takes place. There is also severe heat loss from the burn area, as shown by the rate of oxygen consumption. The energy losses may be as crucial to the ultimate survival of the patient as the loss of protein.

The early part of treatment consists of the intravenous administration of dextrose and electrolyte solutions and blood plasma. When the patient can take oral feeding, he is given a high-calorie, high-protein diet or tube feeding or both. Greatly increased amounts of ascorbic acid (to aid in wound healing) and the B vitamins (to meet tremendously increased metabolic demands) and two times the allowance of the fat-soluble vitamins should be given as medication.

If flames or fumes have been inhaled, injuring the respiratory and the gastrointestinal tracts, or if there are burns about the mouth and the face, the oral route of feeding may at first be impossible. Oral or tube feeding may be further contraindicated, as badly burned patients frequently have gastrointestinal atony the first few days after injury.

If tube feeding is used as the first oral feeding, excessive protein without adequate water intake, especially in children, should be avoided (see Hazards of Tube Feeding in this chapter).

When food can be eaten in adequate quantities, between-meal feedings of high-calorie, high-protein beverages are used (see Table 26-3). Because the burn patient may develop gastric hemorrhage, it is advisable to give tube feedings spread evenly over the 24-hour period or serve frequent small meals and between-meal beverages.

To estimate the energy needs of adults Curreri and coworkers recommend 25 kcal. times weight in kilograms plus 40 kcal. times percent of total body surface burned.[14] Using this formula a 70-kg. man with a 40 percent burn would require 3350 kcal. per day. $(25 \times 70 + 40 \times 40 = 3350$ kcal.) Depending on the severity and extent of the burn and on age, a child may require 70 to 100 calories per kilogram and 3 to 5 g. of protein per kilogram of body weight.

There is a tremendous need for supportive care of the severely burned patient by nurses, doctors, dietitians, and all others with whom he comes in contact. The importance of the greatly increased need for food must be carefully explained to the patient. The diet particularly must be individualized to meet his needs and desires, and close cooperation by all who care for him is essential to meet his nutritional and emotional needs.

STUDY QUESTIONS AND ACTIVITIES

1. With the help of members of the nursing team, keep a record of the kinds and amounts of clear liquids consumed in a 24-hour period by a postoperative patient. Using Table 1 in Section 4, estimate this patient's 24-hour energy and nutrient intake. Was it nutritionally adequate for him?
2. Using Table 26-5, plan eight small meals for a patient who has had gastric surgery. Describe the size of serving of each food item.
3. What food may be poorly tolerated after gastric surgery? Why?
4. What are some possible causes of diarrhea in the tube-fed patient? How may it be prevented?
5. Obtain from the dietitian the kinds and nutrient composition of the high-calorie, high-protein beverages served to burn patients or any other patient receiving a similar beverage. Estimate how much these beverages cost per serving.

SUPPLEMENTARY READINGS

Curreri, P. W., et al: Dietary requirements of patients with major burns. J. Am. Dietet. A. 65:415, 1974.

Christie, D. L., and Ament, M. E.: Dilute elemental diet and continuous infusing technique for management of short bowel syndrome. J. Pediatrics 87:705, 1975.

Daly, J. M., et al: Postoperative oral and intravenous nutrition. Ann. Surg. 180:709, 1974.

Gormican, A., and Liddy, E.: Tube feeding: Practical considerations in prescription and evaluation. Postgrad. Med. 53:71, 1973.

Gormican, A., Liddy, E., and Thrush, L. B., Jr.: Nutritional status of patients after extended tube feeding. J. Am. Dietet. A. 63:247, 1973.

Heird, W. C., and Winters, R. W.: Total parenteral nutrition: The state of the art. J. Pediat. 86:2, 1975.

Hoover, H. C., Jr., et al: Nitrogen-sparing intravenous fluids in postoperative patients. N. Eng. J. Med. 293:172, 1975.

Kark, R. M: Liquid formula and chemically defined diets. J. Am. Dietet. A. 64:476, 1974.

Nealon, T. F., et al: Use of elemental diets to correct catabolic states prior to surgery. Ann. Surg. 180:9, 1974.

Newsome, T., et al: Weight loss following thermal injury. Ann. Surgery 178:215, 1973.

Spivey, J., et al: The effect of environmental temperature and nutritional intake on the metabolic response to abdominal surgery. Br. J. Surg. 59:93, 1974.

Young, E. A., et al: Comparative nutritional analysis of chemically defined diets. Gastroenterology 69:1338, 1975.

For further references see Bibliography in Section 4.

REFERENCES

1. Dudrick, J. S., and Rhoads, J. E.: in *Davis-Christopher Textbook of Surgery*, ed. 10, D. C. Sabison, Jr., ed. Philadelphia, Saunders, 1972, Chapter 7.
2. Heird, W. C., and Winters, R. W.: J. Pediat. 86:2, 1975.
3. Dudrick and Rhoads, op. cit.
4. O'Keefe, S. J. D., and Sender, P. M.: Lancet 2:1035, 1974.
5. Flatt, J. P., and Blackburn, G. L.: Am. J. Clin. Nutr. 27:175, 1974.
6. Moore, F. D.: in Sabison, ed., op. cit., Chapter 2.
7. Butterworth, C. E., Jr.: Nutrition Today 9:4, 1974.
8. Gault, M. H., et al: Ann. Int. Med. 68:788, 1968.
9. Malt, R. A.: Nutrition Today 6:30, 1971.
10. Spiro, H. M.: *Clinical Gastroenterology*. New York, Macmillan, 1970.
11. Malt, op. cit.
12. Personal communication. The Ohio State University Hospital Dietary Department.
13. Spiro, op. cit.
14. Curreri, P. W., et al: J. Am. Dietet. A. 65:415, 1974.

27   weight control

Weight Norms
Obesity
Underweight
Anorexia Nervosa

The *achievement* and the *maintenance* of an appropriate weight status for height, sex, age, and activity throughout the life span are positive approaches to avoiding or delaying many of the health problems associated with obesity. It is estimated that 50 million of the 210 million people in the U. S. are above desirable weight due to overfatness. Some of these individuals are mildly obese while others are moderately to grossly obese. It has been observed that diabetes mellitus and hypertension occur more frequently in obese individuals than in those of normal weight. Although there is not a clear association between obesity and coronary heart disease, the obese individual is apt to experience elevated blood levels of triglycerides and cholesterol. The grossly obese as a group are poor risks for surgery due to adverse reactions to anesthesia. They also experience a variety of skin and skeletal problems. Inappropriate weight status during childhood and adolescence appears to be associated not only with physical problems but also with problems of psychosocial development, and the obese adult in our society faces numerous social pressures. From the magnitude and the complexity of the problems of obesity it is readily apparent that the obese comprise a major portion of the clients served by the nutrition counselor.

At any point in the life-span the achievement and maintenance of an appropriate weight status is client-managed (see Chapter 12). During infancy and childhood weight control is the responsibility of the parents, and throughout the remainder of the life-span it is the responsibility of the individual. From the prevalence and incidence of obesity in our society it is evident that the major task of the nutrition counselor is to affect the food choices of individuals so that they can achieve and maintain an appropriate weight status.

From the formulas and baby foods fed to infants to the meals served older adults in a congregate meals program, the energy value of food is the primary focus in the promotion of proper weight status for any individual. It is also the primary focus in the dietary treatment of individuals with excessive amounts of adipose tissue: i.e., obese individuals with or without diabetes mellitus and/or hyperlipidemias. As pointed out in Chapter 10, the energy value of a food varies primarily according to differences in carbohydrate and fat content. In addition to the total carbohydrate and lipid content of food, the diet therapy for some individuals with obesity requires modifications in the types of carbohydrates and lipids (mono-, di-, and polysaccharides and saturated and polyunsaturated fatty acids and cholesterol) ingested.

Weight norms, obesity, underweight, and anorexia nervosa are discussed in this chapter. Diabetes mellitus and aberrations of lipid metabolism, particularly hyperlipoproteinemia, are presented in Chapters 28 and 29. The reader is advised to review Chapter 8, Energy, and Chapter 9, Nutrient Utilization, particularly the section on the glucose-fatty acid cycle and its hormonal control.

WEIGHT NORMS

The concept of what constitutes correct weight at any point in the life-span has undergone marked revision in recent years. Even today the definition of the terms *normal* or *desirable* weight is sharply debated. To assess the weight status of individuals we have traditionally used height-weight tables as weight norms and continue to do so while numerous investigators attempt to find more precise methods to assess body composition and its relation to weight status.

Height-Weight Tables

The first tables for adults were based on the heights and weights for age of men and women who were life insurance policyholders. The figures in these tables reflected the average weights for height and age of the individuals measured. Since the data showed an increase in weight with age, the recommended weight for height in the tables increased with each age group. For example, it was recommended that a woman 5 feet 4 inches tall weigh 131 pounds at age 30, and 144 pounds at age 55.[1]

In recent years the height-weight tables have been reevaluated and revised. It is now recognized that, when growth in height has been achieved by about age 20, there is no biological need to gain weight in excess of that which is satisfactory for the individual. Also, the best health prognosis is found in individuals who have achieved and maintained a reasonable weight status throughout the life-span.

It must be remembered that body weight is made up of a number of components: fat, muscle, organs, bone, and fluids. In evaluating an individual's weight status the percentage of the weight each one of these components contributes to the total weight is critical. One approach to this problem has been the attempt to classify individuals by body build (frame), using the terms small, medium, and large. These terms reflect Sheldon's somatotypes: the small frame, ectomorphy; the medium frame, mesomorphy; and the large frame, endomorphy.[2] However, as yet there are no commonly accepted clinical criteria for estimating precisely the frame size of an individual to identify his body build. Given two men of the same height, the one with a large frame will normally weigh more than the one with a small frame.

The revised height-weight tables in current use reflect the concern for maintaining over the life-span the weight appropriate for an individual at age 25. The Metropolitan Life Insurance Company's Desirable Weight Tables, published in 1960, give desirable weight ranges for heights for men and women 25 years of age and over, and allow for differences in body frame, which is designated as small, medium, and large. The range for a 5 feet 4 inch woman with a small frame is 108 to 116 pounds; with a medium frame, 113 to 126 pounds; and with a large frame, 121 to 138 pounds (see Table 9, Section 4).

In clinical practice height-weight tables must be used judiciously. For example, a professional football player may be overweight for height due to the size of his muscle mass, while a fifty-year-old woman who is at the correct weight for height and estimated frame may actually be overfat. The measuring equipment must be well maintained and measurements must be taken accurately under standardized conditions (with a minimum of clothes and without shoes).

Growth Charts

Growth charts for children have been discussed in Chapter 18. Growth charts for infants (Fig. 27-1) are also available. As with the adult height-weight tables,

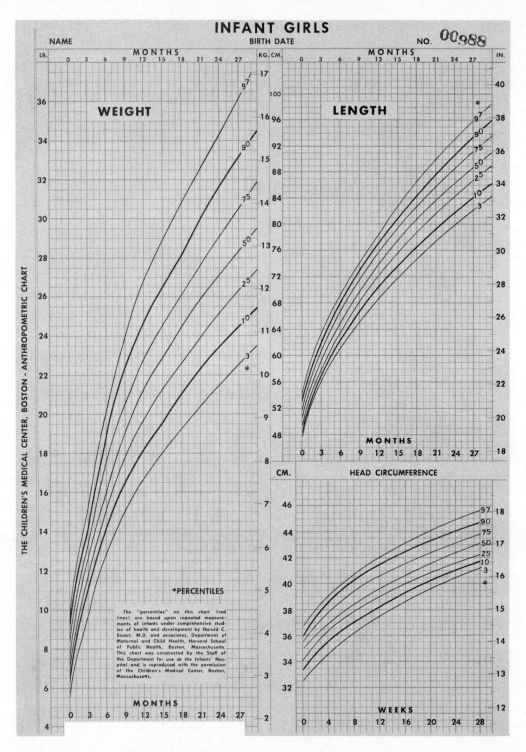

Fig. 27-1. Anthropometric height-weight chart for infant girls. The 50th percentile is the median range. Most infant girls will fall somewhere between the 10th and 90th percentiles. (Children's Medical Center, Boston, Mass.)

the data used to formulate these growth charts were derived from the experiences of healthy infants and children. Up to at least 24 months of age the length of a child is measured in the recumbent (supine) position. The accurate measurement of length, especially in the first months of life, requires the appropriate equipment and two individuals; one to hold the infant's head against the vertical plane of the measuring device and another to extend the normal flexure of an infant's lower extremities and to place the heels against the movable footboard of the measuring device.[3] The scales used to weigh infants (preferably scales which are calibrated in grams and kilograms) must be carefully maintained and accurately read. In addition, the exact age in months derived from the reported birthdate must be used in plotting the data.

Inaccurate data for length, weight, and age plotted on an infant growth chart could create a problem for the clinician where there is none or, equally important, could lead him to missing a problem where there is one. Weighing and measuring an infant or child at appropriate intervals are of more value to the clinician than one set of measurements.

As with adults, the measurement of length and weight of infants and children does not identify body composition or body build. However, when significant discrepancies between length and weight are observed, they must be investigated carefully to identify the cause. For example, it is not unusual to find that an infant at six months of age who is in the 97th percentile for weight and the 30th percentile for length on a growth chart is being overfed. The converse may also be true: a six-month-old infant who is in the 75th percentile for length and below the 10th percentile for weight may have been underfed in the past four to six weeks.

Skinfold Thickness

Brozek and coworkers, Behnke and coworkers, and other investigators are presently studying a variety of sophisticated techniques such as measurements of body density, total body water, or total body potassium to determine body composition.[4] In general these investigations are directed to identifying the nonfat component of the body: that component which is the major determinant of energy and nutrient needs. At present the majority of the techniques used in this research are not adaptable to routine clinical use.

Fat is the component of body composition which has the greatest effect on variations in total body weight during growth in infants and children and after the adult has attained his full growth status. The fat content of individuals of normal weight varies,

according to sex, age, and activity, from 14 to 30 percent of total body weight. Numerous studies have shown that skinfold thickness measurements can be used to estimate the fat content of the body, particularly in adults.

An instrument to measure skinfold thickness is available for clinical use. Calipers are used to measure the thickness of skin and subcutaneous fat, most commonly at the triceps muscle, although other sites may also be used. Figure 27-2 illustrates the measurement of the triceps skinfold thickness at the back of the right upper arm midway between the bony prominence of the shoulder (acromion) and the bony prominence of the elbow (olecranon). Training is required to use the calipers accurately for valid interpretation of the data.

The norms for skinfold thickness measurements are presented in Table 27-1. They are the minimum triceps skinfold thickness measurements, beginning at age five, which indicate obesity. Measurements below these norms indicate the presence of a normal amount of body fat, unless the measurements are very low, which would indicate less than normal amounts of adipose tissue. At present there are no widely accepted norms for infants and children under five years of age in the United States. Karlberg and coworkers in Sweden have developed norms for Swedish children during the first three years of life.[5]

Hopefully in the future more precise height, weight, and skinfold thickness norms will be available which will identify normal weight status with a

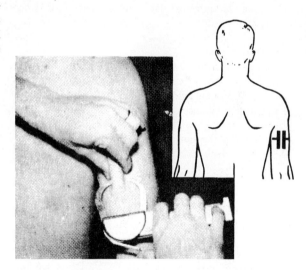

Fig. 27-2. Skinfold measurement at back of upper arm (triceps). (Hertzberg, H. T. E., Churchill, E., Dupertius, C. W., White, R. M., and Damon, A. Aerospace Medical Research Laboratories, U.S.A.F.), *Anthropometric Survey of Turkey, Greece and Italy.* Pergamon Press, 1963, p. 120.

Table 27-1. Obesity Standards in Caucasian Americans*

AGE (Years)	MINIMUM TRICEPS, SKIN FOLD THICKNESS INDICATING OBESITY† (Millimeters)	
	Males	Females
5	12	14
6	12	15
7	13	16
8	14	17
9	15	18
10	16	20
11	17	21
12	18	22
13	18	23
14	17	23
15	16	24
16	15	25
17	14	26
18	15	27
19	15	27
20	16	28
21	17	28
22	18	28
23	18	28
24	19	28
25	20	29
26	20	29
27	21	29
28	22	29
29	22	29
30-50	23	30

*Seltzer, C. C., and Mayer, J.: Postgrad. Med. 38:A101, 1965.
†Figures represent the logarithmic means of the frequency distribution plus one standard deviation.

higher degree of confidence than at present so that the clinician can more readily identify who is, or is not, overfat.

Visual Inspection

In many clinical settings the weight status of an individual can be evaluated by visual inspection. During a physical examination the physician or nurse can observe excessive accumulations of body fat or the lack of body fat. The nutrition counselor can visually identify the overfat or too thin client as he sits beside the desk.

OBESITY

Definition

Although there is as yet no general agreement, the following descriptions of overweight and obesity are being used.

Overweight is "overheaviness," and the term does not carry any direct implication with regard to fatness. *Obesity* is described as a bodily condition marked by excessive generalized deposition or storage of fat in adipose tissue.

Many investigators define obesity as being present in an individual who is 20 percent above the weight for age and sex in the weight tables. Others may use 5 to 10 percent as a criterion. These criteria do not differentiate overfatness from overheaviness. However, until the skinfold thickness measurements are better standardized so that one can estimate the number of pounds or the percentage of total body weight which is fat, we will continue to use weight to define obesity.

Prevalence and Incidence

Obesity is considered a major public health problem today, although there are limited statistics for its general prevalence and incidence in the total population. Mayer observed a 20 percent prevalence of obesity in schoolchildren in a middle-class suburban community.[6] The Ten-State Nutrition Survey reported that the percentage of obese adolescents varied from 11 to 39 percent for white males and from 5 to 33 percent for black males; and from 9 to 19 percent for white females and from 5 to 33 percent for black females.[7]

The highest prevalence in obesity in the Ten-State Nutrition Survey occurred in adult women. Fifty percent of the black women 45 to 55 years of age and 40 percent of the white women 45 to 55 years of age were obese. Obesity was less prevalent in adult males, although 20 percent of white males were found to be obese.

Excessive weight gain occurs more frequently at certain ages or periods in the life-span. As the Ten-State Nutrition Survey indicates, obesity frequently occurs at adolescence in both boys and girls and after age 45 in women. The data collected in 1960-1962 by the National Center for Health Statistics, U. S. Public Health Service, on the heights and weights of adults were not evaluated for desirable, under-, or overweight, but it is interesting to note that the maximum average weight for men occurred between ages 35 to 54 and for women between ages 55 to 64.[8] Of approximately 7500 women 65 years of age and older in the population surveyed, none weighed 230 pounds or over while 208 of approximately 8000 women 55 to 64 years of age weighed 230 pounds or more. Perhaps these statistics are one more piece of evidence of what has already been demonstrated—that overweight shortens life (see Fig. 27-3).

The prevalence of obesity would also appear to be related to social class. The data of Stunkard and coworkers indicates that there is less obesity among the high socioeconomic class, particularly in women, than at a lower socioeconomic level.[9]

It has also been observed that there are two types

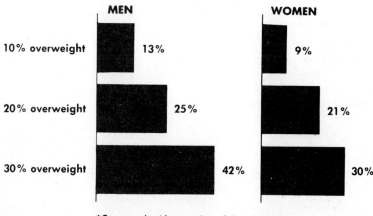

Excess Mortality*

MEN   **WOMEN**

10% overweight   13%   9%

20% overweight   25%   21%

30% overweight   42%   30%

Fig. 27-3. Overweight shortens life. (From Overweight—Its Significance and Prevention. Metropolitan Life Insurance Company. Derived from The Build and Blood Pressure Study, Society of Actuaries, 1959)

*Compared with mortality of Standard risks
(Mortality ratio of Standard risks = 100%)

of obese adults: those who became obese during childhood and adolescence and those who became obese later in life. The time of onset of obesity has implications for therapy and will be discussed later.

Etiology

In previous editions of this book, obesity was attributed with a high degree of confidence to excessive food intake. Today, with the extensive research being reported on ATP utilization and other aspects of energy metabolism,[10] one is less sure of a direct relationship between food intake and obesity. However, if one studies the energy value of the preliminary 1974 figures from the USDA of the food available for civilian consumption (Chapter 10) it is reasonable to equate obesity with food intake.

From the evidence available today it appears that the etiology of obesity is multifactorial. In addition to energy imbalance, derangement of glucose and fat metabolism, genetics, and psychological processes may all contribute to the development of obesity.
ENERGY IMBALANCE (FOOD INTAKE AND PHYSICAL ACTIVITY). Obesity is the result of a positive energy balance and can be due to a daily calorie intake which exceeds the energy needs of an individual. It is generally accepted that a pound of body fat contains approximately 3500 calories. Theoretically an intake in excess of need of even 100 calories a day will add up to 3000 calories a month, or almost one pound of body weight. Over a year this will amount to a weight gain of 10 pounds.

However, not every obese client will report an excessive calorie intake. Energy expenditure is as important as food intake in the development of obesity.

In the past 25 to 50 years, life in the highly developed areas of the world has undergone great changes. Work hours have been shortened, laborsaving machinery has been installed in homes and factories, transportation is easier, homes are well heated, and even our leisure-time activities are sedentary rather than active. This has reduced the energy needs of the body markedly, but, by and large, food habits have not changed sufficiently to offset the decreased need. Although the American breakfast is considerably smaller today than that which our ancestors were accustomed to eating, the coffee break, morning and afternoon, the increased use of sugar, the ubiquitous candy bar, and the TV "snack" (see Table 27-2) have more than compensated for the change in breakfast patterns. Perhaps the energy crises and the inflation of the 1970s will reverse these trends to some extent (see Fig. 27-4).

A number of investigators have observed that the obese person, and particularly the obese child or adolescent, is less active than his counterpart of the same age. Whether this is due to his inability to keep pace with other children or to apathy born of emotional conflict, the inactivity lowers the energy need of the body and in this way contributes to the overweight. This situation is also true of obese women as compared to women of normal weight. In obese men the difference in activity is less striking but still of significance.
METABOLIC AND ENDOCRINE ABERRATIONS (HYPERCELLULARITY AND HYPERINSULINISM). In the past numerous attempts have been made to relate obesity to a disturbance of function of one or more of the endocrine glands, such as the thyroid or

Table 27-2. Energy Values for Common "Snack" Foods*

	AMOUNT OR AVERAGE SERVING	ENERGY (kcal.)
"Just a Little Sandwich"		
Hamburger on bun	3-in. patty	330
Peanut butter sandwich	2 tbsp.	330
Cheese sandwich	1 oz. cheese	280
Ham sandwich	1 oz. ham	320
TV Snack		
Pizza (cheese)	⅛ of 14-in. diam. pie	185
Popcorn with oil and salt	1 c.	40
Pretzel, thin, twisted	1	25
Cheese fondue	½ c.	265
Dips (sour cream)	½ c.	248
Chippers	10	150
Beverages		
Carbonated drinks, soda, root beer, etc.	6-oz. glass	80
Cola beverages	12-oz. glass (Pepsi)	150
Club soda	8-oz. glass	5
Chocolate malted milk	10-oz. glass (1¾ c.)	500
Ginger ale	6-oz. glass	60
Tea or coffee, straight	1 c.	0
Tea or coffee, with 2 tablespoons cream and 2 teaspoons sugar	1 c.	90
Alcoholic Drinks		
Ale	8-oz. glass	155
Beer	8-oz. glass	110
Highball (with ginger ale—ladies' style)	8-oz. glass	185
Manhattan	Average	165
Martini	Average	140
Wine, Muscatel or Port	2-oz. glass	95
Sherry	2-oz. glass	75
Scotch, bourbon, rye	1½-oz. jigger	130
Fruits		
Apple	1 3-in.	75
Banana	1 6-in.	130
Grapes	30 medium	75
Orange	1 2¾-in.	70
Pear	1	65
Salted Nuts		
Almonds, filberts, hazelnuts	12-15	95
Cashews	6-8	90
Peanuts	15-17	85
Pecans, walnuts	10-15 halves	100
Candies		
Chocolate bars,		
Plain, sweet milk	1 bar (1 oz.)	155
With almonds	1 bar (1 oz.)	140
Chocolate-covered bar	1 bar	270
Chocolate cream, bon bon, fudge	1 piece 1-in. square	90-120
Caramels, plain	2 medium	85
Hard candies, Lifesaver type	1 roll	95
Peanut brittle	1 piece 2½ x 2½ x ⅜ in.	110

*Adapted from Smith Kline and French Laboratories

the pituitary. Patients with insufficient thyroid function (hypothyroidism) are usually overweight. However, part of the excess weight is due to fluid retention. These individuals contribute only a small percentage to the total number of overweight persons, and their condition responds to treatment with thyroid hormone.

Following the work of Winick on the effect of an inadequate intake of energy and nutrients on cell division and cell size during infancy (see Chapter 15),

Hirsch and Knittle studied the number and size of adipose cells in obese and nonobese children.[11] They have demonstrated that at all ages obese children have larger and more numerous adipose cells compared to the adipose cells in nonobese children. In similar work with adults Hirsch and Knittle have shown that those subjects with onset of obesity in childhood had significantly more adipose cells than adults who were not obese and who had never been obese at any time in their lives. Some but not all of

Table 27–2. Energy Values for Common "Snack" Foods (Continued)

	AMOUNT OR AVERAGE SERVING	ENERGY (kcal.)
Desserts		
Pie:		
Fruit—apple, etc.	⅙ pie 1 average serving	410
Custard	⅙ pie 1 average serving	265
Mince	⅙ pie 1 average serving	400
Pumpkin pie with whipped cream	⅙ pie 1 average serving	460
Cake:		
Chocolate layer	3-in. section	350
Doughnut, sugared	1 average	150
Sweets		
Ice Cream:		
Plain vanilla	⅙ qt. serving	200
Chocolate and other flavors	⅙ qt., ⅔ c.	260
Orange sherbet	½ c.	120
Sundaes, small chocolate nut with whipped cream	Average	400
Ice-cream sodas, chocolate	10-oz. glass	270
Midnight Snacks for Icebox Raiders		
Cold potato	½ medium	65
Chicken leg (fried)	1 average	88
Glass milk	7-oz. glass	140
Mouthful of roast	½ in. x 2 in. x 3 in.	130
Piece of cheese	¼ in. x 2 in. x 3 in.	120
Leftover beans	½ c.	105
Brownie	¾ in. x 1¾ in. x 2¼ in.	140
Cream puff	4 in. diam.	450

these subjects also had more lipid per cell. These researchers have also demonstrated that with significant weight loss there is a significant decrease in adipose cell size due to loss of lipid, but there is not a concomitant loss in numbers of adipose cells.

The data of Hirsch and Knittle are less clear as to whether or not the onset of obesity in adulthood results in an increase in adipose cell size only or an increase in both size and number. However, the data of Sims and coworkers suggest that the onset of obesity in adults results in an increase in adipose cell size but not in cell number.[12]

The quantity and quality of adipose tissue in obese children and adults have important metabolic consequences. Many obese adults experience elevated blood glucose levels and excessive quantities of insulin in the blood (hyperinsulinemia) in the fasting and postprandial state.[13] The same metabolic aberrations have also been observed in obese children.[14] The prevalence of these occurrences is not known at this time. The analysis of blood insulin levels is a complex and costly laboratory procedure and at present is a research tool that is not widely used in clinical medicine diagnostically.

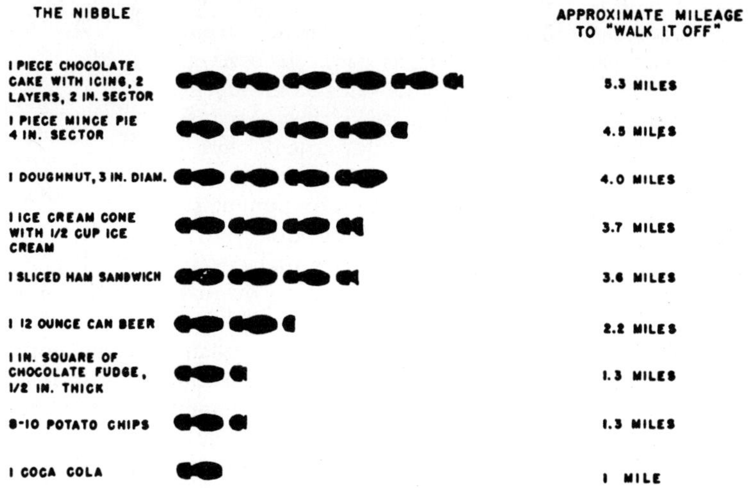

Fig. 27–4. Mileage to walk off that nibble. (Peyton, A. B., *Practical Nutrition*, ed. 2. Philadelphia, Lippincott; adapted from Hauck, H. M., How to control your weight. Ithaca, N. Y., New York State College of Home Economics)

It appears that a significant number of obese subjects with hyperinsulinemia also experience glucose intolerance. Knittle and other investigators suggest that the glucose intolerance is due to an unresponsiveness or resistance to insulin by the muscle and adipose cells.[15] The pathophysiology of this unresponsiveness to insulin is not well understood. The size of the adipose cell in the obese person may be the cause. It has been observed that following significant weight loss with reduction of adipose cell size due to loss of lipid the glucose intolerance improves and the blood levels of insulin return to normal. Sims and coworkers observed the development of glucose intolerance and hyperinsulinemia in a group of healthy men of normal weight after a period of high calorie feeding which led to weight gain and measurable deposition of body fat.[16] When Sims' subjects returned to their usual food practices and lost weight the blood glucose and insulin levels returned to normal. Grey and Kipnis concluded from their observations of a group of hyperinsulinemic obese women that the carbohydrate composition of the diet may be a significant factor in the elevation of blood glucose levels.[17]

It has also been observed that although the glucose-intolerant obese subject is hyperinsulinemic, there is a delayed early secretion of insulin in response to a glucose challenge. The characteristics of blood glucose and insulin levels in response to a glucose challenge (the glucose tolerance test) are discussed in Chapter 28, Diabetes Mellitus.

GENETICS. Genetic factors responsible for the development of obesity have been established in animals but not in humans. However, studies show that overweight and obesity tend to exist as a family pattern. Mayer found that 8 to 9 percent of children of normal weight parents became obese.[18] When one parent is obese, the likelihood of the child's becoming obese is 40 percent; this proportion rises to 80 percent when both parents are obese. It has also been observed that identical twins reared in the same environment have less difference in weight than do fraternal twins; and that the weights of adopted children do not correlate with the weights of their adoptive parents.

While there may be a genetic component in human obesity, in those families where both parents and children are obese the pattern of food intake tends to be excessive and the body image of an overfed person is the preferred one. Such families may eat because excessive food intake has become an established pattern of recreation and sociability, or excessive food intake is used to relieve anxiety or boredom or is a social status symbol.

EMOTIONAL PROBLEMS. The contribution of psychological factors to the etiology of obesity varies with the individual. In some situations psychological characteristics play little or no role while in others they are a major factor. In the latter case it is difficult to discover whether the psychological factors cause the obesity or the obesity causes the psychological problems. For example, does the obese adolescent feel worthless because she is obese or does she become obese because she feels worthless? The most comprehensive presentation of the emotional problems of obesity is found in Bruch's book, *Eating Disorders*.[19]

Stunkard and his coworkers have described a so-called *night-eating* syndrome which occurs in some gravely obese patients.[20] Such patients eat little during the day, but in the evening and in the early night hours they consume large quantities of food. Some of these patients exhibited symptoms of severe emotional stress when an attempt was made to reduce their weight. The investigators concluded that it might be wiser to allow such patients to remain obese than to precipitate an emotional illness with a weight reduction program.

BALANCE BETWEEN HUNGER AND SATIETY. In recent years there has been renewed interest in the physiological control of hunger and satiety. Many individuals maintain a balance between food intake and energy expenditure which keeps their weight comparatively stable over a period of many years. The work of Schachter indicates that eating is triggered by a different set of signals in the obese than in those individuals of normal weight.[21] His experience seems to indicate that in the obese there is no relationship between the state of hunger and eating behavior. Instead such external factors as smell, sight, taste, and other people's actions determine what and when the obese eat.

Campbell, Hashim, and Van Itallie have studied the responses of lean and obese young adults to variation in the nutrient density of a machine-dispensed liquid diet.[22] They observed that the lean subjects adjusted their intake to maintain weight when, unknown to the subjects, the energy content of the diet was adjusted. In contrast, the obese subjects were not able to adjust intake to physiological need when the nutrient density varied. They consumed the same amount of the diet whether it was diluted or concentrated.

Prevention

Successful weight reduction and the maintenance of weight loss are not easily achieved. It is hoped that as we learn more about the causes of obesity, health workers will focus their attention on its prevention at all stages in the life-span.

INFANTS AND CHILDREN. Prevention of obesity begins with the careful supervision of the feeding of infants and children. The physician and other health workers involved with infants and children can all play a role in prevention. The plotting of accurate weights and lengths on a growth chart combined with a dietary interview of the mother gives clues to the development of weight problems in infants and children. During the first year of life weight and length should be plotted on the infant growth chart every six weeks to two months, and at least every six months during childhood.

Effective nutrition counseling of the mother can correct the problem in its earliest stages. At the same time it must be remembered that the weight status of a child may reflect a problem of mother-child interaction and not solely a nutrition problem. Overfeeding in infancy may reflect a mother's inability to differentiate between fussiness and hunger in her infant.

For the school-age child the physical education programs in elementary and secondary schools and in youth groups should be directed to helping all boys and girls develop a lifetime pattern of physical activity. The present emphasis on team sports, which provide activity for only a few students, does not always help the individual to be active in his adult years. Hiking, bicycle tours, cross-country skiing, tennis, and swimming are just five examples of individual activities (see Table 27-3).

Nutrition education including home economics courses can also focus on the prevention of obesity. The recipes used in foods classes should reflect society's need to control the intake of fats and refined sugar. And biology courses which introduce the role of DNA and RNA in human metabolism should also introduce cellular energy metabolism.

ADOLESCENTS. The adolescent presents a special challenge. This is a period in life when peer group behavior competes with parental advice; food plays an important role in the adolescent's socialization. Overly weight-conscious adolescent girls are prone to try crash dieting to control their weight while others establish a lifelong pattern of obesity during this period.

ADULTS. As adults settle into a routine of daily living in their late twenties and early thirties, and if physical activity is limited because of the demands of their employment, a conscious effort should be made to limit energy intake. For many adults this means decreasing their intakes of fats and sugars in such foods as gravies and sauces and high-calorie desserts and snacks, and carefully monitoring their intakes of alcohol and sweetened carbonated beverages. For example, a man who maintained his normal weight at

Table 27-3. Kilocalorie Expenditure for Some Types of Activity*

	70-KG. MAN KCAL./HOUR	58-KG. WOMAN KCAL./HOUR
Painting furniture	200	160
Walking (3 mi./hr.)	240	190
Skating	340	285
Swimming (2 mi./hr.)	685	570

age 20 with a daily intake of 3000 calories may find at age 30 he will maintain his weight on 2500 calories (See NAS-NRC RDA, Table 10-1). The Pattern Dietary (Table 22-1) with reasonable additions of food to maintain weight provides a guide for these individuals.

Both the activity and the time devoted to exercise must be taken into consideration when it is combined with food intake to control body weight. It is a consistent daily pattern of physical activity rather than occasional vigorous activity which is effective in controlling weight. Table 27-3 shows the calories expended by the 70-kg. man (154 pounds) or the 58-kg. woman (128 pounds) in a few activities. It must be noted that these figures apply to a *full hour* of continuous activity. For many adults in our society it is difficult to devote one hour every day to some form of physical activity. A conscious effort to increase activity throughout the day may be possible; for example, walking to a nearby grocery store or newspaper vending machine instead of driving the car, or walking up one or two flights of stairs instead of taking the elevator. In the 1970s to conserve one form of energy one might expend another form of energy by using public transportation, bicycling, or walking. In our society today, however, finding a safe place to walk is often a real problem; many suburban areas have no sidewalks. And bicycling in heavy traffic may also be hazardous.

Controlling weight by diet and exercise is a family affair. Parents have the responsibility for planning and carrying out family activities which promote exercise. The homemaker is often the one who bears the major responsibility for food. If her family has a tendency to gain weight easily or a family history of diabetes mellitus or coronary artery disease, she will have to pass up the recipes in gourmet cookbooks or in the daily newspaper which require ½ pint of whipping cream, 1 pint of sour cream, 12 ounces of cream cheese, or ½ to ¾ pound of butter combined with 1 to 2 cups of sugar. She can, on the other hand, control calories behind the scene by reducing the fat she uses in food preparation by substituting skim milk for whole milk in sauces and puddings and by broiling rather than frying meat with added fat.

The nutrition counselor in a health maintenance organization or any other health-care agency which focuses on preventive health-care services is responsible for reviewing annually the height, weight, and skinfold thickness status of all adults who entered the health-care plan at their desirable weights. Any adult whose measurements show an increase in body weight due to fat in any one year should be scheduled for either individual or group counseling and be helped to lose the excess weight. This approach may uncover problems other than excessive food intake, such as emotional problems or the beginning phase of alcoholism.

Whenever an individual enters the hospital for any reason his height and weight should be measured and recorded as one item in his admission data base. Whenever the weight is 5 percent above ideal weight, the dietitian should identify the cause for this discrepancy in height and weight and, if appropriate, assist this individual to lose weight.

Dietary Treatment

The discussion of the dietary treatment of obesity in this section refers to the adult patient only. Obesity in infants and children is discussed in Chapter 34, Nutrition in Diseases of Infancy and Childhood.

Designing the Diet Order

The diet order is prescribed by the physician and is designed for the individual. It reflects metabolic needs by height, sex, age, and life-style.

PRINCIPLE. Since obesity represents the storage of an excess of energy as lipid in adipose cells, the energy intake must be less than the actual daily expenditure of energy if the body is to draw upon and reduce its surplus of energy stores. To maintain the weight loss, *continuous surveillance* of energy intake is required or the adipose cells will be refilled with excess lipid.

DETERMINATION OF PRESENT PRACTICES. The first step in designing the diet order for an obese patient is to determine how he lives his day, specifically his food and beverage intake and his pattern of physical activity. With the hospitalized patient this information can be obtained, usually by the clinical dietitian, through individual interview (see Chapter 12). The interviewer should schedule one half to three quarters of an hour to collect the information required to appraise the patient's present practices. During the interview, the interviewer can also discover the patient's past experiences with energy-restricted diets and his knowledge of the energy value of foods. In some hospitals the patient is given a self-administered diet history which the nutrition counselor reviews with the patient for clarification. This method cannot be used by patients with visual handicaps or by patients who are functional illiterates.

In the ambulatory care setting, more complete information can be obtained by having the patient who is able keep a detailed diary for one or two weeks. In this diary he should record all his activities of daily living: what he does each hour, when he eats, what and how much he eats, where he eats, with whom he eats, and what he does during mealtime. For example, does he read? watch television? On the patient's return to the ambulatory care facility the nutrition counselor should carefully review the diary with the patient.

With the information gained through interview combined with a self-administered diet history or diary, one can estimate the energy value of the patient's usual food practices and the level of his physical activity. These estimates of energy intake and physical activity are used to design a diet which should promote weight loss.

CALORIES. Considerable difficulty may be encountered in determining the appropriate level of reduced energy intake for an individual patient. His previous intake may have been underestimated, or his energy expenditure overestimated. Because it is difficult to estimate correctly the quantity of fat in meals or the amounts added to season food, 200 to 300 calories should be added to the estimate of a patient's usual calorie intake to prevent underestimation. For example, if the appraisal of a patient's usual food intake is 2300 calories per day, it is probable that his actual intake is 2500 to 2600 calories.

In theory, without an increase in activity, a deficit in intake of 500 calories per day, compared with previous intake, should promote a weight loss of approximately 1 pound per week. (500 calories × 7 = 3500 calories = 1 pound of fat.) A relatively sedentary obese woman 55 years old and 5 feet 4 inches tall, who has been consuming approximately 1700 calories per day, should lose weight on a 1200-calorie diet, while a sedentary obese business executive 35 years old and 6 feet tall, who has been consuming 2500 to 3000 calories should lose weight on a 2000-calorie diet. Unfortunately the rate of weight loss tends to decrease with the duration of the restriction of energy intake because reduced energy intake produces some loss of lean body mass as well as fat. At this point energy expenditure tends to equal energy intake. Therefore, it can be anticipated that a patient may need to reduce his energy intake further to reach his goal.

A deficit of 1000 calories per day should promote a loss of 2 pounds per week. It is considered unwise for an individual to lose more than 2 pounds per week unless he is under the close supervision of the physician. It is also considered unwise for a patient to attempt to maintain a diet of less than 1000 calories per day unless he is hospitalized.

Some physicians will calculate the level of calorie restriction for a patient by multiplying the patient's ideal weight, obtained from a height-weight table, by a factor of 10 calories. For example, the physician would prescribe a 1500-calorie diet for a patient whose ideal weight is 150 pounds.

Regardless of the level of calorie restriction prescribed by the physician, it must be recognized that, through variations in daily food selection and serving size, the actual calorie intake at home will not be exactly the number of calories ordered. For example a 1200-calorie diet may vary by chance from 1000 to 1400 calories. Also, physical activity will vary from day to day.

PROTEIN. For adults, 20 percent of calories from protein is recommended to supply the body's needs for this nutrient in 1000- to 1500-calorie diets (50 to 75 g. of protein). Or, the diet may be planned to provide 1 to 1½ g. of protein per kg. of body weight. In the diet pattern this allows for a more liberal, and usually more satisfying, use of very lean meat, poultry, and fish, and low-fat cheeses.

FAT AND CARBOHYDRATE. Since these two nutrients constitute the greatest source of energy in the average diet, they are limited in amount in the energy-restricted diet. The 1200-calorie diet pattern in Table 27–4 derives approximately 20 percent of its calories from protein, or 68 g. of protein; 35 percent from fat or 45 g. of fat; and approximately 45 percent

from carbohydrate or 121 g. of carbohydrate. The usual 2400-calorie diet with 35 percent of its calories from fat would contain about 95 g. of fat; and with 50 percent of its calories from carbohydrate it would contain 300 g. of carbohydrate.

There is considerable difference of opinion today as to whether carbohydrate or fat should be reduced to a minimum in an energy-restricted diet. Individuals have reported significant weight losses in the first few days on a practically carbohydrate-free diet. This is probably a loss of body water since Keys and Grande estimate that each gram of glycogen binds 3 to 4 grams of water.[23] Without carbohydrate in the diet the glycogen stores in the body are reduced and utilized to maintain normal blood glucose levels while the bound water and electrolytes will be excreted by the kidneys.

Practically carbohydrate-free and, therefore, high-protein and high-fat-reducing diets, consisting mainly of meat, poultry, fish, eggs, and butter, have been in and out of vogue since Banting published his "Letter on Corpulence" in 1860.[24] Up to the present time no carefully controlled studies have been conducted to prove their worth. The Council of Foods and Nutrition of the American Medical Association reminds us of the hazards of the intake of excessive amounts of saturated fatty acids and cholesterol from a diet of meats and eggs[25] (see Chapter 29). Until well-controlled research has proven otherwise, the energy-reduced diet should contain a reasonable distribution of protein, fat, and carbohydrate, so that the energy-controlled diet can serve as a basis for the maintenance diet after weight loss has been achieved.

MINERALS AND VITAMINS. Care should be taken to see that the energy-restricted diet plan provides all the other essentials of a normal diet, such as minerals and vitamins, in quantities at least equivalent to the Recommended Dietary Allowances. If the calorie intake is very restricted (less than 1000 calories), vitamin and mineral supplements may be needed.

ALCOHOL. One gram of alcohol provides 7 calories. Also, in some alcoholic beverages such as beer and wines, carbohydrate contributes calories. If these beverages are to be used, their calorie value must be calculated in the energy-restricted diet plan. For some patients the calories from the alcoholic beverages they consume may be the difference between losing and not losing weight (see Table 6, Section 4).

WATER. Water and other nonnutritive fluids are not restricted unless there are heart or kidney complications. Sometimes there is fluid retention prior to menstruation, which may temporarily mask the real loss of body fat in women.

Table 27–4. Nutrient Composition of a 1200-Kcal. Diet Pattern

FOOD EXCHANGES*	AMOUNT		PROTEIN (g.)	FAT (g.)	CARBO-HYDRATE (g.)	ENERGY (kcal.)
	NUM-BER	HOUSE-HOLD MEASURE				
Milk, skim	2	1 pint	16	..	24	160
Vegetables, Group A	as desired		..	..	..	..
Vegetables, Group B	1	½ cup	2	..	7	35
Fruit	3	varies	..	..	30	120
Bread	4	varies	8	..	60	280
Meat	6	6 oz.	42	30	..	450
Fat	3	3 tsp.	..	15	..	135
TOTALS†			68	45	121	1180

*See Table 23–2, Nutrient Composition of Food Exchanges.
†20 percent kcal. protein, 25 percent fat, and 45 percent carbohydrate.

Food Selection and Preparation for Energy-Restricted Diets

The following discussion on food selection and preparation is organized around the Exchange System of food groups (see Chapter 23, Tables 23–2 and 23–4) and applies primarily to 1000- to 1500-calorie diets for adults. Much of the information is also applicable to the planning of diets for patients with diabetes and/or hyperlipoproteinemia (Chapters 28 and 29), and it will not be repeated in subsequent chapters. Rather, additional information will be given where necessary. In the following discussions of the exchange food groups, the reader is advised to refer to Table 27–4, an example of the food used in a 1200-calorie diet pattern.

MILK EXCHANGE. In the milk exchange group, skim milk (nonfat dried milk solids or fluid) fortified with vitamins A and D is the only item which can be used in a 1000- to 1500-calorie diet pattern. If a patient chooses to have more limited or no fat exchanges calculated in his pattern (see Table 27–4), then 2 percent or whole milk may be included. One pint of milk should be included to insure an adequate calcium and riboflavin intake unless the patient selects adequate amounts of leafy green vegetables from the Group A vegetable exchange and cheddar cheese from the meat exchange food groups. In this case a minimum of ½ pint of skim milk should be included in the diet pattern.

Buttermilk made from skim milk is a possible choice but, if the information is not on the carton, the patient must check with local dairies to be sure it is made from skim milk. One-half pint (8 ounces) of yogurt made from skim milk can be substituted for ½ pint (8 ounces) of skim milk. Sweetened flavored yogurt cannot be substituted for skim milk.

The milk exchanges included in a 1000- to 1500-calorie diet can be used as a beverage, in tea and coffee, as whipped topping sweetened with an artificial sweetener, or in mixed dishes (see section on mixed dishes).

VEGETABLE EXCHANGE, GROUP A. Vegetables in this food group can be used in amounts as desired by the patient. At levels of 1000 to 1200 calories the amount should be limited to 2 cups because amounts in excess of this could contribute an excess of 100 to 150 calories per day depending on the items and amounts selected.

These vegetables may be used raw, as garnishes or in salads, or cooked. Salt, pepper, herbs, low or no-calorie salad dressings, vinegar, or lemon juice may be used to flavor them. Any fat added for flavoring must be the fat included in the diet pattern. The low caloric density of the items in this food group can easily be changed to a higher density by the addition of fat. (One tsp. fat equals 45 calories.) For example, four spears (60 g.) of asparagus contains 60 calories, while the same amount of asparagus with one teaspoon of margarine contains 105 calories.

VEGETABLE EXCHANGE, GROUP B. A defined amount (½ cup per serving) of this group of vegetables is identified in an energy-restricted diet pattern. As with vegetables in Group A, no fat, other than that planned in the diet pattern, can be added to these vegetables during preparation or at the table. It should be pointed out to the patient that corn, a very popular vegetable, parsnips, and potatoes are listed in the bread exchange food group because of their higher carbohydrate content, and that one vegetable exchange, Group B, is equivalent to one half of a bread exchange.

FRUIT EXCHANGE. The serving size of the items in the fruit exchange food group identifies that amount of fruit which contains 10 grams of carbohydrate. These are fresh fruits served or processed without added sugar. Most of the canned fruits in the diet section of supermarkets today have some sugar added and contain approximately 12 grams of carbohydrate per size serving as listed in the fruit exchanges, Table 23–4. Depending on the frequency of use these canned fruits can be eaten in place of fresh ones if they are well drained and the syrup is not used. Many older patients prefer canned fruits and in some small communities a wide variety of fresh fruits is not available throughout the year. Also, the cost of fresh fruits at certain times of the year often prohibits the use of three or four servings per day.

At least one serving of fruit should be included in the diet pattern with emphasis placed on the selection of a fruit that is a good source vitamin C. If the patient prefers vegetables and selects two or three items such as tomatoes and cabbage from the vegetable exchange, Group A, and potatoes from the bread exchange food group each day, he may have an adequate intake of vitamin C without a serving of fruit.

BREAD EXCHANGE. The serving sizes of the items listed in the bread exchange food group vary considerably. One slice of bread refers to the usual slice which weighs approximately 23 grams. One and one-third slices of diet bread, which weighs 18 grams per slice, are equal in calories to one slice of bread weighing 23 grams.

The biscuits, muffins, and cornbread listed in the bread exchanges are products made from standard homestyle recipes, not the mixes widely available in the supermarket. The recipes used by patients who frequently make these hot breads should be checked for the amount of fat included. Some cooks make tender biscuits, muffins, or cornbread because they add more fat than stated in the recipe.

The use of a wider variety of crackers than listed in the bread exchange food group may be possible if the package includes a nutrient label. However, the amount of fat listed on the nutrient label must be checked in order to avoid a daily intake of fat in excess of 35 percent of the total calories.

The vegetables, potatoes, dried beans, and pasta listed in the bread exchange food group are prepared and served without added fat. If any fat is added to these items, it must be some of the fat included in the diet pattern. Some patients use part of the milk and margarine in their diet patterns to season mashed potatoes. Others remove the contents of a baked potato, mix it with some of their milk and margarine, return the mixture to the shell, and reheat the stuffed baked potato. French-fried, pan-fried or hash-brown potatoes are excluded because these methods of preparation call for more fat than can be included in a 1000- to 1500-calorie diet pattern.

The ice cream listed in the bread exchange food group in Table 23–4 cannot be used as an exchange for one slice of bread in a 1000- to 1500-calorie diet unless two fat exchanges are also included in this substitution.

MEAT EXCHANGE. Any serving of meat, poultry, or fish must be prepared and served without the addition of *any* fat, and no visible fat should be eaten. Only lean meats should be selected, for example, ground beef with less than 20 percent fat. The patient must be counseled to bake, broil, braise, or pan fry meat, poultry, and fish without adding fat and to carefully drain off all fat after cooking.

The most efficient way to remove fat from the juices which collect when meat is roasted is to add a small amount of water to dissolve all the material in the bottom of the pan, put this fluid in a container and refrigerate overnight. The next day the hardened fat can be removed and discarded and the remaining juice, now fat-free, can be seasoned and heated to be served with meat or to season vegetables. This juice can also be used to make a gravy thickened with flour but without added fat. Two and one-half tablespoons of flour are equivalent to one bread exchange. Two and one-half tablespoons of presifted flour will thicken one to two cups of liquid. One-fourth cup of this gravy will contain approximately 20 calories compared with 100 or more calories in one fourth of a cup of gravy made with flour and fat.

Eggs, cottage cheese, and cheddar type but not processed cheese or cheese spread can be used as meat exchanges unless blood lipid levels indicate that their use should be restricted. For example, in an individual with an elevated blood cholesterol level, eggs may be excluded or limited to no more than three per week.

FAT EXCHANGE. For many obese clients the items selected from this food group should be limited to those made from oils and fats with a significant amount of polyunsaturated fatty acids. The items in the fat exchange list which fit this criterion are margarine and mayonnaise or French dressing made with vegetable oils—safflower, soy, or corn oils. This limitation is recommended since many obese persons demonstrate abnormalities of lipid, as well as of glucose, metabolism (see Chapter 29).

MIXED DISHES. The amounts of food in a diet pattern may be combined in mixed dishes. For example, if an individual selected three meat exchanges, one vegetable exchange, Group B, and one bread exchange for his evening meal, he could combine in a casserole dish 3 ounces cooked lean stew beef, ½ cup mixed onions and carrots, and ½ cup cooked rice. Tomatoes, a vegetable exchange, Group A, and herbs and other seasoning can be added as desired.

A number of cookbooks which give the exchange values of one serving of a recipe are available. Patients who are interested and skilled in food preparation often find that these cookbooks help relieve the monotony of an energy-restricted diet. A list of these cookbooks is included at the end of this chapter.

CONVENIENCE FOODS. The majority of convenience foods such as TV dinners, precooked frozen meats in gravy, and frozen vegetables in butter or other sauces cannot be used in energy-restricted diets. Exceptions to this list are the calorie-restricted TV dinners, available in most supermarkets, which give the calorie and nutrient value per dinner on the label.

It is possible that in the future with the increasing use of nutrient labeling by food manufacturers more of the convenience foods can be used. However, one is cautioned to check the distribution of nutrients in these products so that the total fat in the diet does not exceed 35 percent of the total calories in the diet order, even though calories in excess of the diet order are not consumed.

DIETETIC FOODS. Other than saccharin for sweetening beverages and other foods and an unsweetened gelatin desert (D'Zerta) there are very few other "diet foods" which can be used in an energy-restricted diet. (See the discussion of dietetic foods in Chapter 23).

MEALS:	AMT.	P	F	C	kcal	AMT.	P	F	C	kcal	AMT.	P	F	C	kcal
MILK															
VEG. B															
VEG. A															
FRUIT															
BREAD															
MEAT															
FAT															
SUB-TOTAL	(M)					(N)					(E)				
BETWEEN MEALS															
SUB-TOTAL	(IO)					(2)					(HS)				

PT. NAME _____ DIET _____
INSULIN _____

TOTALS P ___ F ___ C ___ kcal ___

Fig. 27–5. Form for calculating diet patterns (8 x 5 Kardex card).

Planning the Energy-Restricted Diet Pattern

The clinical dietitian will need a form on which to calculate a client's diet pattern. Figure 27–5 is one example of a form for calculation. A copy of the calculation should be included in the client's medical record and a new one added whenever the pattern is revised so that other members of the health-care team have access to the plan.

STEP 1. The first step in calculating an energy-restricted diet pattern is to identify those items from the client's diet history which can be included in the pattern. For example, if a client usually has fruit juice, toast, and coffee for breakfast, his energy-restricted diet pattern will contain fruit and bread exchanges in the breakfast pattern.

The serving size or method of preparation of the foods as reported in the diet history may need to be modified when calculated in the energy-restricted diet pattern. Eight ounces of orange juice may be modified to 4 ounces; French toast served with butter and syrup may be modified to one egg poached in water and served on unbuttered toast; and coffee with sugar and cream may be modified to coffee with saccharin and some of the skim milk calculated in the pattern.

STEP 2. The second step is to complete the calculation of the energy-restricted pattern with the client. The calories should be distributed reasonably in three meals. If the client wishes, a bedtime snack can be calculated. A pattern which provides one half or more of the calories in one meal should be avoided, especially if the individual has hyperinsulinemia, because the quantity of insulin secreted is related to the quantity of food consumed at a meal.

Table 27–5 illustrates the nutrient composition of a 1200-calorie diet pattern, and Table 27–6 shows how the 1200 calories were distributed in three meals

Table 27–5. 1200-Kcal. Diet Pattern (Three Meals and a Bedtime Snack)

MEAL	FOOD EXCHANGES	NUM-BER	PRO-TEIN (g.)	FAT (g.)	CAR-BOHY-DRATE (g.)	ENER-GY (kcal.)
Morning	Fruit	1	—	—	10	40
	Bread	1	2	—	15	70
	Milk, skim	1	8	—	12	80
TOTAL			10	—	37	190
Noon	Meat	2	14	10		150
	Vegetables, Group A	as desired	—		—	—
	Bread	1	2		15	70
	Fruit	1	—	—	10	40
	Fat	1	—	5	—	45
TOTAL			16	15	25	305
Evening	Meat	4	28	20	—	300
	Vegetables, Group A	as desired	—		—	—
	Vegetables, Group B	1	2	—	7	35
	Bread	1	2	—	15	70
	Fruit	1	—	—	10	40
	Fat	1	—	5	—	45
TOTAL			32	25	32	490
Bedtime	Milk, skim	1	8	—	12	80
	Bread	1	2	—	15	70
	Fat	1	—	5	—	45
TOTAL			10	5	27	195
	TOTALS		68	45	121	1180

and a bedtime snack. This pattern was calculated with a 50-year-old woman who was 30 pounds above her ideal weight and who was limited in activity because of arthritis in one hip. This client preferred fruit juice and cereal with milk at breakfast; a salad and fruit at noontime; and meat, vegetables, and salad at the evening meal, which she eats with her husband. The major modifications in her usual food practices were the omission of desserts, frequent snacks of cookies and candy during the day, and a sandwich at bedtime.

Table 27-7 shows a 1500-calorie diet pattern calculated with a young businessman who was 20 pounds overweight. In addition to decreasing his daily energy intake, he also increased his energy expenditure by walking 10 blocks to work each morning.

Counseling the Obese Individual

APPROACHES TO THE PATIENT. In 1960, Feinstein reviewed the literature of the treatment of obesity published in professional journals from 1940 to 1959.[26] He carried out a critical analysis of the methods used and the results obtained by numerous investigators. From his analysis of various approaches to the treatment of obese patients, he concluded that successful weight reduction involves the interaction of three sets of factors: (1) the patient himself; (2) the therapeutic relationship between patient and clinician; and (3) the dietary program. The patient himself and the therapeutic relationship appeared to be the most significant factors, while the type of energy-restricted diet program was of lesser significance in promoting successful weight reduction.

The evidence available to Feinstein demonstrated that any obese patient could lose weight on an energy-restricted diet with varying proportions of protein, fat, and carbohydrate, with or without therapeutic adjuncts such as appetite-depressant drugs, in an environment which restricted the patient's access to food, usually the hospital environment. Comparable success was not observed in patients being treated in an ambulatory care setting.

Since the restriction of the obese patient to hospitalization for treatment is unrealistic and expensive, Feinstein pointed out the patient characteristics which are related to success in any setting. A small group of obese patients are capable of losing weight when they decide to do so and are provided with the information which helps them to control their food intake. On the other hand, the majority of obese patients, even though they are knowledgeable about the energy value of foods, are unable to resist food intake. Within this category of obese patients there are two subgroups: one, the smaller of the two, requires psychiatric help because they are truly compulsive eaters; and the other, the majority of obese patients, do not have severe psychiatric problems yet have difficulty depriving themselves of food.

Feinstein points out that an external source of motivation may be the decisive factor in assisting the majority of obese patients to lose weight. The external source of motivation for many of these individuals is an ongoing therapeutic relationship with a clinician. Feinstein identified the clinician as the physician or

Table 27-7. Nutrient Composition of a 1500-Kcal. Diet Pattern

FOOD EXCHANGES*	AMOUNT NUM-BER	AMOUNT HOUSE-HOLD MEASURE	PRO-TEIN (g.)	FAT (g.)	CAR-BOHY-DRATE (g.)	ENER-GY (kcal.)
Milk, skim	2	1 pint	16	..	24	160
Vegetables, Group A	as desired		..	..	..	..
Vegetables, Group B	1	½ cup	2	..	7	35
Fruit	3	varies	..	..	30	120
Bread	7	varies	14	..	105	490
Meat	6	6 oz.	42	30	..	450
Fat	6	6 tsp.	..	30	..	270
TOTALS†			76	60	166	1525

*See Table 23-2, Nutrient Composition of Food Exchanges.
†20 percent kcal. protein, 35 percent fat, and 45 percent carbohydrate.

Table 27-6. Suggested Menu—1200-Kcal. Diet

Breakfast
½ cup unsweetened orange juice
½ cup cornflakes
½ cup skim milk
Coffee, black or with skim milk and saccharin

Noon Meal
Tuna salad plate
  2 ounces water-packed tuna
  1 tsp. mayonnaise
  cucumber wedges marinated in herb vinegar
  tomato wedges
  celery curls
  salad greens
6 rye rounds
1 cup fresh strawberries
Coffee, black or with skim milk and saccharin

Evening Meal
4 ounces broiled sirloin steak
½ cup corn
½ cup green peas
  flavored with 1 tsp. margarine
Green salad with no-calorie dressing
Fruit cup parfait—½ cup of fruit cup canned
  without sugar in D'Zerta with whipped skim milk
  topping

Bedtime Snack
8 oz. of skim milk
6 rye rounds
1 tsp. margarine

other individual with an adequate knowledge of the energy value of foods and the ability to establish a positive relationship with the client. Feinstein emphasized that the clinician must see the patient frequently, or, as it is described today, there must be "continuity of care;" and that the clinician must be accepting of the patient's needs and problems.

Regarding the third factor, the dietary program, Feinstein pointed out that his data demonstrate that any patient will lose weight if he controls energy intake adequately and that some patients are more successful with unusual diet programs such as liquid formulas or limited choices of foods.

Bruch's recently published book, *Eating Disorders*, reinforces many of Feinstein's conclusions. Bruch points out:

> Among the many factors that need to be evaluated before a reducing regimen is prescribed, there is no one aspect more important than the patient's motive for wanting to lose weight, or conversely, for not being interested in it. [27]

In addition, Bruch shows from her experience that there are those patients who prefer to be obese and who meet the stresses of daily living more successfully when they are obese.[28]

Since Feinstein's review of the literature, self-help organizations such as TOPS (Take Off Pounds Sensibly) and Weight Watchers have been organized. The participants in these groups have had varying success in achieving and maintaining weight reduction, but this approach has not proved any more effective than the client-clinician approach.

Recently the disciplines of psychiatry and psychology have been studying behavior modification as an approach to the treatment of obesity. At present the reports in the literature do not indicate that behavior modification is any more successful than other approaches to prompting a *significant* weight loss.[29,30] Only reports of long-term follow-up will demonstrate whether or not this approach will be effective in achieving and maintaining weight loss.

From the evidence available today the person who is most likely to lose weight successfully:

1. Is slightly to moderately above a desirable weight for him, due to excess adipose tissue;
2. Gained weight as an adult;
3. Never attempted to lose weight as an adult;
4. Is well adjusted emotionally;
5. Accepts weight reduction as a realistic goal.[31]

THE NUTRITION COUNSELOR'S ROLE. The first responsibiltiy of the nutrition counselor, as in any counseling situation, is to establish communication with the client so that together they can explore all aspects of the problem, and he can arrive at his own decision to lose weight and maintain his weight loss. This implies that the counselor must accept the client and his problem and be willing to help, not ridicule, him. In other words, the counselor must establish a helping relationship with the client (see Chapter 12).

Within this relationship the counselor is responsible for assisting the patient to plan a diet pattern compatible with his life-style and the constraints of the diet order, and assisting him to achieve a level of knowledge of the energy composition of foods so that his food choices will be consistent with his goal to lose weight. This includes such instructional aids as pamphlets, cookbooks, and if necessary, a scale to help him become familiar with the weights of portions of food.

Other Approaches To Weight Reduction

STARVATION REGIMENS. In 1964 Drenick and co-workers reported on the use of starvation to promote weight reduction.[32] Water and other noncaloric fluids together with vitamin and mineral supplements are used during the starvation period. The body conserves glucose to meet the metabolic needs of the brain by utilizing adipose triglyceride and muscle protein to meet its energy needs. Ketoacidosis rarely occurs but the increase in purine degredation to uric acid when muscle protein is utilized for fuel can result in gout, an abnormality of uric acid metabolism.

During fasting, weight loss is rapid, averaging 1 to 3 pounds per day. Hospitalized patients appear to tolerate this approach for periods of 30 days or more. However, long-term follow-up reports of patients who have used this regimen indicate that weight loss is not easily maintained, and that it is no more effective than other approaches to the treatment of obesity. It should never be self-administered and should be carried out only in a hospital setting where medical personnel can monitor the patient's clinical progress. Episodes of hypoglycemia with loss of consciousness, which are hazardous to the patient and perhaps to others (e.g., if he were driving a car), can occur.

FORMULA DIETS. Liquid formula diets fortified with vitamins and minerals are now available in most supermarkets. They contain approximately 225 calories per 8-ounce serving; and four 8-ounce servings per day yield 900 calories. Their advantage lies in the fact that they provide a specific number of calories per serving; their disadvantage is the monotony of a bland liquid diet.

Some people have found it helpful to use the formula diet for one meal a day and eat a calorie-restricted diet at other meal's. These formulas, generally made from nonfat dry skim milk with vitamins and minerals added, are relatively expensive.

ANOREXIGENIC AGENTS. The amphetamines and other drugs have been used to promote weight loss. They depress appetite, but it has been observed that their effectiveness decreases after about six weeks of use. In increasing doses they have unpleasant side effects. In the obese person who also has cardiac disease these drugs are dangerous. Anorexigenic drugs should be taken only under the supervision of the physician. With the recent abuse of amphetamines, physicians today rarely prescribe these drugs for obese patients.

HORMONES. Thyroid hormone has been used as an adjunct to diet therapy on the grounds that obese patients are in a hypometabolic state and need this metabolic stimulant if weight loss is to be accomplished. When an individual has hypothyroidism, hormone preparations are required to achieve a weight loss. For obese individuals with normal thyroid function—the majority of patients—thyroid hormone can be dangerous.

Injections of human chorionic gonadotrophin, a glycoprotein hormone produced by the trophoblasts of the placenta, have been used to treat obese women. In work with rats it has been observed that this hormone decreases the level of enzymes involved in fatty acid synthesis. The reports of clinical trials with humans are equivocal and its future as an agent in the treatment of obesity is uncertain at this time.

DIURETICS AND LAXATIVES. The indiscriminate use of diuretics and laxatives, which promote fluid loss, may give the patient a false sense of accomplishment when he weighs himself. His weight loss will reflect a water loss, not a decrease in adipose tissue. Only when the physician observes abnormal fluid retention in a patient will a diuretic be part of the patient's therapy.

Obese patients have used excessive amounts of laxatives to promote malabsorption of nutrients. This is usually achieved by taking a laxative after every meal. This practice not only interferes with the absorption of nutrients by increasing the transit time of food in the gastrointestinal tract but also can lead to fluid and electrolyte imbalance due to the diarrhea-type stools caused by the laxative.

ILEAL-BYPASS SURGERY.* Morbid obesity refers to a weight of two or three times the ideal which has been maintained in spite of all efforts to reduce it. In an attempt to find a solution to this problem Varco suggested a surgical short-circuiting of the small intestine to reduce the available absorptive area.[33] Currently the most satisfactory procedure is the anas-

*With the assistance of B.A. Ashcraft, Senior Student, Medical Dietetics, Ohio State University.

tomosis of 10 inches of the proximal jejunum to the terminal 8 inches of the ileum.[34] The bypassed segments of the jejunum and ileum are left in place. Theoretically the advantage of bypass surgery is that it allows the patient to continue to eat those foods which satisfy his needs and at the same time to lose weight.

The absorptive and metabolic effects of ileal bypass vary widely from individual to individual. Some are able to eat anything in any amount, while others have many food intolerances.[35] Diarrhea is the most significant problem following surgery and is in part related to diet. The unabsorbed nutrients, particularly carbohydrate and fat, have a strong osmotic effect, drawing fluid into the lumen of the intestine instead of allowing normal fluid absorption. Significant amounts of potassium are lost in the diarrheal fluid. However, it has been observed that the diarrhea can be reduced by decreasing fat and mono- and disaccharide intake.[36] The patient soon learns which foods he can and cannot tolerate.

Fatty degeneration of the liver has been observed in some patients after surgery.[37] There appears to be no correlation between the degree of fatty infiltration or liver damage and the amount or rapidity of weight loss, or the degree of obesity at the time of surgery.[38] Some report that the abnormal liver function tests return to normal within 6 to 12 months postsurgery[39] while others report much more devastating and permanent damage.[40]

The selection of patients for this surgery must be done carefully. The patient must be physically and psychologically able to withstand the procedure and accept the possible complications.[41] At present the results are unpredictable; some will benefit and others will have continuous problems or minimal weight loss.

UNDERWEIGHT

Underweight, like overweight, is a relative term, being based on the ideal weight for a given height, build, and sex. Weight more than 10 percent below the ideal is usually considered to be abnormal, especially in persons under 25, and is worthy of medical investigation.

Leanness or underweight may be due to an inadequate energy intake, to excessive bodily activity, or to both; or it may be familial. Physical disease such as malignancy, gastrointestinal disorders, chronic infectious disease, or endocrine disturbances such as hyperthyroidism may be a cause of progressive weight loss.

Underweight due to an inadequate caloric intake may be a serious condition, especially in the young.

Resistance to infection, particularly to tuberculosis, may be lowered; and the occurrence of the complications of pregnancy in young women may result from malnutrition due to an inadequate energy intake.

Nutritional Care of the Underweight Patient

Table 27-8 shows the kinds of foods used to increase calorie intake. Reasonable goals that take into consideration the individual's age, height, and previous weight status must be set with each underweight patient. For example, a high-calorie diet for a 5 feet 4 inch 40-year-old woman may be 2500 calories, while a high-calorie diet for a 6 foot 3 inch 19-year-old boy may be 3500 calories.

The diet must be built up gradually, otherwise the individual may not be able to tolerate the sudden increase. Care must be taken to ascertain his likes and dislikes and to prepare the food as appetizingly as possible, both as to methods of cooking and appearance when served. Above all, he must be encouraged to accept the necessity for his cooperating by consuming all food served to him.

Some guidelines for assisting the underweight individual are:

1. An adequate diet as described in Chapter 10;

Table 27-8. Kinds of Foods Used for Increased Energy Intake

PRINCIPLES

1. High in caloric value: 25-50 percent above normal
2. High in protein: 90-100 g. for adults
3. High in vitamins, especially in the vitamin B complex
4. Nourishment may be served between meals and before retiring

FOODS USED

Milk
  Milk and yogurt
Cheese
  All kinds
Fats
  Butter and margarine; all other fats
Eggs
  Cooked in all ways
Meats, fish and fowl
  All varieties; bacon and fat meats are indicated if the patient tolerates them
Soups
  Preferably creamed or thick soups
Bread, cereals, macaroni products
  All kinds; preferably whole grain or enriched
Vegetables
  All vegetables, including potatoes
Salads
  All kinds; oil dressings especially desirable
Fruits
  All fresh and cooked fruits and juices, jellies, jams and marmalades
Desserts
  Ice cream, custards, tapioca and rice puddings, cake, fruit desserts, other desserts
Beverages
  Tea, coffee, cocoa; served with cream and sugar; fruit juices; malted preparations
Vitamin concentrates
  If ordered by the physician

2. Adequate energy intake that may be obtained by: (a) increasing the quantity of food eaten at each meal, (b) increasing the carbohydrate and, to some extent, the fat intake, and (c) adjusting the frequency of feedings. For some this last recommendation may be achieved by offering nourishments between meals, for others it may be more appropriate to offer a hearty bedtime snack of a sandwich or a dessert plus a beverage;
3. One to 1½ g. of protein per kilogram of body weight to combat any previous inadequate intake;
4. Adequate intake of vitamins and minerals;
5. Reduction in bulk from excessive servings of fruits and vegetables in favor of foods with more concentrated energy value. Low-calorie soups, salads, and beverages should not be eaten at the beginning of a meal, as they tend to give temporary satiety and to diminish appetite for the more substantial part of the meal.
6. Easily digested foods. Carbohydrate is both easily digested and quickly converted into body fat. Foods rich in fat may be used to increase the energy value without unduly increasing bulk, but they must be used with discretion. Fat-rich foods lessen the appetite of many patients, and too much fat in any form is frequently distasteful unless cleverly disguised. The uncooked fats, such as cream, butter, and salad oils are usually better tolerated than the fat in fried foods.

ANOREXIA NERVOSA

Anorexia nervosa is a physiological disorder which derives from psychological problems. It manifests itself as self-induced starvation resulting in marked cachexia and severe metabolic defects. If not treated, the starvation leads to death. The term anorexia is not truly descriptive of the problem. The patient does not lose her appetite. Rather she does not permit herself to eat. Many of the patients are expert calorie counters and frequently place themselves on 600- to 900-calorie diets. For example, one 16-year-old high school girl whose ideal weight was 104 pounds consistently consumed 900 calories per day. She weighed 76 pounds when seen by the physician.

The typical patient is a teen-age girl. Prior to the onset of their illness many have been overweight and were teased or ridiculed about their weight status by family, friends, or teachers. Parents usually report that in the past the patient was cooperative and easy to get along with. Silverman describes the behavior of these patients at the time they come to medical treatment for significant weight loss as greedy, envious, narcissistic, and with desire to control the family.[42] Dally has noted in his series of patients that the major emotional problem is a poor mother-daughter relationship.[43]

In addition to marked underweight (10 to 50 percent of previous weight), Silverman has observed that a significant number of his 29 subjects exhibited dry, scaly skin, abnormal glucose tolerance tests (either a diabetic type or a flat curve), and elevated blood urea nitrogen (BUN) levels. The elevated BUN probably reflects an inadequate fluid intake in most instances; and the flat glucose tolerance curve, functional malabsorption.

The treatment of the anorexia nervosa patient requires the intensive intervention of both medical and psychiatric personnel. The representatives of these two disciplines must work closely together. They establish their approach to treatment and must orient the other health disciplines such as nursing and dietetics to their treatment plan because these patients act in a manipulative way toward all staff. For the benefit of the patient all the staff involved must consistently exhibit the same behavior in their contacts with her. For example, Silverman has a very precise routine for the care of his patients when they are admitted to the hospital which the staff together with him must implement without any variations. One of his requirements is that the patient will drink a minimum of one liter of calorie-containing fluids each day.

In some situations it is necessary to institute tube feeding as a first step in treatment in order to correct fluid and electrolyte imbalance and to begin nutritional rehabilitation. One should begin with a dilute feeding and increase the caloric density as tolerated (see discussion of tube feedings, Chapter 26). An estimation of energy and nutrient intake should be recorded daily in the patient's medical record. It is interesting to note that Dally has observed that as these patients improve they talk freely about food and frequently request recipes and other instruction in food preparation.

Anorexia nervosa is an example of a nutritional problem which is secondary to another problem: in this case an emotional one. As Silverman has demonstrated, psychiatric as well as medical therapy is required if these patients are to achieve and maintain a reasonable weight status.

STUDY QUESTIONS AND ACTIVITIES

1. In conversation with adult patients ask each patient to recall what he or she weighed at age 12, 18, 25, 35, 45, and 55. For some patients it will be easier for them to relate weight to some event in their lives—e.g., graduation from high school, the time of marriage, induction into the armed forces, or, the time of birth of the first baby. Do any of these patients illustrate: (1) normal weight over their life-span thus far; (2) obesity throughout their life-span; (3) obesity which developed during their adult years?

2. In conversation with adult patients discover what foods they consider "fattening." In clinical conference with your classmates and instructor discuss these ideas.

3. Calculate a 1500 calorie diet pattern for yourself. For three days, use this pattern to select your foods for each meal. Record all food and beverages you consume each day. Appraise the calorie value of each day's intake. In clinical conference with your instructor discuss the problems you met and your feelings about "counting" calories each day.

4. Make an appointment to accompany the clinical dietitian when she conducts the diet interview and when she gives diet instruction to an obese patient. Observe and talk with this patient at one mealtime for at least three days and report your observations to the dietitian. Summarize this experience and with the dietitian report to your classmates in clinical conference.

5. How were today's weight tables established? What criteria were used?

6. What does the skinfold thickness measurement reveal? How is it done?

7. Why is obesity considered a public health problem?

8. What is the direct cause of overweight? What are some of the factors which may play a role in the development of obesity?

9. What role does exercise play in weight control? What factors militate today against maintaining desirable weight?

10. What are the criteria for successful weight reduction?

11. In teaching a patient, what should be the attitude of the nutrition counselor?

12. What are some methods of weight control besides food limitation? Why are most of these considered dangerous?

13. How can an underweight patient be helped to gain weight?

SUPPLEMENTARY READINGS

BODY COMPOSITION
Crawford, P. B., et al: An obesity index for six-month-old children. Am. J. Clin. Nutr. 27:706, 1974.
Kryzywicki, H. J., et al: A comparison of methods for estimating human body composition. Am. J. Clin. Nutr. 27:1380, 1974.

Ward, G. M., et al: Relationship of anthropometric measurements to body fat as determined by densitometry, potassium-40, and body water. Am. J. Clin. Nutr. 28:162, 1975.

OBESITY–ETIOLOGY

Archer, J. A., et al: Defect in insulin binding to receptors in obese man: Amelioration with calorie restriction. J. Clin. Invest. 55:166, 1975.

Buskirk, E. R.: Obesity: A brief overview with emphasis on exercise. Fed. Proc 33:1948, 1974.

Gates, J. C., et al: Food choices of obese and non-obese persons. J. Am. Dietet. A. 67:339, 1975.

Stern, J. S., and Greenwood, M. R. C.: A review of development of adipose cellularity in man and animals. Fed. Proc. 33:1952, 1974.

OBESITY–TREATMENT

Council on Food and Nutrition: A critique of low carbohydrate ketogenic weight reduction regimens. JAMA 224:1415, 1973.

Holzbach, R. T., et al: Hepatic lipids in morbid obesity: Assessment at and subsequent to jejunoileal bypass. N. Eng. J. Med. 290:296, 1974.

Jordan, H. A.: In defense of body weight. J. Am. Dietet. A. 62:17, 1973.

Levitz, L. S.: Behavior therapy in treating obesity. J. Am. Dietet. A. 62:22, 1973.

Mann, G. V.: The influence of obesity on health. N. Eng. J. Med. 291:178, 226, 1974.

New restrictions on diet pills. FDA, Consumer 7:18, 1973.

Rivlin, R. S.: Therapy of obesity with hormones. N. Eng. J. Med. 292:26, 1975.

ANOREXIA NERVOSA

Halmi, K. A.: Anorexia nervosa: Demographic and clinical features in 94 cases. Psychosomatic Med. 36:18, 1974.

Schmidt, M. P. W., and Duncan, B. A. B.: Modifying eating behavior in anorexia nervosa. Am. J. Nurs. 74:1646, 1974.

Silverman, J. A.: Anorexia nervosa: Clinical observations in a successful treatment plan. J. Pediat. 84:68, 1974.

PATIENT RESOURCES

Better Homes and Gardens Calorie Counter's Cookbook. Des Moines, Iowa, Better Homes and Gardens Books, 1970.

Calories and Weight: The USDA Pocket Guide. USDA Agri. Information Bull. No. 364, 1974.

Danowski, T. S.: Sustained Weight Control, ed. 2. Philadelphia, Davis, 1973.

Food and Fitness, Chicago, Blue Cross Plans, 1973.

Netzer, C. T.: The Brand-Name Calorie Counter. New York, Dell, 1969.

®Nidetch, J.: Weight Watchers[R] Program Cookbook. Great Neck, N. Y., Hearthside, 1973.

Zane, P.: The Jack Sprat Cookbook. New York, Harper, 1973.

For further references see Bibliography in Section 4.

REFERENCES

1. Cooper, et al: Nutrition in Health and Disease, ed. 7. Philadelphia, J. B. Lippincott, 1940.
2. Sheldon, W., et al: Varieties of Human Physique, New York, Harper, 1940.
3. Fomon, S. J.: Infant Nutrition, ed. 2. Philadelphia, Saunders, 1974.
4. Keys, A., and Grande, F.: in Modern Nutrition in Health and Disease, ed. 5, R. S. Goodhart and M. E. Shils, eds. Philadelphia, Lea and Febiger, 1973, Chapter 1.
5. Karlberg, et al: Acta Pediat. Scand. (Suppl. 187):48, 1968.
6. Mayer, J.: in Goodhart and Shils, eds., op. cit., Chap. 22.
7. Ten-State Nutrition Survey, 1968-1970. III. Clinical Anthropometry, Dental. DHEW Pub. No. (HSM) 72-8131.
8. Weight by Height and Age of Adults. National Center for Health Statistics, Series 11, No. 14, DHEW, 1966.
9. Stunkard, A., et al: JAMA 221:579, 1972.
10. Hegsted, D. M.: Nutr. Rev. 32:33, 1974.
11. Hirsch, J., and Knittle, J. L.: Fed. Proc. 29:1516, 1970.
12. Sims, E. A. H., et al: Ann. Rev. Med. 22:235, 1971.
13. Rabinowitz, D.: Ann. Rev. Med. 21:241, 1971.
14. Martin, M. M., and Martin, L. A.: Pediatrics 82:192, 1974.
15. Knittle, J. L.: J. Pediat. 81:1048, 1972.
16. Sims, E. A. H., et al: in Treatment and Management of Obesity, G. A. Bray and J. E. Bethune, eds. New York, Harper, 1974.
17. Grey, N., and Kipnis, D. M.: N. Eng. J. Med. 285:827, 1971.
18. Mayer, J.: Am. J. Clin. Nutr. 9:530, 1961.
19. Bruch, H.: Eating Disorders. New York, Basic Books, 1973.
20. Stunkard, A. et al: Am. J. Med. 19:78, 1955.
21. Schachter, S.: Science 161:751, 1968.
22. Campbell, R. G., et al: N. Eng. J. Med. 285:1402,1971.
23. Keys and Grande, op. cit.
24. Bruch, op. cit.
25. Council on Food and Nutrition: JAMA 224:1415, 1973.
26. Feinstein, A.: J. Chronic Dis. 11:349, 1960.
27. Bruch, op. cit., p. 325.
28. Bruch, H.: Am. J. Clin. Nutr. 5:192, 1957.
29. Jordan, H. A., and Levitz, L. S.: J. Am. Dietet. A. 62:27, 1973.
30. Levitz, L. S., and Strunkard, A.: Am. J. Psychiatry 131:423, 1974.
31. Young, C. M.: Am. J. Clin. Nutr. 8:896, 1960.
32. Drenick, E. J., et al: JAMA 187:100, 1964.
33. Scott, H. W., Jr., et al: Ann. Surg. 171:770, 1970.
34. Payne, J. H., et al: Arch. Surg. 106:432, 1973.
35. Salmon, P. A.: Surg. Gyn. Obst. 132:965, 1971.
36. Moxley, R. L., et al: N. Eng. J. Med. 290:921, 1974.
37. Maxwell, J. G., et al: Am. J. Surg. 116:648, 1968.
38. Holzbach, R. T., et al: N. Eng J. Med. 290:296, 1974.
39. Juhl, E., et al: N. Eng. J. Med. 285:543, 1971.
40. McGill, D. B., et al: Gastroenterology 63:872, 1972.
41. Solow, C., et al: N. Eng. J. Med. 290:300, 1974.
42. Silverman, J. A.: J. Pediat. 84:68, 1974.
43. Dally, P.: Anorexia Nervosa. New York, Grune & Stratton, 1969.

28   diabetes mellitus

Diabetes mellitus is a chronic, hereditary disease characterized by an abnormally elevated level of blood glucose (hyperglycemia) and by the excretion of the excess glucose in the urine (glycosuria). The basic defect appears to be an absolute or relative lack of insulin which leads to abnormalities in carbohydrate (glucose) metabolism as well as in the metabolism of protein and fat. Therefore, any patient with diabetes mellitus needs help in planning and accepting a daily diet containing the appropriate amounts of carbohydrate, protein, and fat, together with adequate amounts of vitamins and minerals. In severe, untreated diabetes mellitus abnormalities of fluid and electrolyte metabolism may also occur.

The history of diabetes mellitus goes back many centuries. The word *diabetes* was derived from the Greek word meaning "to siphon; to pass through," and *mellitus* came from the Latin word "honey." Thus two characteristic symptoms, copious urination (polyuria) and glucose in the urine (glycosuria), gave the name to the disease. It was not until 1921 that Banting and Best, working in

Canada, demonstrated that the substance insulin, extracted from the pancreas lowered blood sugar in their experimental animals. Following this research, insulin extracted from the islet cells of the pancreas of animals became available for the treatment of diabetes mellitus in man.

Today it is generally agreed that the hormone insulin, secreted by the beta cells (islets of Langerhans) of the pancreas, controls glucose metabolism by mediating the transfer of glucose from the spaces around the cell (extracellular) into the cell interior (intracellular), particularly the cells of adipose tissue and muscle. Insulin also appears to mediate the transfer of amino acids from the extracellular spaces into the cells, especially in muscle. Present research indicates that in some individuals with diabetes mellitus there is an absolute lack of insulin, or an insufficient amount, secreted by the beta cells of the pancreas. In other individuals, such as the obese hyperglycemic, there is an elevated amount of insulin secreted but tissue resistance interferes with the action of insulin, which leads ultimately to hyperglycemia and glycosuria. The work of Unger and his associates[1] indicates that a relative excess of another pancreatic hormone, glucagon, is involved in the incidence of hyperglycemia in diabetes.

EPIDEMIOLOGY
Predisposing Factors

It is generally accepted that diabetes mellitus is inherited. Some investigators have concluded that it is inherited as an autosomal recessive trait, while others have proposed other modes of inherited transmission.[2] It is likely that a patient with diabetes will know of other members of his family who have had the disease. It has also been observed that the disease occurs at a progressively earlier age with each passing generation of affected individuals.[3] Diabetes in adults is frequently associated with obesity. It is possible that the susceptibility to diabetes mellitus is enhanced by obesity combined with inactivity. Weight reduction alone often results in improvement in obese adult diabetes.

Prevalence and Incidence

It is estimated that there are approximately 3½ to 4 million individuals in the United States who have diabetes mellitus, and according to the National Health Survey, about 60 percent are known and 40 percent are undiagnosed cases. At present, there is no mechanism for reporting the national annual incidence of diabetes mellitus; however, it is estimated that between 200,000 and 300,000 new cases are diagnosed each year. The World Health Organization has observed signs of the increasing prevalence of diabetes mellitus around the world, particularly in areas where there has been economic improvement due to industrialization and a more generous food supply.

Diabetes occurs in all age groups from young infants to the elderly. The greatest incidence occurs in middle or older aged adults. It is estimated that 80 to 85 percent of all individuals with diabetes mellitus are 45 years of age or older. In the United States as a whole there appears to be a sex difference in the incidence of the disease. More women than men, and more women over 45 years of age who have had children have the disease. The higher incidence in women who have had children may reflect factors related to pregnancy. Today's longer life expectancy and the reduced mortality rate for infants of diabetic mothers results in the "seeding" of the diabetic potential, therefore, the number of people who will develop the disease is expected to increase.

Detection and Preventive Intervention

Case-finding programs conducted by health departments and the local chapters of the American Diabetes Association seek to discover individuals who are unaware that they have the disease and to guide them to treatment in the hope of retarding possible complications. Those individuals who are relatives of known diabetics are strongly advised to be tested by their physicians each year; in this way, if they do develop the disease they can be identified and treated early. Also, members of families with a history of diabetes are advised to maintain their weight at desirable or slightly below desirable levels throughout the life span because of the association of obesity with the disease.

Classification by Types

Diabetes mellitus may be classified as (1) growth or juvenile onset, and (2) maturity or adult onset. These two types of diabetes vary not only by age of onset but also in the characteristics of the disease process.

GROWTH ONSET DIABETES. The terms growth onset or juvenile diabetes usually apply to the onset of the disease in children 0 to 14 years of age. However, this type of diabetes may also be observed in older adolescents and in young adults approximately up to the age of 35 to 40. It rarely occurs under one year of age and there appears to be no special frequency of occurrence by age in the younger group.

The onset of the disease is sudden and the patient is frequently in ketoacidosis at the time of diagnosis.

The majority of patients have lost weight prior to diagnosis due to glucose wastage (glycosuria) and most are underweight to some degree. Insulin secretion by the pancreas is minimal or lacking and, therefore, these patients are *insulin dependent* and require diet plus insulin to control the disease. The course of the disease can be unstable, characterized by episodes of hypoglycemia (low blood sugar), hyperglycemia, and their sequelae.

MATURITY ONSET DIABETES. Maturity onset diabetes usually occurs in individuals over age 40 and most frequently in the older age group, 55 and over. In the oldest group the age-related increase in normal fasting blood glucose levels must be differentiated from the elevated blood glucose levels of diabetes mellitus.

The onset of the disease is gradual and may not be diagnosed until years after onset. The course of the disease in many instances is stable and the patients are not prone to develop ketoacidosis except during a severe illness such as a myocardial infarction (heart attack) or cerebral vascular accident (stroke). Approximately 85 percent of patients with maturity onset diabetes are obese at the time of diagnosis. Although adequate insulin may be produced by the pancreas, the secretion of insulin may be delayed in response to a glucose challenge, or there may be peripheral resistance (muscle and adipose cell) to the action of insulin with overproduction by the islet cells of the pancreas. It is possible that, over time, the ability of the pancreas to secrete insulin may decrease and, as a result, some patients may require exogenous insulin to control glucose metabolism. Otherwise, maturity onset diabetes can be controlled by diet or diet plus oral agents.

SECONDARY DIABETES MELLITUS. Diabetes mellitus can occur secondary to other disease states such as pancreatitis, cirrhosis of the liver, cystic fibrosis of the pancreas, tumors of the pancreas (insulinomas), or disorders of other endocrine glands, e.g., the pituitary, the adrenals, or the thyroid.

METABOLIC ABERRATIONS

In Chapter 9, Nutrient Utilization, it was pointed out that insulin may be regarded as the hormone of energy storage. In the immediate postprandial (postfed) state it mediates the synthesis of glycogen and the glycolysis of glucose-6-PO_4 in the liver to provide substrate for the tricarboxylic acid cycle or for triglyceride synthesis. Insulin also mediates the translocation of glucose and amino acids into muscle cells where glucose can be synthesized into glycogen; and it is the medium for the translocation of glucose

and triglycerides into the adipose cells where the glucose provides substrate for further triglyceride synthesis.

Metabolic Consequences of Insulin Deficiency

Without insulin the synthesis of glycogen in the liver is depressed and there is an increase in glucose synthesis through the gluconeogenic pathway. At the same time there is a decreased uptake of glucose by the muscle and adipose cells and an increased catabolism of glycogen in muscle cells. An increase in proteolysis also occurs, with the release of amino acids from muscle cells and an increase in lipolysis, with the release of fatty acids and glycerol from the adipose cells. Certain amino acids and the glycerol released from the cells serve as substrate for gluconeogenesis in the liver. Therefore, hyperglycemia together with hyperlipemia occur in the absence of insulin (Fig. 28-1); such hyperglycemia may result in part from excessive amounts of glucagon.

Without insulin fatty acids become the major fuel for energy metabolism in the tricarboxylic acid (TCA) cycle. However, when an excess of acetyl CoA accumulates due to the lack of other substrate required by the TCA cycle, cholesterol and ketone bodies are synthesized in the liver. The ketone bodies are acetoacetic and betahydroxy butyric acids and acetone. Acetoacetic acid and betahydroxy butyric acids can be metabolized for energy to some extent by brain and muscle cells. However, in the absence of insulin the quantity in the circulation exceeds the body's capacity to metabolize them, leading to ketonemia.

When the amount of glucose filtered by the glomeruli of the kidney exceeds the capacity of the renal tubules to reabsorb it, it is excreted in the urine. This usually occurs at blood glucose levels of 160 mg. per 100 ml. or higher. Since glucose requires water for excretion, an increase in urine volume results, with the loss of body water and the electrolyte sodium.

At the same time, there is an increase in the amount of urea nitrogen to be excreted due to the deamination of amino acids, so that their carbon structures can serve as substrate for gluconeogenesis. Also, when cellular proteins are catabolized and their amino acids transported to the liver for gluconeogenesis, potassium is lost from the cells. The increasing amounts of both urea and potassium in the circulation again require water for excretion by the kidneys.

Finally the ketone bodies, betahydroxy butyric acid, acetoacetic acid, and acetone, in excess of what the body can use in the TCA cycle require water for excretion by the kidney. Acetone is volatile and is

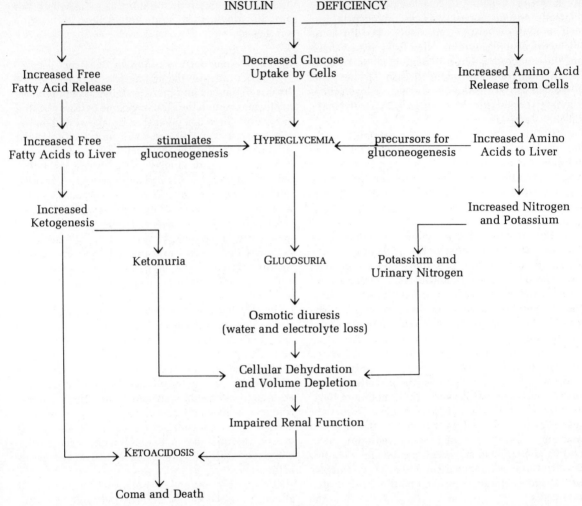

Fig. 28-1. Metabolic consequences of insulin deficiency. (Adapted from Tepperman, J., *Metabolic and Endocrine Physiology*, ed. 3. Chicago, Year Book Medical Publishers, 1973.)

also excreted by the lungs. This attempt by the kidney to excrete an abnormal quantity of metabolites leads to cellular dehydration and the depletion of body water and electrolytes. At the same time there is an increase in blood hydrogen ion concentration (metabolic acidosis). All of these metabolic events lead to circulatory failure. If treatment is not instituted promptly to reestablish carbohydrate metabolism and fluid and electrolyte balance, death may ensue.

Patients with maturity onset diabetes do not usually develop ketoacidosis. It appears that, since these patients frequently have hyperinsulinism and insulin is antilipolytic, excessive amounts of fatty acids are not released from the adipose cell for TCA cycle metabolism. However, this does not mean that maturity onset diabetics do not experience hyperlipemia. In the presence of insulin and excessive amounts of glucose, there is an increase of triglyceride synthesis in the liver with secretion into the circulation.

Other Metabolic Problems

Its been observed that disease of the small and large blood vessels occurs more frequently in diabetics than in nondiabetics. In the diabetic there is a tendency to recurrent myocardial infarction with an increase in the incidence of congestive heart failure. Small blood vessel diseases such as retinopathy, peripheral vascular disease and nephropathy also occur more frequently than in the nondiabetic. Diabetic retinopathy was the fourth cause of legal blindness in 1967, accounting for 11 percent of all patients added to the register in that year.[4] Diabetic nephropathy and atherosclerosis are the major causes of death among diabetics. Siperstein[5] has observed a thickening in the capillary basement membrane in diabetics, and Spiro[6] has identified an abnormality in the mucopolysaccharides in the basement membrane which may account for the vascular complications of diabetes. The polyol pathway of glucose metabolism is also involved in some of the complications of the disease.

CAPILLARY BASEMENT MEMBRANE. The glomerular membranes of the kidney have been extensively studied because of the serious complications of the renal disease associated with long-standing diabetes mellitus.

Spiro[7] has observed that the normal glomerular basement membrane consists of a glycoprotein material made up of peptide chains to which carbohydrate is attached. An important unit in the membrane consists of a disaccharide containing glucose and galactose linked to hydroxylysine. In the glomerular basement membrane of diabetics Spiro has observed a significant increase of the glucosylgalactose units attached to hydroxylysine with a proportional decrease in lysine. This change in composition changes the structure and function of the basement membrane.

At the present time the implications of this aberration to the treatment of diabetes mellitus are not clear. However, future research in this area may identify the real hazard of hyperglycemia in any individual and have a significant effect on therapy, including diet.

POLYOL PATHWAY OF GLUCOSE METABOLISM. Polyols are organic compounds containing multiple alcohol groups that are derived from sugars by the reduction of their aldo or keto groups. Sorbitol is the polyol that results from the reduction of glucose in mammalian tissues.

There seems to be some evidence that the cataracts which are associated with diabetes mellitus may result from an increased concentration of sorbitol in the lens. The lens does not require insulin for the intracellular transport of glucose. The presence of hyperglycemia, therefore, increases the concentration of sorbitol. The polyol pathway of glucose metabolism may also be involved in the neuropathy of diabetes mellitus.

Symptoms

The onset of the symptoms of the metabolic aberrations in juvenile diabetes is usually abrupt. Ketoacidosis with nausea, vomiting, and lethargy is present at the time of diagnosis. Two to three weeks prior to this, the classical symptoms—polydipsia, polyphagia, polyuria, and weight loss—are observed.

Usually an infectious disease or other illness occurs just before the onset of symptoms.

In maturity onset, nonketotic diabetes mellitus, the onset of symptoms is usually slow and the disease may go undetected for as long as ten years.[8] Although many of these patients have glycosuria, they are not aware that they are experiencing polydipsia and polyuria with nocturia. If they are hyperinsulinemic, they may also experience the symptoms of reactive hypoglycemia such as sweating, tremor, and palpitation three to four hours after a meal. They do not often lose weight or develop spontaneous ketoacidosis. However, with a severe infection ketoacidosis may develop. The disease is often detected when patients participate in a community screening program, or when they seek medical care for the symptoms of diseases associated with diabetes such as obesity, hypertension, heart disease, visual difficulties, and skin infections.

SCREENING AND DIAGNOSTIC TESTS

The diagnosis of diabetes mellitus can be made with a fair degree of confidence in individuals with the classical symptoms of the disease and elevated fasting or postprandial levels of blood glucose and glycosuria. Ketonemia and ketonuria may or may not be present. In other individuals a glucose challenge administered under defined conditions is used for the clinical diagnosis of the disease. It can be anticipated that if an inexpensive clinical laboratory method is developed, the determination of blood insulin levels will also be used in the diagnostic workup of patients who are suspected diabetics.

Tests

The most commonly used screening tests are the determination of the fasting blood glucose level or the two-hour postprandial (after a meal) blood glucose level, while the most common diagnostic one is the oral glucose tolerance test (OGTT).

The normal levels for fasting blood glucose vary between 70 to 100 mg. per 100 ml. of blood (ferricyanide auto-analyzer method). For both the fasting and two-hour postprandial tests levels in excess of 120 mg. of glucose per 100 ml. of blood are indicative of diabetes mellitus, while values between 110 to 120 mg. are equivocal. In the untreated diabetic patient without complications, the fasting level will range from 180 to 300 mg. per 100 ml.; and in an individual approaching or in ketoacidosis, the fasting blood glucose level will exceed 300 mg.

When the fasting or 2-hour postprandial blood glucose levels are equivocal, an oral glucose tolerance

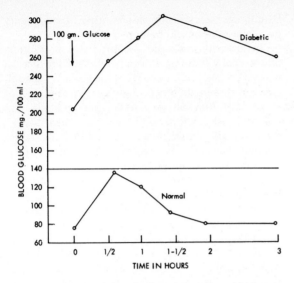

Fig. 28-2. Results of glucose tolerance tests in a normal person and a diabetic.

test is done. Following an overnight fast the patient is given a solution of glucose to drink. This contains 75 to 100 g. of glucose for adults and less for children, depending on body size. Just prior to drinking the glucose solution, blood is drawn and a specimen of urine is collected. Blood and urine samples are obtained at ½, 1, 1½, 2 and 3 hours after the glucose solution is consumed. In some instances blood and urine are also obtained at 4 and 5 hours. In a normal person the blood glucose values will not exceed 100 mg. per 100 ml. at zero time, 140 mg. at ½ hour, and will return to the fasting level at 2 hours (see Fig. 28-2). The urine will be free of glucose.

Table 28-1 gives the minimum criteria and interpretation of the oral glucose tolerance test formulated by the United States Public Health Service and by Fajans and Conn at the University of Michigan. It will be noted that the USPHS uses a point system, while Fajans and Conn use specific blood glucose levels to identify diabetes mellitus.

Preparation for Tests

There is dietary preparation of the patient for the two-hour postprandial blood glucose test and the oral glucose tolerance test, but not for the fasting blood glucose test. For three days prior to the first two tests, the patient must consume an adequate diet containing at least 300 g. of carbohydrate daily. An inadequate carbohydrate intake prior to the test can influence the results. A person consuming a low or no carbohydrate diet would have an increase above normal limits in blood glucose after ingestion of the glucose challenge for either test, which would reflect previous intake, not the presence of diabetes. The patient should be carefully instructed in preparation for these tests especially if he suspects he has diabetes and has restricted his carbohydrate intake.

THERAPY

The goals of the treatment of diabetes mellitus are to: (1) prevent excessive postprandial hyperglycemia and, therefore, the symptoms of glucose wastage; (2) prevent hypoglycemia if the patient is using insulin or an oral agent; (3) achieve and maintain ideal body weight in adults and normal growth and development in children; (4) return serum triglycerides and cholesterol to normal levels; and (5) prevent or delay large and small blood vessel disease.

Depending on the needs of the patient, the goals of therapy may be achieved by: (1) *diet*; (2) *diet* plus insulin; or (3) *diet* plus oral hypoglycemic agents. In the obese diabetic without symptoms both the hyperglycemia and hyperinsulinemia may be corrected by an energy-restricted diet resulting in weight loss. The insulin dependent diabetic will need a diet appropriate to maintain ideal weight status and/or growth combined with daily insulin injections. The obese diabetic with symptoms usually responds to an energy-restricted diet to promote weight loss and an oral hypoglycemic agent. However, some of the pa-

Table 28-1. Minimum Criteria and Interpretation of Oral Glucose Tolerance Test. Glucose Values in MG. Percent*

| | UNITED STATES PUBLIC HEALTH SERVICE** | | | FAJANS AND CONN† | |
	Whole Blood	Serum or Plasma		Whole Blood	Serum or Plasma
Fasting	110	130	1 point	———	———
One Hour	170	195	½ point	160	185
One and one-half hours	———	———	———	140	165
Two hours	120	140	½ point	120	140
Three hours	110	130	1 point	———	———

*Skillman, T. G., and Tzagournis, M.: Diabetes Mellitus. Kalamazoo, Mi., The Upjohn Co., 1973.
**Two or more points is definite diabetes, one point is possible diabetes.
†One- and two-hour levels at or exceeding the stated values represents diabetes; 1½ hour level must be reached or exceeded in borderline cases.

tients in this last group may finally require insulin to treat their disease.

Insulin

Since the discovery of insulin, many advances have been made in its commercial preparation from the pancreas of animals, primarily cattle and swine. Its production is carefully controlled to assure the number of units of insulin per volume when the product is purchased by the diabetic patient. Insulin can only be administered hypodermically because it is a protein and, if taken orally, would undergo enzymatic digestion in the gastrointestinal tract and be absorbed as its constituent amino acids, not as the intact, active hormone.

TYPES OF INSULIN. There are several types of insulins available for the treatment of the insulin dependent diabetic patient. They differ primarily in the rate of onset and duration of action which is reflected in the three classifications; rapid, intermediate, and long-acting (see Table 28–2). The most commonly used insulins today are the two intermediate acting ones, Lente and NPH (Neutral Protamine Hagedorn). They are stable solutions of insulin that possess the desirable properties of relatively rapid onset (two to eight hours) and moderately prolonged duration of action (24 to 28 hours). Regular insulin is used in the treatment of ketoacidosis because its rapid onset of action permits the physician to monitor blood glucose levels and adjust insulin injections to the need of the patient.

It must be recognized that the action of exogenous insulin injected hypodermically, usually once a day, is not the same physiologically as that of endogenous insulin released by the beta cells of the pancreas in response to the ingestion of food. Exogenous insulin is continuously available in the bloodstream and, therefore, the patient must adjust to it by consuming properly spaced meals. Although the mechanism which causes this is not understood, it has been observed that exercise enhances glucose utilization in the diabetic. Therefore, if an insulin dependent diabetic patient increases his activity significantly on any one day, he must increase his food intake or decrease his usual insulin dose for that day.

The stable insulin dependent diabetic patient usually requires one injection before breakfast of intermediate acting insulin to achieve reasonable control of blood sugar. However, some labile insulin dependent diabetics require two injections to achieve reasonable control during the day and to avoid nocturnal hyperglycemia. One injection is given in the morning before breakfast and the second one preceding the evening meal or a feeding at bedtime. The quantity of insulin injected will vary with each patient.

INSULIN REACTIONS. Hypoglycemic episodes in the diabetic due to excess insulin are to be avoided because prolonged and repeated insulin reactions lead to irreversible damage to the cortical neurons. Most of these reactions occur because the patient has not properly spaced his food intake or has omitted a meal entirely. They can also occur because of an unplanned increase in activity or the injection of the wrong dose of insulin.

Intermediate and long acting insulins in excess produce a gradual decrease in blood glucose levels. The patient experiences headache, blurred or double vision, fine tremors, uncontrollable yawning, mental confusion, and incoordination. If these symptoms are not treated, unconsciousness ensues. The insulin reaction in a patient who is conscious can be treated by an oral glucose solution such as fruit juice and sweetened carbonated beverages or with sugar. Diabetic patients using intermediate or long-acting insulin are advised to carry with them at all times a source of glucose such as sugar cubes, candy, or a special tube of concentrated glucose.

Whenever the ability of the patient to swallow without aspiration is in question or he is unconscious, the hormone glucagon is injected subcutaneously to stimulate gluconeogenesis. When conscious, the patient is offered an oral glucose solution. If the patient is in a hospital, the glucagon injection may be followed by intravenous dextrose in water.

HYPOGLYCEMIC HYPERGLYCEMIA. Episodes of mild hypoglycemia followed almost immediately by hyperglycemia have been observed in patients with growth onset diabetes using intermediate-acting insulin. The hypoglycemia, a reaction occurring at the peak time of insulin action, activates a counter-regulatory hormonal response characterized by the release of epinephrine, adrenal corticosteroids, and growth hormone. This hormonal release is a strong stimulus to gluconeogenesis, with the result that rebound hyperglycemia occurs. In other words "hypo-

Table 28–2. Insulin Action*

TYPE	ACTION	PEAK ACTION (Hours)	DURATION (Hours)
Regular	Rapid	1-2	5-6
Semilente	Rapid	1-2	12-16
Globin	Intermediate	2-4	18-24
NPH	Intermediate	2-8	24-28
Lente	Intermediate	2-8	24-28
PZI	Long-acting	8-12	36
Ultralente	Long-acting	8-14	36

*Adapted from Skillman, T. G., and Tzagournis, M.: Diabetes Mellitus. Kalamazoo, Mi., The Upjohn Co., 1975.

glycemia begets hyperglycemia." This swing in blood glucose is also known as the Symogyi effect. The problem is caused by too much insulin and is treated by slowly reducing the daily dose of insulin.

Oral Hypoglycemic Agents

There are two types of synthetic compounds, the sulfonylureas and the biguanides, which can enhance glucose utilization in maturity onset diabetic patients who can secrete reasonable amounts of endogenous insulin. They are not effective in the treatment of the insulin dependent diabetic patient.

Either drug has been proven effective in the treatment of patients with maturity onset diabetes. In some of these patients a sulfonylurea is used in combination with a biguanide, since one stimulates the secretion of insulin and the other appears to enhance the uptake of insulin by the muscle cells. These drugs can be taken by mouth, which relieves some patients of daily insulin injections. However, it has been observed that after an initially good response, the drugs are not effective in the control of blood glucose in some maturity onset diabetics and, as a result, insulin therapy must be used.

A recent study, the University Group Diabetes Program (UGDP), indicates that patients using oral agents appear to experience a greater number of deaths from atherosclerosis than patients treated with insulin.[9] There is considerable controversy about the outcomes of the UGDP study. Some clinicians hesitate to use oral hypoglycemic agents while others have continued to use them in the treatment of maturity onset diabetes.

Patients using oral hypoglycemic agents must space their meals properly because hypoglycemic reactions can occur, although not as commonly as they do in those using insulin. Hypoglycemia can occur in patients with uremia who are taking sulfonylureas because the drug is excreted by the kidney and in uremia (kidney failure) excretion is limited due to decreased kidney function. Alcohol intolerance has also been observed in some patients using the sulfonylureas.

Approaches to Therapy

There is a sharp controversy among physicians in the United States as to the best method of treating the patient with diabetes mellitus. The disagreement centers on the control of blood glucose levels. A group of conservative physicians believe that blood glucose levels higher than normal, resulting in the presence of glucose in the urine, contribute to the onset and the severity of vascular disease in diabetes. Hence, diet and insulin or oral hypoglycemic therapy are regulated carefully so that the blood glucose levels will be kept within normal limits and no glucose will be found in the urine. This careful treatment of diabetes is known as chemical regulation; it is achieved by the use of a weighed diet, repeated urine testing throughout the day, and frequent adjustments in the dose of insulin or oral agents.

A group of liberal physicians believe, from the evidence available to them, that careful regulation does not delay the onset of vascular disease. They treat their patients with insulin, if needed, and a liberal diet as long as no symptoms of diabetes other than glycosuria, without ketonuria and weight loss, are present. The physicians who advocate this approach to treatment claim that the patient lives a more nearly normal and satisfying life. This regimen is called the clinical method of regulation. The patient is placed on an unmeasured or "free" diet, restricting only sugar and foods high in sugar.

A third group, the majority of physicians who treat diabetic patients, have adopted a middle-of-the-road approach. Their treatment plan is neither as limiting as the chemical method nor as liberal as the clinical method. They use the Exchange Method of diet planning, a somewhat liberal yet moderately accurate method, which is based on standard household measures (see Chapter 23, Tables 23–2 and 23–4).

Regardless of the approach to therapy, the diet is an integral part of the treatment of any patient with diabetes mellitus. Every diabetic patient must consume daily the quantity of energy and nutrients he needs. There cannot be wide variations in intake from day to day. At the same time he must space his meals properly whether his treatment is diet or diet combined with insulin or the oral agents. To avoid variations in blood glucose levels, sugar and foods high in sugar content must be excluded from the diet. For some individuals the diagnosis diabetes mellitus will require a drastic and unavoidable change in lifestyle if they are to achieve a reasonable degree of control.

DIET THERAPY

The diet prescription for a patient with diabetes mellitus must be translated into a diet pattern acceptable to the patient. The diet must be nutritionally adequate; maintain, in so far as possible, normal blood glucose levels throughout 24 hours; and promote desirable weight status in the adult and normal growth and development in children and adolescents. This applies even in those situations where the diet prescription is regular (free) diet without added sugar or, as for children, diet-for-age without added sugar.

The Diet Prescription

ENERGY. The energy requirement for the nonobese adult diabetic is the same as that for normal individuals of the same sex, age, height, and activity. However, the diabetic is cautioned to maintain weight status slightly below his desirable weight. If his daily energy expenditure is significantly less than a normal individual, his calorie prescription may be somewhat less. For example, a 55-year-old-woman who is a secretary may require 25 calories per kilogram, not the 30 calories per kilogram recommended for a more active woman. The calorie prescription for an obese adult diabetic is designed to promote weight loss and is based on the criteria used to establish the calorie level of any energy-restricted diet (see Chapter 27).

The energy requirement for a child or an adolescent diabetic, neither of whom is usually obese, is the same as for others of his age group. The energy requirements for growth must be met to prevent growth retardation. Since insulin is lipogenic, it has been observed that energy intake may need to be reduced after adolescence to avoid an increase in body fat, especially in girls.

CARBOHYDRATE. The American Diabetes Association recommends that 40 percent of one's total calories should be derived from carbohydrate. For example, at 40 percent a 1500 calorie diet contains 150 g. of carbohydrate.

$$\frac{40 \times 1500}{100} = 600 \text{ cal}:4 = 150 \text{ g. cho.}$$

Recent research reported by Bunzell and coworkers[10] indicates that a higher percent of calories from carbohydrate can be used by insulin dependent patients without compromising the control of blood glucose levels. Therefore, some physicians are ordering diets which contain 50 percent or more of calories from carbohydrate. For example, at 50 percent a 1500 calorie diet contains approximately 190 g. carbohydrate.

$$\frac{50 \times 1500}{100} = 750 \text{ cal}:4 = 190 \text{ g. cho.}$$

This permits a reduction in total calories from fat (see the following discussion). However, for patients with carbohydrate induced hyperlipidemia it is recommended that carbohydrate be restricted to 40% of total calories (see Chapter 29).

The type of carbohydrate to be used, simple vs. complex, has also been under consideration. The simple carbohydrates are mono- and disaccharides, and the complex ones, polysaccharides. The disaccharide sucrose is severely limited as a source of carbohydrate in any diabetic diet because it is readily hydrolyzed and absorbed in the gastrointestinal tract, especially when consumed without other foods, and has an adverse effect on blood glucose levels. Drash[11] has recommended 55 percent of total calories from carbohydrates for children, with 65 percent of the carbohydrate to be derived from complex carbohydrates and 35 percent from simple carbohydrates. The complex carbohydrate is derived from cereal grains, root vegetables, and dried seeds, while the simple carbohydrate is derived from the lactose in milk and the naturally occurring mono- and disaccharides in fruits and vegetables. This modification in the type of carbohydrate is also being used by clinicians who treat adult diabetics, especially patients with vascular complications. The rationale for this change is derived from the recommendations for the dietary treatment of hyperlipidemias (see Chapter 29).

PROTEIN. The American Diabetes Association recommends that 15 to 20 percent of the total calories should be derived from protein. For example, at 20 percent a 1500 calorie diet will contain 75 g. of protein.

$$\frac{20 \times 1500}{100} = 300 \text{ cal}:4 = 75 \text{ g. protein}$$

This is greater than the average protein intake of nondiabetics, which varies from 10 to 13 percent of total calories from protein. Drash[12] recommends 15 percent protein for children.

For diabetic patients with chronic renal failure (Kimmelsteil-Wilson or other renal disease) the protein will be limited to what they can tolerate and the total calories derived from carbohydrate will be increased. (See Chapter 31, Renal Disease.)

FAT. The American Diabetes Association recommends that 40 to 45 percent of the total calories be derived from fat. For example, at 40 percent a 1500 calorie diet contains approximately 65 g. of fat.

$$\frac{40 \times 1500}{100} = 600 \text{ cal}:9 = 65 \text{ g. fat}$$

In view of the possible association of fat intake and vascular disease, some clinicians are ordering diets for adults which derive 35 percent of total calories from fat. For children with diabetes Drash[13] recommends 30 percent of total calories from fat.

Since the kind of fat in the diet—i.e., saturated vs. polyunsaturated fatty acids and cholesterol—may have a relationship to the development of atherosclerosis, the clinician may also order a modification in the type of fat and the amount of cholesterol included in the diet of the diabetic. (See Chapter 29, Hyperlipoproteinemias.)

DAILY DISTRIBUTION OF ENERGY INTAKE. The diabetic patient who is dependent on exogenous insulin or an oral hypoglycemic agent to control blood glucose must distribute his energy intake in some reasonable fashion. Table 28–3 shows a commonly recommended distribution of energy intake by type of patient using intermediate-acting insulin or diet with or without an oral agent.

It will be observed that both stable and labile insulin dependent diabetic patients using intermediate-acting insulin must consume approximately one-half their energy intake during the hours of peak action of the insulin (two to eight hours after injection or between 7 to 8 A.M. and 3 to 4 P.M.) and the remainder to provide for the total duration of insulin activity.

The stable, insulin dependent diabetic type is usually the patient with maturity onset diabetes and the labile insulin dependent is most apt to be the patient with growth onset diabetes. For this latter type, frequent snacks in addition to meals are customary for the preschool child and, fortunately, the same pattern of eating can be established for children and adolescents attending school.

The noninsulin dependent, stable diabetic patient is also advised to distribute his energy intake reasonably throughout the day. He may or may not be using oral hypoglycemic agents. Table 28–3 recommends a 2/7, 2/7, 3/7 distribution. Some clinicians recommend a 1/3, 1/3, 1/3 distribution for these patients. If desired these patients can also use a 2/7, 2/7, 2/7,1/7 distribution.

Because it has been shown that total energy intake determines insulin requirements more than carbohydrate per se, emphasis has been placed on the daily distribution of energy intake; a reasonable distribution of carbohydrate, protein, and fat to supply the energy should be included in each feeding. For example, a bedtime snack might consist of an apple and cheese, not just an apple or other food which is primarily carbohydrate.

Table 28–3. Examples for Daily Distribution of Caloric Content of Energy Intake*

TYPE OF DIABETIC PATIENT	TIME OF DAY AND FRACTION OF TOTAL CALORIES					
	Break-fast	Mid-morning	Noon	After-noon	Supper	Bed-time
Stable, Insulin-Requiring	2/7		2/7		2/7	1/7
Labile, Insulin-Requiring	2/10	1/10	2/10	1/10	3/10	1/10
Noninsulin-Requiring, Stable	2/7		2/7		3/7	

*Skillman, T. G., and Tzagournis, M.: Diabetes Mellitus, Kalamazoo, Mi., The Upjohn Co., 1975.

In summary, the diabetic diet prescription for a man 60 years of age who requires 1500 calories per day would contain 75 g. protein, 65 g. of fat and 150 g. of carbohydrate or, 20 percent of calories from protein, 40 percent from fat, and 40 percent from carbohydrate. If this man is a stable, insulin-dependent diabetic his diet pattern would be planned to contain approximately 430 calories in the morning, noon, and evening meals, and 215 calories at bedtime (2/7, 2/7, 2/7, 1/7).

Food Selection and Preparations for Diabetic Diets

The reader is advised to study the section on food selection and preparation for energy-restricted diets in Chapter 27, pp. 286-287. This information applies as well to energy-restricted diabetic diets and is not repeated here. The following discussions of the exchange food groups present additional information related to diabetic diets.

MILK EXCHANGES. All the items in the milk exchange food group (Chapter 23, Table 23–4) can be used in planning a diabetic diet pattern if the energy prescription is 1500 calories or more. However, elevated blood levels of triglycerides and cholesterol occur in some diabetic patients. In this situation only skim milk is used at any calorie level to control the intake of saturated fatty acids and cholesterol.

To accomplish Drash's recommendation that no more than 30 percent of the total calories in a diabetic diet for children should be derived from fat, milk with two percent butterfat* or skim milk must be used. Otherwise only very limited quantities of the fat exchanges such as margarine or vegetable oil can be used in the diet pattern. It is advisable that an adolescent boy who requires 3000 calories per day use milk with 2 percent fat, or skim milk, to provide his calcium and riboflavin allowances without an excessive intake of fat from milk.

VEGETABLE EXCHANGE, GROUP A. Vegetables in this food group can be used as desired by the diabetic patient. However, if the intake of simple carbohydrate is to be limited, use of the items in this food group should be limited to 1 to 1½ cups per day and the patient should be guided to select the deep green vegetables to assure an adequate intake of vitamin A.

VEGETABLE EXCHANGE, GROUP B. Defined amounts (½ cup servings) of the foods in this group are identified in the diabetic diet pattern. As with group A vegetables, if simple carbohydrates are to be limited only one or two servings of vegetables in group B can be included in the diet pattern.

*Whole milk, 3.5 percent butterfat.

FRUIT EXCHANGE. The serving size of the items in the fruit exchange food group specifies the amount of fruit, fresh, dried, or canned, without the addition of sugar which contains 10 grams of carbohydrate. When the intake of simple carbohydrates is restricted, the amount of fruit in the diet pattern will be limited. However, the patient should be guided to select a fruit each day that is a good source of vitamin C. If the total carbohydrate allows it, fresh potatoes (complex carbohydrate) in large enough quantity can be relied on as a significant source of vitamin C. Fruit drinks with vitamin C added should be avoided because the first and, therefore, most important ingredient on labels of these beverages is sugar.

BREAD EXCHANGES. Traditionally, the use of bread exchanges as a source of carbohydrate in the diabetic diet pattern has been limited. In addition to milk, emphasis was placed on using more servings of fruits and vegetables than is commonly consumed by normal, healthy persons. With the present interest in the type of carbohydrate (simple vs. complex), as well as an increase in total energy from carbohydrate, more bread exchanges may be used in diabetic diet patterns than in the past. It can be anticipated that diet prescriptions will reflect this trend. However, one may encounter some difficulty implementing this change particularly in the older patient who has had a long exposure to the concept that, not only sugar, but also bread and potatoes must be excluded from a diabetic or energy-restricted diet. On the other hand most adolescent diabetic boys will readily accept bread and potatoes in preference to excessive quantities of fruits and vegetables.

Items in the bread exchange food group with a high sucrose content, such as ice cream and unfrosted cakes, should be restricted to occasional use. This also applies to other baked products like plain doughnuts, unfrosted cup cakes, and simple cookies. Sugar coated cereals and any cereal product where sugar is the first or second item in the list of ingredients on the package must be excluded from the diet.

Diet cookies and cakes made with artificial sweeteners in place of sugar are not recommended. They are not usually acceptable substitutes due to their flavor and texture, and gram for gram, may contain as much carbohydrate and energy as products made from standard ingredients.

MEAT EXCHANGES. The items in this food group contain primarily protein and fat. The one exception, peanut butter, contains 3 grams of carbohydrate per tablespoon (15 g.). This amount of carbohydrate will be significant only if an individual uses 6 to 8 tablespoons of peanut butter per day (18 to 24 g. carbohydrate).

It is advisable that diabetic patients select lean meats, fish, and poultry, and limit the use of eggs to three a week to control their intake of saturated fatty acids and cholesterol.

FAT EXCHANGES. The best choices in this food group are those items which contain a significant amount of polyunsaturated fatty acids—the margarines and vegetable oils.

MIXED DISHES. Cookbooks which give the exchange values of one serving of the product are available for diabetic patients and a selection of books and publications containing these recipes are listed at the end of this chapter. The exchange values of a serving of the patient's own recipes can also be calculated.

CONVENIENCE FOODS. Unless the nutrient label makes it possible to estimate the exchange values of a serving of the product, convenience foods cannot be used by the diabetic patient. The list of ingredients on the packages of many convenience foods indicates that a variety of food fats, lactose in milk solids, or various forms of sugar, such as refiners syrup and invert sugar and corn syrups, are used by the processors in formulating these foods. Unfortunately, unless the package also has a nutrient label stating the energy, protein, fat, and carbohydrate value of an average serving, it is impossible to tell whether or not fats and sugars are present in significant or insignificant amounts.

ALCOHOL. If alcohol is used by the diabetic patient, the energy value of the amount to be used is subtracted from the calorie intake defined in the diet prescription before the grams of protein, fat, and carbohydrate are calculated. For example, an 1800 calorie diet prescription which includes 150 calories from alcohol becomes a 1650 calorie diet. The decision to include alcohol in the diet plan rests with the physician. It should be remembered that patients using the sulfonylureas may be intolerant of alcohol. Also alcohol should be excluded from the diets of some patients with hyperlipidemias (see Chapter 29).

Distilled spirits—scotch, rye, bourbon, vodka and gin—do not contain carbohydrate, while fermented spirits—beer, ales and wines—contain carbohydrate. Therefore, when alcohol is used the patient should be advised to use distilled spirits. If the energy prescription is 1500 calories or less, alcoholic beverages must be excluded because this source of energy without other nutrients may make it impossible to meet the patient's daily nutrient needs.

Planning the Diabetic Diet Pattern with the Patient
STEP I. The first step in planning the diet pattern with any newly diagnosed patient, either in the hospital or in an ambulatory-care setting, is to obtain a

complete history of the patient's usual food practices and daily activities. At the time of diagnosis many maturity onset diabetics do not require hospitalization. Gathering the data base for assessment prior to planning the diet pattern will probably take from one to one and one-half hours and may require more than one encounter with the patient before a suitable diet pattern can be planned.

The data gathered about food practices should cover the same information one gains from any patient requiring a modified diet: the *when, what, where,* and with *whom* the individual customarily eats. With the diabetic patient it is very important to identify any variation in his daily schedule which may occur on weekends or on his days off from employment. Insulin-dependent patients must establish and maintain a consistent meal schedule every day of the week.

What kinds and amounts of foods consumed at each meal or snack must be determined in detail (see Chapter 12). How foods are prepared and the basic ingredients in commonly used recipes should also be elicited at this time. Knowledge of the methods of food preparation is important because it may be

Table 28–4. Nutrient Composition of 1500 Calorie Diabetic Diet
(50% Simple and 50% Complex Carbohydrate)

FOOD EXCHANGES	AMOUNT Number	AMOUNT Household Measure	PROTEIN (g.)	FAT (g.)	CARBO-HYDRATE (g.)	ENERGY (cal.)
Milk	2	1 pint	16	20	24	340
Vegetables Group A	As desired					
Vegetables Group B	2	1 cup	4		14	70
Fruit	4	varies			40	160
Bread	5	varies	10		75	350
Meat	6	6 oz.	42	30		450
Fat	3	3 tsp.		15		135
TOTALS			72	65	153	1505

Table 28–5. 1500 Calorie Diabetic Diet Pattern
(75 G. Protein, 65 G. Fat, 150 G. Carbohydrate;
50% Simple and 50% Complex Carbohydrate)

MEAL	FOOD EXCHANGE	AMOUNT	PROTEIN (g.)	FAT (g.)	CARBOHYDRATE (g.)	ENERGY (cal.)
Morning						
Milk	1	8 oz.	8	10	12	170
Fruit	1	varies			10	40
Meat	1	1 oz.	7	5		75
Bread	1	varies	2		15	70
Fat	1	1 tsp.		5		45
TOTAL			17	20	37	400
Noon						
Meat	2	2 oz.	14	10		150
Bread	2	varies	4		30	140
Fruit	1	varies			10	40
Fat	1	1 tsp.		5		45
TOTAL			18	15	40	375
Evening						
Meat	3	3 oz.	21	15		225
Bread	2	varies	4		30	140
Vegetable B	2	1 cup	4		14	70
Fruit	1	varies			10	40
Fat	1	1 tsp.		5		45
TOTAL			29	20	54	520
Bedtime						
Milk	1	8 oz.	8	10	12	170
Fruit	1	varies			10	40
TOTAL			8	10	22	210
TOTALS			72	65	153	1505

necessary to make modifications. If the patient is a married man, information about his daily meal pattern and methods of home food preparation is generally obtained from his wife.

The frequency with which a patient's usual meal pattern varies should also be ascertained. For example, routine social engagements such as "bowling night" may modify the patient's usual evening meal pattern and intake of alcoholic beverages. Some patients will report that "bowling night" is also "beer night."

Where and with whom the patient eats is also important information. With the national trend to-ward eating more meals outside the home, it is important to know the restaurants in which the patient eats most frequently and the type of menus offered. Many patients can continue this practice, depending on their diet prescription and the food served by the restaurant. If the patient is the mother, father, or a child in a large family, it is advisable to modify, if necessary, the family's usual food practices, because other members of the family may be high risks for developing diabetes mellitus.

If the diabetic patient is a child, the data is obtained from the mother and any other individual who may be closely involved in the child's care. For exam-

Table 28–6. Nutrient Composition of 1500 Calorie Diabetic Diet
(35% Simple and 65% Complex Carbohydrate)

FOOD EXCHANGES	AMOUNT Number	AMOUNT Household Measure	PROTEIN (g.)	FAT (g.)	CARBO-HYDRATE (g.)	ENERGY (cal.)
Milk	1	8 oz.	8	10	12	170
Vegetables Group A	As desired					
Vegetables Group B	1	½ cup	2		7	35
Fruit	3	varies			30	120
Bread	7	varies	14		105	490
Meat	7	7 oz.	49	35		525
Fat	4	4 tsp.		20		180
TOTALS			73	65	164	1530

Table 28–7. 1500 Calorie Diabetic Diet Pattern
(75 G. Protein, 65 G. Fat, 150 G. Carbohydrate;
35% Simple and 65% Complex Carbohydrate)

MEAL	FOOD EXCHANGE	AMOUNT	PROTEIN (g.)	FAT (g.)	CARBOHYDRATE (g.)	ENERGY (cal.)
Morning						
Fruit	1	varies			10	40
Bread	2	varies	4		30	140
Milk	1	8 oz.	8	10	12	170
Fat	1	1 tsp.		5		45
TOTAL			12	15	52	395
Noon						
Meat	2	2 oz.	14	10		150
Bread	2	varies	4		30	140
Fruit	1	varies			10	40
Fat	1	1 tsp.		5		45
TOTAL			18	15	40	375
Evening						
Meat	4	4 oz.	28	20		300
Bread	2	varies	4		30	140
Vegetable B	1	½ cup	2		7	35
Fruit	1	varies			10	40
Fat	2	1 tsp.		10		90
TOTAL			34	30	47	505
Bedtime						
Meat	1	1 oz.	7	5		75
Bread	1	varies	2		15	70
TOTAL			9	5	15	155
TOTALS			73	65	154	1530

ple, if the mother works, the babysitter should be included in the interview.

During the interview one can also discover what the client knows about diet in the treatment of diabetes mellitus. Some newly diagnosed adult patients have had experience with the diet if another family member also has diabetes. This experience can have a positive or a negative effect on the patient's attitude, depending on a number of factors such as the type of diet and the severity of the relative's condition.

STEP II. The second step is to plan the diabetic diet pattern. It should be planned within the constraints of the diet prescription and incorporate, whenever possible, the usual food practices of the patient. Table 28–4 illustrates the energy and nutrient composition of the quantities of food in a 1500 calorie diabetic diet. Twenty percent of the total calories is derived from protein and 40 percent, from fat and carbohydrate respectively. Approximately 50 percent is simple and 50 percent complex carbohydrate. Table 28–5 illustrates the distribution (2/7, 2/7, 2/7, 1/7) of the exchanges used in Table 28–4 in three meals and a bedtime snack. The food exchanges in each meal reflect the choices of a 55-year-old homemaker who developed this diet pattern with her nutrition counselor.

Tables 28–6 and 28–7 illustrate the same process except that approximately 35 percent is simple and 65 percent is complex carbohydrate. The energy and percentage of protein, fat, and carbohydrate are the same in both diet patterns. The reader is advised to translate both diet patterns into a day's menu using the Exchange Lists on Table 23-4 of Chapter 23, p. 329, and the additional information on food selection and preparation in Chapter 27 (p. 386) and in this chapter. A copy of the diet pattern (see Fig. 27–5) should be entered in the patient's record for use by the health-care team and in follow-up counseling sessions.

Because many Americans omit or eat very little breakfast, one of the major adjustments in food practices which an adult patient may need to be guided toward is accepting an increase in the quantities of foods he consumes at breakfast. The patient who uses intermediate-acting insulin may have an insulin reaction during the morning if he does not have an adequate breakfast.

Regular Diet with No Added Sugar

If the diet prescription is regular (free) diet, or diet-for-age, with no added sugar, the energy and nutrient needs of the patient must be identified and translated into reasonable quantities of foods for the day. This information is used to assist the patient to establish a consistent daily meal schedule. If the mother of a newly diagnosed child is very anxious about her ability to feed her child at home, it may be wise to offer her a meal plan using the Exchange System. As the mother gains confidence in her ability to feed her child, she will need help to liberalize the plan.

Weighted Diets

The physician who uses the chemical method to treat the diabetic will require his patients to purchase a scale which weighs in grams. The patient will weigh each serving of food at each meal. The instruction materials for the patient will give the gram weight of each serving of food. The equivalent household measure may also be included. Many of these physicians have adapted the Exchange System or constructed a similar system for this method of diet instruction. The nutrient values of foods used by physicians may vary to some degree from those used in the Exchange system, therefore the counselor will need to use the nutrient values of the physician when calculating the diet pattern with a patient. As the patient acquires experience in weighing his food he becomes expert in judging serving size and may be advised by his physician to weigh his food only one day a week to check his practices.

Diet Planning for Associated Diseases

In addition to modifying the diabetic diet in the treatment of elevated blood levels of triglycerides and cholesterol, discussed in Chapter 29, the diet may also be modified if other diseases are present. The consistency of the diabetic diet may be modified if there is gastrointestinal disease (see Chapter 25). If hypertension, or cardiac or renal disease is present, the diet may also be restricted in fluids and the electrolyte sodium and, if necessary, in protein (see Chapters 30 and 31).

COUNSELING THE PATIENT

The diabetic patient must be helped to accept the fact that his disease cannot be cured but that he can, with proper dietary care, and the use of insulin or oral hypoglycemic agents, if necessary, live a comfortable and productive life. Explaining to the patient in understandable terms the nature of the disease and why his dietary program is necessary is frequently the responsibility of the physician and the nurse. As soon as the hospitalized patient's diabetes is stabilized, actual dietary counseling should begin, with the physician, nurse, and nutrition counselor working closely together. In many instances a social worker and clinical psychologist should also be members of this team. In the ambulatory care setting, the health care team has an advantage in that the patient's disease is usually stable and he is less anxious and, therefore, better able to learn.

Stone[14] has demonstrated that, given adequate instruction and the time to learn, the majority of diabetic patients can manage their diets successfully: they are capable of client-managed care. No patient can accept the diagnosis of diabetes mellitus and learn to manage its control during hospitalization (an average of seven to eight days) or during two visits to ambulatory care services. Therefore, the health-care team must accept, and plan to meet, his needs for continuity of care.

Gathering the assessment data is the first step in the counseling process. From her appraisal of this data the counselor can plan her program. Also, this process often helps the client identify for himself the adjustments he will need to make in his food practices.

The primary objective of nutrition counseling for the diabetic patient is to help him use his diet pattern correctly. He needs to be able to translate his pattern into daily menus and to identify the correct size portion of each item in his menu. To do this he is given a permanent record of the number of food exchanges in his diet pattern (see Table 28-5 or 28-7) and a copy of the Exchange Lists (see Table 23-4) from which to select his daily menu.

For the hospitalized patient his trays are an important teaching aid. With guidance he can learn the size of food portions and familiarize himself with the items in each exchange food group. The lack of certain foods which do not appear on the tray such as sugar, jelly, pies, cakes, and other desserts can be emphasized. As counseling progresses, the selective menu can be used as a "paper and pencil test" to evaluate the patient's understanding.

In the ambulatory care setting food models are a useful aid in helping patients visualize portion sizes. If a demonstration kitchen and food are available, portion sizes can be demonstrated with real food. It is often helpful to have the patient keep a record of his food intake for one or two days between appointments. These records are used to formulate precise objectives for the counseling session.

Whenever the patient's food choices differ for ethnic reasons from those included in the teaching materials, the materials should be modified to suit his choices.

Other members of the family should be involved in counseling sessions with the patient so that they understand his care and can give him support. If work or other schedules make it impossible for family members to be available during the day, counseling sessions should be scheduled at the convenience of the patient and the relative during a weekend or late in the day. Some ambulatory care facilities schedule clinics at least one evening a week in addition to Saturday morning.

SPECIAL CONCERNS
Ketoacidosis and Coma

Ketoacidosis and coma require emergency treatment to reestablish fluid and electrolyte balance and normal metabolism. If the patient is in coma, or if he is nauseated and vomiting, insulin and intravenous fluids will be used to treat him. As his hyperglycemia and ketonemia decrease, and when he can tolerate it, he will be offered a variety of fluids by mouth. When his condition is stabilized he will be given a diabetic diet and insulin.

When the patient can tolerate fluids it is advisable that, directly after each feeding, the amount and nutrient composition is recorded in his chart so that his information is readily available to the physician and nurse as they monitor the patient's progress. When a known diabetic is able to eat he can assist with his menu selection. The newly diagnosed patient can share his food preferences with the dietitian but she will be responsible for planning his meals.

Replacements

It is expected that diabetic patients receiving insulin or an oral hypoglycemic agent will consume all the food served at each meal to prevent the possibility of insulin reaction. When a patient refuses a food, he should be provided with a substitute equal in nutritional composition to the food refused.

If a patient refuses the major portion of a meal for any reason, the physician may require that the total available glucose of the meal be replaced. Carbohydrate, together with protein and fat, contribute to the total available glucose in a meal. The grams of carbohydrate yield an equal number of grams of glucose, or 100 percent glucose. It is estimated that 58 percent of protein and 10 percent of fat form glucose in intermediary metabolism. Therefore, to calculate the total available glucose (TAG) in a meal, one multiplies the grams of carbohydrate by 1.0, the grams of protein by 0.58, and the grams of fat by 0.10, the results are then added to obtain the total available glucose.

For example: a meal containing 30 g. of protein, 30 g. of fat and 60 g. of carbohydrate has 80 g. of available glucose.

30 g. of protein × 0.58 = 17.4 g. of glucose; 30 g. of fat × 0.1 = 3 g. of glucose; and 60 g. of carbohydrate = 60 g. of glucose.

This amount of carbohydrate may have to be given in several small feedings within the next two or three hours to prevent insulin reaction.

Surgery

Today diabetic individuals undergo surgery with comparative safety. In emergencies, such as an acute appendix, there is usually no reason to delay surgery because of diabetes. In these situations the patient is given insulin and intravenous fluids and glucose.

When there is time to prepare for surgery the status of the patient's diabetes is carefully evaluated and, if his disease is not well-controlled, the proper diet and insulin treatment is instituted before he undergoes surgery. On the day of surgery breakfast is withheld. Part of the usual dose of moderate-acting insulin may be given before surgery. After the operation glucose and fluids with sufficient insulin are given intravenously. Oral feedings of liquids such as fruit juices, broth, tea, and ginger ale are started as early as possible. Later, the patient's usual diet is resumed.

Diabetes in Pregnancy

Diabetes has always been a special hazard in pregnancy. There is increased fetal loss in the course of the pregnancy as well as an increased loss of infants carried to term as compared with the nondiabetic patient. Also, it has been observed that the infants experience more problems in the neonatal period than do infants of nondiabetic mothers. In the past few years, however, by keeping close watch on the mother and infant, physicians have been able to secure a far greater number of successful pregnancies than formerly.

Early prenatal care is an important factor in the salvage of these babies as well as in the maintenance of the health of the mother. The diet during pregnancy must be adjusted to control the mother's diabetes and to provide for the nutritional needs of the developing fetus. As the woman progresses through pregnancy her insulin requirement increases steadily, and decreases dramatically to prepregnancy levels immediately after delivery. In an obstetrical unit food acceptance by the postpartum woman must be closely monitored to avoid insulin reactions.

DIABETES IN CHILDREN

The outlook for children who develop diabetes has changed markedly from the preinsulin days when the disease invariably was fatal. White[15] reported on 1072 patients whose onset of diabetes occurred before the age of 15 and who had had the disease 20 years or more. Of these, 879 were living at the time of the study. Of the 879 patients, 71 percent had had diabetes from 20 to 29 years, 24 percent had had diabetes from 30 to 34 years, and 5 percent had had the disease for more than 35 years.

However, in a large percentage of such patients, complications develop after 15 to 20 years or more of diabetes. These include diminished vision and heart and kidney disease, all attributable to blood vessel changes. In a later paper[16] White states that 90 percent of patients who developed diabetes before the age of 15 and had had the disease for 30 years or more could be shown to have such blood vessel changes. Thus, although gains have been made in increasing the life-span of the young diabetic, much remains to be done in terms of halting the complications of the disease.

Dietary Management

The controversy over the best approach to treatment applies particularly to this younger age group of patients. Clinicians who advocate the "free" diet or diet-for-age without added sugar feel that it promotes a more positive attitude in the family and a more normal psychosocial development in the child. To avoid wide daily variations in blood glucose levels, however, the nutrition counselor is called on to assist the mother with meal planning so that there is a consistent daily intake of energy and nutrients. For example, a four-year-old child cannot consume 1000 calories today and 1600 calories tomorrow and still maintain reasonable control. At the same time, food intake must be spaced throughout the day as with any patient using intermediate-acting insulin to avoid hyper- or hypoglycemic episodes.

Achievement of Genetic Growth Potential

Drash[17] reports that diabetic children attain an adult height which is well within the range of normal but below the mean for the United States population. English observers report that with the onset of diabetes prior to the adolescent growth spurt, full growth potential is not achieved. However, with the use of long- and intermediate-acting insulins and adequate food intake, the diabetic dwarfism of the past does not occur.

Emotional Adjustment

Coping with a chronic disease in childhood such as diabetes mellitus presents a major challenge to both the family and the child. A number of studies show that there is an increased incidence of emotional stress in children with diabetes compared with normal children. They tend to be dependent, anxious, and hostile and have impaired self-images. Acute emotional stress adversely affects diabetic control and can cause ketoacidosis. Rage and extreme anxiety can trigger epinephrine release from the adrenal medulla. Epinephrine stimulates gluconeogenesis which can result in hyperglycemia. Also, emotional stress may lead to episodes of food gorging or omitting insulin injections entirely. The child with diabetes, who experiences episodes of ketoacidosis due to emotional stress, and his family may need the help of a psychiatrist or psychologist to establish an environment within the family that will promote the stabilization of the child's diabetes mellitus.

STUDY QUESTIONS AND ACTIVITIES

1. Check the products on the "diet" shelf in a local supermarket or health food store. Compare the energy and nutrient composition of a dietetic product with the composition of the same amount of a standard product. For example 1 oz. of a dietetic chocolate bar with 1 oz. of a standard chocolate bar.
2. Discover by observation and interview how the mother of a well-controlled school aged diabetic child (who has been hospitalized in a state of ketoacidosis due to overwhelming infection) manages his diet and activities of daily living. What resources has she used for guidance and counseling? What adjustment, if any, has the family made in its lifestyle since the child's diagnosis?
3. Mrs. A. is a 70-year-old diabetic. Her major source of income is her monthly social security check of $145.00. She purchases food stamps to supplement her food budget. Her diet prescription is 1500 calories. Calculate her diet pattern, write up a week's menu and a market order. Price the market order at a store in a neighborhood where many of the elderly in your community live. What percent of her income would she spend on food?
4. Price U-40 and U-100 insulin and the equipment needed to inject insulin at a discount drugstore, an independently owned drugstore, and the hospital pharmacy. How much does it cost a diabetic patient to administer 35 units of insulin per day?
5. Collect menus from a variety of local restaurants. Select a noon and evening meal using the diet pattern which you planned for the diet prescription in question 3.
6. Find out the total number of adult diabetic patients in your hospital today. The therapeutic dietitian's records of diet orders will give you this information most readily. How many of these diets are also calorie restricted (1500 or less)?
7. Record the 24-hour food and nutrient beverage intake of a patient with diabetes. Using the appropriate food value system, appraise his calorie and nutrient intake. Compare his actual intake of calories, protein, fat, and carbohydrate with the diet order prescribed by his physician. Compare his mineral and vitamin intake with guidelines appropriate for him. If there is any significant discrepancy between intake and order, seek the assistance of your instructors in identifying the reason and in solving the problem.
8. Give five substitutes that a diabetic can make for a slice of bread.
9. What is meant by the chemical regulation of diabetes? The clinical regulation? Why is there controversy over these two methods of regulation?
10. What is meant by a "free" diabetic diet? What advantages are claimed for it?

SUPPLEMENTARY READINGS

Backscheider, J. E.: Self-care requirements, self-care capabilities, and nursing systems in the diabetic nurse management clinic. Am. J. Public Health 64:1138, 1974.

Bruck, E., and MacGillivray, M. H.: Posthypoglycemic hyperglycemia in diabetic children. J. Pediat. 84:672, 1974.

Doar, J. W. H., et al: Influence of treatment with diet alone on oral glucose-tolerance test and plasma sugar and insulin levels in patients with maturity-onset diabetes mellitus. Lancet 1:1263, 1975.

Drash, A.: Diabetes mellitus in childhood: a review. J. Pediat. 78:919, 1971.

Felig, P.: Insulin: routes and rates of delivery. N. Eng. J. Med. 291:1031, 1974.

Kaufman, R. L., et al: Plasma lipid levels in diabetic children: Effect of diet restricted in cholesterol and saturated fats. Diabetes 24:672, 1975.

McFarlane, J.: Children with diabetes: special needs during growth years. Am. J. Nurs. 73:1360, 1973.

McFarlane, J., and Hames, C. C.: Children with diabetes: learning self-care in camp. Am. J. Nurs. 73:1362, 1973.

O'Sullivan, J. B.: Age gradient in blood glucose levels: Magnitude and clinical implications. Diabetes 23:713, 1974.

Partridge, J. W., et al: Attitudes of adolescents toward their diabetes. Am. J. Dis. Child. 124:226, 1972.

Paz-Guevara, A. T., et al: Juvenile diabetes mellitus after forty years. Diabetes, 24:559, 1975.

Rosenbloom, A. L.: Advances in commercial insulin preparations. Am. J. Dis. Child. 128:631, 1974.

Salzar, J. E.: Classes to improve diabetic self-care. Am. J. Nurs. 75:1324, 1975.

Schmitt, B. D.: An argument for the unmeasured diet in juvenile diabetes. Clin. Pediatrics 14:68, 1975.

Tattersall, R. B., and Fajans, S. S.: Prevalence of diabetes and glucose intolerance in 199 offspring of thirty-seven conjugal diabetic parents. Diabetes 24:452, 1975.

Unger, R. H., and Orci, L.: Hypothesis: the essential role of glucagon in the pathogenesis of diabetes mellitus. Lancet 1:14, 1975.

West, K. M.: Diet therapy of diabetes: an analysis of failure. Ann. Int. Med. 79:425, 1973.

Rosenthal, H. and Rosenthal, J.: *Diabetic Care in Pictures,* ed. 4. Philadelphia, Lippincott, 1968.

Salmon, M. B. and Quigley, A. E., eds.: *Enjoying Your Restricted Diet.* Springfield, Ill., Thomas, 1972.

For further references see Bibliography in Section 4.

PATIENT RESOURCES

Berman, D. M.: *A Cookbook for Diabetics.* Am. Diabet. Assoc., 1 West 48th St., New York, N. Y. 10020.

Danowski, T. S.: *Diabetes as a Way of Life,* ed. 2. New York, Coward-McCann, 1970.

Diabetes Forecast. Am. Diabet. Assoc., 1 West 48th St. New York, N. Y. 10020 ($3.00/year).

Gibbons, E.: *Feast on a Diabetic Diet,* rev. ed. New York, David McKay, 1973.

Gormican, A.: *Controlling Diabetes with Diet.* Springfield, Ill., Thomas, 1971.

La Dieta Diabetica—The Diabetic Diet in Spanish. California Dietetic Assoc., 1609 Westwood Blvd., Los Angeles, Ca. 90024.

Revell, D. T.: *Gourmet Recipes for Diabetics.* Springfield, Ill., Thomas, 1971.

REFERENCES

1. Unger, R. H. and Orci, L.: Lancet 1:14, 1975.
2. Tattersall, R. B. and Fajans, S. C.: Diabetes, 24:44, 1975.
3. Sunder, J. H.: in *Diabetes Mellitus, Diagnosis and Treatment,* Vol. 2. New York, Am. Diabet. Assoc., 1964.
4. Davis, M. D.: in *Diabetes Mellitus,* Vol. 3. New York, Am. Diabet. Assoc., 1971.
5. Siperstein, M. D.: in *Diabetes Mellitus,* Vol. 3. New York, Am. Diabet. Assoc., 1971.
6. Spiro, R. G.: N. Eng. J. Med. 288:1337, 1973.
7. Ibid.
8. Anderson, T. W.: Diabetes 15:160, 1966.
9. Diabetes (Supplement 2) 19:747, 1970.
10. Bunzell, J. B. et al: Diabetes 23:138, 1974.
11. Drash, A.: J. Pediat. 78:919, 1971.
12. Ibid.
13. Ibid.
14. Stone, D. B.: Am. J. Med. Sci. 241:436, 1961.
15. White, P.: Diabetes 5:445, 1956.
16. White, P.: Diabetes 9:345, 1960.
17. Drash, A., op. cit.

29 atherosclerosis

Prevalence and Incidence
Diagnostic Procedures
Diet Therapy
Patient Counseling
Hypolipidemic Drugs

This chapter could appropriately be subtitled
Hyperlipidemia or Hyperlipoproteinemia (see
Table 29-1, Glossary of Terms). From the available
evidence the incidence of atherosclerosis is
strongly associated with aberrations in the
intermediary metabolism of cholesterol and
triglycerides. Evidence is also available that the
manipulation of the dietary intake of cholesterol,
the type of fatty acids (saturated vs.
polyunsaturated), and sucrose (particularly the
fructose component) can have a positive effect on
the blood lipid abnormalities in hyperlipidemia
from both a preventive and a therapeutic aspect.
Reference was made to these dietary manipulations
in the previous chapters on obesity and diabetes
mellitus, because hyperlipidemia is frequently
associated with these metabolic problems.
However, not all hyperlipidemic patients are obese
or diabetic.

Before proceeding with the following
discussion of atherosclerosis and the dietary
modification recommended for the prevention and
treatment of hyperlipidemia, the reader is advised
to review Chapter 3, Fats and Other Lipids, and
Chapter 9, Nutrient Utilization, in this book, and
the structures and functions of the cardiovascular
system in a basic physiology textbook.

Table 29-1. Glossary of Terms

Hyperlipidemia: an elevation of the concentration of any blood lipid constituent; usually implies elevated cholesterol or triglycerides or both.

Hyperlipoproteinemia (HLP): an elevation of the blood concentration of one or more lipoprotein families; nearly always accompanied by hyperlipidemia.

Hyperlipemia: a lactescent (milky) appearance of blood caused by increased concentration of triglyceride in either very low-density lipoproteins (VLDL) or chylomicrons.

Hyperglyceridemia (or hypertriglyceridemia): an elevation in the blood levels of glycerides, usually triglycerides.

Hyperchylomicronemia: an elevation in the blood levels of chylomicrons.

Hypercholesterolemia: an elevation in the blood level of total cholesterol.

Although atherosclerosis is not the only disease state associated with hyperlipidemia, it is the one which occurs most frequently in the United States and in many other developed countries in the Western world. The term atherosclerosis is derived from two Greek words: *athere*, meaning "porridge" or "mush," and *skleros*, meaning "hard." The atheromatous lesion, which develops in the arterial blood vessels, begins as a soft deposit and hardens as it ages. With time these lesions, known as plaques, gradually grow and thicken the intima of the arterial walls, thus narrowing the lumen of the blood vessels (Fig. 29-1). The atherosclerotic plaque is composed of various substances which include cholesterol, fatty acids, lipoproteins (a complex molecule of protein and fat), calcium deposits, complex carbohydrates, fibrous scar tissue, and blood.[1] How and why these plaques develop is not well understood, and numerous theories have been under intensive study for the past twenty years.

Myocardial infarction, or heart attack, occurs when a blood clot forms suddenly and occludes the lumen of a coronary artery already narrowed by an atheromatous plaque. This event deprives the surrounding tissue of its blood supply. Depending on the extent of damage to the tissue of the heart in the area of the occlusion, the patient may survive or die suddenly. If the occlusion of a blood vessel occurs in the brain, the result is a cerebral hemorrhage, or "stroke." Other arterial blood vessels in the body may also be occluded, causing serious disease or death.

Prevalence and Incidence

Atherosclerosis is a major public health problem because the sequelae to the formation of atheromata—coronary artery disease and cerebral hemorrhage—are the leading causes of disability and death in the United States and Canada. In 1972 more than 600,000 persons in the United States, and 77,000 in Canada, died of coronary heart disease. It is estimated that over 160,000 of the deaths in the United States occurred in persons under 65 years of age, predominantly males in this age group. According to the National Health Examination Survey data, 5 million Americans have atherosclerosis, which makes it the second most prevalent cardiovascular disease. (The most prevalent cardiovascular problem is hypertension.)

Coronary Risk Factors

After 20 years of intensive epidemiologic and laboratory research, the etiology of atherosclerosis is still equivocal. However, there is relatively general agreement that the causation is multifactorial, i.e., that a number of factors interact in determining the inception, rate of progression, and ultimate clinical course of atherosclerosis in an individual. Table 29-2 lists the factors which appear to increase the risk of coronary heart disease, but not all investigators would agree that each item in the table is a risk factor. For example, there is considerable controversy about the role of excessive coffee drinking. However, there is consensus that the major risk factors in coronary heart disease are positive family history, increase in the level of blood cholesterol, excessive cigarette smoking, blood pressure levels above normal, and, for some age groups, increased body weight in relation to height.[2]

In 1973 the Heart and Lung Institute of the National Institutes of Health established the Multiple Risk Factor Intervention Trial (MRFIT) to assess the effectiveness of measures to reduce elevated blood cholesterol, high blood pressure, and cigarette smoking in preventing first heart attacks and reducing death rates from cardiovascular disease.[3] Twenty clinical research centers around the country enroll

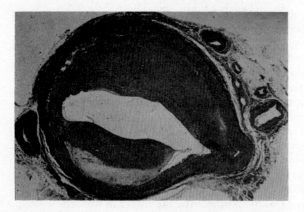

Fig. 29-1. Atherosclerotic obliteration of the lumen of the iliac artery. (Bailey, C. P., et al, *Rheumatic and Coronary Heart Disease*. Philadelphia, Lippincott, 1967)

Table 29-2. Factors Known to Increase the Risk of Coronary Heart Disease*

GROUP 1. (Not amenable to preventive intervention)
Maleness
Age (increased risk with increased age)
Family history (positive for premature vascular disease)
Certain somatotypes
Particular behavior patterns and personality types

GROUP 2. (Associated disease entities)
Hyperlipoproteinemias
Arterial hypertension
Obesity
Diabetes mellitus
Hyperuricemia and gout

GROUP 3. (Primarily due to culture and environment)
Dietary practices (high intake of cholesterol, saturated fats, sucrose[a] and energy)
Sedentary living habits (lack of physical exercise)
Cigarette smoking
Excessive coffee drinking[b]
Soft water for drinking[c]

*Adapted from Brusis, O. A., and McGandy R. B.: Fed. Proc. 30:1417, 1971.
[a]Ahrens, R. A.: Am. J. Clin. Nutr. 27:403, 1974.
[b]Jick, H., et al: N. Eng. J. Med. 289:63, 1973.
[c]Perry, H. M., Jr.: J. Am. Dietet. A. 62:631, 1973.

600 men, ages 35 to 57, who are above average risk for coronary heart disease due to various combinations of these three factors. The subjects studied in each center must commit themselves to six years of participation. Included in the staff of each study center is a nutritionist to assist the subjects to modify their diets; a behavioral scientist to help reduce smoking; and a physician to direct the medical procedures to reduce blood pressure.

Nutritional Research

The relationship to coronary heart disease of the dietary intake of cholesterol, total fat and fatty acids, and carbohydrate, especially sucrose, has been and continues to be under intensive investigation.

CHOLESTEROL. The majority of patients with coronary artery disease have an elevated blood cholesterol level, and researchers are attempting to relate the occurrence of this elevation in cholesterol to the dietary intake of this nutrient in order to design therapeutic as well as preventive nutritional care. Both epidemiologic and clinical research have been used to study this problem.

It has been shown that the usual American diet contains an average of 800 to 1000 mg. of cholesterol per day from meat, eggs, whole milk, and whole-milk products. Depending on food choices, an individual can easily consume more than 1000 mg. per day. For example, one egg contains about 250 mg. of cholesterol. Two or three eggs per day contribute 500 to 750 mg. of cholesterol.

It must be remembered that the cholesterol absorbed from food is not the only source of blood cholesterol. It is synthesized endogenously by the cells of the liver and gastrointestinal tract from the two carbon structure acetate formed in intermediary metabolism (see Chapter 9). Therefore, hexoses, glycerol, fatty acids, and certain deaminized amino acids can contribute carbon atoms for the endogenous synthesis of cholesterol. Research indicates, however, that blood levels do reflect in part the dietary intake of cholesterol. Hegsted has shown that as the intake of cholesterol from food increases from 0 to 800 mg. per day, the blood cholesterol increases progressively.[4]

FATS AND FATTY ACIDS. The information gathered by Keys and coworkers after World War II from the study of food intake and the incidence of coronary heart disease in a number of countries showed that the incidence of disease in the populations studied seemed to be related to the amount of fat in the national diet.[5] For example, the Japanese, who at the time consumed about 10 percent of their total calories as fat (Fig. 29-2), had a low incidence of coronary heart disease compared to Americans, who were consuming about 40 percent of their total

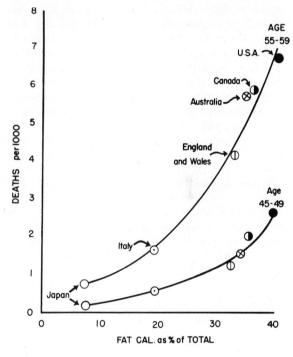

Fig. 29-2. Degenerative heart disease in men. Mortality from degenerative heart disease in two age groups, as related to percentage of fat calories in total calories of the national diet. (From Keys, A., Atherosclerosis: a problem in newer public health. J. Mt. Sinai Hosp., 20:118)

calories as fat. At the same time it was observed that in populations with low fat intakes the serum cholesterol levels were appreciably lower than in Americans with high fat intakes. It was also observed that polyunsaturated fatty acids provided a significant amount of the fat in the low-fat diets.

These observations of the relationship of the amount and type of fat in the diet to coronary heart disease did not apply equally to all the groups studied. For example, certain pastoral tribes in Africa who have a high milk intake and, therefore, a high saturated fat intake have a relatively low serum cholesterol level and incidence of coronary heart disease. It is suspected that physical activity may explain this difference, since the members of these tribes are more active than the other populations which were observed.

Following these population studies, extensive research was done to determine the effect of polyunsaturated fat on serum cholesterol levels in humans and animals. The results of these investigations indicate that saturated fats tend to increase serum cholesterol, while fats containing primarily polyunsaturated fatty acids tend to decrease serum cholesterol.[6] Monounsaturated fats appear to have no effect on serum cholesterol levels. There is, as yet, no agreement on the mechanism(s) by which the degree of saturation of fats affects serum cholesterol levels.

At the same time other investigators studied the effects of modifying the fatty acid composition of usual diets on blood cholesterol levels. They studied individuals, primarily men, under metabolic research conditions, and groups of men living and eating at home with their families.

The work of Page and Brown and their coworkers in Cleveland is one example of the first type of research. These investigators have determined critical limits for the fat and cholesterol composition of a diet effective in reducing serum cholesterol. Their research involved 134 normal, free-living, active subjects who were served test diets prepared in a research kitchen. All but 15 of the subjects were men between the ages of 20 and 55.[7] Table 29-3, based on their work, shows that there are critical limits in the fatty acid and cholesterol composition of diets which had a significant effect on lowering the serum cholesterol

levels of their subjects. A diet with 36 to 40 percent of calories from fat was effective in lowering serum cholesterol when less than 14 percent of total calories were provided by saturated fatty acids, more than 14 percent of total calories were from polyunsaturated fatty acids (linoleic), and the diet contained less than 350 mg. of cholesterol. A diet containing 25 to 30 percent of calories from fat was effective when less than 11 percent of total calories were provided by saturated fatty acids, more than 13 percent by polyunsaturated fatty acids, and the diet contained less than 300 mg. of cholesterol.

Christakis and his group in New York have studied 814 men ages 40 to 59 who were placed on a diet relatively rich in polyunsaturated fatty acids.[8] This diet resulted in a significant decrease in serum cholesterol levels, and the decrease was maintained for as long as five years. A control group of 463 men on nonrestricted diets was also studied. Compared with the control group the diet group had less morbidity from new coronary heart disease.

CARBOHYDRATE. At the same time that Keys and his associates were relating the incidence of coronary heart disease (CHD) to the diets of various populations, Yudkin suggested that the incidence of CHD was associated with the increasing consumption of sucrose in these same populations.[9] In 1961 E. H. Ahrens and his coworkers demonstrated that hypertriglyceridemia can be induced by the carbohydrate in the diet: the higher the carbohydrate intake the higher the blood triglyceride level.[10] It is still uncertain whether or not the type of carbohydrate, simple or complex, is responsible for this effect. There is some evidence that this problem may relate to the metabolism of fructose.[11] The major source of fructose in the Western diet is the disaccharide sucrose, compared with the limited amounts of fructose which occur naturally in commonly used fruits and vegetables.

ENERGY INTAKE. There has been conflicting evidence about the role of obesity per se as a risk factor in coronary heart disease. Bagdade has observed that hyperlipidemia, especially hypertriglyceridemia, frequently occurs in the obese.[12] The data from the Framingham Heart Study, an ongoing study of the development of coronary heart disease in a commun-

Table 29-3. Critical Limits of Dietary Fat Composition for Serum Cholesterol Reduction*

COMPONENT	DIET WITH 30-40 PERCENT FAT CALORIES	DIET WITH 25-30 PERCENT FAT CALORIES
Saturated fatty acids	less than 14% calories	less than 11% calories
Polyunsaturated fatty acids (linoleic)	more than 14% calories	more than 13% calories
Cholesterol	less than 350 mg.	less than 300 mg.

*Brown, H. B., and Farrand, M. E.: J. Am. Dietet. A. 49:303, 1966.

ity, shows that moderately large changes in serum cholesterol and blood pressure were proportional to changes over time in relative body weight.[13] Levy and coworkers have shown that, with restricted total energy intake leading to weight reduction, the cholesterol and triglyceride levels can be normalized in almost all patients with abnormal blood lipid levels.[14]

Hyperlipoproteinemias

At the same time that numerous investigators were studying coronary risk factors and the relationships of lipid, carbohydrate, and energy intake to the problems, Frederickson, Levy and Lee at the National Institutes of Health were studying the mechanisms of fat transport in lipoproteins.[15] In Chapter 3 it was pointed out that lipids are transported in the blood by chylomicrons, very low-density lipoproteins (VLDL), low-density lipoproteins (LDL), and high-density lipoproteins (HDL) (see Table 3–3). Recently an intermediate low-density lipoprotein (ILDL) which is a catabolic product of VLDL has been identified.[16]

Frederickson and coworkers demonstrated that measurements of the lipoproteins per se were better indicators of blood lipid abnormalities than analyses of the concentrations of blood lipid fractions alone. Their original classification of the hyperlipoproteinemias (HLP) into types I, II, III, IV, and V has been modified to: Type I, hyperchylomicronemia (normal or elevated cholesterol with markedly elevated triglyceride); Type IIa, hypercholesterolemia (increased LDL); Type IIb or Type III, hypercholesterolemia with endogenous hyperglyceridemia (Type IIb, increased LDL and VLDL and Type III, increased ILDL); Type IV, endogenous hyperglyceridemia (increased VLDL); and Type V, mixed hyperglyceridemia (increased chylomicrons and VLDL).

They have also demonstrated that HLPs are of two classes: (1) primary or familiar with genetic transmis-

Table 29–4. Five Types of Primary Hyperlipoproteinemia*

FEATURES	TYPE I	TYPE II a	TYPE II b or III	TYPE IV	TYPE V
Incidence	Very rare	Common	Relatively uncommon	Common	Uncommon
Appearance of plasma	Cream layer over clear infranatant fluid on standing	Clear	Clear, cloudy or milky	Slightly turbid to cloudy, unchanged with standing	Cream layer over turbid infranatant on standing
Cholesterol	Normal or elevated	Elevated	Elevated	Normal or elevated	Elevated or normal
Triglyceride	Markedly elevated	Normal or slightly elevated	Usually elevated	Elevated	Elevated to markedly elevated
Lipoprotein family	Elevated chylomicrons	Increased LDL	II b Increased LDL and VLDL III Increased ILDL	Increased VLDL	Increased chylomicrons and VLDL
Clinical presentation	Lipemia retinalis, eruptive xanthomas, hepatosplenomegaly, abdominal pain	Xanthelasma, tendon and tuberous xanthomas, juvenilis corneal arcus, accelerated atherosclerosis	Xanthoma planum; tuberoeruptive and tendon xanthomas; accelerated atherosclerosis of coronary and peripheral vessels	Accelerated coronary vessel disease, abnormal glucose tolerance, hyperuricemia	Lipemia retinalis, eruptive xanthomas, hepatosplenomegaly, abdominal pain, hyperglycemia, hyperuricemia
Origin; possible mechanism	Genetic recessive; deficiency in lipoprotein lipase	When genetic, dominant, sporadic; decreased catabolism of beta-lipoprotein	When genetic, recessive; sporadic?	When genetic, dominant, sporadic; excessive endogenous glyceride synthesis or deficient glyceride clearance?	Probably genetic, dominant, sporadic
Age of detection	Early childhood	Early childhood (in severe cases)	Adulthood (over age 20)	Adulthood	Early adulthood
Conditions to be excluded†	Dysgammaglobulinemia, insulinopenic diabetes	Dietary cholesterol excess, porphyria, myxedema, myeloma, nephrosis, obstructive liver disease	Myxedema, dysgammaglobulinemia	Diabetes, glycogen storage disease, nephrotic syndrome, pregnancy, Werner's syndrome	Myeloma, dysproteinemias, diabetic acidosis, nephrosis, alcoholism, pancreatitis

*Adapted from Levy, R. I.: Fed. Proc., 30:829, 1971, and N. Eng. J. Med. 290:1295, 1974.
†Secondary hyperlipoproteinemias.

Table 29-5. Composition of Fat-Controlled Diets Recommended by the American Heart Association*

NUTRIENT AND DIETARY PATTERN	PREVENTIVE DIET (3)[a]	THERAPEUTIC DIETS			
		1200 calories	1800 calories	2000-2200 calories	2400-2600 calories
Nutrients					
carbohydrate (g.)	273	120	200	270	335
protein (g.)	114	75	85	95	110
fat (g.)	83	42	68	70	84
saturated fatty acids (g.)	18	7	10	11	12
linoleic acid (g.)	26	14	26	26	33
cholesterol (mg.)	356	258	258	279	286
iron (mg.)	21.6	12	14	17	19
Dietary patterns					
% calories from carbohydrate	47	41	45	51	52
% calories from protein	20	26	20	18	17
% calories from fat	33	32	35	30	30
% calories from saturated fatty acids	7	5	5	4	4
% calories from linoleic acid	10	10	13	11	11
P:S ratio[b]	1.4:1	2:1	2.6:1	2.4:1	2.8:1

*Mueller, J. F.: J. Am. Dietet. A. 62:614, 1973
[a]2300 calories.
[b]Ratio of linoleic acid to saturated fatty acids.

Table 29-6. Summary of Diets for Type I-V Hyperlipoproteinemias*

Diet	Diet Prescription	Energy	Protein	Fat
Type I (Diet 1) Hyperchylomicronemia	Low Fat (25-35 g.)	Calories not restricted	Total protein not limited	Restricted to 25-35 g. per day, type of fat not important
Type II a (Diet 2) Hypercholesterolemia	Low Cholesterol Increased poly-unsaturated fat	Calories not restricted	Total protein not limited	Increased polyunsaturated fatty acid. Limited saturated fat
Type II b or III (Diet 3) Hypercholesterolemia and Endogenous Hyperglyceridemia	Low Cholesterol Approximately 20% Cal.-Pro. 40% Cal.-Fat 40% Cal.-Cho.	Achieve and maintain "ideal" weight (Reduction diet if necessary)	1½ to 2 g. per kg. of body weight or 18 to 21% total calories	40% of total calories (polyunsaturated fatty acid in preference to saturated fatty acid)
Type IV (Diet 4) Endogenous Hyperglyceridemia	Controlled Cho., approximately 45% of calories. Moderately restricted cholesterol	Achieve and maintain "ideal" weight (Reduction diet if necessary)	Total protein not limited	Not limited unless reduction diet needed (polyunsaturated fatty acid in preference to saturated fatty acid)
Type V (Diet 5) Mixed Hyperglyceridemia	Restricted fat, 30% of calories Controlled Cho., 50% of calories Moderately restricted cholesterol	Achieve and maintain "ideal" weight (Reduction diet if necessary)	1½ to 2 g. per kg. of body weight or 21-24% total calories	0.9 to 1.3 g. per kg. body weight Polyunsaturated fatty acid in preference to saturated fatty acid

*Adapted from the Dietary Management of Hyperlipoproteinemia: A Handbook for Physicians and Dietitians. DHEW Pub. No. (NIH) 73-110.

Diet	Cholesterol	Carbohydrate	Alcohol
Type I	Not restricted	Not limited	Not recommended
Type IIa	Less than 300 mg. per day (as low as possible 100-200 mg. preferred)	Not limited	May be used with discretion
Type IIb or III	Less than 300 mg. per day	Controlled—sucrose and concentrated sweets are restricted	Limited to 2 oz. of gin, rum, vodka, or whisky
Type IV	300-500 mg. per day	Limited to 4 to 5 g. per kg. body weight Sucrose and concentrated sweets are restricted	Limited to 2 oz. of gin, rum, vodka, or whisky
Type V	300-500 mg. per day	Limited to 5 g. per kg. body weight Sucrose and concentrated sweets are limited	Not recommended

sion; and (2) secondary to other diseases such as diabetes, hypothyroidism, obstructive liver disease, pancreatitis, and alcoholism. Premature atherosclerosis occurs frequently in those individuals with primary Type IIa, IIb, or IV lipoprotein patterns[17] (see Table 29–4). This work also lends support to family history (genetics) as an important risk factor in the development of coronary heart disease. By manipulating the intake of cholesterol, fatty acids, and/or carbohydrate, and total energy when the patient is obese, researchers showed that the blood lipid abnormalities could be modified.

Recommendations for the Prevention of CHD

As a result of research, the Council on Foods and Nutrition of the American Medical Association published in 1972 a council statement on diet and coronary heart disease.[18] It was recommended that: (1) the measurement of the plasma lipid profile [HLP typing] become a part of all health maintenance physical examinations and that all other risk factors be assessed periodically; (2) persons falling into risk categories on the basis of their blood lipid levels receive diet counseling; (3) the dietary advice does not compromise the intake of essential nutrients; and (4) modified and ordinary foods required by the diets be readily available on the market, reasonably priced, and easily identified. Similar statements have also been published by the American Heart Association[19] and the American Dietetic Association.[20]

DIAGNOSTIC PROCEDURES
Blood Lipids

Blood is drawn after a 12- to 14-hour fast for analysis of blood lipids. Correlations of blood cholesterol with the incidence of premature coronary heart disease show that there is an increasing risk when the cholesterol is higher than 220 mg. per 100 ml. of blood. A fasting triglyceride of greater than 150 mg. is also considered a high risk factor.

Lipoprotein Analysis

Lipoprotein analysis is a complex procedure; the reader is referred to a discussion of the method in *The Metabolic Basis of Inherited Disease.*[21] The conditions for the preparation of the subject for drawing blood for lipid analysis are of concern to the nutrition counselor. The subject must fast for 12 to 14 hours; for the preceding two weeks, he must consume his usual diet and neither gain nor lose weight; he must not be taking any medication known to affect plasma lipids; and he must not consume alcoholic beverages or take any other medication in the preceding 24 hours.

DIET THERAPY

The diet recommendations of the American Heart Association and of Frederickson and coworkers for the prevention and/or treatment of various types of HLPs share many characteristics. The American Heart Association recommends: (1) energy intake should be adjusted to achieve and/or maintain ideal weight; (2) no more than 35 percent of total calories should be contributed by fat; (3) saturated fatty acids should be restricted to 10 percent of total calories and polyunsaturated fatty acids should comprise 10 to 11 percent of total calories; and (4) dietary cholesterol should be restricted to less than 300 mg. per day.[22] Table 29–5 gives the nutrient composition of the fat-controlled diets in the pamphlets published by the American Heart Association (see also Patient Resources at the end of this chapter). These recommendations reflect the findings of Brown and Farrand given in Table 29–3.

Table 29–6 summarizes the recommendations of

Table 29-7. Nutrient Composition of Exchange System for Fat-Controlled and HLP Diets*

Food Group	Amount	Weight (g.)	Protein (g.)	Total Fat (g.)	Saturated Fatty acids (g.)	Linoleic Fatty acid (g.)	Choles-terol[a] (mg.)	Carbo-hydrate (g.)	Energy (cal.)
Milk, skim	1/2 pt. (8 oz.)	240	8	tr.	——	——	5	12	80
Vegetables									
Group A	as desired	——	——	——	——	——	——	——	——
Group B	½ cup	100	2	——	——	——	——	7	35
Fruit	varies	——	——	——	——	——	——	10	40
Bread and cereal	varies	——	2	1	——	——	——	15	75
Meat, lean only	1 oz.	30	8	3	0.6	0.1	21	——	60
Egg (3/week)	3/7	21	3	3	0.9	0.2	108	——	35
Fat									
Vegetable oil[b]	1 tbsp.	14	——	14	2.0	8.0	——	——	125
Margarine[c]	1 tbsp.	14	——	11	2.0	4.0	——	——	100

*Compiled with the assistance of M. C. Zuckel.
[a]Feeley, R. M., et al: J. Am. Dietet. A. 61:134, 1972.
[b]Corn, cottonseed, safflower, soybean oils.
[c]Nutrition Label, Chiffon margarine, 1973.

Frederickson and coworkers for the dietary management of hyperlipoproteinemias. It will be noted that in addition to recommendations for energy, fat, and cholesterol, this table includes recommendations for protein, carbohydrate, and alcohol. The National Heart and Lung Institute has also published a series of pamphlets for patients (see Patient Resources at the end of this chapter).

Since the recommendations of the American Heart Association and the National Institutes of Health have many similarities and the nutrition counselor must individualize diet patterns for patients, an Exchange System and Exchange Lists are presented in this section. This Exchange System is based on Tables 23-2 and 23-4 in Chapter 23.

Nutrient Composition of Fat-Controlled or Hyperlipoproteinemia Exchange System

Table 29-7 gives the energy and nutrient composition of the exchange food groups which can be used to calculate a fat-controlled or an HLP diet pattern. It will be noted that in addition to protein, fat, carbohydrate, and energy, values are given for cholesterol and saturated and polyunsaturated (linoleic) fatty acids. The cholesterol figures were derived from those published by Feeley et al in 1972.[23] The fatty acid figures for meat reflect weighted averages derived from values for lean beef, lamb, pork, and ham; poultry without skin; veal; and fish. Poultry and fish, which contain more linoleic acid than the other meats, contributed the greatest number of times to the weightings (weighting factor of 9 for fish and poultry vs. 5 for the meats).[24]

It will be noted that, in comparison with the other food groups in Table 29-7, the one ounce of lean meat and the 3/7 of an egg make the most significant contributions to the saturated fatty acid and cholesterol values and the least significant contributions of linoleic acid. On the other hand, the vegetable oils and margarine contribute the most significant quantities of the polyunsaturated fatty acid, linoleic. The fatty acid values for meat, egg, and vegetable oils and margarine demonstrate the quantitative differences in the types of fatty acids in animal fats and vegetable oils. Table 29-8 also demonstrates this difference.

To satisfy the recommendations of polyunsaturated fatty acids in preference to saturated ones in HLP diets 1 through 5 (see Table 29-6) vegetable oils and margarine are the only food fats which can be used as fat exchanges in the diet patterns. This is shown in Table 29-12, Nutrient Composition of a 1500-Calorie, HLP Diet 4, where about one half of the total grams of fat is contributed by vegetable oils and margarine.

Table 29-8. Fatty Acid and Energy Composition of Selected Foods

Food	Weight (g.)	Total Fat (g.)	Saturated Fatty Acids (g.)	Linoleic Fatty Acid (g.)	Energy (cal.)
Margarine[a]	14	11	2.0	4.0	100
Vegetable oil[b]	14	14	2.0	8.0	125
Butter	14	11	6.5	0.5	100
Milk, whole	240	9	5.0	0.5	170
Beef, rib with fat[c]	30	11	5.4	tr.	60

[a]Nutrition Label, Chiffon Margarine, 1973.
[b]Corn, cottonseed, safflower, soybean oils.
[c]USDA Handbook No. 8, Table 3.

The fatty acid values in Table 29-7 are used to plan a diet pattern with a specific ratio of linoleic to saturated fatty acids (P/S ratio). The calculation of a 1500-calorie, fat-controlled diet pattern with a P/S ratio of 1.5:1 is shown in Table 29-13. Only vegetable oils and margarine are used as fat exchanges.

Compared with Table 23-2 in Chapter 23, the other differences in the HLP Exchange System are: the nutrient values of the milk exchange are for skim milk only; 1 gram of fat has been added to the bread exchange values to reflect the fat used in breadmaking and the quantity of fat in cereal products and, therefore, the energy value of one exchange is 75 calories; meat exchanges are divided into two groups, meat exchanges and egg exchanges; the meat exchange is described as lean and contains 8 g. protein, 3 g. fat, and 60 calories; the nutrient values in the egg exchange are for $3/7$ of an egg or 3 eggs per week; and the amount of a fat exchange has been increased from 1 *teaspoon to 1 tablespoon*, and the energy value for 1 tablespoon of vegetable oil is 125 calories, and for 1 tablespoon of margarine, 100 calories.

Table 29-9. Food Exchange Lists for HLP or Fat-Controlled Diets*

Milk Exchanges
(One serving contains 8 g. of protein, 12 g. of carbohydrate, 7 mg. of cholesterol, and 80 calories.)

Skim milk	1 c.
Nonfat dried milk	¼ c.
Buttermilk (made from skim milk)	1 c.
Yogurt (made from skim milk)	½ c.

Vegetable Exchanges
Groups A and B
See Exchange Lists, Chapter 23, Table 23-4.

Fruit Exchanges
See Exchange Lists, Chapter 23, Table 23-4.

Bread Exchanges
(One serving contains 2 g. of protein, 1 g. of fat, 15 g. of carbohydrate and 75 calories.)

Bread (white, whole wheat, rye, pumpernickel, French, Italian)	1 slice
Melba toast (3½" x 1½" x ⅛")	4
Matzo (5" x 5")	1
Bread sticks, rye wafers	¾ oz.
Cereal, cooked	⅓ c.
dry, flake or puffed	¾ c.
Crackers	
oyster (½ c.)	20
saltines (2" sq.)	5
soda (2½" sq.)	2
Rolls	
hamburger or hot dog	½
hard roll, small	1
large	½
Rice, grits, cooked	½ c.
Spaghetti, noodles, cooked	½ c.
Macaroni, cooked	½ c.
Dry bread crumbs	¼ c.
Flour	3 tbsp.
Cornmeal	2½ tbsp.
Beans, peas, dried, cooked	½ c.
Corn, kernels or creamstyle	⅓ c.
Corn on the cob, medium ear	½ c.
Potatoes, white (2" diam.)	1
Potatoes, sweet	¼ c.

Meat Exchanges
(One ounce contains 8 g. of protein, 3 g. of fat, 21 mg. of cholesterol, and 60 calories. Lean meats only.)

Beef	Fresh fish
Lamb	Cod
Pork	Flounder
Ham	Halibut
Veal	Tuna (canned in water)
Poultry (without skin)	Oysters, clam, lobster

Egg Exchanges
($3/7$ egg contains 3 g. of protein, 3 g. of fat, 108 mg. of cholesterol, and 35 calories.)

Limit to 3 per week
2 oz. of one of the following may be substituted for 1 egg:
Crab, shrimp
Liver, sweetbreads

Fat Exchanges
(One tablespoon of vegetable oils contains 14 g. of fat, 2 g. of saturated fatty acid, 8 g. of linoleic fatty acid, and 125 calories.)

Corn oil	1 tbsp.
Cottonseed oil	1 tbsp.
Safflower oil	1 tbsp.
Soybean oil	1 tbsp.
French dressing (made with any of the oils listed above)	1½ tbsp.
Mayonnaise (made with any of the oils listed above)	1 tbsp.
Margarine (11 g. of fat, 2 g. of saturated fatty acid, 4 g. of linoleic acid, and 100 calories)	1 tbsp.

Sugar and Dessert Exchanges
(One serving contains about 12 g. of carbohydrate and 50 calories.)
Sugars

White, brown or maple	1 tbsp.
Corn syrup or maple syrup	1 tbsp.
Honey	1 tbsp.
Molasses	1 tbsp.
Jelly, jam, or marmalade	1 tbsp.

Desserts

Tapioca or cornstarch pudding (made with fruit and fruit juice or with skim milk from milk calculated in diet plan)	¼ c.
Gelatin dessert	⅓ c.
Fruit whip	¼ c.
(made with egg whites, no cream)	
Water ice	¼ c.
Sweetened canned or frozen fruit	⅓ c.
(equals 1 fruit exchange and 1 tablespoon sugar)	
Angel food cake, plain	1 sm. piece
Sweetened carbonated beverages	6 oz.

Candies

Gumdrops	3 med.
	14 sm.
Marshmallows	3 large
Hard fruit drops	4

*Adapted from The Dietary Management of Hyperlipoproteinemia, A Handbook for Physicians. Bethesda, Maryland, National Heart and Lung Institute, 1973.

Exchange Lists

The HLP Exchange Lists are presented in Table 29-9 and should be compared to the Exchange Lists in Table 23-4 in Chapter 23.

MILK EXCHANGE. Only skim milk products can be used because the fat-controlled or HLP diets restrict total fat or recommend polyunsaturated fatty acids in preference to saturated fatty acids. The fat-controlled diets and HLP diets 2 through 5 also restrict cholesterol. For example, 8 ounces of whole milk contain 34 mg. of cholesterol, while 8 ounces of skim milk contain 5 mg. Yogurt and buttermilk must be made from skim milk.

VEGETABLE EXCHANGES, GROUPS A AND B, AND FRUIT EXCHANGE. The items in the vegetable and fruit exchange lists in Table 23-4, Chapter 23, are used to plan daily menus for fat-controlled or HLP diets and are not reproduced in Table 29-9. If the patient is not obese and the diet is not restricted in sucrose, fruits canned or frozen with sugar may be used, while vegetables frozen in butter sauce or any other sauce must not be used. Any fat exchanges calculated in a diet pattern can be used to season cooked vegetables or in salad dressings. The number of servings of vegetables and fruits will be limited in the diet pattern if the diet prescription limits the amount of simple carbohydrates. (See the discussion of simple vs. complex carbohydrates in Chapter 28, Diabetes Mellitus.)

BREAD EXCHANGE. This list is less extensive than the bread exchange list in Table 23-4, Chapter 23. The breads in Table 29-9 are limited to those made with a minimum amount of added fat.

One biscuit (2-inch diameter), one muffin (3-inch diameter), two pancakes (4-inch diameter) or one-half waffle (7-inch diameter) can be substituted for one bread exchange and one-third fat exchange (1 tsp.)

Table 29-10. Cholesterol Content of Foods* (per exchange serving)

Food	Household Measure	Weight (g.)	Cholesterol (mg.)
Whole milk	8 oz.	240	34
Egg	1	50	242
Meat, fish	1 oz.	30	21
Chicken (with skin)	1 oz.	30	24
Liver	1 oz.	30	131
Sweetbreads	1 oz.	30	140
Shrimp	1 oz.	30	45
Lobster	1 oz.	30	25
Crab	1 oz.	30	30
Oysters, clams	1 oz.	30	15
Cheese, cheddar	1 oz.	30	28
Butter	1 tbsp.	14	35
Margarine (all veg. oil)	1 tbsp.	14	0

*Calculated from Feeley, R. M., et al: J. Am. Dietet. A. 61:134, 1972.

provided they are made with skim milk and vegetable oil or margarine. Muffins, pancakes, and waffles may not be used if sucrose or simple carbohydrates are limited by the diet prescription, because sugar is an ingredient in the recipes for these products.

Only the fat exchanges calculated in the diet pattern can be used as a spread on bread or to season the other items in this list such as the pasta, rice, potatoes, and corn.

MEAT EXCHANGE. The items in this food group vary significantly from the meat exchange list in Table 23-4, Chapter 23, in order to control the total fat, saturated fatty acid, and cholesterol they contribute to the diet pattern. Only well-trimmed, lean meat, poultry without skin, and fish can be used. The skin of poultry is excluded because of the amount of fat it contains. Luncheon meats, frankfurters, and sausage are also excluded because of their fat content.

When the P/S ratio must be calculated, more poultry and fish than the other meats should be used in menu planning so that the quantity of saturated fatty acids in the diet will not be in excess of the figure given in Table 29-7 for 1 ounce of lean meat.

EGG EXCHANGE. It should be carefully noted that eggs are limited to 3 per week and that a list of substitutions for eggs is given. This restriction on the use of eggs reflects their saturated fatty acid and cholesterol content, and the substitutions for eggs reflect their cholesterol content. Table 29-10 lists the cholesterol content of selected foods. Whole-milk cheeses are not included in the meat or egg exchanges food groups because of their saturated fatty acid content. If available, uncreamed (dry cured) cottage cheese can be used.

Since eggs and liver are significant sources of dietary iron and are limited or excluded from the diet patterns, the counselor should check the iron content of a patient's usual menu selections. Iron medication may be required to meet the daily needs for this mineral, especially for children and women of childbearing age.

FAT EXCHANGE. The items in the fat exchange list differ significantly from those in Table 23-4, Chapter 23. Only vegetable oils, salad dressing made with vegetable oils, and margarine are included because of the amount of the polyunsaturated fatty acid, linoleic, which they contain (see Table 29-11). Butter, lard, hydrogenated shortening, and bacon are excluded.

SUGAR AND DESSERT EXCHANGES. This list is included to show the types of sugars and desserts which can be used to meet energy needs when total fat and cholesterol are severely restricted, but total energy is not restricted, in the diet pattern. If simple carbohydrates are also restricted for any reason, the

Table 29–11. Approximate Fatty Acid Composition of Vegetable Oils*

Vegetable Oil	Saturated Fatty Acids†	Monoun-saturated Fatty Acids†	Polyun-saturated Fatty Acids†
Coconut	86	7	—
Cocoa butter	56	37	2
Olive	11	76	7
Peanut	22	43	29
Cottonseed	25	21	50
Soy	15	20	59
Corn	10	28	54
Safflower	8	15	72

*From USDA Home Economics Report No. 7. and Brown, H. B., and Farrand, M. G.: J. Am. Dietet. A. 49:303, 1966.
†Grams per 100 g. ether extract or crude fat.

items in this exchange list cannot be used. It will be noted that only egg whites, which do not contain fat or cholesterol, and skim milk are used to make desserts.

MIXED DISHES. Numerous items included in an HLP or fat-controlled diet pattern can be combined in mixed dishes. For example, a white sauce can be made with skim milk and flour without the addition of any fat, and gravy can be made with fat-free broth or fat-free meat drippings and flour. Tomatoes, tomato juice, or tomato paste can be used in combination with pasta or rice, meat, or uncreamed cottage cheese and other vegetables to make casserole dishes.

CONVENIENCE FOODS. Unless the nutrition label defines the types and amounts of fatty acids and the cholesterol content of a serving of the food, these products cannot be used on fat-controlled or HLP diets. In some cases the quantity of sucrose in the product may also restrict its use.

DIETETIC FOODS. Various egg and cheese products and meat substitutes made from soy protein isolate which are modified in cholesterol and fatty acid composition in comparison with the usual foods are now available in most supermarkets. For example, Cheez-ola* is a filled pasteurized processed cheese which contains corn oil in place of milk fat and has a 4.5:1 P/S ratio. However, the sodium content of this product will limit its use, since the diets for patients with hypertension and edema or for those recovering from myocardial infarction are also restricted in sodium. One ounce of Cheez-ola contains 480 mg. sodium and, therefore, could not be used in planning a 1000- or 2000-mg. sodium-restricted diet pattern (see Chapter 30). The egg and meat substitutes also contain significant amounts of sodium.

*Fisher Cheese Co., Wapakoneta, Ohio.

Planning Diet Patterns

The most frequently prescribed diets for the prevention and treatment of hyperlipidemia are HLP diets 2 and 4 and the energy-restricted fat-controlled diet. It can also be anticipated that diet 4 will be prescribed for patients with diabetes and diet 5 for patients in diabetic ketoacidosis or for patients with alcoholism.

An energy-restricted diet will be a frequent first diet prescription in the treatment of hyperlipidemias because many of the patients with premature atherosclerosis, or who have coronary heart disease and/or diabetes, are overweight due to overfatness. The achievement and maintenance of ideal weight status will correct the hyperlipidemia in many of these patients. In these situations one can use the information in Chapter 27 for planning energy-restricted diets with special emphasis on the use of vegetable oils and margarine and lean meats; and on the restriction in the use of eggs, whole-milk products, and sucrose.

The first step in planning the diet, as with any diet, is to gather extensive information about the patient's usual food practices. In some cases it is also important to know about the total family's food practices, particularly the families of patients with primarily HLP. For example, Glueck and coworkers have reported that in 70 families where one parent had a myocardial infarction before age 50, 31 percent of the children had Type IIa, IIb, or IV lipoprotein patterns. These investigators strongly recommend an early intervention program for these children.[25]

In her contact with the patient and his family, the nutrition counselor should determine how much and what kinds of fats are consumed by the family; the commonly used methods of food preparation which may add fats to an otherwise low-fat food, and the amounts of simple carbohydrate and alcohol consumed daily. Information about snack foods and the frequency of eating outside the home, as well as the usual meal pattern, should be obtained.

HLP DIET 4 AND THE FAT-CONTROLLED DIET. As indicated in Table 29–6, HLP Diet 4 is restricted to 300 to 500 mg. of cholesterol per day; polyunsaturated fatty acids are used in preference to saturated fatty acids; and carbohydrate is limited to 4 to 5 g. per kg. of ideal body weight or approximately 45 percent of total calories. Sucrose and concentrated sweets are also restricted; some physicians will exclude these items entirely. If the energy intake is also restricted, the sugar and dessert exchanges cannot be used in calculating the diet pattern. Table 29–12 illustrates the nutrient composition of a 1500-calorie HLP Diet 4.

The fat-controlled diet (Table 29–5) has restrictions similar to those in HLP Diet 4 but in addition recommends a specific P/S ratio at each energy level. Table 29–13 shows the nutrient composition of a 1500-calorie fat-controlled diet with a P/S ratio of 1.5:1.

Careful inspection of the diet patterns in Tables 29–12 and 29–13 will show that the same number and kinds of exchanges have been used in each. The saturated fatty acids and linoleic acid are estimated in the fat-controlled diet pattern but not in the HLP Diet 4 pattern. At a higher calorie level (1800 to 2000) sugar and dessert exchanges in limited quantities could be included in both diet patterns if permitted by the physician's diet prescription.

Both 1500-calorie diet patterns derive approximately 20 percent of the total calories from protein, 35 percent from fat, and 45 percent from carbohydrate. Approximately 65 percent of the carbohydrate is derived from complex carbohydrates and 35 percent from simple carbohydrates.

A suggested menu for both diet patterns using the foods in the HLP exchange lists is given in Table 29–14. Part of the skim milk in the breakfast menu could be reserved for making whipped topping from skim milk powder to garnish the fruit in the D'Zerta in

Table 29-12. Nutrient Composition of a 1500-Calorie HLP Diet 4

Food Group	Amount	Weight (g.)	Protein (g.)	Total Fat (g.)	Cholesterol (mg.)	Carbohydrate (g.)	Energy (cal.)
Milk, skim	1 pt. (2 c.)	480	16	tr.	10	24	160
Vegetables							
Group A	as desired	varies	—	—	—	—	—
Group B	½ cup	100	2	—	—	7	35
Fruit	3 servings	varies	—	—	—	30	120
Bread and cereal	7	varies	14	7	—	105	525
Meat, lean	6 oz.	180	48	18	126	—	360
Egg	3/wk. (³/₇)	21	3	3	108	—	35
Fat							
Vegetable oils*	1 tbsp.	14	—	14	—	—	125
Margarine†	1½ tbsp.	21	—	16.5	—	—	150
Totals			83	58.5	244	166	1510

*Corn, cottonseed, safflower, soybean oils.
†Nutrition Label, Chiffon margarine, 1973.

Table 29-13. Nutrient Composition of a 1500-Calorie Fat-Controlled Diet (P/S Ratio 1.5:1)

Food Group	Amount	Weight (g.)	Protein (g.)	Total Fat (g.)	Saturated fatty acids (g.)	Linoleic fatty acid (g.)	Cholesterol (g.)	Carbohydrate (g.)	Energy (cal.)
Milk, skim	1 pt. (2 c.)	480	16	tr.	—	—	10	24	160
Vegetables									
Group A	as desired	varies	—	—	—	—	—	—	—
Group B	½ cup	100	2	—	—	—	—	7	35
Fruit	3 servings	varies	—	—	—	—	—	30	120
Bread and cereal	7	varies	14	7	—	—	—	105	525
Meat, lean	6 oz.	180	48	18	3.6	0.6	126	—	360
Egg	3 wk. (³/₇)	21	3	3	0.9	0.2	108	—	35
Fat									
Vegetable oil*	1 tbsp.	14	—	14	2.0	8.0	—	—	125
Margarine†	1½ tbsp.	21	—	16.5	3.0	6.0	—	—	150
Totals			83	58.5	9.5	14.8	244	166	1510

*Corn, cottonseed, safflower, soybean oils.
†Nutrition Label, Chiffon margarine, 1973.

the evening meal. Two teaspoons of margarine are used as an ingredient of the biscuits. Another teaspoon of margarine would be available to season the potatoes and peas if one large hard roll and one teaspoon of margarine were substituted for the two biscuits.

For the hospitalized patient, careful precautions must be taken to insure that the patient who requires a fat-controlled or HLP diet is not served vegetables that have been seasoned with butter, meat that is well-marbled with fat or from which the visible fat has not been removed, or hot breads made with other than vegetable oil shortening. At the same time, relatives and friends should be instructed to avoid offering the patient candies and ice cream or beverages made with whole milk and ice cream.

Other Hyperlipoproteinemia Diets*

HLP DIET 1. The fat in Diet 1 for patients with hyperchylomicronemia is restricted to 25 to 35 g. per day. None of the items in the fat exchange food group can be included in the Diet 1 diet pattern because all long-chain fatty acids, other than those in the meat and bread exchange food groups, are excluded from the diet. For example, six meat exchanges and ten bread exchanges contain 28 g. of fat, primarily long-chain saturated fatty acids. If the patient requires 2000 or more calories per day, he will make extensive use of the sugar and dessert exchanges.

The physician may prescribe the use of medium-chain triglycerides (see Chapter 23) in the Diet 1 pattern because the medium-chain fatty acids in these triglycerides are absorbed into the portal circulation and do not require the synthesis of chylomicrons for transport. Medium-chain triglyceride oil (MCT) can be used in frying and in making hot breads and salad dressings. However, MCT oil is expensive and may not be acceptable to the patient as a substitute for regular food fats and oils.

HLP DIET 2. In this diet the cholesterol is severely limited (preferably to 100 to 200 mg. per day) and the polyunsaturated fatty acid is increased. To achieve the cholesterol restriction, the egg exchange food group cannot be included in the diet pattern (see Table 29–7). Adequate amounts of vegetable oils and margarine must be used to insure an increased intake of linoleic acid. Unless the patient is obese, energy and carbohydrate are not restricted. Therefore, the sugar and dessert exchanges can be included in the diet pattern.

HLP DIET 3. This diet is restricted to less than 300 mg. of cholesterol per day; 20 percent of total calories

*See Table 29–6.

Table 29–14. Suggested Menu for 1500-Calorie HLP Diet 4 or a 1500-Calorie Fat-Controlled Diet

Breakfast

4 oz. orange juice
½ cup cooked oatmeal
1 slice of toast
1 tsp. margarine
8 oz. skim milk

Noon Meal

Chicken sandwich
  2 slices of bread
  2 ounces chicken
  2 tsp. mayonnaise
  lettuce
Fresh peach
8 oz. skim milk

Evening Meal

4 ounces roast veal
1 cup mashed potatoes
½ cup green peas
sliced tomatoes with 1 tsp. French dressing
2 biscuits
  (made with allowed fat)
½ tbsp. margarine
  (for potatoes and biscuits)
½ cup fruit cup, made with fruit canned without sugar
  (in D'Zerta with skim milk whipped topping)

are derived from protein, 40 percent from fat, and 40 percent from carbohydrate. When the 1500-calorie HLP Diet 4 in Table 29–12 is used as a model to achieve the Diet 3 recommendations, the number of bread and/or fruit exchanges would be reduced and the number of the fat exchanges increased. It is advisable to exclude egg exchanges from the diet pattern to control the cholesterol intake. The physician's diet prescription may exclude all sugar and dessert exchanges. Otherwise a sugar or dessert exchange may be substituted for a fruit or bread exchange two or three times a week.

HLP DIET 5. This diet restricts fat to 30 percent of total calories. Fifty percent of total calories is derived from carbohydrate and 20 percent from protein. Because blood triglycerides are markedly elevated, the sugar and dessert exchanges are usually excluded from the diet pattern.

PATIENT COUNSELING

The patient who requires a fat-controlled or HLP diet will need careful, detailed diet instructions because these diets require extensive changes in the use of fats, and usually sugar, compared with the average American diet (see Chapter 10). Since the majority of patients who experience heart attacks are men, it is essential that the patient's wife be present for the diet history interview and during all diet instruction. Many of these patients and their wives will be well motivated to learn how to cope with the HLP or fat-controlled diet. Also, if the children in the family have been screened and are found to have positive lipoprotein patterns, the homemaker will need help in modifying the food practices of the whole family.

The press, popular magazines, and television have all helped to make middle-aged Americans conscious of the need for "polyunsaturates" in their diets. Unfortunately, some of these media have oversimplified the problem by emphasizing only one food—for example, changing from butter to "special" margarines and salad oils—without considering the needs to change to skim milk and skim milk products and lean meat, and to monitor the number of eggs used each week, as well.

It is possible that many food-buying practices and methods of food preparation will need to be changed. For example, if an individual has always made fruit whip with whipped cream, she will need to be instructed to make it with egg whites. Or, if she has found it convenient to use frozen dinners frequently, she may need help in planning the preparation of meals which require more of her time in the kitchen. If she has children, she will need help in planning meals and snacks to meet their energy and nutrient needs for growth, and at the same time modify the types and amounts of fat and sugar in their diets.

Various kinds of cookbooks are available to patients. One of these has been published by the American Heart Association.[26] The recipes in some of the other books are not appropriate for every type of diet. Therefore, the counselor should review any cookbook before recommending it. It would also be advisable to test a few of the recipes in these cookbooks for ease of preparation and the quality and acceptability of the product. With the help of the counselor many homemakers can modify their own favorite recipes.

Resources for patient education, which the clinical dietitian can use to supplement her own educational material, are listed at the end of the chapter. However, as with any complex food modification, continuing contact with the nutrition counselor will be necessary as patients learn to cope with their problems. As the disease progresses in those patients who have had a myocardial infarction, the clinical dietitian can also expect to help them restrict sodium intake as well as fat.

HYPOLIPIDEMIC DRUGS

Two types of hypolipidemic drugs may be used in conjunction with diet to treat hyperlipidemias.[27] One type decreases VLDL synthesis. The two most commonly used agents of this type are nicotinic acid, a B vitamin, and clofibrate, a branched-chain fatty acid.

Both agents may cause nausea and diarrhea. The other type increases LDL catabolism. The two most commonly used agents of this type are the resins, cholestryramine and sitosterol. Cholestyramine frequently causes constipation in older patients and occasionally nausea, vomiting, abdominal distention, and cramps. Sitosterol may have a mild laxative effect or may sometimes produce nausea and diarrhea.

STUDY QUESTIONS AND ACTIVITIES

1. Why is atherosclerosis a public health problem of major importance?
2. List the foods which contain the greatest percentage of linoleic fatty acid.
3. Is it correct to say that all plant oils contain only linoleic fatty acid and that all animal fats contain only saturated fat? (See Chapter 3; and Table 2, Section 4.)
4. List some of the foods commonly used in the American diet which are omitted on the fat-controlled or HLP diets.
5. What epidemiologic study is being carried out to assess the effect of diet on elevated blood cholesterol levels in men?
6. Why should the prevention of coronary artery disease begin in childhood?
7. Can a diet without eggs be adequate in all nutrients?
8. Calculate a 2000-calorie fat-controlled diet containing 38 percent fat, more than 14 percent linoleic fatty acid, and less than 14 percent saturated fat.
9. Estimate the cholesterol in the food you consumed in one day. (see Table 2, Section 4.)
10. Check the supermarkets in your area for the availability and cost of special foods for fat-controlled or HLP diets.

SUPPLEMENTARY READINGS

Ahrens, R. A.: Sucrose, hypertension and heart disease: An historical perspective. Am. J. Clin. Nutr. 27:403, 1974.
Albrink, M. J.: Dietary and drug treatment of hyperlipidemia in diabetes. Diabetes 23:913, 1974.
Bierenbaum, M. L., et al: Ten-year experience of modified diets of younger men with coronary heart disease. Lancet 1:1404, 1973.
Blacket, R. B., et al: Type IV hyperlipidemia and weight-gain after maturity. Lancet 2:517, 1975.
Fristrom, G. A., et al: Comprehensive evaluation of fatty acids in foods. IV. Nuts, peanuts, and soups. J. Am. Dietet. A. 67:351, 1975.
Gangl, A., and Ockner, R. K.: Intestinal metabolism of lipids and lipoproteins. Gastroenterology 68:167, 1975.

Glueck, C. J., et al: Hypercholesterolemia and hypertriglyceridemia in children: A pediatric approach to primary atherosclerosis prevention. Am. J. Dis. Child. 128:569, 1974.

Gotto, A. M., and Scott, L.: Dietary aspects of hyperlipidemia, J. Am. Dietet. A. 62:617, 1973.

Grundy, S. M.: Effect of polyunsaturated fats on lipid metabolism in patients with hypertriglyceridemia. J. Clin. Invest. 551:269, 1975.

Hackett, T. P., and Cassem, N. H.: The psychologic reactions of patients in the pre- and post-hospital phases of myocardial infarction. Postgrad. Med. 57:43, (April) 1975.

Ireton, C. L., et al: Case report: Diagnosis and management of type I hyperlipoproteinemia. J. Am. Dietet. A. 66:42, 1975.

Jansen, C., et al: A tool for individualized management of fat-controlled diets. J. Am. Dietet. A. 67:23, 1975.

Levy, R. I.: The meaning of lipid profiles. Postgrad. Med. 57:35, (April) 1975.

Marshall, M. W., et al: Composition of diets containing 25 and 35 percent calories from fat: Analyzed vs. calculated values. J. Am. Dietet. A. 66:470, 1975.

Nauidi, M. K., and Kummerow, F. A: Nutritional value of Egg Beaters compared with "farm fresh eggs." Pediatrics 53:565, 1974.

Pratt, D. E.: Lipid analysis of a frozen egg substitute. J. Am. Dietet. A. 66:31, 1975.

Salel, A. F., et al: The importance of type IV hyperlipoproteinemia as a predisposing factor in coronary artery disease. Am. J. Med. 57:897, 1974.

Stamler, J.: Major coronary risk factors before and after myocardial infarction. Postgrad. Med. 57:25, (April) 1975.

PATIENT RESOURCES

Planning Fat-Controlled Meals for 1200 and 1800 Calories (Revised). New York, Am. Heart Assoc., 1966.

Planning Fat-Controlled Meals for Approximately 2000-2600 Calories (Revised). New York, Am. Heart Assoc., 1967.

Programmed Instruction for Fat-Controlled Diet, 1800 Calories. New York, Am. Heart Assoc., 1969.

Dietary Management of Hyperlipoproteinemia, Bethesda, Md., National Heart and Lung Institute, NIH, Rev., 1973. Diet 1 for Hyperchylomicronemia. Diet 2 for Hypercholesterolemia. Diet 3 for Hypercholesterolemia with Hyperglyceridemia. Diet 4 for Endogenous Hyperglyceridemia. Diet 5 for Mixed Hyperglyceridemia.

Cutler, C: Haute Cuisine for Your Heart's Delight. New York, Potter, 1973 (dist. by Crown Pub.).

Eskleman, R., and Winston, M.: The American Heart Association Cookbook. New York, McKay, 1973.

Heiss, K. B., and Heiss, C. G.: Eat to Your Heart's Content. San Francisco, Chronicle, 1972.

Keys, M., and Keys, A.: The Benevolent Bean. New York, Farrar, 1972.

Salmon, M. B., and Quigley, A. E., eds.: Enjoying Your Restricted Diet. Springfield, Ill., Thomas, 1972.

Stead, E. A., and Warren, J. V: Low-Fat Cookery, ed. 3. New York, McGraw-Hill, 1975.

Zane, P.: The Jack Sprat Cookbook. New York, Harper, 1973.

For further references see Bibliography in Section 4.

REFERENCES

1. Spain, D. M.: Scientific American 215:48, 1966.
2. Hatch, F. T.: Am. J. Clin. Nutr. 29:80, 1974.
3. Nutrition Today 9:28, 1974.
4. Hegsted, D. M., et al: Am. J. Clin. Nutr. 17:281, 1965.
5. Keys, A.: J. Mt. Sinai Hosp. 20:118, 1953.
6. Mueller, J. F.: J. Am. Dietet. A. 62:613, 1973.
7. Brown, H. B., and Farrand, M. E.: J. Am. Dietet. A. 49:303, 1966.
8. Christakis, G., et al: JAMA 198:129, 1966.
9. Yudkin, J.: Lancet 2:115, 1957.
10. Ahrens, E. H., Jr.: Trans. Assoc. Am. Physicians 74:134, 1961.
11. Ahrens, A. J.: Am. J. Clin. Nutr. 27:403, 1974.
12. Bagdade, J. D.: Lancet 2:630, 1968.
13. Hatch, op. cit.
14. Levy, R. I., et al: J. Am. Dietet. A. 58:406, 1971.
15. Frederickson, D. S., et al: N. Eng. J. Med. 276:32, 94, 148, 215, 273, 1967.
16. Levy, R. I., et al: N. Eng. J. Med. 290:1295, 1974.
17. Frederickson, D. S.: in Harrison's Principles of Internal Medicine, ed. 7. New York, McGraw-Hill, 1974, Chapter 244.
18. JAMA 222:1647, 1972.
19. Preventive Med. 1:255, 1972.
20. J. Am. Dietet. A. 60:503, 1972.
21. Stanbury, J. B., et al, eds: The Metabolic Basis of Inherited Disease, ed. 3. New York, McGraw-Hill, 1972, pp. 548-551.
22. Mueller, op. cit.
23. Feeley, R. M., et al: J. Am. Dietet. A. 61:134, 1972.
24. Zuckel, M. C.: Background information on fat-controlled diets, rev. 1967 (unpublished).
25. Glueck, C. J., et al: Am. J. Dis. Child. 127:70, 1974.
26. Eskleman, R., and Winston, M.: The American Heart Association Cookbook. New York, McKay, 1973.
27. Levy, R. I., et al: N. Eng. J. Med. 290:1295, 1974.

30 cardiovascular disease

The basic metabolic problem in cardiac disease, and the diseases discussed in Chapters 31 and 32, renal and liver disease, is fluid and electrolyte balance. From Chapter 5, Water and Mineral Metabolism, it will be remembered that the maintenance of the appropriate fluid volume in the vascular system and in the spaces surrounding the cell (interstitial) and within the cells (intracellular) is a function not only of the constituents of the blood and the integrity of the vascular tissue but also of the heart, kidneys, liver, and lungs; and all of these interrelated functions are mediated by a variety of hormones.

ETIOLOGY

The focus on fluid and electrolyte metabolism in this chapter is determined by the problems presented by cardiac disease and vascular disease or cardiovascular disease. Cardiac disease may be primary or secondary. The major cause of primary disease is congenital anomalies of the heart, many of which can be corrected by surgery. Secondary cardiac disease is due to: (1) infections such as rheumatic fever (streptoccocal infection) or syphilis; or (2) diseases of the vascular system such as hypertension and arteriosclerosis including atherosclerosis.

Arteriosclerosis is the generic term for any vascular disease characterized by induration or thickening of the arterial wall. Atherosclerosis, a form of arteriosclerosis, involves the intimal layer of the arteries, while arteriosclerosis involves primarily the medial layer. The etiology of primary hypertension, an elevation of arterial blood pressure due to peripheral resistance, cannot be defined at this time, although neurogenic mechanisms are suspected. The major causes of secondary hypertension are diseases of the kidney or the adrenal glands. Secondary hypertension has also been observed in some women taking oral contraceptive agents.

PREVALENCE AND INCIDENCE

Approximately one million deaths due to all cardiovascular diseases occur in the United States each year. After the age of 35, it is the leading cause of death, and over 90 percent of these deaths can be attributed to atherosclerosis and other forms of arteriosclerosis and hypertension. It is estimated that 15 to 20 percent of the adult population in the United States has hypertension, with the highest prevalence among black Americans. Recent studies indicate that hypertension may occur in children more frequently than previously suspected.[1]

The morbidity and mortality from all forms of cardiovascular disease, especially in adults during the productive years from ages 35 to 65, have a major social impact on the individual, his family, and the public at large. If the individual is the wage earner, his income may be reduced as a consequence of his disability. Coronary care units in community hospitals are expensive to staff and maintain, and Medicare and Medicaid in addition to private medical insurance plans are used to finance the acute and continuing care of the patient with cardiovascular disease. In the United States today health agencies and organizations are urging early detection and treatment of cardiovascular disease in the hope of reducing the cost to society.

SEVERITY OF INVOLVEMENT

The severity of cardiovascular disease depends on the degree to which the normal functions of the system are altered and the extent to which this alteration interferes with them. The onset may be sudden, with no previous history of problems, such as may occur in the patient with a myocardial infarction. Or the disease may be chronic, of long standing, with increasing loss of cardiac function, often referred to as cardiac reserve. If the problem is minimal and the heart is able to maintain adequate circulation to all tissues of the body, the disease is classified as mild or "compensated." The patient may have to avoid strenuous activity which increases the oxygen needs of the body, but otherwise he will be able to perform his daily tasks without discomfort.

Decompensation, or severe cardiac disease, is said to occur when the heart is unable to sustain adequate circulation of blood to the tissues. The blood flow to the lungs is slowed, and oxygen uptake and carbon dioxide excretion are inadequate. The patient suffers from shortness of breath and chest pain when he performs any sort of activity. As decompensation progresses, edema may appear in the dependent parts of the body and, sometimes, in the pleural and peritoneal cavities, and the kidneys and the liver may become involved. Severe cardiac disease of this magnitude is called congestive heart failure.

When patients are chronically ill with severe heart disease, their activities must be severely restricted, and they may even have to spend much of their time in bed so that the limited oxygen supply will be sufficient for whatever activity is allowed. Drugs to improve the function of the heart muscle or to reduce blood pressure are commonly prescribed. If edema is present, diuretic drugs to increase sodium and water excretion are usually given, and a diet restricted in sodium is prescribed.

EDEMA

Welt defines edema as an increase in and retention of the extravascular component of the extracellular (interstitial) fluid volume.[2] Sodium is retained with the fluid. Edema in cardiovascular disease is caused primarily by an alteration of the pressure in the vascular system, which permits the outflow of fluids into the interstitial spaces but interferes with the return of the fluids into the vascular system. In addition, the blood flow to the kidney may be involved so that there is a reduction in the glomerular filtration rate with a decrease in the excretion of fluids and sodium. Aldosterone, the adrenal cortical hormone which promotes sodium retention and potassium excretion by the kidney, and the pituitary antidiuretic hormone, which aids the kidney in the reabsorption of water, may also be involved. Hypernatremia, an elevated blood sodium level, may also occur.

Mild edema may cause some swelling of the ankles, puffiness around the eyes, or the tightness of a ring on a finger. The persistence of an indentation of the skin following pressure is known as pitting edema. Ascites and hydrothorax refer to the accumulation of excess fluid in the peritoneal and pleural cavities respectively, and anasarca refers to gross generalized edema.

RATIONALE FOR RESTRICTING DIETARY SODIUM INTAKE

The quantity of extracelluar fluid volume is largely dependent on its sodium content. (See Chapter 5, Water and Mineral Metabolism.) The reduction of the extracellular fluid volume is dependent primarily on reducing total body sodium stores; the restriction of dietary sodium intake is one factor in reducing these stores.

Dietary restriction alone may be effective in reducing fluid volume in patients with mild heart failure. However, patients with moderate or severe heart failure will also require diuretics and a digitalis compound to reestablish normal fluid volume. Diuretics are used to increase the rate of urine formation and decrease sodium reabsorption by the kidney, which leads to increased fluid and electrolyte excretion.[3] Digitalis compounds increase the force of myocardial contractions, which increases cardiac output. As a result of this action there is also an increase in fluid and electrolyte excretion.

Certain diuretics also promote potassium excretion, which can lead to hypokalemia (low blood potassium). This is hazardous for the patient with cardiovascular disease because hypokalemia results in disturbances in neuromuscular function, including the muscles of the heart. The dietary implications of hypokalemia are discussed in the section on special concerns in this chapter.

Average Sodium Intake

It is estimated that the average adult in the United States consumes from 2000 to 7000 mg. (100 to 300 mEq.) of sodium per day, equivalent to 6 to 18 g. of salt (NaCl). However, salt is not the only source of dietary sodium. In addition to the salt added to food during preparation and at mealtimes, certain foods naturally contain some sodium. However, the major source of sodium today in the diets of most Americans is probably the salt and numerous sodium compounds added to foods during production and processing.

Except for the small amount of sodium needed by the body each day—estimated to be equivalent in the adult to the sodium in one gram of salt (400 mg.)—sodium intake in excess of need is excreted by the kidneys in urine or lost in perspiration. Dahl has shown that prolonged feeding of excessive salt to his experimental animals leads to hypertension.[4] However, there is no evidence to show that hypertension can be produced in normal humans by ordinary salt intake. On the other hand, the blood pressure in hypertensive individuals does respond to a restricted sodium intake.

Water Intake

Most patients who require diuretics and a restriction of sodium intake do not require a restriction of water intake. As has been demonstrated, when sodium is excreted from the body, there is a corresponding water loss. (See the discussion of the sodium content of water supplies later in the chapter.)

The Diet Prescription

ENERGY. The achievement and the maintenance of weight status slightly below the ideal are the first goals of diet therapy in the treatment of all patients with cardiovascular disease. Not only does this measure tend to reduce basal metabolism and thus the work of the heart, but it also contributes to the reduction of hyperlipidemia if it is present.

SODIUM. The level of sodium restriction in milligrams is stated in the prescription and will reflect the patient's condition. An intake of 2000 to 3000 mg. (90 to 130 mEq.) of sodium per day is considered a mild restriction; 1000 to 2000 mg. (43 to 90 mEq.) a moderate restriction; and any amount less than 1000 mg. (43 mEq.) a severe restriction. With the effectiveness of the diuretics in current use, the most commonly prescribed restrictions vary from 1000 to 3000 mg. In the past, there was confusion because the diet order restricting sodium intake tended to be general, rather than specific. Such terms as salt-poor, low-salt, or salt-free diet gave little indication of the amount of sodium desired. This confusion has disappeared as we have learned how the body uses sodium and how to analyze foods for their sodium content.

Since diet prescriptions may state the quantity of sodium in milliequivalents (mEq.) rather than milligrams, mEq will have to be converted to milligrams because food composition tables give the sodium content of foods in milligrams. One milliequivalent of sodium is 23 mg., the gram-atomic weight. For example, a diet prescription of 40 mEq. sodium converts to 920 mg. sodium. Sodium chloride is 39.3 percent sodium. Therefore, to convert a specified weight of sodium chloride to sodium, one multiplies the weight in grams by 0.393. For example, 5 g. of sodium chloride contains 1.965 g., or 1965 mg., of sodium.

Whenever necessary, the energy-restricted, the fat-controlled, the hyperlipoproteinemia (HLP), the diabetic diets, and others can also be restricted in sodium. However, a high-protein diet (2 to 3 g. per kg.

of body weight) is not compatible with a restriction of 1000 mg. or less of sodium, unless special sodium-free foods are used.

DIET THERAPY
Sodium in Food

The *sodium* content of food depends on whether the food is from an animal or a plant source. When *produced, processed,* and *prepared without* the addition of salt (NaCl) or any other sodium compound, meat, fish and poultry, milk and milk products, and eggs contain *significant* amounts of sodium. The fluids surrounding the cells of meat are physiological saline solutions just as the fluids surrounding human muscle cells. Animal fats and seed oils contain no, or insignificant amounts of, sodium; cereal grains and fruits and vegetables contain *insignificant* amounts of sodium provided they are produced, processed, or prepared without the addition of salt or any other sodium compound.

If all the foods in the Pattern Dietary (Table 22-1) are produced, processed, or prepared without the addition of any sodium compound, and no salt is added at the table, the sodium content of this 1400-calorie diet pattern is approximately 500 mg. The pint of milk, one egg, and four ounces of cooked meat contribute approximately 400 mg. of sodium; and the cereal, bread, fruits, and vegetables contribute approximately 100 mg. of sodium.

There are two other important sources of dietary sodium: the sodium in the various compounds *added* to foods during processing; and the salt or other flavor enhancers such as monosodium glutamate added to foods during preparation in the home, institution, or restaurant, or by the individual at the time of consumption of the food at the table. The sodium added to some foods during processing is obvious, for example, the salt on crackers and potato chips or the salt used to cure ham. However, some foods can contain a significant amount of added sodium without tasting salty, for example, frozen vegetables with monosodium glutamate added during processing.

Sodium-Restricted Exchange Systems

Table 30-1 gives the sodium composition of the exchange food groups which are used to calculate sodium-restricted diet patterns. The protein, fat, carbohydrate, and energy values in Table 23-2 in Chapter 23 also apply in this Exchange System and are not repeated in Table 30-1. The sodium values apply only to foods *produced, processed,* and *prepared without* the addition of salt or any other sodium compound and reflect the quantities of sodium which foods naturally contain.

Table 30-1. Sodium-Restricted Exchange System

Food Group	Household Measure	Weight (g.)	Sodium* (mg.)
Milk Exchanges	8 oz. (½ pt.)	240	120
Meat Exchanges	1 oz.	30	25
Egg	one	50	70
Vegetable Exchanges	½ cup	100	9
Fruit Exchanges	1 serving	varies	2
Bread Exchanges	1 serving	varies	5
Fat Exchanges	1 tsp.	5	0

*Food produced, processed, or prepared without the addition of any sodium compound.

It will be observed that the milk, meat, and egg exchanges contribute the most significant amounts of sodium, while vegetables, fruits, cereal grains, and fats contribute the least important amounts. The addition of salt or any sodium compound to any exchange will invalidate these figures. For example, 1 teaspoon of unsalted butter contains about ¼ mg. of sodium, while 1 teaspoon of butter with salt added (regular butter) contains 50 mg. of sodium (see Table 4, Section 4).

Sodium-Restricted Exchange Lists

The Sodium-Restricted Exchange Lists are given in Table 30-2. The foods listed in each exchange group apply to the calculation of diet patterns containing 1000 mg. of sodium or less. Some additions can be made to certain lists when the diet prescription for sodium is greater than 1000 mg., and these are included in the discussion of each exchange list.
MILK EXCHANGES. The items in this food group do not differ significantly from those in the milk exchange list in Table 23-4, Chapter 23. One cup (8 ounces) of whole or skim milk contains 120 mg. of sodium. Salt is frequently added to buttermilk; therefore, one must check with the producer before using it. Due to its sodium content, any milk used in food preparation should be part of the milk exchanges calculated in the sodium-restricted diet pattern.
MEAT EXCHANGES. One ounce (30 g.) of the items in this list contains 25 mg. of sodium after cooking. This figure applies to meat, poultry, and fish which is fresh, frozen, or canned without the addition of sodium. The products canned without added salt or sodium in any form are referred to as "dietetic" canned. No meats or fish cured with salt, such as ham, bacon, chipped beef, smoked tongue, or smoked fish, or products such as luncheon meat, frankfurters, or sausage are included in the meat list.

Kosher meat and poultry may present a problem for Jewish patients who follow the orthodox dietary laws. Under the conditions for koshering, freshly slaughtered meat or poultry is salted for one hour to

Table 30-2. Sodium-Restricted Exchange Lists

MILK EXCHANGES
1 cup (8 oz.) contains 120 mg. of sodium
Whole milk
Skim milk
Evaporated milk
Unsalted buttermilk
6 ounces of plain yogurt

MEAT EXCHANGES
Each ounce, cooked, contains 25 mg. of sodium
Fresh or Frozen Meat

Beef	Tongue
Lamb	Liver
Pork	Rabbit
Veal	

Fresh or Frozen Poultry
Chicken
Cornish hens
Duck
Turkey

Fresh or *Dietetic Canned* Fish

Cod	Bass
Flounder	Perch (Lake)
Haddock	Pike
Halibut	Whitefish
Perch (Ocean)	
Salmon	
Tuna	

EGG EXCHANGE
1 egg contains 70 mg. of sodium.

VEGETABLE EXCHANGES
1 serving, ½ cup, contains about 9 mg. of sodium.

Fresh, frozen without any sodium compound, and low-sodium canned dietetic vegetables or vegetable juices.

Group A

Asparagus	Lettuce
Broccoli	Mushrooms
Brussels sprouts	Okra
Cabbage	Peppers
Cauliflower	Radishes
Chicory	String beans
Cucumbers	Squash, summer
Escarole	Tomatoes
Eggplant	Tomato juice
Green beans	Wax beans

VEGETABLE EXCHANGES *(continued)*
Group B

Onions	Pumpkins
Peas, green	Rutabagas
Squash, winter	

FRUIT EXCHANGES
Each serving contains about 2 mg. of sodium.
Fresh, frozen, canned or dried fruit and fruit juices.
See Table 23–4 for complete listing.

BREAD EXCHANGES
Each serving contains about 5 mg. of sodium.

Low-sodium bread, 1 slice
Low-sodium rolls, 1 medium
Crackers
   Low-sodium dietetic melba toast, 4 slices
Cereals, long cooking, ½ cup
   Farina
   Hominy grits
   Oatmeal
   Rolled wheat
   Wheat meal
Dry Cereals, ¾ cup
   Puffed Rice
   Puffed Wheat
Pasta and other cereal products, ½ cup cooked
   Macaroni
   Noodles
   Spaghetti
   Barley
Flour, white or whole wheat, 1 cup
Dried beans and peas, ½ cup cooked
Corn, ⅓ cup cooked
Potato, white, 1 small or ½ cup cooked
Sweet potatoes, ¼ cup cooked

FAT EXCHANGES
1 tsp. contains practically no sodium.
Unsalted butter and margarine
Vegetable oils
Shortenings
Low-sodium mayonnaise and salad dressings

MISCELLANEOUS FOODS
The following foods contain no sodium:

Coffee, no instant	Limes
Tea, no instant	Gelatin
Sugar, white	Vinegar
Honey	Sodium-free
Calcium saccharin	baking powder
Lemons	Yeast

---

remove the blood. Then the meat or poultry is washed thoroughly before cooking. Although this will remove some of the added salt, a good deal will have penetrated the inner portion of the meat. Kaufman states that meat so treated has from 334 to 375 mg. of sodium per 100 g. (90 to 115 mg. per 30 g.), depending on the manner of cooking.[5] She suggests that Jewish patients be taught to salt their meat lightly and allow it to stand for the minimal amount of time. After it has been rinsed and soaked in water, it should be boiled in a generous amount of water and the broth should be discarded. Meat so treated was found to contain 63

mg. of sodium per 100 g. (19 mg. per 30 g.). As an alternative, she suggests the use of ammonium chloride salt in place of sodium chloride for drawing out the blood. Ammonium chloride cannot be used by individuals with advanced cirrhosis of the liver (Chapter 32).

Only fresh or dietetic canned fish is included in the meat exchanges. Fresh fish must be rinsed thoroughly in water because it is sometimes kept in saltwater or temporarily frozen with salt before it reaches the market. Shellfish vary in sodium content. However, at prescriptions of sodium above 3000 mg., it may be possible to show a patient how to include them in his diet pattern (see Table 4, Section 4 or other food composition tables).

Cheeses are not included in the meat exchange list in Table 30-2 because of their sodium content. For example, 1 ounce of cheddar cheese contains approximately 210 mg. of sodium. This amount reflects the sodium in the milk used to make cheese and the sodium in compounds added during processing. Low-sodium dietetic cheeses are available in some markets. The amount of sodium in milligrams per serving is listed on the label. These products are relatively expensive compared to regular cheese. However, some patients use them for variety in menu planning and need directions for calculating the amount of cheese they can substitute for 1 ounce of meat. For example, Low-Sodium Colby cheese, produced by Pauly, a division of Swift and Company, contains 20 mg. per 100 g., or 6 mg. per 30 g. of cheese.* Because of the sodium content, 3 ounces of this cheese can be substituted for 1 ounce of meat, or 1 ounce of cheese could be added to a hamburger patty without increasing sodium significantly.

The low-sodium dietetic cheeses are made from dialyzed milk, a process which removes the sodium. Unfortunately, during dialysis potassium is usually exchanged for the sodium. Since some patients who require sodium-restriction may also require potassium-restriction (see Chapter 31, Renal Disease) not all patients should use these cheeses.

On the other hand, if the diet prescription is 2000 to 3000 mg. of sodium, and the patient customarily uses cheese, he can be shown how to substitute regular cheese for the milk exchanges calculated in his diet pattern. The substitutes can be calculated from the figures for the sodium content of cheese from Table 4, Section 4, or items 643 through 652 in USDA Handbook No. 8 or, if available, from the nutrition label on a package of cheese. If the diet is also fat-controlled, no whole-milk cheese can be used (see Chapter 29).

One-fourth cup (55 g.) of unsalted dry curd cottage cheese contains approximately 30 mg. of sodium, and ¼ cup of creamed cottage cheese contains approximately 150 mg. of sodium. The patient who prefers cottage cheese to milk can be shown how to substitute creamed cottage cheese for the milk exchanges calculated in his diet pattern. Low-sodium peanut butters are also available, and from the label information one can calculate the amount of peanut butter which can be substituted for meat.

EGG EXCHANGE. One egg contains 70 mg. of sodium. Therefore, it cannot be considered an ex-

*Label information, Low-Sodium Colby Cheese, 1973.

change for meat. The major portion of the sodium in an egg is in the white. One egg yolk contains approximately 10 mg. of sodium. However, all the fat and cholesterol in an egg are in the yolk. Therefore, if cholesterol and fat or saturated fatty acids are also restricted, eggs cannot be included in the diet pattern. VEGETABLE EXCHANGES. One serving, ½ cup, of the items in this list contains approximately 9 mg. of sodium if no salt or sodium compound is added during production, processing, or preparation. The items in the Group A and Group B vegetable exchange lists in Table 23-4, Chapter 23, which are not in this vegetable exchange list are excluded because of their natural sodium content. For example, ½ cup of fresh spinach cooked without added salt contains 45 mg. of sodium.

Frozen peas and lima beans cannot be used because during processing the vegetables are put in a brine solution and a significant amount of sodium is picked up. For example, 100 g. of fresh green peas contain about 1 mg. of sodium, while 100 g. of frozen peas contain about 115 mg. of sodium. Frozen vegetables in sauces or those labeled "lightly salted" or "monosodium glutamate added" cannot be used.

The use of low-sodium dietetic canned vegetables should be limited to those listed in Table 30-2. Low-sodium canned carrots are available. However, ½ cup of this product contains approximately 36 mg. of sodium.

When the diet prescription is 2000 mg. of sodium or more, the vegetables which have been excluded from Table 30-2 because they contain more than 9 mg. of sodium per ½-cup serving may be calculated in a diet pattern. Table 30-3 gives the sodium content of these vegetables. It will be observed that they are primarily leaves and roots. The three Group B vegetables could be put in an exchange list containing 35

Table 30-3. Sodium in Selected Fresh Vegetables

VEGETABLE *	SODIUM (mg. per 100 g.)†
Group A	
Beet greens, cooked	76
Celery, raw	126
Chard, cooked	86
Collards, cooked	25
Kale, cooked	43
Mustard greens, cooked	18
Spinach, cooked	45
Group B	
Beets	36
Carrots	33
Turnips	34

*Cooked without added salt.
†Church, C. F., and Church, H. N.: *Food Values of Portions Commonly Used*, ed. 12. Philadelphia, Lippincott, 1975.

mg. of sodium per ½-cup serving. Ten grams of chopped raw celery could be added to the vegetable exchange list in Table 30–2 for those patients who enjoy this in tuna or other salads.

Also, at levels above 2000 mg. of sodium, vegetables canned with salt added, such as string beans, peas, carrots, and beets can be used if the solids are well drained from the liquid in the can. The vegetables should then be rinsed with water in a strainer and heated for serving in unsalted water. This process significantly reduces the amount of sodium in the vegetables.[6]

FRUIT EXCHANGES. Each serving, as described in Table 23–4, contains approximately 2 mg. of sodium. The items in this food group, fresh, frozen, or canned, do not present problems regarding the addition of sodium. However, the labels on cans of synthetic fruit drinks should be carefully checked for food additives containing sodium.

BREAD EXCHANGES. Each serving as described in this food group contains approximately 5 mg. of sodium. The sodium figure applies to one slice of bread made without milk. When low-sodium bread is made with milk, the sodium content increases to approximately 30 mg. per slice. One slice of regular bread contains approximately 150 mg. of sodium, contributed by milk, salt, and other sodium compounds used to prevent staling or molding.

The instant forms of cooked cereals such as instant oatmeal or farina (Cream of Wheat) cannot be used because disodium phosphate is used in the precooking process. Dry cereals, other than the two listed, are also excluded because of their sodium content. For example, ½ cup of wheat flakes contains approximately 200 mg. of sodium. Quick-cooking rice and instant mashed potato cannot be used because they undergo the same precooking with sodium added as the instant cereals.

The commonly used leavening agents used in batters and doughs, yeast and baking powder, differ significantly in the amount of sodium they contain. Yeast does not contain sodium, while baking power does. Products made from yeast doughs, however, must not contain added salt or sodium compounds when used in planning sodium-restricted diets. A low-sodium baking powder* is available for making biscuits or muffins which can be substituted for bread. Any milk or egg used in making these products should be that calculated in the patient's diet pattern. (See Resources for Patients at the end of this chapter for a list of cookbooks with tested recipes using low-sodium baking powder.) It is not wise to substitute the low-sodium baking powder for regular baking powder in a recipe in a standard cookbook.

*Cellu-Featherweight, Chicago Dietetic Supply, Inc., LaGrange, Ill.

Low-sodium bread is not readily available in all communities and is usually more expensive than regular bread. Also, the activity of many patients requiring sodium-restricted diets is limited, and they are not able to expend their limited energy kneading bread dough. Therefore, whenever the sodium level of the diet permits, usually about 1000 mg., regular bread, containing 150 mg. of sodium per slice, is calculated in the diet pattern. The sodium content of regular bread can also be applied to one hamburger or one frankfurter bun.

In addition to low-sodium dietetic melba toast, a variety of crackers with unsalted tops is available in most supermarkets. The list of ingredients on the labels of these products should be read carefully. Although salt has not been added to the tops of these crackers, some are made from a dough which usually contains some sodium compound. This type of cracker was originally called soda cracker.

FAT EXCHANGES. One *teaspoon* of the items listed in this exchange contains practically no sodium. Both unsalted butter and unsalted margarine are widely available. If a blender is available, low-sodium mayonnaise can easily be made in the home using a standard recipe but omitting the salt. However, various low-sodium salad dressings and mayonnaise may also be found in the supermarket.

Whenever the diet is also fat-controlled, only margarine and corn, cottonseed, safflower, or soybean oils are used in calculating the diet pattern.

MIXED DISHES. Any of the exchanges calculated in the diet pattern can be used to prepare mixed dishes. A variety of herbs and spices, other than salt, can be used. (See section on salt substitutes and seasonings.) Many patients requiring sodium-restricted diets become, with guidance, excellent gourmet cooks. However, wines and other alcoholic beverages, common ingredients in gourmet recipes, cannot be used because of their wide variation in sodium content.[7]

CONVENIENCE AND OTHER PROCESSED FOODS. Since many sodium compounds are found in convenience and other processed foods, these cannot be used by patients requiring sodium-restricted diets, unless the milligrams of sodium per serving are clearly stated on the nutrition label. The quantity of sodium in some convenience foods may be minimal, or it may be excessive. One frozen entree, a veal dish, contains 1200 mg. of sodium for each 2-ounce serving of the meat. The same item made at home without salt added would contain approximately 75 mg. of sodium.

A partial list of food additives containing sodium which are commonly used in food processing is given in Table 30–4. The function of the additive and the foods in which it is used are also given. Food addi-

Table 30–4. Food Additives Containing Sodium (Partial List)*

COMPOUND	FUNCTION	FOOD
Sodium bicarbonate	Leavening agent, adjust acidity	Baking powder, tomato soup, ices, sherbets, syrups for frozen products, confections, self-rising flours
Sodium carbonate	Neutralizer	Butter, cream, ice cream, processing olives, cocoa products
Sodium caseinate	Texturizer	Ice cream, frozen custard, ice milk, sherbet
Sodium hexametaphosphate	Emulsifier, sequestrant, texturizer	Breakfast cereals, angel food cake, flaked fish, ice cream, ice milk, bottled beverages, puddings, processed cheeses, artificially sweetened jellies
Sodium hydroxide	Glazing agent, peeling agent, neutralizer	Pretzels, tubers and fruits, sour cream, cocoa products, canned peas
Sodium pectinate	Stabilizer and thickener	Syrups for frozen products, ice cream, ice milk, confections, fruit sherbets, French dressing, other salad dressings, fruit jelly, preserves, jams
Sodium stearoyl-2-lactylate	Emulsifier, plasticizer, surface active agent	Bakery mixes, baked products, cake icings, fillings and toppings, dehydrated fruits and vegetables, frozen desserts, pancake mixes, precooked instant rice, pudding mixes
Monosodium glutamate	Flavor enhancer	Meats, condiments, pickles, soups, candy, baked goods, frozen vegetables

*Adapted from Winter, R.: *A Consumer's Dictionary of Food Additives*. New York, Crown, 1972.

tives may or may not be listed on the product label. The listing of ingredients on the label is not required for processed foods for which the Food and Drug Administration has established standards of identity. The standard specifies the kind and minimum content of each ingredient to be used in processing the product. Therefore, if salt or a food additive containing sodium is included in the standard of identity, it does not have to be listed on the package label.

The listing of the quantity of sodium per serving under the Nutrition Labeling Law is optional and is usually stated only on the labels of dietetic foods (see section on low-sodium dietetic foods).

Some of the commonly used convenience foods which must be excluded from any sodium-restricted diet are TV dinners and frozen entrees; frozen vegetables in seasoned sauce; biscuit, muffin, pancake, cake, and cookie mixes and self-rising flours; seasoned rice; packaged potato dishes; hamburger extenders and seasoned bread stuffings; meat substitutes made from textured soy isolate protein; and snack crackers.

LOW-SODIUM DIETETIC FOODS. Products offered as low-sodium dietetic foods come under the Food and Drug Administration's Nutrition Labeling Law (1973). Under the regulations, the milligrams of sodium per serving size, as defined by the producer, must be listed on the label.

In addition to those products already mentioned such as low-sodium canned vegetables, cheeses, and melba toast, various low-sodium dietetic condiments, entrees, soups, and baked products are available in many supermarkets. Some of these products may not be usable in diets restricted to 2000 mg. or less of sodium because, although reduced in sodium compared with the regular food, they still contain too much sodium per serving. Each product needs to be evaluated before it is used, and patients must be instructed that the symbol Na, rather than the term sodium, may be used on some labels.

SALT SUBSTITUTES AND SEASONINGS. Many patients find a sodium-restricted diet unappetizing because of the flatness or blandness of foods served without added salt. It can be explained that they are experiencing the real flavor of food, but this does not make the food any more appealing to them. Salt substitutes and spices and herbs can be used to make the diet more palatable.

Salt substitutes are available in drugstores and some supermarkets. They usually contain potassium or ammonium in place of sodium. These substitutes are contraindicated if there is renal or liver disease. In the hospital they may be offered to patients on sodium-restricted diets routinely or only by order of the physician. Those patients who use a salt substitute need to be advised to use it sparingly because in

Table 30–5. Seasonings, Extracts, Herbs, and Spices*

Low in Sodium May be used Freely		High in Sodium Do Not Use
Allspice	Mint	Bouillon cubes, regular
Almond extract	Mustard, dry, or mustard seed	Catsup
Anise seed	Nutmeg	Celery flakes, seed, salt
Basil	Onion, onion juice, or onion	Chili sauce
Bay leaf	powder	Garlic salt
Bouillon cube, low-sodium	Orange extract	Horseradish, prepared with salt
dietetic if less than 5 mg.	Oregano	Instant vegetable broth
of sodium per cube	Paprika	Meat extracts
Caraway seed	Parsley	Meat sauces
Cardamon	Pepper, fresh green or red	Meat tenderizers
Catsup, dietetic	Pepper, black, red, or white	Monosodium glutamate
Chili powder	Peppermint extract	Mustard, prepared
Chives	Pimiento peppers for garnish	Olives
Cinnamon	Poppy seed	Onion salt
Cloves	Poultry seasoning	Parsley flakes
Cocoa (1 to 2 teaspoons)	Purslane	Pickles
Coconut	Rosemary	Relishes
Cumin	Saccharin, calcium (sugar	Saccharin, sodium (sugar
Curry	substitute)	substitute)
Dill	Saffron	SALT
Fennel	Sage	Salt substitutes, unless recom-
Garlic, garlic juice, or garlic	Salt substitutes, if recommended	mended by the physician
powder	by the physician	Soy sauce
Ginger	Savory	Tomato paste
Horseradish root or horseradish	Sesame seeds	Worcestershire sauce
prepared without salt	Sorrel	
Juniper	Sugar	
Lemon juice or extract	Tarragon	
Mace	Thyme	
Maple extract	Turmeric	
Marjoram	Vanilla extract	
Meat extract, low-sodium	Vinegar	
dietetic	Wine, if allowed	
Meat tenderizers, low-sodium dietetic	Walnut extract	

*Adapted from "Your 1000-milligram Sodium Diet," The American Heart Association, New York, N. Y. 10010.

excessive amounts some individuals find the taste unpleasant. Also, it may be more acceptable when added to the food at the table, rather than during cooking. One of the substitutes, labeled "seasoned," has a variety of spices added and is very palatable. Lite-Salt* cannot be used in sodium-restricted diets because it contains about one half the sodium chloride content of regular salt.

Various spices and herbs which can be used are listed in Table 30–5. Fortunately, most of these are low in sodium; however, some commonly used seasonings contain a large amount of salt. These are celery, garlic, and onion salt; dried parsley and onion flakes; prepared mustard, Worcestershire sauce, and soy sauce; and monosodium glutamate and meat tenderizers. Patients who have not previously used a variety of spices and herbs should be cautioned to use them sparingly until they are sure they enjoy the new flavors.

DRINKING WATER. In some areas of the country drinking water may present a special hazard because of its high sodium content. This may be due either to

*Morton Salt Co., Chicago, Ill.

the sodium content of the soil from which the water is drawn or to the use of water softener. In one study of over 2000 local water supplies widely distributed throughout the United States and covering approximately 50 percent of the population, great variation in sodium content was found, as shown in Table 30-6.[8]

It will be noted that only 58 percent or a little over one half the water supply was within the range of none to 20 mg. of sodium per liter (approximately a

Table 30–6. Range of Sodium Ion in Drinking Water for a Sampling Period*

Range of Sodium Ion Concentration	Number of Samples	Percent of Total Samples
mg./L.		
0- 19.9	1194	58.2
20- 49.9	391	19.0
50- 99.9	190	9.3
100-249.9	178	8.7
250-399.9	74	3.6
400-499.9	10	0.5
500-999.9	14	0.7
Over 1000	2	0.1

*From White, J. M., et al: Sodium ion in drinking water. J. Am. Dietet. A. 50:32, 1967.

PLATE 2

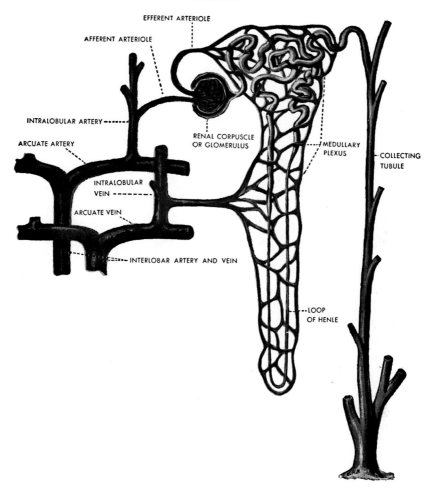

A schematic drawing of the nephron, showing arterial and venous circulation. Water and water-soluble substances are filtered from the glomerular blood capillaries into the tubule. In the tubule, all of the glucose and much of the water, sodium and other components of the glomerular filtrate are reabsorbed into the surrounding capillary bed. The remainder passes from the collecting tubule into the pelvis of the kidney and, finally, by way of the ureters, into the bladder. (Sharp & Dohme's *Seminar*, vol. 9, No. 3, August, 1947.)

Table 30-7. A 1000-mg. Sodium-Restricted, 1500-Calorie Diet Pattern

FOOD GROUP	AMOUNT	SODIUM (mg.)	ENERGY (Calories)
Milk, whole	1 pt.	240	340
Meat	4 oz. cooked	100	300
Egg	1	70	75
Vegetables	4 one-half-cup servings	36	100
Fruit	3 servings	6	120
Bread, unsalted	3 servings	15	210
Bread, salted	3 slices	450	210
Fat, unsalted	3 tsp.	—	135
TOTALS		917	1490

quart). Water used for coffee and tea, for drinking, and for food preparation is estimated at 2½ to 3 liters per person per day. When water contains more than 20 mg. of sodium per liter, it can significantly increase the sodium content of the diet. The patient should obtain information about his community's water supply by contacting the department of health. Also, home water-softening systems should be checked to insure that the sodium content of the water has not been increased.

"SOFT DRINKS." Bottled "soft drinks" may be high in sodium due to the sodium content of the water in the area where they are manufactured. Low caloric beverages may have their sodium content increased still further by the substitution of sodium saccharin, an artificial sweetener, for sugar. They are therefore omitted when careful sodium restriction must be maintained.

Planning the Sodium-Restricted Diet Pattern

The first step in planning any sodium-restricted diet pattern is to estimate, from the patient's diet history, the sodium content of his usual food choices and the amount of salt he customarily adds to foods at the table. Special care should be taken to identify the kinds and amounts of processed and convenience foods eaten at home and the frequency with which meals are eaten in restaurants or in a social setting. This information will help to identify the magnitude of the adjustment facing the patient. Some hospitalized patients will have been advised previously to "cut down on salt," while others may have had no previous diet counseling.

THE MODERATELY SODIUM-RESTRICTED DIET PATTERN, 1000 TO 2000 mg. Table 30-7 shows a diet pattern calculated with Mr. A., a 55-year-old man in moderate congestive failure due to rheumatic fever in childhood. His diet prescription was 1000 mg. of sodium and 1500 calories because he was 30 pounds overweight.

The six bread exchanges in his diet pattern consist of three unsalted ones and three slices of regular bread. The choice of regular bread made the diet more palatable for him. Occasionally he substituted 8 ounces of skim milk for whole milk and added two unsalted fat exchanges. Table 30-8 is a day's menu selected by Mr. A., using his diet pattern in Table 30-7.

In four weeks, when Mr. A.'s condition had improved, his physician increased his sodium allowance to 1500 mg. per day, but continued the restriction in calories to 1500. Table 30-9 shows how his diet pattern was modified. The six bread exchanges now consisted of items with salt added. Mr. A. chose to have four slices of regular bread and 1 cup of mashed potato which Mrs. A. made from potatoes cooked in lightly salted (less than ⅛ teaspoon of salt) water. The fat exchanges were now also salted ones.

Table 30-8. A Day's Menu Selected by Mr. A.

Breakfast
½ cup of orange juice
1 soft poached egg
1 slice of regular bread, toasted
1 cup of decaffeinated coffee

Noon Meal
Sandwich
1 oz. of roast beef, unsalted
lettuce
2 slices of regular bread
8 oz. of whole milk
1 peach

Evening Meal
3 oz. of roast veal, unsalted
1 cup of mashed potato with 1 tsp.
of salt-free butter
1 cup of salt-free string beans with
1 tsp. of salt-free butter
1 cup of salt-free broccoli
with lemon juice

Bedtime
8 oz. of whole milk
10 grapes
4 slices of melba toast

Table 30-9. A 1500-mg. Sodium-Restricted 1500-Calorie Diet Pattern

FOOD GROUP	AMOUNT	SODIUM (mg.)	ENERGY (Calories)
Milk, whole	1 pt.	240	340
Meat	4 oz., cooked	100	300
Egg	1	70	75
Vegetables	4 one-half-cup servings	36	100
Fruit	3 servings	6	120
Bread, salted	6 servings	900	420
Fat, salted	3 tsp.	150	135
TOTALS		1502	1490

cardiovascular disease 437

Mr. A., with Mrs. A.'s help, readily accepted his sodium-restricted diets. Fortunately he had not added excessive amounts of salt to his food, and Mrs. A. used very few convenience or processed foods and salted food lightly during preparation. However, she frequently fried meats and potatoes with fat and had to modify this practice. Mr. A. had to give up three of his favorite foods, bacon, ham, and pretzels.

THE MILDLY SODIUM-RESTRICTED DIET PATTERN, 2000 TO 3000 mg. All highly salted foods and the addition of salt to food at the table are excluded from any mildly sodium-restricted diet. At 2000 mg., foods processed or cooked with moderate amounts of salt can be used. The processed foods include cottage cheese, regular breads without salt toppings, salted butter or margarine, and vegetables canned with added salt. During preparation meats and fresh vegetables can be lightly salted. Otherwise food choices should be restricted to those in the Exchange Lists, Table 30-2.

At 3000 mg. of sodium, regular canned tuna, shellfish, all cereals, and biscuits and muffins made from standard recipes using baking powder can be used. If there is no restriction in energy, doughnuts, sweet rolls, fruit pies, sugar cookies, and ice cream can also be included. Catsup, but not chili sauce or pickles, can be used. The convenience foods previously mentioned and cured meats and fish are excluded at any level of mild sodium restriction.

When Mr. A. had achieved his normal weight status, he underwent surgery for a heart valve replacement. After surgery his physician prescribed a mildly sodium-restricted diet, 2500 to 3000 mg. per day. Mr. A.'s diet was modified by the addition of salt to the preparation of meats and vegetables, and the occasional use of cheddar cheese, shellfish, and homemade biscuits and muffins in place of bread. He continued to monitor his weight status and on special occasions had fruit pies or ice cream for dessert.

THE SEVERELY SODIUM-RESTRICTED DIET PATTERN, LESS THAN 1000 mg. Patients with gross edema due to severe congestive failure frequently require sodium restriction to 500 mg. or less. These patients are hospitalized because they are critically ill and frequently have a very poor appetite. Their nutritional care at this point is primarily practitioner-managed (see Chapter 12).

Table 30-10 shows a 500-mg. sodium-restricted diet pattern. The same quantities of exchanges were used to calculate this pattern as the 1000-mg. sodium-restricted diet pattern in Table 30-7. However, compared with the bread exchanges in Table 30-7, all the bread exchanges in Table 30-10 are salt free. Most critically ill patients will probably not want

Table 30-10. A 500-mg. Sodium-Restricted Diet Pattern

FOOD GROUP	AMOUNT	SODIUM (mg.)	ENERGY (calories)
Milk, whole	1 pt.	240	340
Meat	4 oz., cooked	100	300
Egg	1	70	75
Vegetables	4 one-half-cup servings	36	100
Fruit	3 servings	6	120
Bread, unsalted	6 servings	30	420
Fat, unsalted	3 tsp.	—	135
TOTALS		482	1490

the vegetables calculated in this diet pattern and will prefer fruit juices to fruit, if their fluid intake is not restricted as well.

If the diet prescription were 250 mg. of sodium in place of 500 mg., Lonalac,* a low-sodium milk, can be used in place of whole milk. One pint of Lonalac contains approximately 12 mg. of sodium, which would reduce the sodium content of the diet pattern in Table 30-10 to 254 mg.

Severe restrictions of sodium for patients with cardiovascular disease are usually prescribed as an emergency measure. After fluid and electrolyte balance is reestablished, a more moderate restriction is usually prescribed. The planning and serving of the 500-mg. sodium-restricted diet to hospitalized patients must be carefully monitored so that errors are not made. If two slices of regular bread were served in place of two slices of salt-free bread, the patient would consume 300 mg., not 10 mg., of sodium, and his day's intake of sodium would be far in excess of the amount ordered due to this one error.

COUNSELING THE PATIENT
Patient Problems

The sodium-restricted diet is probably the most difficult therapeutic diet for the patient to accept. In addition to modifying his food choices, he is confronted with a major change in the taste of his food. For the patient who has always added salt liberally at the table, his food now tastes flat and unappetizing. At the same time that he is coping with a sodium-restricted diet, he may also be advised by his physician to modify drastically his total life-style. For example, an aggressive businessman, who may require mild sodium restriction of a fat-controlled diet after a severe myocardial infarction, may encounter difficulty in accepting diet counseling.

*Mead Johnson Laboratories, Evansville, Ind.

As well as helping the patient and his wife to understand the purpose of his sodium-restricted intake, the counselor must also help him identify all dietary sources of sodium. Salt, because of its distinctive taste, is not difficult for the patient to understand. However, food additives with sodium are more difficult to interpret to the patient because many of them do not give a salty taste to food.

With the present interest in the United States in the adoption of the metric system, it can be anticipated that some patients will be better able to understand instructions regarding grams and milligrams of salt and sodium. The patient with a strong science background will readily understand the metric system. The patient who can understand grams and milligrams has an advantage in that he can interpret the information on labels and have a wider selection of foods or be able to avoid those which he cannot use. Figure 30-1 gives some of the types of labels patients will encounter. For the patient who cannot comprehend the metric system, food choices will be limited to the food lists in the instructional materials which he receives, and he will need considerable assistance in making any additions to the lists.

People who eat frequently in restaurants will need help with menu selection. Plain broiled meats, baked potatoes, and green salad with oil and vinegar dressing are three items which can be served without salt added. Unfortunately meat tenderizers are used in many restaurants today. In congregate meal programs for the elderly no highly salted foods such as ham should be served, and foods should be lightly salted during preparation because many of the participants in these programs may have mild cardiovascular disease.

Ethnic food practices also present some problems. Southern patients in the habit of cooking with bacon or salt pork must be warned about this. This is also true for people who eat "soul" foods. Jewish patients, following their dietary laws of heavily salting their meats before cooking (koshering) will need help in readjusting their deeply ingrained convictions (see earlier in this chapter). Italian patients should be warned not to use commercially canned tomato paste, olives, Italian cheese, and Italian bread. Tomato paste can be made at home, omitting salt and spices containing sodium. Occasionally an Italian bakery will make low-sodium bread if there is sufficient demand for it. Japanese and Chinese patients must particularly be cautioned to omit sodium glutamate and soy sauce, both of which are commonly used in the seasoning of their food. Greek patients and those coming from the Near East frequently use heavily salted olives as an accompaniment to meals.

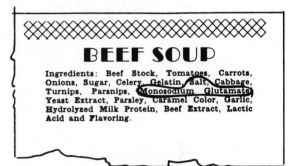

Some cereals have salt added.

Even if this can of soup did not contain salt it should not be used because of the monosodium glutamate.

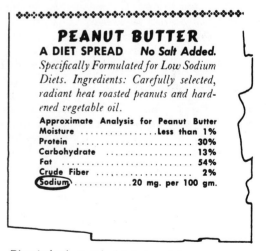

Dietetic foods must be labeled carefully.

Fig. 30-1. Examples of labeling.

Instructional Materials

In addition to the instructional materials developed by a hospital or other health agency for patients requiring sodium-restricted diets, three booklets have been published by the American Heart Association. They are available to the patient only through his physician, who may obtain them from the local heart association, or, where there is no local association, from the national office.* The booklets were prepared by the American Heart Association in conjunction with the American Dietetic Association, the Council on Foods and Nutrition of the American Medical Association, the Nutrition Foundation, and the Public Health Service of the Department of Health, Education, and Welfare. The diets are constructed on the Exchange System similar to the one presented in this chapter. The three booklets are entitled "Your 500 Milligram Sodium Restricted Diet"; "Your 1000 Milligram Sodium Restricted Diet"; and "Your Mild Sodium-Restricted Diet." The first two booklets have also been issued as simplified leaflets.

Any instruction materials for patients on sodium-restricted diets should reflect as much as possible the usual food practices in the area and be reviewed and revised constantly as changes occur in food processing. "New and improved" products may contain more sodium than the original ones.

SPECIAL CONCERNS

The Patient with an Acute Myocardial Infarction

The nutritional care of the patients in a coronary care unit has been reviewed by Christakis and Winston.[9] Table 30–11 presents their recommendations. The nutritional care is usually given by the nursing staff in consultation with the clinical dietitian.

As soon as possible after admission, the patient's likes and dislikes of the fluids used should be ascertained, usually from a relative or close friend in order not to disturb the patient. Special care should be taken to determine if the patient has any intolerance to milk, such as gastric distress or diarrhea, so that this fluid can be avoided, if necessary. In some coronary units the physicians may exclude carbonated beverages since some patients experience epigastric distress after drinking them.

It is also advisable to be sure that fluids, and food when tolerated, are not too hot or too cold because extremes in temperature of fluids and foods may have an adverse effect on the function of cardiac muscle

*American Heart Association, New York, N.Y.

Table 30–11. Suggested Nutritional Pattern for a Coronary Care Unit*

The following nutritional pattern for use in the Coronary Care Unit is suggested for short-term use, i.e., the initial five- to ten-day period, following acute myocardial infarction.

(a) Nothing by mouth prior to evaluation by the physician. In most instances, intravenous solution started to facilitate administration of drugs required if arrhythmias and shock ensue.

(b) Patient to be re-evaluated for dietetic progression after first 24 hr.

(c) For the first 24 hr., 500- to 800-kcal (1000 to 1500 ml.) liquid diet, with only small amounts of liquid taken at a time. Foods which may be offered include: clear soups, broth, skim milk, fruit juices, tea, ginger ale, and water.

(d) Caloric level of 1000 to 1200 kcal to meet patient's basal metabolic requirement. Nutritional proportions should be, approximately: 20 percent protein, 45 percent carbohydrate, and 30 to 35 percent fat (low saturated fat; polyunsaturates as the primary source of dietary fat) with cholesterol limited to 300 mg. per day. Sodium restriction if indicated by patient's condition.

(e) Beverages and other liquids served at body temperatures. Non-caffeine and decaffeinated beverages are preferred. Stimulants and extremes in temperature to be avoided.

(f) Small, frequent meals consisting of foods which are easily digested, free of gastric irritants, soft, and low in roughage.

(g) Foods to be included: tender, lean cuts of meat; fish and poultry; tender, cooked or canned vegetables and fruits; plain breads; cooked cereals; simple puddings and gelatin desserts. Egg yolks limited to three a week.

(h) Nutritional plan to be individualized on basis of patient's clinical status, physiologic and psychologic needs. Areas usually requiring modification are: carbohydrates, protein, fat, total calories, electrolytes, and fluids.

*Christakis, G., and Winston, M,: J. Am. Dietet. A., 63:233, 1973.

(cardiac arrhythmias). Coffee and tea are usually excluded because the stimulants they contain may increase heart rate. Decaffeinated beverages may be substituted. Many physicians advise their patients with heart disease to exclude or strictly limit their consumption of any beverage containing caffeine or other stimulants (coffee, tea, cocoa, chocolate, cola beverages).

Hypokalemia

Three types of diuretics, the thiazides, furosemide, and ethacrynic acid, can promote hypokalemia. In addition to oral intake of potassium chloride or the rotation of diuretics, foods with significant quantities of potassium can also be used to prevent hypokalemia. Potassium is present in all foods, but fruits and fruit juices are significant sources which can be recommended without, at the same time, increasing the sodium intake.

Sodium in Medications

The physician will avoid prescribing medications which contain sodium. The patient should be cautioned to take no medication, "patent" medicine, or home remedy without consulting his physician. Baking soda (sodium bicarbonate) is a popular home remedy for indigestion or "heartburn"; and many alkalizers, antacids, headache remedies, sedatives, and cathartics are high in sodium and should not be used.

The Debilitated Patient

Since many patients with cardiovascular disease, especially arteriosclerosis, are in the older age group, they frequently present special nutritional care problems. A person may be confused and disoriented and require assistance in feeding himself at each meal or may need to be fed by a staff member in an institution or by a relative in his home. If he lacks teeth or has poorly fitting dentures, the consistency of his food should be modified to what he can chew. Not all patients will require the same modification.

Appetite may vary during the day. In the morning, after a night's rest, patients may eat well at breakfast. As the day progresses, they may become progressively weaker and will eat less well at the noon and evening meals. Five small meals a day may be helpful. It is well to avoid those foods which the patient reports give him gastric distress. Frequently these foods are milk, members of the cabbage family, and dried peas and beans.

STUDY QUESTIONS AND ACTIVITIES

1. Why may the patient with cardiac disease develop edema?
2. Why will a diet restricted in sodium aid in preventing or eliminating edema in the cardiac patent?
3. Is low-sodium bread available in your community? How does its price compare with regular bread?
4. What is the sodium content of one slice of regular bread? of one teaspoon of salted butter or margarine? of one tablespoon?
5. Make out a menu for a day for a patient with congestive heart failure whose diet order is: 1000 mg. sodium, soft diet, five meals.
6. Which foods used in planning the sodium-restricted diet contain the most sodium? Which the least?
7. Using Table 4, Section 4, make a list of common beverages which contain a significant amount of potassium for a patient taking a diuretic which promotes potassium excretion.

8. What should a patient on a sodium-restricted diet be taught about convenience foods and the labels on any food package?

SUPPLEMENTARY READINGS

Aagaard, G. N.: The management of hypertension. JAMA 224:329, 1973.

Christakis, G., and Winston, M.: Nutritional therapy in acute myocardial infarction. J. Am. Dietet. A. 63:233, 1973.

Committee on Nutrition: Salt intake and eating patterns of infants and children in relation to blood pressure. Pediatrics 53:115, 1974.

Forster, S. B.: Pump failure. Am. J. Nurs. 74:1830, 1974.

Loggie, J. M. H., et al: Renal function and diuretic therapy in infants and children. J. Pediat. 86:485, 657, 825, 1975.

MacLeod, S. M.: The rational use of potassium supplements. Postgrad. Med. 57:123, 1975.

Spice measurements in grams. J. Am. Dietet. A. 62:290, 1973.

RESOURCES FOR PATIENTS

Dupuy, M. E., and Dupuy, B. J.: Fat-Controlled and Sodium-Restricted Cooking. Garden City, N. Y., Doubleday, 1971.

Payne, A. S., and Callahan, D.: Fat and Sodium Control Cookbook, ed. 4. Boston, Little, Brown, 1975.

Salmon, M. B., and Quigley, A. E.: Enjoying Your Restricted Diet. Springfield, Ill., Thomas, 1972.

Your 500 Milligram Sodium-Restricted Diet (booklet and leaflet); Your 1000 Milligram Sodium-Restricted Diet (booklet and leaflet); Your Mild Sodium-Restricted Diet (booklet); American Heart Association, New York, N. Y.

For further references see Bibliography in Section 4.

REFERENCES

1. Lieberman, E.: J. Pediat. 85:1, 1974.
2. Welt, L. G.: in Harrison's Principles of Medicine, ed. 7. New York, McGraw-Hill, 1974. Chapter 264.
3. Ramires, A., and Abelman, W. H.: N. Eng. J. Med. 290:499, 1974.
4. Dahl, L. K.: J. Exp. Med. 114:231, 1961.
5. Kaufman, M.: Am. J. Clin. Nutr. 5:676, 1957.
6. Sinar, L. J., and Mason, M.: J. Am. Dietet. A. 66:155, 1975.
7. Newburg, B.: Arch. Int. Med. 123:692, 1969.
8. White, J. M., et al: J. Am. Dietet. A. 50:32, 1967.
9. Christakis, G., and Winston, M.: J. Am. Dietet. A. 63:233, 1973.

31

renal disease; nephrolithiasis

The Kidney's Role in Normal Metabolism
Terminology and Metabolic Aberrations
Classification
Hemodialysis and Transplantation
Diet Therapy
Counseling the Patient
Nephrolithiasis

The nutritional care of patients with renal disease focuses on the intake of energy, protein, fluids, and electrolytes. In the early stages of chronic renal disease, the modifications of the dietary intake may be moderate. However, as chronic renal disease progresses to end-stage renal failure, nutrition is one of the most critical components of the medical care plan and requires complex manipulation. The same is true in acute renal failure. The patterns calculated to fulfill the diet prescription for patients in end-stage renal failure with the uremic syndrome generally do not, and cannot, reflect the usual food practices of the well person. Also, as the patient copes with his complex diet modifications, he and his family are faced with the decision to accept maintenance hemodialysis or, depending on his age and condition, a renal transplant.

Before proceeding with the discussions of renal disease and diet therapy, the reader is urged to review Chapter 4, Proteins, Chapter 5, Water and Mineral Metabolism, and Chapter 30, Cardiovascular Disease, especially the sodium restricted diet; and the structure and functions of the normal kidney in a textbook of physiology.[1]

THE KIDNEY'S ROLE IN NORMAL METABOLISM

The normal kidney performs three major interrelated metabolic functions: (1) they *filter* the end products of protein catabolism from the blood and excrete them from the body in the urine; (2) they control the level of constituents of the body fluids by *reabsorbing* them from, or *secreting* them into, the filtrate; and (3) they *maintain* the volume of body fluids by reabsorbing water from the filtrate. The kidney also performs certain endocrine functions. It produces renin which, through its action on angiotensin, profoundly affects the systemic blood pressure. It is indirectly involved in iron metabolism because the hormone erythropoietin, which regulates the formation of red blood cells in the bone marrow, is produced in the kidney. It is also involved in calcium metabolism, because 25-hydroxy-calciferol is hydroxylated in the kidney to 1-25-dihydroxy-calciferol, the active form of vitamin D, which is now considered to be a hormone (see Chapter 6, Fat Soluble Vitamins).

The structural and functional unit of the kidney is the nephron (see Plate 2). It is estimated that each kidney contains about 1 million nephrons, and physiologists favor the view that all nephrons are continuously active. However, there appears to be considerable physiological reserve. For example, after the surgical removal of one kidney, renal function is maintained through the process of compensatory hypertrophy by the nephrons in the remaining kidney.[2] The glomerulus is the filtering unit of the kidney and the tubule is the reabsorptive and secretory unit; both their structure and function are closely interrelated.

Blood from the afferent arteriole (see Plate 2) enters a network of capillaries in the glomerulus, the glomerular tuft, where an essentially protein-free filtrate of plasma is separated from the blood and enters the glomerular space. The filtered blood leaves the network of capillaries through the efferent arterioles and enters a network of capillaries which surround the tubules. The membrane surrounding the glomerular space, Bowman's capsule, merges into the tubule where the filtrate is drastically modified in both volume and composition by the various segments of the tubule—the proximal convoluted tubule, the loop of Henle, and the distal convoluted tubule. Ultimately the concentrated filtrate, containing about 5 percent solids made up of electrolytes, urea, creatinine, and uric acid, flows into the collecting tubules and thence into the urinary bladder for excretion.

The membrane of the glomerular capillaries differs from that of other capillaries in that it is more permeable to water and small blood constituents. The glomerular filtration process is driven by the hydrostatic pressure of the blood within the capillaries. In normal humans, approximately 125 ml. of glomerular filtrate is formed each minute. About 180 liters of fluid are filtered each 24 hours, while approximately 1 to 2 liters of urine of normal concentration are excreted each day. In addition to water the filtrate contains glucose, amino acids, electrolytes such as sodium, potassium, magnesium, chlorides, phosphates, and sulfates, as well as the nitrogenous end products of protein catabolism—urea, uric acid, and creatinine. As the filtrate passes through the tubules, over 99 percent of the water, virtually all of the glucose and amino acids, a major portion of the electrolytes and uric acid, and approximately one half of the urea is reabsorbed into the capillaries surrounding the tubules. Glucose, amino acids, phosphate, sulfate, and possibly uric acid are actively reabsorbed while the other constituents are passively reabsorbed. Creatinine is the only constituent of the filtrate which is not reabsorbed, and potassium is unique in that it is both reabsorbed from, and secreted into, the filtrate by the tubules.

TERMINOLOGY AND METABOLIC ABERRATIONS

Renal failure or renal insufficiency are the terms used to describe altered kidney function. It may be acute or chronic and the acute phases may or may not lead to the chronic one. Acute renal failure includes all forms of the acute cessation of kidney function with the suppression of urine formation; chronic renal failure includes all degrees of the progressive decrease in normal kidney function. The terms uremic syndrome and uremia are used to describe the critical phase of progressive renal failure after 90 percent of kidney function has been lost, or to the critical phase of acute renal failure due to sudden kidney shutdown.

The uremic syndrome is characterized by the presence of excessive quantities of the end products of protein catabolism in the blood and by marked nausea, vomiting, headache, convulsions, and coma. Azotemia refers to an elevation of urea or other nitrogenous end products of protein catabolism in the blood without the symptoms of the uremic syndrome.

Renal disease may destroy nephrons so that a reduced number of nephrons must maintain the functions of the kidney. The remaining functional nephrons hypertrophy to accommodate an increase in both the volume of fluid and the quantity of constituents in the filtrate. However, the tubules may not be able to handle the increased quantity of filtrate completely.

As a result excessive quantities of fluid (polyuria) and electrolytes, particularly sodium, are lost from the body. At the same time urea may be reabsorbed at its usual rate.

Renal disease may affect the permeability of the glomerular membrane or the reabsorptive and secretory functions of the tubules. In many situations the altered functions of the glomeruli lead to progressive tubular involvement and the reverse may also occur. The diseased glomerular membrane may become more permeable and permit the passage of substances larger than those usually filtered, especially blood proteins, resulting in proteinuria. However, the predominant effect appears to be a decrease in the permeability of the glomerular membrane, which results in azotemia. As chronic renal failure progresses to end-stage renal failure, therefore, the rate of glomerular filtration and urinary output decreases. A glomerular filtration rate of 30 ml. per minute (normal, 125 ml. per minute) is considered critical; as the rate decreases hemodialysis, the mechanical filtering of the blood, or kidney transplantation is required to maintain life.

As a result of the altered structures and functions of the kidney in renal disease, the metabolic problems which can be encountered are: (1) excessive fluid and electrolyte losses leading to dehydration or excessive fluid and electrolyte retention leading to edema; (2) proteinuria; and (3) azotemia. At the same time disturbances in hydrogen ion concentration of the blood leading to acidosis or alkalosis can also occur. Anemia occurs in progressive and end-stage renal failure due to altered erythropoiesis: and in end-stage renal failure renal osteodystrophy (faulty nutrition of bone) occurs due to altered calcium metabolism. The diet prescriptions used in the treatment of renal disease reflect these metabolic problems (see later section on Principles of Diet Therapy).

CLASSIFICATION

Renal disease may result from inflammatory or degenerative diseases or congenital abnormalities. Table 31-1 lists by diagnosis the most common renal diseases due to inflammatory or degenerative processes. Renal diseases due to congenital abnormalities such as polycystic kidney, nephrogenic diabetes insipidus, and the aminoacidurias are relatively rare. Polycystic kidney disease involves all the units of the kidney while the others are due to one or more defects in the mechanisms which facilitate active reabsorption by the tubules.

The common renal diseases due to inflammatory processes are glomerulonephritis, pyelonephritis,

and the nephrotic syndrome; arteriolar nephrosclerosis and diabetic nephropathy are due to degenerative processes.

GLOMERULONEPHRITIS. There is considerable evidence that Group A hemolytic streptococcus is the major infectious agent, although syphilis and other infections may also be involved. Recent research has demonstrated that the damage to the glomerulus is the result of immune-complex disease caused by antigen-antibody reactions.[3] It occurs more often in childhood or early adult life than in later years.

Acute glomerulonephritis is characterized by proteinuria, hematuria (red cells in the urine), hypertension, oliguria (deficient secretion of urine), puffy eyes (periorbital edema), swelling of the ankles due to edema, and varying degrees of nitrogen retention. There may be anorexia or nausea and vomiting. If oliguria is present, dietary protein and sodium intakes are restricted. With improvement in kidney function the protein is gradually increased, while the sodium restriction is continued until the edema has subsided. The disease is self-limiting, and complete recovery results in four to six months in the large majority of patients. In a few cases, however, the disease may go on to chronic glomerulonephritis.

Chronic glomerulonephritis may follow an attack of acute nephritis, particularly if repeated infections occur; or it may be insidious in onset, the symptoms being so mild at first that the subject is not aware of his condition until attention is drawn to it, perhaps when he is undergoing a physical examination for life insurance. The volume of urine is usually excessive (polyuria) and of low specific gravity (dilute) and it may show much or comparatively little protein. There may be morning headache and loss of appetite, and the patient may be annoyed by nocturia (the necessity of frequent urination during the night) due to the inability of the kidneys to concentrate the urine. During this phase the intake of fluids and of electrolytes, sodium and potassium, is increased to compensate for excessive urinary losses. The intake of dietary protein may be normal or increased.

As time goes on these symptoms may become more severe. Increased loss of protein in the urine lowers the level of serum albumin, and therefore the osmotic pressure of the blood, resulting in generalized edema. This is called the nephrotic phase of glomerulonephritis. At this time, the intake of dietary sodium is restricted and the dietary protein is increased to compensate for the urinary losses. As the disease progresses toward end-stage renal failure, nitrogen retention occurs, which requires a protein restriction. At the same time the kidney cannot conserve sodium and chloride. Therefore, the diet is no

Table 31-1. Renal Diseases Due to Inflammatory and Degenerative Processes

DIAGNOSIS	PATHOLOGICAL CHARACTERISTICS	CLINICAL CHARACTERISTICS
Inflammatory		
Glomerulonephritis		
Acute	Inflammation of glomeruli	Proteinuria Hematuria Hypertension ↓Renal function*
Chronic	Fibrosis of glomeruli and afferent arterioles with progressive tubular involvement	Proteinuria Hematuria Edema Hypertension ↓Renal function*
Chronic pyelonephritis	Interstitial inflammation leading to fibrosis of tubules and glomeruli	Hypertension Mild proteinuria ↓Renal function*
Nephrotic syndrome	Diffuse injury to glomeruli	Massive proteinuria Hypoalbuminemia Gross edema ↑Blood lipids, especially cholesterol
Degenerative		
Arteriolar nephrosclerosis	Thickening and hyalinization of arterioles due to hypertension leading to progressive loss of glomeruli	Hypertension Proteinuria ↓Renal function*
Diabetic nephropathy	Nodular lesions of the glomeruli	Proteinuria Hypertension Edema ↓Renal function*
Advanced Renal Failure		
Uremic syndrome	Minimal renal function	↑Blood urea nitrogen and electrolytes Gastrointestinal symptoms Anemia Edema Congestive heart failure Renal osteodystrophy

*Varying degress of nitrogen retention (↑BUN) and/or electrolyte retention or loss.

longer restricted in sodium. Many of these patients, both children and young adults, become candidates for maintenance hemodialysis or renal transplantation (see section on dialysis and transplantation).

CHRONIC PYELONEPHRITIS. Chronic pyelonephritis results from bacterial infection of the interstitium of the kidney, which affects the tubules and ultimately the glomeruli. The onset of the disease is insidious and patients often do not seek medical care until they have hypertension or are in renal failure. They will complain of fatigue, which is due to the anemia of renal disease. Because of hypertension the dietary sodium is restricted; if the patient is also retaining nitrogen, the protein and possibly the potassium are restricted.

NEPHROTIC SYNDROME. This syndrome, which is characterized by massive proteinuria, hypoalbuminemia (low blood albumin), and massive edema

is due to diffuse damage to the glomerulus. As previously mentioned it may occur in glomerulonephritis or as a result of allergic reactions to pollens, poisonous plants, and insect stings. It differs from other glomerular disease in that hyperlipemia occurs. The reason for this is unknown at present. Facial edema and loss of appetite are two common symptoms. The diet is restricted in sodium and increased in protein. The nephrosis which occurs in children is discussed in Chapter 34.

ARTERIOLAR NEPHROSCLEROSIS. Nephrosclerosis occurs among older patients and is usually the result of arteriosclerosis and essential hypertension of long standing. The blood supply to the kidneys has decreased gradually because of the thickening of the wall and the narrowing of the lumen of the blood vessels. Usually this is accompanied by increased blood pressure and is characterized by mild retention of nitrogen. In the more severe cases, mild or moderate proteinuria also may be present.

DIABETIC NEPHROPATHY (KIMMELSTEIL-WILSON SYNDROME). Nodular lesions occur in the glomerular capillaries in diabetic nephropathy. The patient presents many of the same problems as does the patient with nephrosclerosis. As the kidney function decreases, urinary glucose may not be an accurate guide to blood glucose because it is not filtered by the glomerulus. In both nephrosclerosis and diabetic nephropathy, the sodium and protein in the diet are restricted; if hyperkalemia is also present, the dietary potassium will be restricted.

UREMIC SYNDROME. In the uremic syndrome, due to either acute or progressive renal failure, the urea nitrogen, creatinine, and potassium blood levels are extremely high while the calcium level is below normal. These patients are usually disoriented, have nausea and vomiting, anemia, and, in the most severe cases, congestive heart failure. Dialysis is frequently used to relieve the symptoms of uremia, and the diet is restricted in protein, sodium, and potassium.

HEMODIALYSIS AND TRANSPLANTATION

HEMODIALYSIS. Dialysis is an artificial method for carrying out the basic functions of the kidneys: the filtration process to remove the end products of protein catabolism and the excess of fluids which accumulate between dialyses. It is used in conjunction with diet therapy to alleviate the symptoms of uremia in acute or end-stage renal failure. Peritoneal dialysis introduces the dialysate directly into the peritoneum, while hemodialysis is performed by running the blood through the artificial kidney.

Hemodialysis is used to prepare those individuals who are candidates for kidney transplant or to stabilize end-stage renal failure in those patients who do not qualify for renal transplantation. Hemodialysis is established during hospitalization and continued two or three times a week on an outpatient basis at a dialysis center. Recent federal legislation has made it possible to establish centers in many cities around the country. Many individuals with renal disease on maintenance hemodialysis return to a reasonable degree of normal living and productive activity.

RENAL TRANSPLANTATIONS. The disciplines of medicine, surgery, and immunology working together have been able to transplant the human kidney relatively successfully. Kidneys for transplantation are obtained from two sources: from a donor who is a relative of the patient or from the donation of kidneys after death from causes other than renal disease. If the transplant is not successful, usually due to the body's rejection of the transplanted kidney, the patient returns to maintenance dialysis.

DIET THERAPY
Principles of Diet Therapy

The following discussion of the principles of diet therapy refers primarily to the metabolic problems of chronic and end-stage renal failure. However, many of the same principles apply in acute renal failure.

ENERGY. All patients with renal failure, whether acute, chronic, or end-stage, require an adequate energy intake (approximately 35 to 40 kcal. per kg. for adults). Without adequate energy supplied by carbohydrate and fat, amino acids from food and body cells will be deaminized in intermediary metabolism to contribute to energy needs through the gluconeogenic pathway. This will decrease the amount of protein available to compensate for the loss of protein in the urine, e.g., massive proteinuria in the nephrotic syndrome; or the catabolism of protein for energy will increase the amount of nitrogen (as ammonia) available for the synthesis of urea, which leads to an increase in the amount of urea to be excreted by the kidneys. Consideration of this critical relationship between energy and protein in intermediary metabolism is the first step in planning diet therapy for the patient with renal disease and is often overlooked.

Patients with primary renal disease are rarely obese, while patients with renal disease secondary to trauma, diabetes, hypertension, or cardiac disease may be obese. A moderate restriction of energy intake (to 1800 calories or less) may be prescribed for the obese adult patient. The energy intake of a child must be adequate to support normal growth insofar as possible. One investigator has reported that growth failure in children with renal disease could be attributed in part to inadequate intakes of energy.[4]

PROTEIN. Proteinuria is a common clinical characteristic of renal disease. When this occurs, the protein in the diet is increased to 1½ to 2 g. per kg. for adults (100 to 140 g. per day for a 70-kg. man) to compensate for the urinary losses, even though the level of blood urea nitrogen (BUN) is moderately elevated (40 to 60 mg. per 100 ml.). When massive proteinuria occurs, as in the nephrotic syndrome, the protein intake is usually increased to 2 to 3 g. per kg. for adults (140 to 200 g. per day for a 70-kg. man). The protein in the diet for children with proteinuria is also increased. Proteins of high biological value should be used to supply 60 to 70 percent of the total protein in the diet pattern.

With increasing nitrogen retention (blood urea nitrogen over 100 mg. per 100 ml.) in end-stage renal failure, the protein in the diet is restricted to control the amount of nitrogen available for urea synthesis. At the same time the body's needs for essential amino acids must be met by proteins of high biological value. Proteins of high biological value: (1) have most of their nitrogen present in their essential amino acids; (2) contain all the essential amino acids; and (3) have a concentration of amino acids roughly proportional to Rose's minimum daily requirements (see below). The foods which best satisfy these criteria are milk and eggs. Meats also satisfy these criteria except that they contain somewhat more nitrogen from nonessential amino acids than do milk and eggs.

The evidence which demonstrated the importance of restricting the intake to proteins of high biological value in uremia was first published by Giordano in 1963.[5] He reported that he fed a group of uremic patients in Italy a diet adequate in energy, vitamins, and minerals with a mixture of synthetic essential amino acids as the sole source of nitrogen. The quantity of nitrogen was adequate to meet the needs of the patients. He observed a decrease in blood urea nitrogen (BUN) levels, positive nitrogen balance, and a decrease in many uremic symptoms such as nausea and vomiting. He postulated that the nitrogen in the BUN was utilized for the synthesis of nonessential amino acids in the body.

In 1967, Richard and coworkers reported that, from their investigations using labeled ammonia, ammonia was the form in which urea nitrogen was used for the endogenous synthesis of nonessential amino acids (see Urea Synthesis, Chapter 9).[6]

In 1964, Giovannetti and Maggiore reported results similar to Giordano's when they used a mixture of the synthetic essential amino acids or two eggs (100 g.) and an adequate energy intake from low-protein wheatstarch and cornstarch.[7]

In 1965, Shaw and his coworkers in England reported on their treatment of uremic patients using a modified Giovannetti diet.[8] Their diet, adequate in energy, minerals, and vitamins, contained 18 to 20 g. of protein, 12 g. of which was supplied by the high biological protein in 50 g. of egg (1 egg) and 200 ml. of milk. These patients also experienced relief from uremic symptoms.

Similar results with a modified Giovannetti diet were reported in the United States.[9] The diet contained 20 g. of protein with 12 to 13 g. provided by 50 g. of egg and 200 ml. of milk. The remainder of the protein was obtained from low-protein cereals and vegetables and fruit. Wheatstarch, sugars, and fats were used to supply an adequate intake of energy.

Table 31–2 shows the essential amino acids in 200 ml. of milk and 50 g. of egg and in 100 g. of egg compared with Rose's minimum requirements for the essential amino acids. Both the Giovannetti and the Shaw diets are in good agreement with Rose's figures with the exception of phenylalanine and methionine.

The modified Giovannetti diet provided approximately 0.28 g. protein per kg. of body weight for a 70-kg. man. The long-term use of this quantity of protein presented problems in maintaining nitrogen balance.[10] Recent research has indicated that the quantity of protein in the diet of the uremic patient should be determined by his glomerular filtration rate as estimated by the creatinine clearance rate plus any amount of protein lost in the urine.[11] Table 31–3 shows the minimal advisable intake of grams of protein per kilogram of body weight according to the degree of renal failure as recommended by Anderson

Table 31–2. Comparison of Shaw and Giovannetti Diets with Rose's Proposed Minimum Requirements of Essential Amino Acids (Male)

FOOD	WEIGHT (g.)	AMINO ACIDS (mg.)[a]								PROTEIN (g.)
		Phe	Ile	Leu	Val	Met	Trp	The	Lys	
Milk, whole[b]	200	340	446	683	480	228	98	322	544	7
Egg (1)[b]	50	369	425	563	475	350	105	318	409	7
Totals		709	871	1251	955	578	203	640	953	14
Eggs (2)[c]	100	739	850	1126	950	700	211	637	819	14
Rose's Proposed Requirements[d]		1110	700	1100	800	1100	250	500	800	

[a]Table 3, Section 4.
[b]Shaw, A. B.: Q. J. Med. 34:237, 1965.
[c]Giovannetti, S., and Maggiore, G.: Lancet 1:100, 1964.
[d]Chapter 4, Proteins.

Table 31-3. Recommended Protein Intake According to Degree of Renal Failure*

Creatinine Clearance (ml./min./1.73 sqm.)	Protein Intake (g./kg. body weight)†
30-20	0.7-0.5
19-5	0.36
5	0.26

*Adapted from Anderson, C. F., et al: JAMA 223:68, 1973.
†Plus amount of protein equal to 24-hour urinary loss.

and his coworkers. The diet should primarily contain proteins of high biological value, preferably from milk and eggs.

When hemodialysis is used either to maintain the patient free of uremic symptoms or to prepare him for renal transplantation, he will require 0.75 to 1.0 g. of protein per kilogram of body weight to maintain nitrogen balance. Because of the size of their molecules, all blood proteins do not pass through the dialyzer membranes and some are removed from the body during dialysis. Therefore, the diet must provide enough protein of high biological value for the replacement of this loss.[12] After successful renal transplantation, it is unnecessary to restrict dietary protein.

SODIUM. Sodium wasting may occur in polyuria when the tubules are unable to conserve sodium. To prevent hyponatremia, additional sodium as sodium chloride is required to compensate for the urinary losses. If it is tolerated, sodium chloride is added to food. Otherwise sodium chloride tablets are taken with meals to avoid gastric irritation. If there is metabolic alkalosis with a fall in hydrogen ion concentration, sodium bicarbonate is used in place of sodium chloride.

As the glomerular filtration rate and daily urinary volume decline, the intake of sodium will be restricted, the level depending on the patient's problems. In the absence of edema and hypertension, the sodium may be mildly restricted (2000 mg. or more). If edema and hypertension are present, a moderate restriction, 1000 to 2000 mg., is often prescribed. With massive edema and hypertension a 500-mg. sodium diet is used. In uremia or acute renal failure, it may be necessary to restrict sodium to 250 mg.

POTASSIUM. When urinary volume is adequate, a normal blood potassium level is usually maintained, while in polyuria there can be an excessive loss of potassium, leading to hypokalemia. The urinary loss of potassium can be corrected by medication supplemented by fruits and fruit and vegetable juices and other foods which are significant sources of potassium (see Table 4, Section 4). When edema is

present, treatment with diuretics can also promote the loss of potassium (see Chapter 30).

In end-stage renal failure, hyperkalemia can occur due to the catabolism of body cells with the release of potassium into the blood. The cell breakdown is due in part to an inadequate energy intake. At this point potassium intake is usually restricted to 1500 mg. (40 mEq.) or less.

PHOSPHATE. Patients with uremia experience hypocalcemia and hyperphosphatemia. Since the uremic patient's diet is restricted in protein, the phosphate intake is also restricted. However, the diet of the patient on hemodialysis is not restricted in protein, but milk may be limited in the diet of these patients because of its phosphate content. They may also be given aluminum hydroxide to promote the excretion of phosphates in the feces. The hypocalcemia is treated by intravenous calcium therapy.

VITAMINS AND OTHER MINERALS. When the intake of dietary protein, sodium, and potassium is severely restricted, an adequate intake of vitamins cannot be achieved and during dialysis water-soluble vitamins can be lost. Therefore, multivitamin capsules and folic acid are given daily to provide an adequate intake.

Protein-restricted diets are also inadequate in iron, and iron supplements may be given. However, this supplementation may not be effective in treating the anemia of chronic renal failure because the anemia is a result of the kidney's role in hemapoiesis and is not solely due to a deficient intake of iron.

WATER. Restriction of fluid intake becomes a critical factor in acute or end-stage renal failure. The daily intake of fluid is restricted to the output and may be as low as 500 to 600 ml. In most situations the fluid intake is distributed between mealtime beverages and water used to take medications. In some situations the water content of the food served may be calculated as part of the total fluid intake.

Diet Therapy in Acute Renal Failure

Acute kidney failure may occur in response to severe hemorrhage, in burns, or in poisoning, especially with heavy metals—such as mercury—which are deposited in the tubules as the kidney tries to excrete them. The onset is usually sudden and the critical phase may last a few days to two or three weeks. The patient is anuric and has an elevated BUN, hyperkalemia, and anemia. He is disoriented and experiences nausea and vomiting. If conditions permit, he may be dialyzed.

In the anuric phase fluid intake is restricted to approximately 600 ml. to replace insensible fluid losses. If the patient can tolerate oral feedings, 100 to

150 g. of carbohydrate, free of nitrogen and electrolytes, is dissolved in the fluid allowed to minimize protein catabolism. Epstein has had clinical success with a solution of 50 g. of lactose, 25 g. of sucrose, and 25 g. of glucose dissolved in the water allowed and flavored with lemon juice to reduce the sweetness.[13] It is possible that the lactose in this solution could cause diarrhea. For this reason, he recommends that the solution be sipped, not taken in quantity at any one time (see Lactose Intolerance, Chapter 25). Epstein feels that the 400 calories from sugars in his formula are adequate and that a higher calorie intake with a mixture of carbohydrate and fat is not required.

Various high-calorie, low-electrolyte, and relatively nitrogen-free products are commercially available. Two of these are Controlyte* and Cal-Power.† Controlyte is a powder which contains per 1 ounce (30 g.) approximately 145 calories, 6.4 g. fat, 20.4 g. carbohydrate, 3 mg. sodium, 1 mg. potassium, and a trace of protein. It is dissolved in the water allowed or, depending on the potassium restriction, in fruit juice. Cal-Power, packaged in 8-ounce containers, is a lemon-flavored beverage which contains per fluid ounce about 70 calories, 4 mg. sodium, and 0.5 mg. potassium. It is relatively sweet to taste but has a pleasant flavor when frozen and served as a sherbet.

A nasogastric feeding of glucose and a vegetable oil in emulsified form (Lipomul**) has been recommended. Earlier, Kolff suggested butter and sugar mixtures to be taken by mouth.[14] Most patients find these butter mixtures distasteful.

If oral fluids cannot be tolerated, intravenous fluid therapy is used. Hyperalimentation with a solution of glucose and the essential l-amino acids has also been used successfully in the treatment of acute renal failure.[15]

When kidney function improves, diuresis takes place. When BUN is less than 80 mg. per 100 ml. and the patient can tolerate it, he is offered a diet containing protein beginning with 10 to 20 g. per day and increasing as kidney function improves.

Diet Therapy In Chronic Renal Failure

The sodium-restricted diet is the therapeutic diet most commonly used in the treatment of chronic renal failure when hypertension and/or edema are present. The sodium-restricted Exchange System and food lists in Chapter 30 are used to calculate these diet patterns. The amount of protein prescribed may be increased, normal, or moderately decreased, depending on kidney function. However, the major portion

*D. M. Doyle Pharmaceutical Co., Minneapolis, Minn.
†General Mills Chemical Co., Minneapolis, Minn.
**Upjohn Company, Kalamazoo, Mich.

should be provided by food proteins of high biological value. When fluid loss is excessive, patients must be helped to increase fluid intake. It is helpful for them to drink fluid each time after urinating.

The protein-restricted, sodium-restricted diet is discussed in the next section. However, in many instances when the diet is restricted in sodium, it is increased in protein to compensate for proteinuria. Table 31-4 shows the calculation of a diet pattern containing 2200 calories, 100 g. of protein, and 800 mg. of sodium. The sodium figures apply to foods produced, processed, and prepared without the addition of any sodium compound and are the same values as those in Table 30-1, Sodium-Restricted Exchange System, in Chapter 30. The values for energy and protein are those in Table 23-2, Chapter 23. The sodium-restricted exchange lists in Table 30-2, Chapter 30, are used to plan daily menus for this diet pattern. If the sodium is restricted to 500 mg., the protein in the diet pattern cannot be greater than 70 g. unless low-sodium milk‡ is used. Dialysed whole fluid milk is not recommended because it contains excessive quantities of potassium.

Diet Therapy in End-Stage Renal Failure

The diet prescription, the potassium content of foods, wheatstarch products, and an exchange system for calculating the protein-, sodium-, and potassium-restricted diet are discussed in this section. The diet is used to relieve the symptoms of uremia before dialysis is started. Although the protein in the diet for the patient on hemodialysis may not be severely restricted, relatively severe restrictions of sodium and potassium intake are usually necessary. It may also be used for a short time as kidney function improves in acute renal failure.

DIET PRESCRIPTION. The amount of protein prescribed will depend on the level of renal function as measured by the glomerular filtration rate (see Table

Table 31-4. 2200-Calorie, 100-g. Protein, 800 mg.-Sodium Diet Pattern

Food Group*	Amount	Protein (g.)	Sodium (mg.)	Energy (calories)
Milk	4 c.	32	480	680
Meat	6 oz. cooked	42	150	450
Egg	2	14	140	150
Fruit	3 servings	——	6	120
Vegetables	1 serving	2	9	35
Bread	8 servings	16	40	560
Fat	6 tsp.	——	——	270
TOTALS		106	825	2265

*Produced, processed, and prepared without the addition of any sodium compound.

‡Lonalac, Mead Johnson, Evansville, Ind.

Table 31-5. Exchange System for Calculating Protein-, Sodium-, and Potassium-Restricted Diets

FOOD EXCHANGES	HOUSEHOLD MEASURE	GRAMS	PROTEIN (g.)	SODIUM (mg.)	POTASSIUM† (mg.)
Milk	½ c.	120	4	60	170
Meat					
Group A	1 oz.	30	7	60	70
Group B	1 oz.	30	7	25	120
Egg	1	50	7	70	100
Vegetables					
Group A	½ c.	100	1	9	150
Group B	½ c.	100	2	9	240
Fruit					
Group A	varies	varies	1	2	100
Group B	varies	varies	1	2	145
Bread, unsalted					
Group A	varies	varies	2	5	25
Group B	varies	varies	3	5	50
Group C*	1 slice	30	0.1	15	8
Fat, salted	1 tsp.	5	0	50	0

*Values for Dietetic Paygel Baking Mix.
†Handbook No. 8, USDA, 1963.

31–3). The amount of sodium, potassium, and fluid prescribed will also reflect the glomerular filtration rate. Protein can vary from 20 to 60 g., sodium from 250 to 2000 mg. (10 to 85 mEq.), potassium from 700 to 2000 mg. (18 to 50 mEq.), and fluid as low as 500 to 600 ml. per day. Unless the individual is obese, the calories are not stated in the diet prescription. It is expected that the diet will provide 35 to 40 cal. per kg. per day for adults and adequate calories for age for children and adolescents.

POTASSIUM IN FOOD. Potassium is found in the cells of all living tissue and is, therefore, widely distributed in all foods with the exception of pure fats and oils. The average adult intake of potassium varies from 2000 to 6000 mg. per day (50 to 150 mEq.). In terminal renal failure the potassium in the diet may be restricted to 2500 to 1500 mg. (60 to 40 mEq.) or less per day.

Because potassium is in the cell, it cannot easily be removed from food. The potassium in vegetables can be reduced to some extent by cooking in water. For example, Louis and Dolan report that soaking raw potatoes before cooking for 30 minutes results in a loss of approximately 75 percent of the potassium— from 387 mg. to 86 mg. per 100 g.[16] The water the potatoes are soaked in is discarded and fresh water is used to boil the potatoes.

Canned vegetables and fruits also appear to lose some potassium in processing. For example, 100 g. of fresh apricots have 281 mg. of potassium and canned apricots, 246 mg.; 100 g. of frozen peas (cooked) have 152 mg. of potassium and canned peas, 95 mg. (see

Table 4, Section 4). Canned vegetables and fruit are drained carefully when served to a patient whose diet is restricted in potassium because the potassium is in the juice. Also, when fluids are restricted, the juice would add to total fluid intake.

The bran layer of grains has a higher concentration of potassium than the endosperm. A 25-g. slice of regular white bread contains 25 mg. of potassium, and a 25-g. slice of whole wheat, 65 mg. of potassium. Highly milled grains, especially cornstarch and wheatstarch, are practically free of potassium. The starches of certain roots, arrowroot and tapioca, are also practically free of potassium. Therefore, these starches—corn, wheat, arrowroot and tapioca—are used in baked products or as thickening agents in puddings in planning renal diets (see section on special starch for renal diets).

Stewing meat and poultry and discarding the water used in cooking will also reduce the potassium to some extent. For example, 100 g. of canned chicken, meat only, contains 138 mg. of potassium, while 100 g. of roasted chicken, white meat, contains 422 mg. of potassium. Chicken or beef broth and meat drippings are significant sources of potassium and cannot be used in a potassium-restricted diet plan.

Tea and coffee, either regular or instant, are significant sources of potassium and, therefore, are excluded or served in very limited amounts in potassium-restricted diets. One level teaspoon of instant coffee contains approximately 45 mg. of potassium; 1 level teaspoon of instant tea contains about 63.4 mg. At a restriction of 1500 mg. or less of potas-

Table 31-6. Protein, Sodium, and Potassium Exchange Lists

Milk Exchange

1 serving contains 4 g. of protein, 60 mg. of sodium, 170 mg. of potassium

Milk, whole	½ cup
Milk, skim	½ cup
Light cream 18%	½ cup
Heavy cream 40%	¾ cup
Half and half	½ cup
Ice cream, regular	½ cup
Sour cream	¾ cup

Meat Exchanges: Group A

1 serving contains 7 g. of protein, 60 mg. of sodium, 70 mg. of potassium

Oysters, raw	4 in number
Lobster, shrimp fresh or canned in water without salt	1 ounce
Tuna, canned in water	¼ cup

Meat Exchanges: Group B

1 serving contains 7 g. of protein, 25 mg. of sodium, 120 mg. of potassium

Beef, lamb, pork, rabbit	1 ounce
Chicken, turkey	1 ounce
Haddock	1 ounce

Egg Exchange

1 egg contains 7 g. of protein, 70 mg. of sodium, 120 mg. of potassium

Vegetable Exchanges: Group A

1 serving contains 1 g. of protein, 9 mg. of sodium, 150 mg. of potassium

Beans, green or wax	½ cup
Beets*	½ cup
Cabbage	½ cup
Corn, whole kernel	½ cup
Eggplant	½ cup
Summer squash	½ cup
Zucchini	½ cup

All vegetables *cooked* or *canned* without salt and *well-drained*.
*Reduce to ⅓ cup if sodium restricted to less than 500 mg.

Vegetable Exchanges: Group B

1 serving contains 2 g. of protein, 9 mg. of sodium, 240 mg. of potassium

Asparagus	½ cup
Broccoli	½ cup
Brussels sprouts	½ cup
Carrots*	½ cup
Potatoes†	½ cup
Pumpkin	½ cup
Winter squash	½ cup
Tomatoes	½ cup
Tomato juice, low-sodium dietetic	½ cup
Turnips	⅓ cup

All vegetables *cooked* or *canned* without salt and *well-drained*.
*Reduce to ⅓ cup if sodium restricted to less than 500 mg.
†Pare, soak in water ½ hour, discard water, cook in fresh water.

Fruit Exchanges: Group A

1 serving contains 1 g. of protein, 2 mg. of sodium, 100 mg. of potassium

Apple, raw	1 small
Apple juice	½ cup
Applesauce	½ cup
Blueberries	⅝ cup
Peach nectar	½ cup
Pears, canned	⅓ cup
Pear nectar	½ cup
Pineapple, canned	1 slice

Fruit Exchanges: Group B

1 serving contains 1 g. of protein, 2 mg. of sodium, 145 mg. of potassium

Blackberries, fresh or frozen	½ cup
Fruit cocktail	⅓ cup
Grape juice, canned	½ cup
Grapefruit, raw	½ medium
Grapefruit, juice	⅓ cup
Grapefruit sections	½ cup
Pear, raw	½ medium
Pineapple juice	⅓ cup
Plums, purple, canned	3 medium

Fruit Exchanges: Group B (continued)

Raspberries, red, fresh, frozen	½ cup
Strawberries, fresh, frozen	½ cup
Tangerine	1 medium
Watermelon, raw, cubed	¾ cup

Bread Exchanges: Group A

1 serving contains 2 g. of protein, 5 mg. of sodium, and 25 mg. of potassium

Low-sodium bread	1 slice
Unsalted cooked cereal	
Rice	½ cup
Farina	¾ cup
Corn grits	¾ cup

Use regular only. Do not use instant or quick-cooking varieties.

Dry cereal	
Puffed rice	1 cup
Unsalted cornflakes	1 cup

Bread Exchanges: Group B

1 serving contains 3 g. of protein, 5 mg. of sodium, 50 mg. of potassium

Dry cereal	
Puffed wheat	½ cup
Unsalted cooked	
Macaroni	½ cup
Noodles	½ cup
Spaghetti	½ cup

Bread Exchanges: Group C

1 serving contains 0.1 g. of protein, 15 mg. of sodium, and 3 mg. of potassium

Bread*	1 slice

*Also applies to Aproten products, Dietetic Paygel Baking Mix

Fat Exchanges

1 serving contains 0 protein, 50 mg. of sodium, 0 potassium

Butter, salted	1 teaspoon
Margarine, salted	1 teaspoon
Mayonnaise, salted	1 teaspoon

Unsalted butter and margarine, and vegetable oil may be used as desired

Beverages

May be used according to fluid allowance.
Pepsi-Cola
Royal Crown Cola
Sodium and potassium may vary according to local water supply.
Juices, milk, ice cream and sherbet must be counted as part of total fluid allowance.

Miscellaneous

These items may be used as desired.

Spices and flavorings

Allspice	Nutmeg
Caraway	Paprika
Cinnamon	Pepper
Curry powder	Peppermint extract
Garlic	Sage
Garlic powder	Thyme
(not salt)	Tumeric
Ginger	Vanilla extract
Mace	Vinegar (limit to
Mustard, dry	1 tablespoon)

Sugars and candies

Hard candies	Lollipops
Honey	Syrup, corn
Jams	Sugar, white
Jellies	

Small amounts of the following may be used in food preparation.

Celery	Mint leaves
Green pepper	Mushrooms
Horseradish, fresh	Onions

sium per day, it is difficult to use more than 4 fluid ounces (120 ml.) of coffee or tea and plan a diet pattern that meets the nutrient needs of an individual.

Water may also be a significant source of potassium. In areas where the water is high in potassium, the renal failure patient may need to use distilled water for cooking and drinking. The local health department has information about the potassium content of the water supply.

Neither salt substitutes nor sodium-free baking powder can be used because of the potassium content. Depending on the level of sodium restriction, an alum type baking powder (Calumet) may be used to make bread and cakes with wheatstarch. This baking powder, compared with other types, is relatively free of potassium. (See footnote, page 557).

LOW-PROTEIN STARCH PRODUCTS. When the protein in the renal diet is restricted, those foods such as cereals, breads, and desserts made with regular flours, which are good sources of calories, cannot be used to meet energy needs. Wheatstarch products that are relatively free of protein are available. Dietetic Paygel-P wheatstarch and Dietetic Paygel Baking Mix* and Cellu wheatstarch and Cellu Low Protein Baking Mix† can be used in making bread, muffins, biscuits, cookies, and pie crust. General Mills has also made available in the United States the Aproten products manufactured in Italy. These include imitation pastas which can be used to make mixed dishes; semolina, a cereal; and rusks.

Each company provides recipes which use the products. The directions for making bread with these wheatstarches must be followed carefully, because the protein (gluten) of regular flour that gives the structure to yeast bread has been removed from the wheatstarch. The structure, texture, and flavor of breads made from these wheatstarches differ from bread made with regular flour. Some patients readily accept the product while others do not. Besides the calories in the wheatstarch bread, the butter, jelly, or jam served with the bread can make significant contributions to total calorie intake. The pies and cookies made from wheatstarch are usually well accepted. Recipes are also available for using the Aproten products in mixed dishes. The manufacturer's materials give the caloric and nutrient composition per serving of the recipes. (See patient resources at the end of this chapter for directions for securing recipes using wheatstarches.)

*General Mills, Minneapolis, Minn. 55435.
†Cellu-Featherweight, Chicago Dietetic Supply, Inc., LaGrange, Ill. 60525.

EXCHANGE SYSTEM. An Exchange System for calculating protein-, sodium-, and potassium-restricted diet patterns is given in Table 31–5. With the exception of the milk and fat exchanges, the exchange food groups in this system contain two or more subdivisions which reflect primarily the variation in the quantity of potassium in foods.

The energy values of the exchanges are not given because the foods in each exchange vary in calorie content. For example, in the milk exchange list (see Table 31–6) there is whole milk, skim milk, light and heavy cream, half and half, ice cream, and sour cream. While the protein, sodium, and potassium in each serving are approximately the same, the energy value varies: ½ cup of whole milk contains 85 calories; ½ cup of skim milk, 40 calories; and ¾ cup of sour cream, 340 calories.

A value for protein is given for each exchange or for each subdivision within each exchange except for the fat exchanges. In Table 23–2, Chapter 23, figures are given for protein in only the milk, meat, bread, and vegetable B exchanges because in calculating most modified diets the concern is with those foods which contribute the most significant amounts of protein. In uremia, however, the total protein is limited and the need for essential amino acids must be met. Specific quantities of milk, eggs, and meat are used to provide the essential amino acids, and the intake of nonessential amino acids is restricted. Therefore, the protein in breads, fruits, and all vegetables is calculated to avoid an excessive amount of nonessential amino acids in the diet. The protein value for the bread exchange, Group C, applies only to bread made with protein-free wheatstarch.

EXCHANGE LISTS. The foods in each Exchange List (Table 31–6) differ significantly from those in Table 23–4, Chapter 23. There is a Group A and a Group B meat exchange, which reflect significant differences in sodium and potassium levels. Potatoes are included in the Group B vegetable exchange, not in the bread exchange, because of their potassium content.

The canned fruits listed in the fruit exchanges are those canned with sugar, while the vegetables are those canned or cooked without salt. If the sodium restriction is 2000 mg., a small amount of salt may be added in cooking fresh vegetables; or well-drained and rinsed vegetables canned with added salt can be used. All canned vegetables should be well-drained before being heated in fresh water in order to avoid any of the potassium in the water in the can.

In the bread exchanges the figures for protein, sodium, and potassium in Group C apply to one slice (30 g.) of bread made with Dietetic Paygel Baking

Table 31-7. Calculation of Diet Pattern for 40 g. Protein, 1000 mg. Sodium, and 1500 mg. Potassium

Food Group	Amount	Protein (g.)	Sodium (mg.)	Potassium (mg.)
Milk	½ c.	4	60	170
Meat–				
Group A	1 oz.	7	60	70
Egg	2	14	140	240
Vegetables				
Group A	1 serving	1	9	150
Group B	1 serving	2	9	240
Fruit				
Group A	2 servings	2	4	200
Group B	1 serving	1	2	145
Bread				
Group A	1 serving	2	5	25
Group B	1 serving	3	5	50
Group C	6 slices	0.6	90	18
Fat, salted	9 tsp.	——	450	——
TOTALS		36.6	834*	1308*

*Does not include other foods made with wheatstarch such as fruit pies, cookies, and puddings which will increase sodium and potassium to the desired levels.

Mix. These figures can also be applied to 100 g. of the cooked Aproten semolina and pasta products. The pasta products can be combined in mixed dishes with the egg or meat and the vegetable exchanges calculated in the diet pattern.

The fat exchanges are those with salt added. Because those foods which are the major contributors of sodium to the diet—milk, meat, and eggs (see Chapter 30, Table 30-1)—must be limited, some salted foods are required when sodium is only moderately restricted. Salted butter also increases the acceptability of the wheatstarch breads. If the sodium is severely restricted (less than 1000 mg. sodium), only unsalted fats are used.

Spices and flavorings in the miscellaneous list, if tolerated, can be used to enhance the flavor of foods. For example, dry mustard and vinegar can be mixed to make mustard to accompany meat. The sugar and candies can be used to supply energy. When corn syrup* is used, the sodium content should be calculated because salt is added during the processing of corn syrup.

CALCULATING THE DIET PATTERN. Table 31-7 demonstrates the calculation of a pattern for a diet prescription of 40 g. protein, 1000 mg. sodium, and 1500 mg. potassium. This diet was prescribed for a woman weighing 58 kg. who required 0.7 g. protein per kg. of body weight per day. The energy value of this diet pattern has not been calculated. The six Group C bread exchanges (6 slices of wheatstarch bread made from Dietetic Paygel Baking Mix) and the

*Karo, Best Foods, Englewood Cliffs, N.J.

nine fat exchanges provide approximately 1150 calories. Each 30-g. slice of bread contains about 125 calories and each fat exchange, 45 calories. The meat, egg, vegetable, fruit and other bread exchanges in the pattern provide approximately 500 calories when fruit canned with sugar is used. Other products made with wheatstarch, such as cookies or pies, using the fruit calculated in the diet pattern, or mixed dishes made with rice or pasta and the meat exchanges in the diet pattern can provide an additional 200 to 400 calories for a total of approximately 1700 to 1900 calories per day.

Foods containing high biological protein contribute about 70 percent of the total protein in the diet pattern. The one Group A meat and the two eggs together with one milk exchange provide an adequate intake of essential amino acids. The use of additional wheatstarch products in fruit pies and cookies will correct the discrepancy between the sodium as prescribed (1000 mg.) and as calculated (834 mg.). Additional wheatstarch and a 4-ounce cup of coffee will correct the discrepancy between the potassium as prescribed (1500 mg.) and as calculated (1308 mg.).

Table 31-8 illustrates a day's menu using the calculated diet pattern in Table 31-7. This menu contains approximately 360 ml. of fluid. If the intake of fluid is restricted to 600 ml. per day and more than 240 ml. of water is needed to take medication, then

Table 31-8. Menu for 40 g. Protein, 100 mg. Sodium, and 1500 mg. Potassium* Diet

Breakfast

½ c. apple juice
1 c. puffed rice
½ c. of milk
2 slices of wheatstarch bread
3 tsp. salted butter
½ c. of coffee (4 oz.)

Noon Meal

1 oz. tuna canned in water
2 slices wheatstarch bread
1 leaf lettuce
1 tsp. salted butter
2 tsp. salted mayonnaise
½ c. unsalted canned green beans (well drained)
½ c. grapefruit sections (well drained)
3 wheatstarch cookies

Evening Meal

Omelet made with 2 eggs
½ c. noodles, seasoned with 1 tsp. salted butter
½ c. tomatoes
2 slices wheatstarch bread
1 tsp. salted butter
1 small apple as apple pie made with wheatstarch crust

*Provides 360 ml. fluid of day's total.

renal disease; nephrolithiasis   453

the fluid in the menu can be reduced by omitting the coffee or substituting applesauce for apple juice.

Special Problems

The patient being prepared for maintenance hemodialysis or kidney transplant, or the patient in end-stage renal failure who is not a candidate for dialysis or transplant, often finds the protein-, sodium-, and potassium-restricted diet difficult to accept. The restriction for some of these patients can be as low as 30 g. of protein, 500 mg. of sodium, and 700 mg. of potassium. At the same time the majority are anorexic and nauseated. Acceptance of the diet can often be improved if the menus are planned daily with the patient. If he is disoriented, a close relative can often make suggestions as to the foods he might accept.

For the hospitalized patient an estimate of the previous 24-hour intake of energy, protein, sodium, and potassium is recorded in the patient's record each morning. The same daily recording is also done for the patient in acute renal failure. To insure a relatively accurate estimate of daily intake, the patient's intake of foods and beverage must be monitored continuously throughout the day. The intake data correlated with the results of blood chemistry data are used to adjust the diet prescription.

Careful communication between dietary and nursing services is required to carry out the fluid orders for any patient with renal disease. Other than water, which may or may not be a significant source of sodium and potassium, many fluids commonly offered to hospitalized patients contain significant amounts of sodium and/or potassium.For example: orange juice and tea contain potassium; and tomato juice canned with salt contains sodium and potassium. If a diet is severely restricted in electrolytes, a 4- to 8-ounce serving of any one of these beverages could contribute to a serious error in therapy. Severe fluid restrictions present special problems. The nurse needs water to give with medications and the dietitian needs fluids to enhance the palatability of the diet. Hourly communication between nursing personnel and the dietitian is needed to carry out a severe fluid restriction.

Diet and the Post-Transplant Patient

After kidney transplant the patient is maintained on steroid therapy, usually prednisone. Therefore, many clinicians order a mildly sodium-restricted diet (see Chapter 30). This diet is also usually bland because individuals on long-term steroid therapy are apt to develop gastrointestinal bleeding (see Chapter 25).

COUNSELING THE PATIENT

The protein-, sodium-, and potassium-restricted diet is one of the most difficult diets for a patient to carry out in his home. The patient being prepared by hemodialysis for kidney transplant may be required to manage his restricted diet on an outpatient basis for as long as three months or more, while the patient on maintenance hemodialysis will require a restricted diet for the remainder of his life. In addition to dietary counseling during hospitalization the patient should have access to counseling services when he returns for dialysis two or three times a week.

Many of these patients will have had previous experience with protein- and sodium-restricted diets and will need help to understand the potassium restriction, while other patients may not have had any previous experience. A careful diet history taken when the patient is comfortable will identify the knowledge he needs. During hospitalization the patient and any close relatives or friends should be counseled daily so that they can ask frequent questions and plan the patient's menus to demonstrate their understanding of the diet. A copy of the diet pattern used to counsel the patient at discharge from the hospital is included in his record for use at any follow-up visit.

The Exchange Lists in this chapter or those designed for the renal diet in any institution should be made available for the patient's use at home. Occasionally a very anxious patient will prefer to develop menus for one or two weeks for use at discharge from the hospital and modify these with the counselor at a future date when he is more confident of his ability to carry out his diet.

The hospital tray becomes the visual aid for teaching not only what foods may be used, but also the portion size. The recipes for any mixed dishes served to the patient in the hospital should be avilable to him. He should also be given the names and addresses of any local stores which sell low-protein wheat products or, if not available locally, the names and addresses of the companies which can supply the products. And he should be advised carefully to follow the recipes which come with the products, including the use of the recommended equipment.

Unless the restrictions are moderate, the patient cannot eat in restaurants or use any convenience foods. This may present a real problem for the individual living alone, especially the individual who experiences fatigue easily because of anemia. Homemaker services may be required to help these individuals with grocery shopping and some food preparation.

NEPHROLITHIASIS

Relatively little is known about the formation of kidney stones or urinary calculi. They may form and grow because the concentration of a particular substance in the urine exceeds its solubility. This is called the precipitation-crystallization theory.[17] A low urine volume and the pH of the urine are also factors.

The stones vary in size from fine gritty particles to those which fill the pelvis of the kidney, and they may form in either the kidney or the bladder. The type of stone from which a patient suffers is determined by careful urinalysis and by the chemical identification of crystals in the urinary sediment.

About 66 percent of all kidney stones contain calcium. They may also contain magnesium and ammonia combined with phosphates, carbonates, and oxalates. Cystine and uric acid stones together account for about 10 percent of all stones.

Calcium Phosphate Stones

These may occur in hyperparathyroidism, in which oversecretion of the parathyroid hormone causes loss of calcium from the bones, resulting in a high blood level of calcium with increased excretion of calcium in the urine. Immobilization for long periods of time, osteoporosis, or an abnormally high intake of milk, alkalis, or vitamin D may also give rise to the formation of calcium phosphate stones.

Dietary Treatment. A moderately low calcium and phosphorus diet and the use of an aluminum hydroxide gel has been successful in controlling the formation of calcium phosphate stones. The aluminum hydroxide, given by mouth, unites with the phosphates present in food to form insoluble aluminum phosphate which is excreted in the feces. Such calcium as is excreted in the urine is now in the form of soluble salts such as calcium chloride and calcium citrate, which are less likely to precipitate. The diet restricts the intake of calcium and phosphates to minimal levels consistent with maintaining nutritional adequacy. The moderately calcium- and phosphorus-restricted diet plan in Table 31–9 contains about 500 to 700 mg. of calcium and 1000 to 1200 mg. of phosphorus. When a greater restriction of calcium is required (200 to 300 mg.) all milk and milk products except butter are excluded from the diet and

Table 31–9. Moderately Calcium- and Phosphorus-Restricted Diet Plan
(This diet will contain from 500 to 700 mg. of calcium and from 1000 to 1200 mg. of phosphorus*)

Foods Used

Milk
Limited to 1 cup (½ pint) a day. Cream may be substituted for part of the milk.

Cheese
Pot or cottage cheese only. Limited to 2 ozs.

Fats
As desired

Eggs
Limited to 1 a day; egg whites as desired.

Meat, fish, fowl
Limited to 4 ozs. daily of beef, lamb, pork, veal, chicken, turkey, fish. See those to be avoided.

Soups and broths
All. Cream soups made with milk allowance only.

Vegetables
At least 3 servings besides potato. One or 2 servings of deep green or deep yellow vegetables to be included daily. See list of those to be avoided.

Fruits
All except rhubarb. Include citrus fruit daily.

Breads, cereals, Italian pastas
White, enriched bread, rolls and crackers except those made from self-rising white flour. Farina (not enriched), cornflakes, corn meal, hominy grits, rice, Rice Krispies, Puffed Rice. Macaroni, spaghetti, noodles.

Desserts
Fruit pies, fruit cobblers, fruit ices, gelatin. Puddings made with allowed milk and egg. Angel food cake. (Do not use packaged mixes.)

Beverages
Coffee, Postum, Sanka, tea, ginger ale

Condiments
Sugar, jellies, honey, salt, pepper, spices

Foods to be Avoided

Cheese
All except pot or cottage cheese.

Meat, fish, fowl
Brains, heart, liver, kidney, sweetbreads. Game (pheasant, rabbit, deer, grouse). Sardines, fish roe.

Vegetables
Beet greens, chard, collards, mustard greens, spinach, turnip greens. Dried beans, peas, lentils, soybeans.

Fruits
Rhubarb

Breads, cereals, Italian pastas
Whole-grain breads, cereals and crackers. Rye bread. All breads made with self-rising flour. Oatmeal, brown and wild rice. Bran, Bran Flakes, wheat germ. All dry cereals except those allowed.

Desserts
All except those allowed.

Beverages
Carbonated "soft" drinks; cocoa.

Miscellaneous
Nuts, peanut butter, chocolate, cocoa. Condiments having a calcium or a phosphate base. (Read labels.)

*Adapted from Shorr, E.: Aluminum hydroxide gels in the management of renal stone. J. Urol. 53:507, 1945.

the amount of bread made with dry milk solids is limited. At this more restricted level of intake vitamin supplementation will be needed to insure an adequate riboflavin intake.

Calcium Oxalate Stones

Until recently this type of kidney stone has been the most resistant to treatment. Calcium oxalate stones tend to recur and may obstruct the urinary tract, necessitating surgery for their removal. A diet limited in oxalic acid, omitting such foods as rhubarb, spinach, cocoa and chocolate, wheat germ and several varieties of nuts, has been prescribed, but has proved relatively ineffective.

A few years ago, Gershoff and his coworkers noted that in the vitamin-B_6-deficient rats with which they were working, there was marked increase in urinary oxalate accompanied by calcium oxalate stone formation similar to that found in humans.[18] The feeding of high levels of magnesium to the experimental animals reduced the formation of calcium oxalate stones but did not affect the oxaluria.

Applying their findings to the treatment of patients with demonstrated calcium oxalate stones, they report on the results with 36 patients, treated for a period of five years. Besides a diet restricted in milk and cheese, which are high in calcium, and the drinking of 2 quarts of water a day, all patients received a daily medication of magnesium oxide and vitamin B_6, both given by mouth. All but five patients in the group have had no further stone formation, or have shown marked improvement.

These investigators postulate that the magnesium aids in keeping the oxalate in solution, and thereby prevents its precipitation and stone formation. Vitamin B_6 increases citric-acid excretion, which may also serve to keep oxalate in solution.

It has been discovered that hyperoxaluria occurs as a result of a hereditary enzymatic defect in the intermedary metabolism of oxalate but at present the mechanism for this defect is unknown. Recurrent renal oxalate stone formation occurs in small-bowel disease, due probably to an increased absorption of dietary oxalate.

Uric Acid Stones

Uric acid stones occur in patients who have an increased level of uric acid in the blood (hyperuricemia), and increased urinary excretion of uric acid. It may or may not be accompanied by symptoms of gout. Since uric acid is an end product of purine metabolism, foods with a high purine content are avoided. This is discussed in Chapter 33, under Gout.

The precipitation of uric acid crystals in the urinary tract occurs most readily when the urine is acid.[19] Medications to keep the urine alkaline together with an increased fluid intake are used in the treatment of uric acid stones.

Cystinuria; Cystine Stones

The only known cause of cystinuria and the formation of cystine stones is an inborn error of metabolism which interferes with both the gastrointestinal and tubular transport of the amino acids cystine, ornithine, lysine, and arginine. Of these, cystine is the least soluble. It will precipitate when there is increased concentration in the urine, and form stones. Hydration, alkalies, and a low-protein diet have been prescribed, but with little success.

In 1965 McDonald and Henneman reported that the administration of d-penicillamine dramatically reduced the amount of cystine in the urine of three patients with cystinuria and kidney stones, preventing further stone formation and, in one of the patients, resulting in complete dissolution of stones already formed.[20] It is postulated that the d-penicillamine keeps the cystine in solution.

Acid and Alkaline Ash Diets

The mineral elements in food are sometimes referred to as "ash" because they are not oxidized in metabolism. They form a residue which is eventually excreted either by the intestinal tract (most of the calcium and the iron) or in the urine. By changing the composition of the diet, the urine may be made either acid or alkaline. An acid urine may act to limit enlargement of already present alkaline stones, or prevent their further formation. Likewise, an alkaline urine may affect the less common acid stones in the same manner.

Most vegetables and fruits will yield an alkaline ash and, therefore, aid in the formation of an alkaline urine. Meats, fish, fowl, eggs, and cereals will give an acid ash when metabolized and cause the urine to be acid. Since much of the calcium of milk is re-excreted in the intestinal tract while the remainder of its mineral content is excreted in the urine, its effect on the acidity or the alkalinity of urine is problematical.

Although most physicians will alter the pH of the urine by prescribing the appropriate medication, occasionally a diet may be ordered to achieve a change in pH. On an alkaline ash diet, sometimes used for oxalate stones, vegetables and fruits should predominate, while meat, eggs, and cereals are somewhat restricted. Conversely, on an acid ash diet, which may be prescribed for calcium phosphate and calcium carbonate stones, meat, eggs, and cereals are liberally included and vegetables and fruits are restricted. On either diet milk is restricted to 1 pint. All foods should be in sufficient quantity for nutritional adequacy.

STUDY QUESTIONS AND ACTIVITIES

1. What are the basic metabolic functions of the kidney? Using Plate 2, explain how they are accomplished.
2. What substances are filtered from the blood? Which are largely reabsorbed? Which are excreted?
3. Plan a day's menu for a 10-year-old boy with acute gomerular nephritis whose diet prescription is 2000 calories, 30 g. of protein, 800 mg. of sodium, and 800 ml. of fluid.
4. In which circumstances is protein usually restricted in the diet of a patient with nephritis? What is the purpose of this restriction? When may the protein in the diet be increased over normal needs? Why?
5. Why may sodium be restricted in kidney disease?
6. What is the danger of an increased potassium level in the blood?
7. What is meant by the sodium depletion syndrome? How may the physician treat it?
8. Why are fluids restricted in kidney failure? On what basis is the amount of fluid allowed calculated?
9. Using the Protein-, Sodium-, and Potassium-Restricted Diet Exchange Lists, make out a Pattern Dietary for a 16-year-old boy who is receiving hemodialysis. His physician has ordered a diet containing 60 g. of protein, 750 mg. of sodium, 2000 mg. of potassium, and fluids restricted to 1000 ml. The boy is in school, continually hungry, and rather anxious.
10. Name some of the seasonings the boy's mother may use on the above diet to make it more palatable. What food combinations can you suggest to use extra fat in the diet?
11. Make out a menu for a day for a patient critically ill with nephrosclerosis and uremia. His physician has ordered: 30 g. of protein, 500 mg. of sodium, 1500 mg. of potassium, fluids restricted to 800 ml. The patient is anorexic and has some nausea. The diet should be bland and semisoft.
12. Look at Table 4 in Section 4. What foods are high in sodium? In potassium? Take average servings of foods into account.
13. Make out a menu for a day for a patient who has a calcium phoshate kidney stone, and who has been placed on a moderately low calcium and phosphorus diet. He is young and somewhat of a gourmet.

SUPPLEMENTARY READINGS

Burton, B. T.: Current concepts of nutrition and diet in diseases of the kidney. I. General principles of dietary management. J. Am. Dietet. A. 65:623, 1974.

————: Current concepts of nutrition and diet in diseases of the kidney. II. Dietary regimen in specific kidney disorders. J. Am. Dietet. A. 65:627, 1974.

Close, J. H.: The use of amino acid precursors in nitrogen accumulation diseases. N. Eng. J. Med. 290:663, 1974.

Coe, F. L., and Kavalach, A. G.: Hypercalcinuria and hyperuricosuria in patients with calcium nephrolithiasis. N. Eng. J. Med. 291:1344, 1974.

Cohodes, A: Better care aim of dialysis network. Hospitals 49:44, Feb. 16, 1975.

Landsman, M. E.: The patient with chronic renal failure, a marginal man. Ann. Int. Med. 82:268, 1975.

Lewy, J. E., and New, M. I.: Growth in children with renal failure. Am. J. Med. 58:65, 1975.

Lindner, A., and Kingsbury, C.: Morbidity and mortality associated with long-term hemodialysis. Hospital Practice 9:143, 1974.

Santopietro, M. C. S.: Meeting the emotional needs of hemodialysis patients and their spouses. Am. J. Nurs. 75:629, 1975.

Schoolwerth, A. C., and Engle, J. E.: Calcium and phosphorus in diet therapy of uremia. J. Am. Dietet. A. 66:460, 1975.

Vetter, L., and Shapiro, R.: An approach to dietary management of the patient with renal disease. J. Am. Dietet. A. 66:158, 1975.

Williams, H. E.: Nephrolithiasis. N. Eng. J. Med. 290:33, 1974.

PATIENT RESOURCES

A Guide to Protein Controlled Diets. California Dietetic Assoc., 1609 Westwood Blvd., No. 101, Los Angeles, Ca. 90024.

Low Protein Diets Made Simple. Dietary Dept., Loma Linda University Medical Center, Loma Linda, Ca. 92354.

Aproten Low Protein Diet Products. General Mills Chemicals, Inc., Minneapolis, Minn. 55435.

Dietetic Paygel Baking Mix. General Mills Chemicals, Inc., Minneapolis, Minn. 55435.

Jolly Ann Baked Low-Protein Bread. Ener-G Foods, Inc., 1526 Utah So., Seattle, Wash. 98134.

Low Protein Baking Mix. Cellu-Featherweight, Chicago Dietetic Supply, Inc., La Grange, Ill. 60525.

For further references see Bibliography in Section 4.

REFERENCES

1. Brobeck, J. R., ed.: *Best and Taylor's Physiological Basis of Medical Practice,* ed. 9. Baltimore, Williams and Wilkins, 1973.
2. Renkin, E. M., and Robinson, R. R.: N. Eng. J. Med. 290:785, 1974.
3. Dixon, F. J.: in Harrison's *Principles of Internal Medicine,* ed. 7. New York, McGraw-Hill, 1974, Chapter 69.
4. Simmons, J. M., et al: N. Eng. J. Med. 285:653, 1971.
5. Giordano, C.: J. Lab. Clin. Med. 62:231, 1963.
6. Richard, P., et al: Lancet 2:845, 1967.
7. Giovannetti, S., and Maggiore, G.: Lancet 1:100, 1964.
8. Shaw, A. B.: Q. J. Med. 34:237, 1965.
9. Bailey, G. L., and Sullivan, N. R.: J. Am. Dietet. A. 52:125, 1968.
10. Kopple, J. D., and Coburn, J. W.: Medicine 52:583, 1973.
11. Anderson, C. F., et al: JAMA 223:68, 1973.
12. Ginn, H. E., et al: Am. J. Clin. Nutr. 21:565, 1968.
13. Epstein, F. H.: in *Harrison's Principles of Internal Medicine,* ed. 7. New York, McGraw-Hill, 1974, Chapter 269.
14. Kolff, W. J.: Am. J. Med. 12:667, 1952.
15. Abel, R. M., et al: N. Eng. J. Med. 288:695, 1973.
16. Louis, C. J., and Dolan, E. M.: J. Am. Dietet. A. 57:42, 1970.
17. Williams, H. E.: N. Eng. J. Med. 290:33, 1974.
18. Gershoff, S. N., and Prien, E. L.: Am. J. Clin. Nutr. 20:393, 1967.
19. Williams, H. E., op. cit.
20. McDonald, J. E., and Henneman, P. H.: N. Eng. J. Med. 273:578, 1965.

32

liver disease

The nutritional care in liver disease shares many of the characteristics of nutritional care in renal disease because the disease process can alter the structure and function of the liver so that its metabolic functions are impaired. These alterations, particularly in progressive chronic liver disease leading to end-stage hepatic failure, also require modifications in the dietary intake of energy, protein, fluid, and electrolytes. Liver disease may be acute or chronic, progressing to end-stage hepatic failure, and the acute phase may or may not progress to the chronic phase. Because the liver is unique in its ability to regenerate cells, the successful treatment (primarily dietary) of the early stages of liver disease usually result in the recovery of adequate liver function.

Many patients with liver disease present the same challenges to nutritional care as those with renal disease because they also experience nausea and vomiting, and fatigue due to anemia; and, in end-stage hepatic failure (hepatic coma), they are often disoriented. In one aspect the medical care of the patient with liver disease differs from the care of the renal patient. For those patients whose liver disease is due to alcoholism, the treatment is both medical and psychiatric because alcoholism is an addictive process.

Before proceeding with the discussion of liver disease and diet therapy, the reader is urged to review Chapter 9, Nutrient Utilization, as well as the metabolism of alcohol in a biochemistry textbook, and the structure and function of the liver in a physiology textbook. Diseases of the gallbladder and pancreas which are usually discussed with liver disease are presented in Chapter 25, Gastrointestinal Disease, because the nutritional problems they present are more directly related to this pathology.

NORMAL METABOLIC FUNCTIONS OF THE LIVER

Because of the diversity of its metabolic functions, the liver is one of the most important glandular organs in the body. All nutrients that are ingested and absorbed are transported directly to the liver by the portal circulation, with the exception of long chain fatty acids and fat soluble vitamins. Through the systemic circulation a portion of the long chain fatty acids and the fat-soluble vitamins are also transported to the liver. It utilizes the nutrients in both synthetic and degradative metabolic processes and also stores nutrients, particularly the fat-soluble vitamins, vitamin B_{12} and glucose as glycogen.

AMINO ACIDS. The liver regulates the distribution of the amino acids to the cells of the body where they are used in the synthesis of cellular proteins. It synthesizes many protein enzymes and the plasma proteins, fibrinogen, prothrombin, albumin, and most of the alpha and beta globulins. Urea, the end product of the degradation of all amino acid nitrogen, is synthesized in the liver (see Chapter 9).

CARBOHYDRATE. The liver converts glucose, fructose, and galactose to glycogen and through glycogenolysis provides glucose to maintain energy metabolism in the brain, muscles, adipose, and other body cells. An excess of the intermediary metabolites of glucose are converted to fats. Through the gluconeogenic pathway it also synthesizes glucose from the deaminized amino acids.

LIPIDS. The liver converts fats to very low density lipoproteins which are transported to other tissues for storage as triglycerides. The liver synthesizes cholesterol from acetyl-CoA through the squalene pathway and is the only organ in the body which synthesizes ketone bodies.

MINERALS AND VITAMINS. An important function of the liver is the storage of iron, as ferritin, and copper which it makes available for the synthesis of the hemoglobin in red blood cells. Other minerals such as zinc and magnesium are also present in the liver where they function as a part of many essential enzymatic reactions in intermediary metabolism. For example, alcohol dehydrogenase in the liver requires zinc for its activity.

Most of the vitamin A stored in the body is found in the liver. Although the major portion of ingested carotene is converted to vitamin A in the cells of the gastrointestinal tract, some carotene is also converted in the liver. The other fat-soluble vitamins, D, E, and K, are stored in the liver. The B vitamins are also found there in considerable amounts, where they function as parts of the enzyme systems in intermediary metabolism.

BILE, which is composed of bile acids, pigments (bilirubin) and salts, cholesterol, and water, is synthesized by the cells of the liver and flows through the bile ducts to the cystic duct to be stored in the gallbladder. (See Chapter 25 for the role of bile in digestion.)

DETOXIFICATION. A major degradative function of the liver is detoxification. It detoxifies many substances such as hormones and drugs. For example, oral contraceptives, morphine, and barbiturates are inactivated by the liver to terminate their effect.

METABOLIC ABERRATIONS

It is not surprising that an organ which performs as many critical metabolic functions as does the liver should cause numerous aberrations in intermediary metabolism when it is diseased. The metabolic aberrations reflect primarily alterations in structure and function due to the disease processes. These alterations can be classified as: (1) fatty infiltration of hepatic cells; (2) diffuse inflammation with hepatic cell necrosis and regenerative activity; and (3) loss of functional liver cells due to necrosis accompanied by fibrosis of supporting tissues and the vascular bed and nodular regeneration of the remaining cell mass.

Fatty Liver

There is an excessive accumulation of lipids in the cytoplasm of the liver cells in fatty liver disease which may result from: (1) an increased influx of fatty acids into the liver; (2) an increase in fatty acid synthesis by the hepatic cells; (3) a decrease in fatty acid oxidation; or (4), a decreased synthesis of protein for triglyceride transport out of the liver. Fatty livers occur in poorly controlled diabetes, obesity, acute and chronic alcoholism, and energy-protein malnutrition in infancy and early childhood, and is frequently a complication of long-standing heart failure. Severe acute fatty liver is produced by hepatotoxins such as carbontetrachloride and DDT.

Removal of alcohol or hepatotoxins, treatment of the underlying disease, and appropriate diet usually result in a decrease in the accumulation of lipids in the hepatic cells. However, there may be some necrosis of liver cells produced by chronic alcohol ingestion or by hepatotoxins. Diet is determined by the underlying disease, e.g., diabetes, obesity, and heart disease. An adequate diet appropriate for age is required for malnourished infants and children and one appropriate for weight, sex, and age should be used for adults whose fatty liver is due to alcoholism.

Diffuse Inflammation (Hepatitis)

There are two forms of hepatitis, acute and chronic. Viral infection is the most common cause of acute hepatitis although it may be induced by drugs, alcohol, and hepatotoxins. The infectious form of acute hepatitis is caused by two different agents, hepatitis A and hepatitis B, and both can be transmitted by the oral or parenteral route. Hepatitis A was formerly called infectious hepatitis and hepatitis B, serum hepatitis. The cause of chronic hepatitis is unknown in most cases, although some individuals with hepatitis B do develop it.

In addition to the inflammatory process in hepatitis, there is necrosis and regenerative activity in the hepatic cells and, in some individuals, bile stasis with jaundice. There is an elevation of serum transaminase and bilirubin and a decrease in plasma prothrombin levels due to hepatic cell necrosis. In acute viral hepatitis the total serum proteins are usually normal or there may be a slight decrease in serum albumin, while in chronic hepatitis there is usually a decrease in serum albumin levels. Anorexia and fatigue followed by nausea, vomiting, and diarrhea are common symptoms with both types of hepatitis. In acute hepatitis the anorexia is often severe with a strong aversion to food.

During the nausea and vomiting phase, a full liquid diet as tolerated is prescribed or, if necessary, a standard tube feeding is used. (See liquid diets and tube feedings, Chapter 26.) When food is tolerated a diet adequate in energy and nutrients is provided to support the regenerative activity of the hepatic cells and to meet the total metabolic needs of the body. For the adult the diet should contain 35 to 40 calories per kilogram of body weight with 12 to 15 percent of the energy from protein, about 35 percent from fat, and the remainder from carbohydrate. The diet contains 75 to 90 g. protein, about 80 g. fat, and 300 g. carbohydrate for an adult requiring 2500 calories per day. It should be adequate in minerals and vitamins. However, depending on the patient's problems, supplementary minerals and vitamins may be required. Davidson has observed that patients with acute hepatitis eat better if they consume frequent small meals rather than three meals a day.[1]

If massive necrosis of the liver cells occurs in severe hepatitis, a high or even normal intake of protein can induce hepatic coma with hyperammonemia. (See discussion of protein in Diet Therapy section in this chapter.) Therefore, the protein in the diet may be severely restricted or excluded in this case until there is improvement in hepatic function.

Loss of Functional Hepatic Cells (Cirrhosis)

Cirrhosis is a generic term used to describe all forms of liver disease characterized by a significant loss of cells.[2] The most common types are Laennec's, postnecrotic, biliary, and cardiac or congestive cirrhosis. Cirrhosis also occurs due to congenital anomalies of the liver, in hemachromatosis (abnormal iron metabolism) and in Wilson's disease (abnormal copper metabolism). Alcoholism is usually, but not always, a factor in the development of Laennec's cirrhosis, while viral hepatitis is a factor in many cases of postnecrotic cirrhosis.

Although regenerative activity occurs in cirrhosis, the progressive loss of liver cells exceeds cell replacement. At the same time there is also progressive distortion of the vascular system which results in interference with the portal blood flow through the liver. In early cirrhosis there is a variable elevation in serum bilirubin and transaminase levels. The serum albumin is usually depressed and anemia is a common problem.

In severe advanced cirrhosis the distortion of the vascular bed of the liver leads to portal hypertension and the shunting of portal blood into the portal-systemic venous collateral circulation. With portal hypertension ascites occurs; there is sodium retention, impaired water excretion, and decreased plasma osmotic pressure because of severe hypoalbuminemia. The shunting of portal blood into the systemic circulation causes the engorgement of the lower esophageal veins (esophageal varices). When the varices rupture, severe hemorrhage occurs. The shunting of the portal blood also causes an elevation of the blood ammonia level with hepatic encephalopathy. At the same time there is a deficiency of prothrombin and the blood urea nitrogen, which is synthesized primarily in the liver, is low normal or low. The progressive degeneration of liver structure and function leads ultimately to hepatic failure and death.

In the treatment of early cirrhosis the diet for

adults should provide 35 to 40 calories or more and 1 g. of protein of high biological value per kilogram of body weight, with an adequate intake of minerals and vitamins. In biliary cirrhosis dietary fat is usually not well-tolerated because of a significant decrease in bile flow, so that the intake should be restricted to 30 to 40 grams daily. (See Low-Fat Diet, Chapter 25.) As the blood ammonia level rises in progressive liver disease, the dietary protein is restricted to tolerance and limited to proteins of high biological value. (See Diet Therapy section in this chapter.) With ascites the sodium is restricted to 200 to 500 mg. (10 to 20 mEq.) and fluid intake is restricted to the amount lost each day. The diet may also be restricted in roughage if esophageal varicies are present but not bleeding. If esophageal bleeding occurs, a liquid diet, restricted in fluid, protein, and sodium, if necessary, may be required.

ALCOHOL AND LIVER DISEASE

In the United States the ingestion of alcohol is one of the most common causes of all categories of liver disease—fatty infiltration, hepatitis, and cirrhosis. It is estimated that one of 12 chronic users of alcohol develops cirrhosis[3] which, if the individual does not abstain from alcohol, can progress to end-stage hepatic failure. The development of alcoholic cirrhosis appears to be related to the duration of alcohol intake and the amount consumed daily. Research indicates that the mean duration of alcohol intake to produce cirrhosis is 10 years and the dose is estimated to be in excess of 160 g. of alcohol daily,[4] e.g., 16 ounces of Scotch whiskey.

For many years it was thought that all forms of alcoholic liver disease were not caused by alcohol per se but by the inadequate diets consumed by many chronic alcoholics, and it has been common practice to advise individuals who drink appreciable amounts of alcohol daily to eat an adequate diet to avoid liver disease. However, the current research of Rubin and Lieber[5] strongly suggests that alcohol is the causative agent. Using baboons, which are phylogenetically closer to man than other laboratory animals, they have observed in their animals the development of fatty livers with progression to alcoholic hepatitis and cirrhosis when fed a nutritionally adequate diet with a daily isocaloric substitution for carbohydrate of 4.5 to 8.3 g. of alcohol per kilogram of body weight. They conclude that adequate nutrient intake with the continued intake of excessive quantities of alcohol will not prevent the development of fatty livers, alcoholic hepatitis, or cirrhosis.

Concurrent with liver disease, the patient who is a chronic alcoholic is likely to exhibit severe malnutrition because he does not eat. Weight loss may not be marked because an individual can derive 1500 to 2500 calories a day from alcoholic beverages. One gram of alcohol yields 7 calories. (See Table 7, Section 4 for energy content of alcoholic beverages.) These patients frequently have the polyneuritis of thiamine deficiency and the cheilosis and beefy red tongue of riboflavin deficiency. The Wernicke-Korsakoff syndrome, an acute form of thiamine deficiency, can also occur. With abstinence from alcohol, adequate energy and nutrient intake corrects the malnutrition of chronic alcoholism and, at the same time, supports the regenerative activity of the liver cells provided the disease process has not progressed to end-stage hepatic failure.

DIET THERAPY
Principles of Diet Therapy

The following discussion focuses primarily on diet therapy in advanced cirrhosis including the complication of ascites, esophageal bleeding, hepatic encephalopathy and coma.

ENERGY. All patients with liver disease require an adequate energy intake (approximately 35 to 40 cal./kg. for adults). Without adequate energy supplied by carbohydrate and fat, amino acids from food and body cells will be deaminized in intermediary metabolism to contribute to energy needs through the gluconeogenic pathway. This will decrease the quantity of amino acids available for liver cell regeneration; and, in advanced cirrhotics, increase the amount of ammonia available for ureagenesis.

In advanced cirrhosis with a decrease in the number of functioning liver cells and with protein intolerance, 50 to 60 percent or more of the calories should be derived from carbohydrate. The research of Walker and his associates[6] suggests that in this situation carbohydrate is important, not only as a source of energy, but also as a depressor of glucagon and, therefore, gluconeogenesis. Walker's group supplemented the diets of five cirrhotics who were moderately protein intolerant (40 to 60 g. per day) with hourly feedings of glucose (amount not stated). Insulin blood levels increased significantly and glucagon levels were significantly depressed; the blood ammonia level did not rise in any of the subjects. This research also suggests that the high carbohydrate diet patterns for advanced cirrhosis should include six to eight or more feedings daily.

PROTEIN. Protein intolerance can develop in acute hepatitis or advanced cirrhosis. The characteristic biochemical aberration is hyperammonemia caused by severe liver cell damage in acute hepatitis and by cell damage and portal blood shunting in advanced cirrhosis. The ability of the damaged cells to synthesize urea for ammonia excretion is decreased. With portal shunting the ammonia absorbed from the gastrointestinal tract enters the systemic circulation and thus contributes to the elevated blood ammonia level. (Normal 80-110 mcg./100 ml.) The sources of ammonia in the gastrointestinal tract are discussed later in this section.

Although the mechanism is not well understood,[7] the elevated blood ammonia level impairs cerebral function which can progress to hepatic coma. The pre-coma phase is characterized by drowsiness and lethargy; and fetor hepaticus (liver breath), asterixis (flapping tremors of hands and tongue when extended), and disorientation occur with progressive coma.

To reduce the blood ammonia levels in pre-coma, dietary protein is restricted to tolerance. The restriction may vary depending on the patient's situation from 0.3 g. to 0.8 g. of protein per kg. of body weight (20 to 60 g. of protein per day for a 70 kg. man). In hepatic coma all protein is excluded from the feedings. A tube feeding of glucose or glucose and fat or intravenous glucose is used to provide energy. As the patient improves small quantities of protein as tolerated are added to the diet. The first addition may be as little as 10 g. of protein per day. Any patient with advanced cirrhosis who has experienced pre-coma or coma may need to restrict protein intake to tolerance for the rest of his life.

The work of Rudman and coworkers[8] suggests that the protein used in the diet of any patient with advanced cirrhosis should be primarily of high biological value not only to supply the essential amino acids but also to control blood ammonia levels. In both cirrhotic patients and in normal individuals, they tested the ammonigenicity of 18 of the 20 amino acids which occur in food. They did not test methionine and cystine, the sulfur containing amino acids. Methionine is known to precipitate coma in cirrhotics with portal shunting even without hyperammonemia.[9]

From the results of their study Rudman and coworkers classified the 18 amino acids into three groups based on the increase observed in blood ammonia levels when the acids were fed to the cirrhotic subjects. Group A, with the highest ammonigenic potency, contains seven amino acids—glycine, serine, threonine, glutamine, histidine, lysine, and asparagine. The other two groups, B and C, containing the other 11 amino acids tested, were significantly less ammonigenic than the seven acids in Group A.

With the exception of threonine and lysine the amino acids in Group A are nonessential amino acids. Rudman and coworkers conclude that the Group A amino acids have a greater ammonigenic potency than those in Groups B and C because they can be deaminated in body tissues which releases ammonia into the circulation; and that the ammonigenicity of the Group A amino acids is directly dependent on the dietary intake. They recommend that, at least theoretically, the results of their study might be applied to planning diets limited in Group A amino acids yet otherwise nutritionally adequate.

Although the evidence is limited, it would appear that a diet reduced in ammonigenicity can be achieved by applying the same principles as those used in planning the protein content in the protein-restricted diet for renal disease (see Chapter 31, Renal Disease). The amino acid content of selected foods is available (see Table 4, Section 4). However, there is limited data on the glutamine and asparagine content of foods. One major food source of glutamine is cereal protein and of asparagine, plant protein. For example, forty percent of the amino acids in the gliadin fraction of the wheat protein, gluten, is glutamine.[10] A significant reduction in glutamine intake can be achieved by using low-protein wheatstarch products (see Chapter 31). The Group A amino acids, exclusive of glutamine and asparagine, in the quantity of milk, egg, and meat containing 7 g. of protein is given in Table 32-1. It will be noted that the total quantity of ammonigenic amino acids in milk is less than in egg or meat. Therefore, the choice of milk or milk and egg would appear to be the best choices when protein is limited to 20 g. or less per day because of severe protein intolerance.

Other measures are also used to control blood ammonia levels in advanced cirrhosis. It is estimated that approximately 25 percent of the blood urea nitrogen normally diffuses into the lumen of the gastrointestinal tract where it is hydrolyzed by urease which is of bacterial origin. The ammonia released by this

Table 32-1. Milligrams of Group A Amino Acids* in Foods Containing 7 Grams of Protein

AMINO ACIDS (mg.)	MILK (whole) (200 g.)	EGG (55 g.)	MEAT† (44 g.)
Glycine	138	249	436
Serine	412	591	285
Threonine	322	350	311
Histidine	184	169	245
Lysine	544	450	615
Totals	1600	1809	1892

*Calculated from Amino Acid Content of Foods, H. Ec. Res. Report #4, USDA, 1957.
†Hamburger

Table 32–2. Protein–Sodium Restricted Exchange System

FOOD GROUP	HOUSE-HOLD MEASURE	WEIGHT (g.)	PRO-TEIN (g.)	SO-DIUM* (mg.)
Milk Exchanges	8 oz.	240	8	120
Meat Exchanges	1 oz.	30	7	25
Egg	one	50	7	70
Vegetable Exchanges	½ cup	100	2	9
Fruit Exchanges	1 serving	varies	1	2
Bread Exchanges	varies	varies	2	5
Fat Exchanges	1 tsp.	5	0	0

*Foods produced, processed, or prepared without the addition of any sodium compound.

process is reabsorbed primarily in the colon. Other sources of ammonia in the gut are amino acids in the colon and possibly ammonia naturally occurring in foods.[11] If gastrointestinal bleeding is present the digested blood may also be a source of ammonia. Neomycin, an antibiotic, is used to sterilize the colon to reduce urease. Lactulose, a nonabsorbable, non-metabolized, synthetic disaccharide which appears to trap ammonia in the colon and, thus, prevent its absorption, has also been used in the treatment of hepatic coma.[12]

VITAMINS AND MINERALS. With the restriction of protein, and, if low protein wheatstarch products are used as a major source of calories, it is strongly recommended that nutrient intake from food be supplemented with vitamin and mineral preparations including all the B vitamins, iron, and trace minerals.

ELECTROLYTES AND FLUIDS. If ascites is present, sodium intake is restricted to 200 to 500 mg. (10 to 20 mEq.) per day and fluid is restricted to the amount lost each day. The limited sodium and fluid intake may also be combined with some level of protein restriction. Sodium-restricted diets are discussed in Chapter 30.

Potassium is usually not a problem in cirrhosis. However, renal failure commonly occurs in end-stage hepatic failure. When this occurs the potassium in the diet may also be limited.

FREQUENCY OF MEALS. From the work of Walker and his associates[13] and the observations of Davidson[14] the patient with advanced cirrhosis should consume frequent small feedings. Also, the patient with severe ascites will need frequent small feedings because the fluid collection in his abdomen makes it impossible for him to eat large quantities of food at a meal.

SUMMARY. Diets for the treatment of advanced cirrhosis are adequate in energy, restricted to tolerance

in protein using food proteins of high biological value, usually restricted in sodium, and, if necessary, limited in fluids. If required, nasogastric feeding may be used in the absence of esophageal bleeding.

Planning the Diet Pattern

PROTEIN-SODIUM-RESTRICTED EXCHANGE SYSTEM. The protein values for the food Exchanges in Table 32-2 are the same as those in the basic Exchange System (see Table 23-2, Chapter 23.) with the exception that a value of 1.0 g. of protein per serving is given for fruit. This is the same protein value for fruit used in the Exchange System for planning renal diets (see Table 31-5, Chapter 31). As in the diet for patients with renal disease, the protein in fruit is calculated in the diet pattern of patients with cirrhosis to reflect the potential nitrogen in all foods. The sodium values in Table 32-2 are the same as those in Table 30-1, Sodium-Restricted Exchange System, Chapter 30, and apply only to foods produced, processed, and prepared without the addition of any sodium compounds.

The Protein-Sodium Exchange System is used to calculate patterns for diet prescriptions ranging from 10 to 60 g. protein and 250 to 500 mg. or more of sodium per day. If the diet prescription specifies only proteins of high biological value, then the low-protein wheatstarch products are used as Bread Exchanges (see Chapter 31, p. 451). In this situation the values for protein and sodium for one Bread Exchange in Table 32-2 do not apply. The values for Group C Bread Exchanges in Table 31-5, 0.1 g. of protein and 15 mg. of sodium, are used.

EXCHANGE LISTS. The Sodium-Restricted Exchange Lists in Table 30-2, Chapter 30, are used to plan the daily menus for protein- and sodium-restricted diets, and the table is not repeated in this

Table 32–3. 1500 Calorie, 75 Gram Protein and 500 Milligram Sodium Diet Pattern*

FOOD GROUP	AMOUNT	PRO-TEIN (g.)	SO-DIUM[a] (mg.)	ENER-GY (cal.)
Milk, Whole	1 pint	16	240	340
Meat	4 oz. cooked	28	100	300
Egg	1	7	70	75
Vegetables	4½ c. servings	8	36	100
Fruit	3 servings	3	6	120
Bread (unsalted)	6 servings	12	30	420
Fat (unsalted)	3 tsp	0	0	135
Totals		74	482	1490[b]

*Table 30-10, Chapter 30, with protein calculation added.
[a]Foods produced, processed or prepared without the addition of any sodium compound.
[b]Add sugar and additional unsalted fat, if tolerated, for 1800 to 2000 calories.

chapter. The discussion in Chapter 30 on the foods used in these diets and the material on convenience foods and sodium in water supplies should be reviewed.

CALCULATING THE DIET PATTERN. Tables 32–3, 32–4, and 32–5 demonstrate the calculation of a 1500 Calorie Diet Pattern with varying amounts of protein and sodium. The diet pattern in Table 32–3 is the same as the one in Table 30–10, Chapter 30. This diet pattern contains approximately 75 g. protein and 500 mg. of sodium. The energy can be increased to 1800 or 2000 calories by the addition of sugar to fruits and cereals and an increase in the quantity of unsalted fat, if tolerated.

Table 32–4 demonstrates a diet pattern containing approximately 60 g. of protein and 500 mg. of sodium, while Table 32–5 demonstrates a 1500 calorie diet containing approximately 35 g. of protein and 250 mg. of sodium. The diet pattern in Table 32–5 will contain 1500 calories only if high calorie, low electrolyte supplements are used. If tolerated, additional unsalted fat can also be used to increase calories. However, the research of Walker and coworkers[15] suggests that patients with advanced cirrhosis might benefit more from the carbohydrate in the high calorie, low electrolyte supplements than the addition of unsalted fats.

If the diet for the patient with cirrhosis is limited in the Group A amino acids (see discussion of protein on p. 463), wheatstarch products are substituted for regular bread exchanges. In this situation the diet pattern is planned using the protein and sodium values in the exchange system in Table 31–5, Chapter 31. The exchange lists in Table 31–6 are used to plan menus. The potassium is not calculated in the diet pattern for the patient with cirrhosis unless renal as well as hepatic failure occurs.

Table 32–4. 1500 Calorie, 60 Gram Protein, 500 Milligram Sodium Diet Pattern

FOOD GROUP	AMOUNT	PRO-TEIN (g.)	SO-DIUM* (mg.)	ENER-GY (cal.)
Milk, Whole	1 pint	16	240	340
Meat	2 oz. cooked	14	50	150
Egg	1	7	70	75
Vegetables	4½ c. servings	8	36	100
Fruit	3 servings	3	6	120
Bread (unsalted)	6 servings	12	30	420
Fat (unsalted)	6 tsp.	0	0	270
Totals		60	432	1475†

*Foods produced, processed, and prepared without the addition of any sodium compound.
†Add sugar and additional unsalted fat, if tolerated, for 1800 to 2000 calories.

Table 32–5. 1500 Calorie, 35 Gram Protein, 250 Milligram Sodium Diet Pattern

FOOD GROUP	AMOUNT	PRO-TEIN (g.)	SO-DIUM* (mg.)	ENER-GY (cal.)
Milk, whole	8 oz.	8	120	170
Meat	0	—	—	—
Egg	1	7	70	75
Vegetables	2½ c. servings	4	18	50
Fruit	3 servings	3	6	120
Bread (unsalted)	6 servings	12	30	420
Fat (unsalted)	6 tsp.	0	0	270
Totals		34	244	1105†

*Foods produced, processed or prepared without the addition of any sodium compound.
†Plus high calorie, low electrolyte supplement and additional unsalted fat, if tolerated, to supply 1500 or more calories.

TUBE FEEDING. Some patients in hepatic coma without esophageal bleeding may be fed by nasogastric tube. When the ammonia blood level is elevated, Tisdale, LaMont, and Isselbacher[16] recommend a tube feeding of 20 to 25 percent glucose solution to provide 2000 calories per day. The high calorie, low electrolyte, relatively nitrogen-free products recommended for the patient in acute renal failure (Chapter 31, p. 448) can also be used as tube feedings for the hepatic coma patient. If sodium is not severely restricted, Polycose, derived from the controlled acid hydrolysis of cornstarch, which contains primarily maltose and dextrins, may be used. However, there are 122 mg. (5.3 mEq.) of sodium in 100 g. (400 calories) of Polycose powder and, therefore its use may be limited when sodium is restricted to 250 mg. (10 mEq.) of sodium per day. According to the research of Walker[17] it is advisable to administer small hourly feedings rather than larger amounts every three or four hours (see Tube Feeding, Chapter 26).

If the patient requiring a tube feeding can tolerate some protein, and the sodium is not severely restricted, whole milk can be used. Eight ounces of whole milk contains 8 g. protein and 120 (5.1 mEq.) of sodium. If sodium is severely restricted, Lonalac (powdered low-sodium milk) can be used as the source of protein without adding significant amounts of sodium to the feeding. There are approximately 3.4 g. protein and 2.5 mg. sodium in 100 ml. of reconstituted Lonalac.

SPECIAL PROBLEMS. Since the majority of hospitalized patients with liver disease are anorexic, their fluid and nutrient intake should be carefully monitored daily. Each morning an estimate of the patient's intake of energy, protein, and sodium for the previous 24 hours should be recorded in his medical record. The physician needs this information so that he can correlate energy and nutrient intake with the patient's symptoms and laboratory data. Some appraisal of the mineral and vitamin intake should also be recorded so that supplementary preparations can be provided if necessary.

A record of the patient's food likes and dislikes should be obtained from the patient or a relative so that in so far as possible he will be served foods and beverages he will consume.

SALT SUBSTITUTES. Salt substitutes containing ammonia are not used to enhance the flavor of the sodium-restricted diets of patients with liver disease because the ammonia in the substitute can increase the quantity absorbed from the gastrointestinal tract. This is hazardous for patients prone to hyperammonemia.

ESOPHAGEAL BLEEDING. In patients with esophageal bleeding due to portal hypertension, surgical intervention may be required. A portacaval shunt is done to relieve the pressure in the esophageal veins. If considerable liver damage has occurred prior to the surgery, the diet will continue to be restricted in protein and sodium after surgery.

COUNSELING THE PATIENT

The patient with liver disease presents the nutrition counselor with numerous challenges, especially the patient with liver disease due to chronic alcoholism. Many of these patients have limited resources, little money and inadequate living quarters; and have frequently alienated themselves from their families. At the same time the health care team often has difficulty accepting them unconditionally.

If the patient has liver damage complicated by ascites, his diet will be severely restricted in sodium for six months or more to resolve the ascites. It may also be restricted in protein to some extent. Therefore, he will need help over time to learn how to manage his diet, and information regarding where to buy sodium-restricted foods in his community (see Counseling the Patient, Chapter 31).

At the same time that the patient is accommodating himself to a restricted diet, he is also trying to cope with abstinence from alcohol. If receptive, the patient can often be helped by a psychiatric counselor or by a community self-help group such as Alcoholics Anonymous.

WILSON'S DISEASE

Wilson's disease (hepatolenticular degeneration) is a degenerative disease characterized by the storage of excessive amounts of copper in the liver and other tissues. It is inherited as an autosomal recessive trait and the disease is not detected until young adulthood, usually between 20 and 30 years of age. Approximately 98 percent of serum copper is bound normally to a specific protein, ceruloplasmin. It has been demonstrated that patients with Wilson's disease have a decreased amount of ceruloplasmin with which to bind serum copper, with the result that toxic amounts of copper are stored in the liver and other tissues.

Wilson's disease is treated with chelating agents to increase the urinary excretion of copper; the intake of dietary copper is also restricted to 1.0 mg. per day. At this point there is limited data on the copper content of foods. Pennington and Calloway[18] have recently published a review of the factors effecting the copper content of food and have compiled a table showing the range of values for copper as reported by various investigators. The information in this publication may be useful in designing a copper-restricted diet pattern and exchange lists for a patient with Wilson's disease.

STUDY QUESTIONS AND ACTIVITIES

1. How does the liver function in the metabolism of nutrients? As an organ of storage? In detoxification?
2. Why may a diet increased in protein be a source of danger to the patient with severe liver disease?
3. How may hepatic coma develop? Why is a diet devoid or severely restricted in protein essential?
4. Calculate a diet pattern for a 2000 calorie, 20 g. protein restricted in Group A amino acids, 500 mg. sodium diet.
5. Calculate a diet pattern for an 1800 calorie, 60 g. protein, 1000 mg. sodium diet. Plan menus, a weekly market order, and instructional materials for a man living alone who has a gas stove (top burners only), a sink, limited storage space, and shares a refrigerator with two other men. He has $15.00 a week for food and the nearest supermarket is five blocks from his house.
6. What are the resources in your community for helping the chronic alcoholic?

SUPPLEMENTARY READINGS

Davidson, C. S.: Dietary treatment of hepatic disease. J. Am. Dietet. A. 62:515, 1973.
Pennington, J. T., and Calloway, D. H.: Copper content of foods. J. Am. Dietet. A. 63:143, 1973.

Rubin, E., and Lieber, C. S.: Fatty liver, alcoholic hepatitis and cirrhosis produced by alcohol in primates. N. Eng. J. Med. 290:128, 1974.

Rudman, D., et al: Ammonia content of food. Am. J. Clin. Nutr. 26:487, 1973.

Rudman, D., et al: Comparison of the effect of various amino acids upon the blood ammonia concentration of patients with liver disease. Am. J. Clin. Nutr. 26:916, 1973.

Russell, R. M., et al: Hepatic injury from chronic hypervitaminosis A resulting in portal hypertension and ascites. N. Eng. J. Med. 291:435, 1974.

Schenker, S., et al: Hepatic encephalopathy: current status. Gastroenterology 66:121, 1974.

Sherlock, S. and Scheuer, P. J.: Biliary cirrhosis. N. Eng. J. Med. 289:674, 1973.

Silvis, S. E., et al: Treatment of severe liver failure with hyperalimentation. Am. J. Gastroent. 59:416, 1973.

For further references, see Bibliography in Section 4.

REFERENCES

1. Davidson, C. S.: J. Am. Dietet. A. 62:515, 1973.
2. Tisdale, W. A.: in *Harrison's Principles of Internal Medicine*, ed. 7. New York, McGraw-Hill, 1974, Chapter 296.
3. Spiro, H. M.: *Clinical Gastroenterology*. New York, Macmillan, 1970.
4. Rubin, E., and Lieber, C. S.: N. Eng. J. Med. 290:128, 1974.
5. Ibid.
6. Walker, C., et al: Clin. Research 21:850, 1973.
7. Schenker, S., et al: Gastroenterology 66:121, 1974.
8. Rudman, D., et al: Am. J. Clin. Nutr. 26:916, 1973.
9. Tisdale, op. cit.
10. Patey, A. E.: Lancet 1:722, 1974.
11. Rudman, D., et al: Am. J. Clin. Nutr. 26:190, 1973.
12. Fessel, J. M., and Conn, H. O.: Gastroenterology 64:882, 1973.
13. Walker, op. cit.
14. Davidson, op. cit.
15. Walker, op. cit.
16. Tisdale, op. cit.
17. Walker, op. cit.
18. Pennington, J. T., and Calloway, D. H.: J. Am. Dietet. A. 63:143, 1973.

33   special problems

ALLERGY

Allergy is described as an adverse physiological reaction in various tissues resulting from the interaction of an antigen with an antibody or lymphoid cells.[1] The tissues involved are the skin, mucous membranes, or vascular endothelium. The antibodies are immunoglobulins with immunoglobulin E (IgE) the one most commonly involved. The allergic reactions in mucous membranes are attributable to the IgE antibodies synthesized by plasma cells located predominantly under mucosal surfaces, especially the respiratory and gastrointestinal tracts. There is a significant familial incidence which may aid in diagnosis; and there may be a strong emotional component related to the severity of allergic manifestations.

CAUSES. Allergic reactions are caused by a wide variety of substances and conditions. These include pollens, dust, cosmetics and animal hair; poisonous plants; serums, vaccines and drugs; physical agents such as heat, cold, and sunlight; as well as a variety of foods. Reactions to a particular substance may occur in one individual, and in another person a similar reaction may be caused by an entirely different substance. Or the same substance may cause two widely differing reactions in each of two individuals.

SYMPTOMS. The symptoms of allergy are as varied as the substances causing the reaction. Eczema is most common in infants and young children; rhinitis and asthma occur in both children and adults, and are sometimes preceded by allergic eczema in infancy. Urticaria or hives, physical allergies, and angioneurotic edema are common in adults. Serum sickness and drug reactions are directly related to the administration of vaccines and drugs, and may occur at any age.

Foods and Allergy

This discussion is chiefly concerned with food allergies, but it should be kept in mind that any allergy from whatever cause, if severe, may interfere with the nutrition of the individual due to the effect on appetite and thus on general health. This is often the case with a child, whose growth and development may be retarded seriously unless his diet is evaluated carefully and made as attractive and nutritionally adequate as possible.

The protein component of a food is considered to be the causative factor in food allergy, even though foods which cause an allergic reaction may vary widely in protein content. Reaction to a food such as honey is associated with protein in the pollen grains mixed in the honey, for it has been shown that very minute amounts of a given protein may cause an allergic reaction. Also, allergic responses to a food may be either immediate or delayed.

Among the common allergy-producing foods, particularly in children, are oranges, milk, eggs, and sometimes wheat. Other common food allergens are fish and shellfish, chocolate, tomatoes, and strawberries. It has been found that members of the same botanic family may have a similar allergic effect. Lemons and grapefruit are likely to cause a reaction if oranges are allergenic. Likewise, if cabbage gives rise to an allergic reaction, so may broccoli, brussels sprouts, and cauliflower.

Whether or not an allergic disturbance follows the eating of a specific food depends largely upon the individual's physical and often emotional state. This may make the search for the offending food or foods a difficult process. Moreover, no immunologic mechanisms specific to food allergy have been identified, and symptoms are sometimes ascribed to allergy when their cause is obscure.

Diagnosis

HISTORY. All investigators stress the need for a careful history. This is especially true for the older child and the adult, who eat a variety of foods. In the very young infant ingesting only a limited number of foods, the diagnosis may be more easily established. In all instances a detailed history of recent food intake, appearance of symptoms, and other events and conditions relating to the illness is of utmost importance.

SKIN TESTS. If a careful history does not reveal the cause of the allergic symptoms, the physician may resort to skin tests. Solutions, each containing a small quantity of a common allergen, are applied to a scratched portion of the skin, and then covered with cellophane for two to four days. Interdermal injections of the suspected allergen may also be used.

In the event that welts, wheals, and redness develop from any of these tests, an allergic reaction is indicated. However, it has been observed that many foods may give a positive skin test without causing allergic symptoms.

FOOD CHALLENGE. When a food is suspected of causing an allergic reaction it is excluded from the diet for seven to ten days. Even though the exclusion results in improvement in symptoms the food is reintroduced into the diet in large amounts for several meals. If the suspected food contains the allergen, symptoms will recur in a reasonable period of time, usually within seven days. The testing should be done in a blind manner. For example, if milk is the suspected food it can be hidden in mashed potatoes and breads.

Table 33–1. Rowe's Cereal-Free Elimination Diet*

FOODS USED	
Tapioca (pearl or minute)	Apricots[b]
White potatoes	Grapefruit
Sweet potatoes	Lemon
Breads made with any combination of soy, lima, potato starch, and tapioca flour	Peaches
	Pineapples
	Prunes
Soy milk: Mull-Soy and Neo-Mull Soy[a]	Pears
	Cane or beet sugar
Lamb	Salt
Chicken, fryers, roosters, capon (no hens)	Sesame oil (not Chinese)
	Soybean oil
Bacon	Margarine[c]
Liver (lamb, chicken)	Gelatin (Knox)
	White vinegar
Peas	Vanilla extract
Spinach	Lemon extract
Squash	Corn-starch-free baking powder
String beans	Baking soda
Tomatoes	Cream of tartar
Artichokes	
Asparagus	Maple syrup or syrup made with
Carrots	cane sugar flavored with maple
Lettuce	
Lima Beans	

*Adapted from Rowe, A. H.: Food Allergy. Springfield, Ill., Thomas, 1972.
[a]Free of corn syrup solids and corn oil (Syntex Laboratories, Palo Alto, Ca. 94304).
[b]Fruits, fresh or canned in cane sugar.
[c]Free of milk solids or corn oil.

Table 33–2. Rowe's Fruit-Free, Cereal-Free Elimination Diet*

FOODS USED

Tapioca (pearl only)	Cooked carrots
White potatoes	Squash
Sweet potatoes	Artichokes
Bread made with any combination of soy, lima, potato starch, or tapioca flour	Peas
	Lima Beans
	String beans
Soy milk: Mull-Soy and Neo Mull-Soy[a]	Cane or beet sugar
	Soybean oil
	Margarine[b]
Lamb	Gelatin (Knox)
Chicken, fryers, roosters, capon (no hens)	Salt
	Syrup made from cane sugar (no maple syrup)
Bacon	
Liver, (lamb, chicken)	Corn-free, tartaric acid-free baking powder[c]

*Adapted from Rowe, A. H.: *Food Allergy*. Springfield, Ill,. Thomas, 1972.
[a]Free of corn syrup solids and corn oil (Syntex Laboratories, Palo Alto, Ca. 94304).
[b]Free of milk solids and corn oil.
[c]Tartaric acid is made from grapes.

ELIMINATION TEST DIETS. The Rowe[2] elimination test diets are also used by some physicians to identify food allergies. The foods included in these diets are considered unlikely to produce allergic reactions. Table 33–1 lists the foods used in Rowe's cereal-free elimination diet; and Table 33–2, Rowe's fruit-free, cereal-free elimination diet. Both diets exclude breast and cow's milk. Rowe recommends the use of soy milks free of the sugars derived from cornstarch on the theory that corn sugars could be contaminated with corn protein.

The patient is placed on one of the test diets for a period of a week. If the symptoms do not abate, he is tried on the other diet for the same length of time. If, at the end of the second test diet, relief has not been obtained, it is evident that causes other than food should be sought as allergic agents.

On the other hand, if the patient is relieved of his symptoms on any one of the elimination test diets, he is kept on this diet for another week. Other foods, first chosen from the related test diets and then more generally, are added one by one, with wheat, eggs, and milk last, because these foods are most likely to produce allergy. If the patient shows allergic symptoms after the addition of any one food, that food may be suspected as the cause of the allergic reaction and must be omitted from the diet.

In infants or young children suspected of food allergy, the problem of eliminating the offending foods may be solved by placing the patient, if he is an infant, on nothing by mouth except Mull-Soy or Neo-Mull Soy, or on a simple elimination diet consisting of lamb, rice, carrots, pears, and a soy formula if he is older. If symptoms clear, other foods are added to the child's diet one at a time. As with adults, if there is no improvement on the elimination diet, it may be assumed that the allergic symptoms are due to causes other than food.

Dietary Treatment

MILK ALLERGY. Allergy to cow's milk protein appears to occur most commonly in children under two years of age and, in many of these children, tolerance to milk protein increases as they grow older. The lactoglobulin fraction is considered to be the most common allergen in cow's milk protein.

A variety of milk-free formulas are available for feeding these infants and children. (See Table 34–4, Chapter 34.) The soy-base formulas and those made with casein hydrolysate are commonly used in place of milk-based formulas. These preparations are equal in calorie and nutrient value to other commercial infant formulas and, when used as directed, are well-tolerated and support adequate growth.[3]

Evaporated goat's milk may be used to feed an infant who is allergic to cow's milk. However, some infants have the same reaction to goat's milk protein that they have to that in cow's milk. Also, goat's milk is low in vitamins D, B_{12}, and folic acid and when used, must be supplemented with preparations of these vitamins to supply the infant's needs.

When solid foods are included in the infant's diet, care must be taken to avoid foods that have milk or nonfat dry milk added during processing. The mother must be advised to read labels carefully so that she can avoid these products. The companies that market baby foods make available to the nutrition counselor lists of ingredients in their products.

If the child does not accept special milks when he is older, it is necessary to supplement his diet with calcium pills and also with riboflavin. Even the older child who tolerates limited amounts of milk such as the 2 to 4 percent dry milk solids found in some bread and the milk used in preparation of foods such as cakes and cookies will need calcium pills to meet his calcium need. It may also be advisable for the adult who is allergic to milk to use calcium supplements daily. Vitamin D supplements are also needed.

WHEAT ALLERGY. Because wheat bread and other products made with wheat cereal or flour are basic items in the American diet, the individual who is allergic to wheat finds he cannot eat many common foods. He must learn that baker's rye bread contains some wheat flour; that practically all hot breads, pancakes, pastries, and crackers are made chiefly or partly from wheat products; that bran and gluten are wheat derivatives. Thickened gravies, cream soups, and sauces are to be avoided unless thickened with corn or rice starch. Even meat dishes, such as meat loaf, hamburger, bologna, and sausage may contain wheat flour or bread. All malted beverages must be avoided by the wheat-sensitive individual.

For a complete description of the omissions necessary in wheat sensitivity, see Chapter 25, Gluten-Free Diet. For the patient allergic to wheat only, the restrictions on rye flour and oatmeal do not apply, but the remaining material proves helpful in insuring that all wheat products are eliminated from the diet.

EGG ALLERGY. The patient who is allergic to egg must investigate carefully all commercial products before eating them. He must remember that even the baking powder used in baked goods may contain dried egg white; that egg white may be used in the preparation of foaming beverages; and that most desserts, especially cakes, cookies, pastries, puddings, and ice cream, contain eggs. These patients may also be allergic to chicken, which must then be omitted from the diet.

ALLERGY TO CITRUS FRUIT. The major problem for these individuals is an adequate daily intake of vitamin C. Potatoes, other vegetables, and fruit can provide an adequate intake although some individuals may take 50 mg. of ascorbic acid as medication each day to insure an adequate intake.

RESOURCES FOR PATIENTS. At the end of this chapter is a list of sources of recipes for allergy patients. These recipes may help them discover new dishes because allergy diets can become monotonous and uninteresting.

Desensitizing the Patient

The difficulties inherent in strict avoidance of allergy-causing foods, especially in a child, may cause the physician to try to desensitize him to such food. This treatment should follow a period of complete abstinence from the offending food. Fortunately, it may be possible to desensitize by mouth; and, beginning with doses so minute that they cause no reactions in the person being treated, gradually the amount is increased until ordinary food portions can be tolerated.

To illustrate, one child sensitive to egg white was desensitized in this way over a period of seven months by a dosage beginning with 1 mg. of dry or powdered egg white. Another child could tolerate at first only such small amount of egg white as that present in a teaspoonful of a dilution made by adding one drop of egg white to a pint of water. In three months, however, he was able to include eggs in his diet.

Often adults may desensitize themselves successfully. A man acutely but periodically sensitive to milk

desensitizes himself every three or four years, in the following way. After eliminating milk, he takes daily an increasing number of drops of cream until he can resume the use of both cream and milk in his diet.

ANEMIAS

Anemia may be defined as a condition in which there is a decrease in the quantity of hemoglobin, in the number of red cells, in the volume of packed cells (hematocrit), or in a combination of these. From the strictly nutritional standpoint, anemias may be classified as follows: (1) hypochromic microcytic anemias (too little hemoglobin) due to hemorrhage, acute or chronic, or inadequate intake of iron; and (2) hyperchromic macrocytic anemias, due to deficiency of substances essential to red cell formation, and the release of these cells from the bone marrow.

Acute and Chronic Blood Loss

One of the most frequent causes of anemia in the hospitalized patient is acute or chronic blood loss. Over 60 percent of the body's iron (approximately 2.5 g. of iron in an adult) is in the hemoglobin of the circulating red cells and in each milliliter of whole blood there is, on the average, 0.7 mg. of iron. Therefore, the loss of 500 ml. of blood results in the loss of 350 mg. or about ⅓ gram of iron.

ACUTE BLOOD LOSS. In severe hemorrhage the immediate treatment is restoration of blood volume by transfusion. The blood must be further restored by an increase in the production of red blood cells and hemoglobin. In an otherwise normal individual, recovery is spontaneous, but the red cells are replenished more rapidly than is the hemoglobin. The latter will be restored gradually, but the speed of its restoration seems to depend largely on the diet of the individual. The necessary nutrients must be supplied in the diet in order that each of these red cells may contain the normal amount of hemoglobin. (See, Nutritional Anemia.)

CHRONIC BLOOD LOSS. Chronic blood loss may accompany such conditions as gastric ulcer, colitis, or long untreated hemorrhoids. The important aspect of treatment is to determine the cause of the blood loss and to control it. The dietary care is the same as that described under Nutritional Anemia.

Nutritional Anemia

IRON DEFICIENCY. Hypochromic microcytic anemia in the hospitalized patient is observed most frequently in infants and young children, the adolescent girl, and in women 15 to 45 years of age. It may be due to an inadequate intake of dietary iron or malabsorption. (Malabsorption is discussed in Chapters 25 and 34.)

The dietary treatment of iron deficiency anemia must focus not only on iron intake but also on protein, the B vitamins, and ascorbic acid (see Chapter 5). This also applies to the patient recovering from acute or chronic blood loss. For adults the diet should provide 1½ to 2 g. of protein per kilogram of body weight and adequate energy, as well as B vitamins, ascorbic acid and iron in excess of the recommended allowances.

Besides liver, which should be included at least once a week, lean meat, eggs, whole grain and enriched bread and cereals, and potatoes are common and good food sources of iron and, in the case of meat and eggs, of protein. Other foods valuable for iron content which should appear frequently in the diet are kidney, heart, green leafy vegetables, and legumes.

When necessary, supplemental iron should be used. Since oral iron medication sometimes causes gastric irritation when taken on an empty stomach, it should be taken directly after meals.

During hospitalization the food intake of patients with nutritional anemia should be monitored daily. Before discharge they should be counseled in order to avoid a recurrence of their problem.

FOLIC ACID DEFICIENCY. Hyperchromic macrocytic anemia in the hospitalized patient is observed most frequently in the pregnant woman, in patients with malabsorption, and in patients taking medications which interfere with the metabolism of folic acid, such as the anticonvulsants used in epilepsy (p. 493) and drugs used in the treatment of cancer (p. 475). The absorption and metabolism of folic acid is discussed in Chapter 7.

When the deficiency is due to an inadequate dietary intake, the anemia responds readily to folic acid therapy. An adequate dietary intake of folic acid can be obtained from green leafy vegetables, liver, meat, fish, legumes, and whole grains.

Pernicious Anemia

Pernicious anemia is a macrocytic anemia characterized by a decrease in the number of red blood cells. It is due to a lack of the "intrinsic factor" produced in the gastric mucosa which is essential for the absorption of vitamin B_{12} in the distal ileum. B_{12} absorption and metabolism is discussed in Chapter 7. Anemia due to vitamin B_{12} deficiency can also occur due to malabsorption in the distal ileum in such diseases as regional ileitis.

B_{12} deficiency anemia is treated by injections of B_{12} which promotes a rapid increase in blood cell formation. An adequate intake of all nutrients is required to provide substances for both red blood cell production and maturation. Prior to treatment many of these patients have a poor appetitie and gastrointestinal distress. With treatment their appetite returns and they should be counseled to establish and maintain an adequate intake of food and to continue the B_{12} injections.

DISEASES OF THE MUSCULOSKELETAL SYSTEM
Arthritis

Arthritis is a chronic disease process which involves the joints. Perhaps because of its chronicity and its accompanying discomfort and pain, many arthritics become the victims of food faddists, self-appointed "arthritis experts" or quacks, who advocate quick and miraculous cures with bizarre diet plans. At present there is no known dietary cause or cure for arthritis and the medical treatment is palliative, not curative.

OSTEOARTHRITIS. Osteoarthritis or degenerative joint disease occurs in the older age group, more frequently in women than in men. The disease is due to structural changes in the articular cartilage in the joints, usually those which are weight-bearing such as the spine and knees. As the process progresses the joints become stiff and often painful. For this reason activity may be curtailed, and there is a tendency to overweight in this group of patients, placing additional strain on the affected joints.

The nutritional requirements for the older age individual as described in Chapter 19 are equally important for the person with arthritis. Sufficient protein, calcium, iron, and vitamins are needed to maintain good health. Only the energy needs are somewhat reduced, since activity is lessened.

The overweight arthritic will benefit from a further decrease in calories. Sometimes a moderate reduction in energy intake will accomplish this purpose. A more controlled reduction regimen is detailed in Chapter 27. As his weight approaches the normal range for his height and build, the patient with osteoarthritis may well experience some relief from his discomfort and pain, and achieve an increase in activity.

RHEUMATOID ARTHRITIS. Rheumatoid arthritis occurs more frequently than osteoarthritis. It may be seen in children, but usually appears between the ages of 25 and 50. It is three times more common in women than in men. The disease is due to an inflammatory process of the synovium or lining of the joints, accompanied by swelling and eventual deformity. It is a disfiguring, debilitating, and chronic disease, marked by exacerbations and remissions.

In contrast with the osteoarthritic, the patient with rheumatoid arthritis is frequently underweight. Also, many patients have such severe involvement of the joints of the fingers and hands that they have difficulty feeding themselves. In order to achieve an adequate energy and nutrient intake they often need to be trained to use the adaptive equipment presented in Chapter 24.

OTHER TREATMENT. Therapeutic doses of aspirin are used in the treatment of both types of arthritis. Because aspirin can cause gastric distress it is recommended that it be taken after meals. Occasionally corticosteroids are used in the treatment of rheumatoid arthritis. Since these medications promote sodium retention, the diet may be moderately restricted in sodium. Frequently the patient taking aspirin or steroids is advised to use a bland diet and antacids (see Chapter 25).

Gout

Gout or tophic arthritis is due to an inborn error of purine metabolism, characterized by an increase in blood uric acid levels and the deposition of urate crystals in the soft tissues and in the joints, particularly of the fingers and toes. Very occasionally it appears in children, but the incidence is greatest in men after the age of thirty. It is relatively rare in women.

In primary gout the metabolic error in the majority of subjects results in overproduction of uric acid (hyperuricemia), underexcretion of uric acid or both. Secondary gout due to reduced excretion of uric acid occurs in chronic renal disease, hypertensive cardiovascular disease, and starvation in the treatment of obesity. For many years the excessive intake of alcohol has been associated with gout. From a study of alcoholism and attacks of gout, Maclachlan[4] believes that it is the lack of food intake by the alcoholic that is responsible for the precipitation of an acute attack of gout. Recently gout was found to be associated with chronic lead intoxication due to the excessive consumption of unbonded whiskey (moonshine).[5]

Normal blood levels of uric acid are from 2.5 to 5 mg. per 100 m. A level of 6 mg. percent for men, and 5.5 mg. percent for women is considered hyperuricemia and is indicative of the presence of gout, although no overt symptoms may appear. The clinical course of gout may best be described as having three stages. The first is hyperuricemia without symptoms, perhaps discovered at a routine physical examination. The second is characterized by an acute and painful attack of gouty arthritis. The attack may subside spontaneously in anywhere from two days to two weeks, or respond to treatment with drugs which promote uric acid excretion. There may be a long interval before another attack occurs. Chronic tophaceous gout is the third and most severe form of the disease. Tophi, or accumulations of urate crystals, are present in and around one or more of the joints, causing destruction of bone and deformity (Fig. 33-1). Kidney stones or urate crystals may also occur.

MEDICAL TREATMENT. The source of uric acid arises from the metabolism of purines, a constituent of nucleoproteins found in all cells. Purines are obtained from ingested food and from the breakdown of body protein. Purines are also synthesized in the liver from smaller metabolic fragments. Colchicine, a drug which has been used in the treatment of gout for many years, is thought to inhibit the metabolic reactions by which uric acid is derived from purine compounds. More recently, drugs have been available that facilitate the excretion of uric acid by the kidney. These two

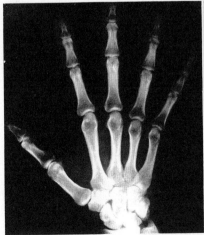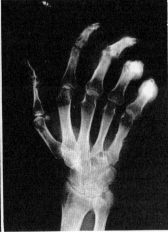

Fig. 33-1. Bones of the hand of a normal person (*left*) and of one with far-advanced gout (*right*), showing marked skeletal changes. (The Department of Radiology, The New York Hospital)

Table 33-3. Purine Content of Foods per 100 Grams*

GROUP I (0-15 mg.)	GROUP II (50-150 mg.)	GROUP III (150-800 mg.)
Vegetables	Meats, poultry	Sweetbreads
Fruits	Fish	Anchovies
Milk	Sea food	Sardines
Cheese	Beans, dry	Liver
Eggs	Peas, dry	Kidney
Cereals, bread	Lentils	Meat extracts
Sugars, fats	Spinach	Brains

*Adapted from Turner, D.: *Handbook of Diet Therapy*, ed. 5. Chicago, University of Chicago Press, 1971.

drugs help to lower the blood uric acid levels in patients with gout.

DIETARY TREATMENT. In the past a purine-restricted diet was used as part of the treatment of gout but it is seldom used routinely today. In the purine-restricted diet, all foods in Group III in Table 33-3, Purine Content of Foods, were excluded and only limited amounts of those in Group II were used.

Today, some physicians restrict foods that are very high in purine content such as liver, kidney, brains and sweetbreads. Otherwise the diet is adequate to meet the individual's needs. Patients with gout should be cautioned about fasting, whether it is practiced to lose weight or, unintentionally, on an alcoholic spree, because it has been observed that fasting, even for 1 or 2 days, leads to an increase in blood uric acid.

Osteoporosis

Osteoporosis is a disease characterized by demineralization of the bone. It occurs in the later decades of life and is much more common in women than in men. There may be back pain due to compression or fracture of the weight-bearing lumbar vertebrae. The frequency with which older women, as compared with men, sustain hip fractures is thought to be due to the greater incidence of osteoporosis in women.

Bone formation and bone resorption (calcium deposition in the bone and calcium loss from the bone) for the maintenance of adequate calcium levels in the blood are part of the normal homeostatic process, regulated by normal activity. It has been shown that parathyroid hormone affects bone resorption, while calcitonin affects bone formation (see Chapter 5). Lutwak[6] suggests that, together with the reciprocal relationship of parathyroid hormone and calcitonin, a long-term inadequate intake of calcium during adult life leads to the development of osteoporosis. He also suggests that

some forms of periodontal disease with resorption of bone may be a preosteoporotic symptom. Therefore, Lutwak recommends an adequate, lifetime, intake of calcium for the prevention of osteoporosis and, from his own observation, the long-term use of a daily supplement of 1 gram of calcium for the treatment of osteoporosis. Some physicians may also use a fluorine supplement.

DIET-MEDICATION INTERRELATIONSHIPS

A variety of commonly used medications can have an effect on the nutritional status of patients. Some medications cause gastric distress, nausea, vomiting, and diarrhea that can lead to a decrease in food intake or to a decrease in nutrient absorption. Others may interfere with nutrient absorption from the gastrointestinal tract or with nutrient utilization at the cellular level. Table 33-4 lists nutrition problems due to various types of commonly used medications. In most, but not all, situations the nutritional problems result from long term use of the medication and can be averted in some instances by use of nutrient supple-

Table 33-4. Nutritional Problems Due to Various Types of Medications

Nutritional Problem	Medications
Stomatitis	Cancer chemotherapeutic agents Antibiotics
Hyperplasia of gums	Anticonvulsants
Nausea, vomiting, gastritis, gastric hemorrhage	Cancer chemotherapeutic agents Antibiotics Salicylates Steroids Potassium and other electrolytes Anticonvulsants
Malabsorption with diarrhea or steatorrhea	Cancer chemotherapeutic agents Antibiotics Laxatives Clofibrate and cholestyramine Antacids Alcohol
Constipation	Anticholinergics Hypnotics, sedatives
Nutrient Utilization Glucose	Steroids
Protein	Cancer chemotherapeutic agents Steroids
Lipids	Steroids
Vitamins and minerals	Cancer chemotherapeutic agents Anticoagulants Anticonvulsives Sedatives
Electrolytes	Diuretics, digitalis Steroids

ments as long as excessive intakes or megadoses of the nutrient are avoided. (See discussion of anticonvulsant medication and folic acid in the treatment of epilepsy in Chapter 34.) The effects of the medication on nutrient intake, absorption, and utilization are so widespread with such medications as cancer chemotherapeutic agents, that the medication may be given intermittently.

In this section cancer therapeutic agents and steroids which have widespread effects on nutritional status are discussed and specific food–drug interactions such as protein intake and levodopa are presented. More extensive information can be found in the fifth edition of A Pharmacological Basis of Therapeutics, edited by Goodman and Gilman,[7] The Physician's Desk Reference (PDR)[8] which cross-references drugs by generic and trade names, or the drug formulary of the pharmacy department of any large hospital.

Cancer Chemotherapeutic Agents

The chemotherapeutic agents used in the treatment of cancer, frequently in combination with other modes of therapy, are cytotoxic drugs. They have an inhibitory effect on the mitotic processes of the cell nucleus and, therefore, inhibit the proliferation of cancer cells. However, the action of the drugs is not limited to cancer cells. They also have adverse effects on other cell nuclei. In relation to nutritional status, the most important cells, which can be classed as continuously mitotic, are the cells of the microvilli and other cells of the gastrointestinal tract and the bone marrow cells, the precursors of red blood cells.

The immediate effect of most chemotherapeutic agents is nausea and vomiting. Therefore, the medication is usually given late in the evening so that the patient is able to consume food during the day. Subsequently, a nonspecific malabsorption of nutrients occurs through the effect of the agents on the microvilli of the gastrointestinal tract. The intermittent use of the drugs reduces the severity of this problem. With some agents stomatitis occurs making it difficult for the patient to eat. In this situation acid foods such as citrus fruits and juices, vinegar, and very salty foods are avoided.

In addition to the general inhibition of bone marrow cell formation by chemotherapy, one agent, methotrexate, is a folic acid antimetabolite. The use of this agent can lead to megaloblastic anemia. Therefore, folinic acid (citrovorum factor) is administered with methotrexate to avoid this type of anemia.

In addition to red blood cell problems, the use of cancer chemotherapeutic agents can also result in a deficiency of immunoglobulins, the blood proteins involved in combating infection. The patient, therefore, is readily susceptible to infection and, when hospitalized, is protected by isolation. All hospital personnel, including food service workers, with upper respiratory or other infections must be excluded from any contact with these patients.

Steroids

Steroids are anti-inflammatory agents which are used in the treatment of a wide variety of disorders. Gastric bleeding is a common complication. When large doses are administered orally, some clinicians advise taking the drug with meals and antacids between meals. Generally, gastric secretagogues are avoided (see Chapter 25).

The majority of steroid preparations promote sodium and, therefore, fluid retention. Depending on the problem, dietary sodium intake may be mildly or moderately restricted. In some situations the sodium intake may be severely restricted (10 mEq.) (See Chapter 30.) Hypokalemia can result with some steroid preparations. If this occurs potassium chloride is used to correct the deficit.

Glucose intolerance develops in some individuals on long-term steroid therapy. This may result in steroid-induced diabetes. These individuals are treated by diet and an oral hypoglycemic agent or insulin (see Chapter 28). The steroid therapy is continued. Osteoporosis is also a frequent complication of steroid therapy. If it develops, therapy may be discontinued.

Specific Food–Drug Problems

TYRAMINE AND MAO INHIBITORS. Monoamine oxidase (MAO) inhibitors used in the treatment of depressed patients interract adversely with tyramine, an amine derived from the amino acid tyrosine. The MAO inhibitor–tyramine interaction results in the release of norepinephrine from the nerve endings which causes a marked rise in blood pressure and other cardiovascular changes. Headache is a common symptom of the elevated blood pressure (hypertension). Intracranial bleeding and death due to the hypertensive crises have been reported.[9]

Tyramine occurs naturally in certain foods such as aged cheeses, liver, dried fish, and in fermented alcoholic beverages such as beer, ale, and some wines (see Table 33–5). The foods listed in Table 33–5 are excluded from the diets of patients taking MAO inhibitors, although yeast bread is not excluded from the diet unless symptoms occur.

PROTEIN INTAKE AND LEVODOPA. Levodopa, a precursor of dopamine, is used in the treatment of parkinsonism, a neurological disorder in which there

Table 33-5. Food Rich in Tyramine*

Dairy Products	Meats
Yogurt	Liver
Aged Cheeses	Game
Cheddar	Dried fish
Gruyere	Herring
Stilton	Cod
Emmentaler	Caplin
Brie	Pickled Herring
Camembert	
Gouda	Vegetables
Mozzarella	Italian Broad Beans with Pods
Parmesan	(fava beans)
Provolone	
Romano	Others
Roquefort	Vanilla
	Chocolate
Alcoholic Beverages	Yeast and Yeast Extracts
Beer and Ale	Soya Sauce
Wine	
Chianti	
Sherry	
Riesling	
Sauterne	

*Adapted from Sen, J. P.: J. Food Science 34:22, 1969.

is a decrease in the dopamine of specific nerve cells. Parkinsonism occurs in the later decades of life and is characterized by involuntary tremulous motion and muscular weakness. Many patients with parkinsonism are markedly improved by daily doses of levodopa.

Mena and Cotzias[10] have observed that a high-protein diet (2 g. protein per kilogram of body weight) can block the effects of levodopa in the treatment of parkinsonism. From their observations they recommend a diet of 0.5 g. protein per kilogram of body weight.[11] Since the majority of these patients are older men and women, beyond the childbearing years, 0.5 g. protein chiefly of high biological value (see Chapter 31) can supply their needs for this nutrient.

SALICYLATE-INDUCED URTICARIA. Salicylate-induced urticaria (hives) responds not only to the avoidance of salicylates in medications (aspirin and other drugs containing salicylate) but also to the exclusion of naturally occuring salicylates in foods and a salicylate-related compound, tartrazine (Yellow No. 5, a food coloring).[12] Table 33-6 lists the foods which contain naturally occurring salicylates. These foods must be avoided by the patient with salicylate-induced urticaria. Tartrazine is widely used in food processing and is not listed on the product label. Unless information is obtained directly from the processor, all processed foods and beverages should be avoided. Noid et al[13] give a list of processed foods free of salicylates and tartrazine up to 1972. However, if any of the products have been modified since then, new information must be obtained from the producer.

Fresh meat, fish and poultry, whole or skim milk, regular bread, unprocessed cereals, butter, sugar, and the fruits and vegetables not listed in Table 33-6 can be used. Because the fruits are limited, a vitamin C supplement free of tartrazine is recommended.

MONOSODIUM GLUTAMATE. It has been observed that some individuals react adversely to monosodium glutamate, a flavor enhancer widely used in food processing. The reaction, known as the "Chinese restaurant syndrome," is characterized by headache, burning sensations of the extremities, facial pressure, and chest pain. It appears to be dose-related although the quantity of monosodium glutamate which stimulates the reaction varies from individual to individual. At this time it is suspected that monosodium glutamate, the sodium salt of glutamic acid, causes a transient hyponatremia.[14]

MISCELLANEOUS METABOLIC PROBLEMS
Hyperthyroidism

The patient with untreated hyperthyroidism, a condition characterized by excessive secretion of the hormone thyroxide that regulates metabolism, experiences hunger and weight loss. Medical or surgical treatment reduces the hypermetabolic state. However, before treatment can effect this change, patients may require 4000 to 5000 calories a day (adequate in all nutrients) to meet their metabolic needs and prevent further weight loss. Supplementary vitamins and minerals may be prescribed, and all stimulants such as tea, coffee, alcohol, and tobacco are limited or omitted.

In addition to regular meal service sizable snacks of sandwiches and other items should be available to the hospitalized patients at their request to avoid hunger.

Table 33-6. Foods Containing Salicylates*

Vegetables	Fruits (cont.)
Potatoes	Lemons
Cucumbers	Melons
Peppers (green, bell,	Nectarines
tobasco)	Oranges
Tomatoes	Peaches
	Plums
Fruits	Prunes
Apples	Raisins
Apricots	Raspberries
Blackberries	Strawberries
Boysenberries	
Cherries	Nuts
Currants	Almonds
Dewberries	
Gooseberries	Beverages
Grapefruit	Root Beer
Grapes	

*Adapted from Noid, H. E., et al: Arch. Dermatol. 109:866, 1974.

Hypoglycemia

Functional hypoglycemia without demonstrable organic disease may occur in adults. The symptoms of an attack are almost identical with those produced by an overdose of insulin and are due to low blood sugar. There is weakness, trembling, sweating, and extreme hunger. In severe cases there may be convulsions, hysterical symptoms, and, eventually, unconsciousness. The attacks do not occur in the fasting state. They are caused by overstimulation of the pancreas resulting in the production of excess insulin following a meal, particularly one high in quickly digested and absorbed carbohydrate. Abdominal discomfort, which is also characteristic, is sometimes ascribed to peptic ulcer because the symptoms are similar.

DIETARY TREATMENT. The objective of dietary treatment is to prevent a marked rise in the blood sugar that stimulates the pancreas to overproduce insulin. For this reason the individual must avoid the quickly digested sugars and limit other carbohydrate foods. The more slowly digested proteins and fats may be ingested freely.

The diet should contain from 120 to 150 g. of protein, from 75 to 100 g. of carbohydrate, and sufficient fat to meet caloric requirements. No candy, sugar, jellies, jams, desserts, and soft drinks containing sugar should be eaten. Saccharin may be substituted for sugar. The low carbohydrate vegetables and fruits (see Chapter 23), and limited quantities of bread, cereal, and potatoes should provide the carbohydrate of the diet. A generous serving of meat, fish, fowl, eggs, or cheese must be included at each meal. Because milk contains the sugar lactose, it must be limited to a pint a day in the adult. Butter or margarine, cream, bacon, mayonnnaise, and other oil dressing and meat fats supply the fat needed for calories. It is best to divide the food intake into five to eight meals a day. The patient may find it useful to carry crackers and a cube of cheese with him to control attacks if they are frequent.

STUDY QUESTIONS AND ACTIVITIES

1. What are some common allergenic foods?
2. Using the producers' literature, make a list of popular baby foods that cannot be fed to an infant who is allergic to cow's milk.
3. Plan an inexpensive dinner menu for a family of four—two adults and two children—with one child who is allergic to wheat.
4. At time of discharge from the obstetrical unit, Mrs. A is advised to be sure to eat high iron foods. She dislikes liver in any form. What foods would you suggest she eat to supply an adequate daily intake of iron? (See Chapter 6.)
5. Why may a patient who needs large doses of aspirin also be taking an antacid medication?

SUPPLEMENTARY READINGS

Berger, H.: Hypoglycemia: a perspective. Postgrad. Med. 57:81 (February), 1975.

Butterworth, C. E., Jr.: Interactions of nutrients with oral contraceptives and other drugs. J. Am. Dietet. A. 62:510, 1973.

Chabner, B. A., et al: The clinical pharmacology of antineoplastic agents. N. Eng. J. Med., 292:1107, 1975.

Gillespie, N. G., et al: Diets affecting treatment of parkinsonism with levodopa. J. Am. Dietet. A. 62:525, 1973.

Hethcox, J. M., and Stanaszek, W. F.: Interaction of drugs and diet. Hospital Pharmacy 9:373, 1974.

Ibarra, J. D., et al: Treatment of hyperthyroidism: panel discussion. Postgrad. Med. 57:84 (June) 1975.

Lutwak, L., et al: Current concepts of bone metabolism. Ann. Int. Med. 80:630, 1974.

Voight, M. N., et al: Tyramine, histamine, and tryptamine content of cheese. J. Milk and Food Tech. 37:377, 1974.

Wittig, H. J.: Diets for children with food allergies. Drug Therapy 5:129, 1975.

SOURCES OF RECIPES: ALLERGY DIETS

Allergy Recipes ($1.00). American Dietetic Association, 620 N. Michigan Avenue, Chicago, Illinois 60611.

Baking for People with Food Allergies ($.10). Superintendent of Documents, U.S. Government Printing Office, Washington, D. C. 20402.

Celiac Disease Recipes ($1.25). Hospital for Sick Children, 555 University, Toronto 5, Ontario, Canada.

Easy, Appealing Milk-Free Recipes. Mead-Johnson and Company, Evansville, Indiana 47221.

Great Recipes for Allergy Diets ($.50), and Helps for Allergics ($.10). Good Housekeeping Institute, 959 Eighth Avenue, New York, New York 10019.

Good Recipes to Brighten the Allergy Diet. Best Foods, Division of Corn Products Company, 10 E. 56th Street, New York, New York 10022.

Low Gluten Diet with Tested Recipes ($1.00). Arthur B. French, M.D., Clinical Research Unit, W 4644 University Hospital, Ann Arbor, Michigan 48104.

Shattuck, R. R.: *Creative Cooking Without Wheat, Milk and Eggs.* Cranbury, N. J., A. S. Barnes & Co., 1974.

Thomas, L. L.: *Caring and Cooking for the Allergic Child.* New York, Drake Publishers Inc., 1974.

For further references see Bibliography in Section 4.

REFERENCES

1. Ellis, E. F.: in *Nelson Textbook of Pediatrics*, ed. 10, V. C. Vaughan III and R. J. McKay, eds. Philadelphia, Saunders, 1975.
2. Rowe, A. H.: *Food Allergy*. Springfield, Thomas, 1972.
3. Lapus, W. E.: in *Nelson Textbook of Pediatrics*, ed. 10, op. cit.
4. Maclachlan, M. J. and Rodnan, G. P.: Am. J. Med. 42:38, 1967.
5. Ball, G. V. and Sorenson, L. B.: N. Eng. J. Med. 280:1199, 1969.
6. Lutwak, L., et al: Ann. Int. Med. 80:630, 1974.
7. Goodman, L. S. and Gilman, A., eds.: *A Pharmacological Basis of Therapeutics*, ed. 5. New York, Macmillan, 1975.
8. *Physician's Desk Reference*. Oradew, N. J., Medical Economics Co. (revised annually).
9. Jarvik, M. E.: in *The Pharmacological Basis of Therapeutics*, ed. 4, L. S. Goodman and A. Gilman, eds. New York, Macmillan, 1970.
10. Mena, I. and Cotzias, G. C: N. Eng. J. Med. 292:181, 1975.
11. Gillespie, N. G., et al: J. Am. Dietet. A. 62:525, 1973.
12. Noid, H. E., et al: Arch. Dermatol. 109:866, 1974.
13. Ibid.
14. Lambert, M. J.: Am. J. Nursing 75:403, 1975.

nutrition in diseases of infancy and childhood

34

Feeding the Sick Child

General Principles of Diet Therapy in Pediatric Nutrition

The Acutely Ill Infant or Young Child

Nutritional Problems in Otherwise Normal Infants and Children

Malabsorption Syndromes

Long-Term Illnesses

There are two major categories of illness presented by the infant or child admitted to the pediatric unit of a general hospital or to a pediatric hospital. The illness may be caused by extrinsic or environmental factors; or it may be related to intrinsic factors, problems existing at or before birth. Some of the problems which derive from extrinsic factors are acute infections, those not controlled by immunization, such as respiratory or gastrointestinal infections; accidents either within or outside the home, including burns; child abuse, including physical injury or underfeeding; and emotional problems. Some of the intrinsic problems which may be present at birth or expressed at a later time are congenital anomalies of various structures such as the heart, kidneys, palate, esophagus, intestines, skeleton, and neurologic system; and inborn errors of metabolism. Some of the malignancies of early childhood are also categorized as intrinsic in origin.

The majority of infants and children whether they are at home or in the hospital need a diet which supplies the energy and nutrients appropriate to the age of the child. This applies even to the acutely ill child after the treatment of the critical problem, such as the correction of dehydration due to infectious diarrhea, or to the child who has undergone surgery. Some children with a birth defect or long-term illness may need modifications in the consistency of food or in the feeding method, such as the child with a cleft palate or the child with cerebral palsy. Other children may need modifications in nutrient intake, such as a sodium-restricted diet for the child with a congenital anomaly of the heart or the restriction of phenylalanine, an essential amino acid, in phenylketonuria, an inborn error of metabolism. Normal diet for age is presented in Chapters 17 and 18. The information in these chapters should be reviewed for it applies to the sick infant or child as well.

Although the sick infant or child is the primary focus of the health care team, they must also meet the needs of the parents. During the acute illness of their child, parents are anxious and their anxieties can often be relieved if the health-care team takes time to communicate with them. When the child with either an acute or a long-term illness is hospitalized, many mothers will want to be involved in their rhildren's care, especially at meal times. These women need to be accepted as members of the health-care team. On the other hand a woman who cannot be at the hospital with her child because she has other children at home or has to work to support her family should not be slighted by the team. Rather, they should accept her situation and communicate with her whenever she is available. And, in some situations, it may be the father or grandparents who join the team.

The families of children with handicaps or long-term illnesses present special problems. Handicaps and long-term illnesses often demand major adjustments in a family's life-style and the continuing care of the child may take a significant portion of the income for such items as drugs, food, and special equipment. For example, one quart (approximately one liter) of medium-chain triglyceride oil costs approximately seven times as much as one quart of vegetable oil. The needs of other children in the family may not be met because of the time, energy, and money expended by the parents in caring for the ill child.

At the same time parents may have strong feelings of anxiety and guilt at having produced a child who is handicapped or has a long-term illness. As a result they may overprotect or completely reject the child. They may also reject genetic counseling in applicable situations. As the child grows into adolescence, questions may arise in his mind about his future, about marriage, about supporting himself, and always, about being different.

These are problems the health-care team will share with the families of these children. The team must be able to cope with the family's anxieties, to counsel the parents on how to care for the child, and to build the parents' confidence in their ability to carry out the program of care. The family must also be informed of where to find financial help and other community resources. Financial aid is available through Medicaid and other federal funding for the costs of medical care for many sick children.

Organizations of parents, professional persons, and other interested individuals, such as the American Diabetes Association, the United Cerebral Palsy Association, and the National Cystic Fibrosis Research Foundation, among others, were founded to stimulate research and to promote knowledge of the disease and care of the afflicted child. Local chapters of the national associations are often of great help to parents by enabling them to share their anxieties and fears with others facing the same problems, and to channel their feelings into constructive action.

FEEDING THE SICK CHILD
Food and Illness

When children become ill they tend to regress to an earlier developmental level. A 13-month-old-baby who has been drinking from a cup may only accept fluids from a nursing bottle, or a two and one-half year old who has been doing a good job of feeding himself may now want to be fed. Also, the type of food the sick child will accept is often limited. The wisest response in a short-term illness such as a cold or minor gastrointestinal upset is to let him have his way, but be sure his fluid intake is adequate. When he feels better, he will return quickly to his more recently acquired food practices and will make up, both in quantity and in quality, the nutrients that were missing in his diet during his illness.

Food intake may become a serious problem in the child who has a long-term illness. Enough food must be eaten to provide his nutritional needs for growth and development. If a modified diet is not required as part of his treatment, he should be offered the normal diet-for-age (see Chapters 17 and 18.) If he has a poor appetite, it may be easier for him to eat smaller, more frequent meals and occasional surprises may help him look forward to mealtimes. However, it may not be wise to offer the very young child who is ill a meal of totally unfamiliar foods or new combinations of his favorite foods. For the child restricted to bed at home, a picnic lunch with his family or a special afternoon snack with his friends in the neighborhood may stimulate him to eat more than he would otherwise. In some situations poor food acceptance by the child with a long-term illness may be a symptom of a poor relationship between the mother and child and the mother may need counseling to solve the problem.

Some children with long-term illnesses will overeat, with the result that they may become obese. Eating is the only recreation for some of these children. They need help in developing new hobbies and activities.

The Child in the Hospital

The sick child who must be hospitalized finds himself in strange surroundings among strange people. In the midst of all this strangeness the one experience he may recognize and enjoy is food. In this new setting the child must be given a great deal of freedom about his food, even to the point of being allowed to refuse it. Some children will eat only bread and butter and drink milk for the first few days in the hospital, as these foods are most reminiscent of home. Children from homes with ethnic food patterns which differ from those of the community at large may have considerable difficulty accepting unfamiliar foods.

In so far as possible, the food served by the dietary department should reflect the usual food practices of the community. It is helpful if, on admission or as soon as possible after admission, the staff obtains from the mother of the young child or directly from the older child a list of his food preferences in order to avoid serving him foods which he dislikes even when well. This will help to bridge the gap between home and hospital. This does not solve the problem, however, because the methods of food preparation vary and the taste of a food prepared in the hospital may differ from the same dish prepared at home. Also, today's child may not be comparing the food served in the hospital with that served at home, but with his

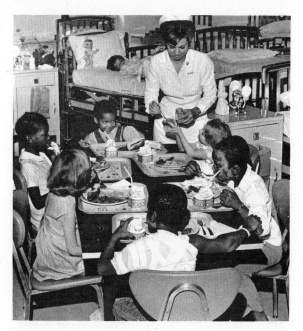

Fig. 34-1. Meals taste better when they are eaten in company with other children in the hospital. (Arkansas Children's Hospital, Little Rock, Arkansas)

past experiences of eating away from home in fast-food service chains, or in preschool or school feeding programs.

Another way of helping the child to feel at home in the hospital is to have him eat at a table with other children of his age as soon as this is feasible (Fig. 34-1). Children often eat better around a table with other children. Also, it takes the time of only one staff member to help these children in a group as compared with the number of staff required to serve individual children in their rooms or at bedside in a ward. When a hospitalized child has a birthday, a birthday cake shared with other patients his age helps to relieve the unpleasantness of illness.

Table 34-1. Daily Amounts of Foods to Meet Energy Needs of 2- to 6-Year-Old Children

FOOD EXCHANGES	2 TO 3 YEARS AMT.	ENERGY (kcal.)*	3 to 4 YEARS AMT.	ENERGY (kcal.)	4 to 6 YEARS AMT.	ENERGY (kcal.)
Milk	3 c. (750 ml.)	510	3 c. (750 ml.)	510	4 c. (1000 ml.)	680
Meat	1 oz. (30 g.)	75	2 oz. (60 g.)	150	2 oz. (60 g.)	150
Egg	1	75	1	75	1	75
Bread	4 Exchanges	280	4 Exchanges	280	5 Exchanges	350
Fruit	2 servings	80	2 servings	80	2 servings	80
Vegetables B	1 serving	35	1 serving	35	1 serving	35
Fat	2 tsp.	90	3 tsp.	135	3 tsp.	135
Dessert†	2/3 serving	100	1 serving	150	1 serving	150
Totals		1245		1415		1655
NRC-RDA	1250 kcal.		1400 kcal.		1600 kcal.	

*Exchange System. Chapter 23.
†Chocolate Pudding. Table 1, Section 4.

Most of all, it is important that mealtime be a happy time, with no pressures about cleaning up plates, drinking all the milk, or not being allowed dessert because not all the other food served was eaten. The dessert should be as important a source of nutrients as any other item on the menu. An illness is not the time for a child to have to learn to eat new foods or to acquire new skills in eating unless he does this on his own initiative. Also, mealtimes should *never* be interrupted to draw blood, change dressings, or to do other painful procedures; and treatments such as physiotherapy and postural drainage should be scheduled so that the child has a rest period before his meals.

The size of a serving offered the child is also important. "Appetite poor" recorded in the nursing notes may mean that a child was served too much food. A serving of 4 ounces (120 ml.) of soup and half a sandwich is adequate for many two to three year olds, while a 12-year-old boy may need a "man size" serving. Table 34–1, using the Exchange System, illustrates the amount of food needed in a day to meet the energy needs of children two to six years old. When this food is distributed over three meals and two or three between meal feedings, the servings are small by adult standards.

Finally, parents have rights. The mother who spends the day with her hospitalized child usually wants to contribute to his care. Choosing the food and feeding the child may be the only contribution she can make. This is especially true if the child has a terminal illness. These mothers may be demanding: they have a right to be demanding and their demands should be met if possible.

GENERAL PRINCIPLES OF DIET THERAPY IN PEDIATRIC NUTRITION

Whenever the diet must be modified as part of the treatment of illness in an infant or child, the following general principles must be considered in each situation. In this way, the therapeutic diet plan will not only contribute to the treatment of the specific problem but also promote, in so far as possible, the normal growth and development of the child.

Energy–Protein

In order to support normal growth the energy and protein needs of the child must be met. For example, the dwarfism in children with diabetes which occurred in the 1930s was due more to inadequate energy intakes than to poor control of the disease with regular insulin.

Table 34–2 is a guide to the energy and protein

Table 34–2. Guide for Calculating Energy and Protein Needs for Infants and Children*

AGE (years)	ENERGY (kcal./kg.)	PROTEIN (g./kg.)
0.0-0.5	117	2.2
0.5-1.0	108	2.0
1-3	100	1.8
4-6	90	1.5
7-10	80	1.2
Males		
11-14	65	1.0
15-18	50	0.9
Females		
11-14	55	1.0
15-18	40	0.9

*Calculated from NAS-NRC, Recommended Dietary Allowances, ed. 8. Washington, D. C., 1974.

needs per kilogram of body weight for infants and children by age; and for adolescents by age and sex. The energy figures in this table can be used to estimate reasonable goals for daily calorie intakes. The estimate may need to be revised because the rate of growth and the energy expenditure due to the level of activity varies with each infant and child. However, the energy intake should not be significantly less than recommended, since, without an adequate energy intake from fat and carbohydrate, the protein in the diet will be utilized for energy rather than for the synthesis of cellular proteins. One seven-month-old infant boy was significantly underweight due to a daily energy deficit of 400 kcal. with no deficit in protein intake.

If the infant or child has experienced growth retardation due to his illness, the estimate of daily energy and total nutrient intake may need to be adjusted upward for a period of time to support catch-up growth. A formula containing 24 kcal. per ounce (30 ml.) may be used for an infant under two months of age, while increased quantities of a formula containing 20 kcal. per ounce (30 ml.) plus infant foods such as cereal may be adequate for the older infant. The older child will need larger servings of an adequate diet-for-age to catch up. Daily weighing of infants and weekly weighing of very young children is used to monitor the adequacy of energy intake.

When the protein is adjusted for therapeutic reasons two important factors must be considered. If total protein intake is limited, proteins of high biological value must be supplied to support the infant's or child's requirement of essential amino acids. For example, the order for 1.5 g. of protein per kilogram of body weight for a two-week-old infant with an inborn error of metabolism in the urea cycle must provide the infant's requirement for the essential amino acids without an excessive quantity of nonessential nitrogen.

The essential amino acid requirements of infants two to four months of age as determined by Holt and Snyderman and coworkers are listed in Chapter 35, Table 35-1, in the section on inborn errors of amino acid metabolism. These investigators[1] have also shown that the infants they studied grew well on an intake of 1.3 g. of cow's milk protein per kilogram of body weight with supplemental nitrogen. This quantity of milk protein supplied the amount of essential amino acids required by their subjects. In clinical practice one can determine the amount of cow's milk protein required to supply an infant's essential amino acid requirement and supplement this with cereal for an adequate nitrogen supply.

Although the infant and the young child require more protein per kilogram of body weight than do adults to support cellular growth, excessive intakes of protein can be hazardous. In early infancy an intake in excess of 4 to 5 g. of protein per kilogram of body weight per day should be carefully monitored because kidney, and possibly liver, function is immature at this age. Excessive blood levels of the endproducts of protein catabolism, particularly ammonia, can be detrimental to the developing central nervous system. In any child excessive intakes of protein without adequate fluid intake can lead to dehydration.

Fluids

Unless contraindicated by a medical problem such as renal failure, the normal fluid requirements of the infant and the child must be taken into consideration when planning therapeutic diets. Table 34-3 gives the range of average fluid requirements for infants and children under ordinary conditions. Until the infant is introduced to table foods, formula and infant foods generally supply the daily fluid needs. In the older child fluid needs can be met by water and a variety of other fluids including milk and fruit juices.

Fats

Fats supply approximately 50 percent of the total energy intake of the breast fed infant. The energy from fat in the commonly used infant formulas varies from 45 to 50 percent. As the child grows older fat usually supplies 35 to 45 percent of the total energy intake. The diet of an infant or young child must contain one to two percent of total calories from linoleic acid, the essential fatty acid (see Chapter 3, Fats). When

Table 34-3. Range of Average Daily Fluid Requirements of Infants and Children Under Ordinary Conditions*

Age	Average Body Weight (kg.)	Fluid per kg. of Body Weight (ml.)
3 days	3.0	80-100
10 days	3.2	125-150
3 months	5.4	140-160
6 months	7.3	130-155
9 months	8.6	125-145
1 year	9.5	120-135
2 years	11.8	115-125
4 years	16.2	100-110
6 years	20.0	90-100
10 years	28.7	70-85
14 years	45.0	50-60
18 years	54.0	40-50

*Adapted from Nelson Textbook of Pediatrics, ed. 10, Phila., Saunders, 1975, pg. 147.

medium-chain triglycerides are used as the major source of fat in a formula for an infant with malabsorption problems, a source of linoleic acid must be included, since medium-chain triglyceride oils do not contain linoleic acid. Corn oil, which contains linoleic acid, is added to special infant formulas which derive their fat content primarily from medium-chain triglycerides (see Table 34-4, Special Infant Formulas). The older child can use the appropriate amounts of margarine or mayonnaise made with corn oil if the diet pattern does not include linoleic acid from other sources.

If a child has a familial hyperlipoproteinemia, the type of fatty acid and/or the cholesterol will be modified as recommended for the type of lipid problem (see Chapter 29, Atherosclerosis).

Carbohydrate

Carbohydrate usually supplies 45 to 50 percent of the total energy intake of infants and young children. Without a source of carbohydrate in the diet, infants will develop hypoglycemia. One formula, CHO-Free*, is available for infants with carbohydrate malabsorption problems. The formula contains protein and fat, but a carbohydrate which is tolerated by the infant must be added to prevent hypoglycemia and ketosis.[2]

The amount of sucrose should be limited in any therapeutic diet, as in any normal diet-for-age, to prevent dental caries. In hyperlipoproteinemias and diabetes mellitus the type of carbohydrate, simple vs. complex, may also be modified.

*Syntex Laboratories, Palo Alto, Ca., 94304

Table 34–4. Special Formulas with Vitamins and Minerals Added*

Product and Producer	Protein	Carbohydrate	Fat	Special Comments	Uses
SOY-BASED LACTOSE-FREE					
Cho-Free Formula Base, Syntex Laboratories, Palo Alto, Ca. 94304	Soy Isolate	To be added	Soy oil	Carbohydrate *must* be added, concentrate†	Diarrhea, disaccharidase intolerance
Isomil, Ross Laboratories, Columbus, Ohio 43216	Soy Isolate	Corn syrup, sucrose, modified cornstarch	Soy, coconut, and corn oil	Concentrate or ready to feed	Diarrhea, cow's milk allergy, lactase deficiency
Mull-Soy, Syntex Laboratories	Soy Flour	Sucrose	Soy oil	Concentrate	For older infants, children, and adults with cow's milk allergy
Neo-Mull Soy, Syntex Laboratories	Soy Isolate	Sucrose	Soy oil	Concentrate	Cow's milk allergy, lactase deficiency
Prosobee, Mead-Johnson Laboratories, Evansville, Ind. 47721	Soy Isolate	Sucrose, corn syrup solids	Soy oil	Concentrate	Cow's milk allergy, lactase deficiency, galactosemia (see Chapter 35)
Soyalac, Loma Linda Food, Riverside, Ca. 92505	Soybean solids and methionine	Dextrins, maltose, dextrose from cornstarch, beet sugar	Soybean oil	Concentrate, 13 percent of total calories from protein	Cow's milk allergy
NON-SOY, LACTOSE-FREE					
Nutramigen, Mead-Johnson Laboratories	Enzymatically hydrolyzed and charcoal-treated casein	Sucrose, tapioca starch	Corn oil	Powder[a] (9.5 g./2 oz. water = 20 kcal./oz.) 15 percent of calories from protein	Diarrhea, cow's milk allergy, galactosemia
MBF (meat base formula), Gerber Products Co. Fremont, Mich. 49412	Beef hearts	Sucrose, tapioca starch	Sesame oil	Concentrate	Cow's milk allergies
Pregestimil, Mead-Johnson Laboratories	Enzymatically hydrolyzed and charcoal-treated casein	Dextrose, tapioca starch	Medium-chain triglycerides, corn oil	Powder (9.5 g./2 oz. water = 20 kcal./oz. 13 percent of calories from protein	Diarrhea, disaccharidase deficiency, steatorrhea
OTHER SPECIAL FORMULAS					
Lofenalac, Mead-Johnson Laboratories	Casein hydrolysate processed to remove most of the phenylalanine, amino acids added	Corn syrup solids, tapioca starch	Corn oil	Powder (9.5 g./2 oz. water = 20 kcal./oz. and approximately 7.9 mg. phenylalanine) 15 percent of calories from protein	Phenylketonuria
Portagen, Mead-Johnson Laboratories	Sodium Caseinate	Sucrose, maltodextrins	Medium-chain triglycerides, corn oil	Powder (8.5 g./2 oz. water = 20 kcal./oz.) 14 percent of calories from protein	Fat malabsorption
Probana, Mead-Johnson Laboratories	Whole milk curd with skim milk curd with added lactic acid, enzymatic casein hydrolysate	Banana powder, dextrose, lactose	Corn oil	Powder (9.5 g./2 oz. water = 20 kcal./oz.) 24 percent of calories from protein and 29 percent from fat	Diarrhea, steatorrhea

*From producer's information.
†Liquid, to be diluted as directed.
[a]Powder, to be reconstituted as directed.

Table 34–4. *(continued)*

Product and Producer	Protein	Carbohydrate	Fat	Special Comments	Uses
Similac PM 60/40, Ross Laboratories	Partially demineralized whey, partially demineralized nonfat milk	Lactose	Corn, coconut oil	Powder (8.56 g./2 oz. water = 20 kcal./oz.) 60/40 ratio lactalbumin: casein, electrolyte content similar to human milk	Renal and cardiac disease
SMA, S-29, Wyeth Laboratories Phila., Pa. 19101	Demineralized whey	Lactose	Oleo, coconut, safflower, and soy oil	Powder (8.5 g./2 oz. water = 20 kcal./oz.) very low in electrolytes	Acute congestive heart failure and acute renal failure
SMA, S-14, Wyeth Laboratories	Nonfat milk	Lactose	Oleo, coconut, safflower, and soy oil	Powder (7.5 g./2 oz. water = 20 kcal./oz.) 7 percent of calories from protein, low in leucine	Leucine-induced hypoglycemia (see Chapter 35)
OTHER PRODUCTS					
Casec, Mead-Johnson Laboratories	Dried, soluble calcium caseinate derived from skim milk curd	Trace	None	Powder (4.7 g. contains 4 g. protein, 75 mg. calcium, 2.7 mg. sodium, and 17 kcal.)	Protein supplement or for designing individualized formulas
Dextri-Maltose, Mead-Johnson Laboratories	None	Glucose, maltose, and oligosaccharides derived from cornstarch by controlled acid/enzyme hydrolysis	None	Powder (7 g. = 27 kcal.)	Carbohydrate supplement for formulas
MCT Oil, Mead-Johnson Laboratories	None	None	Triglycerides of medium-chain fatty acids	Liquid (14 g. = 115 kcal.) 71 percent C8 and 23 percent C10	Substitution for energy from long-chain fatty acids
Polycose, Ross Laboratories	None	Primarily maltose and oligosaccharides derived from cornstarch by controlled hydrolysis	None	Powder (8 g. = 30 kcal. and 10 mg. sodium), liquid (1 oz. = 60 kcal. and 21 mg. sodium)	Carbohydrate supplement for formulas

Electrolytes

With problems of excessive fluid and electrolyte loss in infancy and early childhood, oral solutions of electrolytes may be required (see discussion of diarrhea in next section). In other situations, especially in renal and cardiac disease, the intake of sodium and potassium may be modified.

Vitamins

If the therapeutic diet cannot supply an adequate intake of vitamins, supplements are used. However, excessive intakes of vitamins, especially the fat-soluble ones, must be avoided. When fat malabsorption occurs, as in cystic fibrosis, water-soluble preparations of the fat-soluble vitamins are used.

Minerals

Care must be taken to assure that therapeutic diets for infants and children contain adequate amounts of minerals. It must be remembered that the quantity of a mineral required at one age may not be adequate as the child grows older. For example at one month of age Fomon[3] advises a daily iron intake of 7 mg. and at two to three months, 8 mg. The trace mineral composition of synthetic formulas used in the treatment of inborn errors of amino acid metabolism must be checked carefully to assure adequate intakes.

Special Infant Formulas

Special infant formulas, which vary from the standard ones (see Table 17–4, Chapter 17) in the kinds and amounts of ingredients, are widely available to meet the nutrient needs of infants with metabolic problems. Although the majority of special formulas have the same energy content as the standard ones (20 kcal./30 ml., normal dilution) the food sources of protein, fat, and carbohydrate differ. For example, some formulas have soy isolate as the source of protein for infants who are allergic to milk protein. (see Table 34–4).

Special infant formulas can also be prepared from basic ingredients: casein, dextrin, sugars, and fats (see Table 34–4). Formulas prepared from basic ingredients must contain a reasonable distribution of protein, fat, and carbohydrate, and usually require the addition of minerals, vitamins, and electrolytes. Because all special formulas (concentrates or powders) must be mixed with water to normal dilution they must be terminally sterilized before they can be fed to an infant.

THE ACUTELY ILL INFANT OR YOUNG CHILD
Diarrhea

Mild or acute diarrhea may occur in infants and young children for a variety of reasons. A major cause is bacterial or viral infection in the gastrointestinal tract or infection in another part of the body such as the respiratory tract. Noninfectious diarrhea may be caused by food allergies, emotional problems, excessive ingestion of certain foods and unripe fruits, starvation, or malabsorption syndromes such as celiac sprue and cystic fibrosis. Celiac sprue is discussed in Chapter 25 and cystic fibrosis, later in this chapter. Chronic intractable diarrhea in the newborn is a serious problem and may be treated by hyperalimentation[4] to support growth and development in the first weeks or months of life.

ACUTE DIARRHEA. Severe dehydration with electrolyte imbalance due to diarrhea is life-threatening to the infant. Also, severe dehydration and febrile seizures may damage his central nervous system. The first need of these patients is to reestablish fluid and electroylte balance. If the child is vomiting, intravenous fluids with dextrose and electrolytes are used. If the infant is not vomiting an oral electrolyte solution* may be used. After reestablishing fluid and electrolyte balance, the nutrient and energy needs of each patient must be met by oral feeding to make up for losses during the acute phase of illness and to support normal growth and development.

When the diarrhea has subsided and the infant is ready for oral feeding, a dilute formula is offered, usually 10 to 13 Kcal. per ounce (30 ml.). After the infant has demonstrated tolerance for oral feeding with the dilute formula, one of normal dilution of 20 Kcal. per ounce (30 ml.) is used and, depending on age, cereals and vegetables can be included in the diet. The quantity of any foods taken and retained are recorded after each feeding. Every 24 hours the Kcal. per kilogram consumed are estimated and recorded. This information is correlated with daily weights to

*Lytren, Mead Johnson, Evansville, Ind. 47721
 Pedialyte, Ross Laboratories, Columbus, Ohio 43216

assess the infant's progress. An infant can be expected to take 100 to 120 Kcal. per kilogram per day or more if required for catch-up growth.

Following diarrhea many infants are lactose intolerant[5] and require a lactose-free formula such as Isomil, Pregestimil, or CHO-Free, with carbohydrate other than lactose added. (See Table 34–4 for listing of special formulas.) In about four months after recovery from diarrhea most infants will tolerate lactose. The electrolyte composition, especially sodium and potassium, may also be a factor in prescribing a formula for an infant recovering from diarrhea.

In the past, boiled skim milk was offered infants with diarrhea. This is no longer recommended because the boiling reduces the total water content of the milk, which results in an increase in the total amount of protein, sodium, and potassium per ounce. This concentration of protein and electrolytes may be hazardous in the very young infant because of his immature kidney function or he may be hypernatremic.

Acute diarrhea with dehydration is critical in the young child, ages one to four; however, it is not as devastating as it is in the infant unless it is accompanied by meningitis or encephalitis. Children one to two years of age who have previously been weaned may prefer to take fluids from a nursing bottle and older children may more readily accept fluids other than milk. In addition to water and milk, fruit juices, fruit drinks fortified with vitamin C, popsicles, and carbonated beverages are commonly used to meet fluid needs. Some clinicians use cola syrups to supply glucose and potassium.

Carbonated beverages are usually more acceptable to the yearling if the beverage is poured in advance of offering, to reduce the fizziness. Before offering carbonated beverages to a child, it is a good idea to check with the parents. They may not serve these beverages to the child at home and may not want them used in the hospital. Because there are various other fluids with which the child is familiar and which he usually accepts, there is no reason why the parent's wishes cannot be met.

As these children recover they usually tolerate a soft or simple regular diet adequate to support the nutritional needs of their age group (see Chapter 17). Fluid and food intake, both in kind and amount, should be recorded after each meal.

MILD DIARRHEA. Infants and children with mild diarrhea of one to three or four days duration are usually treated in the home, especially if the problem is not complicated by continued vomiting. Food is withheld for no longer than 24 hours but fluid and electrolyte intake must be maintained. If required,

Lytren* or Pedialyte†, water and electrolyte solutions with minimal amounts of glucose, are available for home use with infants. Mothers need precise directions for using these products. They should keep accurate records of the amount taken and retained and report this information to the pediatrician as requested; also they should discontinue use when advised to do so.

In the past, mothers were advised to offer their infants a homemade glucose and electrolyte solution containing water, Karo Syrup, and a specified amount of salt (NaCl). This practice has been discontinued because it is hazardous. If the salt is not measured carefully and too much is given, the infant can develop hypernatremia.

When an infant's diarrhea subsides, the mother may be advised to offer a dilute (10 to 13 cal./30 ml.) lactose-free formula. At this point the mother also needs precise directions and follow-up. Growth retardation has been noted in infants who were still on the dilute formula two weeks or more after recovery from diarrhea. The mother did not understand that she should resume the normal feeding program.

Water and electrolyte intake can be maintained in the one- to four-year-old child with mild diarrhea by use of such fluids as fruit juice or plain tomato juice, carbonated beverages, dilute tea made from instant tea with sugar added, dilute broth from meat, vegetable soups, or milk, if tolerated. Broth made from bouillon cubes is to be avoided because they contain excessive amounts of sodium and no carbohydrate. Other than the dilute broths from soups, tomato juice, and milk, all other fluids contain potassium and carbohydrate but no sodium. Therefore, a varied selection of fluids, with the addition of saltines or potato chips if tolerated, should be used to assure an intake of sodium as well as potassium and carbohydrate.

Within 24 hours most young children with mild diarrhea will accept a diet-for-age containing their usual food choices. If the diarrhea continues for more than four days, it may be indicative of a malabsorption syndrome requiring dietary treatment.

Surgery or Trauma

After minor surgery most infants and children will be offered diet-for-age when they recover from anesthesia. There are a variety of regimens for feeding the child after a tonsillectomy. These regimens, in general, avoid very hot or cold fluids and any acid juices such as orange, grapefruit, or tomato juice. Milk is usually avoided immediately after surgery because it coats the incision and causes discomfort.

*Mead Johnson, Evansville, Ind. 47721
†Ross Laboratories, Columbus, Ohio 43216

BURNS. After fluid and electrolyte balance has been established and the burned child can tolerate oral feedings, the most important factor in his recovery is his food intake. A goal should be set to provide him with energy and all nutrients in excess of his normal allowances to compensate for losses from the burn surface area and to support wound healing. At this time there is no generally accepted formula for estimating a burned child's specific needs for energy and nutrients comparable to that of adults (see Chapter 26, Surgery: Burns). However, energy and nutrient needs will vary not only by age but also by the amount and degree of surface area burned. Excessive intakes of protein without adequate energy and fluids should be avoided.

Children with burns need the support and acceptance of every member of the health care team.[6] The child's food likes and dislikes should be respected as much as possible. High calorie-high protein supplements acceptable to the child are usually needed to add to his food intake at mealtimes. Milk shakes made from milk, nonfat skim milk, and ice cream can be used to make such supplements, or the child may be offered a commercial supplement (see Table 26–3, Chapter 26). Since these children may be hospitalized from six weeks to as long as six months, there should be considerable variation in the menu from day to day, taking into consideration their food likes and dislikes. Mothers can often contribute to food intake by making a child's favorite dish or bringing him a pizza from the shop in his neighborhood.

TUBE FEEDINGS. The infant who requires a tube feeding can be fed a formula of standard dilution (20 Kcal./30 ml) by nasogastric or gastrostomy tube. When the volume of formula cannot provide an adequate energy intake as the infant grows, cereal can be added to the formula. Since a nasogastric tube has a smaller bore than a gastrostomy tube because of the size of an infant's nasal passage, the amount of cereal which can be added to a nasogastric feeding will be limited. With too much cereal the mixture will be too thick to pass through the tube into the stomach.

For the older infant and the young child it is necessary to design a tube feeding which meets an individual's specific energy and nutrient needs. Most standard tube feedings, whether commercial products or prepared in the hospital, are designed for adults and cannot be used for the child under three years of age. The protein and electrolyte content of most of these formulas may be too high for children under three.

Tube feedings can be formulated for individual children from powdered or concentrated infant formulas which permits the adjustment of the amount of nutrients and the total fluid used. Casec*, dried soluble calcium caseinate made from skim milk curd, can also be used as a source of protein. Dextri-Maltose†, Karo Syrup**, or Polycose††, together with infant fruits and cereals, can be used as additional sources of energy from carbohydrate. Dextri-Maltose and Polycose are derived from the acid hydrolysis of corn starch while Karo Syrup contains hydrolyzed cornstarch with sucrose and salt added.

The tube feeding should contain approximately 100 Kcal. per 100 ml. For example, a two-year-old child weighing 12 kg. requires about 1200 Kcal. per day

(100 Kcal./kg. × 12 kg. = 1200 Kcal.) and about 1500 ml. of fluid per day (125 ml./kg. × 12 kg. = 1500 ml.).

(see Tables 34–2 and 34–3.) Therefore, 1200 ml. of formula containing 1200 Kcal. plus 300 ml. of water for giving medication and for testing the patency of the feeding tube will supply both the fluid and energy needs of this child every 24 hours. Unless otherwise ordered protein should provide no more than 10 to 12 percent of total Kcal.; fat, about 35 percent; and carbohydrate, the rest, about 50 percent. The composition per 100 ml. of Kcal., protein, fat, carbohydrate, sodium, potassium, chloride, and phosphorus should be recorded in the patient's record and the recipe of ingredients should be readily available to the health care team.

NUTRITIONAL PROBLEMS IN OTHERWISE NORMAL INFANTS AND CHILDREN
Underweight

Children vary greatly in their rate of growth. If a child gains weight and grows in height at a regular rate, even though he is somewhat thinner than other children of his height and age, there is no cause for concern. Mothers should be reminded that a child's growth rate declines in velocity at the end of the first year of life and that the child's appetite compensates for this decrease. The child who fails to grow and gain regularly should have his food habits and home environment investigated. Poor housing, inadequate sleeping space, a mother who cannot remain at home, and poverty may contribute to the child's failure to gain.

The school breakfast and lunch programs available in most urban areas can help the child improve his food habits and provide him with as much as half or more of the needed nutrients each day. Under the guidance of the teacher and the school health counselor, children and parents may be helped to achieve better nutrition as well as better patterns of rest and sleep for the underweight child.

Occasionally, one sees a child who is anorexic as a result of the mother's anxiety about his food intake. If the child is otherwise well, the mother needs to be reassured that he will eat eventually if tensions are relieved and he is allowed some choice in deciding how much and what he can eat. For the child who has limited himself to a very few foods this may mean an inadequate diet for a while, but variety in preparation may help to introduce other foods. When the child's appetite has returned to some extent and he begins to look forward to his meals, small quantities of new foods may be tried one at a time. It is always best to serve very small portions and let the child ask for a second helping. Eventually such a child will eat a varied and adequate diet if the tensions about food intake are not renewed.

Growth Failure Due to Underfeeding

When the physician records an infant's or child's "failure-to-thrive" he is dealing with unknown or unrecognized factors. Many of these are being identified, such as inborn errors of metabolism discussed in Chapter 35.

Other factors besides disease may be responsible for a child's failure-to-thrive. The problem of the severely growth-retarded infant, usually under 18 months of age, who has no disease or birth defect, has been called emotional, environmental, or maternal deprivation. When these infants are admitted to the hospital they may be severely dehydrated due to infection, and obviously malnourished. Some may even be marasmic. They may also be retarded in motor development, and most of them take very little interest in their environment.

Bowlby[7] and others have shown that if the infant is to reach the developmental milestones of the first year of life, there must be social interaction between the mother and infant as well as routine physical care. This applies to the infant's own mother or any other persons taking care of him. It has been observed that the infant with growth failure without disease has not experienced adequate mother-child interaction; and that the mothers of these infants are overburdened with personal problems and are unable to meet the physical or psychosocial needs of their infants. Whitten[8] and coworkers have shown that the physical growth failure of these infants is due to underfeeding, while the mothers are not even aware that they are underfeeding them.

*Mead Johnson, Evansville, Ind. 47721.
†Mead Johnson, Evansville, Ind. 47721.
**Best Foods, Englewood Cliffs, N. J. 07632.
††Ross Laboratories, Columbus, Ohio 43216.

On admission to the hospital these infants require the same care as any acutely ill infant with diarrhea. Given a normal diet for age when fluid and electrolyte balance has been reestablished, the infant will increase his intake in three to five days to the point where he will be consuming more food and gaining more weight than expected for his age. For example, one five-month-old infant consumed 150 to 170 Kcal. per kg. (normal, 100 to 120 Kcal.) and gained an average of 70 g. weight per day (normal, about 20 g.) for a two week period.

In addition, it is advisable that these infants be fed and played with by one caretaking person as frequently as possible within the staffing schedules of the nursing unit. A volunteer, or a student, with a particular interest in this problem may be willing to commit herself for eight or nine consecutive days to give intensive care to such an infant and to help him achieve his developmental milestones.

The future of these children depends on two factors: (1) the age at which the underfeeding occurs; and (2), the help the mother and the family receive to solve their problems. Chase and coworkers[9] indicate that the longer the nutritional deprivation exists in early infancy, the less likely the infant is to achieve his growth potential. At the same time the infant is being rehabilitated in the hospital, the family should be receiving intensive counseling. This counseling needs to be continued if the child is to be protected from future episodes of nutritional deprivation.

Obesity

With the realization that much adult obesity has its origins in infancy, childhood, and adolescence, the prevention of obesity begins in infancy (see Chapter 27). At present there is no generally accepted method for identifying the obese infant although a significant discrepancy in percentiles between the length and weight of an infant plotted on a growth chart does indicate a potential problem. For example, a five-month-old infant whose weight is in the ninetieth percentile and whose length is in the tenth percentile is probably obese. Crawford and coworkers[10] concluded from their study that the best obesity index for infants six months of age is a weight gain greater than 5.34 kg. during the period from birth to six months of age. The actual birth weight and date the infant was born must be known in order to apply this index.

As with an obese adult, an obese infant may be overfed or underactive.[11] In any contact with infants and their mothers throughout the first year of life in a health care setting, it is strongly recommended that the daily food intake and activity and sleep pattern of the infant be appraised at each visit. No more than 120 Kcal. per kilogram per day is appropriate for the very young infant and no more than 100 Kcal. per kilogram, for the older infant. The food intake correlated with the activity and sleep pattern should be used as the basis for counseling the mother. She may be overfeeding her infant because she cannot distinguish between a hunger cry or other crying. On the other hand she may not be offering him adequate stimulation to expend a reasonable amount of energy.

Severely energy-restricted diets are not advised for children prior to the completion of the adolescent growth spurt. An inadequate energy intake before and during the growth spurt can lead to growth retardation. Both the food intake and activity pattern of an obese child should be carefully evaluated to serve as the basis for counseling the mother. If the actual energy and nutrient intake is greatly in excess of that recommended for age, the mother should be guided to plan a diet containing energy and nutrients appropriate for age. For example, if an obese five-year-old is consuming 90 to 100 Kcal. per kg. per day, his intake can be reduced to not less than 60 Kcal. per kilogram. At the same time the child's energy expenditure may need to be increased. Mothers of obese children may need considerable help not only in coping with the obese child's problem but, also, in modifying their usual food buying practices and preparation methods (see Chapter 27).

Boys and girls who are entering the adolescent growth spurt and are not excessively obese should be helped to avoid any further weight gain. For example, one 13-year-old boy, just entering his growth spurt and weighing 157 pounds was helped to maintain this weight, his correct weight, when the growth spurt was completed. He did not require a severely restricted energy intake: he reduced his afternoon and evening snacks and increased his activity.

EXERCISE. The obese child or adolescent frequently withdraws from active play rather than participate in it. He should be encouraged to reverse this tendency, not only because it will help to expend some of his stored energy and contribute to weight loss, but also to give him a sense of acceptance and accomplishment within his age group.

EMOTIONAL SUPPORT. There are psychological and emotional factors which play a role in childhood obesity. Bruch[12] warns that we must not look on obesity as "all of one piece," and suggests that there is great need for a differential diagnosis of the underlying causes of obesity in each individual.

One of the problems which the obese child or adolescent faces is the derogatory and rejecting attitudes often exhibited by playmates, parents, and other adults. All who deal with these children should have a supportive approach. The nutrition counselor working with such a child should give him understanding and encouragement, even when the diet has not been strictly followed, so that he may find his own ways of developing mature and independent behavior in his choices of food. The counselor must also be supportive of the mother and elicit her help with the child's problems.

Iron Deficiency Anemia

Iron deficiency anemia may occur in premature infants, in twins, or in infants whose mothers had an inadequate diet during pregnancy. It is also prevalent in infants six to 18 months of age. It has been observed in all socioeconomic classes but is more prevalent in infants from families with inadequate incomes.

Infant formulas which supply the nutrients in early infancy have been poor sources of iron. Infant cereals, the first solid foods added to an infant's diet, are fortified with iron to compensate for the lack of iron in the formula. However, after he has reached six to eight months of age, regular cereals, which may or may not be good sources of iron, are used in place of infant cereals, with the result that the infant's diet may not provide adequate iron intake. Concern for this problem has led the Committee on Nutrition of the American Academy of Pediatrics[13] to recommend the use of iron fortified formulas for the first year of life. Iron fortified formulas containing 8 to 12 mg. of iron per quart, normal dilution, are available. The committee's statement is a controversial issue among pediatricians and has not been accepted by all.

Anemia is observed in older infants and young children who have been consuming excessive quantities of milk and limited amounts of solid food. One 13-month-old girl was admitted to the hospital in impending cardiac failure with a hemoglobin of 3.7 g. and an hematocrit of 15. (Normals: hemoglobin, 11-16 g./100 ml., hematocrit, 31-43 percent.) The child had been drinking over 1½ quarts of whole milk a day, plus carbonated beverages. The only solid foods consumed occasionally were potato chips and crackers. The anemia responded to treatment with iron medication and a diet-for-age limited to ½ pint of milk per day during the first two weeks of treatment. With the child's acceptance of an adequate diet-for-age, the milk was increased to one pint a day.

In the past few years it has been observed that some infants and young children with hypochromic, microcytic anemia show blood loss from the intestinal tract. However, the exact nature of the syndrome and the site of the intestinal bleeding have not yet been determined. Woodruff and Clark[14] have noted

low levels of serum albumin and copper in some anemic infants and have suggested that these findings may be the result of altered intestinal physiology induced by cow's milk (homogenized whole milk). They found decreased albumin turnover rates in anemic infants fed cow's milk, and the turnover rates returned to normal when their subjects were fed heat-treated evaporated milk or soy base formula. In another study Woodruff and coworkers[15] found a greater incidence of iron deficiency anemia in infants fed cow's milk beginning at two months of age than in infants fed a commercial formula for the first year of life.

Other Nutritional Deficiency Diseases

Frank scurvy and rickets, which were prevalent nutritional deficiency diseases in infants and children in the United States prior to World War II, are seen infrequently today. Today infant formulas and homogenized milk are fortified with vitamin D, and infant formulas and many fruit drinks readily accepted by young children are fortified with vitamin C. However, continuous surveillance by health counselors of the intake of both of these vitamins by infants and children is required to avoid a recurrence of these deficiency diseases.

A rare form of rickets, known as vitamin D resistant, hypophosphatic rickets, is a familial disease. It is not due to deficiency in any of the nutrients needed for bone formation, but to inability of the kidney tubule to reabsorb phosphate. Since bone consists largely of calcium phosphate, the mineralization of bone is decreased in infants with this disease, with the resultant lesions of rickets and osteomalacia. The problem is medical rather than nutritional, although the disease may be treated with large amounts of vitamin D. This treatment has not been entirely effective. It is possible that the rickets may respond to the 1,25 dihydroxy form of vitamin D when it becomes commercially available. (See Chapter 6, Fat-Soluble Vitamins.)

MALABSORPTION SYNDROMES

In this section the malabsorption syndromes with onset in infancy such as cystic fibrosis, sucrase-isomaltase deficiency, and glucose-galactose malabsorption are discussed. Lactose intolerance and celiac sprue (gluten-induced enteropathy) are discussed in Chapter 25.

Cystic Fibrosis

Cystic fibrosis, which occurs in approximately one in every 1500 live births, is an inherited disease affecting the mucous and sweat glands of the body. The mucous glands secrete an abnormally thick mucus and the sweat glands produce sweat higher in sodium chloride than normal. The disease may first manifest itself in the lungs where the thick mucus obstructs air passages. There may also be malabsorption with fatty stools due to mucous plugs in the fine pancreatic ducts blocking the release of pancreatic digestive enzymes. Failure to gain weight is a common problem in the infant with cystic fibrosis before the disease is diagnosed. The abnormality in the consistency of mucus is not known but it is suspected to be an inborn error of glycoprotein metabolism. Also, the abnormally high level of sodium chloride is not understood, although it is thought due to a defect in sodium and chloride reabsorption by the sweat glands.[16] Elevated sweat chlorides, which are present at birth, and chronic pulmonary disease occur in all infants with cystic fibrosis, while about 10 percent of affected infants have no insufficiency of pancreatic digestive enzymes.

Until recently, cystic fibrosis was considered a fatal childhood disease. Patients who are diagnosed in early infancy now survive to 20 to 30 years of age or longer. This increase in longevity is attributed to physiotherapeutic techniques used to clear the lungs of mucus, to antibiotics which control secondary infections, and to oral pancreatic enzymes and an adequate diet moderately restricted in fat which reduce malabsorption. However, some patients still die in infancy and early childhood due primarily to the lung problem; those who survive childhood may develop diabetes secondary to destruction of the insulin-secreting cells of the pancreas or cirrhosis of the liver due to biliary obstructions.

Even with effective treatment mild to moderate growth retardation occurs in most children with cystic fibrosis; and Lapey and coworkers[17] have shown that adolescents and young adults excrete significant quantities of fat and nitrogen in their stools. At this time the two problems of malabsorption of nutrients and poor utilization of nutrients in intermediary metabolism are being carefully studied in various research centers.

DIETARY TREATMENT. In cystic fibrosis the digestion of fats presents more problems than the digestion of protein and carbohydrates, For the infant either a formula high in protein and containing long-chain triglycerides, or one containing medium-chain triglycerides (MCT) may be used. Probana* is one example of the former (24% of total calories from protein and 29% from fat) and Portagen* and Pregestimil* are examples of the latter (14 to 15% of total calories from protein and 35 to 40% from fat). In the older child, the diet is increased in protein and carbohydrate and restricted in fat. Excessively fatty foods such as peanut butter, cream, ice cream, fatty meats, mayonnaise, fried foods, and pastry rich in shortening are avoided. Moderate amounts of butter or margarine and homogenized whole milk, if tolerated, may be used.

Berry and coworkers[18] recommend the use of medium-chain triglycerides in the diets of all children with cystic fibrosis to provide an adequate energy intake. However the work of Partin and coworkers[19] suggests that MCT should not be used by children with liver damage. Since the older child with cystic fibrosis may also develop cirrhosis, the long-term use of MCT may be contraindicated in cystic fibrosis.

Preparations of the water-soluble forms of fat-soluble vitamins and the water-soluble vitamins, together with supplementary iron, are prescribed. Whenever there is excessive loss of sodium chloride in the sweat due to activity or climate, extra salt must be added to the food to compensate for the loss.

Pancreatic enzymes must be given with each infant feeding or each meal or snack for the older child. Powdered forms of the enzymes can be added to fruits such as applesauce for the infant and young child, while the older child can take the enzymes in capsule form. The powdered forms should not be added to protein foods since they will change the consistency of the food if the infant or child is a slow eater.

The child with cystic fibrosis hospitalized for the treatment of an acute infection presents numerous problems. A major one is the scheduling of meals and physiotherapy treatments, especially postural drainage. To prevent regurgitation when the child is clearing mucus from his lungs, postural drainage should not be done too soon after a meal. Also food and beverages should be available whenever these children request them because they are often anorexic. The diet may need to be modified in the older patient if he also has diabetes or cirrhosis. (See Chapter 28, Diabetes Mellitus and Chapter 32, Liver Disease.)

The team responsible for helping the patient with cystic fibrosis and his family should include the physician, the nurse, the physiotherapist, the dietitian, and the social worker. The team must communicate not only with the family but also with the school teacher or nurse, and any community agencies working with the child and his family. In many instances a psychologist or psychiatrist is needed to help the family and the patient cope with what may be a fatal illness.

*Mead Johnson, Evansville, Ind. 47721.

Sucrase–Isomaltase Deficiency

This is a rare inherited disorder of infancy in which there is a lack both of sucrase and isomaltase. Sucrase is required to hydrolyze sucrose and isomaltase, to hydrolyze the 1-6 linkage in the amylopectin of starches. The infant develops a watery diarrhea when sucrose, dextrin, or starch is introduced into the diet.

Breast milk or formulas free of sucrose or starch such as Enfamil or Similac are used to feed these infants. All fruits, vegetables and cereals, naturally contain some sucrose or starch.[20] Ament and co-workers[21] report that fruits and vegetables with less than 2 percent sucrose are usually tolerated by these infants. Donaldson and Gryboski[22] have observed that with age, the tolerance for amylopectin improves and small quantities of starch can be added to the diet. Strained meats, without sugar or starch added, and eggs can be used.

Glucose–Galactose Malabsorption

In this very rare genetic disorder the mechanism for the active transport of glucose and galactose through the intestinal mucosa is impaired. The hydrolysis of starch yields *glucose*. Lactose is hydrolyzed to *glucose* and *galactose*, and sucrose is hydrolyzed to *glucose* and fructose. Therefore, all sources of carbohydrate with the exception of pure fructose must be excluded from the diets of these infants.

Cho-Free Formula Base* with fructose added is used to feed the infant. As the infant grows older, meat, fish, and eggs are added to the diet and limited amounts of carbohydrates containing glucose and galactose can be added without producing symptoms.[23]

LONG-TERM ILLNESSES

Diabetes Mellitus

The dietary treatment of diabetes mellitus in children is discussed in Chapter 28.

Cardiac Disease

Infants with congenital cardiac anomalies are frequently growth retarded for reasons which are not well understood at present. Since some of these infants are unable to take adequate amounts of formula containing 67 Kcal. per 100 ml., they may be given a formula containing 100 Kcal. per 100 ml. (30 Kcal./30 ml.). Three parts of a commercial concentrated liquid

*Syntex Laboratories, Palo Alto, Ca. 94304.

formula (133 Kcal./100 ml.) and one part of water will yield a formula containing 100 Kcal. per 100 ml.

Many cardiac anomalies can be corrected by surgery after infancy. Prior to surgery the child may also require a moderately sodium-restricted diet. The sodium-restricted diet is discussed in Chapter 30.

Mothers need guidance in feeding infants with this condition because they become tired easily and need to rest frequently during a feeding. Therefore, the mother must devote more time to feeding her infant than is usual and may need help in planning a daily schedule so that she can give adequate care to the other members of her family.

Renal Disease

NEPHROSIS. Nephrosis, also known as lipid nephrosis or idiopathic nephrotic syndrome of childhood, is a relatively uncommon disease of childhood with onset between two and seven years of age. It is characterized by proteinuria, hypoalbuminemia, hyperlipidemia, and edema. Hematuria and hypertension, which occur in nephritis, is uncommon in nephrosis. Its etiology is unknown although it is suspected that some metabolic disturbance in the glomerular basement membrane leads to increased permeability of the glomeruli to protein.

About 90 percent of patients respond to prednisone (a steroid) therapy, in about two weeks with a significant decrease in proteinuria in four weeks. If a relapse occurs prednisone is given on alternate days because long-term steroid therapy has undesirable side effects, such as the development of cushingoid features, depression, and poor intellectual performance. More serious is the appearance of osteoporosis, gastrointestinal bleeding, growth retardation, and convulsions.

The untreated child with nephrosis is anorexic, irritable, and, if massive edema is present, he is uncomfortable due to ascites and limited vision, which is the result of severe periorbital edema. Since steroid therapy accentuates the retention of sodium in the nephrotic state, Drummond[24] recommends restricting sodium intake to 400 mg. per day as long as there is significant edema and proteinuria. When the edema subsides the sodium intake can be liberalized. Because of their poor appetites these children's food preferences should be respected and the food served should be attractive and as palatable as possible. During recovery the child's appetite will improve and he should be given a diet-for-age with some increase over normal in protein (2 to 3 g./kg.) to compensate for protein losses in the urine and to correct the albuminemia.

KIDNEY DIALYSIS. Many children with congenital renal anomalies or end-state renal failure due to infectious diseases (see Chapter 31) are hemodialyzed. The length of time on dialysis may depend on finding a suitable kidney donor or, especially in infants, waiting until they are large enough to accept an adult-size kidney. The diet for the infant or child on hemodialysis must provide an adequate energy intake and his requirement of the essential amino acids, and must be restricted in electrolytes as required.
NEPHRITIS. The dietary treatment of nephritis is discussed in Chapter 31.

Allergy

Allergy in infants and children is discussed in Chapter 33.

Epilepsy

Epilepsy is a disease of the central nervous system. It occurs in both children and adults, although it is more frequent in children. The chief symptom is momentary loss of consciousness in petit mal seizures, so short they may hardly be noticed; or the loss of consciousness may be of longer duration, accompanied by convulsions, as in grand mal seizures.
DRUG THERAPY. The majority of patients with epilepsy respond to therapy with phenobarbital and anticonvulsant drugs. Low serum folate levels with or without megaloblastic anemia have been observed in patients with epilepsy taking dilantin, an anticonvulsant drug, over long periods of time. It is suspected that dilantin impairs the activity of folic acid. Large doses of folic acid are contraindicated, however, in the patient controlled by dilantin therapy because they have been observed to induce seizures. Patients taking dilantin should be advised to have a diet which supplies the recommended daily amount of folic acid.
THE KETOGENIC DIET. Before anticonvulsant drugs were available it was observed that starvation with ketosis had a favorable effect on epileptic seizures. From this observation a diet high in fat which promotes mild ketosis was used in the treatment of epilepsy prior to the development of drug therapy. Today, when epileptic seizures cannot be controlled by anticonvulsant drugs, a ketogenic diet may be used. It is most effective in controlling petit mal seizures in the preschool and early school-aged child.

There are many drawbacks to the use of the diet, however, and these should be considered before the regimen is attempted. The high fat content of the diet makes it unacceptable to many patients. It demands the use of gram scales for the weighing of all food, careful menu planning, and rigid control. The diet should not be instituted until the parents are carefully assessed for their emotional stability and their ability to follow directions and to accept the restrictions of the diet. Much time must be alotted to instructing them in the details of the diet if it is to be successful.

To produce ketosis, the usual ratio of protein and carbohydrate to fat in the normal diet must be sharply reversed. Fifty percent of protein is glucogenic, and all of the carbohydrate becomes glucose, as does 10 percent of the fat via the glycerol molecule. The remainder of the fat and approximately 50 percent of the protein are ketogenic. Normally fatty acids are metabolized to carbon dioxide and water. When the ratio of fatty acids to available glucose exceeds 2:1, ketosis occurs. However, the ketogenic-antiketogenic (K-AK) ratio of the diet to control seizures must be at least 3:1 at the beginning of treatment and be maintained at a ratio of 4:1 if it is to be successful.

The method for calculating such a diet to meet the individual child's needs is given by Mike.[25] Table 34-5, from Mike's article, shows that the first step in calculating the ketogenic diet is to identify the energy and protein needs of the child. The table also demonstrates a method for calculating the protein, fat, and carbohydrate in a 3:1 or 4:1 ketogenic diet.

Mike's article[26] also includes a Table of Food Values, a table of allowed foods, and many suggestions for using the fats to make the diet as palatable as possible. She warns that the Exchange Lists for diabetic diets are not suitable and should not be used. However, more recently Lasser and Brush[27] have published a system of equivalents comparable to an exchange system which can be used to plan menus for ketogenic diets. Table 34-6 shows a menu using Mike's food tables for an 18-g. protein, 130-g. fat, and 14.5-g. carbohydrate diet, with a K-AK ratio of 4:1. It illustrates some of the difficulties presented by a ketogenic diet.

It can readily be seen from the menu in Table 34-6 that milk, due to its carbohydrate content, cannot be used. All protein foods have to be sharply limited. Carbohydrate foods other than fruits and vegetables must be omitted. Butter, heavy cream, mayonnaise, and oil form the main part of the diet. The protein, fat, and carbohydrate should be equally divided among the three meals, and are calculated to the first decimal point. All foods should be eaten at each meal to maintain ketonuria.

The diet is supplemented with an aqueous solution of multiple vitamins; with calcium gluconate or calcium lactate (not as a syrup which contains carbohydrate); and with an iron medication to provide a daily amount of iron.

Recently, a ketogenic diet using medium-chain triglyceride oil has been developed.[28] It appears that

Table 34–5. Method for Calculating a Ketogenic Diet*

Calorie requirements, rounded to the nearest 100

Age (years)	Cal./kg. body weight
2-3	100-80
3-5	80-60
5-10	75-55

Protein requirement
1 g./kg. body weight for young children
1.5 g./kg. body weight for older children

To calculate for a 3:1 ratio	To calculate for a 4:1 ratio
1 g. fat = 9 cal. × 3 = 27 cal.	1 g. fat = 9 cal. × 4 = 36 cal.
1 g. P + C = 4 cal. × 1 = 4 cal.	1 g. P + C = 4 cal. × 1 = 4 cal.
31 cal. per unit	40 cal. per unit

Example: 4-year-old child, weighing 18 kg. × 70 cal. = 1260 or 1300 cal.

For a 3:1 K-AK ratio (31 cal./unit)	For a 4:1 K-AK ratio (40 cal./unit)
1300 cal: 31 cal. = 42 units	1300 cal.: 40 cal. = 32.5 units
Fat 42 × 3 = 126 g.	Fat 32.5 × 4 = 130 g.
P + C 42 × 1 = 42 g.	P + C 32.5 × 1 = 32.5 g.
P (1 gm./kg.) 18 g.	P (1 gm./kg.) = 18 g.
C (by difference) 24 g.	C (by difference) = 14.5 g.
The diet prescription with a 3:1 K-AK ratio will therefore contain 18 Gm. of protein, 126 Gm. of fat and 24 Gm. of carbohydrate	The diet prescription for a 4:1 K-AK ratio will contain 18 Gm. of protein, 130 Gm. of fat and 14.5 Gm. of carbohydrate See menu in Table 34–6

*From Mike, E. M.: Practical Guide and Dietary Management of Children with Seizures Using the Ketogenic Diet. Am. J. Clin. Nutr. 17:399, 1965.

Table 34–6. Menu for a Ketogenic Diet with a 4:1 K-AK Ratio, Containing 18 g. of Protein, 130 g. of Fat, and 14.5 g. of Carbohydrate*

Food	Weight (Gm.)	Protein	Fat	Carbohydrate
Breakfast				
Orange	30	0.3	0.1	3.0
Heavy cream (diluted with water for drinking)	75	1.6	28.1	2.3
Egg, cooked in	25	3.2	2.9	—
Butter	15	—	12.0	—
		5.1	43.1	5.3
Dinner				
Meat, medium fat, cooked in	20	5.6	3.2	—
Butter	15	—	12.0	—
Asparagus	30	.6	—	1.5
Lettuce	20	.4	—	1.0
Mayonnaise	20	.2	16.0	—
Oil (added to mayonnaise)	10	—	10.0	—
Cantaloupe	20	.2	—	2.0
		7.0	41.2	4.5
Supper				
Egg, hard cooked	25	3.2	2.9	—
Spinach, cooked in	30	.6	—	1.5
Butter	10	—	8.1	—
Lettuce	20	.4	—	1.0
Mayonnaise	20	.2	16.0	—
Heavy cream, whipped with	50	1.1	18.8	1.5
Applesauce	10	.1	—	.5
		5.6	45.8	4.5
Totals for the day		17.7	130.1	14.3

*All figures obtained from Mike, E. M.: Practical Guide and Dietary Management of Children with Seizures Using the Ketogenic Diet. Am. J. Clin. Nutr. 17:399, 1965.

Table 34–7. Comparison of Approximate Composition of 1600 Kcal. MCT Ketogenic Diet with 1600 Kcal. Traditional Ketogenic Diet (3:1 ratio)*

Factor	MCT diet			traditional ketogenic diet		
	g.	Kcal.	% Kcal.	g.	Kcal.	% Kcal.
protein	41	160	10	29	116	7
carbo-hydrate	74	296	19	23	92	6
fat	20	180	11	156	1404	87
MCT	116	963	60	0	0	0
total		1609	100		1612	100

*Signore, J. M.: J. Am. Dietet. A. 62:285, 1973.

medium-chain triglycerides induce ketosis more readily than regular fats containing primarily long-chain triglycerides. Therefore, the total quantity of fat can be reduced and the total quantity of protein and carbohydrate can be increased in the diet compared with the calculations in Table 34–5. A comparison of the approximate composition of a 1600 Kcal., MCT ketogenic diet with a 1600 Kcal. traditional ketogenic diet is given in Table 34–7. Signore's article also gives detailed instructions for calculating a ketogenic diet using MCT oil. She reports that the MCT ketogenic diet is more palatable and requires less rigid control than the traditional ketogenic diet. Also, because of the quantity of protein and carbohydrate which can be used in calculating the diet pattern, milk and larger servings of meat can be used.

Hosptalization of the child is necessary to establish the ketosis and to allow time for observation and for instruction of the parents. Nothing is given by mouth except 500 to 1000 ml. of water daily for 24 to 72 hours. Hunger disappears as ketosis develops. When a high degree of ketosis has been achieved, the diet is begun with a 3:1 K-AK ratio, then changed to the 4:1 K-AK ratio for the duration of treatment. There may be nausea or vomiting at first, but this disappears. A strongly positive ketonuria should be maintained at all times.

The diet is continued for one to three years, then a gradual return to a normal diet is made by slowly reducing the fat and increasing protein and carbohydrate.

STUDY QUESTIONS AND ACTIVITIES

1. Using the information in Table 34–1 plan a day's menu for a 2½-year-old hospitalized child. Do your food selections meet this child's Recommended Dietary Allowance of protein? (See Chapter 10 for NRC-RDA.)

2. Using the recordings in the nursing notes of formula and food intake, estimate the 24-hour calorie intake of an infant. Record the infant's length, daily weight, and head circumference on a growth chart. Is the infant progressing normally?

3. What effect may an emotionally disturbed mother have on the nutritional status of her infant?

4. What may one expect of a child's food habits when he is ill?

5. How can a child be helped to adjust to eating his food in the hospital?

6. What is a common cause of nutritional anemia in young children? How may it be prevented?

7. What should be the relationship between the obese child and the person treating him?

8. Plan a day's diet for a 5-year-old child with celiac disease on a gluten-free diet. See Chapter 25.

9. Why should calories and protein be increased in the diet of a child with cystic fibrosis?

10. When may a ketogenic diet be ordered for epilepsy? How is a condition of ketosis established and maintained?

11. What are some of the difficulties inherent in this diet?

SUPPLEMENTARY READINGS

GENERAL

Authausen, T. R., and Lesh, D.: Parents need TLC too. Hospitals 47:88 (April) 1973.

Mead, J.: The lemonade party. Nursing Outlook 21:104, 1973.

DIET THERAPY

Barness, L. A., et al: Calcium and fat absorption from infant formulas with different fat blends. Pediatrics 54:217, 1974.

DeVizia, B., et al: Digestibility of starches in infants and children. J. Pediat. 86:50, 1975.

THE ACUTELY ILL CHILD

Heird, W. C., and Winters, R. W.: Total parenteral nutrition: the state of the art. J. Pediat. 86:2, 1975.

Rickard, K., and Gresham, E.: Nutritional considerations for the newborn requiring intensive care. J. Am. Dietet. A. 66:592, 1975.

WEIGHT STATUS

Dobbing, J.: The later growth of the brain and its vulnerability. Pediatrics 53:2, 1974.

Fisch, R. O., et al: Obesity and leanness at birth and their relationship to body habitus in later children. Pediatrics 56:521, 1975.

Forbes, G. B.: Stature and lean body mass. Am. J. Clin. Nutr. 27:595, 1974.

Martin, H. P.: Nutrition: its relationship to children's physical, mental and emotional development. Am. J. Clin. Nutr. 26:766, 1973.

Pollitt, E.: Failure to thrive: socioeconomic, dietary intake and mother-child interaction data. Fed. Proc. 34:1593, 1975.

ANEMIA

Macdougall, L. G., et al: The immune response in iron-deficient children: impaired cellular defense mechanisms with altered humoral components. J. Pediat. 86:833, 1975.

Shott, R. J., and Andrews, B. F.: Iron status of a high-risk population at delivery. A. J. Dis. Child. 124:369, 1974.

Williams, M. L., et al: Role of dietary iron and fat on vitamin E deficiency anemia of infancy. N. Eng. J. Med. 292:887, 1975.

Wilson, J. F., et al: Studies on iron metabolism. V. Further observations on cow's milk-induced gastrointestinal bleeding in infants with iron-deficiency anemia. J. Pediatrics 84:335, 1974.

MALABSORPTION

Ament, M. E., et al: Sucrase-isomaltase deficiency: a frequently misdiagnosed disease. J. Pediat. 83:721, 1973.

Burnette, B. A.: Family adjustment to cystic fibrosis. Am. J. Nursing 75:1986, 1975.

Gayton, W. F., and Friedman, S. B.: Psychological aspects of C. F.: a review of the literature. A. J. Dis. Child. 126:856, 1973.

Grossman, M. L.: The psychosocial approach to the medical management of patients with cystic fibrosis. Clin. Pediat. 9:830, 1975.

Lilibridge, C. B., and Townes, P. L.: Physiologic deficiency of pancreatic amylase in infancy: a factor in iatrogenic diarrhea. J. Pediat. 82:279, 1973.

Shwachman, H.: Changing concepts of cystic fibrosis. Hospital Practice 9:143, 1974.

CARDIAC DISEASE

Husc, D. M., et al: Infants with congenital heart disease: food intake, body weight, and energy metabolism. A. J. Dis. Child. 129:65, 1975.

Larson, R., et al: Special diet for familial Type II hyperlipoproteinemia. A. J. Dis. Child. 128:67, 1974.

McBean, L. D., and Speckman, E. W.: An interpretive review: diet in early life and the prevention of atherosclerosis. Pediat. Res. 8:837, 1974.

Tsang, R. C., et al: Neonatal familial hypercholesterolemia. A. J. Dis. Child. 129:83, 1975.

RENAL DISEASE

Giangiacomo, J., et al: Serum immunoglobulins in nephrotic syndrome: a possible cause of minimal-change nephrotic syndrome. N. Eng. J. Med. 293:8, 1975.

Holiday, M. A.: Caloric deficiency in children with uremia: effect upon growth. Pediatrics 50:590, 1972.

EPILEPSY

Livingston, A.: Diagnosis and treatment of childhood myoclonic seizures. Pediatrics 53:542, 1974.

Ch'ien, L. T., et al: Harmful effect of megadoses of vitamins: electroencephalogram abnormalities and seizures induced by intravenous folate in drug-treated epileptics. Am. J. Clin. Nutr. 28:51, 1975.

For further references see Bibliography in Section 4.

REFERENCES

1. Snyderman, S. E., et al: J. Nutrition 78:75, 1962.
2. Fomon, S. J.: *Infant Nutrition*, ed. 2. Philadelphia. Saunders, 1974.
3. Fomon, S. J., op. cit., p. 310.
4. Heird, W. C., and Winters, R. W.: J. Pediat. 86:2, 1975.
5. Lifshitz, F., et al: J. Pediat. 79:760, 1971.
6. Loomis, W. G.: Clin. Pediat. 9:362, 1970.
7. Bowlby, J.: *Attachment and Loss*. Vol. I. New York: Basic Books, 1969.
8. Whitten, F., et al: JAMA 209:1675, 1969.
9. Chase, H. P., and Martin, H. P.: N. Eng. J. Med. 282:933, 1970.
10. Crawford, P. B., et al: Am. J. Clin. Nutr. 27:706, 1974.
11. Rose, H. E., and Mayer, J.: Pediatrics 41:13, 1968.
12. Bruch, H.: Am. J. Public Health 48:1349, 1958.
13. Committee on Nutrition, American Academy of Pediatrics: Pediatrics 47:786, 1971.
14. Woodruff, C. W., and Clark, J. L.: A. J. Dis. Child. 124:18, 1972.
15. Woodruff, C. W., et al: A. J. Dis. Child. 124:26, 1972.
16. diSant'Agnese, P. A.: in *Nelson Textbook of Pediatrics*, ed. 10. V. C. Vaughan III and R. J. McKay, eds. Philadelphia, Saunders, 1975.
17. Lapey, A., et al: J. Pediat. 84:328, 1974.
18. Berry, H. K., et al: A. J. Dis. Child. 129:165, 1975.
19. Partin, J. C., et al: Pediat. Res., 8:384, 1974.
20. Hardinge, M. E., et al: J. Am. Dietet. A. 46:197, 1965.
21. Ament, M. E., et al: J. Pediat. 83:721, 1973.
22. Donaldson, R. M., Jr., and Gryboski, J. D.: in *Gastrointestinal Disease—Pathophysiology—Diagnosis—Management*, M. H. Sleisenger and J. S. Fordtran, eds. Philadelphia, Saunders, 1973.
23. Ibid.
24. Drummond, K. N., in Nelson, op. cit.
25. Mike, E. M.: Am. J. Clin. Nutr. 17:399, 1965.
26. Ibid.
27. Lasser, J. L., and Brush, M. K.: J. Am. Dietet. A. 62:281, 1973.
28. Signore, J. M.: J. Am. Dietet. A. 62:285, 1973.

35 inborn errors of metabolism

Galactosemia
Phenylketonuria (PKU)
Maple Syrup Urine Disease (MSUD)
Other Inborn Errors of Metabolism

In the past 40 years, as more has been learned about the genetic control of metabolism, disorders of carbohydrate, amino acids, lipid, and mineral and vitamin metabolism have been identified. The more common diseases such as diabetes mellitus, familial hyperlipoproteinemia and cystic fibrosis have been discussed in other chapters in this book. Those relatively rare metabolic disorders with onset in early infancy which respond to dietary management are presented in this chapter.

A specific metabolic defect is caused by one, or possibly more than one, mutant gene, and there is considerable variation in the effects of the mutations on the affected individual. Some conditions such as Tay-Sachs disease, an abnormality of glycosphingolipid metabolism, are incompatible with life and death occurs in early childhood. In other conditions such as phenylketonuria, discussed later, the abnormality in intermediary metabolism can be modified by manipulating the exogenous (dietary) source of the metabolite(s) throughout infancy and childhood. In a few conditions such as alcaptonuria, due to the lack of homogentisic acid oxidase, the effects of the mutant gene are minimal in infancy, although some effects may be observed in later life. A common problem of infants and children with inborn errors of metabolism is damage to the

497

developing central nervous system resulting in mental retardation, accompanied in some conditions by growth retardation. It is suspected that central nervous system damage is caused by the biochemical abnormality.

The prevention of mental retardation and growth failure is the goal of therapy in inborn errors of metabolism. In the conditions which respond to diet therapy, the best results have been reported in those infants who were diagnosed during the first week of life with treatment instituted at the time of, or shortly after, diagnosis. Newborn screening programs and positive family histories for mental retardation or early infant deaths are used to identify the newborn infant at risk for a metabolic defect. In some instances the abnormality of the infant can be identified before birth by amniocentesis.

The treatment of these infants and their families is carried out in major medical centers. These centers have a team of specialists in their areas with resources for diagnosing genetic diseases and for monitoring the infant's response to therapy. The team consists of physician and biochemist who are experts in genetics, nutrition counselor, pediatric nurse practitioner, social worker, and psychologist. Such teams also need access to a psychiatrist and genetic counselor. The team works not only with the family but also with the family physician and other health resources in the community.

In those conditions in which diet therapy has proven to be effective, the intake of a specific nutrient is manipulated but, at the same time, the diet must be adequate in energy and all essential nutrients to support normal growth and development. Infants with

1. Galactose + ATP $\xrightarrow{\blacksquare A}$ Galactose-1-Phosphate + ADP

2. Galactose-1-Phosphate + UDP Glucose $\xrightarrow{\blacksquare B}$ UDP Galactose + Glucose-1-Phosphate

3. UDP Galactose $\xrightarrow{C}$ UDP Glucose

4. UDP Glucose + PP $\xrightarrow{D}$ UTP + Glucose-1-Phosphate

A = Galactokinase
B = Galactose-1-Phosphate Uridyltransferase
C = UPD Galactose-4-Epimerase
D = UDP Glucose Pyrophosphorylase

Fig. 35-1. Metabolic reactions for the interconversion of galactose and glucose. ∎ A = galactokinase deficiency galactosemia. ∎ B = transferase deficiency galactosemia.

inborn errors of metabolism present a special challenge to the nutrition counselor and an even greater challenge to their families. The results of the treatment of an infant will depend, in many instances, on the relationship which the nutrition counselor establishes and maintains with the mother.

Galactosemia, phenylketonuria, maple syrup urine disease, homocystinuria and leucine-sensitive hypoglycemia are discussed in the following sections. For more detailed information on these and other inborn errors the reader is referred to the supplementary readings at the end of this chapter and the Bibliography in Section 4.

GALACTOSEMIA

Galactosemia is a term used to describe a syndrome of inherited disorders involving the utilization of galactose. Galactose is required for the synthesis of cerebrosides, certain mucopolysaccharides, and lactose by the mammary glands of lactating women. However, a dietary source of galactose is not required because UDP glucose can be converted to UDP galactose in the body (Fig. 35-1, Reaction 3); and the UDP galactose can supply the body's needs for galactose.

Types of Galactosemia

There are two known types of galactosemia; transferase deficiency galactosemia, and galactokinase deficiency galactosemia[1] (Fig. 35-1, Reactions 1 and 2). Both types are transmitted by autosomal recessive genes and, at present, the transferase type appears to be more prevalent than the galactokinase type. The major alternate pathway of galactose metabolism in both types of galactosemia is the conversion of galactose by aldose reductase to the polyol, galactitol.
TRANSFERASE DEFICIENCY GALACTOSEMIA. Vomiting and diarrhea with growth failure start a few days after birth with the ingestion of human or cow milk. This is followed in approximately one week by disordered liver function which can progress to hepatomegaly and ascites. The infants have high blood galactose levels and intermittent galactosuria. Infantile cataracts have been observed within a few days of birth and, if the infant is not treated, mental retardation can develop. Cataracts develop due to the collection of galactitol in the lens. Galactitol has also been found in brain tissue, which may account for the mental retardation. Early diagnosis and treatment with a galactose-restricted diet reduces the possibility of the complications of the disease.[2] The galactose-restricted diet is discussed later in this section.
KINASE DEFICIENCY GALACTOSEMIA. Infants

with kinase deficiency do not present all the same symptoms as those observed in transferase deficiency. They do not have vomiting and diarrhea with growth retardation or liver disease. They have high blood galactose levels and galactosuria; and cataracts appear later in childhood. Present evidence, although not extensive, suggests that children with this deficiency are not mentally retarded. These children are also treated with a galactose-restricted diet.

Galactose-Restricted Diets

FOOD SOURCES OF GALACTOSE. The major dietary source of galactose is the disaccharide lactose in mammalian milk; human, cow, goat, and the milk of any other mammal used by humans any place in the world. Therefore, all forms of milk—whole milk, nonfat milk, buttermilk, cream, cheese, yogurt, ice cream, and milk sherbets—must be excluded from the diet. Also excluded are foods made with milk—breads, some breakfast cereals, rolls, muffins, biscuits, doughnuts, pastries, cookies, pies, puddings, pancakes, waffles, pizza with cheese, cheese sauces, salad dressings, milk sauces and gravies, margarine, and lunch meats and frankfurters with milk solids added. Liver, pancreas, and brain, animal organs which contain galactose, are excluded. The labels on convenience foods, infant foods, and any other packaged foods must be inspected carefully for the words milk, milk solids, or lactose. Medications containing lactose as a filler must also be avoided.

Foods other than milk also contain galactose. Peaches, pears, and apples contain 0.2 g. galactose per 100 g. edible portion.[3] Cow peas, chick peas, lentils, lima beans, defatted wheat germ, and dry mung beans contain raffinose and stachyose, two sugars containing galactose, while rutabagas, navy beans and soybeans contain galactan, a polysaccharide containing galactose.[4] Pectin used in jelly-making also contains galactose. Some clinicians responsible for the treatment of galactosemic children will exclude the fruits, vegetables, and legumes listed previously, while other clinicians will not. Gitzelman and Auricchio[5] have demonstrated that the raffinose and stachyose in soybean are not hydrolyzed in the gastrointestinal tract and, therefore, the galactose in these two sugars is not available for absorption.

THE INFANT'S DIET. Formulas made with soy-isolate or casein hydrolysate without lactose added are essentially galactose-free. These are Isomil, Neo-Mull Soy, Prosobee and Nutramigen (see Table 34-4). The labels on all infant foods must be inspected carefully because some of these products are unexpected sources of galactose. For example, Gerber High Protein Cereal with Peaches contains nonfat dry milk while Gerber High Protein Cereal does not.* The producers of infant foods make available information about the ingredients in their products* and up-date this information whenever they change their recipes. Rusks, or teething biscuits, for the older infant can be made by drying slices of bread made without milk in a 200° oven until done. Some crackers and simple cookies are also made without milk.

THE OLDER CHILD AND ADULT. As the child grows older he will eat foods from the family table. All foods considered sources of galactose must be avoided. In addition to meat, fish, poultry and eggs, and fruits and vegetables, bread made without milk and cereal products such as rice, macaroni, noodles, and spaghetti can be used to provide an adequate energy and protein intake. Italian and French breads are usually, but not always, made with water rather than milk or nonfat milk solids. Butter is used because margarines, other than Kosher margarine, have nonfat dry milk added. Angel cake and sponge cake and sugar cookies made without milk, as well as gelatin can be used for desserts.

NUTRITIONAL ADEQUACY OF THE DIET. Through the use of a galactose-free infant formula with minerals and vitamins added and infant foods free of galactose, the energy and nutrient needs of the infant can be met. Unless the formula is continued as a beverage or in food preparation as the child grows older, the diet can be inadequate in calcium and riboflavin because it is difficult to achieve an adequate intake of these two nutrients without some milk in the diet. Supplements of calcium and riboflavin may be needed to insure an adequate intake.

LIBERALIZATION OF THE DIET. Segal[6] points out that the ability to metabolize galactose through an alternative pathway, except through galactitol, does not develop with age. Therefore, galactose must be excluded from the diet throughout life.

PHENYLKETONURIA (PKU)

Phenylketonuria (PKU) is an inborn error in the metabolism of the essential amino acid phenylalanine (Phe) and is transmitted through an autosomal recessive gene. The incidence of PKU is estimated to be about 1 in 18,500 live births. Affected individuals lack the hepatic enzyme phenylalanine hydroxylase which converts Phe, in excess of the quantity required for structural proteins, to tyrosine. The alternate pathway of Phe metabolism is phenylpyruvic acid, the keto acid of Phe; hence, the name phenylketonuria (Fig. 35-2).

*Ingredients, Gerber Baby Foods, March 1974. Gerber Products Co., Fremont, Michigan 49412.

The defect is present at birth and the metabolic abnormalities occur when the infant begins to ingest protein (milk). The abnormalities are elevated blood levels of Phe in excess of 20 mg./100 ml. (normal 1 to 3 mg./100 ml.) and of phenylpyruvic acid (normal, O-trace). Subsequently, phenylalanine, phenyl-pyruvic acid, phenyllactic acid and other metabolites are excreted in the urine.[7] These metabolites give a musty odor to the urine.

The infant appears normal at birth but, if the disease goes undetected and untreated, neurological symptoms such as irritability, hyperactivity, and convulsive seizures usually develop between six to 18 months of age, and more than 90 percent will be moderately to severely mentally retarded. The continued high blood levels of Phe and its metabolites are believed to be responsible for the damage to the neurological system during its development in infancy and early childhood. Because melanin, the pigment of hair and skin, is derived from tyrosine (see Fig. 35-2) the untreated infant with PKU will have a lighter coloration of skin and hair than the unaffected members of his family.

The disease was first described by Følling in 1934 but its treatment was delayed for many years because there was no method for limiting the dietary intake of Phe to an infant's requirements and providing an otherwise adequate nutritional intake. At the same time it was not possible to identify these infants at birth. During the late 1950s, with the development of a special formula, Lofenalac, (see Table 34-4) it became possible to limit an infant's intake of Phe. The phenylalanine-restricted diet is discussed later in this section. It was observed that if the dietary treatment was started in the first months of life it was possible for the child to achieve his growth potential both mentally and physically. When the disease is discovered later, dietary treatment is not effective in preventing mental retardation, although the behavior of the child appears to improve with such treatment.

In the early 1960s Guthrie developed an inhibition assay test which detected elevated blood levels of phenylalanine in the newborn. This test gives qualitative, not quantitative, results. Since it has been proven that early treatment of PKU prevents mental retardation, today more than 40 states have compulsory PKU screening programs which use the Guthrie test. Blood is drawn from the infant after feeding has been started and before discharge from the newborn nursery. The result of the test is reported to the infant's physician. Prior to the development of methods to detect and treat the disease, it was estimated that ½ to 1 percent of all patients in institutions for the mentally retarded were phenylketonurics. A recent sur-

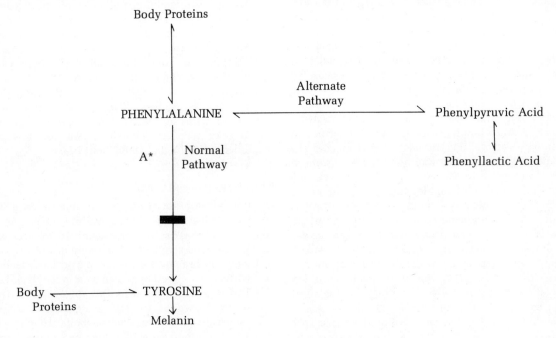

* A = Phenylalanine hydroxylase

Fig. 35-2. Normal pathway of phenylalanine metabolism showing block (■■■■) in PKU due to lack of phenylalanine hydroxylase.

vey[8] indicates there has been a significant reduction in the past ten years in the admission of individuals with PKU to institutions for the mentally retarded.

Types of PKU

The Guthrie Screening Test is confirmed by the quantitative analysis of blood Phe by column chromatography before diet therapy is initiated. From experience it has been discovered that not all infants with a positive Guthrie test have classical phenylketonuria. Three types of hyperphenylalaninemia (elevated Phe levels) have been identified. Type I, classical PKU, is characterized by a Phe blood level persistently greater than 20 mg./100 ml., with the excretion of Phe and its metabolites in the urine. Type II hyperphenylalaninemia is characterized by a Phe blood level less than 20 mg. but greater than 4 mg./100 ml. and near normal levels, or only a slight increase, in Phe metabolites in the urine. Type III, transient mild hyperphenylalaninemia, is characterized by an elevated Phe level above 20 mg./100 ml. which eventually approaches normal. It is suspected that Type II may be due to an isozyme defect and Type III to a possible delay in the development of hepatic Phe hydroxylase.

About 25 per cent of premature and low birthweight infants on a high protein diet will have transient elevations of blood Phe and tyrosine levels with transient excretion of tyrosine in the urine. It is suspected that the defect is the inhibition of p-hydroxyphenylpyruvic oxidase activity. These infants respond to vitamin C therapy.

All infants with a persistent elevation of blood Phe levels above 20 mg./100 ml. have PKU and are treated with a phenylalanine-restricted diet. Generally, with Phe blood levels between 10 to 20 mg./100 ml., Type II patients are treated by diet. At present there is some controversy about treating these Type II patients in this way. Before the types of hyperphenylalaninemia were identified Type III patients treated with a Phe-restricted diet failed to gain weight and were developmentally delayed. They gained weight with a normal infant diet.[9]

The Phenylalanine-Restricted Diet

PRINCIPLES OF DIET THERAPY. Phenylalanine is an essential amino acid required for the synthesis of structural proteins. As one example, the B-chain of insulin contains 3 molecules of Phe, therefore, Phe must be available for the continous synthesis of insulin. The diet for a PKU infant is planned to provide his daily requirement of Phe without an excess to be metabolized through the phenylpyruvic acid pathway. At the same time, an adequate intake of energy,

protein, and all other nutrients must be provided by the diet to support growth and development.

The diet is planned, and continuously revised as the infant grows, to maintain a blood level of 5 to 10 mg. of Phe per 100 ml. The quantity of Phe required to maintain this level will vary with each infant, depending on his size and rate of growth. The Phe requirement of infants two to four months of age, as defined by Holt and Snyderman (see Table 35–1), is used as a guide for determining the amount of Phe to be included in the first feedings. In general, the newly diagnosed PKU infant under two months of age is offered 70 mg. of Phe per kilogram of body weight per day. Seventy mg. of Phe is the midpoint in the range of values given by Holt and Snyderman and comparable with Fomon's preliminary estimates of the amino acid requirements of infants.[10] Weekly monitoring of the blood levels of Phe by column chromatography will indicate whether or not this quantity is appropriate for a particular infant and if not, the diet is adjusted accordingly.

As the infant progresses through the first year of life, the quantity of Phe per kilogram of body weight will decrease because the rate of growth decreases. By two years of age the Phe requirement decreases to 25 to 35 mg. per kilogram of body weight and children 2 to 10 years of age require on the average 30 mg. of Phe per kilogram.[11] At this time experience with the treatment of adolescents is limited. However, the work of Nakagawa and coworkers suggests that the Phe requirement of children 10 to 12 years old is approximately 27 mg. per kilogram.[12]

THE DIET PRESCRIPTION. The diet prescription defines the calories, grams of protein and the milligrams of phenylalanine required by the infant. For example, the diet order for a two-month-old infant weighing 4.5 kg. requiring 70 mg. Phe per kg. would be: 510 Kcal. (120 Kcal. × 4.5 kg. = 510 Kcal.), 10 g. protein (2.2 × 4.5 kg. = 10 protein), and 315 mg. Phe (70 mg. Phe × 4.5 kg. = 315 mg. Phe).

Table 35–1. Essential Amino Acid Daily Requirements of Infants Two to Four Months of Age*

Amino Acid	Requirement (mg./kg./per day)
Histidine	16-34
Isoleucine	80-100
Leucine	76-150
Lysine	88-103
Methionine (in presence of cystine)	33-45
Phenylalanine (in presence of tyrosine)	47-90
Threonine	45-87
Tryptophan	15-22
Valine	85-105

*Adapted from Snyderman, S.: in *Heritable Disorders of Amino Acid Metabolism*, W. L. Nyhan, ed., New York, Wiley, 1974.

As the child grows, the diet prescription will be modified according to his blood Phe level and his changing requirements for energy, protein and Phe. Early in infancy the diet prescription may be changed as frequently as every two weeks and during later infancy, every month.

FOOD FOR THE PHENYLALANINE-RESTRICTED DIET. All foods, with exception of fats and sugars, contain protein, and 3 to 5 percent of the protein is phenylalanine. Five percent of the protein is phenylalanine in foods of animal origin and in cereals, dry legumes, nuts, potatoes, sweet potatoes, and fresh vegetables that are immature seeds such as lima beans, sweet corn, peas, cow peas, and other fresh shelled beans. The protein in dark green leaves contains 4 percent Phe and, in other fruits and vegetables, 3 percent phenylalanine.[13]

Since Phe is present to some extent in all food proteins whether amimal or vegetable, it is not possible to design a diet using only normal foods which is restricted in Phe yet adequate in total protein, energy, and all other nutrients. A specially formulated food, Lofenalac* (low-phenylalanine-milk), is available in the United States for feeding infants and children with PKU. A similar product, Albumaid, is available in England and, to a limited extent, for research purposes in the United States. The protein equivalents in Lofenalac are supplied by an enzymatically digested casein hydrolysate from which most of the Phe has been removed by charcoal filtration. This process also removes the aromatic amino acid, tyrosine. Tyrosine together with tryptophan, histidine, and methionine are added to give an adequate mixture of amino acids. Some amino acids are present in small peptides. Carbohydrate is supplied by corn syrup solids and tapioca starch and fat, by corn oil. Minerals and vitamins are also added to meet an infant's needs for these nutrients.

Lofenalac is marketed as a powder to which water is added to prepare a formula. When reconstituted, it has almost the same appearance and consistency as milk, but a markedly different flavor, which is typical of any amino acid mixture. Most infants and children accept it without difficulty. It is the main source of energy and protein throughout the years of treatment.

The quantity of 9.5 g. of Lofenalac powder (or one packed scoop supplied by the manufacturer) contains 43 Kcal., nitrogen equivalent to 1.4 g. protein, and approximately 7.5 mg. Phe. Due to the processing method, the amount of Phe in Lofenalac can vary from 0.06 to 0.1 percent, or from 5.7 mg. to 9.5 mg. Phe per 9.5 g. powder. A formula of normal dilution (20 Kcal./30 ml.) can be prepared by adding 9.5 g. of

*Mead Johnson, Evansville, Ind. 47721.

Lofenalac to 60 ml. of water. However, it may not be reconstituted routinely to this dilution, but, rather, mixed according to the amount of Phe required and the volume of formula an infant will drink. In this situation, total fluid intake must be checked daily to prevent dehydration due to an inadequate fluid intake.

Although Lofenalac can supply an infant's energy and protein needs, it cannot supply the Phe requirement. This is discussed later in the section on calculating the diet. Cow's milk, which contains 50 mg. Phe per 30 ml., and other foods of known Phe content but of low protein content are used with Lofenalac to provide the Phe requirement.

A modification of the Exchange System has been designed for planning phenylalanine-restricted diets. In this system foods are listed by groups in the amounts which provide approximately 15 mg. or 30 mg. Phe. Table 35-2 gives the average content of Phe, protein, and energy for the food groups used and Table 35-3 gives the serving lists of the foods within each group. No serving lists are given for meat, egg, or milk. If a child's Phe requirement permits the limited use of these foods, the amount to be used can be calculated from Table 3, Section 4. The Bread and Cereal List in Table 35-3 does not include bread per se. One slice of bread made with 4 percent milk solids contains approximately 105 mg. Phe. If the Phe requirement permits, bread can be calculated in the diet pattern.

In addition to the information in Tables 35-2 and 35-3 and Table 3, Section 4, there are other sources of the Phe content of foods. The Phe content of some foods is available from the producers. Many state health departments have published guides for the management of PKU, including tables of the Phe content of foods. PKU treatment centers also make available their materials.*

Table 35-2. Average Nutrient Content Of Serving Lists*

List	Phenyl-alanine mg.	Protein g.	Energy Kcal.
Vegetables	15	0.5	10
Fruits			
Strained and junior	15	0.6	150
Table and juices	15	0.6	70
Breads and Cereals	30	0.6	30
Fats	5	0.1	60
Desserts†	30	varies	varies

*From The Phenylalanine-Restricted Diet—for Professional Use, 1966. The Bureau of Public Health Nutrition of the California State Department of Public Health.
†Average of dessert recipes in Phenylalanine-Restricted Diet Recipe Book, The Bureau of Public Health Nutrition of the California State Department of Health.

*Phenylalanine Content of Foods, Children's Hospital Research Foundation, Cincinnati, Ohio 45229.

Table 35-3. Serving Lists for Phenylalanine-Restricted Diet*

Food	Amount	Phenyl-alanine mg.	Protein g.	Energy Kcal.
Vegetables Each serving as listed contains 15 milligrams of phenylalanine				
Baby and Junior				
Beets	7 tbsp.	15	1.1	35
Carrots	7 tbsp.	15	0.7	28
Creamed Spinach	1 tbsp.	16	0.4	6
Green Beans	2 tbsp.	15	0.3	7
Squash	4 tbsp.	14	0.4	14
Table Vegetables				
Asparagus, cooked	1 stalk	12	0.6	4
Beans, green, cooked	4 tbsp. (¼ cup)	14	0.6	9
Beans, yellow, wax, cooked	4 tbsp. (¼ cup)	15	0.6	9
Bean sprouts, mung, cooked	2 tbsp.	18	0.6	5
Beets, cooked	8 tbsp. (½ cup)	14	0.8	34
Beet greens, cooked	1 tbsp.	14	0.2	3
Broccoli, cooked	1 tbsp.	11	0.3	3
Brussels sprouts, cooked	1 medium	16	0.6	5
Cabbage, raw, shredded	8 tbsp. (½ cup)	15	0.7	12
Cabbage, cooked	5 tbsp. (⅓ cup)	16	0.8	12
Carrots, raw	⅙ large (¼ cup)	16	0.5	16
Carrots, cooked	8 tbsp. (½ cup)	17	0.5	23
Cauliflower, cooked	3 tbsp.	18	0.6	6
Celery, cooked, diced†	4 tbsp. (¼ cup)	15	0.4	6
Celery, raw†	1—8 inch stalk	16	0.5	7
Chard leaves, cooked	2 tbsp.	19	0.6	6
Collards, cooked	1 tbsp.	16	0.5	5
Cucumber slices, raw	8 slices, ⅛" thick	16	0.7	12
Eggplant, diced, raw	3 tbsp.	18	0.4	9
Kale, cooked	2 tbsp.	20	0.5	5
Lettuce†	3 small leaves	13	0.4	5
Mushrooms, cooked†	2 tbsp.	14	0.4	35
Mushrooms, fresh†	2 small	16	0.5	3
Mustard greens, cooked	2 tbsp.	18	0.6	6
Okra, cooked†	2—3" pods	13	0.4	7
Onion, raw, chopped	5 tbsp. (⅓ cup)	14	0.5	20
Onion, cooked	4 tbsp. (¼ cup)	14	0.5	19
Onion, young scallion	5—5" long	14	0.5	23
Parsley, raw, chopped†	3 tbsp.	13	0.4	5
Parsnips, cooked, diced†	3 tbsp.	13	0.3	18
Peppers, raw, chopped†	4 tbsp.	13	0.4	12
Pickles, Dill	8 slices—⅛" thick	16	0.7	12
Pumpkin, cooked	4 tbsp. (¼ cup)	14	0.5	16
Radishes, red, small†	4	13	0.4	8
Rutabagas, cooked	2 tbsp.	16	0.3	10
Soups				
Beef broth (Campbell's condensed)	1 tbsp.	14	0.5	3
Celery (Campbell's condensed)	2 tbsp.	18	0.4	19
Minestrone (Campbell's condensed)	1 tbsp.	17	1.5	25
Mushroom (Campbell's condensed)	1 tbsp.	11	0.2	17
Onion (Campbell's condensed)	1 tbsp.	14	0.6	8
Tomato (Campbell's condensed)	1 tbsp.	11	0.2	11
Vegetarian Veg. (Campbell's condensed)	1½ tbsp.	17	0.4	14
Spinach cooked	1 tbsp.	15	0.4	3
Squash, summer, cooked	8 tbsp. (½ cup)	16	0.6	16
Squash, winter, cooked	3 tbsp.	16	0.6	14
Tomato, raw	½ small	14	0.5	10
Tomato, cooked	4 tbsp. (¼ cup)	15	0.6	10
Tomato juice	4 tbsp. (¼ cup)	17	0.6	12
Tomato catsup	2 tbsp.	17	0.6	34
Turnip greens, cooked	1 tbsp.	18	0.4	4
Turnips, diced, cooked	5 tbsp. (⅓ cup)	16	0.4	12

*From The Phenylalanine-Restricted Diet—for Professional Use, 1966. The Bureau of Public Health Nutrition of the California State Department of Public Health.
†Phenylalanine calculated at 3.3 percent of total protein.

Table 35-3. Serving Lists for Phenylalanine-Restricted Diet (Continued)

Fruits
Each serving as listed contains 15 milligrams of phenylalanine

Food	Amount	Phenyl-alanine mg.	Protein g.	Energy Kcal.
Baby and Junior				
Applesauce and apricots	16 tbsp. (1 cup)	15	0.6	205
Applesauce and pineapple	16 tbsp. (1 cup)	11	0.5	176
Apricots with tapioca	16 tbsp. (1 cup)	16	0.6	187
Bananas	8 tbsp. (½ cup)	14	0.6	97
Bananas and pineapple	16 tbsp. (1 cup)	18	0.6	187
Peaches	10 tbsp.	15	0.7	124
Pears	12 tbsp. (¾ cup)	16	0.5	106
Pears and pineapple	16 tbsp. (1 cup)	17	1.0	166
Plums with tapioca	12 tbsp. (¾ cup)	16	0.5	163
Prunes with tapioca	12 tbsp. (¾ cup)	16	0.5	152
Fruit Juices				
Apricot nectar	6 oz. (¾ cup)	14	0.6	102
Cranberry juice	12 oz. (1½ cup)	15	0.6	39
Grape juice	4 oz. (½ cup)	14	0.5	80
Grapefruit juice	8 oz. (1 cup)	16	1.2	104
Orange juice	6 oz. (¾ cup)	16	1.2	84
Peach nectar	5 oz. (⅔ cup)	15	0.5	75
Pineapple juice	6 oz. (¾ cup)	16	0.6	90
Prune juice	4 oz. (½ cup)	16	0.5	84
Table Fruits				
Apple, raw	4 small 2½" diam.	16	0.8	176
Applesauce	16 tbsp. (1 cup)	12	0.6	192
Apricots, raw	1 medium	12	0.5	25
Apricots, canned	2 medium 2 tbsp. syrup	14	0.6	80
Avocado, cubed or mashed†	5 tbsp. (⅓ cup)	16	0.6	80
Banana, raw, sliced	4 tbsp. (¼ cup)	15	0.4	32
Blackberries, raw†	5 tbsp. (⅓ cup)	14	0.6	25
Blackberries, canned, in syrup†	5 tbsp. (⅓ cup)	13	0.5	55
Blueberries, raw or frozen†	12 tbsp. (¾ cup)	16	0.6	60
Blueberries, canned, in syrup†	10 tbsp.	16	0.6	140
Boysenberries, frozen, sweetened†	8 tbsp. (½ cup)	16	0.6	72
Cantaloupe	5 tbsp. (⅓ cup)	16	0.4	15
Cherries, sweet, canned in syrup†	8 tbsp. (½ cup)	16	0.6	104
Dates, pitted, chopped	3 tbsp.	18	0.7	96
Figs, raw†	1 large	18	0.7	40
Figs, canned, in syrup†	2 figs 4 tsp. syrup	16	0.6	90
Figs, dried†	1 small	16	0.6	40
Fruit cocktail†	12 tbsp. (¾ cup)	16	0.6	120
Grapes, American type	8 grapes	14	0.5	24
Grapes, American slipskin	5 tbsp. (⅓ cup)	16	0.6	25
Grapes, Thompson seedless	8 tbsp. (½ cup)	13	0.8	64
Guava, raw†	½ medium	13	0.5	35
Honeydew melon†	¼ small 5" melon	13	0.5	32
Mango, raw†	1 small	18	0.7	66
Nectarines, raw	1—2" high, 2" diam.	15	0.4	45
Oranges, raw	1 medium 3" diam. or ⅔ cup sections	15	1.1	60
Papayas, raw†	¼ med. or ½ cup	14	0.6	36
Peaches, raw	1 medium	15	0.5	46
Peaches, canned, in syrup	2 medium halves	18	0.6	88
Pears, raw	1—3" x 2½"	14	1.3	100
Pears, canned, in syrup	2 med. halves 2 tbsp. syrup	14	1.3	78
Pineapple, raw†	16 tbsp. (1 cup)	16	0.6	80
Pineapple, canned, in syrup†	2 small slices	13	0.5	93
Plums, raw	½—2" plum	12	0.3	15
Plums, canned, in syrup	3—2 tbsp. syrup	16	0.5	91
Prunes, dried	2 large	14	0.4	54
Raisins, dried seedless	2 tbsp.	14	0.5	54
Raspberries, raw†	5 tbsp. (⅓ cup)	13	0.5	25
Raspberries, canned, in syrup†	6 tbsp.	14	0.5	78
Strawberries, raw†	8 large	16	0.6	32
Strawberries, frozen†	6 tbsp.	14	0.5	108
Tangerines	1½ large	15	1.2	66
Watermelon†	½ cup cubes	13	0.5	28

†Phenylalanine calculated as 2.6 percent of total protein.

Table 35-3. Serving Lists for Phenylalanine-Restricted Diet (Continued)

Food	Amount	Phenyl-alanine mg.	Protein gm.	Energy Kcal.
Breads and Cereals				
Each serving as listed contains 30 milligrams of phenylalanine				
Baby and Junior				
Cereals, ready to serve				
Barley	3 tbsp.	32	0.8	24
Oatmeal	2 tbsp.	34	0.8	16
Rice	5 tbsp. (⅓ cup)	30	0.6	40
Wheat	2 tbsp.	30	0.6	17
Creamed corn	3 tbsp.	30	0.5	27
Sweet Potatoes (Gerber's)	3 tbsp.	32	0.5	31
Table Foods				
Cereals, cooked				
Cornmeal	4 tbsp. (¼ cup)	29	0.6	29
Cream of rice	4 tbsp. (¼ cup)	35	0.7	34
Cream of wheat	2 tbsp.	27	0.6	16
Farina	2 tbsp.	25	0.5	18
Malt-o-meal	2 tbsp.	27	0.5	17
Oatmeal	2 tbsp.	32	0.7	18
Pettijohns	2 tbsp.	24	0.5	19
Ralstons	2 tbsp.	34	0.7	18
Rice, brown or white	4 tbsp. (¼ cup)	35	0.7	34
Wheatena	2 tbsp.	27	0.5	19
Cereals, ready to serve				
Alpha bits	4 tbsp. (¼ cup)	32	0.6	28
Cheerios	3 tbsp.	32	0.6	20
Corn Chex	4 tbsp. (¼ cup)	29	0.6	32
Cornflakes	5 tbsp.	29	0.6	30
Kix	5 tbsp. (⅓ cup)	31	0.6	31
Krumbles	3 tbsp.	32	0.7	26
Rice Chex	6 tbsp.	32	0.7	49
Rice flakes	5 tbsp. (⅓ cup)	33	0.6	32
Rice Krispies	6 tbsp.	30	0.6	40
Rice, puffed	12 tbsp. (¾ cup)	30	0.6	38
Sugar Crisp, puffed wheat	4 tbsp. (¼ cup)	30	0.6	46
Sugar sparkled flakes	5 tbsp. (⅓ cup)	29	0.6	55
Wheat Chex	10 biscuits	30	0.6	22
Wheaties	3 tbsp.	26	0.5	20
Wheat, puffed	6 tbsp.	30	0.6	16
Crackers				
Barnum Animal	5	30	0.6	45
Graham (65/lb.)	1	26	0.5	30
Ritz (no cheese)	2	24	0.5	34
Saltines (140/lb.)	2	29	0.6	28
Soda (63/lb.)	1	36	0.7	30
Wheat thins (248/lb.)	5	30	0.6	45
Others				
Corn, cooked	2 tbsp.	32	0.7	17
Hominy	2 tbsp.	32	0.7	17
Macaroni, cooked	1½ tbsp.	31	0.7	20
Noodles, cooked	3 tbsp.	32	0.7	20
Popcorn, popped	5 tbsp. (⅓ cup)	31	0.6	17
Potato chips	4—2" diam.	30	0.6	44
Potato, Irish, cooked	3 tbsp.	33	0.8	31
Spaghetti, cooked	1 tbsp.	24	0.5	14
Sweet potato, cooked	2 tbsp.	25	0.4	31
Tortilla, corn	1½—6" diam.	30	0.8	31
Fats				
Each serving as listed contains 5 milligrams of phenylalanine				
Butter	1 tbsp.	5	0.1	100
French dressing, commercial	1 tbsp.	5	0.1	59
Mayonnaise, commercial	1 tbsp.	5	0.1	100
Margarine	½ tbsp.	5	0.1	30
Olives, green or ripe	1 medium	5	0.1	12

†Phenylalanine calculated as 2.6 percent of total protein.

Table 35-3.   Serving Lists for Phenylalanine-Restricted Diet (Continued)

Food	Amount
Desserts Each serving as listed contains 30 milligrams of phenylalanine	
Cake†	1/12 of cake
Cookies—Rice flour†	2
Corn starch†	2
Cookies, Arrowroot	1½
Ice Cream—Chocolate†	⅔ cup
Pineapple†	⅔ cup
Strawberry†	⅔ cup
Jello	⅓ cup
Puddings†	½ cup
Sauce, Hershey	2 tbsp.
Wafers, sugar, Nabisco	5

Free Foods
Contain little or no phenylalanine. May be used as desired.

Apple juice	Cherries, Maraschino	Popsicles, with artificial fruit
Beverages, carbonated	Fruit ices (if no more than ½	flavor
Gingerbread‡	cup used daily)	Rich's Topping
Guava Butter	Cornstarch	Salt
Candy	Jell-quik	Shortening, vegetable
Butterscotch	Jellies	Soy sauce
Cream Mints	Kool-ade	Sugar, brown, white, or
Fondant	Lemonade	confectioner's
Gum drops	Molasses	Syrups, corn or maple
Hard	Oil	Tang
Jelly beans	Pepper, black, ground	Tapioca
Lollipops		

†Low phenylalanine recipes—in Phenylalanine-Restricted Diet Recipe Book.
‡Special recipe must be used—in Phenylalanine-Restricted Diet Recipe Book.

CALCULATING THE DIET PATTERN. When formula is the only source of energy and nutrients for an infant, Lofenalac, cow's milk, and Karo Syrup or other sources of carbohydrate are used. For example, an infant weighing 3.5 kg. needs 420 Kcal., 7.7 g. protein and 240 mg. Phe per day. The quantity of formula ingredients would be:

	Kcal.	Protein (g.)	Phe (mg.)
57 g. Lofenalac	258	8.4	45
4 oz. (120 ml.) cow's milk	80	4.4	200
1 tbsp. Karo Syrup	60	—	
water			
	398	12.8	245

As the child grows and solids are added to his diet, cereals, fruits, and vegetables will supply some Phe and energy while Lofenalac and milk continue to be his major source of energy, protein, and Phe. For example, a two-month-old infant weighing 4.5 kg. needs approximately 500 kcal., 10 g. protein and 315 mg. Phe. The quantity of formula ingredients and baby foods would be:

	Kcal.	Protein (g.)	Phe (mg.)
72 g. Lofenalac	340	11.2	60
4 oz. (120 ml.) milk	80	4.4	200
1 tbsp. Karo Syrup	60		
water			
5 tbsp. rice cereal	40	0.6	30
3 tbsp. applesauce	31	0.1	4
3 tbsp. carrots	12	0.3	9
	563	16.6	303

The older infant will gradually increase his intake of cereals, fruits, and vegetables. At this time, Lofenalac will be his major source of protein and the amount of cow's milk in the formula will decrease as the intake of Phe from other foods increases. With each revision in the calculation of the diet pattern, the mineral and vitamin content must be checked for adequacy because an infant's needs for these nutrients will increase as he grows larger.

As the very young child progresses to table foods, Lofenalac continues to be the major source of dietary protein and will supply part of the energy needs.

Cereals, fruits, vegetables, sugars and fats, with small amounts of animal protein if the diet prescription permits, are used to provide Phe and energy. At this stage, part of the Lofenalac is usually reconstituted for drinking and part may be used in making puddings, cookies, and white sauce.[14,15] If the Phe prescription requires it, cornstarch or low-protein wheat starch (see Chapter 31) are used in place of wheat flour in these dishes.

Special Problems in Dietary Treatment

FIRST FEEDINGS. When the first feedings are initiated, the quantity of Phe in the diet may be less than the estimated requirement for an infant. The Phe blood levels are monitored daily and as the level approaches 20 mg./100 ml. or less, the Phe in the feedings will be increased to meet the infant's requirement. This can be achieved most readily by adjusting the quantity of cow's milk in the formula.

EXCURSIONS IN THE PHE BLOOD LEVELS IN THE TREATED PKU PATIENT. An elevated Phe blood level in a treated PKU infant or child may reflect an excessive intake of Phe or an inadequate energy intake. Without an adequate energy intake from fats and carbohydrates, body proteins are catabolized to provide energy. Also, an elevated Phe level may be due to a hypermetabolic state caused by infection. Therefore, not only dietary management but, also, the infant's or child's physical condition must be assessed when blood Phe levels are elevated in a previously well-controlled patient.

Very low blood Phe levels, less than 2 mg./100 ml., are avoided because a blood level this low can result in a condition similar to kwashiorkor or energy-protein malnutrition (see Chapter 20).

EXPENSE OF THE DIET. In some treatment centers funding is available to provide Lofenalac free of cost to the family. In other situations funding is not available and the family must purchase the product. In 1975 a 2½ pound can cost approximately $12.50 or $.90 each day for a three-month-old infant. If any of the wheat starch products are used, these will also increase the cost of feeding the infant or child with PKU.

LIBERALIZATION OF THE DIET. There are no well-controlled studies at this time which indicate whether or not the diet of the PKU child can be liberalized without adverse effects on intellectual development. Koch[16] points out that, probably at age eight, when myelination and brain mass have reached maturity, the diet can be terminated.

PKU treatment centers are especially concerned about the liberalization of the diet of PKU girls. It has been observed that mothers with untreated PKU produce nonphenylketonuric children who are mentally retarded.[17] Therefore, it is possible that the diet for PKU girls may not be liberalized until after the child-bearing years.

Counseling the Mother

The mother and, whenever possible, the father of the infant with PKU needs to be seen by the same nutrition counselor at each visit to the treatment center and have access to the counselor between visits either by telephone or correspondence. If the blood Phe analysis is not available during the time the mother is at the center, the counselor may need to adjust the diet after the visit. If someone other than the mother is responsible for the child's care, that individual should also be instructed by telephone and correspondence.

When the dietary treatment is initiated, the mother will need careful instruction in formula preparation. Errors in the proportions of Lofenalac powder, water, and cow's milk can be hazardous to the infant. It is strongly recommended that the complete preparation of the formula be demonstrated to the mother and that, under supervision, she return the demonstration. If the mother does not have a standard measuring cup and a set of standard measuring spoons, these should be provided and their correct use in measuring infant foods should be demonstrated.

A copy of the calculated diet pattern with the date noted should be typed so that no error can be made in interpreting the counselor's handwriting. If diet adjustments are made by telephone, a written copy should be mailed immediately to avoid any error in interpreting the oral instructions.

The mother should be helped to understand that the infant must consume the prescribed formula each day and that the quantity of each feeding should be as consistent as possible. For example, if at all possible, she should avoid feeding the infant 90 ml. of formula at one feeding and 200 ml. at the next, especially when formula is the most significant dietary source of energy, protein, and Phe.

Between visits to the treatment center the mother records the quantity and kind of formula and foods consumed by the infant each day. A form which simplifies this task for the mother should be supplied by the center. At each visit the nutrition counselor reviews the record with the mother and correlates the estimation of the infant's daily energy, protein, and Phe intakes with the Phe blood levels. This information is shared with the physician so that, if necessary, adjustments can be made in the diet prescription.

Some mothers prefer an exchange system such as

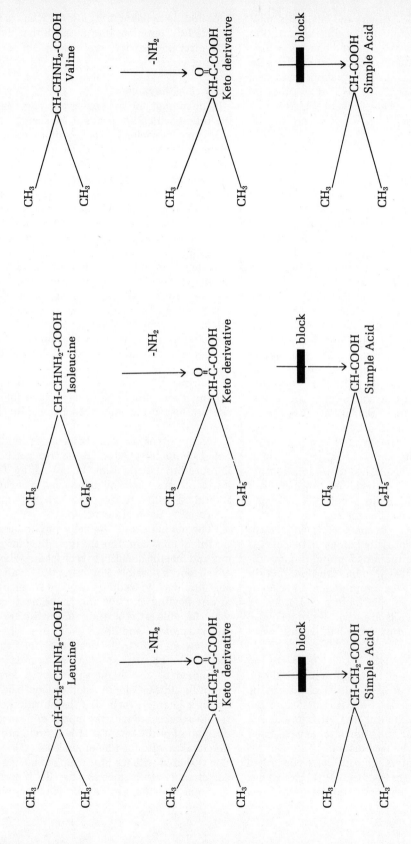

Fig. 35–3. Metabolism of branched-chain amino acids showing the site of block in maple syrup urine disease.

the one in Table 35–3 to plan daily menus. Others prefer to have the values per average serving of food* for older infants and toddlers, in order to calculate the energy, protein, and Phe of the daily menus. With this method a mother can adjust her plans more readily to the child's appetite. For example, on the day a child seems to have a small appetite the mother can offer foods which have more energy and Phe per serving and thus achieve the recommended intake. Also, some mothers will be more comfortable using a scale to weigh foods as the child progresses to table foods.

The mother will also need help to prevent other children in the family, or relatives, friends, and neighbors, from offering the child with PKU any kinds of food or beverages without her knowledge. As the child enters kindergarten or elementary school, the mother will need to communicate with teachers about the child's dietary restrictions.

The instructional methods and materials will vary with each mother depending on her ability to learn and to cope with her infant's diet. Many mothers will need practical suggestions for organizing their daily schedules so that other members of the family as well as the infant with PKU receive her attention and care.

MAPLE SYRUP URINE DISEASE (MSUD)

Maple syrup urine disease is a rare inborn error in the metabolism of the keto acids of the three branched-chain essential amino acids leucine, isoleucine, and valine. The name derives from the maple syrup-like odor of the urine. MSUD is transmitted through an autosomal recessive gene of unknown frequency. Approximately 50 cases have been reported in the literature. However, it is suspected that the diagnosis is often missed because of early infant deaths. The affected individual appears to lack the three decarboxylases required by the three keto acids derived from the transamination of branched-chain amino acids (Fig. 35–3).

The defect is present at birth and the biochemical abnormalities occur as soon as the infant begins to take food protein (milk). The abnormalities are elevated blood levels of the branched-chain amino acids and the three keto acids. The keto acids are also excreted in the urine, hence, another term for the disease, branched-chain ketoaciduria.

The infant is normal at birth but at the end of the first week of life the first symptoms of poor feeding and apathy occur. As early as the fifth day of life the maple syrup-like odor of the urine is detectable. Neurological symptoms with convulsions appear early and, if the disease in untreated, death occurs

*Calculated by the nutrition counselor using Table 35–3, Table 3, Section 4 or other resources.

during the first year of life, sometimes as early as the first week. To avoid neurological damage, diet therapy must be initiated in the first week of life and from present experience it appears that the dietary restrictions must be maintained throughout life.

Types of MSUD

In addition to the classical form of MSUD described above there are two variant forms: one is episodic in nature and the other is a milder form of the classical type. In the episodic form the biochemical abnormalities are only present during major stress such as infection. These children do well on a normal diet without excessive protein. In the mild form, the infant responds to a protein intake limited to requirement. One case of a third variant has been reported.[18] The biochemical abnormality in this child responded to massive doses of thiamine.

Dietary Treatment

PRINCIPLES OF DIET THERAPY: Leucine, isoleucine and valine are essential amino acids. Therefore, in the treatment of MSUD the diet must supply the infant's requirement of these three amino acids without an excess for it to be catabolized through the branched-chain keto acid pathway. At the same time, the diet, as in PKU, must supply adequate energy, total protein, and all other nutrients required for normal growth.

The normal blood levels are: leucine, 1.5 to 3.0 mg./100 ml.; isoleucine, 0.8 to 1.5 mg./100 ml.; and valine, 2.0 to 3.0 mg./100 ml. Smith and Waisman[19] report good control in one patient as measured by normal growth when blood levels of leucine were maintained between 3 to 9 mg./100 ml. With this range in leucine levels the blood level of isoleucine is between 1.5 to 3.0 mg./100 ml. and of valine, between 3 to 6 mg./100 ml. The amino acid requirements of infants as defined by Holt and Snyderman (see Table 35–1) are used as guides in establishing therapy. Smith and Waisman[20] report that in infancy their patient required 130 mg. of leucine per kilogram of body weight during the first months of life and this decreased to 80 mg. per kilogram by the first year.

It has been observed that, to support normal growth, the MSUD infant has a higher energy requirement than normal infants. For example, the patient described above required 160 Kcal. per kilogram of body weight per day during the first year of life instead of 120 to 100 Kcal.

FOOD FOR THE MSUD DIET. All food proteins contain the branched-chain amino acids (BCAA) with a greater percent in animal than vegetable protein. As in the treatment of PKU, a special formula and low-protein foods are used to feed these infants and children.

The formula is a mixture of synthetic amino acids combined with carbohydrate and fat to supply energy. No product similar to Lofenalac is available. A dry base* for special diets is available for research purposes. It contains corn syrup solids, corn oil, and tapioca starch with added minerals and vitamins. There is no source of nitrogen or protein in this mixture. For the MSUD infant a mixture of synthetic amino acids† free of leucine, isoleucine, and valine is added. These two products, the dry base formula and the appropriate mixtures of synthetic amino acids, are used in the treatment of other inborn errors of amino acid metabolism such as isovaleric acidemia and methylmalonic acidemia.

The amino acid mixture for infants with MSUD usually contains the quantity of amino acids in human milk other than BCAA. Appropriate quantities of cow's milk are added to the special formula to supply the BCAA. One hundred ml. of homogenized milk contains 344 mg. of leucine, 223 mg. of isoleucine, and 240 mg. of valine (see Table 3, Section 4). Snyderman[21] reports that without a source of natural protein added to the synthetic amino acid mixture, the infant does not gain weight.

The low-protein foods used can be identified by their leucine content per serving without calculating the isoleucine and valine content because the three BCAA occur in about the same quantity in foods with leucine content usually slightly higher than the other two (see Table 3, Section 4). Also an infant's requirement for the three BCAA are similar (see Table 35–1).

Various investigators[22,23] have developed leucine equivalent tables comparable to an Exchange System. These systems have equated a serving of food with either 15 mg. or 30 mg. of leucine. Table 35–4 gives a list of vegetables equivalent to 15 mg. of leucine per serving, calculated from the leucine values in Table 3, Section 4. Other food lists can also be calculated from Table 3. Rice cereal, low protein fruits, and vegetables are the foods used to supplement the infant's formula. Low-protein wheat starch products (see Chapter 31) may be used as the child grows older as a source of energy.

The MSUD diet is expensive. In 1975 the amino acid mixture for a five-month-old infant with MSUD cost approximately $66 per month compared with the cost of approximately $10 a month for a standard formula. If low-protein wheat starch products are used, this also increases the cost of the diet. As in PKU, some states provide the special foods, while others do not.

*Mead Johnson, Evansville, Ind. 47721
†Grand Island Biological Co., Grand Island, N.Y. 14072.

Table 35-4. Leucine Equivalents (15 mg.) of Selected Vegetables*

Vegetable	Gram Weight	Household Measure
Asparagus	18	1 spear
Beans, snap	26	¼ cup
Beets	50	½ cup
Cabbage	24	½ cup, raw
		¼ cup, cooked
Carrots, raw	23	½ cup
Potatoes, cooked	17	2 tbsp.
Pumpkin	24	¼ cup
Tomatoes	52	½ cup

*Calculated from Table 3, Section 4.

CALCULATING THE DIET. The first feedings for the infant with MSUD are made using a formula consisting of the dry base and synthetic amino acids containing approximately 20 Kcal. per 30 ml. When the elevated BCAA blood levels return to normal, cow's milk is added to the formula to supply the infant's requirement for these essential amino acids. For example, an infant weighting 3.5 kg. requires approximately 445 mg. leucine per day (3.5 kg. × 130 mg.). This amount of leucine can be supplied by 132 ml. (4 oz.) of homogenized milk.

When the child is ready for infant foods, low-protein cereals, fruits, and vegetables can be used, in addition to homogenized milk, to supply the daily requirements of BCAA. The formula of dry base and synthetic amino acids is continued to meet the infant's needs for energy, protein, and all other nutrients.

Counseling the Mother

The mother of the infant with MSUD needs the same assistance as the mother of an infant with PKU (see p. 507).

The formula for the infant with MSUD is more complicated to prepare than Lofenalac. The mother needs a demonstration on its preparation and a written recipe at the beginning and with every change in formula. She may need to be cautioned to shake the bottle with each feeding, especially the first formula without milk added, because the ingredients may settle to the bottom of the bottle on standing.

OTHER INBORN ERRORS OF METABOLISM
Homocystinuria

Homocystinuria is an inborn error in the metabolism of the essential sulfur-containing amino acid methionine due to a marked deficiency in the activity of the hepatic enzyme cystathionine synthase. In the untreated patient the disease is characterized by skeletal and ocular abnormalities and mental retardation. There is an elevated blood level of both methionine and homocystine, with the urinary excretion of significant amounts of homocystine and lesser amounts of methionine.

There are two types of homocystinuric patients. One group responds to massive doses of pyridoxine (vitamin B₆), possibly due to the stimulation of hepatic cystathionine synthase by pyridoxine. These patients can tolerate a diet with a moderate reduction in methionine.[24]

Another group of patients responds to a diet low in methionine with supplemental L-cystine added. Perry recommends[25] Metinaid*, a product low in methione, as the major source of dietary protein for the homocystinuric patient. The Metinaid is dissolved in orange juice or lemonade. Fruits, vegetables, bread, cereals, and fats are used to supply energy (see Table 3, Section 4). One infant with homocystinuria, reported by Perry,[26] required 40 mg. of methionine per kg. of body weight. This value is in good agreement with the figure of Holt and Snyderman of 45 mg./kg. in the presence of cystine in the diet (see Table 35-1). As the child grows, the requirement per kilogram of body weight will decrease.

Leucine-Sensitive Hypoglycemia

Hypoglycemic reactions in infancy induced by the essential amino acid leucine may be another inborn error of metabolism. The evidence for genetic transmission is not well established at present. In normal children the administration of leucine stimulates a small rise in circulating blood insulin and a small decrease in blood glucose. In leucine-sensitive infants with hypoglycemia there is some evidence that the infant has an increased number of pancreatic beta cells which may respond to an increase in insulin release when stimulated by leucine, e.g. a high-protein diet.

The condition may be manifested from birth, or it may appear later in the first year of life. The symptoms are precipitated by a high-protein meal or a state of fast. In the early stages there are irritability and twitching movements of the extremities, and, if the disease is not treated, hypoglycemic convulsions, with blood sugar levels as low as 20 mg. percent. Eventually, failure to thrive and mental and psychomotor retardation occur.

The infant with leucine-sensitive hypoglycemia responds to a diet restricted in leucine, although not as restricted as in the treatment of maple syrup urine disease. Hsia[27] suggests 150 to 230 mg. of leucine per kilogram of body weight. A special formula, SMA

*Milner Scientific and Medical Research Co., Ltd., 37 Ganung Dr., Ossining, N.Y.

S-14* (see Table 34-4), is restricted in leucine and is used to feed these infants. As the child grows older, foods of low leucine content are added to the diet (see Table 3, Section 4).

Roth and Segal have devised a dietary regimen for older children consisting of a leucine restricted diet with extra carbohydrate (between 10 to 30 g. carbohydrate) after each meal to prevent hypoglycemic reactions. This regimen has controlled the symptoms and the children have developed normally.[28,29] By the time the child is five or six years old, he is usually able to tolerate a normal diet.

Histidinemia

Histidinemia is an inborn error of the metabolism of the amino acid histidine due to a deficiency of the enzyme histidase. High levels of histidine are found in the blood and urine. Clinical symptoms are manifested in speech disorders, both in articulation and language, though not in all of the patients known to have this disease. There is mental retardation in some patients, although again, not in all. A diet restricted in protein was not effective in lowering histidine in the blood or urine. However, a high-protein diet should be avoided in infancy.[30]

STUDY QUESTIONS

1. What is the metabolic defect in phenylketonuria? Why is it important that it be treated early?
2. List some of the problems that a family may encounter daily in maintaining a three-year-old child with PKU on a phenylalanine-restricted diet.
3. Why must the energy intake be adequate in an infant with an inborn error of amino acid metabolism?
4. Plan the formula demonstration for a mother with a PKU infant.
5. Why must medications be closely scrutinized when an infant or child is on a galactose-free diet?

SUPPLEMENTARY READINGS

GENERAL

Brady, R. O.: The lipid storage diseases: new concepts and control. Ann. Int. Med. 82:257, 1975.

Erbe, R. W.: Inborn errors of folate metabolism. N. Eng. J. Med. 293:753; 807, 1975.

Frimpter, G. W.: Aminoacidurias due to inherited disorders of metabolism. N. Eng. J. Med. 289:835; 895, 1973.

Hsia, Y. E.: Inherited hyperammonemic syndromes. Gastroent. 67:347, 1974.

GALACTOSEMIA

Applebaum, M. N., and Thaler, M. M.: Reversibility of extensive liver damage in galactosemia Gastroent. 69:496, 1975.

*Wyeth Laboratories, Philadelphia, Pa. 19101.

Beutler, E. M., et al: Galactokinase deficiency as a cause of cataracts. N. Eng. J. Med. 288:1203, 1973.

Cohn, R. M., and Segal, S: Galactose metabolism and its regulation. Metabolism 22:627, 1973.

Fisher, K., et al: Intellectual and personality development in children with galactosemia. Pediatrics 50:412, 1972.

Tedesco, T. A., et al: The genetic defect in galactosemia. N. Eng. J. Med. 292:737, 1975.

PHENYLKETONURIA

Holtzman, N. A., et al: Termination of restricted diet in children with phenylketonuria: a randomized controlled study. N. Eng. J. Med. 293:1121, 1975.

Justice, P., and Smith, G. F.: Phenylketonuria. Am. J. Nurs. 75:1303, 1975.

McCarthy, M. A., Orr, M. L., and Watt, B. K.: Phenylalanine and tyrosine in vegetables and fruits. J. Am. Dietet. A. 52:130, 1968.

McCready, R. A.: Admissions of phenylketonuric patients to residential institutions before and after screening programs of the newborn infant. J. Pediat. 85:383, 1974.

Smith, B. A., and Waisman, H. A.: Adequate phenylalanine intake for optimum growth and development in the treatment of phenylketonuria. Am. J. Clin. Nutr. 24:423, 1971.

Smith, I., and Wolff, O. H.: Natural history of phenylketonuria and influence of early treatment. Lancet 2:540, 1974.

MAPLE SYRUP URINE DISEASE

Levy, H. L., et al: Folic acid deficiency secondary to diet for maple syrup urine disease. J. Pediat. 77:294, 1970.

Smith, B. A., and Waisman, H. A.: Leucine equivalency system in managing branched chain ketoacidurias. J. Am. Dietet. A. 59:342, 1971.

Snyderman, S. E.: The therapy of maple syrup urine disease. A. J. Dis. Child., 113:68, 1967.

OTHER INBORN ERRORS OF METABOLISM

Batshaw, M., et al: Treatment of carbamyl synthetase deficiency with keto analogues of essential amino acids. N. Eng. J. Med. 292:1085, 1975.

Brandt, I. K., et al: Propionicacidemia (ketotic hyperglycinemia): dietary treatment resulting in normal growth and development. Pediatrics 53:391, 1974.

Levy, H. L., et al: Isovaleric acidemia: results of family study and dietary treatment. Pediatrics 52:83, 1973.

Poole, J. H., et al: Homocystinuria due to cystathione synthase deficiency. Studies of nitrogen balance and sulfur excretion. J. Clin. Invest. 55:1033, 1975.

RESOURCES FOR PARENTS OF CHILDREN WITH PKU

PKU — A Diet Guide, 1970. Available from Chief Nutritionist, Division of Child Development, Children's Hospital at Los Angeles, 4650 Sunset Boulevard, Los Angeles, California 90054.

The Low Phenylalanine Diet ($1.00 per copy). Available from Bureau of Public Health Nutrition, Michigan Department of Public Health, Lansing, Michigan.

A Diet Guide for Parents of Children with Phenylketonuria, 1966. Available to residents of the State of California only from Bureau of Public Health Nutrition, California Department of Public Health, 2151 Berkeley Way, Berkeley, California 94704.

Other treatment centers and state departments of public health have materials for parents of children with PKU. Check the nearest resource.

For further references see Bibliography, Section 4.

REFERENCES

1. Segal, S: in *The Metabolic Basis of Inherited Disease*, ed. 3, J. B. Stanbury, J. B. Wyngaarden, and D. S. Fredrickson, eds. New York, McGraw-Hill, 1972, Chapter 8.
2. Ibid.
3. Hardinge, M. G., et al: J. Am. Dietet. A. 46:197, 1965.
4. Ibid.
5. Gitzelman, R. and Auricchio, S.: Pediatrics 36:231, 1965.
6. Segal, S., op. cit.
7. Knox, W. E.: in *The Metabolic Basis of Inherited Disease*.
8. McCready, R. A.: Pediatrics 85:383, 1974.
9. Rouse, B. M.: J. Pediat. 69:246, 1966.
10. Fomon, S. J.: *Infant Nutrition*, ed. 2. Philadelphia, Saunders, 1974, p. 143.
11. Hunt, M. H., et al: A. J. Dis. Child. 122:1, 1971.
12. Nakagawa, I., et al: J. Nutrition 77:61, 1962.
13. McCarthy, M. A., et al: J. Am. Dietet. A. 52:130, 1968.
14. Diet Guide for Parents of Children with Phenylketonuria. Berkeley, Ca., California Department of Health, 1966.
15. Rinic, M. M. and Rogers, P. J.: J. Am. Dietet. A. 55:353, 1969.
16. Koch, R., et al: in *Heritable Disorders of Amino Acid Metabolism*, W. L. Nyhan, ed. New York, Wiley, 1974.
17. Mabry, C. C., et al: N. Eng. J. Med. 275:1331, 1966.
18. Scriver, C. R., et al: Lancet 1:310, 1971.
19. Smith, B. A. and Waisman, H. A.: J. Am. Dietet. A. 59:342, 1971.
20. Ibid.
21. Snyderman, S. E.: in *Heritable Disorders of Amino Acid Metabolism*.
22. Smith, B. A. and Waisman, H. A., op. cit.
23. Levy, H. L. and Erickson, A. M.: in *Heritable Disorders of Amino Acid Metabolism*.
24. Mudd, S. H., et al: J. Clin. Invest. 49:1762, 1970.
25. Perry, T. L.: in *Heritable Disorders of Amino Acid Metabolism*.
26. Ibid.
27. Hsia, D. Y-Y.: *Inborn Errors of Metabolism, Part I, Clinical Aspects*, ed. 2. Chicago, Year Book Medical Pub., 1966.
28. Roth, H., et al: Pediatrics 34: 831, 1964.
29. Snyder, R. D. and Robinson, A.: A. J. Dis. Child. 113:566, 1967.
30. Ghadmi, H.: in *Heritable Disorders of Amino Acid Metabolism*.

tabular material
and bibliography

tables

explanation of tables

TABLE 1. COMPOSITION OF FOODS— EDIBLE PORTION

This table of food values gives proximate composition and mineral and vitamin content of most foods in common use in the United States. It includes processed and prepared foods where such foods would not be consumed in the natural state. The foods have been arranged alphabetically for convenience. The values for 100-g. portions are given for all natural foods, but for some processed foods the common unit of package or can is given where a 100-g. portion would seldom be used.

515

Most of the values are taken from the second edition of Handbook No. 8[1] and a few values from other sources.[2,3,4,5,6]

Reliability of Data

Research in food values has demonstrated repeatedly that the composition of foods is variable, due to differences in variety, soil, and climate in which they are grown, and the methods of handling, sampling, and analyzing. The values given are usually averages of several determinations on a variety of samples and frequently include a wide range of values; therefore, it seems unnecessary to retain decimals where they are of questionable significance. Thus, the values for calories and for grams of protein, fat, carbohydrate, and water are given in whole numbers, and fiber is carried to one decimal place only.

Minerals and vitamins are all measured in milligrams (mg.), except for vitamin A, which is still usually given in International Units (I.U.). In order to be consistent in the use of mg., it is necessary to use decimals for measuring the B complex vitamins because they are present in such small amounts.

The common measures for 100 g. or other quantities commonly used are only approximate. For instance, 100 g. of most liquids would measure about ²/₅ of a cup. Since this is not a convenient fraction for measuring, the designation ½ *cup scant* has been used. This would mean about 1½ tbsp. less than ½ cup.

The individual nutrients in foods have been determined by many different laboratories and the data assembled by the Department of Agriculture or other agencies.

Food Energy

Kcal. values have been calculated by using specific factors for individual foods, taking into consideration the digestibility and the physiologic value of nutrients. It is still possible to estimate caloric value of a food by applying the factors 4, 9, and 4 kcal. per gram of protein, fat and carbohydrate, respectively, but the values will be slightly different from those calculated by the more accurate method mentioned. One kilocalorie (kcal.) is equivalent to 4.186 kilojoules (KJ).

Niacin Values

The values for niacin are for the preformed niacin present in the food. Since niacin may be formed in the body from tryptophan in food protein, the total niacin will be larger than the figure given in most cases. "The average diet in the United States, which con-tains a generous amount of protein, provides enough tryptophan to increase the niacin value by about a third."[7]

TABLE 2. SELECTED FATTY ACIDS AND CHOLESTEROL IN COMMON FOODS

This table gives the total fat; the total saturated fat; the unsaturated fatty acids, oleic (monounsaturated), and linoleic (polyunsaturated); and the cholesterol content of common foods. Values are taken from Handbook No. 8,[8] Hardinge and Crooks,[9] Feeley, et al,[10] Anderson, et al,[11] and Posati, et al.[12]

TABLE 3. AMINO ACID CONTENT OF FOODS PER 100 GRAMS—EDIBLE PORTION

The essential amino acid content of selected foods is listed in an order convenient for nurses and dietitians dealing with inborn errors of metabolism. The values are given in micrograms rather than milligrams to avoid the use of decimals.

TABLE 4. SODIUM, POTASSIUM AND MAGNESIUM CONTENT OF FOODS

Table 4 gives sodium, potassium and magnesium content of foods. Copper values are omitted because the values given in the literature are conflicting and incomplete. References to pertinent articles are given at the end of Table 4.

TABLE 5. ZINC CONTENT OF FOODS PER 100 GRAMS—EDIBLE PORTION

This table lists the total zinc content in milligrams of 100 g. edible portions of raw and cooked foods. It includes the foods which are consumed in greatest quantities by U.S. households and certain other foods which are important sources of zinc. Many values in this table were derived from a limited number of analyses and hence are called provisional.[13]

TABLE 6. ALCOHOLIC AND CARBONATED BEVERAGES

The calorie, carbohydrate, and alcohol content of common alcoholic and carbonated beverages are listed in this table to assist the nutrition counselor in planning and assessing dietary intake.

TABLE 7. EQUIVALENT WEIGHTS AND MEASURES

This table which lists weight, volume, and linear equivalents; comparative temperatures for centigrade and Fahrenheit scales; and approximate weights for common measures, should serve as a ready reference.

TABLE 8. HEIGHT AND WEIGHT FOR AGE— PERCENTILE STANDARDS—BOYS AND GIRLS

Heights and weights for boys and girls for each year from age 2 to 18 are listed according to their percentile standards. This table permits the nutrition counselor to compare and evaluate height and weight in terms of percentile when assessing growth.

TABLE 9. DESIRABLE WEIGHTS FOR MEN AND WOMEN AGED 25 AND OVER

This table gives the desirable adult weight for height according to the size of the individual's frame—small, medium, or large. It is based on the concept that there is no need for an increase in weight once adult height is achieved.

TABLE 10. CURRENT GUIDELINES FOR CRITERIA OF NUTRITIONAL STATUS FOR LABORATORY EVALUATION

Laboratory methods for evaluating nutritional status include biochemical tests which measure levels of nutrients in blood or urine or biochemical functions which are dependent on an adequate supply of essential nutrients. These tests vary in their reproducibility and nutrient levels may vary from time to time reflecting immediate rather than usual intake. The "cut-off points" used in the table "as representing some degree of deficiency are, and will presumably always be a matter of some argument and arbitrary decision."[14] However, evaluating nutritional status by biochemical tests is recognized as a more precise approach than dietary intake studies or clinical examinations.[15]

Signs and Symbols Used in Tables

An asterisk in a table indicates an item for which the composition has been calculated from a recipe.

Dots (. .) show that no basis could be found for imputing a value, although there was some reason to believe that a measurable amount of the constituent might be present.

The designation Tr. (trace) is used to indicate values that would round to zero when calculated to the number of decimal places used in each column.

REFERENCES

1. Watt, B. K., and Merrill, A. L.: Composition of Foods— Raw, Processed, Prepared. Agr. Handbook No. 8, ed. 2. Washington, D. C., USDA, 1963.
2. Burger, M., et al: J. Agr. & Food Chem., 4:417, 1956.
3. Church, C. E., and Church, H. N.: *Food Values of Portions Commonly Used*, ed. 12. Philadelphia, Lippincott, 1975.
4. Hardinge, M. G., and Crooks, H.: J. Am. Dietet. A. 34:1065, 1958.
5. Orr, M. L., and Watt, B. K.: Home Econ. Res. Report No. 4. Washington, D. C., USDA, 1957.
6. Nutrition Value of Foods. Home and Garden Bulletin No. 72. Washington, D. C., Agricultural Research Service, USDA, 1960.
7. Ibid.
8. Watt, op. cit.
9. Hardinge, op. cit.
10. Feeley, R. M., Criner, P. E., and Watt, B. K.: J. Am. Dietet. A. 61:134, 1972.
11. Anderson, B. A., Kinsella, J. E., and Watt, B. K.: J. Am. Dietet. A., 67:35, 1975.
12. Posati, L. P., Kinsella, J. E., and Watt, B. K.: J. Am. Dietet. A. 66:482, 1975.
13. Murphy, E. W., Willis, B. W., and Watt, B. K.: J. Am. Dietet. A. 66:345, 1975.
14. Christakis, G.: Nutritional assessment in health programs. Am. J. Public Health, 63: Supplement (November) 1973.
15. Ibid.

TABLE 1. Composition of Foods—Edible Portion

Food and Description	Wt. Gm.	Approximate Measure	Food Energy K Cal.[a]	Protein Gm.	Fat Gm.	Carbohydrate Total Gm.	Carbohydrate Fiber Gm.	Water Gm.	Minerals Ca Mg.	Minerals P Mg.	Minerals Fe Mg.	Vitamins Vitamin A I.U.	Vitamins Thiamine Mg.	Vitamins Riboflavin Mg.	Vitamins Niacin Mg.	Vitamins Ascorbic Acid Mg.
Acerola (West Indian cherry) raw	100	1 c.	28	Tr.	Tr.	7	0.4	92	12	11	0.2	..	0.02	0.06	0.4	1,300†
Almonds, dried	100	⅔ c.	598	19	54	20	2.6	5	234	504	4.7	0	0.24	0.92	3.5	Tr.
salted	15	12-15	94	3	9	3	0.4	1	35	75	0.7	0	0.04	0.14	0.5	Tr.
Apples:																
Raw, pared	100	medium	54	Tr.	Tr.	14	0.6	85	6	10	0.3	40	0.03	0.02	0.1	2
Frozen, sliced, sweetened	100	⅔ c.	93	Tr.	Tr.	24	0.7	75	5	6	0.5	20	0.01	0.03	0.2	7
Apple Betty*	100	½ c. scant	151	2	4	30	0.5	64	18	22	0.6	100	0.06	0.04	0.4	1
Apple juice, bottled or canned	100	½ c. scant	47	Tr.	0	12	0.1	88	6	9	0.6	..	0.01	0.02	0.1	1
	250	1 c.	120	Tr.	0	30	..	220	15	22	1.5	..	0.03	0.05	0.3	3
Apple sauce, canned:																
Unsweetened	100	½ c. scant	41	Tr.	Tr.	11	0.6	88	4	5	0.5	40	0.02	0.01	Tr.	1
Sweetened	100	½ c. scant	91	Tr.	Tr.	24	0.5	76	4	5	0.5	40	0.02	0.01	Tr.	1
Apricots:																
Raw	100	3 medium	51	1	Tr.	13	0.6	85	17	23	0.5	2,700	0.03	0.04	0.6	10
Canned:																
Solids and liquid water pack	100	½ c. scant	38	1	Tr.	10	0.4	89	12	16	0.3	1,830	0.02	0.02	0.4	4
Syrup pack (heavy syrup)	100	½ c. scant	86	1	Tr.	22	0.4	77	11	15	0.3	1,740	0.02	0.02	0.4	4
Dried, sulfured uncooked	100	{20 large or 30 small halves	260	5	Tr.	67	3.0	25	67	108	5.5	10,900	0.01	0.16	3.3	12
Cooked, sweetened fruit and liquid*	100	⅓ c.	122	1	Tr.	31	0.9	66	19	31	1.6	2,600	Tr.	0.04	0.9	2
Frozen, sweetened	100	½ c.	98	1	Tr.	25	0.6	73	10	19	0.9	1,680	0.02	0.04	0.8	28‡

Tr. (trace) is used to indicate values that would round to zero with the number of decimal places carried in this table. Thus Tr. means 0.4 Gm. or less of protein, fat, carbohydrate or water.

a 1 K Cal. = 4.186 K Joules.

* Values are calculated from a recipe.
† Value for fully ripe fruit. Av. for firm ripe is 1,900; Av. for partially ripe is 2,500.
‡ Varying amounts of ascorbic acid are added in processing.

TABLE 1. COMPOSITION OF FOODS—EDIBLE PORTION (*Continued*)

FOOD AND DESCRIPTION	APPROXIMATE MEASURE	Wt. Gm.	FOOD ENERGY K Cal.[a]	PROTEIN Gm.	FAT Gm.	CARBOHYDRATE Total Gm.	Fiber Gm.	WATER Gm.	MINERALS Ca Mg.	P Mg.	Fe Mg.	VITAMINS Vita-min A I.U.	Thia-mine Mg.	Ribo-flavin Mg.	Nia-cin Mg.	Ascorbic Acid Mg.
Asparagus:																
Fresh, cooked	6-7 spears	100	20	2	Tr.	4	0.7	94	21	50	0.6	900	0.16	0.18	1.4	26
Frozen, cooked	6-7 spears	100	22	3	Tr.	4	0.8	92	22	67	1.1	780	0.16	0.14	1.1	26
Canned:																
Green, drained, solids	½ c. cut or 6-7 spears	100	21	2	Tr.	3	0.8	93	19	53	1.9	800	0.06	0.10	0.8	15
Avocados, raw commercial varieties	½ peeled	100	167	2	16	6	1.6	74	10	42	0.6	290	0.11	0.20	1.6	14
Baby Foods:																
Cereals, pre-cooked:																
Mixed, dry, with added nutrients	3½ ozs.	100	368	15	3	71	1.1	7	820	741	56.4	..	3.15	1.35	22.3	0
Dessert:																
Custard pudding	3½ ozs.	100	100	2	2	19	0.2	77	64	62	0.3	100	0.02	0.12	0.1	1
Fruits:																
Apple sauce	3½ ozs.	100	72	Tr.	Tr.	19	0.5	81	4	7	0.4	40	0.01	0.02	0.1	Tr.
Apple sauce and apricot	3½ ozs.	100	86	Tr.	Tr.	23	0.5	77	4	14	0.3	600	0.01	0.02	0.1	2
Apricot, pineapple, and/or orange with tapioca	3½ ozs.	100	84	Tr.	Tr.	22	0.2	78	15	9	0.4	450	0.02	0.01	0.2	4
Peaches	3½ ozs.	100	81	1	Tr.	21	0.5	78	6	14	0.3	500	0.01	0.02	0.7	3
Pears	3½ ozs.	100	66	Tr.	Tr.	17	1.0	82	7	8	0.2	30	0.02	0.02	0.2	2
Prunes with tapioca	3½ ozs.	100	86	Tr.	Tr.	22	0.3	77	7	21	0.9	400	0.02	0.06	0.4	4
Meats, Poultry and Eggs:																
Beef, strained	3½ ozs.	100	99	15	4	0	0	80	8	127	2.0	..	0.01	0.16	3.5	0
junior	3½ ozs.	100	118	19	4	0	0	76	8	163	2.5	..	0.02	0.20	4.3	0
Beef heart	3½ ozs.	100	93	14	4	Tr.	0	81	5	155	3.7	..	0.06	0.62	3.6	0
Chicken	3½ ozs.	100	127	14	8	0	0	77	..	129	1.9	..	0.02	0.16	3.5	0
Egg yolk, strained	3½ ozs.	100	210	10	18	Tr.	0	70	81	256	3.0	1,900	0.12	0.22	Tr.	Tr.
Lamb, strained	3½ ozs.	100	107	15	5	0	0	79	9	124	2.1	..	0.02	0.17	3.3	..
junior	3½ ozs.	100	121	18	5	0	0	76	13	156	2.7	..	0.02	0.21	4.1	..
Liver, strained	3½ ozs.	100	97	14	3	2	0	80	6	182	5.6	24,000	0.05	2.00	7.6	10
Pork, strained	3½ ozs.	100	118	15	6	0	0	78	8	130	1.5	..	0.19	0.20	2.7	..
junior	3½ ozs.	100	107	19	3	0	0	74	8	144	1.2	..	0.23	0.23	2.8	..
Veal, strained	3½ ozs.	100	91	16	3	0	0	81	10	145	1.7	..	0.03	0.20	4.3	..
junior	3½ ozs.	100	134	19	6	0	0	77	8	157	1.6	..	0.03	0.22	6.0	..

Vegetables:

Food	g	Measure														
Beans, green	100	3½ ozs.	22	1	Tr.	5	0.8	93	33	25	1.1	400	0.02	0.06	0.3	3
Beets	100	3½ ozs.	37	1	Tr.	8	0.6	89	18	27	0.7	20	0.02	0.03	0.1	3
Carrots	100	3½ ozs.	29	1	Tr.	7	0.6	92	23	21	0.5	13,000	0.02	0.03	0.1	3
Mixed vegetables	100	3½ ozs.	37	2	Tr.	9	0.5	89	22	36	0.9	4,700	0.05	0.04	0.6	2
Peas	100	3½ ozs.	54	4	Tr.	9	0.8	86	11	63	1.2	500	0.08	0.09	1.2	10
Spinach, creamed	100	3½ ozs.	43	2	1	8	0.4	88	64	63	0.6	5,000	0.02	0.13	0.3	6
Squash	100	3½ ozs.	25	1	Tr.	6	0.8	92	24	17	0.4	2,400	0.02	0.04	0.3	8
Sweet potatoes	100	3½ ozs.	67	1	Tr.	16	0.5	82	16	34	0.4	4,900	0.04	0.03	0.4	8
Tomato soup	100	3½ ozs.	54	2	Tr.	14	0.2	83	24	52	0.4	1,000	0.05	0.12	0.7	3
Bacon, broiled or fried	100	12 strips	611	30	52	3	0	8	14	224	3.3	0	0.51	0.34	5.2	0
	16	2 strips	100	5	8	1	0	1	2	37	0.5	0	0.08	0.06	0.8	0
Bacon, Canadian, broiled or fried	100	3½ ozs.	277	28	18	Tr.	0	50	19	218	4.1	0	0.92	0.17	5.0	0
Bananas, raw	100	1 small	85	1	Tr.	22	0.5	76	8	26	0.7	190	0.05	0.06	0.7	10
Barley, pearled, light uncooked	100	½ c.	349	8	1	79	0.5	11	16	189	2.0	0	0.12	0.05	3.1	0
Beans, common or kidney: Red kidney, canned or cooked, solids and liquids	100	½ c. scant	90	6	Tr.	16	0.9	76	29	109	1.8	0	0.05	0.04	0.6	..
Canned, baked: Pork and molasses	100	½ c. scant	150	6	5	21	1.7	66	63	114	2.3	..	0.06	0.04	0.5	..
Pork and tomato sauce	100	½ c. scant	122	6	3	19	1.4	71	54	92	1.8	130	0.08	0.03	0.6	2
Beans, Lima: Fresh, cooked	100	⅔ c.	111	8	Tr.	20	1.8	71	47	121	2.5	280	0.18	0.10	1.3	17
Frozen, cooked	100	⅔ c.	99	6	Tr.	19	1.6	74	20	90	1.7	230	0.07	0.05	1.0	17
Canned, drained solids	100	½ c. scant	96	5	Tr.	18	1.8	75	28	70	2.4	190	0.03	0.05	0.5	6
Beans: Snap green: Cooked, fresh or frozen	100	¾ c.	25	2	Tr.	5	1.0	92	50	37	0.6	540	0.07	0.09	0.5	12
Canned, drained solids	100	¾ c.	24	1	Tr.	5	1.0	92	45	25	1.5	470	0.03	0.05	0.3	4
Wax or yellow: Canned, drained solids	100	½ c.	22	1	Tr.	5	1.0	93	50	37	0.6	230	0.07	0.09	0.5	13
Bean Sprouts, mung, raw	100	1 c.	35	4	Tr.	7	0.7	89	19	64	1.3	20	0.13	0.13	0.8	19
Beef, trimmed to retail basis, cooked: Cuts, braised, simmered or pot-roasted: Lean and fat	100	3½ ozs.	289	27	19	0	0	53	12	134	3.4	30	0.05	0.21	4.2	0

TABLE 1. COMPOSITION OF FOODS—EDIBLE PORTION (Continued)

FOOD AND DESCRIPTION	WT. Gm.	APPROXIMATE MEASURE	FOOD ENERGY K Cal.[a]	PROTEIN Gm.	FAT Gm.	CARBOHYDRATE TOTAL Gm.	CARBOHYDRATE FIBER Gm.	WATER Gm.	MINERALS CA Mg.	MINERALS P Mg.	MINERALS FE Mg.	VITAMINS VITAMIN A I.U.	VITAMINS THIAMINE Mg.	VITAMINS RIBOFLAVIN Mg.	VITAMINS NIACIN Mg.	VITAMINS ASCORBIC ACID Mg.
Beef: (Continued)																
Lean only (from above serving)	85	3 ozs.	165	26	6	0	0	52	12	128	3.2	10	0.05	0.19	3.2	0
Hamburger, broiled:																
Market ground	100	3½ ozs.	286	25	20	0	0	54	11	194	3.2	40	0.09	0.21	5.4	0
	100	or 2 patties	219	27	11	0	0	60	12	230	3.5	20	0.09	0.23	6.0	0
Ground lean	50	1 patty	109	14	6	0	0	30	6	115	1.8	10	0.05	0.12	3.0	0
Roast, oven-cooked no water added																
Relatively fat such as rib:																
Lean and fat	100	3½ ozs.	417	21	36	0	0	42	9	175	2.7	70	0.06	0.16	3.8	0
Lean only (from above serving)	63	2.2 ozs.	135	18	6	0	0	38	7	153	2.3	12	0.04	0.14	3.3	0
Relatively lean such as round:																
Lean and fat	100	3½ ozs.	317	25	23	0	0	51	11	207	3.1	40	0.06	0.19	4.5	0
Lean only (from above serving)	76	2.8 ozs.	145	23	5	0	0	47	10	186	2.8	7	0.06	0.17	4.0	0
Steak, broiled																
Relatively fat such as sirloin:																
Lean and fat	100	3½ ozs.	387	23	32	0	0	44	10	191	2.9	50	0.06	0.18	4.7	0
Lean only (from above serving)	66	2.3 ozs.	136	21	5	0	0	39	8	173	2.6	7	0.06	0.17	4.2	0
Relatively lean such as round:																
Lean and fat	100	3½ ozs.	261	29	15	0	0	55	12	250	3.5	30	0.08	0.22	5.6	0
Lean only (from above serving)	81	2.9 ozs.	152	25	5	0	0	50	11	218	3.0	8	0.07	0.19	4.9	0
Beef, canned:																
Corned beef	100	3½ ozs.	185	26	8	0	0	62	21	110	4.5	..	0.02	0.25	3.5	0
Corned beef hash	100	3½ ozs.	181	9	11	11	1	67	13	67	2.0	..	0.01	0.09	2.1	..
Beef, dried or chipped	100	3½ ozs.	203	34	6	0	0	48	20	404	5.1	0	0.07	0.32	3.8	0
cooked, creamed	100	3½ ozs.	154	8	10	7	0	72	105	140	0.8	360	0.06	0.19	2.6	Tr.
Beef and vegetable stew canned	100	½ c.	79	6	3	7	0.3	83	12	45	0.9	970	0.03	0.05	1.0	3

Food		Measure													
Beets, cooked, drained	100	½ c.	32	1	Tr.	7	0.8	91	14	23	0.5	20	0.03	0.04	0.3	6
canned, solids	100	½ c.	37	1	Tr.	9	0.8	90	19	18	0.7	20	0.01	0.03	0.1	3
Beet greens, cooked	100	⅔ c.	18	2	Tr.	3	1.1	94	99†	25	1.9	5,100	0.07	0.15	0.3	15
Beverages, carbonated:																
Ginger ale	100	3½ ozs.	31	..	..	8	..	92	..	..	..	..	..	..	..	..
Other, including cola type	100	3½ ozs.	40	..	..	10	..	90	..	..	..	..	..	..	..	..
Biscuits, baking powder, made with enriched flour*	100	3 biscuits 2-in. diam.	369	7	17	46	0.2	27	121	175	1.6	Tr.	0.21	0.21	1.8	Tr.
Blackberries: including dewberries, boysenberries																
Raw	100	⅔ c.	58	1	1	13	4.2	85	32	19	0.9	200	0.03	0.04	0.4	21
Canned, solids and liquids:																
Water pack	100	½ c. scant	40	1	1	9	2.8	89	22	13	0.6	140	0.02	0.02	0.2	7
Syrup pack	100	½ c. scant	91	1	1	22	2.6	76	21	12	0.6	130	0.01	0.02	0.2	7
Blueberries:																
Raw	100	⅔ c.	62	1	1	15	1.5	83	15	13	1.0	100	0.03	0.06	0.5	14
Frozen without sugar	100	⅔ c.	55	1	Tr.	14	1.5	85	10	13	0.8	70	0.03	0.06	0.5	7
Canned, solids and liquids:																
Water pack	100	½ c. scant	39	Tr.	Tr.	10	1.0	89	10	9	0.7	40	0.01	0.01	0.2	7
Syrup pack	100	½ c. scant	101	Tr.	Tr.	26	1.0	73	9	8	0.6	40	0.01	0.01	0.2	6
Bouillon cubes	100	25 cubes	120	20	5	5	0	4	..	..	..	..	..	..	..	..
	4	1 cube	2	Tr.	Tr.	Tr.	0	Tr.	..	..	..	..	..	..	..	..
Brains, all kinds, raw	100	3½ ozs.	125	10	9	1	0	79	10	312	2.4	0	0.23	0.26	4.4	18
Bran (breakfast cereal, almost wholly bran)	28	1 oz.	95	3	1	21	2.0	1	24	350	2.9	0	0.11	0.09	5.0	0
Bran flakes (40 percent bran) with added thiamine	100	2½ c.	303	10	2	81	3.6	3	71	495	4.4	0	0.40	0.17	6.2	0
	28	¾ c. 1 oz.	85	3	1	23	1.0	1	20	138	1.2	0	0.11	0.05	1.7	0
Bran flakes with raisins added thiamine	100	2 c.	287	8	1	79	3.0	7	56	396	4.0	0	0.32	0.13	5.3	0
Brazil nuts, shelled	100	⅔ c.	654	14	67	11	3.1	5	186	693	3.4	Tr.	0.96	0.12	1.6	0

* Values are calculated from a recipe.

† Calcium may not be available because of the presence of oxalic acid.

TABLE 1. COMPOSITION OF FOODS—EDIBLE PORTION (Continued)

FOOD AND DESCRIPTION	WT. Gm.	APPROXIMATE MEASURE	FOOD ENERGY K Cal.[a]	PROTEIN Gm.	FAT Gm.	CARBOHYDRATE Total Gm.	Fiber Gm.	WATER Gm.	Ca Mg.	P Mg.	Fe Mg.	VITAMIN A I.U.	THIAMINE Mg.	RIBOFLAVIN Mg.	NIACIN Mg.	ASCORBIC ACID Mg.
Breads:*																
Boston brown bread made with degermed corn meal, enriched	100	2 sl. 3 x ¾ in.	211	6	1	46	0.7	45	90	160	1.9	..	0.11	0.06	1.2	0
Cracked wheat bread made with enriched flour	100	4 sl.	263	9	2	52	0.5	35	88	128	1.1	0	0.12	0.09	1.3	Tr.
	23	1 sl.	60	2	Tr.	12	0.1	8	20	29	0.3	0	0.03	0.02	0.3	Tr.
French or Vienna breads: unenriched	100	3½ ozs.	290	9	3	55	0.2	31	43	85	0.7	0	0.08	0.08	0.8	Tr.
enriched	100	3½ ozs.	290	9	3	55	0.2	31	43	85	2.2	0	0.28	0.22	2.5	Tr.
Italian bread: unenriched	100	3½ ozs.	276	9	1	56	0.2	32	17	77	0.7	0	0.09	0.06	0.8	0
enriched	100	3½ ozs.	276	9	1	56	0.2	32	17	77	2.2	0	0.29	0.20	2.6	0
Raisin bread	100	4 sl.	262	7	3	54	0.2	35	71	87	1.3	Tr.	0.05	0.09	0.7	Tr.
	23	1 sl.	60	2	1	13	Tr.	7	16	20	0.3	Tr.	0.01	0.02	0.2	0
Rye bread, American (⅓ rye, ⅔ wheat flour)	100	4 sl.	243	9	1	52	0.4	36	75	147	1.6	0	0.18	0.07	1.4	0
	23	1 sl.	56	2	Tr.	12	0.1	9	17	34	0.4	0	0.04	0.02	0.3	0
White bread, unenriched: 4 percent nonfat dry milk	100	4 sl.	270	9	3	51	0.2	36	84	97	0.7	Tr.	0.07	0.09	1.1	Tr.
	23	1 sl.	62	2	1	12	Tr.	8	19	22	0.2	Tr.	0.02	0.02	0.3	Tr.
White bread, enriched: 1-2 percent nonfat dry milk	100	4 sl.	269	9	3	50	0.2	36	70	87	2.4	Tr.	0.25	0.17	2.3	Tr.
	23	1 sl.	62	2	1	12	0.1	9	16	20	0.6	Tr.	0.06	0.04	0.5	Tr.
3-4 percent nonfat dry milk†	100	4 sl.	270	9	3	50	0.2	36	84	97	2.5	Tr.	0.25	0.21	2.4	Tr.
	23	1 sl.	62	2	1	12	0.1	9	19	22	0.6	Tr.	0.06	0.05	0.6	Tr.
5-6 percent nonfat dry milk	100	4 sl.	275	9	4	50	0.2	35	96	102	2.5	Tr.	0.27	0.20	2.4	Tr.
	23	1 sl.	63	2	1	12	0.1	9	22	24	0.6	Tr.	0.06	0.05	0.6	Tr.
Whole wheat, graham, entire wheat bread, 2 percent dry milk	100	4 sl.	243	10	3	48	1.6	37	99	228	2.3	Tr.	0.26	0.12	2.8	Tr.
	23	1 sl.	56	2	1	11	0.4	9	23	53	0.6	Tr.	0.06	0.03	0.6	Tr.
Bread crumbs, dry	100	1 c.	392	13	5	73	0.3	7	122	141	3.6	Tr.	0.22	0.30	3.5	Tr.

Food	g	Measure														
Breakfast foods. See individual grain, as corn, oatmeal, etc.																
Broccoli, flower stalks,																
fresh or frozen	100	⅔ c.	32	4	Tr.	6	1.5	89	103	78	1.1	2,500	0.10	0.23	0.9	113
cooked	100	⅔ c.	26	3	Tr.	5	1.5	91	88	62	0.8	2,500	0.09	0.20	0.8	90
Brussels sprouts,																
fresh or frozen, cooked	100	¾ c.	36	4	Tr.	6	1.6	88	32	72	1.1	520	0.08	0.14	0.8	87
Buckwheat flour, light	100	1 c. sifted	347	6	1	80	0.5	12	11	88	1.0	0	0.08	0.04	0.4	0
Bun, hamburger. See Rolls.																
Butter	100	½ c. scant	716	1	81	Tr.	0	16	20	16	0	3,300‡	Tr.	..	..	0
	14	1 tbsp.	100	Tr.	11	Tr.	0	2	3	2	0	460‡	..	..	..	0
Buttermilk, cultured (made from skim milk)	100	½ c. scant	36	4	Tr.	5	0	91	121	95	Tr.	Tr.	0.04	0.18	0.1	1
Cabbage:																
Raw	100	wedge 3½ x 4½ in.	24	1	Tr.	5	0.8	92	49	29	0.4	130	0.05	0.05	0.3	47§
Cooked (short time)	100	1⅔ c.	20	1	Tr.	4	0.8	94	44	20	0.3	130	0.04	0.04	0.3	33
Cabbage, celery or Chinese, raw	100	1 c., 1-in. pieces	14	1	Tr.	3	0.6	95	43	40	0.6	150	0.05	0.04	0.6	25
Cakes: home recipes:																
Chocolate (devil's food with icing)	100	1 piece	369	4	16	56	0.3	22	70	131	1.0	160	0.02	0.10	0.2	Tr.
Fruit cake, dark type	100	3 pieces, 2 x 2 x ½ in.	379	5	15	60	0.6	18	72	113	2.6	120	0.13	0.14	0.8	Tr.
Plain or cup cake, no icing	100	2 cupcakes	364	5	14	56	0.1	25	64	102	0.4	170	0.02	0.09	0.2	Tr.
Sponge cake	100	2 pieces	297	8	6	54	0	32	30	112	1.2	450	0.05	0.05	0.2	Tr.
Cakes: made from mixes:																
Angel food	100	2 pieces	259	6	Tr.	59	Tr.	34	95	119	0.3	0	Tr.	0.11	0.1	0
Coffee cake	100	2 pieces	322	6	10	52	0.1	30	61	174	1.6	160	0.18	0.16	1.4	Tr.
Yellow cake, chocolate icing	100	3-in. piece	337	4	11	58	0.2	26	91	182	0.6	140	0.02	0.08	0.2	Tr.
Cake icing, mix:																
Chocolate fudge	100	3½ ozs.	378	2	14	67	0.5	15	16	66	1.0	270	0.01	0.04	0.2	0

* Values are calculated from a recipe.

† When the amount of nonfat milk solids in commercial bread is unknown, use bread with 3 to 4 percent nonfat milk solids.

‡ Year-round average.

§ Freshly harvested av. 51 Mg.; stored av. 42 Mg.

TABLE 1. COMPOSITION OF FOODS—EDIBLE PORTION (Continued)

Food and Description	Wt. Gm.	Approximate Measure	Food Energy K Cal.[a]	Protein Gm.	Fat Gm.	Carbohydrate Total Gm.	Carbohydrate Fiber Gm.	Water Gm.	Ca Mg.	P Mg.	Fe Mg.	Vitamin A I.U.	Thiamine Mg.	Riboflavin Mg.	Niacin Mg.	Ascorbic Acid Mg.
Candy:																
Candied or glacé peel—lemon, orange or grapefruit peel	100	3½ ozs.	316	Tr.	Tr.	81	..	17	..	..	..	..	..	..	..	0
Butterscotch	28	1 oz.	111	..	1	26	0	..	5	2	0.4	40	0	0	0	0
Caramels, plain	28	1 oz.	109	1	3	27	0.1	2	42	34	0.4	3	0.01	0.05	0.1	Tr.
Chocolate, plain, milk	28	1 oz.	146	2	9	16	0.1	Tr.	64	65	0.3	75	0.02	0.10	0.1	Tr.
Chocolate, milk with almonds	28	1 oz.	150	3	10	14	0.2	Tr.	64	76	0.4	64	0.02	0.11	0.2	Tr.
Chocolate covered peanuts	28	1 oz.	157	4	12	11	0.3	Tr.	32	84	0.4	Tr.	0.10	0.05	2.4	Tr.
Fudge, plain chocolate	28	1 oz.	112	1	3	21	Tr.	2	22	24	0.3	Tr.	0.01	0.03	0.1	Tr.
Hard candy	28	1 oz.	108	0	Tr.	27	0	Tr.	7	2	0.7	0	0	0	0	0
Marshmallows	28	1 oz.	85	1	Tr.	22	0	5	5	2	0.4	0	0	0	0	0
Peanut bar	28	1 oz.	144	5	9	13	0.3	Tr.	12	74	0.5	0	0.12	0.02	2.6	0
Peanut brittle	28	1 oz.	118	2	3	22	0.1	Tr.	10	28	0.6	0	0.04	0.01	0.9	0
Cantaloupe, raw netted type	100	⅓ melon, 5 in. diam.	30	1	Tr.	8	0.3	91	14	16	0.4	3,400	0.04	0.03	0.6	33
Carrots:																
Raw	100	2 carrots, 5½ x 1 in. or 1 c. grated	42	1	Tr.	10	1.0	88	37	36	0.7	11,000	0.06	0.05	0.6	8
Cooked, drained	100	⅔ c.	31	1	Tr.	7	1.0	92	33	31	0.6	10,500	0.05	0.05	0.5	6
Canned: Drained solids	100	⅔ c.	30	1	Tr.	7	0.8	92	30	22	0.7	15,000	0.02	0.03	0.4	2
Cashew nuts, roasted or cooked	100	3½ ozs.	561	17	46	29	1.4	5	38	373	3.8	100	0.43	0.25	1.8	0
	28	1 oz.	168	5	14	9	0.4	1	11	112	1.1	30	0.13	0.08	0.5	0
Cauliflower:																
Raw	100	1 c. flower buds	27	3	Tr.	5	0.9	91	25	56	1.1	60	0.11	0.10	0.7	78
Cooked, drained	100	1 c. scant	22	2	Tr.	4	0.9	93	21	42	0.7	60	0.09	0.08	0.6	55
Frozen, raw	100	1 c. scant	22	2	Tr.	4	0.8	93	19	42	0.6	30	0.06	0.06	0.5	56
Celery, bleached:																
Raw	100	2 large stalks or 1 c. diced	17	1	Tr.	4	0.6	94	39	28	0.3	240	0.03	0.03	0.3	9
Cooked	100	¾ c. diced	14	1	Tr.	3	0.6	95	31	22	0.2	230	0.02	0.03	0.3	6

Food	g	Measure														
Chard, leaves and stalks, cooked	100	⅔ c.	18	2	Tr.	3	0.7	94	73†	24	1.8	5,400	0.04	0.11	0.4	16
Cheeses:																
Blue mold, or Roquefort	100	3½ ozs.	368	22	31	2	0	40	315	339	0.5	1,240	0.03	0.61	1.2	0
	28	1 oz.	110	6	9	1	0	11	88	95	0.1	343	0.01	0.18	0.4	0
Camembert	100	3½ ozs.	299	18	25	2	0	52	105	184	0.5	1,010	0.04	0.75	0.8	0
	28	1 oz.	84	5	7	1	0	15	29	52	0.2	282	0.01	0.22	0.2	0
Cheddar, American, regular	100	3½ ozs.	398	25	32	2	0	37	750	478	1.0	2,310	0.03	0.46	0.1	0
	28	1 oz.	120	7	9	1	0	10	210	134	0.3	650	0.01	0.14	Tr.	0
Cheddar, American, processed	100	3½ ozs.	370	23	30	2	0	40	697	771	0.9	1,220	0.02	0.41	Tr.	0
	28	1 oz.	107	6	8	1	0	11	195	218	0.3	340	0.01	0.11	Tr.	0
Cottage, from skim milk, creamed	100	3½ ozs.	106	14	4	3	0	78	94	152	0.3	170	0.03	0.25	0.1	0
	28	1 oz.	30	4	1	1	0	23	28	43	0.1	48	0.01	0.07	Tr.	0
Cream cheese	100	3½ ozs.	374	8	38	2	0	51	62	95	0.2	1,540	0.02	0.24	0.1	0
	28	1 oz.	113	2	10	1	0	14	17	27	0.1	430	0.01	0.07	Tr.	0
Parmesan	100	3½ ozs.	393	36	26	3	0	30	1,140	781	0.4	1,060	0.02	0.73	0.2	0
	28	1 oz.	110	11	8	1	0	9	312	218	0.1	296	0.01	0.20	0.1	0
Pimiento, American, processed	100	3½ ozs.	371	23	30	2	Tr.	40	..	..	..	..	..	..	..	..
	28	1 oz.	103	6	8	1	Tr.	11	..	..	..	..	..	..	0.1	0
Swiss, processed	100	3½ ozs.	355	26	27	2	0	40	887	867	0.9	1,100	0.01	0.40	0.1	0
	28	1 oz.	99	7	8	1	0	11	245	240	0.3	310	Tr.	0.11	Tr.	0
Cherries:																
Sour, red, raw	100	1 c. whole or	58	1	Tr.	14	0.2	84	22	19	0.4	1,000	0.05	0.06	0.4	10
Sweet, raw	100	⅔ c. pitted	70	1	Tr.	17	0.4	80	22	19	0.4	110	0.05	0.06	0.4	10
Red, sour, canned, heavy syrup	100	½ c. scant	89	1	Tr.	23	0.1	76	14	12	0.3	650	0.03	0.02	0.2	5
Maraschino	100	½ c. scant	116	Tr.	Tr.	29	0.3	70	..	..	..	..	..	..	..	..
Chicken, cooked																
Light meat	100	3½ ozs.	166	32	3	0	0	64	11	265	1.3	60	0.04	0.10	11.6	0
no skin, roasted, fried	100	3½ ozs.	197	32	6	1	0	60	12	280	1.3	50	0.05	0.25	12.9	0
Dark meat	100	3½ ozs.	176	28	6	0	0	64	13	229	1.7	150	0.07	0.23	5.6	0
no skin, roasted, fried	100	3½ ozs.	220	30	9	2	0	58	14	225	1.8	130	0.07	0.45	6.8	0
Canned, boneless	100	3½ ozs.	198	22	12	0	0	65	21	247	1.5	230	0.04	0.12	4.4	4
Chickpeas or garbanzos, dry, whole seed, raw	100	½ c.	360	21	5	61	5.3	11	150	331	6.9	50	0.31	0.15	2.0	..
Chili sauce	100	½ c. scant	104	3	Tr.	25	0.7	68	20	52	0.8	1,400	0.09	0.07	1.6	..
	17	1 tbsp.	18	1	Tr.	4	0.1	11	3	9	0.1	238	0.02	0.01	0.3	..

† Calcium may not be available because of the presence of oxalic acid.

TABLE 1. COMPOSITION OF FOODS—EDIBLE PORTION (*Continued*)

FOOD AND DESCRIPTION	WT. Gm.	APPROXIMATE MEASURE	FOOD ENERGY K Cal.ᵃ	PRO-TEIN Gm.	FAT Gm.	CARBO-HYDRATE TOTAL Gm.	FIBER Gm.	WATER Gm.	MINERALS CA Mg.	P Mg.	FE Mg.	VITAMINS VITA-MIN A I.U.	THIA-MINE Mg.	RIBO-FLAVIN Mg.	NIA-CIN Mg.	ASCORBIC ACID Mg.
Chocolate:																
Bitter or unsweetened	100	3½ ozs.	505	11	53	29	2.5	2	78‖	384	6.7	60	0.05	0.24	1.5	0
	28	1 oz. square	142	3	15	8	0.8	1	23‖	116	2.0	18	0.01	0.07	0.5	0
Bittersweet	100	3½ ozs.	477	8	40	47	1.8	2	58‖	284	5.0	40	0.03	0.17	1.0	0
	28	1 oz.	143	2	12	14	0.5	1	17‖	85	1.5	12	0.01	0.05	0.3	0
Chocolate syrup, thin type ...	100	⅓ c.	245	2	2	63	0.6	32	17‖	92	1.6	Tr.	0.02	0.07	0.4	0
	20	1 tbsp.	49	Tr.	Tr.	13	0.1	6	3‖	18	0.3	Tr.	Tr.	0.01	0.1	0
Clams, long and round:																
Raw, meat only	100	3½ ozs.	76	13	2	2	..	82	69	162	6.1	100	0.10	0.18	1.3	10
Canned, solids and liquid ..	100	3½ ozs.	52	8	1	3	..	86	55	137	4.1	..	0.01	0.10	1.1	..
Cocoa beverage, made																
with all milk*	100	½ c. scant	95	4	5	11	0.1	79	119	114	0.4	160	0.04	0.19	0.2	1
	250	1 c.	236	10	12	27	0.3	198	298	285	1.0	400	0.10	0.46	0.5	3
Coconut:																
Fresh, meat	100	1 c. shredded	346	4	35	9	4.0	51	13	95	1.7	0	0.05	0.02	0.5	3
Dried, shredded (sweetened)	100	3½ ozs.	548	4	39	53	4.1	3	16	112	2.0	0	0.04	0.03	0.4	0
Coleslaw, French dressing ...	100	¾ c.	95	1	7	8	0.7	84	42	26	0.4	110	0.04	0.04	0.3	29
Collards: leaves only																
Cooked (boiled in small amount of water)	100	½ c.	33	4	1	5	1.0	90	188	52	0.8	7,800	0.11	0.20	1.2	76
Cookies:*																
Assorted, commercial	25	1 cookie	120	1	5	18	Tr.	1	9	41	0.2	20	0.01	0.01	0.1	Tr.
Brownie with nuts	50	1 bar	242	3	16	25	0.5	5	20	74	1.0	100	0.10	0.06	0.4	Tr.
Chocolate chip	25	3 small	129	1	8	15	0.1	1	8	25	0.5	28	0.03	0.03	0.2	Tr.
Macaroons, coconut	20	1 cookie	95	1	5	13	0.4	1	5	17	0.2	0	0.01	0.03	0.1	0
Oatmeal with raisins	20	1 cookie	90	1	3	15	0.1	1	4	20	0.6	10	0.02	0.02	0.1	Tr.
Sandwich type, commercial	20	1 cookie	99	1	5	14	Tr.	Tr.	5	48	0.1	0	0.01	0.01	0.1	0
Corn, sweet:																
Cooked, fresh on cob	100	1 small ear	91	3	1	21	0.7	74	3	89	0.6	400†	0.11	0.10	1.4	9
Canned:																
Cream style	100	½ c. scant	82	2	1	20	1.0	76	3	56	0.6	330†	0.03	0.05	1.0	5
Whole kernel	100	½ c. scant	66	2	1	16	0.8	81	4	50	0.4	270†	0.03	0.05	0.9	5

Corn bread or muffins* made with:

Food	g	Measure														
Whole ground corn meal	100	2 muffins, 2¾ in. diam.	215	7	6	35	0.6	49	141	216	1.7	130‡	0.15	0.18	0.8	0
Enriched, degermed corn meal	100	2 muffins, 2¾ in. diam.	219	7	5	37	0.2	49	139	155	1.9	130§	0.17	0.23	1.3	0
Corn Cereals:																
Cornflakes (added thiamine, niacin and iron)	100	4 c.	386	8	Tr.	86	0.6	4	17	45	1.4	0	0	0.07	2.1	0
	28	1 c., 1 oz. pkg.	108	2	Tr.	24	0.2	1	5	13	0.4	0	0	0.02	0.6	0
Corn, puffed, sweetened	100	4 c.	379	4	Tr.	90	0.3	5	11	28	1.8	0	0	0.17	2.1	0
	28	1 oz. package	106	1	Tr.	25	0.1	1	3	8	0.5	0	0	0.05	0.6	0
Corn shredded (added thiamine and niacin)	100	2½ c.	389	7	Tr.	87	0.6	3	5	39	2.4	0	0	0.18	2.1	0
	28	¾ c., 1 oz. pkg.	109	2	Tr.	25	0.2	1	1	11	0.7	0	0	0.05	0.6	0
Corn grits, degermed, white:																
Unenriched, cooked*	100	½ c. scant	51	1	Tr.	11	0.1	87	1	10	0.1	Tr.	0.02	0.01	0.2	0
Enriched, cooked*	100	½ c. scant	51	1	Tr.	11	0.1	87	1	10	0.3	Tr.	0.04	0.03	0.4	0
Corn meal, white or yellow:																
Degermed, unenriched, cooked*	100	½ c. scant	50	1	Tr.	11	0.1	88	1	14	0.2	60†	0.02	0.01	0.1	0
Degermed, enriched, cooked*	100	½ c. scant	50	1	Tr.	11	0.1	88	1	14	0.4	60†	0.06	0.04	0.5	0
Cowpeas, immature seeds, cooked	100	⅔ c.	108	8	1	18	1.8	72	24	146	2.1	350	0.30	0.11	1.4	17
Crabs, Atlantic and Pacific, hard shell, steamed	100	3½ ozs.	93	17	2	1	0.1	79	43	175	0.8	2,170	0.16	0.08	2.8	2
Canned, meat only	100	3½ ozs.	101	17	3	1	..	77	45	182	0.8	..	0.08	0.08	1.9	..
Crackers:																
Graham	14	2 medium	55	1	1	10	0.1	1	3	28	0.3	0	0.04	0.02	0.2	0
Saltines	8	2 crackers	34	1	1	6	Tr.	1	2	7	0.1	0	Tr.	Tr.	0.1	0
Soda, plain or oyster crackers	14	2 crackers	60	1	1	5	..	..	..	..	..	..	..	..	..	..
Ritz type	7	1 cracker	34	2	2	4	..	..	..	..	..	..	..	..	..	..

* Values are calculated from a recipe.
† Vitamin A based on yellow corn: white corn contains only a trace.
‡ Based on recipe using white corn meal: if yellow, the vitamin A value is 330 I.U.
§ Based on recipe using white corn meal: if yellow, the vitamin A value is 250 I.U.
|| Calcium may not be available because of the presence of oxalic acid.

TABLE 1. COMPOSITION OF FOODS—EDIBLE PORTION (*Continued*)

FOOD AND DESCRIPTION		WT. Gm.	APPROXIMATE MEASURE	FOOD ENERGY K Cal.ª	PROTEIN Gm.	FAT Gm.	CARBOHYDRATE Total Gm.	FIBER Gm.	WATER Gm.	CA Mg.	P Mg.	FE Mg.	VITAMIN A I.U.	THIAMINE Mg.	RIBOFLAVIN Mg.	NIACIN Mg.	ASCORBIC ACID Mg.
Cranberries:																	
Raw		100	1 c.	46	Tr.	1	11	1.4	88	14	11	0.5	40	0.03	0.02	0.1	11
Juice, cocktail		100	½ c. scant	65	Tr.	Tr.	17	Tr.	83	5	3	0.3	Tr.	0.01	0.01	Tr.	40†
Sauce, sweetened, canned strained		100	½ c. scant	146	Tr.	Tr.	38	0.2	62	6	4	0.2	20	0.01	0.01	Tr.	2
Cream:																	
Light, table or coffee		100	½ c. scant	211	3	21	4	0	72	102	80	Tr.	840	0.03	0.15	0.1	1
		15	1 tbsp.	31	Tr.	3	1	0	11	15	12	0	125	Tr.	0.02	Tr.	Tr.
Heavy or whipping		15	1 tbsp.	53	Tr.	6	1	0	8	12	9	0	230	Tr.	0.02	Tr.	Tr.
Cucumbers, raw pared		100	⅓ of 7-8 in. cucumber	14	1	Tr.	3	0.3	96	17	18	0.3	Tr.	0.03	0.04	0.2	11
Currants, red & white, raw		100	1 c.	50	1	Tr.	12	3.4	86	32	23	1.0	120	0.04	0.05	0.1	41
Custard, baked*		100	½ c. scant	115	5	6	11	0	77	112	117	0.4	350	0.04	0.19	0.1	Tr.
Dandelion greens, raw		100	1 c.	45	3	1	9	1.6	86	187	66	3.1	14,000	0.19	0.26	..	35
cooked		100	½ c.	33	2	1	6	1.3	90	140	42	1.8	11,700	0.13	0.16	..	18
Dates, "fresh" and dried		100	½ c. pitted	274	2	1	73	2.4	23	59	63	3.0	50	0.09	0.10	2.2	0
Doughnuts, cake type made with enriched flour*		100	2 or 3 doughnuts	391	5	19	51	0.1	24	40	190	1.4	80	0.16	0.16	1.2	Tr.
Duck, domestic raw, flesh only		100	3½ ozs.	165	21	8	0	0	69	12	203	1.3	..	0.10	0.12	7.7	..
Eels, raw, American		100	3½ ozs.	233	16	18	0	0	66	18	202	0.7	1,610	0.22	0.36	1.4	..
Eggplant, boiled, drained		100	3½ ozs.	19	1	Tr.	4	0.9	94	11	21	0.6	10	0.05	0.04	0.5	3
Eggs, fresh, stored or frozen:																	
Raw or cooked:																	
Whole		100	2 medium	163	13	12	1	0	74	54	205	2.3	1,180	0.10	0.29	0.1	0
		50	1 medium	81	7	6	Tr.	0	38	27	102	1.2	590	0.05	0.15	Tr.	0
White		100	3 medium	51	11	0	1	0	89	9	15	0.1	0	0	0.27	0.1	0
		31	1 medium	16	3	0	Tr.	0	27	3	5	Tr.	0	0	0.08	Tr.	0
Yolk		100	6 medium	348	16	31	1	0	51	141	569	5.5	3,400	0.27	0.44	0.1	0
		17	1 medium	58	3	5	Tr.	0	9	24	96	0.9	580	0.05	0.07	Tr.	0

Cooked, omelet or scrambled*	100	made with 2 small eggs	173	11	13	2	0	73	80	189	1.7	1,080	0.08	0.28	0.1	0
Dried, whole	100	1 c.	592	47	41	4	0	5	187	800	8.7	4,290	0.33	1.20	0.2	0
Endive or escarole, raw	100	3½ ozs.	20	2	Tr.	4	0.9	93	81	54	1.7	3,300	0.07	0.14	0.5	10
Evaporated milk. See milk.																
Farina: quick cooking																
Unenriched, cooked*	100	½ c. scant	43	1	Tr.	9	0	89	4	13	0.2	0	0.01	0.01	0.1	0
Enriched, cooked	100	½ c. scant	43	1	Tr.	9	0	89	60	13	5.0	0	0.05	0.03	0.4	0
Fats, cooking (vegetable fat or oil)	100	½ c.	884	0	100	0	0	0	0	0	0	0	0	0	0	0
	12.5	1 tbsp.	110	0	13	0	0	0	0	0	0	0	0	0	0	0
Figs:																
Raw	100	3 small	80	1	Tr.	20	1.2	78	35	22	0.6	80	0.06	0.05	0.4	2
Canned, heavy syrup, solids and liquid	100	3 figs and 2 tbsp. syrup	84	1	Tr.	22	0.7	77	13	13	0.4	30	0.03	0.03	0.2	1
Dried	100	5 figs	274	4	1	69	5.6	23	126	77	3.0	80	0.10	0.10	0.7	0
Filberts or hazelnuts	100		634	13	62	17	3.0	6	209	337	3.4	..	0.46	..	0.9	Tr.
Fig Bars																
	100	4 large	350	4	5	76	1.7	14	69	69	1.3	0	0.02	0.06	0.9	0
	25	1 large	88	1	1	19	0.4	3	17	17	0.3	0	0.01	0.01	0.2	0
Fish:																
Bluefish:																
Baked or broiled	100	3½ ozs.	159	26	5	0	0	68	29	287	0.7	50	0.11	0.10	1.9	..
Fried	100	3½ ozs.	205	23	10	5	0	61	35	257	0.9	..	0.11	0.11	1.8	..
Cod:																
Broiled	100	3½ ozs.	170	29	5	0	0	65	31	274	1.0	180	0.08	0.11	3.0	..
Dried	100	3½ ozs.	375	82	3	0	0	12	..	891	3.6	0	0.08	0.45	10.9	0
Flounder, baked	100	3½ ozs.	202	30	8	0	0	58	23	344	1.4	..	0.07	0.08	2.5	..
Haddock, fried	100	3½ ozs.	165	20	6	6	..	67	40	247	1.2	..	0.04	0.07	3.2	2
Halibut, broiled	100	3½ ozs.	171	25	7	0	0	67	16	248	0.8	680	0.05	0.07	8.3	..
Herring:																
Atlantic, raw	100	3½ ozs.	176	17	11	0	0	69	..	256	1.1	110	0.02	0.15	3.6	..
Pacific, raw	100	3½ ozs.	98	18	3	0	0	79	..	225	1.3	100	0.02	0.16	3.5	..
Canned in tomato sauce	100	3½ ozs.	176	16	11	4	0	67	..	243	..	..	..	0.11	3.5	..
Smoked, kippered	100	3½ ozs.	211	22	13	0	0	61	66	254	1.4	30	..	0.28	3.3	..

* Values are calculated from a recipe.

† Ascorbic acid added in processing.

TABLE 1. COMPOSITION OF FOODS—EDIBLE PORTION (Continued)

FOOD AND DESCRIPTION	WT. Gm.	APPROXIMATE MEASURE	FOOD ENERGY K Cal.[a]	PROTEIN Gm.	FAT Gm.	CARBOHYDRATE TOTAL Gm.	FIBER Gm.	WATER Gm.	CA Mg.	P Mg.	FE Mg.	VITAMIN A I.U.	THIAMINE Mg.	RIBOFLAVIN Mg.	NIACIN Mg.	ASCORBIC ACID Mg.
Fish: (*Continued*)																
Mackerel:																
Atlantic, broiled	100	3½ ozs.	236	22	16	0	0	62	6	280	1.2	530	0.15	0.27	7.6	..
Pacific, canned,																
solids and liquid ..	100	3½ ozs.	180	21	10	0	0	66	260	288	2.2	30	0.03	0.33	8.8	..
Salmon:																
Cooked, broiled or baked	100	3½ ozs.	182	27	7	0	0	63	..	414	1.2	160	0.16	0.06	9.8	..
Canned: solid & liquid																
Chinook or King ..	100	3½ ozs.	210	20	14	0	0	65	154	289	0.9	230	0.03	0.14	7.3	..
Pink or humpback ..	100	3½ ozs.	141	21	6	0	0	70	196	286	0.8	70	0.03	0.18	8.0	..
Sockeye or red	100	3½ ozs.	171	20	9	0	0	67	259	344	1.2	230	0.04	0.16	7.3	..
Smoked	100	3½ ozs.	176	22	9	0	0	59	14	245	..	..	..	..	..	..
Sardines:																
Atlantic type, canned in oil,																
drained solids	100	3½ ozs.	203	24	11	0	Tr.	62	437‡	499‡	2.9	220	0.03	0.20	5.4	..
Pacific type,																
In brine or mustard ..	100	3½ ozs.	196	19	12	2	..	64	303	354	5.2	30	0.01	0.30	7.4	..
In tomato sauce	100	3½ ozs.	197	19	12	2	..	64	449	478‡	4.1	30	0.01	0.27	5.3	..
Shad, baked	100	3½ ozs.	201	23	11	0	0	64	24	313	0.6	30	0.13	0.26	8.6	..
Swordfish, broiled ...	100	3½ ozs.	174	28	7	0	0	65	27	275	1.3	2,050	0.04	0.05	10.9	..
Tuna fish, canned in oil drained solids	100	3½ ozs.	197	29	8	0	0	61	8	234	1.9	80	0.05	0.12	11.9	0
Canned in water solids and liquid	100	3½ ozs.	127	28	1	0	0	70	16	190	1.6	..	..	0.10	13.3	..
White fish, cooked baked, stuffed	100	3½ ozs.	215	15	14	6	..	63	..	246	0.5	2,000	0.11	0.11	2.3	Tr.
Frog legs, raw	100	3½ ozs.	73	16	Tr.	0	0	82	18	147	1.5	0	0.14	0.25	1.2	..
Fruit cocktail, canned, light syrup solids and liquids	100	½ c. scant	60	Tr.	Tr.	16	0.4	84	9	12	0.4	140	0.02	0.01	0.5	2
Gelatin, dry:																
Plain	100	⅔ c.	335	86	Tr.	0	0	13	0	0	0	0	0	0	0	0
....	10	1 tbsp.	34	9	0	0	0	1	0	0	0	0	0	0	0	0

	Gm.	Approximate measure														
Gelatin dessert, ready to serve:																
Plain	100	½ c. heaping	59	2	0	14	0	84	0	0	0	0	0	0	0	0
With fruit added	100	½ c. heaping	67	1	Tr.	16	0.2	82	6	11	3	110	0.03	0.02	0.2	3
Gingerbread from a mix	100	2 pieces, 2 x 2 x 2 in.	276	3	7	51	Tr.	37	90	100	1.6	Tr.	0.03	0.09	0.8	Tr.
Grapefruit: white																
Raw, pulp only	100	½ small	41	1	Tr.	11	0.2	88	16	16	0.4	80	0.04	0.02	0.2	38
Canned in syrup, solids and liquid	100	½ c. scant	70	1	Tr.	18	0.2	81	13	14	0.3	10	0.03	0.02	0.2	30
Grapefruit juice:																
Fresh or frozen reconstituted	100	½ c. scant	41	1	Tr.	10	Tr.	90	10	17	0.1	10	0.04	0.02	0.2	38
Canned: Unsweetened	100	½ c. scant	41	1	Tr.	10	Tr.	89	8	14	0.4	10	0.03	0.02	0.2	34
Canned: Sweetened	100	½ c. scant	53	1	Tr.	13	Tr.	86	8	14	0.4	10	0.03	0.02	0.2	31
Grapefruit-orange juice blend, canned or frozen reconstituted:																
Unsweetened	100	½ c. scant	43	1	Tr.	10	0.1	89	10	15	0.3	100	0.05	0.02	0.2	34
Sweetened	100	½ c. scant	50	1	Tr.	12	0.1	87	9	15	0.3	100	0.05	0.02	0.2	34
Grapes, raw:																
American type (slip skin) as Concord, Delaware, Niagara and Scuppernong	100	1 bunch 3½ x 3 in.	69	1	1	16	0.6	82	16	12	0.4	100	0.05	0.03	0.3	4
European type (adherent skin) as Malaga, muscat, sultana, Thompson seedless and Tokay	100	⅔ c.	67	1	Tr.	17	0.5	82	12	20	0.4	100	0.05	0.03	0.4	4
Grape juice, bottled, commercial	100	3½ ozs.	66	Tr.	0	17	..	83	11	12	0.3	..	0.04	0.02	0.3	Tr.
Guavas, common, raw	100	1 large	62	1	1	15	5.5	83	23	42	0.9	280	0.05	0.05	1.2	242†
Heart:																
Beef, lean, braised	100	3½ ozs.	188	31	6	1	0	61	6	181	5.9	30	0.25	1.22	7.6	1
Chicken, cooked	100	3½ ozs.	173	25	7	Tr.	0	67	4	107	3.6	30	0.06	0.92	5.3	4
Pork, cooked	100	3½ ozs.	195	31	7	Tr.	0	61	4	121	4.9	40	0.20	1.72	6.7	1

‡ Includes skin and bones; if discarded, Ca 54 mg.; P 319 per 100 Gm.

† Range for varieties grown in U.S.—23 to 1,160 mg.

534

TABLE 1. COMPOSITION OF FOODS—EDIBLE PORTION (Continued)

Food and Description	Wt. Gm.	Approximate Measure	Food Energy K Cal.[a]	Protein Gm.	Fat Gm.	Carbohydrate Total Gm.	Fiber Gm.	Water Gm.	Ca Mg.	P Mg.	Fe Mg.	Vitamin A I.U.	Thiamine Mg.	Riboflavin Mg.	Niacin Mg.	Ascorbic Acid Mg.
Honey, strained or extracted	21	1 tbsp.	64	Tr.	0	17	..	4	1	1	0.1	0	Tr.	0.01	Tr.	Tr.
Honeydew melon, raw	100	wedge 1½ x 7 in.	33	1	Tr.	8	0.6	91	14	16	0.4	40	0.05	0.03	0.6	23
Ice cream, plain, 12 percent fat	100	¾ c.	207	4	13	21	0	62	123	99	0.1	520	0.04	0.19	0.1	1
	62	1 container	129	3	8	13	0	37	76	61	0.1	320	0.03	0.12	0.1	1
Ice milk	100	⅔ c.	152	5	5	22	0	67	156	124	0.1	210	0.05	0.22	0.1	1
Infant Foods See Baby Foods.																
Jams, marmalades, preserves	20	1 tbsp.	55	Tr.	Tr.	14	0.2	6	4	2	0.2	Tr.	Tr.	Tr.	Tr.	2†
Jellies	20	1 tbsp.	50	0	0	14	0	7	4	2	0.3	Tr.	Tr.	Tr.	Tr.	1†
Kale: leaves only Cooked, fresh	100	1 c.	39	5	1	6	..	87	187	58	1.6	8,300	0.10	0.18	1.6	93
Frozen, boiled, drained	100	1 c.	31	3	1	5	0.9	90	121	48	1.0	8,200	0.06	0.15	0.7	38
Kidneys, raw: Beef	100	3½ ozs.	130	15	7	1	0	76	11	219	7.4	690	0.36	2.55	6.4	15
Lamb	100	3½ ozs.	105	17	3	1	0	78	13	218	7.6	690	0.51	2.42	7.4	15
Pork	100	3½ ozs.	106	16	4	1	0	78	11	218	6.7	130	0.58	1.73	9.8	12
Kohlrabi: Raw	100	¾ c. diced	29	2	Tr.	7	1.1	90	41	51	0.5	20	0.06	0.05	0.2	66
Cooked	100	⅔ c.	24	2	Tr.	7	1.1	92	33	41	0.3	20	0.06	0.03	0.2	43
Lamb, trimmed to retail basis, cooked: Chop, thick, broiled Lean and fat	100	3½ ozs.	359	22	29	0	0	47	9	172	1.3	..	0.12	0.23	5.0	..
Lean only (from above serving)	66	2.4 ozs.	125	19	5	0	0	41	8	145	1.3	..	0.10	0.18	4.1	..
Leg, roasted Lean and fat	100	3½ ozs.	266	26	17	0	0	55	11	212	1.8	..	0.15	0.27	5.6	..
Lean only (from above serving)	85	3 ozs.	121	19	4	0	0	41	8	157	1.5	..	0.11	0.20	4.1	..

	g	Measure													
Shoulder, roasted																
Lean and fat	100	3½ oz.	338	22	27	0	0	50	10	172	1.2	..	0.13	0.23	4.7	..
Lean only (from above serving)	74	2.7 ozs.	150	20	7	0	0	46	9	162	1.4	..	0.11	0.21	4.3	..
Lard	100	½ c.	902	0	100	0	0	0	0	0	0	0	0	0	0	0
	14	1 tbsp.	126	0	14	0	0	0	0	0	0	0	0	0	0	0
Lemons, peeled fruit	100	1 medium, 2¾ x 2 in.	27	1	Tr.	8	0.4	90	26	16	0.6	20	0.04	0.02	0.1	53
Lemon juice, fresh and canned, unsweetened	100	½ c. scant	24	Tr.	Tr.	8	0	91	7	10	0.2	20	0.03	0.01	0.1	42
Lentils, mature, cooked	100	3½ ozs.	106	8	Tr.	19	1.2	72	25	119	2.1	20	0.07	0.06	0.6	0
Lettuce, crisp, headed	100	¼ head	13	1	Tr.	3	0.6	96	20	22	0.5	330	0.06	0.06	0.3	6
leafy types, Boston, Bibb	100	4 large leaves	14	1	Tr.	3	0.5	95	35	26	2.0	970	0.06	0.06	0.3	8
Limes, peeled fruit	100	2 medium	28	1	Tr.	10	0.5	89	33	18	0.6	10	0.03	0.02	0.2	37
Lime juice, fresh	100	½ c. scant	26	Tr.	0	9	0	90	9	11	0.2	10	0.02	0.01	0.1	32
Liver:																
Beef: Raw	100	3½ ozs.	140	20	4	5	0	70	8	352	6.5	43,900	0.25	3.26	13.6	31
Fried	100	3½ ozs.	229	26	11	5	0	56	11	476	8.8	53,400	0.26	4.19	15.6	27
Calf, fried	100	3½ ozs.	261	30	13	4	0	51	13	537	14.2	32,700	0.24	4.17	16.5	37
Chicken, simmered	100	3½ ozs.	165	27	4	3	0	65	11	159	8.5	12,300	0.17	2.69	11.7	16
Lamb, broiled	100	3½ ozs.	261	32	12	3	0	50	16	572	17.9	74,500	0.49	5.11	24.9	36
Pork, fried	100	3½ ozs.	241	30	12	3	0	54	15	539	29.1	14,900	0.34	4.36	22.3	22
Lobster: Raw	100	3½ ozs. meat	91	17	2	1	0	79	29	183	0.6	..	0.40	0.05	1.5	..
Canned or cooked	100	3½ ozs.	95	19	2	Tr.	0	77	65	192	0.8	..	0.10	0.07	..	..
Loganberries, raw	100	⅔ c.	62	1	1	15	3.0	83	35	17	1.2	200	0.03	0.04	0.4	24
Luncheon meat: Canned, ham or pork	100	3½ oz. slice	294	15	25	1	0	55	9	108	2.2	0	0.31	0.21	3.0	..
Macaroni: Unenriched: Cooked,* firm	100	⅔ c. elbow type	148	5	1	30	0.1	64	11	65	0.5	0	0.02	0.02	0.4	0
Enriched: Cooked,* firm	100	⅔ c. elbow type	148	5	1	30	0.1	64	11	65	1.1	0	0.18	0.10	1.4	0

† Variable according to fruit used.
* Values are calculated from a recipe.

TABLE 1. COMPOSITION OF FOODS—EDIBLE PORTION (Continued)

FOOD AND DESCRIPTION	WT. Gm.	APPROXIMATE MEASURE	FOOD ENERGY K Cal.a	PROTEIN Gm.	FAT Gm.	CARBOHYDRATE TOTAL Gm.	CARBOHYDRATE FIBER Gm.	WATER Gm.	MINERALS CA Mg.	MINERALS P Mg.	MINERALS FE Mg.	VITAMINS VITAMIN A I.U.	VITAMINS THIAMINE Mg.	VITAMINS RIBOFLAVIN Mg.	VITAMINS NIACIN Mg.	VITAMINS ASCORBIC ACID Mg.
Macaroni and cheese, baked* made with enriched macaroni	100	½ c.	215	8	11	20	0.1	58	181	161	0.9	430	0.10	0.20	0.9	Tr.
Mangos, raw	100	½ medium	66	1	Tr.	17	0.9	81	10	13	0.4	4,800	0.05	0.05	1.1	35
Margarine, fortified	100	½ c. scant	720	1	81	Tr.	0	16	20	16	0	3,300	..	..	..	0
	14	1 tbsp.	101	Tr.	11	Tr.	0	2	3	2	0	460	..	..	..	0
Marmalades. See Jams.																
citrus	100	½ c. scant	257	1	Tr.	70	0.4	29	35	9	0.6	..	0.02	0.02	0.1	6
	14	1 tbsp.	36	Tr.	Tr.	10	0.1	4	5	1	0.1	..	Tr.	Tr.	Tr.	1
Mayonnaise. See Salad dressings.																
Meat. See Beef, Lamb, Pork, Veal.																
Milk, cow:																
Fluid (pasteurized and raw):																
Whole	100	½ c. scant	65	3.5	3.5	5	0	87	118	93	Tr.	140	0.03	0.17	0.1	1
	244	1 c.	160	8.5	8.5	12	0	212	288	226	0.2	350	0.08	0.42	0.2	2
Nonfat (skim)	100	½ c. scant	36	3.6	Tr.	5	0	91	121	95	Tr.	Tr.	0.04	0.18	0.1	1
	246	1 c.	88	8.8	Tr.	13	0	224	297	234	0.2	Tr.	0.10	0.44	0.2	2
Canned:																
Evaporated (unsweetened)	100	½ c. scant	137	7	8	10	0	74	252	205	0.1	320	0.04	0.34	0.2	1
Condensed (sweetened)	100	⅓ c.	321	8	9	54	0	27	262	206	0.1	360	0.08	0.38	0.2	1
Dried:																
Whole	100	1 c. scant	502	26	28	38	0	2	909	708	0.5	1,130	0.29	1.46	0.7	6
	8	1 tbsp.	40	2	2	3	0	Tr.	72	56	0.1	90	0.02	0.12	0.1	1
Skim, instant	100	1¼ c.	359	36	1	52	0	4	1,293	1,005	0.6	30	0.35	1.78	0.9	7
	8	1 tbsp.	29	3	Tr.	4	0	Tr.	103	80	0.1	2	0.03	0.31	0.1	1
Malted†																
Dry powder	30	1 oz.	115	4	2	20	0	Tr.	81	107	0.6	285	0.09	0.15	..	0
Beverage with whole milk powder	270	1 c.	281	12	12	32	0	210	364	328	0.8	670	0.17	0.56	..	2

Food	Measure	g														
Chocolate flavored*	½ c. scant	100	76	3	2	11	0	83	108	91	0.2	80	0.04	0.16	0.1	1
made with skim milk	1 c.	250	190	7	6	27	0	207	272	228	0.5	200	0.10	0.40	0.2	2
Milk, goat, fluid	½ c. scant	100	67	3	4	5	0	87	129	106	0.1	160	0.04	0.11	0.3	1
	1 c.	244	164	7	10	12	0	212	315	259	0.2	390	0.10	0.26	0.7	2
Molasses, cane:																
First extraction or light	⅓ c.	100	252	··	··	65	··	24	165	45	4.3	··	0.07	0.06	0.2	··
Second extraction or medium	⅓ c.	100	232	··	··	60	··	24	290	69	6.0	··	··	0.12	1.2	··
Third extraction or blackstrap	⅓ c.	100	213	··	··	55	··	24	579	85	11.3	··	0.12	0.18	2.0	··
Muffins, made with enriched wheat flour*	2 muffins, 3¾-in. diam.	100	294	8	10	42	0.1	38	104	151	1.6	100	0.17	0.23	1.4	Tr.
Corn, enriched, ungerminated meal		100	314	7	10	48	0.2	33	105	169	1.7	300	0.20	0.23	1.6	Tr.
Mushrooms, cultivated, raw	½ c.	100	28	3	Tr.	4	0.8	90	6	116	0.8	Tr.	0.10	0.46	4.2	3
canned, solids and liquid	½ c.	100	17	2	Tr.	2	0.6	93	6	68	0.5	Tr.	0.02	0.25	2.0	2
Muskmelons See Cantaloupe.																
Mustard greens: Cooked	⅔ c.	100	23	2	Tr.	4	0.9	92	138	32	1.8	5,800	0.08	0.14	0.6	48
Frozen, cooked	⅔ c.	100	20	2	Tr.	3	0.9	93	104	43	1.5	6,000	0.03	0.10	0.4	20
Nectarines, raw	1 small	100	64	1	Tr.	17	0.4	82	4	24	0.5	1,650	··	··	··	3
Noodles (containing egg), enriched, cooked*	⅔ c.	100	125	4	2	23	0.1	70	10	59	0.9	70	0.14	0.08	1.2	0
Oat cereal, ready-to-eat (added vitamins and minerals)	4 c.	100	397	12	6	75	1.1	3	177	408	4.7	0	0.98	0.18	1.9	0
	1 c.	25	100	3	2	19	0.3	1	44	102	1.2	0	0.25	0.04	0.5	0
Oatmeal or rolled oats: Cooked*	⅔ c.	100	55	2	2	10	0.2	87	9	57	0.6	0	0.08	0.02	0.1	0
Oils, salad or cooking	½ c.	100	884	0	100	0	0	0	0	0	0	0	0	0	0	0
	1 tbsp.	14	124	0	14	0	0	0	0	0	0	0	0	0	0	0
Okra, cooked	9 pods	100	29	2	Tr.	6	1.0	90	92	41	0.5	490	0.13	0.18	0.9	20

* Values are calculated from a recipe. † Based on unfortified products.

TABLE 1. COMPOSITION OF FOODS—EDIBLE PORTION (*Continued*)

Food and Description	Wt. Gm.	Approximate Measure	Food Energy K Cal.[a]	Protein Gm.	Fat Gm.	Carbohydrate Total Gm.	Carbohydrate Fiber Gm.	Water Gm.	Minerals Ca Mg.	Minerals P Mg.	Minerals Fe Mg.	Vitamins Vitamin A I.U.	Vitamins Thiamine Mg.	Vitamins Riboflavin Mg.	Vitamins Niacin Mg.	Vitamins Ascorbic Acid Mg.
Olives, pickled:																
Green	100	16 olives	116	1	13	1	1.3	78	61	17	1.6	300	..	..	..	..
Ripe, Mission	100	10 olives	184	1	20	3	1.5	73	106	17	1.7	70	Tr.	Tr.	..	..
	20	2 olives	37	Tr.	2	Tr.	0.3	15	21	3	0.3	14	..	..	..	..
Onions:																
Mature:																
Raw	100	1 onion, 2½-in. diam.	38	2	Tr.	9	0.6	89	27	36	0.5	40	0.03	0.04	0.2	10
Cooked, drained	100	½ c.	29	1	Tr.	7	0.6	92	24	29	0.4	40	0.03	0.03	0.2	7
Young, green, raw bulb and white top	100	12 small, without tops	45	1	Tr.	11	1.8	88	40	39	0.6	Tr.	0.05	0.04	0.4	25
Oranges, all varieties peeled fruit	100	1 small	49	1	Tr.	12	0.6	86	41	20	0.4	200	0.10	0.04	0.4	50‡
Orange juice:																
Fresh	100	½ c. scant	45	1	Tr.	11	0.1	88	11	17	0.2	200	0.09	0.03	0.4	50‡
Canned, unsweetened	100	½ c. scant	48	1	Tr.	11	0.1	88	10	18	0.4	200	0.07	0.02	0.3	40
Orange juice, concentrate, Frozen:																
Undiluted	100	3½ ozs.	158	2	Tr.	38	0.2	58	33	55	0.4	710	0.30	0.05	1.2	158
Reconstituted, 3 parts water	100	3½ ozs.	45	1	Tr.	11	Tr.	88	9	16	0.1	200	0.09	0.01	0.3	45
Oysters, meat only, raw Av. Eastern	100	5-8 medium	66	8	2	3	..	85	94	143	5.5	310	0.14	0.18	2.5	..
Oyster stew:																
1 part oysters to 3 parts milk by volume	100	½ c. scant	86	5	5	5	..	84	117	109	1.4	280	0.06	0.18	0.7	..
Pancakes (griddlecakes):*																
Wheat (home recipe), with enriched flour	100	4 cakes, 4 in. diam.	231	7	7	34	0.1	50	101	139	1.3	120	0.17	0.22	1.3	Tr.
Buckwheat, with milk and egg pancake mix	100	4 cakes	200	7	9	24	0.4	58	220	337	1.3	230	0.12	0.16	0.7	Tr.

Food	Grams	Measure	Food energy (cal.)	Protein (g)	Fat (g)	Carbohydrate (g)	Fiber (g)	Water (g)	Calcium (mg)	Phosphorus (mg)	Iron (mg)	Vitamin A (I.U.)	Thiamine (mg)	Riboflavin (mg)	Niacin (mg)	Ascorbic acid (mg)
Papayas, raw	100	½ c., ½ in. cubes	39	1	Tr.	10	0.9	89	20	16	0.3	1,750	0.04	0.04	0.3	56
Parsley, common, raw	3½	1 tbsp. chopped	1	Tr.	0	Tr.	Tr.	3	7†	2	0.2	300	Tr.	0.01	0.1	7
Parsnips, cooked	100	⅔ c.	66	2	1	15	2.0	82	45	62	0.6	30	0.07	0.08	0.1	10
Peaches: Raw	100	1 peach, 2½ x 2 in. diam.	38	1	Tr.	10	0.6	89	8	19	0.5	1,330§	0.02	0.05	1.0	7
Canned, solids and liquid: Water pack	100	½ c. scant	31	Tr.	Tr.	8	0.4	91	4	13	0.3	450	0.01	0.03	0.6	3
Syrup pack, heavy	100	½ c. scant	79	Tr.	Tr.	20	0.4	79	4	12	0.3	430	0.01	0.02	0.6	3
Frozen, sliced	100	3½ ozs.	88	Tr.	Tr.	23	0.4	77	4	13	0.5	650	0.01	0.03	0.7	40‖
Dried, sulfured: Uncooked	100	⅔ c.	262	3	1	68	3.1	25	48	117	6.0	3,900	0.01	0.19	5.3	18
Cooked, sugar added*	100	4-5 halves, 2 tbsp. fluid	119	1	Tr.	31	0.8	67	13	32	1.6	1,070	Tr.	0.05	1.4	2
Peanuts: roasted and salted	100	⅔ c.	585	26	50	19	2.4	2	74	401	2.1	0	0.32	0.13	17.2	0
	9	1 tbsp. chopped	52	2	5	2	0.2	Tr.	7	36	0.2	0	0.03	0.01	1.6	0
Peanut butter, made with small am't added fat	100		581	28	49	17	1.9	2	63	407	2.0	0	0.13	0.13	15.7	0
	15	1 tbsp.	87	4	7	3	0.3	Tr.	10	61	0.3	0	0.02	0.02	2.3	0
Pears: Raw, including skin	100	1 med. pear, 2½ x 2 in.	61	1	Tr.	15	1.4	83	8	11	0.3	20	0.02	0.04	0.1	4
Canned, solids and liquid: Water pack	100	½ c. scant	32	Tr.	Tr.	8	0.7	91	5	7	0.2	Tr.	0.01	0.02	0.1	1
Syrup pack, light	100	2 med. halves	61	Tr.	Tr.	16	0.7	84	5	7	0.2	Tr.	0.01	0.02	0.1	1
Peas, green: Immature: Cooked fresh or frozen	100	⅔ c. drained	72	5	Tr.	12	2.0	82	22	93	1.9	610	0.27	0.10	2.0	16
Canned: Solids and liquid	100	½ c. scant	66	4	Tr.	13	1.5	83	20	66	1.7	450	0.09	0.05	0.9	9
Drained solids	100	⅔ c.	88	5	1	17	2.3	77	26	76	1.9	690	0.09	0.06	0.8	8
Mature dry seeds, split	100	½ c.	348	24	1	62	1.2	9	33	268	5.1	120	0.74	0.28	3.0	..
Pecans, shelled	100	1 c. halves	687	9	71	15	2.3	3	73	289	2.4	130	0.86	0.13	0.9	2
	7½	1 tbsp. chopped	51	1	5	1	0.2	Tr.	5	22	0.2	10	0.06	0.01	0.1	Tr.

* Values are calculated from a recipe.
‡ Year-round average.
† Calcium may not be available because of the presence of oxalic acid.
‖ Ascorbic acid added in processing.
§ Based on yellow varieties; White types 50 I.U. 100 Gm.

TABLE 1. COMPOSITION OF FOODS—EDIBLE PORTION (Continued)

FOOD AND DESCRIPTION	WT. Gm.	APPROXIMATE MEASURE	FOOD ENERGY K Cal.a	PROTEIN Gm.	FAT Gm.	CARBOHYDRATE TOTAL Gm.	FIBER Gm.	WATER Gm.	MINERALS CA Mg.	P Mg.	FE Mg.	VITAMINS VITAMIN A I.U.	THIAMINE Mg.	RIBOFLAVIN Mg.	NIACIN Mg.	ASCORBIC ACID Mg.
Peppers, green:																
Raw	100	1 large	22	1	Tr.	5	1.4	93	9	22	0.7	420	0.08	0.08	0.5	128
Cooked, boiled and drained	100	1 large or 2 small	18	1	Tr.	4	1.4	95	9	16	0.5	420	0.06	0.07	0.5	96
Persimmons, Japanese, raw	100	1 medium	77	1	Tr.	20	1.6	79	6	26	0.3	2,710	0.03	0.02	Tr.	11
Pickles:																
Dill, cucumber	100	1 large	11	1	Tr.	2	0.5	93	26	21	1.0	100	Tr.	0.02	Tr.	6
Fresh, cucumber (as bread and butter pickles)	100	½ c.	73	1	Tr.	18	0.5	79	32	27	1.8	140	Tr.	0.03	Tr.	9
Sour, cucumber or mixed	100	½ c.	10	1	Tr.	2	0.5	95	17	15	3.2	100	Tr.	0.02	Tr.	7
Sweet, cucumber or mixed	100	½ c.	146	1	Tr.	37	..	61	12	16	1.2	90	Tr.	0.02	Tr.	6
Pies: *		⅙ of 9-in. pie														
Apple	160		410	3	18	61	0.6	76	1	35	0.5	48	0.03	0.03	0.6	2
Blueberry	160		387	4	17	56	1.1	82	18	37	1.0	48	0.03	0.03	0.5	5
Cherry	160		418	4	18	62	0.2	74	22	40	0.5	705	0.03	0.03	0.8	Tr.
Chocolate chiffon	160		525	11	25	70	0.3	53	38	155	1.9	496	0.05	0.16	0.3	0
Custard	150		327	9	17	35	Tr.	87	144	170	0.9	345	0.08	0.24	0.4	0
Mince	160		434	4	18	66	0.6	69	45	61	1.6	Tr.	0.11	0.06	0.6	2
Pecan	160		668	8	37	82	0.8	31	75	165	4.5	256	0.25	0.11	0.5	Tr.
Pumpkin	150		317	6	17	37	0.8	94	76	104	0.8	3,700	0.04	0.15	0.8	Tr.
Pimientos, canned solid and liquid	38	1 medium	10	Tr.	Tr.	2	0.2	35	3	6	0.6	875	0.01	0.02	0.1	36
Pizza:																
Cheese topping	100	⅛ of 14-in. pie	236	12	8	28	0.3	48	221	195	1.0	630	0.06	0.20	1.0	8
Sausage topping	100		234	8	9	30	0.3	51	17	92	1.2	560	0.09	0.12	1.5	9
Pineapple:																
Raw	100	¾ c. diced or 1 med. slice	52	Tr.	Tr.	14	0.4	85	17	8	0.5	70	0.09	0.03	0.2	17
Canned, solids and liquid																
in juice	100	1 med. slice	58	Tr.	Tr.	15	0.3	84	16	8	0.4	60	0.10	0.03	0.3	10
in heavy syrup	100	1 med. slice	74	Tr.	Tr.	19	0.3	80	11	5	0.3	50	0.08	0.02	0.2	7
Frozen, chunks	100	3½ ozs.	86	Tr.	Tr.	22	0.3	77	9	4	0.4	30	0.10	0.03	0.3	8

Pineapple juice, canned																
unsweetened	100	½ c. scant	55	Tr.	Tr.	14	0.1	86	15	9	0.3	50	0.05	0.02	0.2	9
Frozen, reconstituted	100	½ c. scant	52	Tr.	Tr.	13	0.1	87	11	8	0.3	10	0.07	0.02	0.2	12
Pine nuts:																
Pignolias	100	3½ ozs.	552	31	47	12	0.9	6	..	..	..	..	0.62	..	..	..
Piñon	100	3½ ozs.	635	13	61	21	1.1	3	12	604	5.2	30	1.28	0.23	4.5	Tr.
Pistachio nuts	100	3½ ozs.	594	19	54	19	1.9	5	131	500	7.3	230	0.67	..	1.4	0
Plantain, raw, baking banana	100	1 small	119	1	Tr.	31	0.4	66	7	30	0.7	..	0.06	0.04	0.6	14
Plums:																
All, excluding prunes, raw	100	2 medium	48	1	Tr.	12	0.6	87	12	18	0.5	250	0.03	0.03	0.5	6
Italian prunes, canned, syrup pack, solids and liquid	100	½ c. scant or 3 med. prunes	83	Tr.	Tr.	22	0.3	77	9	10	0.9	1,210	0.02	0.02	0.4	2
Popcorn, popped	14	1 c.	54	2	1	10	0.3	1	2	39	0.4	0	..	0.02	0.3	0
Pork, fresh, trimmed to retail basis, cooked:																
Chop, thick:																
Lean and fat	100	1 large chop 3½ ozs.	391	25	32	0	0	42	12	268	3.4	0	0.96	0.28	5.6	..
Lean only from 1 chop	72	2.6 ozs.	195	22	11	0	0	38	9	248	2.7	0	0.82	0.24	4.9	..
Roast, loin or shoulder	100	3½ ozs.	373	23	31	0	0	45	10	232	2.9	0	0.50	0.23	4.9	..
Lean only from above serving	77	2.9 ozs.	182	22	10	0	0	44	9	226	2.8	0	0.46	0.22	4.2	..
Picnic cut simmered																
Lean and fat	100	3½ ozs.	374	23	31	0	0	46	10	139	3.0	0	0.54	0.25	4.8	..
Lean only from above serving	74	2.6 ozs.	157	21	7	0	0	45	9	130	2.7	0	0.49	0.22	4.4	..
Pork, smoked ham																
Ham, cooked																
Lean and fat	100	3½ ozs.	289	21	22	0	0	54	9	172	2.6	0	0.47	0.18	3.6	..
Lean only from above serving	84	3 ozs.	157	21	7	0	0	52	9	170	2.7	0	0.49	0.19	3.8	..
Ham, canned	100	3½ ozs.	193	18	12	1	0	65	11	156	2.7	0	0.53	0.19	3.8	..
Pork, fat, salted raw	100	3½ ozs.	783	4	85	0	0	8	Tr.	Tr.	0.6	0	0.18	0.04	0.9	..

* Values are calculated from a recipe.

TABLE 1. COMPOSITION OF FOODS—EDIBLE PORTION (*Continued*)

Food and Description	Wt. Gm.	Approximate Measure	Food Energy K Cal.ª	Protein Gm.	Fat Gm.	Carbohydrate Total Gm.	Carbohydrate Fiber Gm.	Water Gm.	Minerals Ca Mg.	Minerals P Mg.	Minerals Fe Mg.	Vitamins Vitamin A I.U.	Vitamins Thiamine Mg.	Vitamins Riboflavin Mg.	Vitamins Niacin Mg.	Vitamins Ascorbic Acid Mg.
Potatoes:																
Baked in skin	100	1 med.	93	3	Tr.	21	0.6	75	9	65	0.7	Tr.	0.10	0.04	1.7	20‡
Boiled, pared before cooking	100	1 med.	65	2	Tr.	15	0.5	83	6	48	0.5	Tr.	0.09	0.03	1.2	16
French fried	100	20 pieces 2 x ½ x ½ in.	274	4	13	36	1.0	45	15	111	1.3	Tr.	0.13	0.08	3.1	21
Fried from raw	100	⅔ c.	268	4	14	33	1.0	47	15	101	1.1	Tr.	0.12	0.07	2.8	19
Hash brown after holding overnight	100	½ c.	229	3	12	29	0.8	54	12	79	0.9	Tr.	0.08	0.05	2.1	9
Mashed, milk and table fat added	100	½ c.	94	2	4	12	0.4	80	24	53	0.4	170	0.08	0.05	1.0	9
Dehydrated Flakes, prep. with water, milk and butter added	100	3½ ozs.	93	2	3	15	0.3	79	31	47	0.3	130	0.04	0.04	0.9	5
Potato chips	20	10 med. or 7 large	114	1	8	10	0.1	1	8	28	0.4	Tr.	0.04	0.02	1.0	3
Potato flour	100	1 c. sifted	351	8	1	80	1.6	8	33	178	17.2	Tr.	0.42	0.14	3.4	19
Pretzels	5	5 small sticks	19	Tr.	Tr.	4	Tr.	Tr.	1	6	Tr.	0	Tr.	Tr.	Tr.	0
Prunes:																
Dried, softenized uncooked	100	⅔ c. medium	255	2	1	67	1.6	28	51	79	3.9	1,600	0.09	0.17	1.6	3
Cooked, no sugar added	100	6 prunes, 2 tbsp. juice	119	1	Tr.	31	0.8	66	24	37	1.8	750	0.03	0.07	0.7	1
Cooked, sugar added	100	6 prunes, 2 tbsp. juice	172	1	Tr.	45	0.6	53	19	30	1.5	600	0.03	0.06	0.6	1
Prune juice, canned	100	½ c. scant	77	Tr.	0	19	..	80	14	20	4.1	..	0.01	0.01	0.4	2
Prune whip*	100	¾ c.	148	3	Tr.	37	0.7	59	26	42	1.8	460	0.04	0.11	0.7	2
Pudding, chocolate*	100	½ c.	148	3	5	26	0.2	66	96	98	0.5	150	0.02	0.14	0.1	Tr.
Pumpkin, canned	100	⅞ c.	33	1	Tr.	8	1.2	90	25	26	0.4	6,400	0.03	0.05	0.6	5
Radishes, raw	40	4 small	7	Tr.	Tr.	1	0.1	37	12	12	0.4	Tr.	0.01	0.01	0.1	10

Food	Gm.	Measure													
Raisins, natural dried, seedless (unbleached)	100	2/3 c.	18	289	3	Tr.	77	0.9	62	101	3.5	20	0.11	0.08	0.5	1
	10	1 tbsp.	2	29	Tr.	Tr.	8	0.1	6	10	0.3	Tr.	0.01	0.01	Tr.	Tr.
Raspberries:																
Black, raw	100	3/4 c.	81	73	2	1	16	5.1	30	22	0.9	0	0.03	0.09	0.9	18
Red:																
Raw	100	3/4 c.	84	57	1	1	14	3.0	22	22	0.9	130	0.03	0.09	0.9	25
Frozen, sweetened	100	3½ ozs.	74	98	1	Tr.	25	2.2	13	17	0.6	70	0.02	0.06	0.6	21
Rhubarb, stems only:																
Raw	100	3/4 c. diced	95	16	1	Tr.	4	0.7	96†	18	0.8	100	0.03	0.07	0.3	9
Cooked, sugar added or canned in syrup*	100	1/3 c.	63	141	Tr.	Tr.	36	0.6	78†	15	0.6	80	0.02	0.05	0.3	6
Rice:																
Brown, cooked	100	2/3 c.	70	119	3	1	26	0.3	12	73	0.5	0	0.09	0.02	1.4	0
White, milled enriched, cooked	100	2/3 c.	73	109	2	Tr.	24	0.1	10	28	0.9§	0	0.11§	0.01	1.0§	0
Parboiled, converted, cooked	100	2/3 c.	73	106	2	Tr.	23	0.1	19	57	0.8	0	0.11§	0.03	1.2	0
Precooked, instant, cooked	100	2/3 c.	73	109	2	Tr.	24	0.1	3	19	0.8	0	0.13§	0.01	1.0§	0
Rice products (added thiamine and niacin):																
Flakes	30	1 c.	1	118	2	Tr.	26	0.2	9	40	0.5	0	0.11	0.02	1.6	0
Krispies	30	1 c.	Tr.	107	2	Tr.	25	0.1	7	33	0.5	0	0.11	0.01	2.0	0
Puffed, presweetened	14	1 c.	Tr.	55	1	Tr.	12	Tr.	6	10	0.3	0	0.05	.	0.6	0
Rice pudding with raisins	100	2/3 c.	66	146	4	3	27	0.1	98	94	0.4	110	0.03	0.14	0.2	Tr.
Rolls:*		one roll														
Hard, enriched	35	average	9	109	3	1	21	0.1	16	32	0.8§	Tr.	0.09§	0.08§	0.9§	Tr.
Plain, enriched (pan roll)	38	average	12	113	3	2	20	0.1	28	32	0.7§	Tr.	0.11§	0.07§	0.8§	Tr.
Hamburg bun	30	1 large	10	89	3	2	16	0.1	22	26	0.6§	Tr.	0.08§	0.05§	0.7§	Tr.
Sweet roll, enriched	55	average	16	178	5	4	30	0.3	35	57	0.3	0	0.03	0.07	0.6	0
Danish pastry	35	1 small	8	148	3	8	16	Tr.	17	38	0.3	108	0.02	0.05	0.3	Tr.
Rutabagas, boiled, drained	100	2/3 c. diced	91	35	1	Tr.	8	1.4	59	31	0.3	550	0.06	0.06	0.8	26
Rye wafers or "Swedish health bread" or Rye Krisp	13	2 wafers 1⅛ x 3½ in.	1	43	2	Tr.	10	0.3	6	52	0.6	0	0.04	0.03	0.2	0

* Values are calculated from a recipe.

† Calcium may not be available because of the presence of oxalic acid.

‡ Year-round average. Recently dug potatoes contain about 24 mg. of ascorbic acid per 100 Gm. The value is only half as high after 3 months of storage and about one third as high when potatoes have been stored as long as 6 months.

§ Based on minimum levels of enrichment specified in standard of identity, F.D.A., for iron, thiamine, riboflavin and niacin.

TABLE 1. COMPOSITION OF FOODS—EDIBLE PORTION (*Continued*)

FOOD AND DESCRIPTION	WT. Gm.	APPROXIMATE MEASURE	FOOD ENERGY K Cal.[a]	PROTEIN Gm.	FAT Gm.	CARBOHYDRATE TOTAL Gm.	FIBER Gm.	WATER Gm.	CA Mg.	P Mg.	FE Mg.	VITAMIN A I.U.	THIAMINE Mg.	RIBOFLAVIN Mg.	NIACIN Mg.	ASCORBIC ACID Mg.
Salad dressings:																
French, commercial	100	½ c.	410	1	39	18	0.3	39	11	14	0.4	..	..	..	..	..
	15	1 tbsp.	61	Tr.	6	3	Tr.	6	2	2	0.1	..	..	..	..	..
Italian	15	1 tbsp.	83	Tr.	9	1	Tr.	4	2	1	Tr.	..	..	..	..	..
Mayonnaise, commercial	100	½ c.	718	1	80	2	Tr.	15	18	28	0.5	280	0.02	0.04	Tr.	..
	13	1 tbsp.	93	Tr.	10	Tr.	Tr.	2	2	4	0.1	36	Tr.	0.01	Tr.	..
Salad dressing, Mayonnaise type	100	½ c.	435	1	42	14	..	41	14	26	0.2	220	0.01	0.03	Tr.	..
	15	1 tbsp.	65	Tr.	6	2	..	6	2	4	Tr.	33	Tr.	Tr.	Tr.	..
Homemade, cooked	100	½ c. scant	164	4	10	15	0	68	89	93	0.6	490	0.05	0.16	0.2	Tr.
	17	1 tbsp.	28	1	2	3	0	12	15	16	0.1	83	0.01	0.03	Tr.	Tr.
Thousand Island	100	½ c.	502	1	50	15	0.3	32	11	17	0.6	320	0.02	0.03	0.2	3
	15	1 tbsp.	75	Tr.	8	2	Tr.	5	2	3	0.1	48	Tr.	Tr.	Tr.	Tr.
Sauerkraut, canned, drained solids	100	⅔ c.	18	1	Tr.	4	0.7	93	36	18	0.5	50	0.03	0.04	0.2	14
Sausage:																
Bologna	100	3½ ozs.	304	12	28	1	0	56	7	128	1.8	..	0.16	0.22	2.6	..
Frankfurter, cooked	100	2 medium	309	13	28	2	0	56	7	133	1.9	..	0.16	0.20	2.7	..
Liver, liverwurst	100	3½ ozs.	307	16	26	2	0	54	9	238	5.4	6,350	0.20	1.30	5.7	..
Pork, links or bulk, cooked	100	3½ ozs.	476	18	44	0	0	35	7	162	2.4	0	0.79	0.34	3.7	..
Pork, bulk, canned	100	3½ ozs.	381	18	33	0	0	43	11	210	2.8	0	0.20	0.24	3.0	..
Vienna sausage, canned	100	3½ ozs.	240	14	20	0	0	63	8	153	2.1	0	0.08	0.13	2.6	..
Scallops, cooked, steamed	100	3½ ozs.	112	23	1	..	..	73	115	338	3.0	..	..	..	..	..
Sherbet,* orange	100	½ c.	134	1	1	31	0	67	16	13	0	60	0.01	0.03	Tr.	2
Shortbread*	16	2 squares, 1¾ x 1¾ in.	81	1	4	10	Tr.	1	2	9	0.1	0	0.01	Tr.	0.1	0
Shrimp, French fried	100	3½ ozs.	225	20	11	10	..	57	72	191	2.0	..	0.04	0.08	2.7	0
Canned, dry pack or drained	100	3½ ozs.	116	24	1	1	..	70	115	263	3.1	60	0.01	0.03	1.8	0
Soups, canned:†† prepared to serve																
Bean with pork	100	⅖ c.§	67	3	2	9	0.6	84	25	51	0.9	260	0.05	0.03	0.4	1
Beef bouillon	100	⅖ c.	13	2	0	1	Tr.	96	Tr.	13	0.2	Tr.	Tr.	0.01	0.5	..

Celery, cream of	100	2/5 c.	69	3	4	6	0.2	86	81	63	0.3	160	0.02	0.11	0.3	1
Chicken, cream of	100	2/5 c.	73	3	4	6	0.1	85	70	62	0.2	250	0.02	0.11	0.3	Tr.
Chicken noodle	100	2/5 c.	26	1	1	3	0.1	93	4	15	0.2	20	0.01	0.01	0.3	Tr.
Clam chowder, Manhattan with tomato, no milk ...	100	2/5 c.	33	1	1	5	0.2	92	14	19	0.4	360	0.01	0.01	0.4	..
Minestrone	100	2/5 c.	43	2	1	6	0.3	90	15	24	0.4	960	0.03	0.02	0.4	..
Mushroom, cream of	100	2/5 c.	88	3	6	7	0.1	83	78	69	0.2	100	0.02	0.14	0.3	Tr.
Onion	100	2/5 c.	27	2	1	2	0.2	93	12	11	0.2	Tr.	Tr.	0.01	Tr.	..
Pea (green), made with water	100	2/5 c.	53	2	1	9	0.4	86	18	46	0.4	140	0.02	0.02	0.4	3
Tomato, with water	100	2/5 c.	36	1	1	6	0.2	91	6	14	0.3	410	0.02	0.02	0.5	5
Made with milk	100	2/5 c.	69	3	3	9	0.2	84	67	62	0.3	480	0.04	0.10	0.5	6
Vegetable beef	100	2/5 c.	32	2	1	4	0.2	92	5	20	0.3	1,100	0.02	0.02	0.4	..
Soups, frozen: prepared Clam chowder, N.E. style with milk	100	2/5 c.	86	4	5	7	0.1	83	98	82	0.4	100	0.03	0.12	0.2	Tr.
Shrimp, cream of	100	2/5 c.	99	4	7	6	0.2	82	77	68	0.2	120	0.03	0.11	0.2	Tr.
Soybeans, canned, immature, boiled	100	3½ ozs.	103	9	5	7	1.4	77	67	114	2.8	340	0.06	..	..	2
Soybean flour or grits: High fat	100	1 c.	380	41	12	33**	2.2	8	240	650	9.0	..	0.89	0.36	2.3	0
Low fat	100	1 c.	356	43	7	37**	2.5	8	263	634	9.1	80	0.83	0.36	2.6	0
Defatted	100	1 c.	326	47	1	38**	2.3	8	265	655	11.1	40	1.09	0.34	2.6	0
Soybean Products: Soybean milk, fluid	100	½ c. scant	33	3	2	2	0	92	21	48	0.8	40	0.08	0.03	0.2	0
Soybean curd (Tofu)	100	3½ ozs.	72	8	4	2	0.1	85	128	126	1.9	0	0.06	0.03	0.1	0
Fermented (Natto)	100	3½ ozs.	167	17	7	12	3.2	63	103	182	3.7	0	0.07	0.05	..	0
Soy sauce	15	1 tbsp.	10	1	Tr.	1	0	10	12	16	0.7	0	Tr.	0.04	0.1	0
Soybean sprouts, cooked boiled, drained	100	1 c.	38	5	1	4	0.8	89	43	50	0.7	80	0.16	0.15	0.7	4
Spaghetti: Enriched: Cooked* plain	100	⅔ c.	149	5	1	30	0.2	61	9	65	1.1	0	0.18	0.10	1.4	0
With tomato and cheese sauce*	100	⅔ c.	104	4	4	15	0.2	77	32	54	0.9	430	0.10	0.07	0.9	5

* Values are calculated from a recipe.

† All ready-to-serve soups are calculated from equal weights of the condensed soup and water, except cream soup, which is based on equal weights of the condensed soups and milk.

‡ Dehydrated soups have about the same nutritive values as canned soups when each is prepared as directed on can or package.

§ Usual serving of soups is 1 cup, 2½ times amount given here.

** Approximately 40 percent of this total amount of carbohydrate calculated by difference is sugar, starch and dextrin. The remaining portion is made up of materials thought to be utilized only poorly, if at all, by the body.

TABLE 1. COMPOSITION OF FOODS—EDIBLE PORTION (Continued)

FOOD AND DESCRIPTION	WT. Gm.	APPROXIMATE MEASURE	FOOD ENERGY K Cal.[a]	PROTEIN Gm.	FAT Gm.	CARBOHYDRATE TOTAL Gm.	CARBOHYDRATE FIBER Gm.	WATER Gm.	MINERALS CA Mg.	MINERALS P Mg.	MINERALS FE Mg.	VITAMINS VITAMIN A I.U.	VITAMINS THIAMINE Mg.	VITAMINS RIBOFLAVIN Mg.	VITAMINS NIACIN Mg.	VITAMINS ASCORBIC ACID Mg.
Spaghetti: (*Continued*)																
With meat balls in tomato sauce, canned	100	⅔ c.	103	5	4	11	0.1	78	21	45	1.3	400	0.06	0.07	0.9	2
Spinach:																
Raw	100	3½ ozs.	26	3	Tr.	4	0.6	91	93‖	51	3.1	8,100	0.10	0.20	0.6	51
Cooked	100	½ c. packed	23	3	Tr.	4	0.6	91	93‖	38	2.2	8,100	0.07	0.14	0.5	28
Canned:																
Drained solids	100	½ c. packed	24	3	1	4	1.0	91	118‖	26	2.6	8,000	0.02	0.12	0.3	14
Frozen, cooked drained	100	3½ ozs.	23	3	Tr.	4	0.8	92	113‖	44	2.1	7,900	0.07	0.15	0.4	19
Squash:																
Summer:																
Cooked, diced, fresh or frozen	100	½ c.	15	1	Tr.	3	0.6	95	25	25	0.4	440	0.05	0.08	0.8	11
Winter:																
Baked	100	3½ ozs.	63	2	Tr.	15	1.8	86	28	48	0.8	4,200	0.05	0.13	0.7	13
Boiled, mashed	100	½ c.	38	2	Tr.	9	1.4	89	19	32	0.5	3,500	0.04	0.10	0.4	8
Starch, pure (including arrowroot, corn, etc.)	100	¾ c.	362	Tr.	Tr.	87	0.1	12	0	0	0	0	0	0	0	0
	8	1 tbsp.	29	0	0	7	Tr.	1	0	0	0	0	0	0	0	0
Strawberries:																
Raw	100	⅔ c.	37	1	1	8	1.4	90	21	21	1.0	60	0.03	0.07	0.6	59
Frozen, sugar added	100	3½ ozs.	109	1	Tr.	28	0.8	71	14	17	0.7	30	0.02	0.06	0.5	53
Sugars:																
Granulated, cane or beet	100	½ c.	385	0	0	100	0	1	..	..	..	0	0	0	0	0
	12	1 tbsp.	46	0	0	12	0	..	..	..	..	0	0	0	0	0
Powdered	100	¾ c.	385	0	0	100	0	1	..	..	3.4	0	0	0	0	0
Brown	100	½ c.	373	0	0	96	0	3	88	19	2.6	0	0	0.03	0.2	0
Maple	100	3½ ozs.	348	..	..	90	0	8	143	11	1.4	..	..	..	..	..
Sweet potatoes:																
Baked in skin	100	1 small	141	2	1	33	0.9	64	40	58	0.9	8,100	0.09	0.07	0.7	22
Boiled in skin	100	½ medium	114	2	Tr.	26	0.7	71	32	47	0.7	7,900	0.09	0.06	0.6	17
Candied	100	½ medium	168	1	3	34	0.6	60	37	43	0.9	6,300	0.06	0.04	0.4	10

Food	g	Measure														
Canned, vacuum or solid pack	100	½ c.	108	2	Tr.	25	1.0	72	25	41	0.8	7,800	0.05	0.04	0.5	14
Syrup, table blends (chiefly corn syrup)	100	⅓ c.	290	0	0	75	..	24	46	16	4.1	0	0	0	0	0
	20	1 tbsp.	58	0	0	15	..	5	9	3	0.8	0	0	..	..	0
Tangerines (including other Mandarin type oranges)	100	1 medium	46	1	Tr.	11	0.5	87	40	18	0.4	420	0.06	0.02	0.1	31
Tangerine juice, unsweetened: Fresh or frozen reconstituted	100	½ c. scant	43	1	Tr.	10	..	89	18	14	0.2	420	0.06	0.02	0.1	31
Canned, unsweetened	100	½ c. scant	43	1	Tr.	10	..	89	18	14	0.2	420	0.06	0.02	0.1	22
Tapioca, cream pudding	100	½ c.	134	5	5	17	0	72	105	109	0.4	290	0.04	0.18	0.1	1
Tomatoes: Raw	100	1 small	22	1	Tr.	5	0.5	94	13	27	0.5	900	0.06	0.04	0.7	23
Canned or cooked	100	½ c.	23	1	Tr.	5	0.4	94	6	19	0.5	900	0.05	0.03	0.7	20
Tomato juice, canned	100	½ c. scant	19	1	Tr.	4	0.2	94	7	18	0.9	800	0.05	0.03	0.8	16
Tomato ketchup	17	1 tbsp.	18	Tr.	Tr.	4	0.1	12	4	5	0.1	340	0.02	0.01	0.3	3
Tomato purée, canned	100	½ c. scant	39	2	Tr.	9	0.4	87	13	34	1.7	1,000	0.09	0.05	1.4	33
Tongue beef, canned	100	3½ ozs.	267	19	20	Tr.	0	57	10	180	2.5	0	0.05	0.22	2.5	0
Tortillas	30	1 tortilla	63	2	Tr.	13	0.3	8	35	57	0.3	0	0.03	0.07	0.6	..
Tuna fish. See Fish.																
Turkey, total edible roasted	100	3½ ozs.	263	27	16	0	0	55	..	..	..	Tr.	0.09	0.14	8.0	0
Flesh only, roasted	100	3½ ozs.	190	32	6	0	0	61	8	251	1.8	..	0.05	0.18	7.7	0
Turnips: Raw	100	¾ c. diced	30	1	Tr.	7	0.9	92	39	30	0.5	Tr.	0.04	0.07	0.6	36
Cooked, boiled, drained	100	⅔ c. diced	23	1	Tr.	5	0.9	94	35	24	0.4	Tr.	0.04	0.05	0.3	22
Turnip greens, boiled in small amount of water, short time	100	⅔ c.	20	2	Tr.	4	0.7	93	184	37	1.1	6,300	0.15	0.24	0.6	69

|| Calcium may not be available because of presence of oxalic acid.

TABLE 1. COMPOSITION OF FOODS—EDIBLE PORTION (Continued)

FOOD AND DESCRIPTION	WT. Gm.	APPROXIMATE MEASURE	FOOD ENERGY K Cal.a	PROTEIN Gm.	FAT Gm.	CARBOHYDRATE TOTAL Gm.	CARBOHYDRATE FIBER Gm.	WATER Gm.	MINERALS CA Mg.	MINERALS P Mg.	MINERALS FE Mg.	VITAMINS VITAMIN A I.U.	VITAMINS THIAMINE Mg.	VITAMINS RIBOFLAVIN Mg.	VITAMINS NIACIN Mg.	VITAMINS ASCORBIC ACID Mg.
Veal, cooked:																
Cutlet, broiled	100	3½ ozs.	234	26	13	0	0	59	11	225	3.2	..	0.07	0.25	5.4	..
Roast, medium fat, rib 82 percent lean	100	3½ ozs.	269	27	17	0	0	55	12	248	3.4	..	0.13	0.31	7.8	..
Stew meat without bone medium fat, cooked	100	3½ ozs.	303	26	21	0	0	52	12	138	3.3	..	0.05	0.24	4.6	..
Vinegar, distilled	100	½ c. scant	12	0	..	5	0	95	..	..	..	..	..	..	..	..
Waffles, made with enriched flour*, egg and milk	100	2 small waffles, 4½ x 5½ x ½ in.	279	9	10	38	0.1	41	113	173	1.7	330	0.17	0.25	1.3	Tr.
Walnuts, Persian or English	100	1 c. of halves	651	15	64	16	2.1	4	99	380	3.1	30	0.33	0.13	0.9	2
	8	1 tbsp. chopped	52	1	5	1	0.2	Tr.	8	31	0.2	Tr.	0.03	0.01	0.1	Tr.
Watermelons	100	3½ oz. portion	26	1	Tr.	6	0.3	92	7	10	0.5	590	0.03	0.03	0.2	7
Wheat flours:																
Whole (from hard wheat)	100	1 c. scant	333	13	0	71	2.3	12	41	372	3.3	0	0.55	0.12	4.3	0
Self-rising, enriched	100	1 c. scant	352	9	1	74	0.4	12	265	466	2.9†	0	0.44	0.26	3.5	0
Patent:																
All purpose or family flour:																
Unenriched	100	1 c. scant	364	11	1	76	0.3	12	16	87	0.8	0	0.06	0.05	0.9	0
Enriched	100	1 c. scant	364	11	1	76	0.3	12	16	87	2.9†	0	0.44	0.26	3.5	0
Bread flour:																
Unenriched	100	1 c. scant	365	12	1	75	0.3	12	16	95	0.9	0	0.08	0.06	1.0	0
Enriched	100	1 c. scant	365	12	1	75	0.3	12	16	95	2.9†	0	0.44	0.26	3.5	0
Cake or pastry flour	100	1 c. level	364	8	1	79	0.2	12	17	73	0.5	0	0.03	0.03	0.7	0
Wheat products:																
Flakes (added iron, thiamine and niacin)	100	4 c.	354	10	2	81	1.6	4	41	309	4.4	0	0.64	0.14	4.9	0
	35	1 c.	125	4	1	28	0.6	1	..	107	1.5	0	0.22	0.05	1.7	0
Germ, commercially milled	100	3½ ozs., 1 c.	363	27	11	47	2.5	12	72	1,118	9.4	0	2.01	0.68	4.2	0
Germ cereal with added nutrients	28	1 oz.	110	8	3	14	0.5	1	13	310	2.5	0	0.55	0.27	1.5	0

Food	gm	Measure														
Puffed (added iron, thiamine and niacin)	100	8 c.	363	15	2	79	2.0	3	28	322	4.2	0	0.55	0.23	7.8	0
	12	1 c.	43	2	Tr.	10	0.2	Tr.	3	39	0.5	0	0.07	0.03	0.9	0
Rolled, cooked*	100	½ c. scant	75	2	Tr.	17	0.5	80	8	76	0.7	0	0.07	0.03	0.9	0
Shredded, plain	30	1 large biscuit, 4 x 2¼ in.	107	3	1	24	0.7	2	13	117	1.0	0	0.07	0.03	1.3	0
Wheat, whole meal cooked*	100	⅓ c. scant	45	2	Tr.	9	0.3	88	7	52	0.5	0	0.06	0.02	0.6	0
Wheat and malted barley cereal quick cooking, cooked	100	½ c. scant	65	2	Tr.	13	0.2	84	9	59	0.4	0	0.05	0.01	..	0
White sauce, medium*	100	½ c. scant	162	4	13	9	0	73	115	93	0.2	460	0.04	0.17	0.2	Tr.
Wild rice, parched, raw	100	⅔ c.	353	14	1	75	1.0	9	19	339	..	0	0.45	0.63	6.2	0
Yeast: Dried, brewer's	8	1 tbsp.	22	3	Tr.	3	0.1	1	16	141	1.4	0	1.24	0.35	3.0	0
Yoghurt, from partially skimmed milk	100	⅓ c.	50	3	2	5	0	89	120	94	Tr.	70	0.04	0.18	0.1	1
	246	1 c.	123	8	4	13	0	218	295	230	Tr.	170	0.10	0.43	0.2	2

* Values are calculated from a recipe.

† Based on the minimum level of enrichment specified under the Food, Drug and Cosmetic Act.

TABLE 2. SELECTED FATTY ACIDS AND CHOLESTEROL IN COMMON FOODS

ITEM AND DESCRIPTION	TOTAL FAT G.	TOTAL SATURATED FAT G.	UNSATURATED FATTY ACIDS		CHOLESTEROL Mg.
			OLEIC G.	LINOLEIC G.	
Almonds, shelled	54.2	4	36	11	0
Avocado, raw	16.4	3	7	2	0
Bacon, broiled or fried	52.0	17	25	5	100
Beef, edible, raw, chuck	31.4	13	13	1	68
Porterhouse steak	36.2	15	15	1	68
Round, entire	11.9	5	5	Tr.	68
Round, separable lean	4.9	2	2	Tr.	65
Rump, total edible	25.3	11	10	1	68
Hamburger, regular	21.2	9	9	Tr.	68
cooked, pan broiled	22.7	10	9	1	91
Beef, corned, canned	12.0	6	5	Tr.	..
Brazil nuts, shelled	66.9	13	32	17	..
Bread, white, 3-4% milk solids	3.2	1	2	Tr.	..
Butter	81.0	46	27	2	250
Cake, yellow, from mix with eggs, water, and chocolate frosting	11.3	3	7	1	48
Candy, made with chocolate, nuts and vegetable shortening Chocolate-coated peanuts	41.3	11	22	7	..
Fudge with walnuts	17.4	6	5	6	..
Cashew nuts	45.7	8	32	3	..
Cheese, cheddar, natural	32.8	20	8	1	99
cottage, creamed	4.2	3	1	Tr.	19
Chicken, raw, edible portion Fryer	7.2	2	2	2	67-88
Roasting	12.6	4	6	2	67-88
Stewing	25.0	6	11	6	67-88

	AMOUNT IN 100 G. EDIBLE PORTION				
ITEM AND DESCRIPTION	TOTAL FAT G.	TOTAL SATURATED FAT G.	UNSATURATED FATTY ACIDS		CHOLESTEROL Mg.
			OLEIC G.	LINOLEIC G.	
Chocolate, bitter, cooking	53.0	30	20	1	0
Coconut, shredded, sweetened	39.1	34	3	Tr.	0
Cookies, sugar, with v. f.*	16.8	4	10	1	50
Cornbread or muffins, v. f.*	8.4	3	4	1	46
Crackers, Graham, v. f.*	10.0	2	6	1	0
plain soda, v. f.*	10.2	2	6	1	0
Cream, light, coffee	20.6	13	5	Tr.	67
Cream, heavy whipping	36.7	23	9	1	133
Custard, baked, milk and egg	5.0	3	2	Tr.	105
Duck, raw, whole, fresh	14.5	4	6	1	..
Eggs, whole	11.3	3	4	1	504
yolks only	30.6	10	13	2	1,480
Filberts, shelled	62.4	3	34	10	0
Herring, raw	11.3	2	Tr.	2	85
Ice cream, 10% fat	10.6	7	4	Tr.	40
Ice milk	5.1	3	2	Tr.	20
Lamb, raw, leg, edible portion	16.2	9	6	Tr.	71
shoulder, edible portion	23.9	13	9	1	71
Lard	100	38	46	10	75
Liver, pork, raw	3.7	1	1	Tr.	300
Luncheon meat	24.2	9	10	2	..
Margarine, hydrogenated, all vegetable oil	81.0	18	47	14	0
Milk, whole, cow's	3.7	2	1	Tr.	14
canned, evaporated	7.9	4	3	Tr.	31
dry, whole	27.5	15	9	1	109

* v.f.—vegetable fat.

	AMOUNT IN 100 G. EDIBLE PORTION				
			UNSATURATED FATTY ACIDS		
ITEM AND DESCRIPTION	TOTAL FAT G.	TOTAL SATURATED FAT G.	OLEIC G.	LINOLEIC G.	CHOLESTEROL Mg.
Noodles, egg, dry form	4.6	1	2	Tr.	94
Oils: corn	100	10	28	53	0
cottonseed	100	25	21	50	0
olive	100	11	76	7	0
peanut	100	18	47	29	0
safflower seed	100	8	15	72	0
soybean	100	15	20	52	0
Olives, ripe, Mission type	20.1	2	15	1	0
Oysters, raw or canned	2.0	..	..	..	50
Peanuts, roasted, shelled	48.7	11	21	14	0
Peanut butter, oil added	50.6	9	25	14	0
Pecans, shelled	71.2	5	45	14	0
Pistachio nuts, shelled	53.7	5	35	10	0
Popcorn, popped, plain	5.0	1	1	3	0
Pork, fresh, raw ham, edible portion	26.6	10	11	2	60-90
Pork, loin, edible portion	24.9	9	10	2	60-90
cured, ham, edible portion	23.0	8	10	2	60-90
canned	12.3	4	5	1	60-90
Potatoes, French-fried, vegetable oil	13.2	3	3	7	0
scalloped, milk and margarine	3.9	2	1	Tr.	6
Potato chips, vegetable oil	39.8	10	8	20	0
Salad dressings: made with soybean, cottonseed or corn oil French, commercial	38.9	7	8	20	0
Italian, commercial	60.0	10	13	31	0
Mayonnaise, with egg	79.9	14	17	40	70

TABLE 2. SELECTED FATTY ACIDS AND CHOLESTEROL IN COMMON FOODS (*Continued*)

| | AMOUNT IN 100 G. EDIBLE PORTION | | | | |
| ITEM AND DESCRIPTION | TOTAL FAT G. | TOTAL SATURATED FAT G. | UNSATURATED FATTY ACIDS | | CHOLESTEROL Mg. |
			OLEIC G.	LINOLEIC G.	
Russian	50.8	9	11	26	..
Salmon, canned, pink	5.9	2	1	Tr.	35
Salt pork	85.0	32	39	5	60-90
Sausage, country style	31.1	11	13	3	60-90
pork, link, cooked	44.2	16	19	4	60-90
Shrimp, raw	.8	..	..	..	150
Tuna fish, canned in oil, drained solids	8.2	3	2	2	65
Turkey, dark meat, cooked	8.3	3	4	2	101
light meat, cooked	3.9	1	2	1	77
Veal, total edible, raw Chuck, medium fat	10.0	5	4	Tr.	70
Rib, medium fat	14.0	7	6	Tr.	70
Walnuts, shelled, black	59.3	4	21	28	0
English type	64.0	4	10	40	0
Wheat germ, commercial	11.5	2	3	6	0

Figures in this table are taken from Table 3, Handbook No. 8. Washington, U.S.D.A., 1963, and from Hardinge, M. G., and Crooks, H.: J. Am. Dietet. A., 34:1065, 1958; Feeley, R. M., Criner, P. E., Watt, B. K.: J. Am. Dietet. A., 61:134, 1972; Anderson, B. A., Kinsella, J. E., Watt, B. K.: J. Am. Dietet. A., 67:35, 1975; Posati, L. P., Kinsella, J. E., Watt, B. K.: J. Am. Dietet. A., 66:482, 1975.

TABLE 3. AMINO ACID CONTENT OF FOODS PER 100 GRAMS—EDIBLE PORTION*

Food Item	Nitrogen Conversion Factor	Protein Content Percent	Phenyl-alanine Mg.	Iso-leucine Mg.	Leucine Mg.	Valine Mg.	Sulfur Containing			Trypto-phan Mg.	Threo-nine Mg.	Lysine Mg.	Tyro-sine Mg.	Argi-nine Mg.	Histi-dine Mg.
							Methio-nine Mg.	Cystine Mg.	Total Mg.						
Milk, Milk Products															
Fluid, whole	6.38	3.5	170	223	344	240	86	31	117	49	161	272	178	128	92
Canned, evap. unsweetened	6.38	7.0	340	447	688	481	171	63	234	99	323	545	357	256	185
Dried, non-fat	6.38	35.6	1,724	2,271	3,493	2,444	870	318	1,188	502	1,641	2,768	1,814	1,300	937
Cheese, Cheddar, processed	6.38	23.2	1,244	1,563	2,262	1,665	604	131	735	316	862	1,702	1,109	847	756
Cottage	6.38	17.0	917	989	1,826	978	469	147	616	179	794	1,428	917	802	549
Eggs, whole															
fresh or stored	6.25	12.8	739	850	1,126	950	401	299	700	211	637	819	551	840	307
Meat, Poultry, Fish															
Beef, chuck, med. fat	6.25	18.6	765	973	1,524	1,033	461	235	696	217	821	1,625	631	1,199	646
Hamburg, reg.	6.25	16.0	658	837	1,311	888	397	202	599	187	707	1,398	543	1,032	556
Rib roast	6.25	17.4	715	910	1,425	590	432	220	652	203	768	1,520	590	1,122	604
Round	6.25	19.5	802	1,020	1,597	1,083	484	246	730	228	861	1,704	661	1,257	677
Rump	6.25	16.2	666	848	1,327	899	402	205	607	189	715	1,415	550	1,045	562
Lamb, med. fat															
Leg	6.25	18.0	732	933	1,394	887	432	236	668	233	824	1,457	625	1,172	501
Rib	6.25	14.9	606	772	1,154	734	358	195	553	193	682	1,206	517	970	415
Pork, fresh, med. fat															
Ham	6.25	15.2	598	781	1,119	790	379	178	557	197	705	1,248	542	931	525
Loin	6.25	16.4	646	842	1,207	853	409	192	601	213	761	1,346	585	1,005	567
Pork, cured															
Bacon, med. fat	6.25	9.1	434	399	728	434	141	106	247	95	306	587	234	622	246
Ham	6.25	16.9	646	841	1,306	879	411	273	684	162	692	1,420	652	1,068	544
Luncheon meat, canned, spiced	6.25	14.9	570	741	1,151	775	362	241	603	143	610	1,252	879	942	479
Veal, med. fat															
Round	6.25	19.5	792	1,030	1,429	1,008	446	231	677	256	846	1,629	702	1,270	627
Poultry, flesh only															
Chicken, fryer	6.25	20.6	811	1,088	1,490	1,012	537	277	814	250	877	1,810	725	1,302	593
Turkey	6.25	24.0	960	1,260	1,836	1,187	664	330	994	..	1,014	2,173	..	1,513	649
Fish															
Cod, fresh, raw	6.25	16.5	612	837	1,246	879	480	222	702	164	715	1,447	446	929	..
Haddock, raw	6.25	18.2	676	923	1,374	930	530	245	775	181	789	1,596	492	1,025	..

Food	Factor	Protein													
Halibut, raw	6.25	18.6	690	943	1,405	991	542	250	792	185	806	1,631	503	1,048	...
Salmon, Pacific, raw	6.25	17.4	646	883	1,314	927	507	234	741	173	754	1,526	470	980	...
Canned, sockeye or red	6.25	20.2	750	1,025	1,526	1,076	588	271	859	200	876	1,771	546	1,138	...
Meat Products	6.25														
Liver, calf	6.25	19.0	958	994	1,754	1,195	447	234	681	286	903	447	711	1,158	505
Bologna sausage	6.25	14.8	540	718	1,061	744	313	185	498	126	606	1,191	481	1,028	398
Frankfurters	6.25	14.2	518	688	1,018	713	300	177	477	120	582	1,143	461	986	382
Liverwurst	6.25	16.7	759	818	1,400	1,037	347	203	550	187	724	1,301	510	1,034	497
Legumes, dry and Nuts															
Bean, red kidney, canned	6.25	5.7	315	324	490	346	57	57	114	53	247	423	220	343	162
Peanuts	5.46	26.9	1,557	1,266	1,872	1,532	271	463	734	340	828	1,099	1,104	3,296	749
Peanut Butter	5.46	26.1	1,510	1,228	1,816	1,487	263	449	712	330	803	1,066	1,071	3,198	727
Pecans	5.30	9.4	564	553	773	525	153	216	369	138	389	435	316	1,185	273
Walnuts	5.30	15.0	767	767	1,228	974	306	320	626	175	589	441	583	2,287	405
Grains and Their Products															
Bread, white 4% milk solids	5.70	8.5	465	429	668	435	142	200	342	91	282	225	243	340	192
Cereal combinations															
Infant food, precooked mixed cereal & dry milk	6.25	19.4	543	...	...	...	310	137	447	118	...	273	447	447	233
Oat-corn-rye, puffed	5.83	14.5	933	841	1,368	900	388	234	622	172	545	343	622	776	326
Corn Products	6.25														
Corn grits	6.25	8.7	395	402	1,128	444	161	113	274	53	347	251	532	306	180
Corn meal, degermed	6.25	7.9	359	365	1,024	403	147	102	249	48	315	228	483	278	163
Cornflakes	6.25	8.1	354	306	1,047	386	135	152	287	52	275	154	283	231	226
Hominy	6.25	8.7	333	349	810	398	99	...	...	84	316	358	331	444	203
Oatmeal, rolled oats	5.83	14.2	758	733	1,065	845	209	309	518	183	470	521	524	935	261
Rice, white or converted	5.95	7.6	382	356	655	531	137	103	240	82	298	300	347	438	128
Rice, products flakes or puffed	5.95	5.9	286	...	...	...	...	44	...	46	...	56	124	137	137
Wheat products	5.70														
Farina	5.70	10.9	579	...	...	...	143	184	327	124	...	199	447	424	268
Flakes	5.70	10.8	478	496	891	572	127	191	318	121	356	360	311	559	231
Macaroni or Spaghetti	5.70	12.8	669	642	849	728	193	243	436	150	499	413	422	582	303

* Figures for the amino acid content of foods are taken from Orr, M. L., and Watt, B. K.: Amino Acid Content of Foods. Home Economics Research Report No. 4. Washington, U.S.D.A., 1957. Amino acid content is given in milligrams, using whole numbers, rather than in grams, using decimals. The order of listing the amino acids has been arranged for the convenience of dietitians dealing with inborn errors of metabolism. For further explanation of the nitrogen conversion factors see reference above.

TABLE 3. AMINO ACID CONTENT OF FOODS PER 100 GRAMS—EDIBLE PORTION* (Continued)

Food Item	Nitrogen Conversion Factor	Protein Content Percent	Phenyl-alanine Mg.	Iso-leucine Mg.	Leucine Mg.	Valine Mg.	Methionine Mg.	Cystine Mg.	Total Mg.	Trypto-phan Mg.	Threonine Mg.	Lysine Mg.	Tyrosine Mg.	Arginine Mg.	Histidine Mg.
Grains and Their Products (Continued)															
Noodles, made with															
egg	5.70	12.6	610	621	834	745	212	245	457	133	533	411	312	621	301
Shredded wheat	5.83	12.8	755	..	..	..	..	246	..	136	..	466	481	742	371
Fruits															
Bananas, ripe	6.25	1.2	..	..	..	..	11	..	..	18	..	55	31	..	31
Grapefruit	6.25	0.5	..	..	..	..	10	..	..	1	..	30	..	..	19
Muskmelon	6.35	0.6	..	..	..	..	2	..	..	1	..	15	..	..	125
Oranges or orange juice	6.25	0.9	..	..	..	..	2	..	..	3	..	22	..	..	..
Pineapple	6.25	0.4	..	..	..	..	1	..	..	5	..	9	..	..	..
Vegetables															
Asparagus, canned	6.25	1.9	60	69	83	92	27	..	..	23	57	89	..	106	31
Beans, snap, canned	6.25	1.0	24	45	58	48	14	10	24	14	38	52	21	42	19
lima, canned	6.25	3.8	197	233	306	246	41	42	83	49	171	240	131	230	125
Beets, canned	6.25	0.9	15	29	31	28	3	..	..	8	19	48	..	16	12
Beet greens	6.25	2.0	116	84	129	101	34	..	..	24	76	108	..	83	26
Broccoli	6.25	3.3	119	126	163	170	50	..	..	37	122	147	..	192	63
Cabbage	6.25	1.4	30	40	57	43	13	28	41	11	39	66	30	105	25
Carrots, raw	6.25	1.2	42	46	65	56	10	29	39	10	43	52	20	41	17
Cauliflower	6.25	2.4	75	104	162	144	47	..	..	33	102	134	34	110	48
Celery	6.25	1.3	..	..	..	..	15	6	21	12	..	..	..	..	..
Corn, sweet, white or yellow, canned	6.25	2.0	112	74	220	125	39	33	72	12	82	74	67	94	52
Cucumber	6.25	0.7	..	..	..	..	8	..	..	14	..	..	..	..	..
Eggplant	6.25	1.1	48	56	68	65	6	..	..	10	38	30	..	37	19
Lettuce	6.25	1.2	..	..	..	..	4	..	..	..	..	70	..	..	..
Onions, mature	6.25	1.4	39	21	37	31	13	..	..	21	22	64	46	180	14
Peas, canned	6.25	3.4	131	156	212	139	27	37	64	28	125	160	83	302	55
Potatoes cooked or canned	6.25	1.7	75	75	85	91	21	16	37	18	67	91	30	84	24
Pumpkin	6.25	1.2	32	44	63	45	11	..	..	16	28	58	16	43	19
Radishes	6.25	1.2	..	..	..	30	2	..	..	5	59	34	..	..	..
Spinach	6.25	2.3	99	107	176	126	39	46	85	37	102	142	73	116	49
Squash, summer	6.25	0.6	16	19	27	22	8	..	..	5	14	23	..	27	9
Tomatoes, all types	6.25	1.0	28	29	41	28	7	..	..	9	33	42	14	29	15
Turnips	6.25	1.1	20	20	..	..	12	..	..	..	..	57	29	..	..

TABLE 4. SODIUM, POTASSIUM AND MAGNESIUM CONTENT OF FOODS

Food	NA	K	MG
	Mg. per 100 Grams		
Acerola	8	83	..
Almonds, shelled	4	773	270
Apples:			
Raw, pared	1	110	5
Frozen slices, sweetened	14	68	4
Apple juice, canned	1	101	4
Applesauce, canned, sweetened	2	65	5
Apricots:			
Raw	1	281	12
Canned	1	246	7
Dried	26	979	62
Frozen	4	229	9
Nectar	Tr.	151	..
Asparagus:			
Fresh, cooked	1	183	20
Frozen, cooked	1	238	14
Avocados	4	604	45
Bacon:			
Broiled or fried	1,021	236	25
Canadian, broiled or fried	2,555	432	24
Baking powders*			
Bananas	1	370	33
Barley, pearled	3	160	37
Beans, baked canned, no pork	338	268	37
Beans:			
Snap, canned	236	95	14
Canned, low-sodium	2	95	14
Frozen, cooked	1	152	21
Lima, cooked, frozen	101	426	48
Beef:			
Lean, cooked	60	370	29
Heart, raw	86	193	18
Liver, cooked	184	380	18
Tongue, raw	73	197	16
Beets:			
Canned, solids	236	167	15
Cooked, unsalted	46	167	15
Beet greens, raw	130	570	106
Beverages, carbonated†			
Blackberries	1	170	30
Blueberries, raw or frozen	1	81	6
Boysenberries, frozen	1	153	18
Brazil nuts	1	715	225
Breads:			
Boston, brown	251	292	..
Cracked, wheat	529	134	35
Rye, regular	557	145	42
unsalted	30	115	42
White, enriched	507	105	22
unsalted	30	180	22
Whole wheat, regular	527	273	78
unsalted	30	230	78
Raisin	365	233	24
Broccoli, frozen	13	244	21
Brussels sprouts, raw	14	390	29
Butter:			
Salted	987	23	2
Unsalted	10	23	2
Buttermilk, cultured	130	140	14
Cabbage:			
Common	20	233	13
Chinese	23	253	14
Candy:			
Butterscotch	66	2	..
Caramels	226	192	..
Chocolate, milk	94	384	..
Fudge	190	147	..
Hard candy	32	4	Tr.
Peanut brittle	31	151	..
Cantaloupe or honeydew	12	251	16
Carrots, raw	47	341	23
Cashew nuts	15	464	267
Cauliflower, raw	13	295	24
Celery, raw	126	341	22
Cereals:			
Corn flakes	1,005	120	16
Corn grits, cooked	..	11	3
Cornmeal, yellow or white	1	120	106
Farina, cooked	690	188	3
Oatmeal, cooked	218	61	21
Rice, puffed, unsalted	2	100	..
Wheat, shredded, unsalted	3	348	133
Wheat, puffed, unsalted	4	340	..
Chard, raw	147	550	65
Cheese:			
Cheddar	700	82	45
Cottage, creamed	229	85	..
Parmesan	734	149	48
Cherries, sweet or sour	2	191	8-14
Chestnuts, fresh	6	454	41
Chicken, cooked,			
white meat	64	441	19
dark meat	86	321	..
liver	61	151	16
Chicory greens, raw	..	420	13

* Baking powders vary greatly in sodium and potassium content. The label on the package tells the type. One tsp. or 5 Gm. of baking powder contains:

	Mg. NA	Mg. K
Alum type	500	8
Phosphate type	450	9
Tartrate type	360	250
Low-sodium type	2	500

† The sodium content of carbonated beverages depends upon the sodium content of the water in the area where they are manufactured. See JAMA, 195:236, 1966.

TABLE 4. SODIUM, POTASSIUM AND MAGNESIUM CONTENT OF FOODS (*Continued*)

FOOD	NA	K	MG	FOOD	NA	K	MG
	Mg. per 100 Grams				Mg. per 100 Grams		
Chives, raw	..	250	32	Lobster, cooked	210	180	22
Chocolate, bitter	4	830	292	Loganberries, raw	1	170	25
Chocolate syrup	52	282	63	Macaroni, plain, cooked	1	61	18
Clams, meat only	120	181	..	Mangos, raw	7	189	18
Coconut, shredded	..	353	77	Margarine:			
Coffee, instant dry powder	72	3,256	456	Regular	987	23	..
Collards, raw	43	401	57	Unsalted	10 or less	10	..
Corn: sweet, cooked	15	165	..				
frozen, cooked	1	184	22	Marmalade, citrus	14	33	4
canned	236	97	19	Milk:			
Cornbread, from mix	744	127	13	Whole or skim	50	144	13
Crab, cooked meat, canned	1,000	110	34	Evap., unsweetened	118	303	25
Crackers:				Molasses, light	15	917	46
Graham	670	384	51	Mushrooms:			
Soda	1,100	120	29	Canned	400	197	8
Cranberries:				Fresh	15	414	13
Juice	1	10	2	Mussels	289	315	24
Sauce	1	30	2	Mustard greens, cooked	18	220	25
Cream, light, coffee	43	122	11	Nectarines	6	294	13
Cress, garden	14	606	..	Noodles, cooked	2	44	..
Cucumbers	6	160	11	Okra, fresh or frozen	2	168	47
Currants, raw, red	2	257	15	Olives:			
Dates, natural and dry	1	648	58	Green	2,400	55	22
Eggplant, cooked	1	150	16	Ripe	750	27	..
Eggs:				Onions, mature, raw	10	157	12
Whole	122	129	11	Oranges or orange juice	1	200	11
Whites	146	139	9	Oysters, raw	73	121	32
Yolk	52	98	16	Pancakes, from mix	451	156	..
Endive or Escarole	14	294	10	Papaya, raw	3	234	..
Figs, dried	34	640	71	Parsley	45	727	41
Filberts (hazelnuts)	2	704	184	Parsnips, cooked	8	379	32
Fish:				Peaches:			
Cod, broiled	110	407	28	Raw	1	202	10
Haddock, fried	177	348	24	Canned	2	130	6
Halibut, broiled	134	525	..	Peanuts, roasted, unsalted	5	701	175
Salmon, baked, broiled	116	443	30	Peanut butter	606	652	173
Sardines, canned in oil	823	590	24	Pears:			
Tuna, canned, water	41	279	..	Raw	2	130	7
Gooseberries	1	155	9	Canned	1	84	5
Grapefruit:				Peas:			
Pulp	1	135	12	Canned, regular	236	96	20
Juice	1	162	12	Frozen	115	135	24
Grapes:				Low sodium, canned	3	96	24
American type	3	158	13	Pecans	Tr.	603	142
European type	3	173	6	Peppers, raw	13	213	18
Grape juice, canned	2	116	12	Persimmons	6	174	8
Guava, common, raw	4	289	13	Pickles:			
Honey, strained	5	51	3	Dill	1,428	200	12
Ice cream, regular	63	181	14	Sweet	527	..	1
Ice milk	68	195	..	Pineapple:			
Jams, jellies, average	15	81	12	Raw	1	146	13
Lamb, any cut, broiled or				Canned, heavy syrup	1	96	8
roasted	70	290	19	Juice, unsweetened	1	149	12
Leeks, raw	5	347	23	Pistachio nuts	..	972	158
Lemon juice, fresh or frozen	1	141	7	Plums:			
Lettuce, iceberg	9	175	11	Raw	1	170	9
Lime juice	1	104	..	Purple, canned, in syrup	1	142	5

Table 4. Sodium, Potassium and Magnesium Content of Foods (*Continued*)

Food	NA	K	MG	Food	NA	K	MG
	Mg. per 100 Grams				Mg. per 100 Grams		
Pork:				Soybean curd (tofu)	7	42	111
All cuts, fresh cooked	65	390	23	Spinach, cooked	50	324	63
Ham, cured, cooked	930	326	17	**Squash:**			
Sausage, pork, cooked	958	269	16	Summer, cooked, unsalted ...	1	141	16
Potatoes:				Winter, cooked, unsalted	1	141	17
Peeled, boiled, unsalted	2	285	22	Strawberries, raw	1	164	12
French fried, unsalted	6	853	25	Sweet potato, baked	12	300	31
Mashed, milk added	301	261	12	Tangerine, raw	1	126	..
Potato chips	1,000‡	1,130	..	Tomatoes, raw	3	244	14
Pretzels	1,680	130	..	**Tomato juice:**			
Prunes:				Canned	200	227	10
Dried, uncooked	8	694	40	Canned, low sodium	3	227	10
Cooked	4	327	20	**Tomato catsup:**			
Pumpkin, canned, unsalted	2	240	12	Regular	1,338	370	21
Radishes, raw	18	322	15	Low sodium	5-35	370	21
Raisins, uncooked	27	763	35	Turkey, roasted	130	367	28
Raspberries:				**Turnips:**			
Raw, red	1	168	20	Raw	49	268	20
Black	1	199	30	Cooked, unsalted	34	188	20
Rhubard, cooked	2	203	13	Turnip greens, frozen	17	149	26
Rice:				Veal, all cuts, cooked	80	500	18
Cooked, regular, salted	374	28	8	Walnuts, English	2	450	131
Cooked without salt	2	28	8	Watercress	52	282	20
Rutabagas, cooked, unsalted ...	4	167	15	Watermelon	1	100	8
Salad dressings:				**Wheat:**			
French	1,370	79	10	Flour	2	95	25
Italian	2,092	15	..	Bran	9	1,121	490
Mayonnaise	597	34	2	Germ	3	827	336
Russian	868	157	..	Yams	..	600	..
Scallops, cooked	265	476	..	Yogurt	51	143	..
Shrimp, cooked	186	229	51	Zweiback	250	150	..
Syrup, maple	10	176	11				

‡ Potato chips vary in sodium according to amount of salt added.

Sodium, potassium and magnesium figures from Composition of Food, Raw, Processed Prepared. Agr. Handbook No. 8. U.S.D.A., Washington, D.C., 1963; or from Church, C. E., and Church, H. N.: Food Values of Portions Commonly Used, ed. 11. Philadelphia, J. B. Lippincott, 1970.

Values for these minerals in canned and processed foods subject to variation because of methods of processing.

Additional References on Sodium, Potassium and Magnesium Content of Foods

Cancio, M.: Sodium and potassium in Puerto Rican meats and fish. J. Am. Dietet. A., 38:341, 1961.

Cancio, M., and Leon, J. M.: Sodium and potassium in Puerto Rican foods and waters. J. Am. Dietet. A., 35: 1165, 1959.

Chan, S. L., and Kennedy, B. M.: Sodium in Chinese vegetables. J. Am. Dietet. A., 37:573, 1960.

Clifford, P. A.: Sodium content of food. J. Am. Dietet. A., 31:21, 1955.

Dahl, L. K.: Sodium in foods for a 100 Mg. diet. J. Am. Dietet. A., 34:717, 1958.

Davidson, C. S., *et al.*: Sodium-restricted diets. The rationale, complications, and practical aspects of their use. National Academy of Science–National Research Council Publ. No. 325. Washington, D.C., 1954.

Holinger, B. W., *et al.*: Analyzed sodium values in foods ready to serve. J. Am. Dietet. A., 48:501, 1966.

Hopkins, H. T.: Minerals and proximate composition of organ meats. J. Am. Dietet. A., 38:344, 1961.

Hopkins, H. T., and Eisen, J.: Mineral elements in fresh vegetables from different geographical areas. J. Agr. Food Chem., 7:633, 1959.

Nelson, G. Y., and Gram, M. R.: Magnesium content of accessory foods. J. Am. Dietet. A., 38:437, 1961.

Oglesby, L. M., and Bannister, A. C.: Sodium and potassium in salt-water fish. J. Am. Dietet. A., 35:1163, 1959.

Thurston, C. E.: Sodium and potassium content of 34 species of fish. J. Am. Dietet. A., 34:396, 1958.

Thurston, C. E., and Osterhaug, K. L.: Sodium content of fish flesh. J. Am. Dietet. A., 36:212, 1960.

Copper Content of Foods

Tables giving the copper content of certain foods are too conflicting and incomplete to be included in the above table. For persons interested in the copper content of foods in dealing with Wilson's Disease the following references are listed:

Silverberg, M., and Gellis, S. S.: Wilson's Disease. Am. J. Dis. Child., 113:178, 1967 (Lists foods to be avoided).

————: Preventing Wilson's Disease Sequelae. JAMA, 200:41, 1967.

Hook, L., and Brandt, I. K.: Copper content of some low copper foods. J. Am. Dietet. A., 49:202, 1966.

Pennington, J. T., and Calloway, D. H.: Copper content of foods. Factors affecting reported values. J. Am. Dietet. A., 63:143, 1973.

Review: Dietary copper in Wilson's Disease. Nutr. Rev., 23:301, 1965.

TABLE 5. ZINC CONTENT OF FOODS PER 100 GRAMS—EDIBLE PORTION

(Data are given to two decimal places if food contains less than 0.1 mg. zinc)

Item No.	Food and Description	Zinc Mg.	Item No.	Food and Description	Zinc Mg.
1	Apples, raw	.05		Drumstick, thigh, back, meat only:	
2	Applesauce, unsweetened	.1	34	Raw	1.8
3	Bananas, raw	.2	35	Cooked, dry heat	2.8
	Beans, common, mature, dry:			Drumstick:	
4	Raw	2.8	36	Raw (85% meat, 13% skin, 2% fat)	1.7
5	Boiled, drained	1.0			
	Beans, lima, mature, dry:		37	Cooked, dry heat (84% meat, 16% skin)	2.5
6	Raw	2.8			
7	Boiled, drained	.9		Wing, meat only:	
	Beans, snap, green:		38	Raw	1.6
8	Raw	.4	39	Cooked, dry heat	2.4
9	Boiled, drained	.3		Neck, meat only:	
10	Canned, solids and liquid	.2	40	Raw	2.7
11	Canned, drained solids	.3	41	Cooked, moist heat	3.0
	Beef, separable lean:			Skin:	
12	Raw	4.2	42	Raw	1.0
13	Cooked, dry heat	5.8	43	Cooked, dry heat	1.2
14	Cooked, moist heat	6.2		Chickpeas or garbanzos, mature seeds, dry:	
15	Beef, separable fat, raw	.5			
	Beef, ground (77% lean):		44	Raw	2.7
16	Raw	3.4	45	Boiled, drained	1.4
17	Cooked	4.4	46	Chocolate sirup	.9
	Beverages, carbonated, nonalcoholic:			Clams:	
18	Bottled	.01		Soft shell:	
19	Canned	.08	47	Raw	1.5
	Bran, see wheat		48	Cooked	1.7
	Breads:			Hard shell:	
20	Rye	1.6	49	Raw	1.5
21	White	.6	50	Cooked	1.7
22	Whole wheat	1.8	51	Surf, canned, solids and liquid	1.2
23	Butter	.1	52	Cocoa, dry powder	5.6
	Cabbage, common:			Coffee:	
24	Raw	.4	53	Dry, instant	.6
25	Boiled, drained	.4	54	Fluid beverage	.03
26	Cake, white, without icing	.2	55	Cookies, vanilla wafers	.3
	Carrots:			Cooking oil, see oils	
27	Raw	.4	56	Corn, field, whole-grain, yellow, or white	2.1
28	Cooked or canned, drained solids	.3			
29	Cheese, cheddar type	4.0		Corn, sweet, yellow:	
	Chicken, broiler-fryer:		57	Raw	.5
	Breast, meat only:		58	Boiled, drained	.4
30	Raw	.7		Corn, canned, whole kernel, yellow:	
31	Cooked, dry heat	.9	59	Brine pack, solids and liquid	.3
	Breast:		60	Brine pack, drained solids	.4
32	Raw (81% meat, 12% skin, 7% fat)	.7	61	Vacuum pack, solids and liquid	.4
			62	Corn chips	1.5
33	Cooked, dry heat (89% meat, 11% skin)	.9	63	Corn grits, white, degermed, dry form	.4
			64	Corn flakes	.3

Provisional table prepared by E. W. Murphy, B. W. Willis, and B. K. Watt: J. Am. Dietet. A., 66:345, 1975.

TABLE 5. ZINC CONTENT OF FOODS PER 100 GRAMS—EDIBLE PORTION (*Continued*)

(Data are given to two decimal places if food contains less than 0.1 mg. zinc)

Item No.	Food and Description	Zinc Mg.	Item No.	Food and Description	Zinc Mg.
	Cornmeal, white or yellow:			Lentils, mature, dry:	
65	Bolted (nearly whole grain)	1.8	99	Raw	3.1
	Degermed:		100	Boiled, drained	1.0
66	Dry form	.8	101	Lettuce, head or leaf	.4
67	Cooked	.1		Liver:	
68	Cornstarch	.03		Beef:	
	Cowpeas (blackeyes), mature, dry:		102	Raw	3.8
69	Raw	2.9	103	Cooked	5.1
70	Boiled, drained	1.2		Calf:	
	Crabs, blue and Dungeness:		104	Raw	3.8
71	Raw	4.0	105	Cooked	6.1
72	Steamed	4.3		Chicken:	
	Crackers:		106	Raw	2.4
73	Graham	1.1	107	Cooked	3.4
74	Saltines	.5		Turkey:	
75	Doughnuts, cake-type	.5	108	Raw	2.7
	Eggs, fresh:		109	Cooked	3.4
76	Whites	.02		Lobster, crayfish:	
77	Yolks	3.0	110	Raw	1.8
78	Whole	1.0	111	Cooked or canned	2.2
	Farina, regular:			Macaroni:	
79	Dry form	.5	112	Dry form	1.5
80	Cooked	.06	113	Cooked, tender stage	.5
	Fish, white varieties, flesh only:		114	Margarine	.2
81	Raw	.7		Milk:	
82	Cooked, fillet	1.0	115	Fluid, whole or skim	.4
83	Cooked, steak	.8	116	Canned, evaporated	.8
	Gizzard:		117	Dry, non-fat	4.5
	Chicken:			Oatmeal or rolled oats:	
84	Raw	2.9	118	Dry form	3.4
85	Cooked, drained	4.3	119	Cooked	.5
	Turkey:		120	Oat cereal, puffed, ready-to-eat	3.0
86	Raw	2.8	121	Oil, salad or cooking	.2
87	Cooked, drained	4.1	122	Onions, mature or green, raw	.3
88	Granola	2.1	123	Oranges, raw	.2
	Heart:			Orange juice:	
	Chicken:		124	Canned, unsweetened	.07
89	Raw	2.9	125	Fresh or frozen	.02
90	Cooked, drained	4.8		Oysters, raw or frozen:	
	Turkey:		126	Atlantic	74.7
91	Raw	2.8	127	Pacific	9.0
92	Cooked, drained	4.8		Peaches:	
93	Ice Cream	.5	128	Raw	.2
	Lamb:		129	Canned, drained slices	.1
	Separable lean:			Peanuts:	
94	Raw	3.0	130	Raw	2.9
95	Cooked, dry heat	4.3	131	Roasted	3.0
96	Cooked, moist heat	5.0	132	Peanut butter	2.9
97	Separable fat, raw	.5		Peas, green, immature:	
98	Lard	.2	133	Raw	.9

TABLE 5. ZINC CONTENT OF FOODS PER 100 GRAMS—EDIBLE PORTION (*Continued*)

(Data are given to two decimal places if food contains less than 0.1 mg. zinc)

ITEM No.	FOOD AND DESCRIPTION	ZINC Mg.	ITEM No.	FOOD AND DESCRIPTION	ZINC Mg.
134	Boiled, drained	.7		Frankfurters:	
135	Canned, drained solids	.8	166	Made with beef	2.0
	Peas, green, mature seeds, dry:		167	Made with beef and pork	1.6
136	Raw	3.2		Shrimp:	
137	Boiled, drained	1.1	168	Raw	1.5
	Popcorn:		169	Boiled, peeled, deveined	2.1
138	Unpopped	3.9	170	Canned, drained solids	2.1
	Popped:			Spinach:	
139	Plain	4.1	171	Raw	.8
140	Oil and salt added	3.0	172	Boiled, drained	.7
	Pork:			Canned:	
	Trimmed lean cuts, separable lean:		173	Solids and liquid	.6
141	Raw	2.7	174	Drained solids	.8
142	Cooked	3.8	175	Sugar, white, granulated	.06
	Boston butt, separable lean:			Tea:	
143	Raw	3.2	176	Dry leaves	3.3
144	Cooked	4.5	177	Fluid beverage	.02
	Ham or picnic, separable lean:			Tomatoes, ripe:	
145	Raw	2.8	178	Raw	.2
146	Cooked	4.0	179	Boiled, solids and liquid	.2
	Loin, separable lean:		180	Canned, solids and liquid	.2
147	Raw	2.2		Tunafish, canned in oil:	
148	Cooked	3.1	181	85% solids, 15% oil	1.0
149	Separable fat, raw	.5	182	Drained solids	1.1
	Potatoes:			Turkey:	
150	Raw	.3		Light meat:	
151	Boiled, drained	.3	183	Raw	1.6
	Rice:		184	Cooked, dry heat	2.1
	Brown:			Dark meat:	
152	Dry form	1.8	185	Raw	3.1
153	Cooked	.6	186	Cooked, dry heat	4.4
	White, regular:			Neck meat:	
154	Dry form	1.3	187	Raw	5.0
155	Cooked	.4	188	Cooked	6.4
	White, parboiled:			Skin:	
156	Dry form	1.1	189	Raw	1.3
157	Cooked	.3	190	Cooked	2.1
	White, precooked, quick:			Veal:	
158	Dry form	.7		Separable lean:	
159	Cooked	.2	191	Raw	2.8
160	Cereal, ready-to-eat, puffed, or flakes	1.4	192	Cooked, dry heat	4.1
161	Rolls, hamburger	.6	193	Cooked, moist heat	4.2
162	Salad dressing	.2	194	Separable fat, raw	.5
163	Salmon, canned (77% solids, 23% liquid)	.9		Wheat, whole grain:	
	Sausages and cold cuts:		195	Hard	3.4
164	Bologna, beef	1.8	196	Soft	2.7
165	Braunschweiger	2.8	197	White	2.2
			198	Durum	2.7

TABLE 5. ZINC CONTENT OF FOODS PER 100 GRAMS—EDIBLE PORTION (*Continued*)

(Data are given to two decimal places if food contains less than 0.1 mg. zinc)

ITEM No.	FOOD AND DESCRIPTION	ZINC Mg.	ITEM No.	FOOD AND DESCRIPTION	ZINC Mg.
	Wheat flours:		207	Cooked	.5
199	Whole	2.4		Also see Farina	
200	80% extraction	1.5		Wheat cereals, ready-to-eat:	
201	All-purpose	.7	208	Bran flakes, 40%	3.6
202	Bread flour	.8	209	Flakes	2.3
203	Cake or pastry flour	.3	210	Germ, toasted	15.4
204	Wheat bran, crude	9.8	211	Puffed	2.6
205	Wheat germ, crude	14.3	212	Shredded	2.8
	Wheat cereal, whole-meal:				
206	Dry form	3.6			

TABLE 6. ALCOHOLIC AND CARBONATED BEVERAGES

BEVERAGE	AVERAGE PORTION	WEIGHT Gm.	ENERGY (CALORIES)	CARBO-HYDRATE Gm.	ALCOHOL* Gm.
Alcoholic Beverages:					
Ale, mild	8 oz. glass	230	98	8	9
Beer, average	8 oz. glass	240	114	11	9
Benedictine	cordial glass	20	69	7	7
Brandy, California	brandy glass	30	73	0	11
Cider, fermented	6 oz. glass	180	71	2	9
Cordial, anisette	cordial glass	20	74	7	7
Creme de menthe	cordial glass	20	67	6	7
Curaçao	cordial glass	20	54	6	6
Daiquiri	cocktail glass	100	122	5	15
Eggnog, Christmas	4 oz. punch cup	123	335	18	15
Gin Rickey	4 oz. glass	120	150	1	21
Gin, dry	1 jigger, 1 to 1½ oz.	43	105	0	15
Highball, average	8 oz. glass	240	166	0	24
Manhattan	cocktail glass, 3½ oz.	100	164	8	19
Old Fashioned	4 oz. glass	100	179	4	24
Planter's punch	3½ oz. glass	100	175	8	22
Rum	1 jigger, 1 to 1½ oz.	43	105	0	15
Tom Collins	10 oz. glass	300	180	9	22
Whiskey, rye	1 jigger, 1 to 1½ oz.	43	119	0	17
Scotch	1 jigger, 1 to 1½ oz.	43	105	0	15
Wines:					
Champagne	4 oz. glass	120	84	3	11
Muscatel or port	3½ oz. glass	100	158	14	15
Sauterne	3½ oz. glass	100	84	4	10
Sherry, domestic	2 oz. glass	60	84	5	9
Vermouth, dry	3½ oz. glass	100	105	1	15
Vermouth, sweet	3½ oz. glass	100	167	12	18
Carbonated Beverages:					
Coca-cola	6 oz. bottle	170	78	20	0
Ginger ale	6 oz. bottle	230	80	21	0
Pepsi-cola	8 oz. bottle	230	106	28	0
Soda, fruit flavor	8 oz. bottle	230	94	24	0
Root beer	8 oz. bottle	230	106	28	0

Values taken from Church, C. F., and Church, H. N.: Food Values of Portions Commonly Used. ed. 12. Philadelphia. J. B. Lippincott. 1975.

* Alcohol yields 7 calories per gram.

TABLE 7. EQUIVALENT WEIGHTS AND MEASURES

Weight Equivalents

	MILLIGRAM	GRAM	KILOGRAM	GRAIN	OUNCE	POUND
1 microgram (mcg.)	0.001	0.000001				
1 milligram (mg.)	1.	0.001		0.0154		
1 gram (Gm.)	1,000.	1.	0.001	15.4	0.035	0.0022
1 kilogram (Kg.)	1,000,000.	1,000.	1.	15,400.	35.2	2.2
1 grain (gr.)	64.8	0.065		1.		
1 ounce (oz.)		28.3		437.5	1.	0.063
1 pound (lb.)		453.6	0.454		16.0	1.

Volume Equivalents

	CUBIC MILLIMETER	CUBIC CENTIMETER	LITER	FLUID OUNCE	PINT	QUART
1 cubic millimeter (cu. mm.)	1.	0.001				
1 cubic centimeter (cc.)	1,000.		0.001			
1 liter (L.)	1,000,000.	1,000.	1.	33.8	2.1	1.05
1 fluid ounce		30.(29.57)	0.03	1.		
1 pint (pt.)		473.	0.473	16.	1.	
1 quart (qt.)		946.	0.946	32.	2.	1.

Linear Equivalents

	MILLIMETER	CENTIMETER	METER	INCH	FOOT	YARD
1 millimeter (mm.)	1.	0.1	0.001	0.039	0.00325	0.0011
1 centimeter (cm.)	10.	1.		0.39	0.0325	0.011
1 meter (M.)	1,000.	100.	1.	39.37	3.25	1.08
1 inch (in.)	25.4	2.54	0.025	1.	0.083	0.028
1 foot (ft.)	304.8	30.48	0.305	1.12	1.	0.33
1 yard (yd.)	914.4	91.44	0.914	36.0	3.	1.

Comparative Values of Weight and Volume of Water

1 liter	=	1 kilo. = 2.2 lbs.
1 fluid ounce =	30 Gm. = 1.04 ozs.
1 pint	= 473 Gm. = 1.04 lbs.
1 quart	= .946 kilo. = 2.1 lbs.

Table of Common Measures and Metric Equivalents

1 tsp. = 5 cc.
1 tbsp. = 14 cc. (approx. 15 Gm.)
1 cup = 225 cc. (approx. 240 Gm.)

Comparative Temperatures

	CENTIGRADE	FAHRENHEIT
Boiling water, sea level	100	212
Body temperature	37	98.6
Tropical temperature	30	89
Room temperature, average	20	70
Freezing	0	32

Table of Measures and Approximate Weights

3 teaspoons .... 1 tbsp.	*1 tablespoon liquid .... ½ oz.
16 tablespoons .... 1 cup	1 tablespoon flour .... ¼ oz.
½ cup .... 1 gill	1 tablespoon sugar .... ⅜ oz.
2 cups .... 1 pt.	*1 cup liquid .... 8 ozs.
4 cups .... 1 qt.	1 cup flour ....4½ ozs.
2 pints .... 1 qt.	1 cup butter .... 8 ozs.
4 quarts .... 1 gal.	1 cup sugar .... 10 ozs.
1 tablespoon butter ....½ oz.	

* Water or milk.

TABLE 8. HEIGHT AND WEIGHT FOR AGE—PERCENTILE STANDARDS—BOYS AND GIRLS

AGE YEARS	HEIGHT PERCENTILES					WEIGHT PERCENTILES				
	10	25	50	75	90	10	25	50	75	90

BOYS

AGE YEARS	Ins.	Ins.	Ins.	Ins.	Ins.	Lbs.	Lbs.	Lbs.	Lbs.	Lbs.
2	32.7	33.2	33.8	34.3	34.6	24.2	25.8	27.3	28.7	30.6
3	36.0	36.6	37.2	37.6	38.1	28.9	30.4	31.7	33.5	35.5
4	39.0	39.7	40.2	40.8	41.4	30.0	33.1	34.8	35.9	37.9
5	41.7	42.4	43.0	43.6	44.3	37.3	38.8	40.6	42.8	45.4
6	44.1	44.9	45.7	46.3	47.0	41.7	43.2	45.4	48.3	51.6
7	46.3	47.2	48.1	48.9	49.9	46.1	47.8	50.9	54.7	58.6
8	48.5	49.4	50.5	51.4	52.6	50.5	52.9	57.4	61.9	66.6
9	50.6	51.7	52.8	53.8	54.8	55.1	58.6	64.4	70.1	75.2
10	52.5	53.7	54.9	56.1	57.0	60.4	64.8	71.4	78.0	84.2
11	54.3	55.4	56.7	58.2	59.1	65.7	71.2	78.9	86.4	93.5
12	56.0	57.1	58.7	60.3	61.5	71.0	77.8	86.0	94.8	102.7
13	58.1	59.3	61.2	62.6	64.3	76.9	85.3	95.7	105.8	114.6
14	60.4	62.1	64.1	65.5	67.2	88.0	98.5	111.1	119.5	128.7
15	63.0	65.0	66.9	68.3	69.8	101.6	112.2	124.3	134.5	143.3
16	65.6	67.3	68.9	70.4	71.7	112.4	122.6	133.8	146.4	157.4
17	66.5	68.2	69.8	71.2	72.4	120.4	130.1	139.8	153.9	169.3
18	67.1	68.6	70.2	71.5	72.7	127.0	134.3	142.4	158.7	173.3

GIRLS

AGE YEARS	10	25	50	75	90	10	25	50	75	90
2	31.8	32.7	33.5	34.3	34.9	21.6	23.6	25.8	27.6	29.1
3	34.9	35.8	37.0	38.0	38.7	25.6	27.3	30.6	32.4	34.4
4	37.8	38.9	40.4	41.3	42.0	29.3	31.3	35.5	37.5	40.1
5	40.5	41.6	43.3	44.3	45.0	33.1	35.9	40.3	43.4	45.9
6	43.1	44.0	45.9	47.2	47.7	37.0	40.6	45.4	49.6	51.6
7	45.4	46.2	48.5	49.8	50.3	41.4	45.2	51.1	55.8	60.0
8	47.7	48.4	51.0	52.2	52.8	46.2	50.0	58.0	61.9	70.5
9	49.8	50.7	53.5	54.6	55.2	51.1	56.0	65.7	70.5	82.5
10	51.9	53.1	55.6	56.9	58.0	56.0	62.2	74.3	81.8	93.9
11	53.7	55.7	58.1	59.7	60.9	60.8	69.4	83.8	94.6	104.7
12	55.5	59.0	61.3	62.6	63.6	70.5	80.9	96.1	106.5	115.1
13	58.3	61.0	63.9	65.1	65.9	79.4	91.5	108.9	114.9	124.8
14	60.5	62.2	65.0	66.1	67.2	85.5	98.3	116.6	121.7	133.6
15	61.8	63.2	65.6	66.5	67.7	89.1	102.7	121.0	127.0	140.7
16	62.4	63.8	65.9	66.8	68.0	91.5	106.0	123.9	131.0	144.2
17	62.6	64.1	66.1	67.0	68.3	93.0	108.5	125.7	133.8	145.9
18	62.7	64.3	66.2	67.6	68.9	93.7	110.0	126.1	135.4	146.8

From Hathaway, M. L.: Heights and Weights of Children and Youth in the United States. Home Economics Res. Bulletin No. 2. U.S.D.A., Washington, D.C., 1957.

TABLE 9. DESIRABLE WEIGHTS FOR MEN AND WOMEN AGED 25 AND OVER*

Weight in Pounds According to Frame (In Indoor Clothing)

Height		Small Frame	Medium Frame	Large Frame	Height		Small Frame	Medium Frame	Large Frame
		MEN					WOMEN†		
Feet	Inches				Feet	Inches			
5	2	112–120	118–129	126–141	4	10	92– 98	96–107	104–119
5	3	115–123	121–133	129–144	4	11	94–101	98–110	106–122
5	4	118–126	124–136	132–148	5	0	96–104	101–113	109–125
5	5	121–129	127–139	135–152	5	1	99–107	104–116	112–128
5	6	124–133	130–143	138–156	5	2	102–110	107–119	115–131
5	7	128–137	134–147	142–161	5	3	105–113	110–122	118–134
5	8	132–141	138–152	147–166	5	4	108–116	113–126	121–138
5	9	136–145	142–156	151–170	5	5	111–119	116–130	125–142
5	10	140–150	146–160	155–174	5	6	114–123	120–135	129–146
5	11	144–154	150–165	159–179	5	7	118–127	124–139	133–150
6	0	148–158	154–170	164–184	5	8	122–131	128–143	137–154
6	1	152–162	158–175	168–189	5	9	126–135	132–147	141–158
6	2	156–167	162–180	173–194	5	10	130–140	136–151	145–163
6	3	160–171	167–185	178–199	5	11	134–144	140–155	149–168
6	4	164–175	172–190	182–204	6	0	138–148	144–159	153–173

* Metropolitan Life Insurance Company.
† For girls between 18 and 25, subtract 1 pound for each year under 25.

TABLE 10. CURRENT GUIDELINES FOR CRITERIA OF NUTRITIONAL STATUS
FOR LABORATORY EVALUATION[a]

NUTRIENT AND UNITS	AGE OF SUBJECT (YEARS)	CRITERIA OF STATUS		
		DEFICIENT	MARGINAL	ACCEPTABLE
*Hemoglobin (gm./100ml.)	6-23 mos.	Up to 9.0	9.0- 9.9	10.0+
	2-5	Up to 10.0	10.0-10.9	11.0+
	6-12	Up to 10.0	10.0-11.4	11.5+
	13-16M	Up to 12.0	12.0-12.9	13.0+
	13-16F	Up to 10.0	10.0-11.4	11.5+
	16+M	Up to 12.0	12.0-13.9	14.0+
	16+F	Up to 10.0	10.0-11.9	12.0+
	Pregnant (after 6+ mos.)	Up to 9.5	9.5-10.9	11.0+
*Hematocrit (Packed cell volume in percent)	Up to 2	Up to 28	28-30	31+
	2-5	Up to 30	30-33	34+
	6-12	Up to 30	30-35	36+
	13-16M	Up to 37	37-39	40+
	13-16F	Up to 31	31-35	36+
	16+M	Up to 37	37-43	44+
	16+F	Up to 31	31-37	33+
	Pregnant	Up to 30	30-32	33+
*Serum Albumin (gm./100ml.)	Up to 1	—	Up to 2.5	2.5+
	1-5	—	Up to 3.0	3.0+
	6-16	—	Up to 3.5	3.5+
	16+	Up to 2.8	2.8-3.4	3.5+
	Pregnant	Up to 3.0	3.0-3.4	3.5+
*Serum Protein (gm./100ml.)	Up to 1	—	Up to 5.0	5.0+
	1-5	—	Up to 5.5	5.5+
	6-16	—	Up to 6.0	6.0+
	16+	Up to 6.0	6.0-6.4	6.5+
	Pregnant	Up to 5.5	5.5-5.9	6.0+
*Serum Ascorbic Acid (mg./100ml.)	All ages	Up to 0.1	0.1-0.19	0.2+
*Plasma vitamin A (mcg./100ml.)	All ages	Up to 10	10-19	20+
*Plasma Carotene (mcg./100ml.)	All ages	Up to 20	20-39	40+
	Pregnant	—	40-79	80+
*Serum Iron (mcg./100ml.)	Up to 2	Up to 30	—	30+
	2-5	Up to 40	—	40+
	6-12	Up to 50	—	50+
	12+M	Up to 60	—	60+
	12+F	Up to 40	—	40+
*Transferrin Saturation (percent)	Up to 2	Up to 15.0	—	15.0+
	2-12	Up to 20.0	—	20.0+
	12+M	Up to 20.0	—	20.0+
	12+F	Up to 15.0	—	15.0+
†Serum Folacin (ng./ml.)	All ages	Up to 2.0	2.1-5.9	6.0+

* Adapted from the Ten-State Nutrition Survey.
† Criteria may vary with different methodology.
[a] AJPH Supplement, Vol. 63, November, 1973.

NUTRIENT AND UNITS	AGE OF SUBJECT (YEARS)	CRITERIA OF STATUS		
		DEFICIENT	MARGINAL	ACCEPTABLE
†Serum vitamin B_{12} (pg./ml.)	All ages	Up to 100	—	100+
*Thiamine in Urine (mcg./g. creatinine)	1-3	Up to 120	120-175	175+
	4-5	Up to 85	85-120	120+
	6-9	Up to 70	70-180	180+
	10-15	Up to 55	55-150	150+
	16+	Up to 27	27- 65	65+
	Pregnant	Up to 21	21- 49	50+
*Riboflavin in Urine (mcg./g. creatinine)	1-3	Up to 150	150-499	500+
	4-5	Up to 100	100-299	300+
	6-9	Up to 85	85-269	270+
	10-16	Up to 70	70-199	200+
	16+	Up to 27	27- 79	80+
	Pregnant	Up to 30	30- 89	90+
†RBC Transketolase-TPP-effect (ratio)	All ages	25+	15- 25	Up to 15
†RBC Glutathione Reductase-FAD-effect (ratio)	All ages	1.2+	—	Up to 1.2
†Tryptophan Load (mg. Xanthurenic acid excreted)	Adults (Dose: 100mg./kg. body weight)	25+(6 hrs.) 75+(24 hrs.)	— —	Up to 25 Up to 75
†Urinary Pyridoxine (mcg./g. creatinine)	1-3	Up to 90	—	90+
	4-6	Up to 80	—	80+
	7-9	Up to 60	—	60+
	10-12	Up to 40	—	40+
	13-15	Up to 30	—	30+
	16+	Up to 20	—	20+
*Urinary N'methyl nicotinamide (mg./g. creatinine)	All ages	Up to 0.2	0.2-5.59	0.6+
	Pregnant	Up to 0.8	0.8-2.49	2.5+
†Urinary Pantothenic Acid (mcg.)	All ages	Up to 200	—	200+
†Plasma vitamin E (mg./100ml.)	All ages	Up to 0.2	0.2-0.6	0.6+
†Transaminase Index (ratio)				
**EGOT	Adult	2.0 +	—	Up to 2.0
‡EGPT	Adult	1.25+	—	Up to 1.25

* Adapted from the Ten-State Nutrition Survey.
† Criteria may vary with different methodology.
** Erythrocyte Glutamic Oxalacetic Transaminase.
‡ Erythrocyte Glutamic Pyruvic Transaminase.

bibliography

section one
principles of nutrition

GENERAL REFERENCES

Books:

Anderson, L. and Browe, J. H.: *Nutrition and Family Health Services.* Philadelphia, Saunders, 1960.

Anderson, L., Dibble, M. V., Mitchell, H. S., Arlin, M. T.: *The Science of Nutrition.* New York, Macmillan, 1972.

Beaton, G. H. and McHenry, E. W.: *Nutrition. A Comprehensive Treatise,* Vol. III, Nutritional Status, Assessment and Application. New York, Academic Press, 1966.

Berg, A., Scrimshaw, N. S., and Call, D. L.: *International Conference on Nutrition, National Development and Planning.* Cambridge, Mass., MIT Press, 1973.

Birch, F. G., Green, L. F., Plaskett, L. G.: Health and Food. New York: Wiley, 1972.

Bogert, L. J., Briggs, G. M., and Calloway, D. H.: *Nutrition and Physical Fitness,* ed. 9. Philadelphia, Saunders, 1973.

Chaney, M. S. and Ross, M. L.: *Nutrition,* ed. 8. Boston, Houghton Mifflin, 1971.

Davidson, S., Passmore, R., and Brock, J. F.: *Human Nutrition and Dietetics,* ed. 5. Baltimore, Williams, 1973.

Fleck, H. C.: *Introduction to Nutrition,* ed. 2. New York, Macmillan, 1971.

Gifft, H. H., Washbon, M. B., and Harrison G. G.: *Nutrition, Behavior and Change.* Englewood Cliffs, N.J. Prentice-Hall, 1972.

Goodhart, R. S. and Shils, M. E.: *Modern Nutrition in Health and Disease,* ed. 5. Philadelphia, Lea and Febiger, 1973.

Guthrie, H. A.: *Introductory Nutrition,* ed. 2. St. Louis, Mosby, 1971.

Guthrie, H. A. and Braddock, K. S.: *Programmed Nutrition.* St. Louis, Mosby, 1971.

Heinz Handbook of Nutrition, ed. 3. New York, McGraw-Hill, 1967.

Krause, M. V. and Hunscher, M. A.: *Food, Nutrition and Diet Therapy,* ed. 5. Philadelphia, Saunders, 1972.

Kutsky, R. J.: *Handbook of Vitamins and Hormones.* New York, Van Nostrand, 1973.

Lagua, R. T., Claudio, V. S., and Thiele, V. F.: *Nutrition and Diet Therapy. Reference Dictionary.* St. Louis, Mosby, 1974.

Margolius, Sidney: *Health Foods: Facts and Fakes.* New York, Walker, 1973.

Martin, E. A.: *Nutrition in Action,* ed. 3. New York, Holt, Rinehart & Winston, 1971.

Mayer, J.: *Human Nutrition—Its Physiological, Medical and Social Aspects.* Springfield, Ill., Thomas, 1972.

Pike, R. L. and Brown, M. L.: *Nutrition: An Integrated Approach,* ed. 2. New York, Wiley, 1975.

Robinson, C. H.: *Basic Nutrition and Diet Therapy,* ed. 2. Riverside, N.J., Macmillan, 1970.

———:*Fundamentals of Normal Nutrition,* ed. 2. Riverside, N.J., Macmillan, 1973.

———: *Normal and Therapeutic Nutrition,* ed. 14. New York, Macmillan, 1972.

Stare, F. J., and McWilliams, M.:*Living Nutrition.* New York, Wiley, 1973.

Tannahill, R.: *Food in History.* New York, Stein, 1973.

Taylor, C. M., and Pye, O. F.:*Foundations of Nutrition,* ed. 6. New York, Macmillan, 1966.

Williams, R. J.: *Nutrition against Disease: Environmental Prevention.* New York, Pitman, 1971.

Williams, S. R.:*Nutrition and Diet Therapy,* ed. 2. St. Louis, Mosby, 1973.

Wilson, E. D., Fisher, K. H., and Fuqua, M. E.: *Principles of Nutrition,* ed. 3. New York, Wiley, 1975.

Journal Articles:

American Dietetic Association: Position paper on nutrition education for the public. J. Am. Dietet. A. 62:429, 1973.

Benson, E. M., et al: Nutritive values: wild edible plants of the Pacific Northwest. J. Am. Dietet. A. 62:143, 1973.

Goldsmith, G. A.: Clinical nutritional problems in the United States today. Nutr. Rev. 23:1, 1965.

Hagler, L. and Herman, R. H.: Oxalate metabolism IV., V. Am. J. Clin. Nutr. 26:1073, 1242, 1973.

Hodges, R. E.: Nutrition and "The Pill." J. Am. Dietet. A. 59:212, 1971.

King, C. G.: Notes on the history of Nutrition in America. J. Am. Dietet. A. 56:188, 1970.

Leverton, R.: Tools for teaching food needs. J. Home Econ. 65:37, 1973.

Ross, M. L.: The long view. J. Am. Dietet. A. 56:295, 1970.

Sebrell, W. H.: Changing concepts of malnutrition. Am. J. Clin. Nutr. 20:653, 1969.

Todhunter, E. N.: The evolution of nutrition concepts. J. Am. Dietet. A. 46:120, 1965.

Other Journals and Annuals:

American Journal of Nursing
American Journal of Public Health
American Journal of Clinical Nutrition
Borden's Review of Nutrition Research
Family Economics Review
Journal of the American Dietetic Association
Journal of Home Economics
Journal of Nutrition
Journal of Nutrition Education
Metabolism
National Food Situation Economic Research Service (Quarterly)
Nutrition Abstracts and Reviews
Nutrition Reviews
Nutrition Today
World Review of Nutrition and Dietetics

RELIABLE SOURCES FOR NUTRITION INFORMATION

American Dietetic Ass., 420 N. Michigan Ave., Chicago, Ill. 60611.

American Home Economics Ass., 1600 Twentieth St., Washington, D.C. 20009.

Cooperative Extension—State and Federal (USDA) State and County Cooperative Extension Service.

Council on Foods and Nutrition, or Bureau of Investigation, American Medical Ass., 535 N. Dearborn St., Chicago, Ill. 60610.

Food and Nutrition Board, National Academy of Sciences—National Research Council, 2101 Constitution Ave., Washington, D.C. 20418.

Food and Nutrition Departments of State University.

Food and Nutrition Section, American Public Health Ass., 1740 Broadway, New York, N.Y. 10019.

Food and Drug Administration, U.S. Dept. H.E.W., Washington, D.C. 20204.

Federal Trade Commission, Bureau of Investigation, State and Local Health Departments, Washington, D.C.

The Nutrition Foundation, Inc., 99 Park Ave., New York, N.Y. 10016.

United States Department of Agriculture, Washington, D.C.

United States Department of Health, Education and Welfare, Washington, D.C.

Better Business Bureaus.

NATIONAL NUTRITION POLICIES AND NUTRITIONAL STATUS SURVEYS

Books and Pamphlets:

Berg, A.: *The Nutrition Factor.* Washington, D.C., Brookings Institution, 1973.

Food Intake and Nutritive Value of Diets of Men, Women and Children in the United States, Spring 1965. Agr. Research Service, USDA, Washington, D.C., 1969.

Household Food Consumption Survey 1965-66, Report No. 6: Dietary Levels of Households in the United States, Spring 1965. Agr. Research Service, USDA, Washington, D.C., 1969.

Hunger U.S.A. A Report of the Citizen's Board of Inquiry into Hunger and Malnutrition in the U.S. Washington, D.C., New Community Press, 1968.

Mayer, J.: *U.S. Nutrition Policies in the Seventies.* San Francisco, Freeman, 1973.

Nutrition and Human Needs Hearings before the Select Committee on Nutrition and Human Needs of the U.S. Senate, Parts I et seq. Washington, D.C., U.S. Gov't Print. Off., 1969.

Stewart, M. S.: *Hunger in America.*, Public Affairs Pamphlet 457. New York, Public Affairs Committee, 1970.

White House Conference on Food, Nutrition and Health— Final Report. Washington, D.C., U.S. Gov't Print. Off., 1970.

Journal Articles:

Beloian, A. M.: Seasonal variations in U.S. diets. Family Economics Rev. (March) 1971.

Council on Foods and Nutrition: Malnutrition and hunger in the United States. JAMA 213:272, 1970.

Davis, T. R. A., et al: Review of studies of vitamin and mineral nutrition in the United States (1950-1968). J. Nutr. Educa. 1:41 (Supplement), 1969.

Gussow, J. D.: Improving the American diet. J. Home Econ. 65:6, 1973.

Hegsted, D. M.: The development of a national nutrition policy. J. Am. Dietet. A. 62:394, 1973.

Hueneman, R. L.: Interpretation of nutritional status. J. Am. Dietet. A. 63:123, 1973.

Kelsay, J. L.: A compendium of nutritional status studies and dietary evaluation studies conducted in the United States. J. Nutrition 99:123 (Supplement I, Part II), 1969.

Mayer, J.: One year later. J. Am. Dietet. A. 58:300, 1971.

Pimentel, D., et al: Food production and the energy crisis. Science 182:443, 1973.

Plan and Operation of the Health and Nutrition Examination Survey. U.S. 1971-3. Vital and Health Statistics Series 1, Nos. 10a and 10b. DHEW Publ. No (HSM) 73-1310, 1973.

Sabry, Z. I., et al: Nutrition Canada—A national nutrition survey. Nutr. Rev., 32:105, 1974.

Schneider, H. A. and Hesla, J. T.: The way it is. Nutr. Rev. 31:233, 1973.

Scrimshaw, N. S.: Meeting future food needs. J. Canad. Diet. A. 32:117, 1971.

Senti, F. R.: Nutrition awareness in the U.S.D.A. J. Am. Dietet. A. 61:17, 1972.

Symposium—National Nutrition Survey. Viewpoint of a public administrator; Viewpoint of a U.S. Senator; Viewpoint of a nutritionist. Am. J. Clin. Nutr. 25:956, 961, 964, 1972.

Ten-State Nutrition Survey, 1968-70. Highlights. DHEW Pub. No. (HSM) 72-8134, 1972.

The state of nutrition today. FDA Consumer, 7:13 (November), 1973.

Undernutrition in Massachusetts. N. Eng. J. Med. 287:886 (October), 1972.

White, P. L.: National Nutrition Survey. JAMA 223:1272, 1973.

carbohydrates

Journal Articles:

Ad Hoc Committee on Hypoglycemia: Statement on Hypoglycemia. Archives Int. Med. 131:591, 1973.

Anderson, J. T.: Dietary carbohydrate and serum triglycerides. Am. J. Clin. Nutr. 20:168, 1967.

Asano, T., Levitt, M. D., and Goetz, F. C.: Xylitol absorption in healthy men. Diabetes, 22:279, 1973.

Ayres, J. C.: Manioc. Food Tech. 26:128, 1972.

Bebb, H. T., et al: Caloric and nutrient contribution of alcoholic beverages to the usual diets of 155 adults. Am. J. Clin. Nutr. 24:1042, 1971.

Bloom, W. L.: Carbohydrates and water balance. Am. J. Clin. Nutr. 20:157, 1967.

Cohn, R. M. and Segal, S.: Galactose metabolism and its regulation. Metabolism 22:627, 1973.

Dreizer, S.: The importance of nutrition in tooth development. J. School Health 43:114, 1973.

Gallagher, C. R., et al: Lactose intolerance and fermented dairy products. J. Am. Dietet. A. 65:418, 1974.

Goldstein, F.: Diet and colonic disease. J. Am. Dietet. A. 60:499, 1972.

Gryboski, J. D.: Diarrhea from dietetic candies (sorbitol). N. Eng. J. Med. 275:718, 1966.

Hamed, M. G. E., et al: Preparation and chemical composition of sweet potato flour. Cereal Chem. 50:133, 1973.

Hardinge, M. G., et al: Carbohydrates in foods. J. Am. Dietet. A. 46:197, 1965.

Hartles, R. L.: Carbohydrate consumption and dental caries. Am. J. Clin. Nutr. 20:152, 1967.

Hodges, R. E.: Present knowledge of carbohydrates. Nutr. Rev. 24:65, 1966.

Hodges, R. E. and Krehl, W. A.: The role of carbohydrates in lipid metabolism. Am. J. Clin. Nutr. 17:334, 1965.

Lorenz, K.: Food uses of triticale. Food Tech. 26:66, 1972.

McGandy, R. B., et al: Dietary carbohydrate and serum cholesterol levels in man. Am. J. Clin. Nutr. 18:237, 1966.

Nandi, M. A. and Parham, E. S.: Milk drinking by the lactose intolerant. J. Am. Dietet. A. 61:258, 1972.

O'Brien, P. J.: The sweet potato: Its origin and dispersal. Am. Anthropologist 74:342, 1972.

Review: Blood lipids and various dietary carbohydrates. Nutr. Rev. 24:35, 1966.

————: Diet and cancer of the colon. Nutr. Rev. 31:110, 1973.

————: Diet, intestinal flora and colon cancer. Nutr. Rev. 33:136, 1975.

————: Dietary fiber and colonic function—an effect of particle size. Nutr. Rev. 33:70, 1975.

Robbins, G. S. and Pomeranz, Y.: Composition and utilization of milled barley products. Cereal Chem. 49:240, 1972.

Stephenson, L. S. and Latham, M. C.: Lactose intolerance and milk consumption: the relation of tolerance to symptoms. Am. J. Clin. Nutr. 27:296, 1974.

Stevens, H. A. and Ohlson, M. A.: Estimated intake of simple and complex carbohydrates. Am. J. Clin. Nutr. 20:108, 1967.

Trowell, H.: Ischemic heart disease and dietary fiber. Am. J. Clin. Nutr. 25:926, 1972.

Toepfer, E. W., et al: Nutrient composition of selected wheats and wheat products, II, Summary. Cereal Chem. 49:173, 1972.

Yudkin, J.: Evolutionary and historical changes in dietary carbohydrates. Am. J. Clin. Nutr. 20:108, 1967.

fats and other lipids

Books and Pamphlets:

Beaton, G. H. and McHenry, E. W.: Nutrition—A Comprehensive Treatise, Vol. I. Macronutrients and Nutrient Elements, Chapter 2. New York, Academic Press, 1964.

Fisher, H., et al: Fat and cholesterol content of domestic and imported cheeses, Bull. 832-A, New Jersey Agricultural Experiment Station. New Brunswick, Rutgers University.

Food and Nutrition Board: Dietary Fat and Human Health. National Academy of Science—National Research Council Publ. No. 1147. Washington, D.C., 1966.

Home Economics Research Report, No. 7: Fatty Acids in Food Fats. Agr. Research Service, USDA. Washington, D.C., 1959.

Senior, J. R., ed.: Medium Chain Triglycerides. Philadelphia, University of Pennsylvania Press, 1968.

Journal Articles:

Alfin-Slater, R. B.: Fats, essential fatty acids, and ascorbic acid—three essential nutrients. J. Am. Dietet. A., 64:168, 1974.

Ascorbic acid and the catabolism of cholesterol. Nutr. Rev. 31:154, 1973.

Babayan, V. K.: Medium-chain triglycerides. Their composition, preparation and application. J. Am. Oil Chem. Soc. 45:23, 1968.

Bieri, J. G.: Fat-soluble vitamins in the eighth revision of the Recommended Dietary Allowances. J. Am. Dietet. A. 64:171, 1974.

Clegg, A. J.: Composition and related nutritional and organoleptic aspects of palm oil. J. Am. Oil Chem. Soc. 50:321, 1973.

Feeley, R. M., Criner, P. E., and Watt, B. K.: Cholesterol content of foods. J. Am. Dietet. A. 61:134, 1972.

Genetic factors in fat mobilization. Nutr. Rev. 31:157, 1973.

Ginter, E.: Cholesterol: vitamin C controls its transformation to bile acids. Science 179:702, 1973.

Guild, L., Deethardt, D., and Rust, E.: Fatty acids in foods served in a university food service. J. Am. Dietet. A. 61:149, 1972.

Harkins, R. W. and Sarett, H. P.: Medium-chain triglycerides. JAMA 203:272, 1968.

Hashim, S. A.: Medium-chain triglycerides. Clinical and metabolic aspects. J. Am. Dietet. A. 51:221, 1967.

Havel, J.: Caloric homeostasis and disorders of fuel transport. N. Eng. J. Med. 287:1186, 1972.

Itoh, T., Tamura, T., and Matsumoto, T.: Sterol composition of 19 vegetable oils. J. Am. Oil Chem. Soc. 50:122, 1973.

Jensen, R. G.: Composition of bovine milk lipids. J. Amer. Oil Chem. Soc. 50:186, 1973.

Lacroix, D. E., et al: Cholesterol, fat, and protein in dairy products. J. Am. Dietet. A. 62:275, 1973.

Lipoproteins. J. Am. Dietet. A. 60:44, 1972.

McIntyre, N. and Isselbacher, K. J.: Role of the small intestine in cholesterol metabolism. Am. J. Clin. Nutr. 26:647, 1973.

Paulsrud, J. R., et al: Essential fatty acid deficiency in infants induced by fat-free intravenous feeding. Am. J. Clin. Nutr. 25:897, 1972.

Podell, R. N.: Cholesterol and the law. Circulation 48:225, 1973.

Reiser, R.: Saturated fat in the diet and serum cholesterol concentration. A critical examination of the literature. Am. J. Clin. Nutr. 26:524, 1973.

Review: Essential fatty acid deficiency in continuous-drip alimentation. Nutr. Rev. 33:329, 1975.

Schlenk, H.: Odd numbered and new essential fatty acids. Fed. Proc. 31:1430, 1972.

Subbiah, M. T. R.: Dietary plant sterols: current status in human and animal sterol metabolism. Am. J. Clin. Nutr. 26:219, 1973.

Wein, E. and Wilcox, E. B.: Serum cholesterol from pre-adolescence through young adulthood. J. Am. Dietet. A. 61:155, 1972.

Wilson, J. D.: The role of bile acids in the overall regulation of steroid metabolism. Arch. Int. Med. 130:493, 1972.

proteins

(SEE ALSO REFERENCES UNDER DIGESTION, ABSORPTION AND METABOLISM)

Books and Pamphlets:

FAO: *Protein–At the Heart of the World Food Problem.* Rome, FAO, 1967.

———: *Amino Acid Content of Foods and Biological Data on Proteins,* Nutr. Studies No. 24. Rome, FAO, 1970.

FAO/WHO Joint Expert Group: *Protein Requirements.* Rome, FAO, 1965.

Food and Nutrition Board: *Evaluation of Protein Nutrition.* National Academy of Science–National Research Council Publ. No. 711. Washington, D.C., 1959.

———: *Evaluation of Protein Quality.* National Academy of Science—National Research Council Publ. No. 1100. Washington, D.C., 1963.

———: *Improvement of Protein Nutriture.* National Academy of Science—National Research Council, 1975.

———: *Progress in Meeting Protein Needs of Infants and Children.* National Academy of Science-National Research Council Publ. No. 843. Washington, D.C., 1961.

Orr, M. L. and Watt, B. K.: *Amino Acid Content of Food.* Home Econ. Res. Report No. 4 USDA. Washington, D.C., 1957.

Journal Articles:

Amino acid, dipeptide and protein absorption in human beings. Nutr. Rev. 31:272, 1973.

Bradfield, R. B.: Protein deprivation: comparative response of hair roots, serum protein and urinary nitrogen. Am. J. Clin. Nutr. 24:405, 1971.

Calloway, D. H.: Recommended Dietary Allowances for protein and energy, 1973. J. Am. Dietet. A. 64:157, 1974.

Clark, H. E., et al: Requirements of adult human subjects for methionine and cystine. Am. J. Clin. Nutr. 23:731, 1970.

Coltman, C. A., et al: The amino acid content of sweat in normal adults. Am. J. Clin. Nutr. 18:373, 1966.

Committee Report: Assessment of protein nutritional status. Am. J. Clin. Nutr. 23:803, 1970.

Fisher, H., et al: Reassessment of amino acid requirements of young women on low nitrogen diets. I. Lysine and tryptophan. Am. J. Clin. Nutr. 22:1190, 1969.

Fleck, A.: Protein metabolism after injury. Proc. Nutr. Soc. 30:152, 1971.

Hackler, L. R.: Nutritional evaluation of protein quality in breakfast foods. Cereal Chem. 49:677, 1972.

Hardinge, M. G., et al: Nutritional studies of vegetarians. J. Am. Dietet. A. 48:25, 1966.

Hegsted, D. M.: Amino acid fortification and the protein problem. Am. J. Clin. Nutr. 21:688, 1968.

———: Minimum protein requirements of adults. Am. J. Clin. Nutr. 21:352, 1968.

Hegsted, D. M. and Irwin, M. I.: A conspectus of research on protein requirements of man. J. Nutrition 101:385, 1971.

Holt, L. E. and Snyderman, S. E.: Protein and amino acid requirements of infants and children. Nutr. Abstr. Rev. 35:1, 1965.

Huang, P. C., Chong, H. E., and Rand, W. M.: Obligatory urinary and fecal nitrogen losses in young Chinese men. J. Nutrition 102:1605, 1972.

Kelman, L., et al: Effects of dietary protein restriction on albumin synthesis, albumin catabolism and the plasma aminogram. Am. J. Clin. Nutr. 25:1174, 1972.

Kies, C.: Nonspecific nitrogen in the nutrition of human beings. Fed. Proc. 31:1172, 1972.

Kies, C. and Fox, H. M.: Comparisons of dry breakfast cereals as protein resources: human biological assay at equal intakes of cereal. Cereal Chem. 50:233, 1973.

Kopple, J. D. and Swendseid, M. E.: Evidence for a dietary histidine requirement in normal man. Fed. Proc. 33:671A, 1973.

Lockmiller, N. R.: What are textured protein products? Food Tech. 26:59, 1972.

Mattil, K. F.: Composition, nutritional and functional properties and quality criteria of soy protein concentrates and soy protein isolates. J. Am. Oil Chem. Soc. 51:81A (January), 1974.

Mitchell, H. S.: Protein limitation and human growth. J. Am. Dietet. A. 44:165, 1966.

Ozalp, L., et al: Plasma amino acid response in young men given diets devoid of single essential amino acids. J. Nutr. 102:1147, 1972.

Review: Evaluation of a peanut-soybean mixture. Nutr. Rev. 23:75, 1965.

———: Histidine: An essential amino acid for normal adults. Nutr. Rev. 33:200, 1975.

———: Histidine requirements in infancy. Nutr. Rev. 22:114, 1964.

Robinson, R. F.: What is the future of textured protein products? Food Tech. 26:59, 1972.

Roels, O. A.: Marine proteins. Nutr. Rev. 27:35, 1969.

Rose, W. C.: Amino acid requirements of adult man. Nutr. Abstr. & Rev. 27:631, 1957.

Scrimshaw, N. S., et al: Protein requirements of man: variations in obligatory urinary and fecal nitrogen loses in young men. J. Nutrition 102:1595, 1972.

Stegink, L. D. and Besten, L. D.: Synthesis of cysteine from methionine in normal adult subjects: effect of route of alimentation. Science 178:514, 1972.

Taylor, Y. S. M., et al: Daily protein and meal patterns affecting young men fed adequate and restricted energy intakes. Am. J. Clin. Nutr. 26:1216, 1973.

Treonine requirements in young and elderly. Nutr. Rev. 32:234, 1974.

Turk, R. E., et al: Adequacy of spun-soy protein containing egg albumin for human nutrition. J. Am. Dietet. A. 63:519, 1973.

Ultschul, A. M.: Texture adds new dimension to soy products. School Foodservice J. 26:27, 1972.

Walker, R. M. and Linkswiler, H. M.: Calcium retention in the adult human male as affected by protein intake. J. Nutrition 102:1297, 1972.

Waters, E. F.: Plentiful protein from the sea. FDA Consumer 7:10, (November), 1973.

Watts, J. H.: Evaluation of protein in selected American diets. J. Am. Dietet. A. 46:116, 1965.

Wolford, K. M.: Beef/soy: Consumer acceptance. J. Am. Oil Chem. Soc. 51:131A, (January), 1974.

Wolf, W. J.: What is soy protein? Food Tech. 26:44, 1972.

Young, V. R., et al: Plasma tryptophan response curve and its relation to tryptophan requirements in young adult men. J. Nutrition 101:45, 1971.

Young, V. R., et al: Protein requirements of man: efficiency of egg protein utilization at maintenance levels in young men. J. Nutrition 103:1164, 1973.

Young, V. R., et al: Plasma amino acid response curve and amino acid requirements in young men: Valine and lysine. J. Nutrition 102:1159, 1972.

water and mineral metabolism

Andersson, B.: Thirst and brain control of water balance. Am. Scient. 59:408, 1971.

Baker, E. M., et al: Water requirements of men as related to salt intake. Am. J. Clin. Nutr. 12:394, 1963.

Clarkson, E. M., et al: Slow Sodium: An oral slowly released sodium chloride preparation. Brit. Med. J. 5775:604, 1971.

Consolazio, C. F., et al: Excretion of sodium, potassium, magnesium and iron in human sweat and the relation of each to balance requirements. J. Nutrition 79:407, 1963.

Cooper, G. R. and Heap, B.: Sodium ion in drinking water, II, Importance, problems, and potential applications of sodium-ion-restricted therapy. J. Am. Dietet. A. 50:37, 1967.

Food and Nutrition Board: Water deprivation and performance of athletes. Nutr. Rev. 32:314, 1974.

Gundersen, K. and Shen, G.: Total body water in obesity. Am. J. Clin. Nutr. 19:77, 1966.

Klahr, S. and Slatopolsky, E.: Renal regulation of sodium excretion. Arch. Int. Med. 131:780, 1973.

Klahr, S., Wessler, S., and Avioli, L. V.: Acid-base disorders in health and disease. JAMA 222:567, 1972.

Krehl, W. A.: The potassium depletion syndrome. Nutrition Today 1:20, (June) 1966.

_____: Sodium: a most extraordinary dietary essential. Nutrition Today 1:16, 1966.

Potassium imbalance: programmed instruction. Am. J. Nurs. 67:343, 1967.

Review: Dietary sodium and experimental dental caries. Nutr. Rev. 23:117, 1965.

_____: Salt supplementation during fasting in the cold. Nutr. Rev. 23:45, 1965.

Robinson, J. B.: Water, the indispensible nutrient. Nutrition Today 5:16, 1970.

Segar, W. E.: Multiple episodes of potassium deficiency. Am. J. Dis. Child. 109:295, 1965.

White, J. M., et al: Sodium ion in drinking water, I, Properties, analysis, and occurrence. J. Am. Dietet. A. 50:32, 1967.

CALCIUM, PHOSPHORUS AND MAGNESIUM
Books and Pamphlets:
FAO/WHO Expert Committee on Calcium Requirements: *Calicum Requirements.* Rome, FAO, 1962.

Hathaway, M. L.: *Magnesium in Human Nutrition.* Home Econ. Res. Report No. 19. Washington, D.C., Agr. Research Service, USDA. 1962.

Swanson, P. P.: *Calcium in Nutrition.* Chicago, National Dairy Council, 1963.

Journal Articles:
Alvarez, W. C.: Osteoporosis, a disease that attacks millions. Geriatrics 25:77, 1970.

Barzel, U. S.: Symposium Report: Osteoporosis: The state of the art. Am. J. Clin. Nutr. 23:833, 1970.

Birge, S. J., Jr., et al: Osteoporosis, intestinal lactase deficiency and low dietary calcium intake. N. Eng. J. Med. 276:445, 1967.

Birge, S. J., Jr., Gilbert, H. R., and Avioli, L. V.: Intestinal calcium transport: the role of sodium. Science 176:168, 1972.

Briscoe, A. and Ragan, C.: Bile and endogenous calcium in man. Am. J. Clin. Nutr. 16:281, 1965.

_____: Effect of magnesium on calcium metabolism in man. Am. J. Clin. Nutr. 19:296, 1966.

Caddell, J. L. and Goddard, D. R.: Studies in protein-calorie malnutrition, I, Chemical evidence for magnesium deficiency. N. Eng. J. Med. 276:533, 1967.

Caniggia, A.: Medical problems in senile osteoporosis. Geriatrics 20:300, 1965.

Copp, D. H.: Endocrine control of calcium metabolism. Physiol. Rev. 32:61, 1970.

Coulston, A. and Lutwak, L.: Dietary calcium deficiency and human periodontal disease. Fed. Proc. 31:721, 1972.

Dunn, M. M. and Walser, M.: Magnesium depletion in normal man. Metabolism 15:884, 1966.

Exton-Smith, A. N.: Osteoporosis. Nutrition 27:116, 1973.

Garn, S. M.: Adult bone loss, fracture epidemiology and nutritional implications. Nutrition 27:107, 1973.

Hankin, J. H., et al: Contributions of hard water to calcium and magnesium intakes of adults. J. Am. Dietet. A. 56:212, 1970.

Harris, I., Wilkinson, A. W.: Magnesium depletion in children. Lancet 7727:745, (October 2) 1971.

Heaney, R. P.: A unified concept of osteoporosis. Am. J. Med. 36:877, 1965.

Hegsted, D. M.: Nutrition, bone and calcified tissue. J. Am. Dietet. A. 50:105, 1967.

———: Present knowledge of calcium, phosphorus and magnesium. Nutr. Rev. 25:65, 1968.

Hersh, T. and Siddiqui, D. A.: Magnesium and the pancreas. Am. J. Clin. Nutr. 26:362, 1973.

Ho, M. L., Farmer, F. A., and Neilson, H. R.: Sodium, potassium and magnesium content of birds, fish and mammals of northern Canada. J. Canad. Diet. A. 33:164, 1972.

Irwin, M. I. and Keinholz, E. W.: Monograph: A conspectus of research on calcium requirements of man. J. Nutrition 103:1019, 1973.

Kenny, A. D. and Dacke, C. G.: Parathyroid hormone and calcium metabolism. World Rev. Dietet. 20:231, 1975.

Krehl, W. A.: Magnesium. Nutrition Today 2:16, (September) 1967.

Latorre, H. and Kenny, T. M.: Experience and Reason— High-dosage intravenous calcium therapy for osteoporosis and osteomalacia in anticonvulsant therapy with hypomobilization. Pediatrics 53:100, 1974.

Lim, P. and Jacob, E.: Magnesium status of alcoholic patients. Metabolism 21:1045, 1972.

Lotz, M.: Evidence for a phosphorus-depletion syndrome in man. N. Eng. J. Med. 278:409, 1968.

Lutwak, L.: Nutritional aspects of osteoporosis. J. Am. Geriatrics Soc. 17:115, 1969.

———: Osteoporosis—a mineral deficiency disease? J. Am. Dietet. A. 44:173, 1964.

Mahan, K.: Does low calcium intake cause osteoporosis? JAMA 218:263, 1971.

Margen, S., et al: Studies in calcium metabolism, I, The calciuretic effect of dietary protein. Am. J. Clin. Nutr. 27:584, 1974.

Massry, S. G., Freidler, R. M., and Coburn, J. W.: Excretion of phosphate and calcium. Arch. Int. Med. 131:885, 1973.

Munson, P. L. and Gray, T. K.: Function of thyrocalcitonin in normal physiology. Fed. Proc. 29:1206, 1970.

Review: Calcium in sweat. Nutr. Rev. 21:13, 1963.

———: Exercise and calcium utilization. Nutr. Rev. 19:42, 1961.

———: Intestinal calcium and bone formation. Nutr. Rev. 23:6, 1965.

———: Human renal calculus formation and magnesium. Nutr. Rev. 24:43, 1966.

———: Phosphate influence on experimental dental caries. Nutr. Rev. 22:311, 1964.

Seelig, M. S.: The requirement of magnesium by the normal adult. Summary and analysis of published data. Am. J. Clin. Nutr. 14:342, 1964.

Seelig, M. S. and Heggtveit, H. A.: Magnesium interrelationships in ischemic heart disease: A review. Am. J. Clin. Nutr. 27:59, 1974.

Socka, C.: Combatting osteoporosis. Am. J. Nurs. 73:1193, (July) 1973.

Stamp, T. C. B.: Rickets and osteomalacis. Nutrition 27:97, 1973.

Sullivan, J. F., et al: Magnesium metabolism in alcoholism. Am. J. Clin. Nutr. 13:297, 1963.

Tanaka, Y., Frank, H., and DeLuca, H. F.: Intestinal calcium transport: stimulation by low phosphorus diet. Science 181:564, 1973.

Tewell, J. E., Clark, H., and Howe, J. M.: Phosphorus balances of adults fed rice, milk and wheat flour mixtures. J. Am. Dietet. A. 63:530, 1973.

Wacker, W. E. and Parisis, A. F.: Magnesium metabolism. N. Eng. J. Med., 278:658, 712, 772, 1968.

Walker, R. M. and Linkswiler, H. M.: Calcium retention in the adult human male as affected by protein intake. J. Nutrition 102:1297, 1972.

IRON AND COPPER

Books and Pamphlets:

Bothwell, T. H. and Finch, C. A.: Iron Metabolism. Boston, Little, Brown, 1962.

Journal Articles:

Anderson, T. A., Kim, I. and Fomon, S. J.: Iron status of anemic rats fed iron-fortified cereal-milk diets. Nutr. Metab. 6:355, 1972.

Ausman, D. C.: Cobalt-iron therapy for iron-deficiency anemia. J. Am. Geriat. Soc. 13:425, 1965.

Bates, G. W., et al: Facilitation of iron absorption by ferric fructose. Am. J. Clin. Nutr. 25:983, 1972.

Bothwell, T. H.: The control of iron absorption. Brit. J. Haematology 14:453, 1968.

Bothwell, T. H., et al: Iron overload in Bantu subjects: studies on the availability of iron in Bantu beer. Am. J. Clin. Nutr. 14:47, 1964.

Butler, L. C. and Daniel, J. M.: Copper metabolism in young women fed two levels of copper and two protein sources. Am. J. Clin. Nutr. 26:744, 1973.

Butterworth, C. E.: Iron undercontamination? JAMA 220:581, 1972.

Callender, S. T.: Iron absorption. Proc. Nutr. Soc. 26:59, 1967.

Callender, S. T. and Warner, G. T.: Iron absorption from bread. Am. J. Clin. Nutr. 21:1170, 1968.

Cartwright, G. E. and Wintrobe, M. M.: Copper metabolism in normal subjects. Am. J. Clin. Nutr. 14:224, 1964.

———: The question of copper deficiency in man. Am. J. Clin. Nutr. 15:94, 1964.

Coltman, C. and Rowe, N.: The iron content of sweat in normal adults. Am. J. Clin. Nutr. 18:270, 1966.

Conrad, M. W.: Iron balance and iron deficiency anemia. Borden's Rev. Nutr. Res. 28 (No. 3):49, (July-September) 1967.

Cook, J. D., et al: Absorption of fortification iron in bread. Am. J. Clin. Nutr. 26:861, 1973.

Council on Foods and Nutrition: Iron in enriched wheat flour, farina, bread, buns, and rolls. JAMA 220:855, 1972.

Council on Foods and Nutrition: Iron deficiency in the U.S. JAMA 203:407, 1968.

Crosby, W. H.: Control of iron absorption by intestinal luminal factor. Am. J. Clin. Nutr. 21:1189, 1968.

_____: Food pica and iron deficiency. Arch. Int. Med. 127:960, 1971.

_____: Intestinal response to the body's requirement for iron: Control of iron absorption. JAMA 208:347, 1969.

Dowdy, R. P.: Copper metabolism. Am. J. Clin. Nutr. 22:887, 1969.

Elwood, P. C., et al: Absorption of iron from bread. Am. J. Clin. Nutr. 21:1162, 1968.

Evans, G. W.: Function and nomenclature for two mammalian copper proteins. Nutr. Rev. 29:195, 1971.

Filer, L. J., Jr.: The United States today: Is it free of public health nutrition problems?—Anemia. Am. J. Public Health 59:327, 1969.

Finch, C. A.: Iron balance in man. Nutr. Rev. 23:129, 1965.

_____: Iron-defiency anemia. Am. J. Clin. Nutr. 22:512, 1969.

_____: Iron metabolism. Nutrition Today 4:2 (Summer), 1969.

Freiman, H. D., et al: Iron absorption in healthy aged. Geriatrics 18:716, 1963.

Frieden, E.: The ferrous to ferric cycles in iron metabolism. Nutr. Rev. 31:41, 1973.

Greenberger, N. J.: Effects of antibiotics and other agents on the intestinal transport of iron. Am. J. Clin. Nutr. 26:104, 1973.

Hambidge, K. M.: Increase in hair copper concentration with increasing distance from the scalp. Am. J. Clin. Nutr. 26:1212, 1973.

Heinrich, H. C.: Iron deficiency without anemia. Lancet 2:460, 1968.

Hook, L. and Brandt, K.: Copper content of some low-copper foods. J. Am. Dietet. A. 49:202, 1966.

Houston, R. G.: Sickle cell anemia and dietary precursors of cyanate. Am. J. Clin. Nutr. 26:1261, 1973.

Jacobs, A. and Greenman, D. A.: Availability of food iron. Brit. Med. J. 1:673, 1969.

Katzman, R., Novack, A., Pearson, A.: Nutritional anemia in an inner-city community. Relationship to ages and ethnic group. JAMA 222:670, 1972.

Layrisse, M., et al: Effect of interaction of various foods on iron absorption. Am. J. Clin. Nutr. 21:1175, 1968.

Monsen, E. R.: The need for iron fortification. J. Nutr. Educa. 2:152, 1971.

Pearson, H. A., et al: Anemia related to age. Study of a community of young black Americans. JAMA 215:1982, 1971.

Peden, J.: Present knowledge of iron and copper. Nutr. Rev. 25:321, 1967.

Pennington, J. T., Calloway, D. H. and Howes, D.: Copper content of foods. Factors affecting reported values. J. Am. Dietet. A. 63:143, 1973.

Peters, T., Jr., Apt, L., and Ross, J. F.: Effect of phosphates upon iron absorption studied in normal human subjects and in an experimental model using dialysis. Gastroenterology 61:315, 1971.

Prockop, D. J.: Role of iron in the synthesis of collagen in connective tissue. Fed. Proc. 30:984, 1971.

Review: Copper deficiency in malnourished infants. Nutr. Rev. 23:164, 1965.

_____: Fortification of bread with iron. Nutr. Rev. 27:138, 1969.

_____: Gastric function and structure in iron deficiency. Nutr. Rev. 24:326, 1966.

_____: Iron absorption. Nutr. Rev. 24:247, 1967.

_____: Iron metabolism in renal failure. Nutr. Rev. 30:110, 1972.

_____: Symptoms of iron deficiency anemia. Nutr. Rev. 25:86, 1967.

_____: The therapeutic effectiveness of various compounds containing iron. Nutr. Rev. 24:232, 1966.

Schaffrin, R. M., et al: The effects of blood donation on serum iron and hemoglobin in young women. Canad. Med. A. J. 104:229, 1971.

Schroeder, H. A., et al: Essential trace metals in man. Copper. J. Chron. Dis. 19:1007, 1966.

Scott, D. E. and Pritchard, J. A.: Iron deficiency in healthy young college women. JAMA 199:897, 1967.

Seelig, M. S.: Proposed role of copper-molybdenum interaction in iron-deficiency and iron-storage diseases. Am. J. Clin. Nutr. 26:657, 1973.

Seelig, M. S.: Review: Relationship of copper and molybdenum to iron metabolism. Am. J. Clin. Nutr. 25:1022, 1972.

Senchak, M. M., Howe, J. M., and Clark, H. E.: Iron absorption by adults fed mixtures of rice, milk and wheat flour. J. Am. Dietet. A. 62:272, 1973.

Sturgeon, P. and Shoden, A.: Total liver storage iron in normal populations of the U.S.A. Am. J. Clin. Nutr. 24:469, 1971.

Todhunter, E. N.: Iron, blood and nutrition. J. Am. Dietet. A. 61:121, 1972.

Van Campen, D.: Regulation of iron absorption. Fed. Proc. 33:100, 1974.

White, H. S.: Iron deficiency in young women. Am. J. Public Health 60:659, 1970.

White, H. S. and Synne, T. M.: Utilization of inorganic elements by young women eating iron-fortified foods. J. Am. Dietet. A. 59:27, 1971.

IODINE

Journal Articles:

Harrison, M. T., et al: Nature and availability of iodine in fish. Am. J. Clin. Nutr. 17:73, 1965.

Kidd, P. S., et al: Sources of dietary iodine. J. Am. Dietet. A. 65:420, 1974.

Kuhajek, E. J. and Fiedelman, H. W.: Nutritional iodine in processed foods. Food Tech. 27:52, 1973.

Lowenstein, F. W.: Iodized salt in the prevention of endemic goiter: a world wide survey of present programs. Am. J. Public Health 57:1815, 1967.

Review: Goiter and iodine deficiency. Nutr. Rev. 22:169, 1964.

Vought, R. L. and London, W. T.: Dietary sources of iodine. Am. J. Clin. Nutr. 14:186, 1964.

OTHER MINERALS

Books:

Gedalia, I. and Zipkin, I.: *The Role of Fluoride in Bone Structure.* St. Louis, Green, 1973.

Mertz, W. and Cornatzer, W. E.: *Newer Trace Elements in Nutrition.* New York, Marcel Dekkar, 1971.

Prasad, A. S.: *Zinc Metabolism.* Springfield, Ill. Thomas, 1966.

Journal Articles:

A new essential trace element—vanadium. JAMA. 222:255, 1972.

Carlisle, E. M.: Silicon as an essential element. Fed. Proc. 33:1758, 1974.

Chatterjee, P., and Gettman, J. H.: Lead poisoning subculture as a facilitating agent. Am. J. Clin. Nutr. 25:324, 1972.

Food and Nutrition Board: Zinc in human nutrition. National Research Council, Washington, D.C., 1970.

Forssen, A.: Inorganic elements in the human body 1. Occurrence of Ba, Br, Ca, Cd, Cu, K, Mn, Ni, Sn, Sr, Y and Zn in the human body. Annales Medicinae Experimentalis et Biologiae Fenniae 50, Fasc. 3:99, 1972.

Glinsman, W. H., et al: Plasma chromium after glucose administration. Science 152:1243, 1966.

Hadjimarkos, D. M. and Shearer, T. R.: Selenium in mature human milk. Am. J. Clin. Nutr. 26:583, 1973.

Hambidge, K. M.: Chromium nutrition in man. Am. J. Clin. Nutr. 27:505, 1974.

Hambidge, H. M. and Baum, J. D.: Hair chromium concentration of human newborns and changes during infancy. Am. J. Clin. Nutr. 25:376, 1972.

Hopkins, L. L., Jr., and Majaj, A. S.: Normalization of impaired glucose utilization and hypoglycemia by Cr (III) in malnourished infants. Fed. Proc. 25:303, 1966.

Klevay, L. M.: Hypercholesterolemia in rats produced by an increase in the ratio of zinc to copper ingested. Am. J. Clin. Nutr. 26:1060, 1973.

Lanier, V. C., Jr., et al: Zinc and wound healing. Am. J. Clin. Nutr. 23:514, 1970.

Leach, R. M.: Role of manganese in mucopolysaccharide metabolism. Fed. Proc. 30:991, 1971.

Luecke, R. W.: The significance of zinc in nutrition. Borden's Rev. Nutr. Res. 20:45, 1965.

Mayer, J.: Zinc deficiency: a cause of growth retardation. Postgrad. Med. 35:206, 1964.

McBean, L. D., et al: Correlation of zinc concentrations in human plasma and hair. Am. J. Clin. Nutr. 24:509, 1971.

Mertz, W.: Effects and metabolism of glucose tolerance factor. Nutr. Rev. 33:129, 1975.

Mertz, W.: Recommended dietary allowances up to date—trace minerals. J. Am. Dietet. A. 64:163, 1974.

Mills, C. F., et al: Metabolic role of zinc. Am. J. Clin. Nutr. 22:1240, 1969.

Murphy, E. W., et al: Provisional tables on the zinc content of foods. J. Am. Dietet. A. 66:345, 1975.

Nielson, F. H.: "Newer" trace elements in human nutrition. Food Tech. 28:38, 1974.

Nielson, F. H. and Sanstead, H. H.: Are nickel, vanadium, silicon, fluorine, and tin essential for man? Am. J. Clin. Nutr. 27:515, 1974.

O'Dell, B. L.: Effect of dietary components upon zinc availability: A review with original data. J. Nutrition 102:653, 1972.

O'Dell, B. L., Burpo, C. E., and Savage, J. E.: Evaluation of zinc availability in foodstuffs of plant and animal origin. J. Nutrition 102:653, 1972.

Reinhold, J. G., et al: Zinc and copper concentrations in hair of Iranian villagers. Am. J. Clin. Nutr. 18:294, 1966.

Review: Relation of zinc metabolism to a syndrome characterized by anemia, dwarfism, and hypogonadism. Nutr. Rev. 21:264, 1963.

————: Manganese balance in children. Nutr. Rev. 23:236, 1965.

————: Studies on selenium. Nutr. Rev. 33:138, 1975.

————: Trivalent chromium in human nutrition. Nutr. Rev. 25:50, 1967.

Sandstead, H. H.: Zinc nutrition in the United States. Am. J. Clin. Nutr. 26:1251, 1973.

Scott, M. L.: The selenium dilemma. J. Nutrition 103:803, 1973.

Schroeder, H. A.: Renal cadmium and essential hypertension. JAMA. 187:358, 1964.

————: Cadmium as a factor in hypertension. J. Chron. Dis. 18:647, 1965.

Stadtman, T. C.: Selenium biochemistry. Science 183:915, 1974.

Sullivan, J. F., and Lankford, H. G.: Zinc metabolism and chronic alcoholism. Am. J. Clin. Nutr. 17:57, 1965.

Trauma leads to loss of body zinc and other metals. JAMA. 222:253, 1972.

Underwood, E. J.: Cobalt. Nutr. Rev. 33:65, 1975.

vitamins

GENERAL

Books and Pamphlets:

Conserving the Nutritive Values in Foods. Home and Garden Bulletin, No. 90. USDA Washington, D.C., U.S. Gov't Print. Off., 1963.

DeLuca, H. G. and Suttie, J. W. (eds.): *The Fat-Soluble Vitamins.* Madison, University of Wisconsin Press, 1970.

Kutsky, R. J.: *Handbook of Vitamins and Hormones.* New York, VanNostrand Reinhold, 1973.

Report of a Joint FAO/WHO Expert Group: *Requirements of Ascorbic Acid, Vitamin D, Vitamin B_{12}, Folate, and Iron.* Rome, FAO, 1967.

Wagner, A. D. and Folkers, K.: *Vitamins and Coenzymes.* New York, Interscience Publishers, 1964.

Journal Articles:

Bieri, J. G.: Effect of excessive vitamin C and E on vitamin A status. Letters. Am. J. Clin. Nutr. 26:382, 1973.

————: Fat-soluble vitamins in the eighth revision of the Recommended Dietary Allowances. J. Am. Dietet. A. 64:171, 1974.

Campbell, J. A., and Morrison, A. B.: Some factors affecting the absorption of vitamins. Am. J. Clin. Nutr. 12:162, 1963.

Consolazio, C. F., et al: Thiamin, riboflavin, and pyridoxine excretion during acute starvation and caloric restriction. Am. J. Clin. Nutr. 24:1060, 1971.

Gershoff, S. N.: Effects of dietary levels of macronutrients on vitamin requirements. Fed. Proc. 23:1077, 1964.

Herbert, V.: The five possible causes of all nutrient deficiency: illustrated by deficiencies of vitamin B_{12} and folic acid. Am. J. Clin. Nutr. 26:77, 1973.

Levy, G., and Hewitt, R. R.: Evidence in man for different specialized intestinal transport mechanisms for riboflavin and thiamine. Am. J. Clin. Nutr. 24:401, 1971.

Mayer, J.: Vitamins and mental disorders. Postgrad. Med. 45:268, 1969.

New Regulations on Vitamins A and D. FDA Consumer, 7:14, (October) 1972.

Review: Lipids and fat-soluble vitamins in cellular metabolism. Nutr. Rev. 24:272, 1966.

Roe, D. A.: Nutrient toxicity with excessive intake, I, Vitamins. N.Y. State J. Med. 66:869, 1966.

Symposium: Advances in the detection of nutrition deficiences in man. Am. J. Clin. Nutr. 20, (June) 1967.

fat-soluble vitamins

VITAMIN A

Pamphlets:

Agency for International Development: *Vitamin A, Xerophthalmia and Blindness: A Status Report in Three Volumes*, I, A Global Survey of Mass Vitamin A Programs, W. W. Kamel; II, Vitamin A Problems with Special Reference to Less Developed Countries, A. G. van Veen and M. S. van Veen; III, Vitamin A Technology, J. C. Bauernfernd. Washington, D.C., Office of Nutrition, Technical Assistance Bureau, Agency for International Development, U.S. Dept. of State, 1973.

Journal Articles:

Ames, S. R.: Factors affecting absorption, transport and storage of vitamin A. Am. J. Clin. Nutr. 22:934, 1969.

Bondi, A., et al: Effect of vitamin A deficiency on some enzymes involved in protein and vitamin A metabolism. Nutr. Metab. 15:246, No. 4-5, 1973.

Canadian Pediatric Society: The use and abuse of vitamin A. Canad. Med. J. 104:521, 1971.

Council on Foods and Nutrition: Fortification of non-fat milk solids with vitamins A and D. JAMA 198:1107, 1966.

DeLuca, L., et al: Maintenance of epithelial cell differentiation: the mode of action of vitamin A. Cancer 30:1326, 1972.

DiBenedetto, R. J.: Chronic hypervitaminosis A in an adult. JAMA 201:130, 1967.

Goodman, D. S.: Biosynthesis of vitamin A from β-carotene. Am. J. Clin. Nutr. 22:963, 1969.

Hughes, J. D. and Wooten, R. L.: The orange people. JAMA 197:730, 1966.

Katz, C. M. and Tzagournis, M.: Chronic adult hypervitaminosis A with hypercalcemia. Metabolism 21:1171, 1972.

Matte, P. J. (Letters): Bear meat and hypervitaminosis A. JAMA 222:835, 1972.

McLaren, D. S.: Nutritional Disease and the Eye. Borden's Rev. Nutr. Res. 25:1, 1964.

————: Xerophthalmia: a neglected problem. Nutr. Rev. 22:289, 1964.

————: Xerophthalmia in Jordan. Am. J. Clin. Nutrition 17:117, 1965.

Muenter, M. D., et al: Chronic vitamin A intoxication in adults. Am. J. Med. 50:129, 1971.

Olson, J. A.: Metabolism and function of vitamin A. Fed. Proc. 28:1670, 1969.

————: Reddy, V. and Srikantia, S. G.: Serum vitamin A in kwashiorkor. Am. J. Clin. Nutr. 18:105, 1966.

Review: An active metabolite of retinoic acid. Nutr. Rev. 24:113, 1966.

————: Etiology of follicular hyperkeratosis. Nutr. Rev. 21:106, 1963.

————: The influence of vitamin A on sulfate and hexosamine metabolism. Nutr. Rev. 24:204, 1966.

————: Interrelationships between vitamins A and E. Nutr. Rev. 23:82, 1965.

————: Intestinal absorption of vitamin A. Nutr. Rev. 22:86, 1964.

————: Toxic reactions of vitamin A. Nutr. Rev. 22:109, 1964.

————: Transport of vitamin A in the lymphatic system. Nutr. Rev. 24:16, 1966.

————: Vitamin A intoxication in infancy. Nutr. Rev. 23:263, 1965.

————: Vitamin A transport in man. Nutr. Rev. 25:199, 1967.

————: Vitamin A and vascularization. Nutr. Rev. 23:248, 1965.

Rodriguez, M. E. and Irwin, M. I.: A conspectus of research on vitamin A requirements in man. J. Nutrition 102:909, 1972.

Roels, O. A.: Present knowledge of vitamin A. Nutr. Rev. 24:129, 1966.

————: Vitamin A and protein metabolism. N.Y. State J. Med. 64:288, 1964.

————: Vitamin A physiology. JAMA 214:1097, 1970.

Underwood, B. A.: The determination of vitamin A and some aspects of its distribution, mobilization and transport in health and disease. World Rev. Nutr. Dietet. 19:123, 1974.

Wolf, G.: International symposium on metabolic function of vitamin A. Am. J. Clin. Nutr. 22:903, 1969.

VITAMIN D

Journal Articles:

Avioli, L. V. and Haddad, J. G.: Vitamin D: Current concepts. Metabolism 22:507, 1973.

Broadfoot, B. V. R., et al: Vitamin D intakes of Canadian children. Canad. Med. A. J. 94:332, 1966.

Committee on Nutrition: The prophylactic requirement and toxicity of vitamin D. Pediatrics 31:512, 1963.

_____: Vitamin D intake and the hypercalcemic syndrome. Pediatrics 35:1022, 1965.

Dale, A. E. and Lowenberg, M. E.: Consumption of vitamin D in fortified and natural foods and in vitamin preparations. J. Pediat. 70:952, 1967.

DeLuca, H. F.: Recent advances in the metabolism and function of vitamin D. Fed. Proc. 28:1678, 1969.

Favus, M. J.: Treatment of vitamin D intoxication. New Eng. J. Med. 283:1468, 1970.

Fomon, S. J., et al: Vitamin D and growth of infants. J. Nutrition 88:345, 1965.

Fraser, D., et al: Pathogenesis of hereditary vitamin-D-dependent rickets. N. Eng. J. Med. 289:817, 1973.

Harrison, H. E.: The disappearance of rickets. Am. J. Public Health 56:734, 1966.

Haussler, M. M.: Vitamin D: Mode of action and biomedical applications. Nutr. Rev. 32:257, 1974.

Hurwitz, S., et al: Role of vitamin D in plasma calcium regulation. Am. J. Physiol. 216:354, 1969.

Kodicek, E.: The story of vitamin D from vitamin to hormone. Lancet 1:325, 1974.

Lawson, D. E. M.: Metabolites of vitamin D. Nutrition 27:79, 1973.

Medlinsky, H. L.: Rickets associated with anticonvulsant medication. Pediatrics 53:91, 1974.

New ideas on vitamin D. Brit. Med. J. 1:629, (March 17) 1973.

Nichols, B. L., et al: Nutritional rickets among indigent children in Houston. Texas Med. 66:74, 1970.

Norman, A. W.: Problems relating to the definition of an International Unit for vitamin D and its metabolites. J. Nutrition 102:1243, 1972.

Omdahl, J. L. and DeLuca, H. F.: Regulation of vitamin D metabolism and function. Physiol. Rev. 53:327, 1973.

Palmisano, P. A.: Vitamin D: a reawakening. JAMA 224:1526, (June 11) 1973.

Paterson, C. R.: The causes of vitamin D deficiency. Nutrition 27:90, 1973.

Review: Effect of vitamin A on vitamin D toxicity. Nutr. Rev. 20:315, 1962.

_____: Nutritional rickets and parathyroid function. Nutr. Rev. 21:271, 1963.

_____: Safe levels of vitamin D intake for infants. Nutr. Rev. 24:230, 1966.

_____: Serum transport of vitamin D. Nutr. Rev. 24:149, 1966.

_____: Vitamin D and protein synthesis. Nutr. Rev. 24:18, 1966.

Seelig, M. S.: Vitamin D and cardiovascular renal and brain damage in infancy and childhood. Ann. N.Y. Acad. Sci. 147:537, 1969.

Special Report: Hazards of overdose of vitamin D. Nutr. Rev. 33:61, 1975.

Taylor, A. N. and Wasserman, R. H.: Correlations between vitamin D-induced calcium binding protein and intestinal absorption of calcium. Fed. Proc. 28:1834, 1969.

VITAMIN E

Journal Articles:

Bieri, J. G.: Vitamin E. Nutr. Rev. 33:161, 1975.

Bieri, J. G. and Evarts, R. P.: The recommended allowance for vitamin E: Tocopherols and fatty acids in American diets. J. Am. Dietet. A. 62:147, 1973.

_____: Vitamin E adequacy of vegetable oils. J. Am. Dietet. A. 66:134, 1975.

Bunnell, R. H., et al: Alpha-tocopherol content of foods. Am. J. Clin. Nutr. 17:1, 1965.

Committee on Nutrition: Vitamin E in human nutrition. Pediatrics 31:324, 1963.

Christiansen, M. M. and Wilcox, E. B.: Dietary polyunsaturates and serum alpha-tocopherol in adults. J. Am. Dietet. A. 63:138, 1973.

Davis, K.: Vitamin E, adequacy of infants' diets. Am. J. Clin. Nutr. 25:933, 1972.

Draper, H. H. and Callany, A. S.: Metabolism and function of vitamin E. Fed. Proc. 28:1690, 1969.

Green, J. and Bunyan, J.: Vitamin E and the biological antioxidant theory. Nutr. Abst. Rev. 39:321, 1969.

Gross, S. and Guilford, M. V.: Vitamin E-lipid relationships in premature infants. J. Nutrition 100:1099, 1970.

Herting, D. C.: Perspective on Vitamin E. Am. J. Clin. Nutr. 19:210, 1966.

Herting, D. C. and Drury, E. E.: Plasma tocopherol levels in man. Am. J. Clin. Nutr. 17:351, 1965.

Horwitt, M. K.: Role of vitamin E, selenium, and polyunsaturated fatty acids in clinical and experimental muscle disease. Fed. Proc. 24:68, 1964.

Kelleher, J. and Losowsky, M. S.: The absorption of α-tocopherol in man. Brit. J. Nutr. 24:1033, 1970.

Leonard, P. J. and Losowsky, M. S.: Effect of alpha-tocopherol administration on red cell survival in vitamin E-deficient human subjects. Am. J. Clin. Nutr. 24:388, 1971.

Nair, P. P.: Vitamin E and metabolic regulation. Ann. N.Y. Acad. Sci. 203:53, 1972.

Olson, R. E.: Vitamin E and its relation to heart disease. Circulation 48:179, 1973.

Review: Antioxidant replacements for vitamin E. Nutr. Rev. 19:217, 1961.

_____: Erythrocyte hemolysis, lipid peroxidation, and vitamin E. Nutr. Rev. 20:60, 1962.

_____: Interrelationships between vitamins A and E. Nutr. Rev. 23:82, 1965.

_____: Metabolic role of vitamin E. Nutr. Rev. 23:90, 1965.

_____: Vitamin E and amino acid transport. Nutr. Rev. 24:203, 1966.

_____: Vitamin E status of adults on a vegetable oil diet. Nutr. Rev. 24:41, 1966.

Roels, O. A.: Present knowledge of vitamin E. Nutr. Rev. 25:33, 1967.

Supplementation of human diets with vitamin E. Nutr. Rev. 30:327, 1973.

Tappel, A. L.: Vitamin E and free radical peroxidation in lipids. Ann. N.Y. Acad. Sci. 203:12, 1972.

————: Will antioxidant nutrients slow aging processes? Geriatrics 23:97, 1968.

Vitamin E—miracle or myth. FDA consumer 7:24, 1973.

Witting, L. A.: Recommended dietary allowance for vitamin E. Am. J. Clin. Nutr. 25:257, 1972.

VITAMIN K
Journal Articles:

Aballi, A. J.: The action of vitamin K in the neonatal period. Southern Med. J. 58:1, 48, 1965.

Committee on Nutrition: Vitamin K compounds and the water soluble analogues. Pediatrics 28:501, 1961.

Duello, T. J. and Matschiner, J. T.: Characterization of vitamin K from human liver. J. Nutrition 102:331, 1972.

Goldman, H. I. and Amades, P.: Vitamin K deficiency after the newborn period. Pediatrics 44:745, 1969.

Johnson, B. C.: Dietary factors and vitamin K. Nutr. Rev. 22:225, 1964.

Nammacher, M. A., et al: Vitamin K deficiency in infants beyond the neonatal period. J. Pediat. 76:549, 1970.

Shoshkes, M., et al: Vitamin K₁ in neonatal hypoprothrombinemia. J. Am. Dietet. A. 38:380, 1961.

Suttie, J. W.: Control of clotting factor biosynthesis by vitamin K. Fed. Proc. 28:1696, 1969.

————: Vitamin K and prothrombin synthesis. Nutr. Rev. 31:105, 1973.

Wefring, K. W.: Hemorrhage in the newborn and vitamin K prophylaxis. J. Pediat. 63:663, 1963.

water-soluble vitamins

ASCORBIC ACID
Journal Articles:

Anderson, B. G.: Eye the potato for vitamin C. School Foodservice J. 26:58, 1972.

Anderson, T. W., Reid, D. B., and Beaton, G. H.: Vitamin C and the common cold: a double-blind trial. Canad. Med. A. J. 107:503, 1972.

Baker, E. M.: Vitamin C requirements in stress. Am. J. Clin. Nutr. 20:583, 1967.

Coulihan, J. L., et al: Vitamin C prophylaxis in a boarding school. N. Eng. J. Med. 290:6, 1974.

Croft, L. K., Davis, R. K., and Rose, M. E.: Ascorbic acid status of the drug addict patient. Am. J. Clin. Nutr. 26:1042, 1973.

Grewar, D.: Infantile scurvy. Clin. Pediat. 4:82, 1965.

Hodges, R. E., et al: Clinical manifestations of ascorbic acid deficiency in man. Am. J. Clin. Nutr. 24:423, 1971.

King, C. G.: Practical and novel advances in relation to vitamin C. J. Nutr. Educa. 1:19, 1969.

————: Present knowledge of ascorbic acid. Nutr. Rev. 26:33, 1968.

Kinsman, R. A. and Hood, J.: Some behavioral effects of ascorbic acid deficiency. Am. J. Clin. Nutr. 24:455, 1971.

Lamden, M.: Dangers of massive vitamin C intake. (Correspondence.) N. Eng. J. Med. 284:336, 1971.

Lopez, A., et al: Influence of time and temperature on ascorbic acid stability. J. Am. Dietet. A. 50:308, 1967.

McLeroy, V. J. and Schendel, H. E.: Influence of oral contraceptives on ascorbic acid concentrations in healthy, sexually mature women. Am. J. Clin. Nutr. 26:191, 1973.

Merrill, A. L.: Facts behind the figures—citrus fruit values in "Handbook No. 8," revised. J. Am. Dietet. A. 44:264, 1964.

Noble, I.: Ascorbic acid and color of vegetables. Effect of length of cooking. J. Am. Dietet. A. 50:304, 1967.

Pantos, C. E. and Markakis, P.: Ascorbic acid content of artificially ripened tomatoes. J. Food Science 38:550, 1973.

Pelletier, O.: Vitamin C status of cigarette smokers and nonsmokers. Am. J. Clin. Nutr. 23:520, 1970.

Review: Ascorbic acid and the common cold. Nutr. Rev. 25:288, 1967.

Rivers, J. M.: Ascorbic acid metabolism of connective tissue. N.Y. State J. Med. 65:1235, 1965.

Rivers, J. M. and Devine, M. M.: Plasma ascorbic acid concentrations and oral contraceptives. Am. J. Clin. Nutr. 25:684, 1972.

Schwartz, F. W.: Ascorbic acid in wound healing—a review. J. Am. Dietet. A. 56:497, 1970.

Sherloch, P. and Rothschild, E. O.: Scurvy produced by a Zen macrobiotic diet. JAMA 199:794, 1967.

THIAMINE
Journal Articles:

Dreyfus, P. M.: Thiamine deficiency and the central nervous system, a review of pathophysiological concepts. J. Vitaminol. 15:335, 1969.

McIntyre, S.: Cardiac beriberi: Two modes of presentation. Brit. Med. J. 5774:567, 1971.

Noble, L. I.: Thiamine and riboflavin retention in braised meat. J. Am. Dietet. A. 47:205, 1965.

————: Reversible inactivation of thiaminase I by thiamine. Nutr. Rev. 32:22, 1974.

Review: Carbohydrates and thiamine synthesis. Nutr. Rev. 20:216, 1962.

Rogers, E. F.: Thiamine antagonists. Ann. N.Y. Acad. Sci. 98:412, 1962.

Sebrell, W. H.: A clinical evaluation of thiamine deficiency. Ann. N.Y. Acad. Sci. 98:563, 1962.

Wurst, H. M.: The history of thiamine. Ann. N.Y. Acad. Sci. 98:385, 1962.

Ziporin, Z. Z., et al: Excretion of thiamine and its metabolites in the urine of young adult males receiving restricted intakes of the vitamins. J. Nutrition 85:287, 1965.

————: Thiamine requirement in the adult human as measured by urinary excretion of thiamine metabolites. J. Nutrition 85:297, 1965.

RIBOFLAVIN
Journal Articles:

Horwitt, M. K.: Nutritional requirements of man, with special reference to riboflavin. Am. J. Clin. Nutr. 18:458, 1966.

Jusko, W. J., Levy, G., and Yaffe, S. J.: Effect of age on intestinal absorption of riboflavin in humans. J. Pharm. Sci. 59:487, 1970.

Lane, M. and Alfrey, C. P.: The anemia of human riboflavin deficiency. Blood 25:432, 1970.

McCormick, D. B.: The fate of riboflavin in the mammal. Nutr. Rev. 30:75, 1972.

Review: Genetic differences in riboflavin utilization. Nutr. Rev. 22:273, 1964.

_____: Riboflavin coenzymes and congenital malformations. Nutr. Rev. 21:24, 1963.

Revlin, R. D.: Riboflavin metabolism. N. Eng. J. Med. 13:626, 1970.

Sterner, R. T. and Price, W. R.: Restricted riboflavin: within subject behavioural effects in humans. Am. J. Clin. Nutr. 26:150, 1973.

Tillotson, J. A. and Baker, E. M.: An enzymatic measurement of the riboflavin status in man. Am. J. Clin. Nutr. 25:425, 1972.

Windmueller, H. G., et al: Elevated riboflavin levels in urine of fasting human subjects. Am. J. Clin. Nutr. 15:73, 1964.

NIACIN

Books:

Roe, D. A.: *A Plague of Corn. The Social History of Pellagra*. Ithaca, New York, Cornell Univ. Press, 1973.

Journal Articles:

DeLange, D. J. and Joubert, C. P.: Assessment of nicotinic acid status of population groups. Am. J. Clin. Nutr. 15:169, 1964.

Dietrich, L. S.: Regulation of nicotinamide metabolism. Am. J. Clin. Nutr. 24:800, 1971.

Goldsmith, G. A.: Niacin-antipellagra factor, hypercholesterolemic agent. JAMA 194:167, 1965.

Horwitt, M. K.: Niacin—tryptophan requirements of man, in terms of niacin equivalents. J. Am. Dietet. A. 34:914, 1958.

Nakagawa, I., et al: Efficiency of conversion of trytophan to niacin in humans. J. Nutrition 103:1195, 1973.

Review: Bound niacin. Nutr. Rev. 19:240, 1961.

_____: Fetal death from nicotinamide deficiency. Nutr. Rev. 23:58, 1964.

_____: Nicotinic acid and diabetes mellitus. Nutr. Rev. 22:166, 1964.

PYRIDOXINE
VITAMIN B_6

Journal Articles:

Baker, E. M., et al: Vitamin B_6 requirement for adult man. Am. J. Clin. Nutr. 15:59, 1964.

Bunnell, R. H.: Vitamin B_6. Science 146:674, 1964.

Cinnamon, A. D. and Beaton, J. R.: Biochemical assessment of vitamin B_6 status in man. Am. J. Clin. Nutr. 23:696, 1970.

Committee on Nutrition, American Academy of Pediatrics: Vitamin B_6 requirements in man. Pediatrics 38:75, 1966.

Coursin, D. B.: Vitamin B_6 requirements. JAMA 189:27, 1964.

Donald, E. A., et al: Vitamin B_6 requirement of young adult women. Am. J. Clin. Nutr. 24:1028, 1971.

Engler, P. P. and Bowers, J. A.: Vitamin B_6 in reheated, held, and freshly cooked turkey breast. J. Am. Dietet. A. 67:42, 1975.

Linkswiler, H.: Biochemical and physiological changes in vitamin B_6 deficiency. Am. J. Clin. Nutr. 20:547, 1967.

Mudd, S. H.: Pyridoxine-responsive genetic disease. Fed. Proc. 30:970, 1971.

Nelson, E. M.: Association of vitamin B_6 deficiency with convulsions in infants. Public Health Rep. 71:445, 1956.

Polansky, M. M. and Murphy, E. W.: Vitamin B_6 in fruits and nuts. J. Am. Dietet. A. 48:109, 1966.

Review: Control of enzyme levels in vitamin deficiency. Nutr. Rev. 30:232, 1972.

_____: Conversion of vitamin B_6 compounds in human red blood cells. Nutr. Rev. 30:119, 1972.

_____: Effects of insulin on carbohydrate and fat metabolism in vitamin B_6 deficiency. Nutr. Rev. 22:314, 1964.

_____: Oral contraceptives and vitamin B_6. Nutr. Rev. 31:49, 1973.

_____: Pyridoxine and dental caries; human studies. Nutr. Rev. 21:143, 1963.

_____: Pyridoxine dependency. Nutr. Rev. 25:72, 1967.

_____: Vitamin B_6 deficiency and tryptophan metabolism. Nutr. Rev. 21:89, 1963.

_____: Vitamin B_6 dependency state in infants. Nutr. Rev. 19:229, 1961.

Rose, D. P., et al: Erythrocyte aminotransferase activities in women using oral contraceptives and the effect of vitamin B_6 supplementation. Am. J. Clin. Nutr. 26:48, 1973.

Sauberlich, H. E.: Human requirements for vitamin B_6. Vitamins Hormones 22:807, 1964.

Trimpter, G. W., et al: Vitamin B_6 dependency syndromes: new horizons in nutrition. Am. J. Clin. Nutr. 22:794, 1969.

FOLACIN—FOLIC ACID

Journal Articles:

Bernstein, L. H., et al: The absorption and malabsorption of folic acid and its polyglutamates. Am. J. Med. 48:570, 1970.

Chung, A. S., et al: Folic acid, vitamin B_6, pantothenic acid, and vitamin B_{12} in human dietaries. Am. J. Clin. Nutr. 9:573, 1961.

Dong, F. M., Oace, S. M.: Folate distribution in fruit juices. J. Am. Dietet. A. 62:162, 1973.

Girdwood, R. H.: Nutritional folate deficiency in the United Kingdom. Scott. Med. J. 14:296, 1969.

Grossowicz, N., Rachmilewitz, M., and Izak, G.: Absorption of pteroylglutamate and dietary folates in man. Am. J. Clin. Nutr. 25:1135, 1972.

Herbert, V.: Studies of folate deficiency in man. Proc. Roy. Soc. Med. 57:377, 1964.

_____: Folic acid. Ann. Rev. Med. 16:359, 1965.

Hoppner, K., Lampi, B., and Perrin, D. E.: Folacin activity of frozen convenience foods. J. Am. Dietet. A. 63:536, 1973.

———: The free and total folate activity in foods available on the Canadian market. Can. Inst. Food. Tech. J. 5:60, 1972.

Kane, F. J. and Lipton, M.: Folic acid and mental illness. Southern Med. J. 63:603, 1970.

Klipstein, F. A. and Lindenbaum, J.: Folate deficiency in chronic liver disease. Blood 25:443, 1965.

Review: Folacin activity in U.S. diets. Nutr. Rev. 22:142, 1964.

———: Folic acid restriction and cancer inhibition. Nutr. Rev. 21:82, 1963.

Rose, J. A.: Folic acid deficiency as a cause of angular cheilosis. Lancet 7722:453, 1971.

Steinberg, D. (letters): Folic acid deficiency: early onset of megaloblastosis. JAMA 222:490, 1972.

Streiff, R. R.: Folate deficiency and oral contraceptives. JAMA 214:105, 1970.

Velez, H., et al: Folic acid deficiency secondary to iron deficiency in man. Am. J. Clin. Nutr. 19:27, 1966.

Vilter, R. W., et al: Interrelationships of vitamin B_{12}, folic acid and ascorbic acid in the megaloblastic anemias. Am. J. Clin. Nutr. 12:130, 1963.

Vitale, J. J.: Present knowledge of folacin: Nutr. Rev. 24:289, 1966.

Wadsworth, G. R.: Some historical aspects of knowledge about folate deficiency. Nutrition 27:17, 1973.

VITAMIN B_{12}

Journal Articles:

Discovery and synthesis of vitamin B_{12} celebrated. Nutrition Today 8:24, (January, February) 1973.

Ellis, F. R. and Nasser, S.: A pilot study of vitamin B_{12} in the treatment of tiredness. Brit. J. Nutr. 30:277, 1973.

Halsted, C. H.: The small intestine in vitamin B_{12} and folate deficiency. Nutr. Rev. 33:33, 1975.

Hart, R. J., Jr., McCurdy, P. R.: Psychosis in vitamin B_{12} deficiency. Arch. Int. Med. 128:596, 1971.

Herbert, V. and Castle, W. B.: Intrinsic factor. N. Eng. J. Med. 270:1181, 1964.

Herbert, V.: Nutritional requirements for vitamin B_{12} absorption and folic acid. Am. J. Clin. Nutr. 21:743, 1968.

MacKenzie, I. L., and Donaldson, R. M.: Vitamin B_{12} absorption and the intestinal cell surface. Fed. Proc. 28:41, 1969.

Maugh, T. H.: Vitamin B_{12}: after 25 years, the first synthesis. Science 179:266, 1973.

Miller, D. R., et al: Juvenile "congenital" pernicious anemia. N. Eng. J. Med. 275:978, 1966.

Rare forms of familial vitamin B_{12} malabsorption in children. Nutr. Rev. 31:149, 1973.

Review: B_{12} transport in red cell membranes. Nutr. Rev. 25:248, 1967.

———: Oral B_{12} therapy of pernicious anemia. Nutr. Rev. 22:10, 1964.

———: Vitamin B_{12} deficiency in vegetarians. Nutr. Rev. 14:73, 1956.

Rivera, J. V., et al: Anemia due to vitamin B_{12} deficiency after treatment with folic acid in tropical sprue. Am. J. Clin. Nutr. 18:110, 1966.

Spray, G. H.: Absorption of vitamin B_{12} from the intestines. Proc. Nutr. Soc. 26:55, 1967.

Stadtman, T. C.: Vitamin B_{12}. Science 171:859, 1971.

Sullivan, L. W. and Herbert, V.: Studies on the minimum daily requirements for vitamin B_{12}. N. Eng. J. Med. 272:340, 1965.

Toskes, P. P. and Deren, J. J.: Vitamin B_{12} absorption and malabsorption. Gastroenterology 65:662, 1973.

Wilson, T. H.: Intrinsic factor and B_{12} absorption—a problem in cell physiology. Nutr. Rev. 23:33, 1965.

BIOTIN

Journal Articles:

Bridgers, W. F.: Present knowledge of biotin. Nutr. Rev. 25:65, 1967.

McCormick, D. B.: Biotin. Nutr. Rev. 33:97, 1975.

Ochoa, S. and Kaziro, Y.: Biotin enzymes. Fed. Proc. 20:982, 1961.

Review: Mechanism of action of biotin-enzymes. Nutr. Rev. 21:310, 1963.

———: The role of biotin in lipid metabolism. Nutr. Rev. 20:143, 1962.

PANTOTHENIC ACID

Pamphlet:

Zook, E. G., et al: *Pantothenic acid in foods*. Agr. Handbook No. 97. Washington, D.C., USDA, 1956.

Journal Articles:

Faber, S. R., et al: The effects of an induced pyridoxine and pantothenic acid deficiency on excretions of oxalic and xanthurenic acids in the urine. Am. J. Clin. Nutr. 12:406, 1963.

Ishiguro, K.: Studies on pantothenic acid and age. J. Am. Dietet. A. 40:450, 1962.

Review: Relation of pantothenic acid to adrenal cortical function. Nutr. Rev. 19:79, 1966.

energy

Books and Pamphlets:

FAO/WHO: *Energy and protein requirements*. WHO Tech. Rep. Ser. No. 522, Geneva, 1973.

Richardson, M., and McCracken, E. C.: *Energy Expenditures of Women Performing Selected Activities*. Home Econ. Res. Report No. 11. Washington, D.C., Agr. Research Service, 1960.

Sargent, D. W.: *An Evaluation of Basal Metabolic Data for Children and Youth in the United States*. Home Econ. Res. Report No. 14. Washington, D.C., Agr. Research Service, 1961.

———: *An Evaluation of Basal Metabolic Data for Infants in the United States*. Home Econ. Res. Report No. 18. Washington, D.C., Agr. Research Service, 1962.

Journal Articles:

Ashworth, A.: Malnutrition and metabolic rates. Nutr. Rev. 28:279, 1970.

Bell, F. B.: Hypothalamic control of food intake. Proc. Nutr. Soc. 30:103, 1971.

Bradfield, R. B.: A technique for determination of usual daily energy expenditure in the field. Am. J. Clin. Nutr. 24:1148, 1971.

Bradford, R. B. and Jourdain, M. H.: Relative importance of specific dynamic action in weight-reduction diets. Lancet (September 22):640, 1973.

Buskirk, E. R., et al: Comparison of two assessments of physical activity and a survey method for caloric intake. Am. J. Clin. Nutr. 24:1119, 1971.

Buskirk, E. R., et al: Human energy expenditure studies in the National Institute of Arthritis and Metabolic Disease. I. Interaction of cold environment and special dynamic effect. II. Sleep. Am. J. Clin. Nutr. 8:602, 1960.

Call, D. L.: An examination of calorie availability and consumption in the United States, 1909-1963. Am. J. Clin. Nutr. 16:374, 1965.

Clark, R. G.: Caloric requirements after operation. Proc. Nutr. Soc. 30:158, 1971.

Consolazio, C. F., et al: Body weight, heart rate, and ventilatory volume relationships to oxygen uptakes. Am. J. Clin. Nutr. 24:1180, 1971.

Durnin, J. V.: Energy-requirements intake and balance. Proc. Nutr. Soc. 27:188, 1968.

Haisman, M. F.: Energy expenditure of soldiers in a warm humid climate. Brit. J. Nutr. 27:375, 1972.

Hamilton, C. L.: Physiologic control of food intake. J. Am. Dietet. A. 62:35, 1973.

Havel, R. J.: Caloric homeostasis and disorders of fuel transport. N. Eng. J. Med. 287:1186, 1972.

Hawkins, W. W.: The calorie, the joule. J. Nutrition 102:1553, 1972.

Hegsted, D. M.: Energy needs and energy utilization. Nutr. Rev. 32:33, 1974.

Hervey, G. R.: Physiological mechanisms for the regulation of energy balance. Proc. Nutr. Soc. 30:109, 1971.

Hunscher, H. A.: Pertinent factors in interpreting metabolic data. J. Am. Dietet. A. 39:209, 1961.

Johnson, O. C.: Present knowledge of calories. Nutr. Rev. 25:257, 1967.

Kleiber, M.: Joules vs. Calories in nutrition. J. Nutrition 102:309, 1972.

Konishi, F.: Food energy equivalents of various activities. J. Am. Dietet. A. 46:186, 1965.

Margaria, R.: The sources of muscular energy. Sci. Amer. 226 (3):84, 1972.

Mason, E. D., et al: Racial group differences in basal metabolism and body composition of Indian and European women in Bombay. Human Biol. 26:374, 1964.

Maxfield, M. E.: The indirect measurement of energy expenditure in industrial situations. Am. J. Clin. Nutr. 24:1126, 1971.

Mayer, J.: Why people get hungry. Nutrition Today 1:2, 1966.

McCance, R. A.: The composition of the body: Its maintenance and regulation. Nutr. Abstr. Rev. 42:1269, 1972.

Montoye, H. J.: Estimation of habitual physical activity by questionnaire and interview. Am. J. Clin. Nutr. 24:1113, 1971.

Passmore, R.: The regulation of body-weight in man. Proc. Nutr. Soc. 30:122, 1971.

Payne, P. R., Wheeler, E. F., and Salvosa, C. B.: Prediction of daily energy expenditure from average pulse rate. Am. J. Clin. Nutr. 24:1164, 1971.

Review: Body fat in adolescent boys. Nutr. Rev. 22:72, 1964.

————: Diet, exercise, and endurance. Nutr. Rev. 30:86, 1972.

————: Diet and work metabolism. Nutr. Rev. 21:211, 1963.

————: Eating at various times before exercise. Nutr. Rev. 21:40, 1963.

Sasaki, T.: Relation of basal metabolism to changes in food composition and body composition. Fed. Proc. 25(2):1165, 1966.

Southgate, D. A. T.: Assessing the energy value of the human diet. Nutr. Rev. 29:131, 1971.

Weaver, E. I. and Elliot, D. E.: Factors affecting energy expended in home-making tasks. J. Am. Dietet. A. 39:205, 1961.

Wiepkema, P. R.: Behavioural factors in the regulation of food intake. Proc. Nutr. Soc. 30:142, 1971.

Wilmore, J. H. and Haskell, W. L.: Use of the heart rate-energy relationship in the individualized prescription of exercise. Am. J. Clin. Nutr. 24:1186, 1971.

Yoshimura, M., et al: Climatic adaptation of basal metabolism. Fed. Proc. 25(2):1169, 1966.

nutrient utilization: digestion, absorption, and metabolism

Books:

Davenport, H. W.: *Physiology of the Digestive Tract*, ed. 2. Chicago, Yearbook Medical Publishers, 1966.

Wilson, T. H.: *Intestinal Absorption*. Philadelphia, Saunders, 1962.

Wiseman, G.: *Absorption from the Intestine*. New York, Academic Press, 1964.

Journal Articles:

Adelson, J. W. and Rothman, S. S.: Selective pancreatic enzyme secretion due to a new peptide called chymodenin. Science 183:1087, 1974.

Andersson, S.: Secretion of gastrointestinal hormones. Ann. Rev. Physiol. 35:431, 1973.

Babka, J. C. and Castell, D. O.: On the genesis of heartburn. The effects of specific foods on the lower esophageal sphincter. Am. J. Digestive Diseases 18:391, 1973.

Bayless, T. M. and Huang, S.: Inadequate intestinal digestion of lactose. Am. J. Clin. Nutr. 22:250, 1969.

Bell, R. R., Draper, H. H., and Bergan, J. G.: Sucrose, lactose, and glucose tolerance in northern Alaskan Eskimos. Am. J. Clin. Nutr. 26:1185, 1973.

Bergstrom, B.: Absorption of fats. Proc. Nutr. Soc. 26:34, 1967.

Bernstein, L. and Herbert, V.: The role of pancreatic exocrine secretions in the absorption of vitamin B_{12} and iron. Am. J. Clin. Nutr. 26:340, 1973.

Bortz, W. M.: On control of cholesterol synthesis. Metabolism 22:1507, 1973.

Bowie, M. D., et al: Carbohydrate absorption in malnourished children. Am. J. Clin. Nutr. 20:89, 1967.

Brown, R. R.: Biochemistry and pathology of tryptophan metabolism and its regulation by amino acids, vitamin B_6 and steroid hormones. Am. J. Clin. Nutr. 24:243, 1971.

Brown, W. D.: Present knowledge of protein nutrition, Part 3. Postgrad. Med. 41(A):119, 1967.

Christensen, H. M.: Transport of amino acids. Nutr. Rev. 21:97, 1963.

Cohen, M., et al: Lipolytic activity of human gastric and duodenal juice against medium and long chain triglycerides. Gastroenterology 60:1, 1971.

Cornblath, M., et al (eds.): Carbohydrate and energy metabolism in the newborn—an international exploration. Pediatrics 39:582, 1967.

Crane, R. K.: A perspective of digestive-absorptive function. Am. J. Clin. Nutr. 22:242, 1969.

Davenport, H. W.: Why the stomach does not digest itself. Sci. Amer. 226(1):86, 1972.

Dahlqvist, A.: Disaccharide intolerance. JAMA 195:38, 1966.

————: Localization of the small-intestinal disaccharidases. Am. J. Clin. Nutr. 20:81, 1967.

Danielsson, H.: Influence of bile acids on digestion and absorption of lipids. Am. J. Clin. Nutr. 12:214, 1963.

Dill, J. E., et al: Lactase deficiency in Mexican-American males. Am. J. Clin. Nutr. 25:869, 1972.

Duncan, I. W. and Scott, E.: Lactose intolerance in Alaskan Indians and Eskimos. Am. J. Clin. Nutr. 25:867, 1972.

Exton, J. H.: Gluconeogenesis. Metabolism 21:945, 1972.

Fisher, R. B.: Absorption of proteins. Proc. Nutr. Soc. 26:23, 1967.

Gardner, J. D., et al: Columnar epithelial cell of the small intestine: digestion and transport. N. Eng. J. Med. 283:1196, 1264, 1970.

Gaylor, J. L.: Inhibition and cholesterol biosynthesis. N.Y. State J. Med. 66:1097, 1966.

Go, V. L. W., and Summerskill, W. H. J.: Digestion, maldigestion and the intestinal hormones. Am. J. Clin. Nutr. 24:160, 1971.

Gray, G. M.: Drugs, malnutrition and carbohydrate absorption. Am. J. Clin. Nutr. 26:121, 1973.

Haenel, H.: Human normal and abnormal gastrointestinal flora. Am. J. Clin. Nutr. 23:1433, 1970.

Herman, R. H.: Mannose metabolism, I, II. Am. J. Clin. Nutr. 24:488, 566, 1971.

Herskovic, T.: Protein malnutrition and the small intestine. Am. J. Clin. Nutr. 22:300, 1969.

Ingelfinger, F. J.: Gastrointestinal absorption. Nutrition Today 2:2, (March) 1967.

————: How to swallow, and belch and cope with heartburn. Nutrition Today 8:4, (January-February) 1973.

————: For want of an enzyme. Nutrition Today, 3:2, (September) 1968.

————: Gastric function. Nutrition Today 6:2, (September-October) 1971.

Isselbacher, K. J.: Metabolism and transport of lipids by intestinal mucosa. Fed. Proc. 24:16, 1965.

Jacobs, F. A.: Dietary amino acid transport via lymph. Fed. Proc. 26:302, 1967.

Johnson, L. R. and Grossman, M. L.: Intestinal hormones as inhibitors of gastric secretion. Gastroenterology 60:120, 1971.

Jukes, T. H.: Present status of the amino acid code. J. Am. Dietet. A. 45:517, 1964.

Kenworthy, R.: Influence of bacteria on absorption from the small intestine. Proc. Nutr. Soc. 26:27, 1967.

Kurtzman, N. A. and Pellay, V. K. G.: Renal reabsorption of glucose in health and disease. Arch. Int. Med. 131:901, 1973.

Lepkovsky, S.: Newer concepts in the regulation of food intake. Am. J. Clin. Nutr. 26:271, 1973.

Mansford, R. L.: Recent studies on carbohydrate absorption. Proc. Nutr. Soc. 26:27, 1967.

Mao, C. C. and Jacobson, E. D.: Intestinal absorption and blood flow. Am. J. Clin. Nutr. 23:820, 1970.

Mayer, J.: Why people get hungry. Nutrition Today 1:2 (June), 1966.

Nasset, E. S.: Role of digestive system in protein metabolism. Fed. Proc. 24:953, 1965.

Newey, H. and Smyth, D. H.: Assessment of absorptive capacity. Proc. Nutr. Soc. 26:5, 1967.

Oomen, H. A. P. C.: Interrelationship of the human intestinal flora and protein utilization. Proc. Nutr. Soc. 29:197, 1970.

Raisz, L. G.: Some drugs we would like to have in nutrition and metabolism. Am. J. Clin. Nutr. 26:125, 1973.

Review: Amino acid transport and insulin release. Nutr. Rev. 25:41, 1964.

————: Diarrhea caused by disaccharidase deficiency. Nutr. Rev. 22:43, 1964.

————: Effect of dietary protein on proteolytic enzymes. Nutr. Rev. 22:317, 1964.

————: Factors affecting amino acid absorption. Nutr. Rev. 24:332, 1966.

————: Medium chain triglycerides in tropical sprue. Nutr. Rev. 23:71, 1965.

————: Metabolic interrelationships of dietary carbohydrate and fat. Nutr. Rev. 22:216, 1964.

————: Mobilization of liver lipids by specific plasma proteins. Nutr. Rev. 24:87, 1966.

————: Nutritional state and hormonal regulation of liver enzymes. Nutr. Rev. 24:308, 1966.

————: Regulation of gluconeogenesis. Nutr. Rev. 24:347, 1966.

————: Sucrose intolerance: An enzymatic defect. Nutr. Rev. 23:101, 1965.

————: The effect of pectin on cholesterol absorption. Nutr. Rev. 24:209, 1966.

_____: Transport of amino acids. Nutr. Rev. 21:97, 1963.

Rohrer, G. V.: Human gastric mucosa: correlation of structure and function. Am. J. Clin. Nutr. 24:137, 1971.

Rosenweig, N. S., et al: Dietary regulation of small intestine enzyme activity in man. Am. J. Clin. Nutr. 24:65, 1971.

Shiner, M.: The structure of the small intestine and some interesting relations to its function. Proc. Nutr. Soc. 26:1, 1967.

Spencer, R. P.: Intestinal absorption of amino acids. Current Concepts. Am. J. Clin. Nutr. 22:292, 1969.

Stifel, F. B. and Herman, R. H.: Histidine metabolism. Am. J. Clin. Nutr. 24:207, 1971.

Symposium on mechanisms of gastrointestinal absorption. Am. J. Clin. Nutr. 12:161, 1963.

Tedesco, T. A., et al: Galactokinase: evidence for a new racial polymorphism. Science 178:176, 1972.

To nibble or gorge? Brit. Med. J. 5829:716, (September 23) 1972.

Treadwell, C. R., et al: Factors in sterol absorption. Fed. Proc. 21:903, 1962.

Wadhava, P. S. Sr., et al: Metabolic consequences of feeding frequency in man. Am. J. Clin. Nutr. 26:823, 1973.

meeting nutritional norms and nutrition labeling

Journal Articles:

Babcock, M. J. and Murphy, M. J.: Two nutritional labeling systems. J. Am. Dietet. A. 62:155, 1973.

Beloian, A.: Nutrition labels: a great leap forward. FDA Consumer 7:10, 1973.

Boyde, J.: Food labeling and the marketing of nutrition. J. Home Econ. 65:20, 1973.

Brink, M. E., et al: Nutritional values of milk compared with filled and imitation milks. Am. J. Clin. Nutr. 22:168, 1969.

Bruch, H.: The allure of food cults and nutritional quackery. J. Am. Dietet. A. 57:316, 1970.

Campbell, J. A.: Approaches in revising dietary standards—Canadian, U.S. and international standards compared. J. Am. Dietet. A. 64:175, 1974.

Council on Foods and Nutrition: Iron in enriched wheat flour, farina, bread buns and rolls. JAMA 220, No. 6, (May 8) 1972.

Erhard, D.: Nutrition education for the now generation. J. Nutr. Educa. 2:135, 1971.

Harper, A. E.: Recommended Dietary Allowances: Are they what we think they are? J. Am. Dietet. A. 64:151, 1974.

Kammer, J. B. and Shawhan, G. L.: Comparison of food prices in high and low income areas. J. Home Econ. 62:56, 1970.

Lachance, P. A.: A commentary on the new FDA nutrition labeling regulations. Nutrition Today 8:18, (January-February) 1973.

Lane, M. M.: Food fads. Nursing Homes 20:22, 1971.

Leverton, R. M.: Basic nutrition concepts. J. Home Econ. 59:346, 1967.

Mann, G. V.: Relationship of age to nutrient requirements. Am. J. Clin. Nutr. 26:1096, 1973.

Mertz, W.: Recommended dietary allowances up to date—trace minerals. J. Am. Dietet. A. 64:163, 1974.

Mitchell, H. S.: Recommended Dietary Allowances up to date—a symposium. J. Am. Dietet. A. 64:149, 1974.

Nagy, M.: Nutritive value of breakfast cereals. (Questions and Answers) JAMA 215:1994, 1971.

Ohlson, M. A. and Hart, B. P.: Influence of breakfast on total day's food intake. J. Am. Dietet. A. 47:282, 1965.

Patwardhan, V. N.: Dietary allowances—an international point of view. J. Am. Dietet. A. 56:191, 1970.

Review: Nutrition labeling. Nutr. Rev. 30:247, 1972.

_____: Problems in iron enrichment and fortification of foods. Nutr. Rev. 33:46, 1975.

Rusoff, L. L.: The role of milk in modern nutrition. Borden's Rev. Nutr. Res. 25:17, (April-September), 1964.

Revisions and additions to FDA food labeling program. J. Am. Dietet. A. 62:304, 555, 1973.

Sabry, Z. I.: The Canadian dietary standard. J. Am. Dietet. A. 56:195, 1970.

Sebrell, W. H.: The role of the bread-cereal group in the well-balanced diet. Borden's Rev. Nutr. Res. 27:1, (January-June) 1966.

Seidler, A. J.: Nutritional contributions of the meat groups to an adequate diet. Borden's Rev. Nutr. Res., 24:29, (July-September) 1963.

Stiebling, H. K.: Foods of the vegetable-fruit group—their contributions to nutritionally adequate diets. Borden's Rev. Nutr. Res. 25:51, (October-December) 1964.

Wadsworth, G. R.: Nutrient requirements and the need for the fortification of foods. Food and Nutr. Notes 30:68, (May-June) 1973.

Walker, A. R. P.: Optimal intake of nutrients. Nutr. Rev. 23:321, 1965.

TABLES OF FOOD COMPOSITION

Anderson, B. A., et al: Comprehensive evaluation of fatty acids in foods, II, Beef products. J. Am. Dietet. A. 67:35, 1975.

Church, C. F., and Church, H. N.: Food Values of Portions Commonly Used, ed. 12. Philadelphia, J. B. Lippincott, 1975.

FAO: Review of Food Composition Tables. Rome, Food Consumption and Planning Branch, FAO, 1965. (Food Composition Tables from around the world.)

_____: Amino Acid Content of Foods. Nutr. Studies No. 24, Rome. 1967.

Feeley, R. M., et al: Major fatty acids and approximate composition of dairy products. J. Am. Dietet. A. 66:140, 1975.

Gormican, A.: Inorganic elements in food used in hospital menus. J. Am. Dietet. A. 56:397, 1970.

Hardinge, M. G. and Crooks, H.: Lesser known vitamins in foods. J. Am. Dietet. A. 38:240, 1961.

Orr, M. L., and Watt, B. K.: Amino Acid Content of Foods. USDA. Washington, D.C., U.S. Government Printing Office, 1957.

Posati, L. P., et al: Comprehensive evaluation of fatty acids in foods, I, Dairy products. J. Am. Dietet. A. 66:482, 1975.

Standal, B. R., et al: Fatty acids, cholesterol and proximate analysis of some ready-to-eat foods. J. Am. Dietet. A. 56:392, 1970.

USDA: *Folic Acid Content of Foods*. Handbook No. 29. Washington, D.C., U.S. Government Printing Office, 1951.

⸻: *Nutritive Value of Foods*. Home and Garden Bull. No. 72. Washington, D.C., U.S. Government Printing Office, 1970.

⸻: *Pantothenic Acid, Vitamin B₆, and Vitamin B₁₂ in Food*. Home Econ. Res. Report No. 36. Washington, D.C., 1969.

Watt, B. K., and Merrill, A. L.: *Composition of Foods—Raw, Processed, Prepared*. USDA Handbook No. 8. Washington, D.C., U.S. Government Printing Office, 1963.

Widdowson, E. M.: British Food Composition Tables. J. Am. Dietet. A. 50:363, 1967.

MEAL MANAGEMENT
Books and Pamphlets:
Food for the Young Family. Home and Garden Bull. No. 85, Washington, D.C., USDA, 1971.

Kinder, F.: *Meal Management*, ed. 4. Riverside, N.J., Macmillan, 1973.

Your Money's Worth in Food. Home and Garden Bull. No. 183, Washington, D.C., USDA, 1970.

Journal Articles:
Donovan, W. P. and Appledorf, H.: Protein, fat and mineral analysis of franchise chicken dinners. J. Food Science 38:79, 1973.

Hansen, R. G.: An index of food quality. Nutr. Rev. 31:1, 1973.

Murphy, E. W., Watt, B. K., and Rizek, R. L.: Tables of food composition: availability, uses, and limitations. Food Tech. 27:40, 1973.

nutrition counseling

Books:
Brill, N. I.: *Working with People. The Helping Process.* Philadelphia, Lippincott, 1973.

Journal Articles:
Callan, L. B.: Supervision, the key to success with aides. Public Health Rep. 85:780, 1970.

Cason, D. and Wagner, M. G.: The changing role of the service professional within the ghetto. J. Am. Dietet. A. 60:21, 1972.

Cauffman, J. G., et al: Community health aides: How effective are they? Am. J. Public Health 60:1904, 1970.

Chase, H. P., et al: Effectiveness of nutrition aides in a migrant population. Am. J. Clin. Nutr. 26:849, 1973.

Craig, D. G.: Guiding the change process in people. J. Am. Dietet. A. 58:22, 1971.

Detmer, D. G.: The nutrition component of training for the physician's assistant and his education. J. Am. Dietet. A. 66:269, 1975.

Dahl, T.: The nutritional functional area in comprehensive health care delivery. J. Am. Dietet. A. 61:497, 1972.

D'Onofrio, C. N.: Aides—pain or panacea. Public Health Rep. 85:788, 1970.

Egan, M. C., and Hallstrom, B. J.: Building nutrition services in comprehensive health care. J. Am. Dietet. A. 61:491, 1972.

Erlander, D.: Dietetics—a look at the profession. Am. J. Nurs. 70:2402, (November) 1970.

Flynn, M., et al: Nutrition in the education of the family physician. J. Am. Dietet. A. 65:269, 1974.

Gailbraith, A. L. and Hatch, L.: Diet manual in a large teaching hospital: philosophy and purpose. J. Am. Dietet. A. 62:643, 1973.

Goldberg, J. P.: Some community nutrition services in a Boston program. J. Am. Dietet. A. 62:537, 1973.

Hallstrom, B. J. and Lauber, D. E.: Multidisciplinary manpower in the nutrition component of comprehensive health care delivery. J. Am. Dietet. A. 63:23, 1973.

Heath, A. M. and Pelz, D. R.: Perception of functions of health aides by themselves and by others. Public Health Rep. 85:767, 1970.

Hildebrand, G. I.: Guidelines for effective use of nonprofessionals. Public Health Rep. 85:773, 1970.

Jamann, J. A.: Health as a function of ecology. Am. J. Nurs. 71:970, (May) 1970.

Johnson, D.: Effective diet counseling begins early in hospitalization. Hospitals 41:94, 1967.

Kocher, R. E.: New dimensions for dietetics in today's health care. J. Am. Dietet. A. 60:17, 1972.

Kocher, R. E.: Monitoring nutritional care of the long term patient, I, Policies and systems that support the on-going evaluation of care. J. Am. Dietet. A. 67:45, 1975.

Mathews, G.: Current concerns of the consultant dietitian: III, Contributing information to patient care plans. J. Am. Dietet. A. 63:45, 1973.

Mathews, L. I.: Principles of interviewing and patient counseling. J. Am. Dietet. A. 50:469, 1967.

Nizel, A. E.: Personalized nutrition counseling. J. Dent. Child. 39:19, 1972.

Ohlson, M. A.: The philosophy of dietary counseling. J. Am. Dietet. A. 63:13, 1973.

Ohlson, M. A.: Uses of the dietary manual to promote communication. J. Am. Dietet. A. 62:534, 1973.

Patterson, L., et al: Nutrition service in health care systems. Food and Nutrition Notes and Reviews 30:74, 1973.

Popkin, B. and Ledman, R.: Economics as an aid to nutritional change. Am. J. Clin. Nutr. 25:331, 1972.

Powers, T. F.: The dietetic technician: paraprofessional as knowledge worker. J. Am. Dietet. A. 65:130, 1974.

Robinson, C. H.: Basic considerations in prescribing diets. J. Am. Dietet. A. 65:161, 1974.

Rodgers, T. V. and Clark, M. E.: Current concerns of the consultant dietitian: II, Sharing information by means of the patient's medical record. J. Am. Dietet. A. 63:43, 1973.

Schiller, M. R. and Vivian, V. M.: I, Ideal role perceived by dietitians and physicians. II, Ideal vs. actual role—Role of the clinical dietitian. J. Am. Dietet. A. 65:284, 287, 1974.

Sipple, H. L.: Problems and progress in nutrition education. J. Am. Dietet. A. 59:18, 1971.

Spondnik, J. P.: Nutrition in the health maintenance organization. J. Am. Dietet. A. 61:163, 1972.

Storie, F.: A philosophy of patient teaching. Nurs. Outlook 19:378, 1971.

The American Dietetic Association: Position paper on the nutrition component of health services delivery systems. J. Am. Dietet. A. 58:538, 1971.

Vargas, J. S.: Teaching as changing behavior. J. Am. Dietet. A. 58:512, 1971.

Vaughn, M. E.: The nutrition consultant and the home aide. J. Am. Dietet. A. 43:435, 1963.

Walters, F. M., et al: Nutritional needs of the outpatient—an overview. J. Am. Dietet. A. 61:170, 1972.

factors influencing food habits

Books and Pamphlets:

Lowenberg, M., Todhunter, E. N., and Wilson, E. D.: *Food and Man*. New York, Wiley, 1968.

Mead, M.: *Food Habits Research: Problems of the 60's*. National Academy of Sciences—National Research Council Publ. No. 1225. Washington, D.C., 1964.

Pyke, M.: *Food and Society*. London, Murray, 1968.

Journal Articles:

Adams, R. N.: Nutrition, anthropology, and the study of man. Nutr. Rev. 17:97, 1959.

Babcock, C.: Attitudes and the use of food. J. Am. Dietet. A. 38:546, 1961.

Fathauer, G. H.: Food habits—an anthropologist's view. J. Am. Dietet. A. 37:335, 1960.

Feeding drug addicts. Hospitals 45: (Part I) 80, (August 1) 1971.

Kallen, D. J.: Nutrition and society. JAMA 215:94, 1971.

Lowenberg, M. E.: Socio-cultural bases of food habits. Food Tech. 24:27, 1970.

Manning, M. L.: The psychodynamics of dietetics. Nurs. Outlook 13:57, 1965.

Mead, M.: Changing significance of food. J. Nutr. Educa. 2:17, 1970.

Parrish, J. B.: Implications of changing food habits for nutrition educators. J. Nutr. Educa. 2:140, 1971.

Queen, G. S.: Culture, economics and food habits. J. Am. Dietet. A. 33:1044, 1957.

Simoans, F. J.: The geographic approach to food prejudices. Food Tech. 20:42, 1966.

MEANING OF FOOD

Journal Articles:

Brozek, J.: Research on diet and behavior. J. Am. Dietet. A. 56:321, 1970.

Cassel, J.: Social and cultural implications of food and food habits. Am. J. Public Health 47:732, 1957.

Jerome, N. W.: Northern urbanization and food consumption patterns of southern-born Negroes. Am. J. Clin. Nutr. 22:1667, 1969.

Pumpian-Mindlin, E.: The meanings of food. J. Am. Dietet. A. 30:576, 1954.

regional, cultural, religious, and unusual food patterns

Journal Articles:

Abiaka, M. H.: Japanese-American food equivalents for calculating exchange diets. J. Am. Dietet. A. 62:173, 1973.

Adolph, W. H.: Nutrition in the Near East. J. Am. Dietet. A. 30:753, 1954.

Bailey, M. A.: Nutrition education and the Spanish-speaking American. J. Nutr. Educa. 2:50, 1970.

Buchau, J. W.: America's Health: fallacies, beliefs, practices. FDA Consumer 6:4, (October) 1972.

Council on Foods and Nutrition: Zen macrobiotic diets. JAMA 218:397, (October 18) 1971.

deGarine, I.: The social and cultural background of food habits in developing countries (traditional societies). Food and Nutrition Notes and Reviews 29:81, (July-August) 1972.

Delgado, G., et al: Eating patterns among migrant families. Public Health Rep. 76:349, 1961.

Dwyer, J. T., et al: The new vegetarians: Group affiliation and dietary strictures related to attitudes and life style. J. Am. Dietet. A. 64:376, 1974.

Ellis, F. R., Holesh, S., and Ellis, J. W.: Incidence of osteoporosis in vegetarians and omnivores. Am. J. Clin. Nutr. 25:555, 1972.

Frankle, R. T.: I, The Door—A center of alternatives: The nutritionist in a free clinic for adolescents. II, Observations of a nutritionist in a free clinic. III, Nutrition and contemporary counseling. J. Am. Dietet. A. 63:269, 273, 275, 1973.

Frankle, R. T., and Heussenstamm, F. K.: Food zealotry and youth: New dilemmas for professionals. Am. J. Public Health 64:11, 1974.

Hardinge, M. G., et al: Nutritional studies of vegetarians. J. Am. Dietet. A. 48:25, 1966.

Hardinge, M. G. and Mann, G. V.: Raising an infant on a vegetarian diet. JAMA 227:88, (January 7) 1974.

Henderson, L. M.: Programs to combat nutritional quackery. J. Am. Dietet. A. 64:372, 1974.

Huang, S. S. and Bayless, T. M.: Milk and lactose intolerance in healthy Orientals. Science 160:83, 1968.

Insull, W. and Kenzaburo, T.: Diet and nutritional status of Japanese. Am. J. Clin. Nutr. 21:753, 1968.

Jerome, N. W.: Northern urbanization and food consumption patterns of southern-born Negroes. Am. J. Clin. Nutr. 22:1667, 1969.

Joseph, S., et al: Composition of Israeli mixed dishes. J. Am. Dietet. A. 40:125, 1962.

Kight, M. A., et al: Nutritional influences of Mexican-American foods in Arizona. J. Am. Dietet. A. 55:557, 1969.

Kilby-Kelberg, S.: Aunt Libby and her cure-alls. Am. J. Nurs. 73:1056, (June) 1973.

Korff, S. I.: The Jewish dietary code. Food Tech. 20:76, 1966.

Mayer, J.: The nutritional status of American Negroes. Nutr. Rev. 23:161, 1965.

Nutrition misinformation and food faddism. Nutr. Rev. 32: special supplement, (July) 1974.

Organic Foods. J. Am. Dietet. A. 62:34, 1973.

Our cooking heritage: African foods. What's New in Home Economics 35:28, 1971.

Register, V. D., Sonnenberg, L. M.: Scientific and practical considerations in the vegetarian diet. J. Am. Dietet. A. 62:253, 1973.

Sakr, A. H.: Dietary regulations and food habits of Muslims. J. Am. Dietet. A. 58:123, 1971.

Sanjur, D. and Scoma, A. D.: Food habits of low-income children in northern New York. J. Nutr. Educa. 2:85, 1971.

Schuck, C. and Tartt, J. B.: Food consumption of low-income, rural Negro households in Mississippi. J. Am. Dietet. A. 62:151, 1973.

Soulsby, T.: Russian-American food patterns. J. Nutr. Educa. 4:170, 1972.

White, H. S.: The organic foods movement. Food Tech. 26:29, 1972.

Wolff, R. J.: Who eats for health? Am. J. Clin. Nutr. 26:438, 1973.

Zen macrobiotic diets. J. School Health 42:289, 1972.

the ecology of food

GENERAL

Books and Pamphlets:

Bernarde, M. A.: The Chemicals We Eat. New York, American Heritage, 1971.

Evaluation of Certain Food Additives and the Contaminants Mercury, Lead and Cadmium. Sixteenth Report of the Joint FAO/WHO Expert Committee on Food Additives. WHO Technical Report Series #505. FAO Nutrition Meeting Report Series No. 51, 1972.

Food Protection Committee, Food and Nutrition Board: New Developments in the Use of Pesticides. National Academy of Sciences-National Research Council Publ. No. 1082. Washington, D.C., 1963.

_____: An Evaluation of Public Health Hazards from Microbiological Contamination of Foods. National Academy of Sciences-National Research Council Publ. No. 1195. Washington, D.C., 1964.

_____: Chemicals Used in Food Processing. National Academy of Sciences-National Research Council Publ. No. 1274. Washington, D.C., 1965.

_____: Toxicants Occurring Naturally in Foods. National Academy of Sciences-National Research Council Publ. No. 1354. Washington, D.C., 1966.

National Communicable Disease Center: Salmonella Surveillance. Report 58. Washington, D.C., HEW, 1967.

Protecting Our Food. Yearbook of Agriculture 1967. Washington, D.C., USDA, 1967.

USDA Agricultural Research Service: Consumer Products by Design. Agric. Information Bull. No. 355. Washington, D.C., Government Printing Office, Stock No. 0100-1589, 1972.

GENERAL AND FOODBORNE DISEASES AND TOXINS

Journal Articles:

Aaron, E., et al: Urban salmonellosis. Am. J. Public Health 61:337, 1971.

Adler, H. E.: Salmonella in eggs—an appraisal. Food Tech. 19:191, 1965.

Bird, K.: The food processing front of the seventies. J. Am. Dietet. A. 58:103, 1971.

Bryan, F. L.: New concepts in foodborne illness. J. Environ. Health 31:327, 1969.

Bryan, J. A., and Huff, J. C.: Hepatitis from clams. Letters. JAMA 226:566, 1973.

Cheng, T. C.: Parasitology and food protection. J. Environ. Health 28:208, 1965.

Cliver, D. O.: Implications of foodborne infectious hepatitis. Publ. Health Rep. 81:185, 1966.

Coon, J. M.: Natural food toxicants—a perspective. Nutr. Rev. 32:321, 1974.

Eadie, G. A., et al: Type E botulism. JAMA 187:496, 1964.

Editorial: One man's cured meat. JAMA 224:1756, (June 25) 1973.

_____: Salmonella control. JAMA 189:691, 1964.

_____: The most deadly poison. JAMA 187:530, 1964.

_____: Carcinogen in groundnuts. Brit. Med. J. 5043:204, 1964.

Formal, S. B., et al: Mechanisms of shigella pathogenesis. Am. J. Clin. Nutr. 25:1427, 1972.

Feuell, A. J.: Toxic factors of mould origin. Canad. Med. A. J. 94:574, 1966.

Gearing, J.: Toprina: the marriage of the agricultural and industrial revolutions. Columbia J. World Business 8:39, 1973.

Goddard, J. L.: Incident at Selby Junior High. Nutrition Today 2:2, (September) 1967.

Gortner, W. A.: The impact of food technology on nutrient supplies. Food and Nutrition Notes and Reviews 30:61, (May-June) 1973.

Harsanyi, Y. L.: Paralytic shellfish poisoning. FDA Consumer 7:22, 1973.

Health legislation: Protection against ionizing radiations. WHO Chronicle 26:516, 1972.

Heidelbaugh, N. D., et al: Clinical nutrition applications of space food technology. J. Am. Dietet. A. 62:383, 1973.

Hot dogs a potential source of pathogens. JAMA 222:633, 1972.

IFT Expert Panel on Food Safety and Nutrition: Botulism. A scientific status summary. J. Food Science 37:985, 1972.

Jukes, T. H.: Scientific agriculture at the crossroads. Nutrition Today, 8:31 (January-February) 1973.

Kauter, D. A. and Lynt, R. K.: Botulism. Nutr. Rev. 31:265, 1973.

Koff, R. S., et al: Viral hepatitis from shellfish. N. Eng. J. Med. 276:703, 1967.

Lachance, P. A.: Nutrification—a new nutritional concept for new types of foods. Food Tech. 24:100, 1970.

LaChapelle, N. C., et al: A gastroenteritis outbreak of staphylococcus aureus, Type 29. Am. J. Public Health 56:94, 1966.

Most, H.: Trichinellosis in the United States. JAMA 162:871, 1965.

Note: Limiting temperature and humidity for production of aflatoxin by Aspergillus flavus in peanuts. Nutr. Rev. 25:286, 1967.

_____: Thermostable Clostridium perfringens as the cause of a food poisoning outbreak. Nutr. Rev. 25:287, 1967.

Review: Foods and feeds as sources of carcinogenic factors. Nutr. Rev. 24:321, 1966.

Salmonella and food in your home. FDA Consumer 7:11, 1973.

Salmonella, the ubiquitous bug. FDA Papers 1:13, (February) 1967.

Spensley, P. C.: Mycotoxins—a menace of moulds. Roy. Soc. Health J. 90:248, 1970.

Strong, F. M.: Naturally occurring toxic factors in plants and animals used as food. Canad. Med. A. J. 94:568, 1966.

_____: Toxicants occurring naturally in food. Nutr. Rev. 32:225, 1974.

Symposium on nutrient retention. Food Tech. 27:16, 1973.

Thatcher, F. S.: Food-borne bacterial toxins. Canad. Med. A. J. 94:582, 1966.

U.S.D.A. views, '73 prospects. Food Engineering, 45:54, 1973.

Wadsworth, G. R.: Nutrient requirements and the need for fortification of foods. Food and Nutrition Notes and Reviews, 30:68, (May-June) 1973.

Waters, E. P.: Codex alimentarius. FDA Consumer 6:14, (December-January) 1972-73.

We want you to know what we know about salmonella and food poisoning. DHEW Publ. No. (FDA) 73-2004, Food and Drug Admin., Washington, D.C., 1973.

Wilson, B. J.: 12, 13 epoxytriclothecenes: potential toxic contaminants of food. Nutr. Rev. 31:169, (June) 1973.

Zimmerman, W. J.: Current status of trichiniasis in U.S. swine. Publ. Health Rep. 80:1061, 1965.

Zimmerman, W. J., et al: Trichiniasis in the U.S. population 1966-70: Prevalence and epidemiologic factors. Health Serv. Rep. 88:606, 1973.

food additives, intentional and accidental

Journal Articles:

Angeline, J. F., and Leonardos, G. P.: Food additives: some economic considerations. Food Tech. 27:40, 1973.

Celeste, A. C. and Shane, C. G.: Mercury in fish. FDA Papers 4:27, 1970.

Comment: Calcium protects against lead poisoning. J. Am. Dietet. A. 64:397, 1974.

Committee on Nutrition A.A.P.: Vitamin K content of infant formula products. Pediatrics 48:483, 1971: 53:146, 1974.

Culliton, B. J.: Delaney clause: defended against an uncertain threat of change. Science 179:666, 1973.

Dales, L. G.: The neurotoxicity of alkyl mercury compounds. Am. J. Med. 53:219, 1972.

Damon, G. E.: A primer on food additives. FDA Consumer 7:15, 1973.

Damon, G. E., and Janssen, W. F.: Additives for eye appeal. FDA Consumer 7:15, 1973.

Dickinson, L., et al: Lead poisoning in family due to cocktail glasses. Am. J. Nurs. 52:391, 1972.

Eyl, T. B.: Organic-mercury food poisoning. Current Concepts. N. Eng. J. Med. 284:706, 1971.

Finkel, A. J.: Mercury residue blood levels and tolerance limits in fish eaters. (Questions and Answers) JAMA 216:1208, 1971.

Fitzhugh, O. G.: Problems related to the use of pesticides. Canad. Med. A. J. 94:598, 1966.

Food Additives: Safety of food additives continually evaluated. Publ. Health Rep. 81:244, 1966.

Guinee, V. F.: Lead poisoning. Am. J. Med. 52:283, 1972.

Hodges, R. E.: The toxicity of pesticides and their residues in food. Nutr. Rev. 23:230, 1965.

IFT Expert Panel on Food Safety and Nutrition: Nitrites, nitrates and nitrosamines in foods—a dilemma. J. Food Sci. 37:989, 1972.

Johnson, P. E.: Health aspects of food additives. Am. J. Public Health, 56:948, 1966.

Jukes, T. H.: Chemical residues in foods. J. Am. Dietet. A. 59:203, 1971.

Kevorkian, J., et al: Mercury content of human tissues during the twentieth century. Am. J. Public Health 62:504, 1972.

Krehl, W. A.: Mercury the slippery metal. Nutrition Today 7:4 (November-December) 1972.

Lamm, S. H. and Rosen, J. F.: Lead contamination in milks fed to infants 1972-73. Pediatrics 53:137, 1974.

Leong, L., et al: Methyl mercury and environmental health. J. Environ. Health 35:436, 1973.

Lin-Fu, J. S.: Vulnerability of children to lead exposure and toxicity. N. Eng. J. Med. 289:1289, (December 13) 1974.

Mitchell, D. G.: Increased lead absorption: Paint is not the only problem. Pediatrics 53:142, 1974.

Oser, B. L.: Problems related to the use of food additives. Canad. Med. A. J. 94:604, 1966.

Philip, J. McL.: Toxicity and naturally occurring chemicals. Royal Soc. Health J. 90:237, 1970.

Smith, E. H.: Problems in the safe and effective use of pesticides in agriculture. Nutr. Rev. 22:193, 1964.

Synder, R. D.: Congenital mercury poisoning. N. Eng. J. Med. 284:1014, 1971.

Special Report: The use of chemicals in food production, processing, storage, and distribution. Nutr. Rev. 31:191, 1973.

Takizawa, Y., et al: Studies on the causes of the Niigata episode of Minamata disease outbreak. Acta Medica et Biologica 19:193, 1972.

Whitfield, C. L., et al: Lead encephalopathy in adults. Am. J. Med. 52:289, 1972.

Wogan, G. N.: Current research on toxic food contaminants. J. Am. Dietet. A. 49:95, 1966.

Wolff, S. A.: Nitrosamines. J. Environ. Health 35:114, (September-October) 1972.

REGULATIONS PROTECTING THE FOOD SUPPLY
Journal Articles:
Analysis of pesticide residues. FDA Papers 1:17, (June) 1967.

Beacham, L. M.: Food standards. FDA Papers 1:5, (July-August) 1967.

Breeling, J. L.: Nutritional guidelines. The how, the why and the when. J. Am. Dietet. A. 59:102, 1971.

Cooke, J. A.: Nutritional guidelines and the labeling of foods. J. Am. Dietet. A. 59:99, 1971.

FAO/WHO Committee on Technical Basis for Legislation on Irradiated Foods: The irradiation of food. WHO Chronicle 20:371, 1966.

FDA units and their function. FDA Papers 4:4, (May) 1970.

Grant, J. D.: New issues in consumerism. FDA Papers 4:15, Dec. 1970-Jan. 1971.

Health legislation: Protection against ionizing radiations. WHO Chronicle 26:516, 1972.

Howard, H. W.: Ingredient labeling. Food Tech. 25:18, 1971.

Kingma, F. J.: Establishing and monitoring drug residue levels. FDA Papers 1:9, (July-August) 1967.

Milk surveillance report. J. Environ. Health, 33:350, 1971.

New regulations on vitamins A and D. FDA Consumer 7:14, (October) 1973.

Roe, R. S.: FDA Food additives requirements. FDA Papers 1:25, (May) 1967.

Somers, R. K.: New meat inspection laws for consumer protection. Publ. Health Rep. 84:214, 1969.

Spiher, A. T., Jr.: The GRAS list review. FDA Papers 4:12, Dec. 1970-Jan. 1971.

Vitamins and minerals and FDA. FDA Consumer 7:18, (September) 1973.

What do you need on a can label? What's New in Home Economics 34:44, 1970.

Wodicka, V. O.: The current status of food regulations. FDA Papers 6:10 (March) 1972.

section two
nutrition throughout the life span
growth and development
GENERAL
Books and Pamphlets:
Baer, M. J.: Growth and Maturation—An Introduction to Physical Development. Cambridge, Mass., Doyle, 1973.

Birch, H. G. and Gussow, J. D.: Disadvantaged Children: Health, Nutrition and School Failure. New York, Grune & Stratton, 1970.

Body Dimensions and Proportions, White and Negro Children 6-11 Years, United States. Vital and Health Statistics, Series II, No. 143, DHEW Publ. No. (HRA) 75-1625, Washington, D.C., 1975.

Cheek, D. B.: Human Growth. Philadelphia, Lea & Febiger, 1968.

Height and weight of children in the United States, India, and the United Arab Republic. P.H.S. Publ. 1000, Series 3, No. 14, DHEW, Washington, D.C., 1971.

Manocha, S. L.: Malnutrition and Retarded Human Development. Springfield, Ill., Thomas, 1972.

Mason, M., et al: Nutrition and the Cell: The Inside Story. Chicago. Yearbook Medical Publishers, 1973.

McCammon, R. W.: Human Growth and Development. Springfield, Ill. Thomas, 1970.

Nutrition and Intellectual Growth in Children. Washington, D.C., The Association for Childhood Education International, 1969.

Skeletal Maturity of Children 6-11 Years, United States. Vital and Health Statistics, Series II, No. 140, DHEW Publ. No. (HRA) 75-1622, Washington, D.C., 1975.

Srimshaw, N. S. and Gordon, J. E.: Malnutrition, Learning and Behavior. Cambridge, Mass. M.I.T. Press, 1968.

Springer, N. S.: An Annotated Bibliography—Nutrition and Mental Retardation (1964-1970). Ann Arbor, Mich., ISMR, University of Michigan, 1970.

Winick, M. (ed.): Nutrition and Development, Vol. I of Current Concepts in Nutrition. New York, Wiley, 1972.

————: Nutrition and Fetal Development, Vol. II of Current Concepts in Nutrition, New York, Wiley, 1974.

————: Childhood Obesity, Vol. III of Current Concepts in Nutrition, New York, Wiley, 1975.

Journal Articles:
Bjornstein, I. and Sjostrom, L.: Number and size of adipose tissue fat cells in relation to metabolism in human obesity. Metabolism 20:703, 1971.

Cone, T. E., Jr.: Growth problems of the adolescent. Med. Clin. N. Am. 49:357, 1965.

Corbin, C. B.: Standards of subcutaneous fat applied to percentile norms for elementary school children. Am. J. Clin. Nutr. 22:836, 1969.

Crispen, S., et al: Nutritional status of preschool children. II. Anthropometric measurements and interrelationships. Am. J. Clin. Nutr. 21:1280, 1968.

Dayton, D. H.: Early malnutrition and human development. Children 16:210, 1969.

Deren, J. S.: Development of structure and function in the fetal and newborn stomach. Am. J. Clin. Nutr. 24:144, 1971.

Dugdale, A. E.: An age-independent anthropometric index of nutritional status. Am. J. Clin. Nutr. 24:174, 1971.

Dugdale, A. E., et al: Patterns of growth and nutrition in childhood. Am. J. Clin. Nutr. 23:1280, 1970.

Editorial: Growth after malnutrition. Brit. Med. J. 2:495, (May 30) 1970.

Eid, E. E.: Follow-up study of physical growth of children

who had excessive weight gain in first six months of life. Brit. Med. J. 2:74, (April 11) 1970.

Forbes, G. B.: Growth of lean body mass in man. Growth 36:325, 1972.

Graham, G. G.: Environmental factors affecting growth of children. Am. J. Clin. Nutr. 25:1184, 1972.

Hathaway, M. L.: Overweight in children. J. Am. Dietet. A. 40:511, 1962.

Hurley, L. S.: Nutrients and Genes: Interactions in Development. Nutr. Rev. 27:3, 1969.

McCance, R. A. and Widdowson, E. M.: Review lecture: The determinants of growth and form. Proc. Roy. Soc. Brit. 185:1, 1974.

Review: Intrauterine growth. Nutr. Rev. 22:266, 1964.

―――: Subsequent growth of children treated for malnutrition. Nutr. Rev. 24:267, 1966.

Sjostrom, L., et al: Cellularity in different regions of adipose tissue in young men and women. Metabolism 21-1143, 1972.

Walker, A. R. P. and Richardson, B. D.: International and local growth standards. Am. J. Clin. Nutr. 26:897, 1973.

NUTRITION AND MENTAL DEVELOPMENT
Journal Articles:

Abelson, P. H.: Malnutrition, learning and behavior. Science 164:17, 1969.

Allen, D. E., et al: Nutrition, family commensality and academic performance among high school youth. J. Home Econ. 62:333, 1970.

Barnes, R. H., et al: Learning behavior following nutritional deprivation in early life. J. Am. Dietet. A. 51:34, 1967.

Champakam, S., et al: Kwashiorkor and mental development. Am. J. Clin. Nutr. 21:844, 1968.

Cravioto, J. and Robles, B.: Evolution of adaptive and motor behavior during rehabilitation from kwashiorkor. Am. J. Orthopsychology 35:449, 1965.

Cravioto, J., et al: Nutrition, growth and neurointegrative development; an experimental ecology study. Pediatrics (Suppl.) 38:319, 1966.

Davison, A. N. and Dobbing, J.: Myelination as a vulnerable period in brain development. Brit. Med. Bull. 22:40, 1966.

Dobbing, J.: The developing brain: a plea for more critical interspecies extrapolation. Nutr. Rep. Intern. 7:401, 1973.

Dobbing, J. and Sands, J.: Timing of neuroblast multiplication of developing human brain. Nature 226:639, 1970.

Douglas, J. W. B., et al: The relation between height and measured educational ability in school children of the same social class, family size and stage of sexual development. Human Biol. 37:178, 1965.

Eichenwald, H. G., and Fry, P. C.: Nutrition and learning. Science 163:644, 1969.

Fernstrom, J. D. and Wurtman, R. J.: Nutrition and the brain. Sci. Amer. 230 (2):84, 1974.

Hertzig, E., et al: Intellectual levels of school children severely malnourished during the first two years of life. Pediatrics 49:814, 1972.

Hopwood, H. H. and Van Iden, S. S.: Scholastic underachievement as related to sub-par physical growth. J. School Health 35:377, (October) 1965.

Hsueh, A. M., et al: Perinatal undernutrition and the metabolic and behavioral development of the offspring. Nutr. Rep. Intern. 7:437, 1973.

Kerr, G. R.: The nutritional correlates of life: growth and learning. J. School Health 42:191, 1972.

Liang, P. H., et al: Evaluation of mental development in relation to early malnutrition. Am. J. Clin. Nutr. 20:1290, 1967.

Martin, H. P.: Nutrition: Its relationship to children's physical, mental and emotional development. Am. J. Clin. Nutr. 26:766, 1973.

Medical News: Mental retardation from malnutrition: irreversible. JAMA 206:30, 1968.

Monckeberg, B.: Malnutrition and mental behavior. Nutr. Rev. 27:191, 1969.

Monckeberg, F.: Malnutrition and mental capacity. Boletin De La Oficina Sanitaria Panamericana (Eng. ed.) 7 (1):87, 1973.

Monckeberg, F., et al: Malnutrition and mental development. Am. J. Clin. Nutr. 25:766, 1972.

Mosier, H. D., Jr.: Physical growth in mental defectives. A study in an institutionalized population. Pediatrics (Suppl.) 36:465, 1965.

Read, M. S.: Malnutrition and mental retardation. J. Nutr. Educa. 2:23, 1970.

Read, M. S.: Malnutrition, hunger and behavior. J. Am. Dietet. A. 63:379, 1973.

Review: Behavioral development during recovery from nutritional marasmus. Nutr. Rev. 29:31, 1971.

―――: Mental development following kwashiorkor. Nutr. Rev. 27:46, 1969.

―――: Present knowledge of the relationship of nutrition to brain developmental behavior. Nutr. Rev. 31:242, 1973.

―――: The infant brain following severe malnutrition. Nutr. Rev. 27:251, 1969.

―――: Undernutrition in children and subsequent brain growth and intellectual development. Nutr. Rev. 26:197, 1968.

Rosso, P., et al: Changes in brain weight, cholesterol, phospholipid, and DNA content in marasmic children. Am. J. Clin. Nutr. 23:1275, 1970.

Stein, Z., et al: Nutrition and mental performance. Science 178:708, 1972.

Winick, M.: Malnutrition and brain development J. Pediat. 74:667, 1969.

Winick, M. and Rosso, P.: The effect of severe early malnutrition on cellular growth of human brain. Pediat. Res. 3:181, 1969.

nutrition in pregnancy and lactation

Books and Pamphlets:

Beaton, G. H. and McHenry, E. W.: *Nutrition: A Comprehensive Treatise*, Vol. III New York, Academic Press, 1966, Chapter 3.

Committee on Maternal Nutrition, Food and Nutrition Board: *Maternal Nutrition and the Course of Pregnancy*. Washington, D.C., National Academy of Sciences-National Research Council, 1970.

Committee on Maternal Nutrition: *Nutritional supplementation and the outcome of pregnancy*. Washington, D.C., National Academy of Sciences-National Research Council, 1975.

Giroud, A.: *The Nutrition of the Embryo*. Springfield, Ill., Thomas, 1970.

Prenatal Care. Children's Bureau Publ. No. 4. Washington, D.C., H.E.W., 1962.

WHO: *Nutrition in Pregnancy and Lactation*. Tech. Report Series No. 302. Geneva, Switzerland, 1965.

Journal Articles:

Allen, C. E., et al: Vigorous weight reduction during pregnancy: Nitrogen balance before and during normal gestation. JAMA 188:392, 1964.

Applebaum, R. M.: The physician and a common sense approach to breast-feeding. Southern Med. J. 63:793, 1970.

Apte, S. V. and Lyengar L.: Composition of the human foetus. Brit. J. Nutr. 27:305, 1972.

Bartholomew, M. M. and Poston, F. E.: Effect of food taboos on prenatal nutrition. J. Nutr. Educa. 2:15, 1970.

Beal, V. A.: Breast- and formula-feeding in infants. J. Am. Dietet. A. 55:31, 1969.

———: Nutritional studies during pregnancy. I, Changes in intake of calories, carbohydrate, protein and calcium. II, Dietary intake, maternal weight gain and size of infant. J. Am. Dietet. A. 58:312, 321, 1971.

Beaton, G. H.: Some physiological adjustments relating to nutrition in pregnancy. Canad. Med. A. J. 95:622, 1966.

Beck, J.: Guarding the unborn. Today's Health 46:38, (January) 1968.

Brenner, W. E. and Hendricks, C. H.: Interdependence of blood pressure, weight gain, and fetal weight during normal human pregnancy. Health Service Reports 87:236, 1972.

Bruhn, C. M. and Pangborn, R. M.: Reported incidence of pica among migrant families. J. Am. Dietet. A. 58:417, 1971.

Butler, N. R., Goldstein, M. and Ross, E. M.: Cigarette smoking in pregnancy: Its influence on birth weight and perinatal mortality. Brit. Med. J. 5806:127, (April 15) 1972.

Butterworth, C. E.: Interactions of nutrients with oral contraceptives and other drugs. J. Am. Dietet. A. 62:510, 1973.

Cantlie, G. S. D., et al: Iron and folate nutrition in a group of private obstetrical patients. Am. J. Clin. Nutr. 24:637, 1971.

Chanarin, I.: Folate metabolism in pregnancy. Nutrition 27:7, (February) 1973.

Chopra, J. G.: Effect of steroid contraceptives on lactation. Am. J. Clin. Nutr. 25:1202, 1972.

Crosby, W. H.: Food pica and iron deficiency. Arch. Intern. Med. 127:960, 1971.

Davidoff, F., et al: Marked hyperlipidemia and pancreatitis associated with oral contraceptive therapy. N. Eng. J. Med. 289:552, 1973.

Editorial: Calorie requirements of breast feeding. Brit. Med. J. 3:721, 1970.

Editorial: Pregnant weight watchers wreck harm to babies. Publ. Health Rep. 85:964, 1970.

Edwards, C. H., et al: Effect of clay and cornstarch intake on women and their infants. J. Am. Dietet. A. 44:109, 1964.

Gold, E. M.: Interconceptional care. J. Am. Dietet. A. 55:27, 1969.

Halsted, J. A.: Geophagia in man: its nature and nutritional effects. Am. J. Clin. Nutr. 21:1384, 1968.

Harfouche, J. K.: The importance of breast-feeding. J. Trop. Ped. 16:134, 1970.

Harrill, I., Lynch, L., and L. Shipman, D.: Nutritive value of foods selected during pregnancy. J. Am. Dietet. A. 63:164, 1973.

Hillman, R. W. and Conway, H. C.: Season of birth and relative body weight. Am. J. Clin. Nutr. 25:279, 1972.

Holly, R. G.: Dynamics of iron metabolism in pregnancy. Am. J. Obst. & Gynec. 93:370, 1965.

Jacobson, H. N.: Nutrition and pregnancy. J. Am. Dietet. A. 60:26, 1972.

———: Nutrition in pregnancy—a critique. JAMA 225:634, 1973.

Kagan, B. M., et al: Body composition of premature infants: relation to nutrition. Am. J. Clin. Nutr. 25:1153, 1972.

Kramer, M. E.: Role of nutrition in pre-eclampsia: Correspondence. N. Eng. J. Med. 289:45, (July 5) 1973.

Kroger, M.: Insecticide residues in human milk. J. Pediat. 80:401,1972.

Landesman, R. and Knapp, R. C.: Diagnosis and treatment of toxemias of pregnancy. I and II. N.Y. State J. Med. 60:3830, 1960.

Larson, R. H.: Effect of prenatal nutrition on oral structures. J. Am. Dietet. A. 44:368, 1964.

Lesser, A. J.: Progress in maternal and child health. Children Today, 1:7, (March-April) 1972.

Lindheimer, M. D. and Katz, A. I.: Sodium and diuretics in pregnancy. N. Eng. J. Med. 288:891, 1973.

Little, B.: Current concepts: Treatment of preeclampsia. N. Eng. J. Med. 270:94, 1964.

Lowenstein, L. et al: The incidence and prevention of folate deficiency in a pregnant clinic population. Canad. Med. A. J. 95:797, 1966.

Malnutrition during pregnancy. (Medical News) JAMA 212:44, 1970.

Matoth, Y., et al: Studies on folic acid in infancy. 3, Folates in breast-fed infants and their mothers. Am. J. Clin. Nutr. 16:356, 1965.

McGarry, J. M. and Andrews, J.: Smoking in pregnancy and vitamin B_{12} metabolism. Brit. Med. J. 5805:74 (April 8) 1972.

Metz, J.: Folate deficiency conditioned by lactation. Am. J. Clin. Nutr. 23:843, 1970.

Meyer, H. G.: Breast-feeding in the U.S. Clin. Pediat. 7:708, 1968.

Naeye, R. L., et al: Urban poverty: effects on prenatal nutrition. Science 166:1026, 1969.

Naismith, D. J.: The foetus as a parasite. Proc. Nutr. Soc. 28:25, 1969.

Nausea of pregnancy. (Questions and Answers.) JAMA 187:165, 1964.

Payton, E., et al: Dietary habits of 571 pregnant southern Negro women. J. Am. Dietet. A. 37:129, 1960.

Pike, R. L. and Smiciklas, H. A.: A reappraisal of sodium restriction during pregnancy. Int. J. Gynecol. Obstet. 10:1, 1972.

Pike, R. L.: Sodium intake during pregnancy. J. Am. Dietet. A. 44:176, 1964.

Pike, R. L. and Gursky, D. S.: Further evidence of deleterious effects produced by sodium restriction during pregnancy. Am. J. Clin. Nutr. 23:883, 1970.

Pitkin, R. M., et al: Maternal nutrition: a selective review of clinical topics. J. Obstet. Gynecol. 40:773, 1972.

Review: Diet, detoxification, and toxemia of pregnancy. Nutr. Rev. 21:269, 1963.

———: Intrauterine growth. Nutr. Rev. 22:266, 1964.

———: Lactation and composition of milk in undernourished mothers. Nutr. Rev. 33:42, 1975.

———: Maternal nutrition and fetal growth. Nutr. Rev. 32:241, 1974.

———: Maternity care: The world situation. WHO Chronicle 21:140, 1967.

———: Metabolic adaptation to pregnancy. Nutr. Rev. 32:270, 1974.

———: Paraphagia and anemia. Nutr. Rev. 27:52, 1969.

———: The caloric cost of pregnancy. Nutr. Rev. 31:177, 1973.

———: Vigorous weight reduction during pregnancy. Nutr. Rev. 22:237, 1964.

Robertson, E. G.: The natural history of oedema during pregnancy. J. Obstet. Gynaec. Brit. Commonw. 78:520, 1971.

Roeder, L. M.: Long-term effects of maternal and infant feeding. Am. J. Clin. Nutr. 26:1120, 1973.

Schmitt, M. H.: Superiority of breast feeding—fact or fancy? Am. J. Nursing. 70:1488, 1970.

Semmens, J. P.: Implications of teen-age pregnancy. Obstet. Gynec. 26:77, 1965.

Smith, F.: Dietary habits of girls pregnant at 16 or under. Public Health Rep. 84:213, 1969.

Smoking, pregnancy and development of the offspring. Nutr. Rev., 31:143, 1973.

Sodium intake in pregnancy: two views. JAMA, 200:42, 1967.

Stevens, H. A., and Ohlson, M. A.: Nutritive value of the diets of medically indigent pregnant women. J. Am. Dietet. A., 50:290, 1967.

Streiff, R. R. and Little, A. B.: Folic acid deficiency in pregnancy. N. Eng. J. Med. 276:776, 1967.

Thomson, A. M., et al: The energy cost of human lactation. Brit. J. Nutr. 24:565, 1970.

Widdowson, E. M.: How the foetus is fed. Proc. Nutr. Soc. 28:17, 1969.

Woody, D. C. and Woody, H. B.: Management of breast feeding. J. Pediat. 68:344, 1966.

nutrition during infancy and early childhood

Books and Pamphlets:

A Practical Guide to Combating Malnutrition in the Preschool Child. *Nutritional Rehabilitation through Maternal Education*. New York, Appleton-Century-Crofts, 1970.

Beech-Nut, Inc.: *Nutritive Values and Ingredients of Beech-nut Baby Foods*. Canajoharie, N. Y., Beech-Nut, Inc., 1969.

Fomon, S. J.: *Infant Nutrition*, ed. 2. Philadelphia, Saunders, 1974.

———: *Prevention of Iron-Deficiency Anemia in Infants and Children of Preschool Age*. P.H.S. Publ. No. 2085. Washington, D.C., DHEW, 1970.

Gerber Products Co.: *Nutritive Values of Gerber Baby Foods*. Fremont, Mich., Gerber Products Co., 1966.

How to make a baby's formula: by terminal heat method, by aseptic method, by tap water method. Chicago, Ill., Evaporated Milk Assn.

Hunt, E. P.: *Recent Demographic Trends and Their Effects on Maternal and Child Health Needs and Services*. Children's Bureau, Washington, D.C., DHEW, 1966.

Nelson, W. E., Vaughn, V. C., and McKay, R. J.: *Textbook of Pediatrics*, ed. 9. Philadelphia, Saunders, 1969.

Spock, B.: *Baby and Child Care*, rev. ed. New York, Hawthorn, 1968.

Journal Articles:

Aykroyd, W. R.: Nutrition and mortality in infancy and early childhood: past and present relationships. Am. J. Clin. Nutr. 24:480, 1971.

Beal, V. A.: Termination of night feeding in infancy. J. Pediat. 75:690, 1969.

Brown, R. E.: Breast feeding in modern times. Am. J. Clin. Nutr. 26:556, 1973.

Caldwell, M. D., Jonsson, H. T., and Othersen, H. B.: Essential fatty acid deficiency in an infant receiving prolonged parenteral alimentation. J. Pediat. 81:894, 1972.

Chinn, P. L.: Infant gavage feeding. Am. J. Nurs. 71:1964 (October) 1971.

Committee on Nutrition, American Acad. of Pediatrics: Salt intake and eating patterns of infants and children in relation to blood pressure. Pediatrics 53:115, 1974.

Cowell, C., et al: Survey of infant feeding practices. Am. J. Public Health 63:138, 1973.

Davies, D. P.: Plasma osmolality and feeding practices of healthy infants in first three months. Brit. Med. J. 2:340, (May 12) 1973.

Dreizen, S.: The importance of nutrition in tooth development. J. School Health 43:114, 1973.

Emmons, L. and Hayes, M.: Nutrition knowledge of mothers and children. J. Nutr. Educa. 5:134, 1973.

Filer, L. J., Jr.: Modified food starches for use in infant foods. Nutr. Rev. 29:55, 1971.

——: Salt in infant foods. Nutr. Rev. 29:27, 1971.

French, J. G.: Relationship of morbidity to the feeding patterns of Navajo children from birth through 24 months. Am. J. Clin. Nutr. 20:375, 1967.

Fryer, B. A., et al: Growth of preschool children in the North Central Region. J. Am. Dietet. A. 60:30, 1972.

Gibbs, J. M.: Cleft palate babies: one mother's experience. Bedside Nurse/Nursing Care, 6:19, 1973.

Guthrie, H. A., Owen, G. A. and Guthrie, G. M.: Factor analysis of measures of nutritional status of preschool children. Am. J. Clin. Nutr. 26:497, 1973.

Hepner, R. and Maidin, N. C.: Growth rate, nutrient intake and "mothering" as determinants of malnutrition in disadvantaged children. Nutr. Rev. 29:219, 1971.

Husband, J., et al: Gastric emptying of starch meals in the newborn. Lancet 2:290, 1970.

Icaza, S. J.: The nutritionist caring for malnourished children. J. Am. Dietet. A. 63:130, 1973.

Jelliffe, D. B. and Jelliffe, E. F. P.: A bookshelf of nutrition programs from preschool children—a recent selected bibliography. Am. J. Publ. Health 62:469, 1972.

Juhas, L.: Nutrition education in day care programs. J. Am. Dietet. A. 63:134, 1973.

Kagan, B. M., et al: Body composition of premature infants: relation to nutrition. Am. J. Clin. Nutr. 25:1153, 1972.

Kennel, W. R. and Dawber, T. R.: Atherosclerosis as a pediatric problem. J. Pediat. 80:544, 1972.

Ladas, A.: Breastfeeding: The less available option. Monograph #25. J. Tropical Pediatrics and Environmental Child Health 18:317, 1972.

Lowe, C. V.: Research in infant nutrition: the untapped well. Food and Nutrition Notes and Reviews 30:1, 1973.

Mackenzie, E. P.: Psychologic factors in milk anemia. Amer. Family Physician 7:80, 1973.

Mayer, J.: Hypertension, salt intake, and the infant. Postgrad. Med. 45:229, 1969.

O'Grady, R. S.: Feeding behavior in infants. Am. J. Nurs. 71:736, (April) 1971.

Review: Lactoferrin—a bacteriostatic protein in human milk, Nutr. Rev. 30:225, 1972.

——: Overfeeding in the first year of life. Nutr. Rev. 31:116, 1973.

Rubini, M. E.: The many-faceted mystique of mono-sodium glutamate. (Editorial.) Am. J. Clin. Nutr. 24:169, 1971.

Pildes, R. S.: Infants of diabetic mothers. N. Eng. J. Med. 289:902, 1973.

Pollitt, E.: Behavior of infant in causation of nutritional marasmus. Am. J. Clin. Nutr. 26:264, 1973.

Widdowson, E. M.: Food intake and growth in the newlyborn. Proc. Nutr. Soc. 30:127, 1971.

Whitten, C. F., et al: Evidence that growth failure from maternal deprivation is secondary to undereating. JAMA 209:1675, 1969.

Ziegler, E. G. and Fomon, S. J.: Fluid intake, renal solute load, and water balance in infancy. J. Pediat. 78:561, 1971.

MINERALS IN INFANT NUTRITION

Journal Articles:

Al-Rashid, R. A., and Spangler, J.: Neonatal copper deficiency. N. Eng. J. Med. 285:841, 1971.

Andelman, M. B. and Sered, B. R.: Utilization of dietary iron by term infants. Am. J. Dis. Child. 111:45, 1966; 113:403, 1967.

Beal, V. A., et al: Iron intake, hemoglobin and physical growth during the first two years of life. Pediatrics 30:518, 1962.

Committee on Nutrition: Iron balance and requirements in infancy. Pediatrics 43:134, 1969.

Coussins, H.: Magnesium metabolism in infants and children. Postgrad. Med. 46:135, 1969.

Editorial: Iron deficiency in infants. JAMA 195:175, 1966.

Filer, L. J. and Martinez, G. A.: Calorie and iron intake by infants in the United States: an evaluation of 4000 representative six-month olds. Clin. Pediat. 2:470, 1963.

Hunter, R. E. and Smith, N. J.: Hemoglobin and hematocrit values in iron deficiency in infancy. J. Pediat. 81:710, 1972.

Krupke, S. S. and Sanders, E.: Prevalence of iron-deficiency anemia among infants and young children seen at rural ambulatory clinics. Am. J. Clin. Nutr. 23:716, 1970.

Review: Calcium deficiency in malnourished infants. Nutr. Rev. 23:164, 1965.

VITAMINS IN INFANT NUTRITION

Journal Articles:

Bakwin, M.: The overuse of vitamins in children. J. Pediat. 59:154, 1961.

Committee on Nutrition: Infantile scurvy and nutritional rickets in the U.S. Pediatrics 29:646, 1962.

Davis, K. C.: Vitamin E content of selected baby foods. J. Food Science 38:442, 1973.

Fomon, S. J., et al: Influence of vitamin D on linear growth of normal full-term infants. J. Nutr. 88:345, 1966.

Herting, D. C. and Drury, E. E.: Vitamin E content of milk, milk products and simulated milks: Relevance to infant nutrition. Am. J. Clin. Nutr. 22:147, 1969.

Ossofsky, H. J.: Infantile scurvy. Am. J. Dis. Child. 109:173, 1965.

Samuel, P. D. and Burland, W. L.: Response to oral administration of pteroylmonoglutamic acid or pteroylpolyglutamate in newborn infants of low birth weight. Brit. J. Nutr. 30:165, 1973.

MILKS

Journal Articles:

Berenberg, W., et al: Hazards of skimmed milk, unboiled and boiled. Pediatrics 44:734, 1969.

Committee on Nutrition: Appraisal of nutritional adequacy of infant formulas used as cow milk substitutes. Pediatrics 31:329, 1963.

Fomon, S. J.: Skim milk in infant feeding. J. Am. Dietet. A. 63:156, 1973.

Fomon, S. J., et al: Excretion of fat by normal full-term infants fed various milk and formulas. Am. J. Clin. Nutr. 23:1299, 1970.

Fomon, S. J., et al: Relationship between formula concentration and rate of growth of normal infants. J. Nutrition 98:241, 1969.

Jackson, R. L., et al: Growth of "well-born" American infants fed human and cow's milk. Pediatrics 33:642, 1964.

Lanin, S., et al: Lead content of milk fed to infants: 1971-72. N. Eng. J. Med. 289:574, 1973.

Owen, G. M.: Modification of cow's milk for infant formulas: Current practices. Am. J. Clin. Nutr. 22:1150, 1969.

Rivera, J.: The frequency of use of various kinds of milk during infancy in middle and lower income families. Am. J. Publ. Health 61:277, 1971.

Smith, C. A.: Overuse of milk in the diets of infants. JAMA 172:567, 1960.

ADDITION OF SOLID FOODS

Journal Articles:

Anderson, T. A. and Fomon, S. J.: Commercially prepared infant cereals: Nutritional considerations. J. Pediat. 78:788, 1971.

————: Commercially prepared strained and junior foods for infants: Nutritional considerations. J. Am. Dietet. A. 58:520, 1971.

Beal, V. A.: On the acceptance of solid foods and other food patterns of infants and children. Pediatrics 20:448, 1957.

Committee on Nutrition: On the feeding of solid foods to infants. Pediatrics 21:685, 1958.

Fomon, S. J., et al: Acceptance of unsalted strained foods by normal infants. J. Pediat. 76:242, 1970.

Jelliffe, D. B.: Commerciogenic malnutrition. Food Tech. 25:55, 1971.

McIntosh, E. M.: Let's talk about baby foods. What's New in Home Economics 35:25, 1971.

Review: Solid foods in the nutrition of young infants. Nutr. Rev. 25:233, 1967.

The use and care of baby's food. What's New in Home Economics 35:93, 1971.

nutrition of children and youth

(SEE ALSO REFERENCES UNDER PROTEINS, MINERALS, VITAMINS)

GENERAL

Books and Pamphlets:

David, L.: Slimming for Teenagers. New York, Pocket Books, 1966.

György, P. and Burgess, A.: Protecting the Pre-School Child. London, Tavistock, 1965.

Hamill, P. V.; Johnston, T. E., and Lemeshow, S.: Height and weight of children: socioeconomic status, United States. Vital and Health Statistics, Series II, No. 119 DHEW Publ. No. (HSM) 73-1601, Washington, D.C., 1972.

Heald, F. P. (ed.): Adolescent Nutrition and Growth. New York, Appleton-Century-Crofts, 1969.

Height and Weight of Youths 12-17 Years, U.S. Vital and Health Statistics, Series II, No. 124, DHEW Publ. No. (HSM) 73-1606, Washington, D.C., 1973.

Hill, M. M.: Food Choices of the Teen-age Girl. New York, Nutrition Foundation, 1966.

McWilliams, M.: Nutrition for the Growing Years. New York, Wiley, 1967.

Moore, W. M., Silverberg, M. M., and Read, M. S.: Nutrition, Growth and Development of North American Indian Children. DHEW Publication No. (NIH) 72-26, Washington, D.C., 1972.

Nutrition for Athletes. A Handbook for Coaches. American Association for Health, Physical Education and Recreation, Washington, D.C., 1971.

Preschool Malnutrition: Primary Deterrent to Human Progress. Washington, D.C., National Academy of Sciences-National Research Council Publ. No. 1281, 1966.

Salmon, M. B.: Food Facts for Teenagers. Springfield, Ill., Thomas, 1965.

Selected Body Measurements of Children 6-11 years. U.S. DHEW Publ. (HSM) 73-1605, Series II, No. 123, Washington, D. C., 1973. Skinfold Thickness of Children 6-11 Years. U.S. Vital and Health Statistics Series II No. 12 DHEW Publ. No. (HSM) 73-1602, Washington, D.C., 1973.

Tanner, J. M.: Growth at Adolescence. Oxford, England, Blackwell Scientific Publications, 1962.

WHO Expert Committee: Health Problems of Adolescence. WHO Publ. No. 308. Geneva, Switzerland, 1965.

Journal Articles:

Beal, V. A.: Nutrition in a longitudinal growth study. J. Am. Dietet. A. 46:457, 1965.

Blackburn, M. L.: Who turns the child "off" to nutrition? J. Nutr. Educa. 2:45, 1970.

Cabacungan, N. B., et al: Hydroxyproline excretion and nutritional status of children. Am J. Clin. Nutr. 26:173, 1973.

Chamberlain, V. M. and Kelly, J.: Nutrition and notable characters. What's New in Home Economics 37:77, 1973.

Eliot. M. M.: Six decades of action for children. Children Today, 1:2, (March, April) 1972.

Emmons, L., Hayes, M.: Accuracy of 24-hr. recalls of young children. J. Am. Dietet. A. 62:409, 1973.

Frey, A. L. et al.: Comparison of Type A and nutrient standard menus for school lunch, I, Development of the Nutrient Standard Method (NSM). J. Am. Dietet. A. 66:242, 1975.

Friedman, G. and Goldberg, S. J.: Normal serum cholesterol values. Percentile ranking in a middle-class pediatric population. JAMA 225:610, 1973.

Futrell, M. F., Kilgore, L. T., and Windham, F.: Nutritional status of black preschool children in Mississippi. Influence of income, mother's education and food programs. J. Am. Dietet. A. 66:22, 1975.

Getty, G. and Hollinsworth, M.: Through a child's eye seeing. Nutrition Today 2:17, (June) 1967.

Gussow, J. D.: Improving the American Diet. J. Home Econ. 65:6 (November) 1973.

Harper, J. M., et al: Comparison of Type A and Nutrient Standard Menus for school lunch, II, Management aspects. J. Am. Dietet. A. 66:249, 1975.

Hutcheson, R. H. and Hutcheson, J. K.: Iron and vitamin C and D deficiencies in a large population of children. Health Ser. Rep. 87:232, 1972.

Jansen, G. R., et al: Comparison of Type A and Nutrient Standard Menus for school lunch, III, Nutritive content of menus and acceptability. J. Am. Dietet. A. 66:254, 1975.

Lukaczer, M.: The National School Lunch Program in 1973: Some accomplishments and failures. Nutr. Rev. 31:385, 1973.

Lyng, R. E.: Child nutrition—a proud record. School Foodservice J. 26:21, 1972.

Malina, R. M.: Weight, height, and limb circumference in American Negro and white children: longitudinal observations over a one year period. J. Tropical Pediatrics and Environmental Child Health 18:280, 1972.

Odland, L. M., et al: Bone density and dietary findings of 409 Tennessee subjects, I, Bone density considerations, II, Dietary Considerations, Am. J. Clin. Nutr. 25:905, 908, 1972.

Osman, J. D.: Nutrition education: too much, too little, or too bad? J. School Health 42:592, 1972.

Paige, D. M., Bayless, T. M., and Graham, G. C.: Milk programs: Helpful or harmful to Negro children. Am. J. Publ. Health 62:1486, 1972.

Puffer, R. R., and Serrano, C. V.: The role of nutritional deficiency in mortality in childhood. Boletin de la Oficina Sanitaria Panamericana. English edition, 7 (1):1, 1973.

Read, M. S.: Malnutrition, hunger and behavior, II, J. Am. Dietet. A. 63:386, 1973.

Reasoner, H.: Vitamins vs. vending machines. School Foodservice J. 27:70, 1973.

Wallace, H. M.: Nutrition and handicapped children, J. Am. Dietet. A. 61:127, 1972.

Walter, J. P.: Two poverties equal one hunger. J. Nutr. Educa. 5:129, 1973.

Watt, B., et al: Energy intake of well-nourished children and adolescents. Am. J. Clin. Nutr. 22:1383, 1969.

What is USDA doing about nutrition education. School Foodservice J. 27:31, 1973.

White, P. L.: New thoughts on dietary practices. School Foodservice J. 27:50, 1973.

Youlton, R., et al: Serum growth hormone and growth activity in children and adolescents with present or past malnutrition. Am J. Clin. Nutr. 25:1179, 1972.

PRESCHOOLERS
Journal Articles:

Armstrong, H.: Nutritional status of black preschool children in Mississippi. Assessment by food frequency scale. J. Am. Dietet. A. 66:488, 1975.

Crumrine, J. L. and Fryer, B. A.: Protein components of blood and dietary intake of preschool children. J. Am. Dietet. A. 57:509, 1970.

Dierks, E. C. and Morse, L. M.: Food habits and nutrient intakes of pre-school children. J. Am. Dietet. A. 47:292, 1965.

Driskell, J. A. and Price, C. S.: Nutritional status of preschoolers from low-income Alabama families. J. Am. Dietet. A. 65:280, 1974.

Eppright, E. S., et al: Eating behavior of preschool children. J. Nutr. Educa. 1:16, 1969.

———: The North Central Regional study of diets of preschool. 2. Nutrition knowledge and attitudes of mothers. 3. Frequency of eating. J. Home Econ. 62:372, 407, 1970.

Fox, H. M., et al.: Diets of preschool children in the North Central Region. Calcium, Phosphorus and Iron. J. Am. Dietet. A. 59:233, 1971.

———: The North Central Regional study of diets of preschool children. 1. Family environment. J. Home Econ. 62:241, 1970.

Fryer, B. A., et al.: Diets of preschool children in the North Central Region. Calories, protein, fat and carbohydrate. J. Am. Dietet. A. 59:228, 1971.

Futrell, M. F., et al.: Nutritional status of Negro preschool children in Mississippi. Evaluation of HOP Index. Impact of education and income. J. Am. Dietet. A. 59:218, 224, 1971.

Gutelius, M. F.: The problems of iron deficiency anemia in preschool Negro children. Am. J. Public Health 59:290, 1969.

Harrison, H. E.: The disappearance of rickets. Am. J. Public Health 56:734, 1966.

Hookworm and nutrition. Postgrad. Med. 46:191, 1969.

Juhas, L.: Nutrition education and the development of language, J. Nutr. Educa. 1:12, 1969.

Kerrey, E., et al: Nutritional status of preschool children. I. Dietary and biochemical findings. Am. J. Clin. Nutr. 21:1274, 1968.

Owen, G. M. and Kram, K. M.: Nutritional status of preschool children in Mississippi: Food sources of nutrients in the diets. J. Am. Dietet. A. 54:490, 1969.

Owen, G. M., et al: Nutritional status of Mississippi preschool children. A pilot study. Am. J. Clin. Nutr. 22:1444, 1969.

Owen, G. M., et al: A study of nutritional status of preschool children in the U.S. 1968-70. Pediatrics 53:4 (Part II) Supplement (April) 1974.

Sulby, A. B., et al: Family day care: the nutritional component. Children Today 2:12, (May-June) 1973.

Tepley, L. J.: Nutritional needs of the preschool child. Nutr. Rev. 22:65, 1964.

The American Dietetic Association: Position paper on food and nutrition services in day-care centers. J. Am. Dietet. A. 59:47, 1971.

Van Duzen, J. P., et al: Protein and calorie malnutrition among preschool Navajo Indian children. Am. J. Clin. Nutr. 22:1362, 1969.

THE SCHOOL AGE CHILD
Journal Articles:

Abernathy, R. P., et al: Lack of response to amino acid supplements by preadolescent girls. Am. J. Clin. Nutr. 25:980, 1972.

Agran, P.: The National School Lunch Program. J. School Health 39:440, 1969.

Council on Foods and Nutrition, A.M.A.: Confections and carbonated beverages in schools. JAMA 180:92, 1962.

Eppright, E. S. and LeBaron, H. R.: Our responsibilities to children and youth. J. Am. Dietet. A. 38:354, 1961.

Lantis, M.: The child consumer; cultural factors influencing his food choices. J. Home Econ. 54:370, 1962.

Myers, M. L., et al: A nutrition study of school children in a depressed urban district. I. Dietary findings. J. Am. Dietet. A. 53:226, 1968.

Paige, D. M.: School feeding program: who should receive what? J. School Health 41:261, 1971.

Review: The effects of a balanced lunch program on the growth and nutritional status of school children. Nutr. Rev. 23:35, 1965.

Saratscotis, J. B. and Gordon, J.: Nutritional status of primary school pupils in Baltimore. H.S.M.H. Health Reports 86:302, 1971.

Sodowsky, J. D.: In-service nutrition education for elementary teachers. J. Nutr. Educa. 5:139, 1973.

Todhunter, E. N.: School feeding from a nutritionist's point of view. Am. J. Public Health 60:2302, 1970.

ADOLESCENTS
Journal Articles:

Daniels, A. M.: Training school nurses to work with groups of adolescents. Children 13:210, (Nov.-Dec.) 1966.

Dwyer, J. T., et al: Nutritional literacy of high school students. J. Nutr. Educa. 2:59, 1970.

Edwards, C. H., et al: Nutrition survey of 6200 teenage youth. J. Am. Dietet. A. 45:543, 1964.

Gaines, E. G. and Daniel, W. A.: Dietary iron intakes of adolescents. Relations of sex, race, and sex maturity ratings. J. Am. Dietet. A. 65:275, 1974.

Hampton, M. C., et al: Caloric and nutrient intakes of teenagers. J. Am. Dietet. A. 50:385, 1967.

Heydon, S., et al: Weight reduction in adolescents. Nutr. Metab. 15:45, 1973.

Huenemann, R. L.: A study of teenagers: body size and shape, dietary practices and physical activity. Food and Nutrition News 37:7, (April) 1966. (Nat. Live Stock and Meat Board.)

Huenemann, R. L., et al: Food and eating practices of teenagers. J. Am. Dietet. A. 53:17, 1968.

Huenemann, R. L.: A review of teenage nutrition in the U.S. Health Ser. Rep. 87:823, 1973.

Johnson, J. A.: Nutritional aspects of adolescence. J. Pediatrics 59:741, 1961.

Kaufman, N. A., et al: Eating habits and opinions of teenagers on nutrition and obesity. J. Am. Dietet. A. 66:264, 1975.

King, J. C., et al: Assessment of nutritional status of teenage pregnant girls, I, Nutrient intake and pregnancy. Am. J. Clin. Nutr. 25:916, 1972.

Law, H. M., et al: Sophomore high school students attitudes toward school lunch. J. Am. Dietet. A. 60:38, 1972.

Mitchell, H. S.: Protein limitation and human growth. J. Am. Dietet. A. 44:165, 1964.

Morse, E. H., et al: Changes in blood constituents of adolescents. Am. J. Clin. Nutr. 25:269, 1972.

Nutritional implications of some problems of adolescents. Dairy Council Digest 38:25, (September-October) 1967.

Stare, F. J., and Dwyer, J.: An eye to the future: healthy eating for teenagers. J. School Health 39:595, 1969.

Thomas, J. A. and Call, D. L.: Eating between meals—a nutrition problem among teenagers. Nutr. Rev. 31:137, 1973.

Vande Mark, M. S. and Underwood, V. R. S.: Dietary habits and food consumption patterns of teenage families. J. Home Econ. 63:540, 1971.

Webb, T. E. and Oski, F. A.: Iron deficiency anemia and scholastic achievement in young adolescents. J. Pediat. 82:827, 1973.

Yoshimura, H.: Anemia during physical training (sports anemia). Nutr. Rev. 28:251, 1970.

geriatric nutrition

Books and Pamphlets:

Howell, S. C. and Loeb, M. B.: Nutrition and aging: A Monograph for Practitioners. Washington, D. C., Gerontological Society, 1970.

Institute of Rehabilitative Medicine, New York University Medical Center: Mealtime Manual for the Aged and Handicapped. New York, Simon & Schuster (Essandess Special Editions), 1970.

Mathiasen, G.: The Golden Years—A Tarnished Myth. The National Council on Aging, Washington, D. C., 1970.

Oregon State Univ.: Guide to Effective Project Operations: The Nutrition Program for the Elderly. Administration on Aging, Washington, D.C. DHEW, 1973.

Timiras, P. S.: Developmental Physiology and Aging. New York, Macmillan, 1972.

Journal Articles:

Anderson, E. L.: Eating patterns before and after dentures. J. Am. Dietet. A. 58:421, 1971.

Balabokin, M. E., et al: Health and nutrition, Gerontologist 12:21, 1972.

Balsley, M., et al: Nutrition in disease and stress. Geriatrics 26:87, 1971.

Barrows, C. H.: Nutrition, aging and geriatric programs. Am. J. Clin. Nutr. 25:829, 1972.

Bechill, W. D. and Wolgamat, I.: Nutrition for the Elderly, DHEW Pub. No. (ses) 73-20236, Washington, D. C., 1973.

Berman, P. M. and Kirsner, J. B.: The aging gut. 2. Diseases of the colon, pancreas, liver and gallbladder, functional bowel disease and iatrogenic disease. Geriatrics 27:117, 1972.

Bernstein, D. S.: Prevalence of osteoporosis in high- and low-fluoride areas in North Dakota. JAMA 198:499, 1966.

Bullamore, J. R., et al: Effect of age on calcium absorption. Lancet, No. 7672:535, (September 12) 1970.

Caniggia, A.: Senile osteoporosis, J. Am. Dietet. A. 47:49, 1965.

Cashman, J. W., et al: Nutritionists, dietitians and Medicare. J. Am. Dietet. A. 50:17, 1967.

Cheraskin, E. et al: The exercise profile. J. Am. Geriatrics Soc. 21:208, 1973.

Clark, M., and Wakefield, L. M.: Food choices of institutionalized vs. independent-living elderly. J. Am. Dietet. A. 66:600, 1975.

Cooking classes help older Britons eat better, JAMA 222:523, 1972.

daCosta, F. and Moorhouse, J. A.: Protein malnutrition in aged individuals on self-selected diets. Am. J. Clin. Nutr. 22:1618, 1969.

Dibble, M. V., et al: Evaluation of the nutritional status of elderly subjects, with a comparison of Fall and Spring. J. Am. Geriat. Soc. 15:1031, 1967.

Eccleston, E. M. and Hamilton, L. W.: Guidelines for Meals-on-Wheels and Congregate Meals for the Elderly. Pennsylvania Dietetic Assn., PO Box 608, Camp Hill, PA, 17011.

Eckerstrom, S.: Clinical aspects of metabolism in the elderly. Geriatrics 21:161, 1966.

Exton-Smith, A. N.: Physiological aspects of aging: relationship to nutrition. Am. J. Clin. Nutr. 25:853, 1972.

Gordon, B. M.: A feeding plan for geriatric patients. Hospitals 39:92, (April 16) 1965.

Gorton, L. A.: Feeding the elderly for love or money. Cooking for Profit 41:78, 1972.

Greenberg, B.: Reaction time in the elderly. Am. J. Nurs. 73:2056, (December) 1973.

Gress, L. D.: Sensitizing students to the aged. Am. J. Nurs. 71:1968, (October) 1971.

Guggenheim, K. and Margulee, I.: Factors in the nutrition of elderly people living alone or as couples and receiving community assistance. J. Am. Geriat. Soc. 13:561, 1965.

Guthrie, H. A., Black, K., and Maddan, J. P.: Nutritional practices of elderly citizens in rural Pennsylvania. Gerontologist 12:330, 1972.

Harmon, D.: Free radical theory of aging: dietary implications. Am. J. Clin. Nutr. 25:839, 1972.

Hawthorne, B.: A training program for project directors in the nutrition program for the elderly. J. Home Econ. 65:23, 1973.

Hegsted, D. M.: Nutrition, bone and calcified tissue. J. Am. Dietet. A. 50:105, 1967.

Henriksen, B. and Cate, H. D.: Nutrient content of food served vs. food eaten in nursing homes. J. Am. Dietet. A. 59:126, 1971.

Jackson, M. L.: HUD's role in the interagency action in nutrition and aging. Am. J. Clin. Nutr. 26:1124, 1973.

Jernigan, A. K.: Home delivered meals as a hospital service. Hospitals 43:90, (September 16) 1969.

Joering, E.: Nutrient contribution of a meals program for senior citizens. J. Am. Dietet. A. 59:129, 1971.

Jones, F. A.: The skin: a mirror of the gut. Geriatrics 28:75, 1973.

Jowsey, J., et al: Effect of combined therapy with sodium fluoride, vitamin D and calcium in osteoporosis. Am. J. Med. 53:43, 1972.

Justice, C. L., et al: Dietary intakes and nutritional status of elderly patients. J. Am. Dietet. A. 63:639, 1974.

Kahn, A. J.: Development, aging, and life duration effects of nutrient restriction. Am. J. Clin. Nutr. 25:822, 1972.

Lane, M. M.: A psychiatrist speaks to dietitians: Nursing Homes 21:28, 1973.

Luhrs, R. E.: Feeding the elderly. Am. J. Clin. Nutr. 26:1150, 1973.

Lukaczer, M.: Lessons for the federal effort against hunger and malnutrition—from a case study. Am. J. Publ. Health 61:259, 1971.

Manning, A. M. and Means, J. G.: A self-feeding program for geriatric patients in a skilled nursing facility. J. Am. Dietet. A. 66:275, 1975.

McCarthy, L. W.: Motivate . . . don't manipulate. Nursing Homes 20:36, 1971.

Meals-on-wheels avert hospitalization. JAMA 222:531, 1972.

Nutrition and eating problems of the elderly . . . Current comment. J. Am. Dietet. A. 58:43, 1971.

Patients drink beer in hospital pub. (Medical News.), JAMA 212:1790, (June 15) 1970.

Pelcovits, J.: Nutrition for older Americans. J. Am. Dietet. A. 58:17, 1971.

Roman, E.: New foods to serve. Nursing Homes 20:14, 1971.

Ross, M. H.: Length of life and caloric intake. Am. J. Clin. Nutr. 25:834, 1972.

Schlenker, E. D., et al: Nutrition and health of older people. Am. J. Clin. Nutr. 26:1111, 1973.

Sebrell, W. H.: It's not age that interferes with nutrition of the elderly. Nutrition Today 1:15, (June) 1966.

Settle, E.: Correction of malnutrition in the aged; comparative efficacy of an anabolic hormone and enzyme vitamin complex. Geriatrics 21:173, 1966.

Sherman, E. M. and Brittan, M. R.: Contemporary food gatherers: A study of food shopping habits of an elderly urban population. Gerontologist 13:358, (Autumn) 1973.

Sherwood, S.: Sociology of food and eating: implications for action for the elderly. Am. J. Clin. Nutr. 26:1108, 1973.

Simko, M. D. and Colitz, K.: Nutrition and Aging—A selected Annotated Bibliography, 1964-72. DHEW, Publ. No. (ses) 73-20237. Washington, D. C.

Soika, C.: Combatting osteoporosis. Am. J. Nurs. 73:1193, (July) 1973.

Stone, V.: Give the older person time. Am. J. Nurs. 69:2124, 1969.

Swanson, P.: Adequacy in old age: I, Role of nutrition. II, Nutrition education program for the aging. J. Home Econ. 56:651, 728, 1964.

Symposium on Nutrition and Aging. Guest editor Donald M. Watkins: Am. J. Clin. Nutr. 25:809, (August), 1972, 26:1108 (October) 1973.

Tappel, A. L.: Will antioxidant nutrients slow aging processes? Geriatrics 23:97, 1968.

Todhunter, E. N.: Meaning of food to the consumer. Nursing Homes 22:22, 1973.

Tontisirin, K., et al: Plasma tryptophan response curve and tryptophan requirements of elderly people. J. Nutrition 103:1220, 1973.

Turner, T. B.: Beer and wine for geriatric patients. Editorial. JAMA 226:779, 1973.

Watkin, D. M.: Nutrition of older people. Am. J. Public Health 55:548, 1965.

Weiner, M. F.: A practical approach in encouraging geriatric patients to eat. J. Am. Dietet. A. 55:384, 1969.

Wells, C. E.: Nutrition programs under the older Americans Act. Am. J. Clin. Nutr. 26:1127, 1973.

Wolczuk, P.: The senior chef. J. Nutr. Ed. 5:142, 1973.

malnutrition—a world problem

Books and Pamphlets:

Berg, A. Scrimshaw, N. S., and Call, D. L.: *Nutrition, National Development and Planning.* Cambridge, Massachusetts, MIT Press, 1973.

FAO/WHO: *Handbook on Human Nutrition Requirements*, WHO Monograph Series No. 61, Rome, 1974.

Fitzpatrick, W. H.: *Nutrition Research in the U.S.S.R.*, 1961-1970. DHEW Publ. No. (NIH) 72-57. Washington, D.C., 1972.

May, J. M., and McLellan, D. L.: *The Ecology of Malnutrition in the Caribbean.* New York, Hafner Press, 1973.

_____: *The Ecology of Malnutrition in Seven Countries in Southern Africa and in Portuguese Guinea–Studies in Medical Geography*, Vol. 10. New York, Hafner Press, 1971.

Patwardhan, V. N. and Darby, W. J.: *The State of Nutrition in the Arab Middle East.* Vanderbilt University Press, Nashville, Tenn., 1972.

Robson, J. R. K.: *Malnutrition. Its Causation and Control*, Volumes I and II. New York, Gordon and Breach, 1972.

Western Hemisphere Nutrition Congress III. Mt. Kisco, New York, Futura Publishing Co., 1972.

Journal Articles:

Arena, J. M.: Nutritional status of China's children: an overview. Nutr. Rev. 32:289, 1974.

Berg, A. and Muscat, R.: An approach to nutrition planning. Am. J. Clin. Nutr. 25:939, 1972.

Bradfield, R. B.: A rapid tissue techinque for the field assessment of protein-calorie malnutrition. Am. J. Clin. Nutr. 25:720, 1972.

Committee 4/V, International Union of Nutritional Sciences: Training for dietitians and nutritionists: World survey and future guidelines. J. Am. Dietet. A. 63:157, 1973.

Coward, W. A. and Whitehead, R. G.: Changes in haemoglobin concentrations during the development of kwashiorkor. Brit. J. Nutr. 28:463, 1972.

Glick, Z. and Reshef, A.: Vitamin A status and related nutritional parameters of children in East Jerusalem. Am. J. Clin. Nutr. 26:1229, 1973.

Goldsmith, G. A.: Nutrition and world health. J. Am. Dietet. A. 63:513, 1973.

Habicht, J. A., et al: Biochemical indices of nutrition reflecting ingestion of a high protein supplement in rural Guatemalan children. Am. J. Clin. Nutr. 26:1046, 1973.

Hodges, R. E., et al: Clinical manifestations of ascorbic acid deficiency in man. Am. J. Clin. Nutr. 24:432, 1971.

IUNS Committee III-3-Nutrition programs for pre-school children; Zagreb guidelines. Nutr. Abst. Rev. 43:1, 1973.

Jelliffe, D. B.: Commerciogenic malnutrition. Nutr. Rev. 30:199, 1972.

Jelliffe, D. B. and Patrice, E. F.: Lactation, conception and the nutrition of the nursing mother and child. J. Pediat. 81:829, 1972.

Kinsman, R. A. and Hood, J.: Some behavioral effects of ascorbic acid deficiency. Am. J. Clin. Nutr. 24:444, 1971.

Lu, F. C.: Toxicological evaluation of food additives and pesticide residues: the role of WHO in conjunction with FAO. WHO Chronicle, 27:43, (February) 1973.

Melner, R. D. G.: Endocrine adaptation to malnutrition. Nutr. Rev. 30:103, 1972.

Oiso, R. and Suzue, R.: Topics of nutrition in Japan. Am. J. Clin. Nutr. 25:1215, 1972.

Omoluhi, A.: Nutrition and the African child. J. Tropical Pediatrics and Environmental Child Health 18:144, 1972.

Review: Cellular immunity and malnutrition. Nutr. Rev. 30:523, 1972.

_____: Endemic goiter and antithyroid agents. Nutr. Rev. 33:171, 1975.

_____: Water and electrolytes in malnutrition. Nutr. Rev. 33:74, 1975.

Riley, D. H.: Help for malnourished children in Latin America. J. Home Econ. 65:19, 1973.

Sauberlich, H. E., et al: Biochemical assessment of the nutritional status of the Eskimos of Wainwright, Alaska. Am. J. Clin. Nutr. 25:437, 1972.

Schertz, L. P.: Nutrition realities in the low income countries. Nutr. Rev. 31:201, 1973.

Scrimshaw, N. S., et al: Nutrition and infection field study in Guatemalan villages, 1959-1964. Arch. Environ. Health 18:56, 1969.

Someswara, R. K.: Malnutrition in the Eastern Mediterranean Region. WHO Chronicle 28:172, 1974.

Viteri, F. E., et al: Intestinal malabsorption before and during recovery. Relation between severity of protein deficiency and the malabsorption process. Am. J. Digestive Diseases 18:201, 1973.

Weisberg, S. M.: Exploiting grass-roots food technology in developing countries. Food Tech. 27:70, 1973.

Zaklama, M. S., et al: Serum vitamin A in protein-calorie malnutrition. Am. J. Clin. Nutr. 26:1202, 1973.

section three diet in disease

GENERAL REFERENCES

Books:

Brobeck, J. R., (ed.): *Best & Taylor's Physiological Basis of Medical Practice*, ed. 9. Baltimore, Williams & Wilkins Co., 1973.

Church, C. F. and Church, H. N.: *Food Values of Portions Commonly Used*, ed. 12, Philadelphia, J. B. Lippincott, 1975.

Davenport, H. W.: *Physiology of the Digestive Tract*, ed. 3. Chicago, Year Book Medical Pub., 1971.

Davidson, I. and Henry, J. B., eds.: *Todd-Sanford Clinical Diagnosis*, ed. 15. Philadelphia, Saunders, 1974.

Davidson, S., Passmore, R., and Brock, J. F.: *Human Nutrition and Dietetics*, ed. 6. Baltimore, Williams & Wilkins, 1975.

Dorland's Illustrated Medical Dictionary, ed. 25. Philadelphia, W. B. Saunders, 1974.

Fomon, S. J.: *Infant Nutrition*, ed. 2. Philadelphia, Saunders, 1974.

Goodhart, R. S. and Shils, M. E. (eds.): *Modern Nutrition in Health and Disease*, ed. 5. Philadelphia, Lea & Febiger, 1973.

Goodman, L. and Gilman, A.: *Pharmacological Basis of Therapeutics*, ed. 4. New York, Macmillan, 1970.

Guyton, A. C.: *Textbook of Medical Physiology*, ed. 4. Philadelphia, Saunders, 1971.

Latner, A. L.: *Cantarow and Trumper Clinical Biochemistry*, ed. 7. Philadelphia, Saunders, 1975.

Montgomery, R., et al: *Biochemistry: A Case-Oriented Approach*. St. Louis, Mosby, 1974.

Paul, P. C. and Palmer, H. H., eds.: *Food Theory and Application*. New York, Wiley, 1972.

Pike, R. L. and Brown, M. L.: *Nutrition: An Integrated Approach*, ed. 2. New York, Wiley, 1975.

Sabiston, D. C., Jr. (ed.): *Davis-Christopher Textbook of Surgery*, ed. 10. Philadelphia, Saunders, 1972.

Sleisenger, M. H. and Fordtran, J. S.: *Gastrointestinal Disease*: Pathophysiology, Diagnosis, Management. Philadelphia, Saunders, 1973.

Stanbury, J. B., Wyngaarden, J. B., and Fredrickson, D. S. (eds.): *The Metabolic Basis of Inherited Disease*, ed. 3. New York, McGraw-Hill, 1972.

Tepperman, J.: *Metabolic and Endocrine Physiology*, ed. 3. Chicago, Year Book Medical Pub., 1973.

Turner, D.: *Handbook of Diet Therapy*, ed. 5. Chicago, University of Chicago Press, 1970.

Vaughan, V. C., III, and McKay, R. J. (eds.): *Nelson Textbook of Pediatrics*, ed. 10, Philadelphia, Saunders, 1975.

Williams, R. H. (ed.): *Textbook of Endocrinology*, ed. 5. Philadelphia, Saunders, 1974.

Wintrobe, M. M., et al (eds.): *Harrison's Principles of Internal Medicine*, ed. 7. New York, McGraw-Hill, 1974.

Journals:

American Journal of Clinical Nutrition
American Journal of Digestive Diseases
American Journal of Diseases of Children
American Journal of Medicine
American Journal of Nursing
American Journal of Obstetrics and Gynecology
American Journal of Public Health
Archives of Internal Medicine
Bulletin New York Academy of Medicine
Diabetes
Gastroenterology
Gut
Journal of Clinical Investigation
Journal of Food Science
Journal of Home Economics
Journal of Pediatrics
Journal of the American Dietetic Association
Journal of the American Medical Association
Lancet
Metabolism
New England Journal of Medicine
Nursing Outlook
Nutrition Reviews
Pediatrics
Postgraduate Medicine
Public Health Reports

INTRODUCTION TO DIET THERAPY
Journal Articles:

Schiller M. R., Sr., and Vivian, V. M.: Role of the clinical dietitian. J. Am. Dietet. A. 65:284;287, 1974.

Stone, D. B.: A true role for the dietitian: a scholar in nutrition. J. Am. Dietet. A. 49:26, 1966.

Vargas, J. S.: Teaching as changing behavior. J. Am. Dietet. A. 58:512, 1971.

FEEDING THE HOSPITALIZED PATIENT
Books and Pamphlets:

Neelon, F. A. and Ellis, G. J.: *A Syllabus of Problem-Oriented Patient Care*. Boston, Little, Brown, 1974.

Journal Articles:

Problem-Oriented Record

Chappelle, M. L. and Scholl, R.: Adapting the problem-oriented medical record to the psychiatric hospital. J. Am. Dietet. A. 63:643, 1973.

Matthewson, G. H.: Contributing information to patient care plans. J. Am. Dietet. A. 63:45, 1973.

Rodgers, T. V. and Clark, M. E.: Sharing information by means of the patient's medical record. J. Am. Dietet. A. 63:42, 1973.

Voytovich, A. E.: The dietitian/nutritionist and the problem-oriented medical record, I, A physician's viewpoint. J. Am. Dietet. A. 63:639, 1973.

Walters, F. M. and DeMarco, M.: The dietitian/nutritionist and the problem-oriented medical record, II, The role of the dietitian. J. Am. Dietet. A. 63:641, 1973.

Weed, L. L.: Medical records that guide and teach. N. Eng. J. Med. 278:593; 652, 1968.

Food Service

Ford, M. C., and Neville, J. N.: Nutritive intake of nursing home patients served three or five meals a day. J. Am. Dietet. A. 61:292, 1972.

Moreland, P. L., and Lawson, C. H.: For contract food service management. Hospitals 44:105, (January) 1970.

Myers, W. W.: For the hospital food service manager. Hospitals 44:104, (January) 1970.

Schultz, H. G., et al: Hospital patients' and employees' reactions to food-use combinations. J. Am. Dietet. A. 60:207, 1972.

Systematic Management of Food Service: Special Issue. Hospitals 44: August 1, 1972.

FOOD COMPOSITION TABLES
Journal Articles:
Davis, K. C.: Vitamin E content of selected baby foods. J. Food Science 38:442, 1973.

Della Monica, E. S., et al: The quantitative determination of glucose, fructose and sucrose in fruits and potatoes. J. Food Science 39:1062, 1974.

Hansen, R. G.: An index of food quality. Nutrition Rev. 31:1, 1973.

Hardinge, M. G., Swarner, J. B., and Crooks, S.: Carbohydrates in foods. J. Am. Dietet. A. 46:197, 1965.

Itoh, I., et al: Sterol composition of 19 vegetable oils. J. Am. Oil Chem. Soc. 50:122, 1973.

Merrill, A. L.: Citrus fruit values in "Handbook No. 8," revised. J. Am. Dietet. A. 44:264, 1964.

Nutritive value and composition of cheese. Dairy Council Digest 46:13, 1975.

Stansby, M. E.: Polyunsaturates and fat in fish flesh. J. Am. Dietet. A. 63:625, 1973.

Watt, B. K.: Concepts in developing food composition tables. J. Am. Dietet. A. 40:297, 1962.

————: Revising the tables in Agriculture Handbook No. 8. J. Am. Dietet. A. 44:261, 1964.

Widdowson, E. M.: Development of British food composition tables. J. Am. Dietet. A. 50:363, 1967.

HANDICAPPING PROBLEMS
Books and Pamphlets:
Committee on Children with Handicaps: The Pediatrician and the Child with Mental Retardation. Evanston, Ill., American Academy of Pediarics, 1971.

Klinger, J. L., et al: Mealtime Manual for the Aged and Handicapped. New York, Simon & Schuster, 1970.

Robinault, I. P. (ed.): Functional Aids for the Multiply Handicapped. New York, Harper and Row, 1973.

Journal Articles:
Donaldson, C. L., et al: Effect of prolonged bed rest on bone mineral. Metabotism 19:1071, 1970.

Hyman, L. R., et al: Immobilization hypercalcemia. Am. J. Dis. Child. 124:723, 1972.

Jernigan, A. K.: Diet for the stroke patient. Hospitals 44:66, (June 16) 1970.

Wallace, H. M.: Nutrition and handicapped children. J. Am. Dietet. A. 61:127, 1972.

GASTROINTESTINAL DISEASES
Books and Pamphlets:
Creamer, B. (ed.): The Small Intestine. Chicago, Year Book Medical Pub., 1974.

Davenport, H. W.: Physiology of the Digestive Tract, ed. 3. Chicago, Year Book Medical Pub., 1971.

Sleisenger, M. H. and Fordtran, J. S. eds.: Gastrointestinal Disease. Philadelphia, Saunders, 1973.

Journal Articles:

Peptic Ulcer—Diet
ADA position paper on bland diet in the treatment of chronic duodenal ulcer disease. J. Am. Dietet. A. 59:244, 1971.

Caron, H. S. and Roth, H. P.: Popular beliefs about the peptic ulcer diet. J. Am. Dietet. A. 60:306, 1972.

Flick, A. L.: Acid content of common beverages. Am. J. Dig. Dis. 15:317, 1970.

Ingelfinger, F. J.: Let the ulcer patient enjoy his food. Roth, J. L. A.: The ulcer patient should watch his diet, in Controversy in Internal Medicine, F. J. Ingelfinger, ed., Philadelphia, Saunders, 1966.

Joint Committee, American Dietetic Association and American Medical Association: Diet as related to gastrointestinal function. J. Am. Dietet. A. 38:425, 1961.

Lennard-Jones, J. E. and Barbouris, N.: Effect of different foods on the acidity of the gastric contents in patients with duodenal ulcer: a comparison between two "therapeutic" diets and freely chosen meals. Gut 6:113, 1965.

Spiro, H. M.: The rough and the smooth, some reflections on diet therapy. N. Eng. J. Med. 293:83, 1975.

Peptic Ulcer—Disease
Cooke, A. R.: Control of gastric emptying and motility. Gastroenterology 68:804, 1975.

Czaja, A. J., et al: Acute gastroduodenal disease after thermal injury: an endoscopic evaluation of incidence and natural history. N. Eng. J. Med. 29:925, 1974.

Fordtran, J. S. and Walsh, J. H.: Gastric acid secretion rate and buffer content of the stomach after eating: results in normal subjects and in patients with duodenal ulcer. J. Clin. Invest. 52:645, 1973.

Levy, M.: Aspirin use in patients with major upper gastrointestinal bleeding and peptic ulcer disease. N. Eng. J. Med. 290:1158, 1974.

Stacher, G., et al: Gastric acid secretion and sleep stages during natural night sleep. Gastroenterology 68:1449, 1975.

Walsh, J. H. and Grossman, M. I.: Gastrin. N. Eng. J. Med. 292:1324:1377, 1975.

Walsh, J. H., et al: pH dependence of acid secretion and gastrin release in normal and ulcer subjects. J. Clin. Invest. 55:462, 1975.

Wesdorp, R. I. C. and Fischer, J. E.: Plasma-gastrin and acid secretion in patients with peptic ulceration. Lancet 2:857, 1974.

Other Upper Gastrointestinal Disorders
Babka, J. C. and Castell, D. O.: On the genesis of heartburn. The effects of specific foods on the lower esophageal sphincter. Am. J. Digest. Dis. 18:391, 1973.

Castell, D. O.: Diet and lower esophageal sphincter. Am. J. Clin. Nutr. 28:1296, 1975.

Ellis, F. H., Jr.: Esophageal hiatus hernia. N. Eng. J. Med. 287:646, 1972.

Higgs, R. H., et al: Gastric alkalinization: effect on lower-esophageal sphincter pressure and serum gastrin. N. Eng. J. Med. 291:486, 1974.

Nebel, O. T. and Castell, D. O.: Lower esophageal sphincter pressure changes after food ingestion. Gastroenterology 63:778-783, 1972.

———: Inhibition of the lower esophageal sphincter by fat —a mechanism for fatty food intolerance. Gut 14:270, 1973.

Pope, C. E., II: Esophageal physiology. Med. Clin. N. Am. 58:1181, 1974.

Malabsorption—General

Caspary, W. F., et al: Influence of exocrine and endocrine pancreatic function on intestinal brush border enzymatic activities. Gut 16:89, 1975.

Connell, A. M.: Clinical aspects of motility. Med. Clin. N. Am. 58:1201, 1974.

Horowitz, S., et al: Small intestinal disease in T cell deficiency. J. Pediat. 85:457, 1974.

Jones, F. A.: The skin: a mirror of the gut. Geriatrics 28:75, (April) 1973.

Lundgren, O.: The circulation of the small bowel mucosa. Gut 15:1005, 1974.

Disaccharide Problems

Gallagher, C. R., et al: Lactose intolerance and fermented dairy products. J. Am. Dietet. A. 65:418, 1974.

Levine, G. M., et al: Role of oral intake in maintenance of gut mass and disaccharidase activity. Gastroenterology 67:975, 1974.

Mitchell, K. J., et al: Intolerance of eight ounces of milk in healthy lactose-intolerant teen-agers. Pediatrics 56:718, 1975.

Newcomer, A. D., et al: Prospective comparison of indirect methods for detecting lactase deficiency. N. Eng. J. Med. 293:1232, 1975.

Olsen, W. A.: Carbohydrate absorption. Med. Clin. N. Am. 58:1387, 1974.

Pena, A. S. and Truelove, S. C.: Hypolactasia and ulcerative colitis. Gastroenterology 64:400, 1973.

Ransome-Kuti, O., et al: A genetic study of lactose digestion in Nigerian families. Gastroenterology 68:431, 1975.

Celiac—Sprue

Barr, D. G. D., et al: Catch-up growth in malnutrition, studied in celiac disease after institution of gluten-free diet. Pediat. Res. 6:521, 1972.

Chapman, B. L., et al: Measuring the response of the jejunal mucosa in adult coeliac disease to treatment with a gluten-free diet. Gut 15:870, 1974.

Cornell, H. J. and Townley, R. R. W.: The toxicity of certain cereal proteins in coeliac disease. Gut 15:862, 1974.

Dissanayake, A. S., et al: Identifying toxic fractions of wheat gluten and their effect on the jejunal mucosa in coeliac disease. Gut 15:951, 1974.

Editorial: Facts about gluten. Lancet 2:1081, 1975.

Hamilton, J. R. and McNeill, L. K.: Childhood celiac disease: response of treated patients to a small uniform daily dose of wheat gluten. J. Pediat. 81:885, 1972.

Ranhotra, G. S., et al: Preparation and evaluation of soy-fortified gluten-free bread. J. Food Sci. 40:62, 1975.

Townley, R. R. W., et al: Toxicity of wheat gliadin fractions in coeliac disease. Lancet 1:1363, 1973.

Weijers, H. A. and van de Kamer, J. H.: Celiac disease and wheat sensitivity. Pediatrics 25:127, 1960.

Young, W. F. and Pringle, E. M.: 110 children with coeliac disease, 1950-1969. Arch. Dis. Child. 46:421, 1971.

Pancreatitis

DiMagno, E. P., et al: Relations between pancreatic enzyme outputs and malabsorption in severe pancreatic insufficiency. N. Eng. J. Med. 288:813, 1973.

Farmer, R. G., et al: Hyperlipoproteinemia and pancreatitis. Am. J. Med. 54:161, 1973.

Greenberger, N. J.: Pancreatitis and hyperlipemia. N. Eng. J. Med. 289:586, 1973.

Saunders, J. H. B. and Wormsley, K. G.: Pancreatic extracts in the treatment of pancreatic exocrine insufficiency. Gut 16:157, 1975.

Westergaard, H. and Dietschy, J. M.: Normal mechanisms of fat absorption and derangements induced by various gastrointestinal diseases. Med. Clin. N. A. 58:1413, 1974.

Large Bowel—Dietary Fiber

Albersheim, P.: The walls of growing plant cells. Scientific American 232:80, April, 1975.

Cummings, J. H.: Progress report: dietary fibre. Gut 14:69, 1973.

Painter, N. S., et al: Unprocessed bran in treatment of diverticular disease of the colon. Brit. Med. J. 2:137, 1972.

Payler, D. K., et al: The effect of wheat bran on intestinal transit. Gut 16:209, 1975.

Large Bowel—Disease

Connell, A. M. : The irritable colon syndrome. Postgrad. Med. J. 44:668, 1968.

Cummings, J. H.: Laxative abuse. Gut 15:758, 1974.

Farmer, R. G.: The protein manifestations of Crohn's disease. Postgrad. Med. 57:129, (January) 1975.

Fleischner, F. G.: Diverticular disease of the colon. New observations and revised concepts. Gastroenterology 60:316, 1971.

Frigo, G. M., et al: Some observations on the intrinsic nervous mechanism in Hirschsprung's disease. Gut 14:35, 1973.

Goldstein, F.: Diet and colonic disease. J. Am. Dietetic A. 60:499, 1972.

Levitt, M. D.: Intestinal gas production. J. Am. Dietet. A. 60:487, 1972.

Mendeloff, A. I., et al: Illness experience and life stresses in patients with irritable colon and with ulcerative colitis. N. Eng. J. Med. 282:14, 1970.

surgical nutrition, burns

Journal Articles:

Baker, D. I.: Hyperalimentation at home. Am. J. Nurs. 74:1826, 1974.

Bury, K. D. and Jambunathan, G.: Effects of elemental diets on gastric secretion in man. Am. J. Surg. 127:59, 1974.

Cassim, M. M., et al: Pancreatic secretions in response to jejunal feeding of elemental diet. Ann. Surg. 180:228, 1974.

Clark, H. E., et al: Nitrogen retention and plasma amino acids of men who consumed isonitrogenous diets containing egg albumen or mixtures of amino acids. Am. J. Clin. Nutr. 28:316, 1975.

Daly, J. M., et al: Postoperative oral and intravenous nutrition. Ann. Surg. 180:709, 1974.

Dougherty, J. C.: Influence of high protein diets on renal function. J. Am. Dietet. A. 63:392, 1973.

Freeman, J. B., et al: Evaluation of amino acid infusions as protein-sparing agents in normal adult subjects. Am. J. Clin. Nutr. 28:477, 1975.

Goldmann, D. A. and Maki, D. G.: Infection control in total parenteral nutrition. JAMA 223:1360, 1973.

Kim, Y. S., et al: Intestinal peptide hydrolases: peptide and amino acid absorption. Med. Clin. N. A. 58:1397, 1974.

Miller, J. M. and Taboada, J. C.: Clinical experience with an elemental diet. Am. J. Clin. Nutr. 28:46, 1975.

Moncrief, J. A.: Burns. N. Eng. J. Med. 288:444, 1973.

Newsome, T. W., et al: Weight loss following thermal injury. Ann. Surg. 178:215, 1973.

Richardson, T. J. and Sgoutas, D.: Essential fatty acid deficiency in four adult patients during total parenteral nutrition. Am. J. Clin. Nutr. 28:258, 1975.

Russell, R. I.: Elemental diets. Gut. 16:68, 1975.

Silk, D. B. A., et al: Jejunal absorption of an amino acid mixture simulating casein and an enzymic hydrolysate of casein prepared for oral administration to normal adults. Br. J. Nutr. 33:95, 1975.

Thomford, N. R., et al: Gastric inhibitory polypeptide response to oral glucose after vagotomy and pyloroplasty. Arch. Surg. 109:177, 1974.

Torsvik, H., et al: Effects of intravenous hyperalimentation on plasma-lipoproteins in severe familial hypercholesterolaemia. Lancet 1:601, 1975.

Voitk, A. J., et al: Use of elemental diet during the adaptive stage of short gut syndrome. Gastroenterology 65:419, 1973.

Wilmore, D. W., et al: Catecholamines: mediator of the hypermetabolic response to thermal injury. Ann. Surgery 180:653, 1974.

weight control

Books and Pamphlets:

Asher, W. L., ed: *Treating the Obese*. New York, Medcom Press, 1975.

Berland, T.: *Rating the Diets*. Skokie, Ill., Consumer Guide, 1974.

Bruch, H.: *Eating Disorders: Obesity, Anorexia Nervosa, and the Person Within*. N. Y., Basic Books, 1973.

Konshi, F.: *Exercise Equivalents of Foods*. Carbondale, Ill., So. Illinois Univ. Press, 1973.

Stuart, R. B. and Davis, P.: *Slim Chance in a Fat World: Behavioral control of obesity*. Champaign, Ill., Research Press, 1972.

Journal Articles:

Bjorntorp, P., et al: Effect of an energy-reduced dietary regimen in relation to adipose tissue cellularity in obese women. Am. J. Clin. Nutr. 28:445, 1975.

Brook, C. G. D.: Evidence for a sensitive period in adipose-cell replication in man. Lancet 2:624, 1972.

Brook, C. G. D., et al: Relation between age of onset of obesity and size and number of adipose cells. Br. Med. J. 2:25, 1972.

Grinker, J.: Behavioral and metabolic consequences of weight reduction. J. Am. Dietet. A. 62:30, 1973.

Hamilton, C. L.: Physiologic control of food intake. J. Am. Dietet. A. 62:35, 1973.

Joosten, H. F. P. and van der Kroon, P. H. W.: Enlargement of epididymal adipocytes in relation to hyperinsulinemia in obese hyperglycemic mice (ob/ob). Metabolism 23:59, 1974.

Jourdan, M., et al: The turnover rate of serum glycerides in the lipoproteins of fasting obese women during weight loss. Am. J. Clin. Nutr. 27:850, 1974.

————: Differential effects of diet composition and weight loss on glucose tolerance in obese women. Am. J. Clin. Nutr. 27:1065, 1974.

Kalkhoff, R. K., et al: Metabolic effects of weight loss in obese subjects. Diabetes 20:83, 1971.

Kalkhoff, R. K. and Ferrou, C.: Metabolic differences between obese overweight and muscular overweight men. N. Eng. J. Med. 284:1236, 1971.

Knittle, J. L.: Obesity in childhood: a problem in adipose tissue cellular development. J. Pediat. 81:1048, 1972.

Levitz, L. S.: Behavior therapy in treating obesity. J. Am. Dietet. A. 62:22, 1973.

Levitz, L. S. and Stunkard, A. J.: A therapeutic coalition for obesity: behavior modification and patient self-help. Am. J. Psychiatry 131:423, 1974.

McCance, R. A.: The composition of the body: its maintenance and regulation. Nutr. Abst. Rev. 42:1269, 1972.

Rose, H. E. and Mayer, J.: Activity, calorie intake, fat storage, and the energy balance of infants. Pediatrics 41:18, 1968.

Salans, L. B., et al: Studies on human adipose tissue: Adipose cell size and number in nonobese and obese patients. J. Clin. Invest. 52:929, 1973.

Solow, C., Silberfarb, P. M., and Swift, L.: Psychosocial effects of intestinal bypass surgery for severe obesity. N. Eng. J. Med. 290:300, 1974.

Stunkard, A., et al: Influence of social class on obesity and thinness in childhood. JAMA 221:579, 1972.

Stunkard, A. J. and Rush, J.: Dieting and depression: a critical review of reports of untoward responses during weight reduction for obesity. Ann. Int. Med. 81:526, 1974.

Wagner, M. and Hewitt, M. I.: Oral satiety in obese and nonobese. J. Am. Dietet. A. 67:344, 1975.

Weismann, R. E.: Surgical palliation of massive and severe obesity. Am. J. Surg. 125:437, 1973.

Weisinger, J. R. et al: The nephrotic syndrome: A complication of massive obesity. Ann. Int. Med. 81:440, 1974.

anorexia nervosa

Books:

Dally, P.: *Anorexia Nervosa.* New York, Grune & Stratten, 1969.

Journal Articles:

Halmi, K., et al: Prognosis in anorexianervosa. Ann. Int. Med. 78:671, 1973.

Melton, J. H.: A boy with anorexia nervosa. Am. J. Nurs. 74:1649, (September) 1974.

diabetes mellitus

Books and Pamphlets:

Marble, A., et al:*Joslin's Diabetes Mellitus*, ed. 11. Philadelphia, Lea and Febiger, 1971.

Mazzaferri, E. L.: *Endocrinology*: A Review of Clinical Endocrinology. Flushing, N. Y., Medical Examination Publishing, 1974.

Tepperman, J.: *Metabolic and Endocrine Physiology*, ed. 3. Chicago, Year Book Medical Pub., 1973.

Williams, R. H. and Porte, D., Jr.: The pancreas, in, *Textbook of Endocrinology*, ed. 5. Philadelphia, Saunders, 1974, Chapter 9.

Journal Articles:

Anderson, J. W.: Metabolic abnormalities contributing to diabetic complications, I, Glucose metabolism in insulin-insensitive pathways. Am. J. Clin. Nutr. 28:273, 1975.

Anderson, J. W. and Herman, R. H.: Effects of carbohydrate restriction on glucose tolerance of normal men and reactive hypoglycemic patients. Am. J. Clin. Nutr. 28:748, 1975.

Brunzell, J. D., et al: Improved glucose tolerance with high carbohydrate feeding in mild diabetes. N. Eng. J. Med. 284:521, 1971.

_____: Effect of a fat free, high carbohydrate diet on diabetic subjects with fasting hyperglycemia. Diabetes 23:138, 1974.

Cahill, G. F., Jr.: Physiology of insulin in man. Diabetes 20:785, 1971.

Caso, E. K.: Calculation of diabetic diets. J. Am. Dietet. A. 26:575, 1950.

_____: Supplements to diabetic diet material. J. Am. Dietet. A. 32:929, 1956.

Davenport, B. R., et al: Dietitians, nurses teach diabetic patients. Hospitals 48:61, Dec. 1, 1974.

Drenick, E. J. and Johnson, D.: Evolution of diabetic ketoacidosis in gross obesity. Am. J. Clin. Nutr. 28:264, 1975.

Eaton, R. P.: Evolving role of glucagon in human diabetes mellitus. Diabetes 24:523, 1975.

Felig, P.: Diabetic ketoacidosis. N. Eng. J. Med. 290:1360, 1974.

Fujita, Y., et al: Basal and postprotein insulin and glucagon levels during a high and low carbohydrate intake and their relationships to plasma triglycerides. Diabetes 24:552, 1975.

Garcia, M. J., et al: Morbidity and mortality in diabetics in the Framingham population. Sixteen year follow-up study. Diabetes 23:105, 1974.

Gerich, J. E., et al: Effects of somatostatin on plasma glucose and glucagon levels in human diabetes mellitus: pathophysiologic and therapeutic implications. N. Eng. J. Med. 291:544, 1974.

_____: Prevention of human diabetic ketoacidosis by somatostatin. N. Eng. J. Med. 292:985, 1975.

Hofeldt, F. D.: Reactive hypoglycemia. Metabolism 24:1193, 1975.

Martin, M. M. and Martin, A. L. A.: Obesity, hyperinsulinism, and diabetes mellitus in childhood. J. Pediat. 82:192, 1973.

Odell, A. C., et al: Effect of processed pears on glucose tolerance in diabetes. J. Am. Dietet. A. 63:410, 1973.

O'Sullivan, J. B.: Age gradient in blood glucose levels: magnitude and clinical implications. Diabetes 23:713, 1974.

Pildes, R. S.: Infants of diabetic mothers. N. Eng. J. Med. 289:902, 1973.

Schade, D. S. and Eaton, R. P.: Modulation of fatty acid metabolism by glucagon in man, II, Effects in insulin-deficient diabetics. Diabetes 24:510, 1975.

Schmitt, B. D.: An argument for the unmeasured diet in juvenile diabetes. Clin. Pediat. 14:68, 1975.

Tattersall, R. B. and Fajans, S. S.: A difference between the inheritance of classical juvenile-onset and maturity-onset type diabetes of young people. Diabetes 24:44, 1975.

Takazakura, E., et al: Onset and progression of diabetic glomerulosclerosis: a prospective study based on serial renal biopsies. Diabetes 24:1, 1975.

Unger, R. H.: Alpha- and beta-cell interrelationships in health and disease. Metabolism 23:581, 1974.

University Group Diabetes Program: V, Evaluation of phenformin therapy. Diabetes 24: (Supplement 1), 1975.

Wadsworth, M. E. J. and Jarrett, R. J.: Incidence of diabetes in the first 26 years of life. Lancet 2:1172, 1974.

West, K. M.: Diabetes in American Indians and other native populations of the world. Diabetes 23:844, 1974.

atherosclerosis

Books and Pamphlets:

Frederickson, D. S.: in *Harrison's Principles of Medicine* ed. 7. Wintrobe, M. M., et al., eds. New York, McGraw-Hill, 1974, Chapters 106 and 244.

Frederickson, D. S. and Levy, R. I.: in, *The Metabolic Basis of Inherited Disease*. J. B. Stanbury, J. B. Wyngaarden, and D. S. Frederickson, New York, McGraw-Hill, 1972, Chapter 28.

Friedman, M. and Rosenman, R. H.: *Type A Behavior and Your Heart.* New York, Knopf, 1974.

Journal Articles:

Bernstein, R. S., et al: Hyperinsulinemia and enlarged adipocytes in patients with endogenous hyperlipoproteinemia without obesity or diabetes mellitus. Diabetes 24:207, 1975.

Bortz, W. M.: The pathogenesis of hypercholesterolemia. Ann. Int. Med. 80:738, 1974.

Christakis, G.: Designing a new American nutritional pattern. Food Tech. 28:17, 1974.

Connell, A. M., et al: Absence of effect of bran on blood-lipids. Lancet 1:496, 1975.

Davidoff, F., et al: Marked hyperlipidemia and pancreatitis associated with oral contraceptive therapy. N. Eng. J. Med. 289:552, 1973.

Dawber, T. R., et al: Coffee and cardiovascular disease: observations from the Framingham study. N. Eng. J. Med. 291:871, 1974.

Dustan, H. P.: Atherosclerosis complicating chronic hypertension. Circulation 50:871, 1974.

Einarsson, K., et al: Gallbladder disease in hyperlipoproteinaemia. Lancet 1:484, 1975.

Farmer, R. G., et al: Hyperlipoproteinemia and pancreatitis. Am. J. Med. 54:161, 1973.

Grundy, S. M.: Effect of polyunsaturated fats on lipid metabolism in patients with hypertriglyceridemia. J. Clin. Invest. 55:269, 1975.

Jenkins, D. J. A., et al: Effect of pectin, guar gum, and wheat fibre on serum-cholesterol. Lancet 1: 1116, 1975.

Lauer, R. M., et al: Coronary heart disease risk factors in school children: the Muscatine study. J. Pediat. 86:697, 1975.

Levy, R. I., et al: Drug therapy: treatment of hyperlipidemia. N. Eng. J. Med. 290:1295, 1974.

Levy, R. I.: Triglycerides as a risk factor in coronary artery disease. JAMA 224:1770, 1973.

————: Hyperlipoproteinemias: some basic concepts on diagnosis and management. JAMA 226:648, 1973.

Livingston, G. E.: The prudent diet: what? why? how? Food Tech. 28:16, 1974.

Olefsky, J., et al: Effects of weight reduction on obesity: studies of lipid and carbohydrate metabolism in normal and hyperlipoproteinemic subjects. J. Clin. Invest. 53:64, 1974.

Olson, R. E.: Vitamin E and its relation to heart disease. Circulation 48:179, 1973.

Perry, H. M., Jr.: Minerals in cardiovascular disease. J. Am. Dietet. A. 62:631, 1973.

Sacks, F. M., et al: Plasma lipids and lipoproteins in vegetarians and controls. N. Eng. J. Med. 292:1148, 1975.

Stone, N. J., et al: Coronary artery disease in 116 kindred with familial type II hyperlipoproteinemia. Circulation 49:476, 1974.

Sturdevant, R. A. L., et al: Increased prevalence of cholelithiasis in men ingesting a serum-cholesterol-lowering diet. N. Eng. J. Med. 288:24, 1973.

Wilmore, J. H. and McNamara, J. J.: Prevalence of coronary heart disease risk factors in boys 8 to 12 years of age. J. Pediat. 84:527, 1974.

cardiovascular disease

Books and Pamphlets:

Kraus, B.: *The Dictionary of Sodium, Fats, and Cholesterol.* New York, Grosset and Dunlap, 1974.

Journal Articles:

Adlin, E. V., et al: Dietary salt intake in hypertensive patients with normal and low plasma renin activity. Am. J. Med. Sci. 261:67, 1971.

Brown, W. J. Jr., et al: Exchangeable sodium and blood volume in normotensive and hypertensive humans on high and low sodium intake. Circulation 43:508, 1971.

Brunner, H. R. and Gavras, H.: Vascular damage in hypertension. Hospital Practice 10:97, (March) 1975.

Edmondson, R. P. S., et al: Abnormal leucocyte composition and sodium transport in essential hypertension. Lancet 1:1003, 1975.

Lieberman, E.: Essential hypertension in children and youth: a pediatric perspective. J. Pediat. 85:1, 1974.

Makoff, D. L.: Common fluid and electrolyte disorders in the cardiac patient. Geriatrics 27:76, 1972.

Muirhead, E. E.: The antihypertensive function of the renal medulla. Hospital Practice 10:99, (January) 1975.

Newborg, B.: Sodium-restricted diets: Sodium content of wines and other alcoholic beverages. Arch. Intern. Med. 123:692, 1969.

Peart, W. S.: Renin-angiotensin system. N. Eng. J. Med. 292:302, 1975.

Wiesman, C. K.: The art of seasoning low-sodium diets. Nursing Homes 20:12, February 1971.

Water quality, trace elements and cardiovascular disease. WHO Chronicle 27:534, 1973.

renal disease, nephrolithiasis

Books and Pamphlets:

deWardner, H. E.: *The Kidney: An Outline of Normal and Abnormal Structure and Function*, ed. 4. London, Churchill Livingston, 1973.

Journal Articles:

Beaumont, J. E., et al: Normal serum-lipids in renal-transplant patients. Lancet 1:599, 1975.

DeFronzo, R. A., et al: Carbohydrate metabolism in uremia: a review. Medicine 52:469, 1973.

DeLuca, H. F.: The kidney as an endocrine organ involved in the function of vitamin D. Am. J. Med. 58:39, 1975.

Chan, J. C. M.: Survival of children with severe chronic uremia. Clin. Pediat. 13:737, 1974.

Calloway, D. H.: Nitrogen balance of men with marginal intakes of protein and energy. J. Nutrition 105:914, 1975.

Erslev, A. J.: Renal biogenesis of erythropoietin. Am. J. Med. 58:25, 1975.

Hagler, L. and Herman, R. H.: Oxalate metabolism. Am. J. Clin. Nutr. 26:758; 882; 1006; 1073; 1242, 1973.

Kahn, H. D., et al: Effect of cranberry juice on urine. J. Am. Dietet. A. 51:251, 1967.

Kies, C.: Nonspecific nitrogen in the nutrition of human beings. Fed. Proc. 31:1172, 1972.

Kopple, J. D. and Coburn, J. W.: Metabolic studies of low protein diets in uremia, I, Nitrogen and potassium. Medicine 52:583, 1973.

———: Metabolic studies of low protein diets in uremia, II, Calcium, phosphorus and magnesium. Medicine 52:597, 1973.

Kopple, J. D. and Swendseid, M. E.: Nitrogen balance and plasma amino acid levels in uremic patients fed an essential amino acid diet. Am. J. Clin. Nutr. 27:806, 1974.

———: Evidence that histidine is an essential amino acid in normal and chronically uremic man. J. Clin. Invest. 55:881, 1975.

Kurtzman, N. A. and Pillay, V. K. G.: Renal reabsorption of glucose in health and disease. Arch. Intern. Med. 131:901, 1973.

Levy, N. B. and Wynbrandt, G. D.: The quality of life on maintenance hemodialysis. Lancet 1:1328, 1975.

Oettinger, C. W., et al: Reduced calcium absorption after nephrectomy in uremic patients. N. Eng. J. Med. 291:458, 1974.

Renkin, E. M. and Robinson, R. R.: Glomerular filtration. N. Eng. J. Med. 290:785, 1974.

Saenger, P., et al: Somatomedin and growth after renal transplantation. Pediat. Res. 8:163, 1974.

Schultze, R. G.: Recent advances in the physiology and pathophysiology of potassium excretion. Arch. Intern. Med. 131:885, 1973.

Varcoe, R., et al: Efficiency of utilization of urea nitrogen for albumin synthesis by chronically uremic and normal men. Clin. Sci. Molec. Med. 48:379, 1975.

Walser, M.: Treatment of renal failure with keto acids. Hospital Practice 10:59, (June) 1975.

Young, V. R., et al: Protein requirements of man: comparative nitrogen balance response within the submaintenance-to-maintenance range of intakes of wheat and beef proteins. J. Nutrition 105:534, 1975.

liver disease

Books and Pamphlets:

Schaffner, F., Sherlock, S., and Leevy, C. M. (eds.): The Liver and Its Diseases. New York, Intercontinental Medical Book, 1974.

Journal Articles:

Davidson, C. S. and Mihas, A. A.: Letter to the editor: alcoholic cirrhosis in baboons (cont.). N. Eng. J. Med. 291:50, 1974.

Gabuzda, G. J.: Cirrhosis, ascites, and edema. Gastroenterology 58:546, 1970.

Kappas, A. and Alvares, A. P.: How the liver metabolizes foreign substances. Scientific American 232:22, (June) 1975.

Krasner, N., et al: Ascorbic-acid saturation and ethanol metabolism. Lancet 2:693, 1974.

Marco, J., et al: Elevated plasma glucagon levels in cirrhosis of the liver. N. Eng. J. Med. 289:1107, 1973.

Popper, H., et al: The social impact of liver disease. N. Eng. J. Med. 281:1455, 1969.

Price, J. B., et al: Glucagon as the portal factor modifying hepatic regeneration. Surgery 72:74, 1972.

Sherlock, S.: Progress report: chronic hepatitis. Gut 15:581, 1974.

Walker, C., et al: Inhibition of ammonia generation in cirrhotics by elevating the insulin: glucagon ratio. Clin. Res. 21:850, 1974.

special problems

Journal Articles:

Allergy

Boat, T. F., et al: Hyperreactivity to cow milk in young children with pulmonary hemosiderosis and corpulmonale secondary to nasopharyngeal obstruction. J. Pediat. 87:23, 1975.

Caldwell, J. H., et al: Serum IgE in eosinophilic gastroenteritis: response to intestinal challenge in two cases. N. Eng. J. Med. 292:1388, 1975.

Feeney, M. C.: Nutritional and dietary management of food allergy in children. Am. J. Clin. Nutr. 22:103, 1969.

Rowlands, D. T., Jr., and Daniele, R. P.: Surface receptors in the immune response. N. Eng. J. Med. 293:26, 1975.

Shiner, M., et al: The small-intestinal mucosa in cow's milk allergy. Lancet 1:136, 1975.

Spitz, E., et al: Serum IgE in clinical immunology and allergy. J. Allergy Clin. Immunol. 49:337, 1972.

Anemia

Beutler, E.: Drug-induced anemia. Fed. Proc. 31:141, 1972.

Camitta, B. M. and Nathan, D. G.: Anemias in adolescence, 1. Disturbances of iron balance. Postgrad. Med. 57:143, (February) 1975.

Elwood, P. C.: Evaluation of the clinical importance of anemia. Am. J. Clin. Nutr. 26:958, 1973.

Jacobs, A. and Worwood, M.: Ferritin in serum: clinical and biochemical implications. N. Eng. J. Med. 292:951, 1975.

Arthritis

Borle, A. B.: Calcium metabolism at the cellular level. Fed. Proc. 32:1944, 1973.

Garn, S. M.: Adult bone loss, fracture epidemiology and nutritional implications. Nutrition 27:107, 1973.

Nimni, M. and Deshmukh, K.: Differences in collagen

metabolism between normal and osteoarthritic human articular cartilage. Science 181:751, 1973.

Peacock, M., et al: Action of 1α-hydroxy vitamin D₃ on calcium absorption and bone resorption in man. Lancet 1:385, 1974.

Posner, A. S.: Bone mineral at the molecular level. Fed. Proc. 32:1933, 1973.

Queener, S. F. and Bell, N. H.: Calcitonin: a general survey. Metabolism 24:555, 1975.

Rodan, G. A., et al: Cyclic AMP and cyclic GMP: mediators of the mechanical effects on bone remodeling. Science 189:467, 1975.

Sahud, M. A. and Cohen, R. J.: Effect of aspirin ingestion on ascorbic acid levels in rheumatoid arthritis. Lancet. 1:937, 1971.

Thyroid Problems

Gilliland, P. F.: Myxedema: recognition and treatment. Postgrad. Med. 57:61, (June) 1975.

Hahn, H. B., Jr.: Congenital nongoitrous hypothyroidism. Postgrad. Med. 57:71, (June) 1975.

McMurry, J. F., Jr.: Thyroid function testing. Postgrad. Med. 57:53, (June) 1975.

Food-Drug Interactions

Christakis, G. and Miridjanian, A.: Diets, drugs, and their interrelationships. J. Am. Dietet. A. 52:21, 1968.

Chopra, D. and Clerkin, E. P.: Hypercalcemia and malignant disease. Med. Clin. N. A. 59:441, 1975.

Mena, I. and Cotzias, G. C.: Protein intake and treatment of Parkinson's disease with levodopa. N. Eng. J. Med. 292:181, 1975.

Symposium: Effects of oral contraceptive hormones on nutrient metabolism. Am. J. Clin. Nutr. 28: Part I, 328; Part II, 515, 1975.

Takacs, F. J.: Fluid and electrolyte problems in patients with advanced carcinoma. Med. Clin. N. A. 59:449, 1975.

West, R. J. and Lloyd, J. K.: The effect of cholestyramine on intestinal absorption. Gut 16:93, 1975.

nutrition in diseases of infancy and childhood

Books and Pamphlets:

Fomon, S. J.: *Infant Nutrition*, ed. 2. Philadelphia, Saunders, 1974.

Helfer, R. E. and Kempe, C. H., (eds.): *The Battered Child*, ed. 2. Chicago, University of Chicago Press, 1974.

Vaughan, V. C., III and McKay, R. J.: *Nelson Textbook of Pediatrics*, ed. 10. Philadelphia, Saunders, 1975.

Sinclair, D.: *Human Growth after Birth*, ed. 2. New York, Oxford Univ. Press, 1973.

Wallace, H. M., Gold, E. M., and Lis, E. F.: *Maternal and Child Health Practices*: Problems, Resources, and Methods of Delivery. Springfield, Ill., Thomas, 1973.

Committee on Nutrition Statements:

Committee on Nutrition, American Academy of Pediatrics: Should milk drinking by children be discouraged. Pediatrics 53:576, 1974.

Committee on Nutrition, American Academy of Pediatrics: Filled milks, imitation milks, and coffee whiteners. Pediatrics 49:770, 1972.

Committee on Nutrition, American Academy of Pediatrics: Childhood diet and coronary heart disease. Pediatrics 49:305, 1972.

Committee on Nutrition, American Academy of Pediatrics: Iron fortified formulas. Pediatrics 47:786, 1971.

Committee on Nutrition, American Academy of Pediatrics: Iron balance and requirements in infancy. Pediatrics 43:134, 1969.

Growth

Eid, E. E.: Follow-up study of physical growth of children who had excessive weight gain in first six months of life. Brit. Med. J. 2:74, 1970.

Falkner, F.: Velocity growth. Pediatrics 51:746, 1973.

Frankenburg, W. K., et al: Development of preschool-aged children of different social and ethnic groups: implications for developmental screening. J. Pediat. 87:125, 1975.

Klein, P. S., et al: Effects of starvation in infancy (pyloric stenosis) on subsequent learning abilities. J. Pediat. 87:8, 1975.

Latham, M. C.: Protein-calorie malnutrition in children and its relation to psychological development and behavior. Physiological Reviews 54:541, 1974.

Owen, G. M.: The assessment and recording of measurements of growth of children: report of a small conference. Pediatrics 51:461, 1973.

Rose, H. E. and Mayer, J.: Activity, calorie intake, fat storage, and the energy balance of infants. Pediatrics 41:18, 1968.

Widdowson, E. M. and McCance, R. A.: A review: new thoughts on growth. Pediat. Res. 9:154, 1975.

Feeding Problems

Ball, T. S., et al: A special feeding technique for chronic regurgitation. Am. J. Ment. Deficiency 78:486, 1974.

Castile, R. G., et al: Vitamin D deficiency rickets: Two cases with faulty infant feeding practices. Am. J. Dis. Child. 129:964, 1975.

Chinn, P. L.: Infant gavage feeding. Am. J. Nurs. 71:1964, 1971.

Salisbury, D. M.: Bottle-feeding: influence of teat-hole size on suck volume. Lancet 1:655, 1975.

Low Birth Weight Infants

Cornblath, M., et al: Hypoglycemia in infancy and childhood. J. Pediat. 83:692, 1973.

Katz, L. and Hamilton, J. R.: Fat absorption in infants of birth weight less than 1,300 gm. J. Pediat. 85:608, 1974.

Lechtig, A., et al: Effects of food supplementation during pregnancy on birthweight. Pediatrics 56:508, 1975.

Lubchenco, L. O., et al: Long-term follow-up studies of pre-maturely born infants, II, Influence of birth weight and gestational age on sequelae. J. Pediat. 80:509, 1972.

Tantibhedhyangkul, P. and Hashim, S. A.: Medium-chain triglyceride feeding in premature infants: effects on fat and nitrogen absorption. Pediatrics 55:359, 1975.

Failure to Thrive

Barnard, M. U. and Woil, L.: Psychosocial failure to thrive. Nurs. Clin. N. A. 8:557, 1973.

Chase, H. P. and Martin, H. P.: Undernutrition and child development. N. Eng. J. Med. 282:933, 1970.

Fischoff, J., Whitten, C. F., and Pettit, M. G.: A psychiatric study of mothers of infants with growth failure secondary to maternal deprivation. J. Pediat. 79:209, 1971.

Leonard, M. F. and Solnit, A. J.: Growth failure from maternal deprivation or undereating. JAMA 212:882, 1970.

Pavenstedt, E.: To help infants weather disorganized family life. Am. J. Nurs. 69:1668, 1969.

Whitten, F., et al: Evidence that growth failure from maternal deprivation is secondary to undereating. JAMA 209:1675, 1969.

Acutely Ill Child

Berenberg, W., et al: Hazards of skimmed milk, unboiled and boiled. Pediatrics 44:734, 1969.

Schneider, D. L., et al: Vitamin K in formula products. Pediatrics 53:273, 1974.

Sherman, J. O., et al: Use of an oral elemental diet in infants with severe intractable diarrhea. J. Pediat. 86:518, 1975.

Anemia

Camitta, B. M. and Nathan, D. G.: Anemia in adolescence, 2, Hemoglobinopathies and other causes. Postgrad. Med. 57:151, Feb. 1975.

Lukens, J. M.: Marginal Comments—Iron deficiency and infection: fact or fable. Am. J. Dis. Child. 129:160, 1975.

Theuer, R. C.: Iron undernutrition in infancy. Clin. Pediat. 13:522, 1974.

Vitamin D Resistant Rickets

Brickman, A. S., et al: Actions of 1, 25-dihydroxy-cholecalciferol in patients with hypophosphatemic, vitamin D-resistant rickets. N. Eng. J. Med. 289:495, 1973.

Fraser, D., et al: Pathogenesis of hereditary vitamin D-dependent rickets: an inborn-error of vitamin D metabolism involving defective conversion of 25-hydroxy vitamin D to 1α, 25-dihydroxy vitamin D. N. Eng. J. Med. 289:817, 1973.

Malabsorption Syndromes

Ament, M. E.: Malabsorption syndromes in infancy and childhood. J. Pediat. 81:685; 867, 1972.

Lilibridge, C. B. and Townes, P. L.: Physiologic deficiency of pancreatic amylase in infancy: a factor in iatrogenic diarrhea. J. Pediat. 82:279, 1973.

Low-Beer, T. S., et al: Abnormalities of serum cholecystokinin and gallbladder emptying in celiac disease. N. Eng. J. Med. 292:961, 1975.

Cystic Fibrosis

Athreya, B. H., et al: Cystic fibrosis and hypertrophic osteoarthropathy in children. Am. J. Dis. Child. 129:634, 1975.

Dodge, J. A., et al: Essential fatty acid deficiency due to artificial diet in cystic fibrosis. Brit. Med. J. 129:192, 1975.

Lee, P. A., et al: Hypoproteinemia and anemia in infants with cystic fibrosis. JAMA 228:585, 1974.

Lloyd-Still, J. D., Khaw, K.-T., and Shwachman, H.: Severe respiratory disease in infants with cystic fibrosis. Pediatrics 53:678, 1974.

Oppenheimer, E. H. and Esterly, J. R.: Hepatic changes in young infants with cystic fibrosis: possible relation to focal biliary cirrhosis. J. Pediat. 86:683, 1975.

Shwachman, H., et al: Studies in cystic fibrosis: report of 130 patients diagnosed under 3 months of age over a 20-year period. Pediatrics 46:335, 1970.

Underwood, B. A. and Denning, C. R.: Blood and liver concentrations of vitamins A and E in children with cystic fibrosis of the pancreas. Pediat. Res. 6:26, 1972.

Cardiac Disease

Friedman, G. and Goldberg, S. J.: Concurrent and subsequent serum cholesterols of breast- and formula-fed infants. Am. J. Clin. Nutr. 28:42, 1975.

Glueck, C. J., et al: Pediatric familial Type II hyperlipoproteinemia: therapy with diet and cholestyramine resin. Pediatrics 52:669, 1973.

———: Hyperlipemia in progeny of parents with myocardial infarction before age 50. Am. J. Dis. Child. 127:70, 1974.

———: Plasma vitamin A and E levels in children with familial type II hyperlipoproteinemia during therapy with diet and cholestyramine resin. Pediatrics 54:51, 1974.

Huse, D. M., et al: Infants with congenital heart disease: food intake, body weight, and energy metabolism. Am. J. Dis. Child. 129:65, 1975.

Lieberman, E.: Essential hypertension in chidren and youth: a pediatric perspective. J. Pediat. 85:1, 1974.

Tsang, R. C., et al: Cholesterol at birth and age 1: comparison of normal and hypercholesterolemic neonates. Pediatrics 53:458, 1974.

Epilepsy

Medlinsky, H. L.: Rickets associated with anticonvulsant medication. Pediatrics 53:91, 1974.

inborn errors of metabolism

Books and Pamphlets:

Centerwall, W. R. and Centerwall, S. A.: *Phenylketonuria: an Inherited Metabolic Disorder Associated with Mental Retardation*, revised 1973. (Available Government Printing Office, Washington, D.C. 20402.)

Nyhan, W. L. (ed.): *Heritable Disorders of Amino Acid Metabolism*. New York, Wiley, 1974.

Scriver, C. R. and Rosenberg, L. E.: *Amino Acid Metabolism and Its Disoders*. Philadelphia, Saunders, 1973.

Stanbury, J. B., Wyngaarden, J. B., and Fredrickson, D. S. (eds.): *The Metabolic Basis of Inherited Disease*, ed. 3. New York, McGraw-Hill, 1972

Journal Articles:

Normal Amino Acid Metabolism

Armstrong, M. D. and Stave, U.: A study of plasma free amino acid levels. II, Normal values for children and adults. Metabolism 22:561, 1973.

Leverton, R. M., et al: The quantitative amino acid requirements of young women. J. Nutrition 58:59, 83, 219, 341, 355, 1956.

Nakagawa, I. and Masana, Y.: Assessment of nutritional status of men: protein. J. Nutrition 93:135, 1967.

Rose, W. C., et al: The amino acid requirements of man. J. Biol. Chem. 217:987, 1955.

Galactosemia

Komrower, G. M. and Lee, D. H.: Long-term follow-up of galactosaemia. Arch. Dis. Child. 45:367, 1970.

Segal, S., et al: Liver galactose-1-phosphate uridyl transferase: Activity in normal and galactosemic subjects. J. Clin. Invest. 50:500, 1971.

Shih, V. E., et al: Galactosemia screening of newborns in Massachusetts. N. Eng. J. Med. 284:753, 1971.

Phenylketonuria

Angeli, E., et al: Maternal phenylketonuria: a family with seven mentally retarded siblings. Develop. Med. Child. Neurol. 16:800, 1974.

Acosta, P. B., et al: Serum lipids in children with phenylketonuria (PKU). J. Am. Dietet. A. 63:631, 1973.

Berry, H. K., et al: Amino acid balance in the treatment of phenylketonuria. J. Am. Dietet. A. 58:210, 1971.

Committee on Children with Handicaps, American Academy of Pediatrics: Phenylketonuria and the phenylalaninemias of infancy. Pediatrics 49:628, 1972.

Composition of Lofenalac, J. Am. Dietet. A. 52:48, 1968.

Kaufman, S., et al: Phenylketonuria due to a deficiency of dihydropteridine reductase. N. Eng. J. Med. 293:785, 1975.

O'Grady, D. J., et al: Cognitive development in early treated phenylketonuria. Am. J. Dis. Child. 121:20, 1971.

Patel, M. S. and Arinze, I. J.: Phenylketonuria: metabolic alterations induced by phenylalanine and phenylpyruvate. Am. J. Clin. Nutr. 28:183, 1975.

Perry, T. L., et al: Unrecognized adult phenylketonuria: implications for obstetrics and psychiatry. N. Eng. J. Med. 289:395, 1973.

Rincic, M. M. and Rogers, P. J.: A low-protein, low-phenylalanine vegetable casserole. J. Am. Dietet. A. 55:353, 1969.

Sibinga, M. S. and Friedman, C. J.: Complexities of parental understanding of phenylketonuria. Pediatrics 48:216, 1971.

Smith, I., et al: New variant of phenylketonuria with progressive neurological illness unresponsive to phenylalanine restriction. Lancet 1:1108, 1975.

Starfield, B. and Holtzman, N. A.: A comparison of effectiveness of screening for phenylketonuria in the United States, United Kingdom and Ireland. N. Eng. J. Med. 193:118, 1975.

Maple Syrup Urine Disease

Goodman, S. I., et al: The treatment of maple syrup urine disease. J. Pediat. 75:485, 1969.

Levy, H. L., et al: Folic acid deficiency secondary to a diet for maple syrup urine disease. J. Pediat. 77:294, 1970.

Snyderman, S. E., et al: Maple syrup disease, with particular reference to dietotherapy. Pediatrics 34:454, 1964.

Schwartz, J. F., et al: Maple syrup urine disease. A review with a report of an additional case. Develop. Med. Child. Neurol. 11:460, 1969.

Other Inborn Errors

Avery, M. E., et al: Transient tyrosinemia of the newborn: dietary and clinical aspects. Pediatrics, 39:378, 1967.

Harries, J. T., et al: Low proline diet in Type I hyperprolinemia. Arch. Dis. of Child. 46:72, 1971.

Holmes, L. B.: Inborn errors of morphogenesis. N. Eng. J. Med., 291:763, 1974.

Lott, I. T., et al: Dietary treatment of an infant with isovaleric acidemia. Pediatrics 49:616, 1972.

McCoy, E. E., et al: Decreased ATPase and increased sodium content of platelets in Down's syndrome: in relation to decreased serotonin content. N. Eng. J. Med. 291:950, 1974.

Nyhan, W. L., et al: Response to dietary therapy in B_{12} unresponsive methylmalonic acidemia. Pediatrics. 51:539, 1973.

Shih, V. E.: Early dietary management of an infant with argininosuccinase deficiency: preliminary report. J. Pediat. 80:645, 1972.

Snyder, R. D. and Robinson, A.: Leucine-induced hypoglycemia. Am. J. Dis. Child. 113:566, 1967.

glossary

acidosis (as'ı-do'sis). A pathological condition resulting from an accumulation of acid or loss of base in the body, and characterized by increase in hydrogen ion concentration.

aflatoxins (a'flah-tok'sin). Group of toxic substances produced by certain molds which grow on peanuts and cereals and which have toxic and carcinogenic effects in many animal species.

albuminuria (al'bu-mĭ-nu'ri-ah). The presence of the protein albumin in the urine.

alginate (ăl'jĭ-nāt). A compound made from marine kelp which forms a viscous solution or a gel.

alkalosis (al'kah-lo'sis). A pathological condition resulting from accumulation of base or loss of acid in the body and characterized by a decrease in hydrogen ion in the body.

allele (ah-lēl'). One of two or more contrasting genes, situated at the same locus in homologous chromosomes, which determine alternative characters in inheritance.

allergen (al'er-jen). Any substance capable of inducing allergy.

alpha-ketoglutaric acid (ke'to-gloo-tar'ik). Intermediary product in the Krebs cycle (citric acid cycle).

amino acids (a-me'no as'id). Organic compounds containing nitrogen known as the building blocks of the protein molecule.

amylase (am'i-lās). A pancreatic or salivary enzyme that digests starch.

amylopectin (am'i-lo-pek'tin). The branched chain insoluble form of starch which stains violet red with iodine and forms a paste with hot water.

amylose (am'ĭ-lōs). The straight chain soluble form

of starch which stains blue with iodine and does not form a paste with hot water.

anabolism (ah-nab'o-lizm). Term applied to that phase of metabolism which synthesizes new molecules, especially protoplasm.

anions (an'i-on). An ion carrying a negative charge. Since unlike forms of electricity attract each other, it is attracted by, and travels to, the anode or positive pole. The anions include all the nonmetals, the acid radicals, and the hydroxyl ion.

anticoagulant (an'tĭ-ko-ag'-u-lant). A substance that inhibits or prevents blood coagulation by interfering with the clotting mechanism.

antihemorrhagic (an'ti-hem'o-raj'ik). Preventing hemorrhage. Often applied to vitamin K.

antimetabolite (an'tĭ-mě-tab'o-lit). A substance bearing a close structural resemblance to one required for normal metabolism which interferes with normal metabolic functioning. Also referred to as metabolic antagonist.

antioxidant (an'ti-ok'se-dant). A substance that prevents or delays oxidation. Often applied to vitamin E.

apoenzyme (ap'o-en'zīm). The protein portion of an enzyme to which the prosthetic group or coenzyme is attached. The coenzyme may be a vitamin.

ascorbic acid (a-skor'bik). Vitamin C, deficiency of which is a causative factor in scurvy.

aspergillus flavus (as'per-jil'us fla-vus). A group of molds found on corn, peanuts, and certain grains when improperly dried and stored; source of aflatoxin.

ataxia (ah-tak'sē-ah). Failure of muscular coordination; irregularity of muscular action.

autosomal (au'to-so'mal). Pertaining to an autosome, a paired chromosome, not a sex chromosome.

avidin (av'i-din). A proteinlike antivitamin isolated from egg white; antagonist of biotin.

avitaminosis (a-vi'ta-min-o'sis). A condition due to the lack or the deficiency of a vitamin in the diet, or to lack of absorption or utilization of it.

biotin (bi'o-tin). A member of the vitamin B complex.

botulism (bot'u-lizm). Poisoning from the toxin produced by the organism *Clostridium botulinum*. The toxin has a selective action on the nervous system.

calciferol (kal-sif'er-ol). Vitamin D_2, produced by irradiating ergosterol.

calcification (kal'si-fi-ka'shun). Process by which organic tissue becomes hardened by a deposit of calcium salts.

calcitonin (kal'si-to'nin). A hormone secreted by the thyroid gland which participates with parathyroid hormone in the regulation of calcium ions in the blood.

calorimeter (kal'o-rim'e-ter). An instrument for measuring the heat change in any system (such as the types pictured in Chapter 8, one of which is used to measure the amount of heat produced by the body), and the bomb calorimeter used to measure the calorie (energy) value of foods.

carotene (kar'o-tēn). A yellow pigment which exists in several forms; alpha, beta, and gamma carotene are provitamins which may be converted into vitamin A in the body.

carotenoid (kah-rot'e-noid). Pertaining to a number of compounds related to carotene. They are primarily yellow pigments.

carrageenin (kar'ah-gēn'in). From carrageen (Irish moss); the commercial colloid extract from the moss which forms a gel.

casein (ka'se-in). The principal protein of milk, the basis of cheese.

catabolism (kah-tab'o-lizm). That aspect of metabolism which converts nutrients or complex substances in living cells into simpler compounds, with the release of energy.

cation (kat'i-on). An ion carrying a positive charge which is attracted to the negative pole or cathode. (See anions, above.) Cations include all metals and hydrogen.

cheilosis (ki-lo'sis). A condition marked by lesions on the lips and cracks at the angles of the mouth.

cholecalciferol (ko'le-kal-sif'er-ol). Vitamin D_3 derived from dehydrocholesterol.

cholesterol (ko-les'ter-ol). The most common member of the sterol group, defined below. It is a precursor of vitamin D and closely related to several hormones in the body. It constitutes a large part of the most frequently occurring type of gallstones, and occurs in atheroma of the arteries.

choline (ko'lēn). A component of lecithin. Necessary for fat transport in the body. Prevents the accumulation of fat in the liver.

chromatin (kro'mah-tin). The more stainable portion of the cell nucleus: contains the chromosomes.

chylomicrons (ki'lo-mi'kron). Particles of emulsified lipoproteins containing primarily triglycerides from dietary fat and very little protein.

chymotrypsin (ki'mo-trip'sin). One of the proteolytic enzymes of the pancreatic juice.

citrovorum factor (sit'ro-vo'rum fak'ter). A biologically active form of folic acid (folinic acid).

clostridium (klos-trid'e-um). A genus of schizomycetes, an anaerobic spore-forming rod-shaped bacterium, *C. perfringens* (and other species) a cause of gangrene.

cobalamin (co-bal'a-min). The basic molecule of vitamin B_{12} several compounds of which have vitamin activity.

collagen (kol′a-jen). The main protein constituent of connective tissue and of the organic substance of bones; changed into gelatin by boiling.

colloidal (ko-loi′dal). Pertaining to a colloid, which is a substance containing tiny, solid, evenly dispersed particles not dissolved in the medium, but which will not settle out.

congenital (kon-jen′i-tal). Existing at or before birth.

creatine (kre′a-tin). A nitrogenous end product of muscle metabolism.

creatinine (kre-at′i-nin). A basic substance, creatine anhydride, derived from creatine.

cretinism (kre′tin-izm). A chronic condition due to congenital lack of thyroid secretion.

cyanocobalamin (si′ah-no-ko-bal′ah-men). Vitamin B_{12}, a dark red compound containing cobalt and a cyanide group.

cyclamate (si′kla-māt). Sodium or calcium cyclamate, known as Sucaryl, used as an artificial sweetener. Use prohibited by FDA.

cystine. (sis′tin). A nonessential amino acid containing sulfur.

cystinuria (sis′ti-nu′re-ah). The occurrence of excessive cystine in the urine.

deaminization (de-am′in-i-za′shun). The process of metabolism by which the nitrogen portion (amine group) is removed from amino acids.

dehydration (de′hi-dra′shun). Removal of water from food or tissue; or the condition that results from undue loss of water.

DHEW. United States Department of Health, Education, and Welfare, Washington, D.C. 20852.

disaccharidase (di-sak′ah-ri-das). An enzyme which hydrolyzes disaccharides.

disaccharide (di-sak′a-rid). Any one of the sugars which yields two monosaccharides on hydrolysis.

DNA, deoxyribonucleic acid (de-ok′se-ri′bo-nu-kle′ik). Found in the nucleus of living cells; functions in the transfer of genetic characteristics.

electrolyte (e-lek′tro-līt). The ionized form of an element. Common electrolytes in the body are sodium, potassium, and chloride.

electron transport chain. Process that occurs in the mitochondria of the cell where hydrogen and then electrons from a substrate are passed from nicotinamide adenine dinucleotide (NAD) to flavin adenine dinucleotide (FAD) to coenzyme Q_{10} to cytochromes and then to oxygen to form water. The series of electron carriers are reduced and oxidized and thus provide for the regeneration of NAD and FAD. As this occurs, the energy released is trapped by adenosine diphosphate (ADP) to form adenosine triphosphate (ATP). This is called oxidative phosphorylation.

encephalopathy (en-sef′ah-lop′ah-the). Any degenerative disease of the brain.

endemic (en-dem′ik). A disease of low morbidity that is constantly present in a human community.

endogenous (en-doj′e-nus). Originating within the organism, e.g., nutrients synthesized in intermediary metabolism.

endosperm (en′do-sperm). The nutritive substance within the embryo sac of plants.

enteropathy (en′ter-op′ah-the). Any disease of the intestine.

enzyme (en′zīm). A substance, usually protein in nature and formed in living cells, which brings about chemical changes.

epinephrine (ep′i-nef′rin). A hormone secreted by the adrenal medulla and released predominantly in response to hypoglycemia.

ergocalciferol (er′go-kal-cif′er-ol). Vitamin D_2 derived from ergosterol, (See *calciferol*.)

ergosterol (er-gos′ter-ol). A sterol found in plant and in animal tissues which, on exposure to ultraviolet light, is converted into vitamin D_2. (See *sterol*.)

exogenous (eks-oj′e-nus). Originating outside the organism, e.g., nutrients in food.

FAO. Food and Agriculture Organization of the United Nations, Headquarters in Rome, Italy.

fatty acids (fat′e as′ids). The organic acids which combine with glycerol to form fat.

favism (fa′vism). An acute hemolytic anemia due to contact with the fava or broad bean.

FDA. Food and Drug Administration of the Public Health Service, U. S. Department of Health, Education, and Welfare, Washington, D.C. 20250.

ferritin (fer′i-tin). An iron-containing protein: the form in which iron is stored in the liver, spleen, intestinal mucosa, and reticuloendothelial cells.

flavoproteins (fla′vo-pro′te-ins). Compounds containing riboflavin, certain nucleotides, and proteins. They are important as enzymes in the citric acid cycle.

folacin (fo′la-sin). Another term for folic acid.

folic acid (fo′lic as′id). A vitamin of the B complex group, known also as pteroylglutamic acid or folacin.

folinic acid (fo-lin′ik). A folic acid derivative closely related to the true enzyme, also called "citrovorum factor."

formiminoglutamic acid (FIGLU) (form-im′i-no′glu-ta′mik). Intermediary product of histidine metabolism. Since folic acid is necessary for its breakdown, the urinary excretion of FIGLU may be measured to determine folic acid status.

galactose (gah-lak'tos). A monosaccharide derived from lactose by hydrolysis.

galactosemia (găh-lak'to-se'me-ah). A hereditary condition characterized by excess galactose in the blood.

genes (jēns). Units of hereditary DNA, carried by chromosomes.

gliadin (gli'a-din). One of the proteins found in the gluten of cereal grains.

gluten (gloo'ten; -t'n). A protein found in many cereal grains.

glycogen (gli'ko-jen). A carbohydrate, similar in composition to the amylopectin form of starch. In this form, carbohydrate is stored in the liver and the muscles.

hemicellulose (hem'e-sel'u-los). A complex carbohydrate similar to cellulose found in the cell wall of plants; indigestible but absorbs water, thereby stimulating laxation.

heterozygote (het'er-o-zi'gōt). An individual possessing different alleles in regard to a given characteristic.

hexose (hek'sos). A single sugar containing six carbon atoms.

histidine (his'ti-din). An amino acid required by growing animals.

homogenized (ho-moj'e-nizd). Made homogeneous. Usually applied to dispersing milk fat in such fine globules that cream will not rise to the top.

homozygote (ho' mo-zi' gōt). An individual possessing an identical pair of alleles in regard to a given characteristic or to all characteristics.

hydrogenation (hi'dro-jen-a'shun). The process of introducing hydrogen into a compound, as when oils are hydrogenated to produce solid fats.

hydrolysate (hi-drol'i-sat). A product of hydrolysis. Often applied to protein hydrolysate.

hydrolysis (hi-drol'i-sis). A chemical reaction in which decomposition is due to the incorporation and splitting of water, resulting in the formation of two new compounds.

hydroxyproline (hi-drok'se-pro'lin). An amino acid which occurs in structural proteins, primarily collagen.

hypercalcemia (hi'per-kal-se'me-ah). An excess of calcium in the blood.

hypercholesteremia (hi'per-ko-les'ter-e'me-a). Excess of cholesterol in the blood.

hyperglycemia (hi'per-gli-se'me-a). An increase in the blood sugar level above normal.

hyperplasia (hi'per-pla'zhe-a). Increase in number of normal cells in normal arrangement in a tissue.

hypertrophy (hi-per'tro-fe). Increase in cell size.

hyperuricemia (hi'per-u'ri-se'me-ah). Excess of uric acid in the blood.

hypervitaminosis (hi'per-vi'ta-min-o'sis). A condition due to an excess of one or more vitamins.

hypoalbuminemia (hi'po-al-bu'min-e'me-a). Abnormally low albumin content of the blood.

hypocalcemia (hi'po-kal-se'me-a). Abnormally low blood calcium.

hypoglycemia (hi'po-gli-se'me-a). A decrease in the blood sugar level below normal.

hypoproteinemia (hi'po-pro'te-in-ε'me-a). A decrease in the normal quantity of serum protein in the blood.

iatrogenic (i'at-ro'jen'ik). Resulting from the activity of physicians.

idiopathic (id'i-o-pathʰ'ĭk). Self-originated; occurring without known cause.

inositol (in-o'si-tol). A hexahydroxycyclohexane once considered to be a member of the vitamin B complex.

isoleucine (i'so-lu'sin). An essential amino acid.

isomer (i'so-mer). One of two or more compounds having the same kind and number of atoms but differing in the atomic arrangements in the molecule.

isotopes (i'so-tope). Two or more chemical elements which have the same atomic number and identical chemical properties, but which differ in atomic weight or in the structure of the nucleus.

isozyme (i'so-zim) or isoenzyme. One of multiple forms in which an enzyme may exist in a single species.

keratin (ker'ah-tin). A scleroprotein which is the principal constituent of epidermis, hair, nails, and the organic matrix of the enamel of teeth.

ketogenic (ke'to-jen'ik). Capable of being converted into ketone bodies. Ketogenic substances in metabolism are the fatty acids and certain amino acids.

ketone bodies (ke'tōn). Acetoacetic acid, β-hydroxybutyric acid and acetone.

ketosis (ke-to'sis). A condition in which there is an accumulation in the body of the ketone bodies as a result of incomplete oxidation of the fatty acids.

kwashiorkor (kwa-shi-or'ker). A severe protein-calorie deficiency disease occurring in small children. Endemic in many parts of the world.

lecithin (les'i-thin). A phospholipid containing glycerol, fatty acids, phosphoric acid, and choline.

leucine (lu'sin). An essential amino acid.

linoleic acid (lin'o-le'ik as'id). A polyunsaturated fatty acid essential for nutrition.

linolenic acid (lin'o-le'nik as'id). A polyunsaturated fatty acid.

lipase (li'pās; lip'ās). An enzyme that digests fat.

lipid (lip'id), **lipoid** (lip'oid). Fat or fatlike substances.

lipoprotein (lip'o-pro'te-in). Combination of a protein with a fat, found in both animal and plant tissues.

lipotrophic (lip'o-trof'ik). Applied to substances essential for fat metabolism.

lysosomes (li'so-sōms). Membranous structures in cytoplasm which contain hydrolytic enzymes.

lysozyme (li'so-zim). Enzyme that digests certain high molecular weight carbohydrates and some gram-positive bacteria.

malabsorption syndrome (mal'ab-sorp'shun). A group of symptoms which result from the inability to digest or absorb food in the intestinal tract.

marasmus (ma-raz'mus). Wasting and emaciation, especially in infants due ot underfeeding or disease.

medulla (me-dul'lah). The middle, inmost part.

melanin (mel'ah-nin). The dark amorphous pigment of the skin, hair and certain other tissues which derives from tyrosine metabolism.

menadione (me-an-di'on). Synthetic vitamin K.

metabolism (me-tab'o-lizm). General term to designate all chemical changes which occur in food nutrients after they have been absorbed from the gastrointestinal tract and to the cellular activity involved in utilizing these nutrients.

methionine (meth-i'o-nin). An essential amino acid containing sulfur.

mitochondria (mit'o-kon'dre-ah). Small granules or rod-shaped structures in the cell.

moiety (moi'ĕ-te). Any equal part.

monosaccharide (mon'o-sak'a-rid). A simple sugar which cannot be decomposed by hydrolysis.

mono-unsaturated (mon'o-un-sat'u-rat-ed). An organic compound such as a fatty acid in which two carbon atoms are united by a double bond.

mucopolysaccharide (mu'ko-pol'e-sak'ah-rid). A group of polysaccharides which contains hexosamine, which may or may not be combined with protein and which, dispersed in water, form many of the mucins.

mucoprotein (mu'ko-pro'te-in). Substance containing a polypeptide chain and disaccharides, found in mucous secretions of the digestive glands.

mycotoxin (mi'ko-tox'sin). A fungal or bacterial toxin.

myelin (mi' ĕ-lin). The fat-like substance forming a sheath around certain nerve fibers.

myelination (mi'ĕ-li-na'shun) or myelinization. The act of furnishing with or taking on myelin.

naphthoquinone (naf'tho-kwin'on). A derivative of quinone; some of these derivatives have vitamin K activity.

NAS–NRC. National Academy of Science–National Research Council, Washington, D.C. 20418.

neutropenia (nu'tro-pe'ne-ah). A decrease in the number of neutrophilic leucocytes in the blood.

niacin (ni'a-sin). A member of the vitamin B complex, formerly known as nicotinic acid. An antipellagra factor.

niacinamide (ni'ah-sin-am'id). Nicotinamide, the amide derivative of nicotinic acid (niacin).

NRC-RDA. National Research Council-Recommended Dietary Allowances.

nucleoprotein (nu'kle-o-pro'tein). The conjugated protein found in the nuclei of cells.

nucleotide (nu'kle-o-tid). Compound containing a sugar-phosphate component and a purine or pyrimidine base.

nutrient (nu'tre-ent). An organic or inorganic substance in food which is digested and absorbed in the gastrointestinal tract and utilized in intermediary metabolism.

oleic acid (o-le'ik). A monounsaturated fatty acid.

oligosaccharide (ōl'i-go sak'ah rid). A complex carbohydrate which contains two to ten molecules of monosaccharides combined with each other.

opsin (op'sin). Protein compound which combines with retinal, vitamin A aldehyde, to form rhodopsin, visual purple.

osteoblast (os'te-o-blast). Any one of the cells that are developed into bone.

osteoclast (os'te-o-clast). A cell that assists in the resorption of bone.

osteomalacia (os'te-o-ma-la'she-a). Softening of the bone due to loss of calcium. Occurs chiefly in adults.

osteoporosis (os'te-o-po-ro'sis). Abnormal porousness or rarefaction of bone due to failure of the osteoblasts to lay down bone matrix, and occurring when resorption dominates over mineral deposition.

oxaluria (ok'sah-lu're-ah). The presence of an excess of oxalic acid or of oxalates in the urine.

oxidation (ok'si-da'shun). A chemical process by which a substance combines with oxygen. Chemically it is an increase of positive charges on an atom through the loss of electrons.

pantothenic acid (pan'to-then'ik). A member of the vitamin B complex.

para-aminobenzoic acid (PABA) (par'a-a-men'no-ben-zo'ik as'id). A part of pteroylglutamic acid, one of the forms of folic acid.

pentose (pen'tos). A single sugar containing five carbon atoms. Ribose is a pentose.

peptide (pep'tid). A compound of two or more amino acids containing one or more peptide bonds. Peptides are formed as intermediary products of protein digestion.

pesticide (pes'ti-sid). A poison used to destroy pests of any sort. The term includes fungicides, insecticides, and rodenticides.

phenylalanine (fen'il-al'a-nen; nin). An essential amino acid.

phenylketonuria (PKU) (fen'il-ke'ton-nu're-ah). An inborn error of the metabolism of phenylalanine; phenylpyruvic acid appears in the urine.

phenylpyruvic acid (fen'il-pi-ru'vik). An intermediate product in phenylalanine metabolism.

phospholipid (fos'fo-lip'id). A fat in which one fatty acid is replaced by phosphorus and a nitrogenous compound.

phosphorylation (fos'for-i-la'shun). The process of introducing the trivalent phosphate group into an organic molecule. The phosphate donor is usually ATP.

photosynthesis (fo'to-sin'the-sis). Formation of carbohydrate from carbon dioxide and water in the chlorophyll tissue of plants under the influence of light.

polysaccharide (pol'e-sak'ah-rid). A complex carbohydrate which contains more than ten molecules of monosaccharides combined with each other.

polyunsaturated (pol'e-un-sat'u-rat'ed). An organic compound such as a fatty acid in which there is more than one double bond.

precursor (pre-kur'ser). A substance which is converted into another; e.g., β carotene to vitamin A.

prophylaxis (pro'fi-lak'sis). Preventive treatment.

protaglandins (pro'tah-glan'dins). A group of hormones containing fatty acids with 20 carbon atoms which cause strong contraction of smooth muscle and dilation of certain vascular beds.

protease (pro'te-as). An enzyme that digests protein.

protein hydrolysate (pro'te-in hi-drol'i-zat). A solution containing the constituent amino acids of an artificially digested protein, usually milk or beef protein.

proteinuria (pro'te-i-nu're-a). Presence of protein in the urine.

proteolytic (pro'te-o-lit'ik). Effecting the digestion of proteins.

provitamin (pro-vi'ta-min). The forerunner of a vitamin. Provitamin A is carotene.

pteroylglutamic acid (ter-ol-glu-tam'ic as'id). (See *folic acid*.)

ptyalin (ti'a-lin). The starch splitting enzyme amylase of·saliva.

purine(s) (pu'rēn). A nonprotein heterocyclic nitrogenous base. End products of nucleoprotein metabolism.

pyridoxine (pi'ri-dok'sin). Vitamin B_6, a member of the vitamin B complex.

rachitogenic (rah-kit'o-jen'ik). Capable of causing rickets.

RAD. A unit of measurement of absorbed doses of ionizing radiation.

reticuloendothelial system (re-tik'u-lo-en'do-the' le'al). Group of cells, except leukocytes, with phagocytic properties.

retinal (ret'i-nal). The aldehyde form of vitamin A which is necessary for the synthesis of rhodopsin, visual purple.

retinoic acid (ret'i-no-ic). The acid form of vitamin A.

retinol (ret'i-nol). The chemical term for vitamin A alcohol.

retinyl (ret'i-nel). Refers to the vitamin A portion of the ester form of the vitamin. Retinyl palmitate is hydrolyzed to vitamin A alcohol (retinol) and palmitic acid in the gastrointestinal tract.

rhodopsin (ro-dop'sin). Visual purple, formed in the rods of the retina by combining the protein opsin and vitamin A aldehyde. It is necessary for scotopic vision.

riboflavin (ri'bo-fla'vin). Heat-stable factor of B complex, sometimes called vitamin B_2.

ribonucleic acid (RNA) (ri-bo-nu'kle-ik). A nucleic acid replicated from DNA and found in cytoplasm.

saccharine (sak'ah-rin). An intensely sweet, white crystalline compound used as a substitute for ordinary sugar. It has no food value.

safflower oil (saf'flou'er). An edible oil from the seeds of the safflower plant, *Carthamus tinctorius*; high in linoleic acid.

serotonin (ser'o-to'nin). A derivative of tryptophan which plays a role in brain and nerve function.

sphingomyelin (sfing'go-mi'e-lin). A phospholipid found primarily in brain and lung tissue as a constituent of the myelin sheaths.

stachyose (stak'e-os). An indigestible tetrasaccharide containing galactose.

stearic acid (ste'a-rik). A saturated fatty acid.

steatorrhea (ste'a-to-re'a). Presence of an excess of fat in the stools.

sterol (ster'ol). Fat-soluble substance with a complex molecular structure.

substrate (sub'strāt). A substance upon which an enzyme acts.

succinic acid (suk-sin'ik). Intermediary product in metabolism.

suet (su'et). Hard fat of beef or mutton.

synergism (sin'er-jizm). The joint action of agents so

that their combined effect is greater than the algebraic sum of their individual effects.

synthesis (sin'the-sis). The process of building up a chemical compound.

thermogenesis (ther'mo-jen'e-sis). The production of heat, especially within the animal body.

thyrotoxicosis (thi'ro-tok'sĭ-ko'sis). A morbid condition resulting from overactivity of the thyroid gland.

thiamine (thi'am-in). Vitamin B_1. Antineuritic factor, member of the B complex.

thyrocalcitonin (thi'ro-cal'ci-to'nin). A thyroid hormone which prohibits release of calcium from bone.

tocopherol (to-kof'er-ol). An alcohol-like substance, several forms of which have vitamin E activity.

transamination (trans'am-i-na'shun). The transferring of an amino group from an amino acid to another compound. By this process the body is able to synthesize the nonessential amino acids as well as form urea. A vitamin B_6-containing enzyme is necessary for this reaction.

transferrin (trans-fer'in). A protein compound found in the blood stream which transports iron to the bone marrow for hemoglobin synthesis, to the liver or spleen for storage, or to the other tissues for their use.

trichinosis (trik'i-no'sis). A disease due to infection with trichinae—parasites found in raw pork.

tularemia (too'la-re'me-ah). A disease of rodents, resembling plague, which is transmitted by the bites of flies, fleas, ticks, and lice and may be acquired by man through handling of infected animals.

tyrosine (ti-ro'sin). A nonessential amino acid.

UNESCO. United Nations Educational, Scientific and Cultural Organization. Headquarters, Paris, France.

urea (u-re'a). The chief nitrogenous end product of protein metabolism in the body.

USDA. United States Department of Agriculture. Washington, D.C. 20250.

valine (val'in). An essential amino acid.

viosterol (vi-o'ster-ol). A solution of irradiated ergosterol in oil; vitamin D_2.

Wernicke-Korsakoff syndrome (ver'ni-ke–korsak'of). A psychosis which is usually based on chronic alcoholism, probably due to prolonged thiamine deficiency.

WHO. World Health Organization of the United Nations, Headquarters, Geneva, Switzerland.

xerophthalmia (ze'rof-thal'mi-a). A dry and lusterless condition of the conjunctiva of the eyes resulting from a vitamin A deficiency.

zein (ze'in). A protein obtained from corn.

zygote (zi'-gōt). The cell resulting from the fusion of two gametes.

index

Wilson's disease, 466
Women. *See* Females
World Food Conference (Rome), 8, 286

Xanthin oxidase, 68
Xanthurenic acid, 104
Xerophthalmia, 76, 288, 291-93

Yeast:
   dried, 217
   fermentation action, 16
   food spoilage, 213
   pantothenic acid source, 108

Yeast: (*continued*)
   in sodium-restricted diets, 434
   thiamine source, 99
   and wheat bread, 21
   in vegetarian diet, 209
   vitamin B-complex source, 96

Zinc, 65-66
   and cadmium tolerance, 69
   children's allowances, 267
   pregnancy allowance, 241
   storage of, 460
   in USDA food plan, 175
Zirconium, 69